$\mathcal{M}$ODERN
CYTOPATHOLOGY

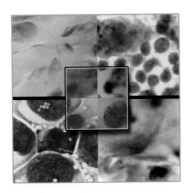

$\mathcal{M}$ODERN CYTOPATHOLOGY

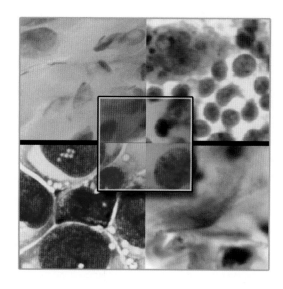

Kim R. Geisinger, MD
Professor of Pathology
Director of Surgical Pathology and Cytopathology
Wake Forest University School of Medicine
North Carolina Baptist Hospital
Winston-Salem, North Carolina

Michael W. Stanley, MD
Professor of Pathology and Laboratory Medicine
The University of Minnesota
Chief, Department of Pathology
Hennepin County Medical Center
Minneapolis, Minnesota

Stephen S. Raab, MD
Professor of Pathology
University of Pittsburgh School of Medicine
Director of Cytology
Director of Pathology Quality and Healthcare Research
University of Pittsburgh Medical Center
Pittsburgh, Pennsylvania

Jan F. Silverman, MD
Professor of Pathology
Drexel University College of Medicine
Chairman and Director of Anatomic Pathology
Allegheny General Hospital
Pittsburgh, Pennsylvania

Andrea Abati, MD
Chief, Cytopathology Section
National Institutes of Health
National Cancer Institute
Bethesda, Maryland

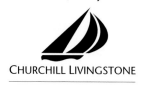

CHURCHILL LIVINGSTONE

An Imprint of Elsevier

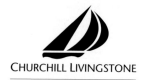

CHURCHILL LIVINGSTONE

An Imprint of Elsevier

The Curtis Center
Independence Square West
Philadelphia, Pennsylvania 19106

NOTICE

Cytopathology is an ever-changing field. Standard safety precautions must be followed, but as new research and clinical experience broaden our knowledge, changes in treatment and drug therapy may become necessary or appropriate. Readers are advised to check the most current product information provided by the manufacturer of each drug to be administered to verify the recommended dose, the method and duration of administration, and contraindications. It is the responsibility of the licensed prescriber, relying on experience and knowledge of the patient, to determine dosages and the best treatment for each individual patient. Neither the publisher nor the author assumes any liability for any injury and/or damage to persons or property arising from this publication.

Library of Congress Cataloging-in-Publication Data

Modern cytopathology / Kim Geisinger . . . [et al].
  p. ; cm.
  Includes bibliographical references and index.
  ISBN 0-443-06598-5 (alk. paper)
  1. Pathology, Cellular. I. Geisinger, Kim R.
  [DNLM: 1. Cytodiagnosis. 2. Cytological Techniques. 3. Pathology—methods. QY 95
M689 2003]
  RB25.M58 2003
  611'.01815—dc21

                                                        2003046201

Acquisitions Editor: Natasha Andjelkovic
Developmental Editor: Kimberley Cox
Publishing Services Manager: Linda McKinley
Project Managers: Kristin Hebberd, Julie Eddy
Editorial Assistant: Jennifer Clark
Designer: Julia Dummitt

Printed in China

Last digit is the print number: 9 8 7 6 5 4 3 2 1

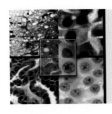

About the Authors

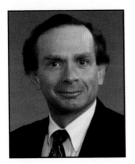

Kim R. Geisinger, M.D.
Dr. Geisinger is Professor of Pathology at Wake Forest University School of Medicine, where he is also Director of Surgical Pathology and Cytopathology. He has published over 150 articles in peer-reviewed journals and 3 cytology books. Dr. Geisinger has given over 100 lectures and workshops in diagnostic cytopathology worldwide. He is the recipient of the American Society for Clinical Pathology (ASCP) George Stevenson Distinguished Service Award for teaching. He served as the Chair of the ASCP's Council on Cytopathology for 4 years. Dr. Geisinger is currently the President of the Papanicolaou Society of Cytopathology.

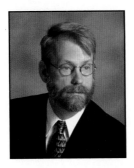

Michael W. Stanley, M.D.
After residency in anatomic pathology and fellowship in surgical pathology at the University of Minnesota, Dr. Stanley studied clinical and interpretive aspects of fine needle aspiration at the Karolinska Hospital, Stockholm, Sweden. He is currently Chief of Pathology at the Hennepin County Medical Center and Professor of Pathology and Laboratory Medicine at the University of Minnesota in Minneapolis. He is past president of the Papanicolaou Society of Cytopathology and recipient of the 2001 Distinguished Service Award from the Commission on Continuing Education of the American Society of Clinical Pathology. Dr. Stanley publishes primarily in the area of cytopathology. He is on editorial boards of 6 pathology journals and is a section or associate editor for 4 journals.

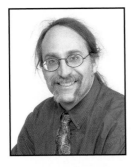

Stephen S. Raab, M.D.
Dr. Raab is Professor of Pathology at the University of Pittsburgh. He did his pathology training at Washington University, completed a fellowship in epidemiology at the University of Pennsylvania, and studied health services research at Stanford University. Dr. Raab currently practices diagnostic cytology and surgical pathology and performs funded research on improving pathology practice and patient outcomes. He was a forum director at the 2001 Bethesda Conference and writes and teaches extensively on gynecologic and nongynecologic cytology. He is a strong advocate for the cytotechnologist profession, cytology education, the role of cytology in patient-centered care, and the advancement of cytology practice. He has contributed to humanitarian medical causes throughout the world and is the Vice President of the Viet American Cervical Cancer Prevention Project, an endeavor aimed at improving the health of women in Vietnam.

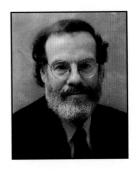

Jan F. Silverman, M.D.
Dr. Silverman is Chairman and Director of Anatomic Pathology at Allegheny General Hospital and Professor of Pathology at the Drexel University College of Medicine. He has authored approximately 425 peer-reviewed articles and abstracts, 29 book chapters, and 7 books. Dr. Silverman has been past President of the Papanicolaou Society of Cytology, Chairman of the Cytopathology Council of the American Society of Clinical Pathology (ASCP), Deputy Commissioner of the ASCP, and currently serves on the Board of Directors of the ASCP. His professional interests are clinicopathologic studies in general cytology, including FNA biopsy and the application of ancillary techniques in surgical pathology and cytology.

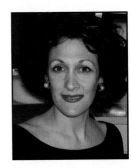

Andrea Abati, M.D.
Dr. Abati trained in Anatomic and Neuropathology at New York University Medical Center and completed a surgical pathology fellowship at Memorial Sloan-Kettering Cancer Center. She is certified by the American Board of Pathology in Anatomic Pathology, Neuropathology, and Cytopathology. The early years of her career were spent as a junior faculty member at New York University Medical Center and Baylor University Medical Center. She has been in the Cytopathology Section of the National Institutes of Health since 1992, serving as the Section Chief since 1996. She originally achieved national recognition through her work organizing the NCI conference, which set forth the current standards of practice for breast FNA. During the 10 years she has been at NIH, she has established herself as a prolific writer, focusing on the application of ancillary techniques for diagnostic enhancement of cytopathology, particularly immunocytochemistry and various molecular techniques. Dr. Abati serves on the Editorial Advisory Boards of Clinical Cancer Research, Cancer Cytopathology, and Diagnostic Cytopathology, where she was recently awarded the section editorship for reviews. In 2003 she was elected to the office of President-Elect of the Papanicolaou Society of Cytopathology.

This to me, which represents the collaborative work of the five authors, is dedicated to our teachers, students, house officers, and professional colleagues who have molded and continually modified our concepts about cytopathology and who have stimulated us to attempt to be better in our diagnostic activities. They have provided the necessary seeds, water, and fertilizer, allowing us to grow and prosper professionally.

Even more so, this work is dedicated to our loved ones, young and old, who have sacrificed by allocating us time away from them to labor on this book. Without their confident support, this end result would never have been achieved.

Thank you all. God bless you!

Kim R. Geisinger
Stephen S. Raab

First to Torsten who, more than any other person worked cytodiagnostic magic and who slapped my inept piano-student hands in every clinic until they pleased him; to my teachers in surgical pathology, especially Pepper and Mark, whose brilliance is always before me; as always, to Chuck whose assessment of me early in my career was that, "He's stable;" to my fallen comrades, Dave, and, probably, Issam; to my coauthors, with warmest loyalty to whom I have tried to imbue every single proofreading—I am the least of these; to the late Stuart Sankey who was the first to teach me that, "Life is too short;" but mostly to my family, whose love daily covers my multitude of follies.

Michael W. Stanley

This book is dedicated to my wonderful and supportive wife, Mary; children, Mischell, Jeff, and Laura, and grandchildren, Jessica, Melissa, and Josh along with my colleagues at Allegheny General Hospital and my authentic friends.

Jan F. Silverman

I was blessed to have been surrounded by truly remarkable people. To those whose love, encouragement, personal strength, and belief in me have brought me to where I am: John and Eleanor Abati; Ernest and Ada Abati; and Lillie and Tony Pappacoda. Also to my children, Hank and Tony, who give true meaning to my life.

Andrea Abati

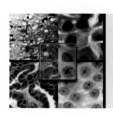

Preface

This text evolved from the authors' common beliefs that a void was waiting to be filled—namely, a need for a comprehensive, yet user-friendly source of diagnostic data for all types of cytologic samples. This work represents the compilation of nearly a century of professional experiences by the five authors, who practice both surgical pathology and cytopathology, and is structured to provide a uniform, practical approach to diagnosis throughout each chapter.

Our nuclear approach recapitulates daily practice in that it is entrenched in the belief that an integration of clinical, radiographic, and cytomorphologic data may render many interpretations. A major attribute of this text is that essential cytomorphologic criteria for a large number of common to infrequent disease entities are distilled into a list format that emphasizes both architectural and individual cellular features associated with each condition. This information is reinforced through lavish illustrations chosen specifically to demonstrate the enumerated attributes. However, as our title implies, when necessary the authors incorporate essential ancillary procedures into the diagnostic scheme. These analyses include immunocytochemistry, electron microscopy, flow cytometry, cytogenetics, and a number of different molecular biological tests.

It is our hope that this book will not sit on a coffee table, but rather be pulled off the shelf for frequent reference by practicing cytologists—with the ultimate goal of enhancing patient care.

Kim R. Geisinger
Michael W. Stanley
Stephen S. Raab
Jan F. Silverman
Andrea Abati

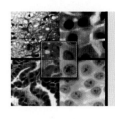

Photo Credits

The authors gratefully acknowledge the following individuals who supplied photographs.

Fadi W. Abdul-Karim, M.D.
Gleb Budzilovich, M.D.
Keith Brosky, C.T., ASCP
Michael Cohen, M.D.
Christie Copeland, C.T., ASCP
Laila Dahmoush, M.D.
Philip Dvoretsky, M.D.
Hormoz Ehya, M.D.
Tarik Elsheikh, M.D.
Andrew S. Field, M.D.
Armando Filie, M.D.
Felicity A. Frost, M.D.
Michael Henry, M.D.
Yasmine Hijazi, M.D.
Terry Johnson, M.D.
Paula R. Larson, M.D.
Britt-Marie Ljung, M.D.
Celeste Powers, M.D.
Diva Salomao, M.D.
Joshua Sickel, M.D.
Aylin Simsir, M.D.
Diane Solomon, M.D.
Charles Sturgis, M.D.
Paul Wakely, M.D.
Anna Maria Wilder, C.T., ASCP

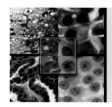

Contents

MODERN CYTOPATHOLOGY

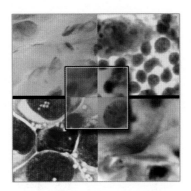

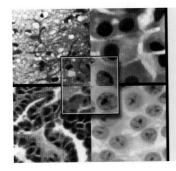

Introduction

CHAPTER
1

Cytopathology is the study of cells for the diagnosis and monitoring of disease and especially to identify primary, recurrent, and metastatic malignant neoplasms and their precursors. For a number of decades, cytopathology was relegated to the bargain basement of medicine because it had been considered by many to be the orphan of pathology. A significant proportion of medical personnel had considered it to be of lesser diagnostic value than surgical pathology and even autopsy pathology. However, during the last 15 years or so, a remarkable, progressive reversal has occurred, with cytology ascending to the upper echelon of the medical department store.

Most cytologic preparations are used to diagnose tumors and a variety of nonneoplastic disease processes. Accordingly, these tests need to possess rather high levels of diagnostic specificity. However, in the minds of many individuals, cytology is equated almost exclusively with cervicovaginal samples (the Papanicolaou [Pap] smear). This test is used to screen for noninvasive precursor lesions to invasive carcinoma of the cervix. As a screening modality, the Pap smear and its more modern monolayer preparations must have relatively high levels of diagnostic sensitivity. If a precursor lesion is identified, then more advanced procedures such as colposcopy with a biopsy can be used to render a definitive diagnosis. Some individuals would also consider the cytologic examination of spontaneously voided urine as a screening procedure. In individuals with abnormal cells in the urine diagnostic or suggestive of tumor, then cystoscopy, often with biopsy, is the next step. Fine-needle aspiration (FNA) biopsy of the thyroid gland serves as both a screening and a diagnostic test. In the former scenario, the aspiration biopsies are identifying the relatively small proportion of patients with thyroid nodules who should undergo surgical removal of the nodules for therapeutic and diagnostic purposes. Thus, a large proportion of patients are saved from unnecessary surgery. On the other hand, aspiration biopsies may yield specific diagnoses (e.g., papillary adenocarcinoma).

SPECIMEN TYPES

The two major types of cytologic samples are exfoliative specimens and aspiration biopsies. *Exfoliative specimens* basically refer to cells that are shed, either spontaneously or after physical sampling, from internal and external body surfaces. The classic exfoliative specimen is the Pap smear, in which both spontaneously exfoliated and physically removed cells are sampled, primarily from the transformation zone of the cervix. For some body sites, several different types of exfoliative cytologic specimens are found. This may be best witnessed in the lung, in which preparations include sputum, bronchial brushings, bronchial washings, and bronchoalveolar lavages. In the vast majority of instances, pathologists are not directly involved in the procurement of exfoliative material.

The other major specimen type is FNA biopsy. The birth of this technique probably occurred at Memorial Hospital in New York City in the early 1920s. However, aspiration biopsies did not gain popularity in the United States until about two decades ago. In the 1940s a new medical specialty evolved in Europe—namely, the cytopathologists who concentrated their efforts in the procurement and interpretation of aspiration specimens. Especially notable for the development of this procedure was the Karolinska Hospital in Stockholm, Sweden.

Aspiration biopsies may be performed on both superficial and deep-seated mass lesions. The latter are typically sampled under radiologic guidance, such as with computed tomography (CT) or ultrasound. In addition, deep organs such as the pancreas may be sampled intraoperatively under direct visualization by the surgeon. Superficial aspiration biopsies target a palpable mass in sites such as the salivary glands, breast, and lymph nodes. Although many of these aspirates are performed by clinicians, whenever possible, this procedure should be done by an experienced pathologist. It is recognized that the quality of the sample obtained is directly related to the experience of the operator. It is certainly believed that whenever possible, the cytology "team" should be present at all aspiration biopsies. However, this may not be logistically, technically, or professionally feasible for many aspirates in some centers.

In any event, the FNA biopsy technique is essentially the same regardless of the target. For superficial masses, the lesion in question should be immobilized by the aspirator's hand that is not holding the needle. Obviously, such immobilization is not the case for the more deeply situated lesions. The needle travels through one or more normal tissues before reaching the mass in question. When the mass is punctured, one can usually note a change in resistance to the needle and possibly feel an actual "popping" quality to the needle passage. When the needle is present within the mass in question, a vacuum is created within the syringe barrel by retraction on the plunger. In general, a negative pressure of 3 ml is considered optimal for sample procurement. This vacuum is not released until just before the needle exits the mass. While in the mass, the needle may be piloted in multiple directions, increasing the proportion of the lesion that is sampled. The aspirator releases the vacuum by letting go of the handle before removing the needle from the mass. Otherwise, some or all of the aspirated cellular material is likely to enter the syringe barrel and thus may not be available for the preparation of a smear. In other words, it is preferable to keep all the aspirated cellular material in the needle hub. It should be emphasized that multiple aspiration biopsy punctures may be performed on the same mass lesion during a single clinic or bedside visit.

The authors are strong advocates of on-site evaluation of the aspiration smears by cytotechnologists and pathologists. This greatly increases the likelihood of obtaining a satisfactory specimen, thus enhancing the ability to make a specific diagnosis. In addition, the pathologist may render an immediate interpretation analogous to frozen sections.

Compared with histologic specimens such as a needle core biopsy, FNA biopsies present several advantages.[1-3] These include more rapid results; a much lower rate of complications, including dissemination of tumor cells along the needle track; the lack of the need of anesthesia in most instances; and in general, lower expenses. In addition, if the pathologist performs the aspirate, the palpatory qualities of the mass can be integrated with all other diagnostic information. Finally, on-site evaluation greatly increases the likelihood of obtaining an adequate and accurate clinical history. Many facets of FNA biopsy are detailed in Chapter 2.

For both exfoliative and aspiration specimens, two major forms in which the slides for microscopic examination can be prepared are direct smears and a number of different concentration techniques. From aspirated samples, smears are prepared through placement of positive pressure on the syringe and expression of the material in the hub onto the slide. The bevel should be face down toward the slide. For direct smears, cytologic material is typically obtained by a brush or other sampling device, such as a swab. The sampling device then is brought into direct contact with and applied along the length of the slide. Such specimens include the conventional cervicovaginal smear, bronchial and gastrointestinal brushings, and direct smears from aspiration biopsies. If the cellular material is to be stained via the Pap technique, it is imperative that the cells be rapidly placed in an ethanol-based fixative. Otherwise, air-drying artifacts are quickly induced, perhaps limiting the diagnostic attributes of the specimen. If the sample is to be stained with a Romanowsky stain, it is imperative that it fully dries before commencement of the staining procedure.

A large number of different forms of concentration techniques have been developed and used successfully in the cytologic evaluation of various types of samples. One of these is the almost-now-defunct filter preparation. Cells suspended in fluid were collected on filters and placed on the tops of vacuum traps. One of their strongest points was

that essentially no cells escaped collection. However, this technique is time consuming and labor intensive. Furthermore, special stains or other diagnostic sampling procedures cannot be performed on cells collected on filters. Other concentration techniques include cytocentrification with smearing of the sediment, cytospins, and the more recently developed monolayer preparations.

The authors are also advocates of the use of cell block preparations in many types of cytologic samples. In a minority of instances, the smears are devoid of neoplastic cells, with all the tumoral elements exclusively present in the cell block. Cell blocks may also better provide the specific histologic attributes of cells that are not evident in the direct smears. For example, true papillary formations tend to be more evident in cell blocks. In some specimen types a direct clot formation may occur rather rapidly. In other instances, clot formation needs to be induced in the laboratory. The addition of plasma and then thrombin to the sample stimulates the production of a clot. The clots are fixed in formalin and then processed like tissue by the histology laboratory, using the routine hematoxylin and eosin stain. Cell blocks often provide the major cellular source for ancillary techniques, particularly immunocytochemistry.

 ## STAINS

The most widely used staining procedure in cytology is the Pap method; it combines the hematoxylin nuclear stain with two subsequent cytoplasmic counterstains, orange G and EA. Its major advantages include excellent nuclear chromatin detail and the orangeophilic staining of cytoplasmic keratin. The Pap stain is the preferred technique for most exfoliated cellular material. However, some pathologists prefer Romanowsky stains for cerebrospinal fluids and effusion specimens. In addition, if a lymphoreticular proliferation is suspected, one or more slides should be stained with a Romanowsky preparation.

For FNA biopsy, many practitioners routinely use two stains, Pap and Romanowsky. The two stains provide complementary diagnostic information in most sample types. However, some pathologists prefer using hematoxylin and eosin on aspirated cellular material. With the Romanowsky stain the initial intended air-drying of the specimen results in cells that are larger than the paired alcohol fixed smear. Differences in sizes are accentuated by this air-drying. Other advantages of the Romanowsky stain include the preservation of potentially suggestive or distinctive cytoplasmic attributes and the metachromatic staining of various types of extracellular matrix material. Air-drying induces a relative roundness to all cellular elements. Finally, air-drying avoids the potential cellular losses that may occur when slides are immersed in alcohol. In general, nuclear detail is better evaluated with the Pap stain.

 ## CYTOLOGIC FEATURES ASSOCIATED WITH MALIGNANCY

In general, no single cytomorphologic attribute determines whether a cell is designated as benign or malignant. Rather, it is the constellation of several features in a specific clinical setting and specimen type that permits the cytologist to ren-

TABLE 1-1		
Morphologic Comparison of Repair and Cancer		
Features	**Repair**	**Cancer**
Cohesion	Well maintained	Reduced with single cells
Polarity	Maintained	Usually disrupted
Aggregates	Flat sheets	Flat to three-dimensional
Pleomorphism	Minimal	Mild to marked
Nuclear membranes	Smooth, thin	Irregularly thickened and shaped
Chromatin staining	Pale	Dark
Chromatin granularity	Fine	Fine to coarse
Chromatin distribution	Even	Irregular
N:C	Normal to slightly increased	Usually increased
Nucleoli	Solitary, round, smooth	One or more, irregular

N:C, Nuclear:cytoplasmic ratio.

der an interpretation of cancer. One feature suggestive of malignancy is variation in cellular size and contour, including the presence of bizarre and giant forms (e.g., pleomorphism). Nuclear enlargement and shape variability are other features characteristic of neoplasia. Increased nuclear staining or hyperchromasia is typically associated with malignant cells. Many but not all cancer cells have high nuclear-to-cytoplasmic ratios, especially when compared with the normal, benign counterparts of the neoplastic cells. Other nuclear features that are in keeping with malignancy include an irregular distribution of the chromatin, coarsely granular chromatin, prominent and/or multiple nucleoli, and abnormal mitotic figures. Compared with benign cellular elements, most cancers are associated with reduced intercellular cohesion. Thus, a proportion of the cells is found individually scattered within smears. Finally, the presence of necrotic debris in the smear background is often associated with a malignant process; although by no means specific to cancers, this process is known as a *tumor diathesis.*

 ## CYTOLOGIC FEATURES OF REPAIR

If all benign cells maintained their normal appearance under all or most circumstances, then distinction from the vast majority of malignant cells would not pose a diagnostic problem in any type of cytologic sample. However, benign cells may undergo morphologic alterations in response to a number of different stimuli, which may create attributes resembling those seen in cancerous elements. The best known of these falls under the rubric of repair or reparative atypia. These morphologic changes may be seen in epithelial or mesenchymal cells in both exfoliative and aspiration samples (Table 1-1). A major pitfall with repair is that the cells and their nuclei are often significantly larger than normal, which is further accentuated by the frequent presence of macronucleoli.

Despite this, microscopic clues to the proper identification of benign repair are usually evident. One of the more important of these is the relative preservation of intercellular cohesion by the benign cellular elements. Characteristically, they are present in large flat sheets in which the cells appear to be spread out and in which the long axes of their nuclei often parallel one another (streaming). In addition,

normal polarity is rather well maintained so that the enlarged nuclei are not especially crowded and cytoplasm is usually evident between the nuclei. At least for epithelial repair, a very helpful feature is the paucity of single, intact atypical cells. Although some variability in cellular and nuclear diameters and configurations is present, marked pleomorphism, as may be seen in cancer, is not evident. Although enlarged, the nuclei tend to have delicate and distinctly smooth membranes, finely granular and often pale-stained chromatin, and a large round nucleolus. Mitotic figures may be evident, but abnormal mitotic configurations are not present. Neutrophils are commonly associated with these benign reparative elements and necrotic material may be seen in the smear background. This is especially true in the face of an ulcer.

 ## GENERAL DIAGNOSTIC APPROACH

Overall, cytopathologic specimens are approached as if they were histopathologic samples. Whenever possible, as specific a diagnosis as possible is attempted, and generally, generic diagnoses such as *malignancy present* are not rendered. For example, if a FNA biopsy of the lung can be diagnosed as a carcinoid tumor, then that diagnosis is rendered in the final report. Similarly, if a pleural fluid contains tumor cells that are compatible with a metastatic colonic adenocarcinoma, then the diagnosis should read as metastatic adenocarcinoma with a comment that the neoplastic cells are morphologically similar to a colonic primary. (The cytologist should always attempt to review the previous surgical pathology specimen.) Whenever possible, using such relatively nonspecific terms as *atypia, atypical cells,* and *consistent with* is avoided.

Similar to tissue specimens, cytopathologic samples should never be diagnosed in a vacuum. Rather, the cytomorphologic features always need to be integrated with pertinent clinical and radiographic attributes. In addition, in a small but significant proportion of all specimens, the results of ancillary diagnostic procedures should be incorporated with the previously mentioned data in the attempt to render the most accurate and specific interpretation. Unfortunately, it must be admitted that in some cytologic specimens, only a more generalized interpretation can be provided along with the offering of a differential diagnosis, usually in the comment section of the official report. The remainder of this chapter is dedicated to previewing some of the basic aspects of the ancillary diagnostic procedures as they may be applied to the many different types of cytopathologic samples.

Immunocytochemistry

Without a doubt, as in surgical pathology, the most widely and extensively used ancillary diagnostic procedure is immunocytochemistry.[4] Immunocytochemistry can be used in essentially every type of cytopathologic specimen. For the most part the major purpose is to determine the exact cell lineage and/or site origin of malignant cells in various types of samples. Additionally, with selected antibodies, immunocytochemistry may provide prognostic and predictive data as it relates to treatment. In some situations, the antibodies chosen can be selectively limited by prior clinical history and histopathologic samples. An example would be a pleural fluid containing abnormal-appearing cells in a patient with a prior diagnosis of ductal carcinoma of the breast; appropriate antibodies in this situation might be directed against gross cystic fluid protein-15 and E-cadherin. Another example is a liver aspirate with a high-grade carcinoma in a patient with a previous diagnosis of rectal adenocarcinoma; in this scenario, antibodies directed against cytokeratins 20 and 7 and carcinoembryonic antigen would seem a prudent initial step. In other cases—for example, a cytologic preparation containing an undifferentiated malignancy in a patient without a prior diagnosis of cancer—a panel of antibodies directed at a large array of cell and organ-specific lineages (e.g., epithelial, mesenchymal, and lymphoid) may be the wisest direction in which to proceed.

In contrast to histopathology, preparation of cytopathologic samples may be much more variable; this may result in potentially nonreproducible and clinically unreliable results. These aberrations in the immunocytochemical staining patterns may be seen within the same sample that is prepared using different techniques.[4] In general, cell block preparations are preferred to direct smears, cytospin samples, and monolayer preparations for immunocytochemistry. It has been the authors' experience that background staining is markedly reduced in cell blocks, compared with other specimen types. Furthermore, it more readily allows an expanded antibody panel to be used. This is especially true in the region of large three-dimensional cellular aggregates in different smear preparations.

Special Stains

Compared with histopathology, histochemical stains have not played as great a role in diagnostic cytopathology. In the authors' experience, the most widely used special stains are those for various microbial organisms. In particular, methenamine silver and acid-fast stains have been heavily emphasized. The silver stain is the most useful in identifying fungus in masses of fibrinopurulent material that may prevent adequate visualization of the organisms in the Pap-stained material. The greatest use has been with various types of pulmonary samples. Acid-fast stains have been most used in pulmonary specimens and lymph node aspi-

rates and in particular after the identification of negative images with the Romanowsky-stained smears. Rare examples of bronchoalveolar lavages have been witnessed, in which false negative direct immunofluorescence examinations for *Pneumocystis carinii* have taken place. In these unusual circumstances the castlike material of pneumocystis may be identified in the Pap-stained smears and confirmed by the methenamine silver reaction.

Epithelial mucin stains continue to be utilized to support the diagnosis of adenocarcinomas in various types of cytologic samples. The greatest use has been in aspiration biopsies, especially of the liver, and serous effusions. In the latter scenario, the mucicarmine stain is highly regarded and the alcian blue stain is more difficult to interpret with the same confidence as the mucicarmine stain. When well-developed intracytoplasmic mucin-positive deposits can be identified, the presence of epithelial glandular cells (generally adenocarcinoma) is well supported.

Although perhaps not used in a widespread fashion, oil red O has been used to detect intracytoplasmic lipids. This has been used largely in bronchoalveolar lavages of young children to identify lipid-laden alveolar macrophages and to semiquantitate the amount of intracytoplasmic lipid.[5] In the proper clinical setting, enumeration of the amount of lipid in the macrophages may correlate with the presence or absence of clinically significant reflux esophagitis with aspiration of gastric contents into the lungs. Much less often, oil red O staining has been used to support the diagnosis of renal cell adenocarcinoma in both exfoliative and aspiration specimens.

In other unusual circumstances, various special histochemical stains may have diagnostic utility. For example, the reticulin stain may prove useful in separating hepatocellular carcinomas from primary hepatocytes in liver aspirates.[6]

Electron Microscopy

Once considered the premier ancillary diagnostic procedure for both surgical pathology and cytopathology, electron microscopy (EM) now has been relegated to the very back of the diagnostic armamentarium shelf. The vast majority of clinical scenarios that use ultrastructural examination of cells have been replaced by more modern procedures, including immunocytochemistry, cytogenetics, and various molecular analyses.

Still, in some specific circumstances, cytopathologic specimens still may be examined by transmission EM. In this setting, a suspension of cellular material is cytocentrifuged to create a cell pellet. This pellet is treated as if it were a small piece of tissue and thus is fixed in glutaraldehyde and then postfixed in osmium tetroxide. The pellet then is thinly sectioned and stained with uranyl acetate and lead citrate. One such situation might be to help differentiate among high-grade malignancies of unknown primary origin. For example, despite negative appropriate immunostaining for melanoma, ultrastructural examination may demonstrate cytoplasmic melanosomes. Uncommon intercellular junctions suggestive of epithelial differentiation of neoplastic cells may be occasionally identified in specimens with negative or equivocal cytokeratin immunostaining. Rarely, EM may also be used to identify microbial organisms, especially viruses, in cytologic material. Although they may create attractive pictures, scanning EM generally serves no pertinent diagnostic purposes.

Flow Cytometry

For flow cytometry a suspension of a large number of the cells to be analyzed is prepared by tagging of the cellular mixture with one or more markers, most often antibodies directed against cell surface antigens.

In its application to cytopathology in the authors' experience, flow cytometry is most commonly used for immunophenotyping lymphoid cellular populations.[7] In its simplest sense, immunophenotyping is the detection of the profile of lymphoid cell surface antigens that characterize a specific population. This is especially useful in distinguishing benign lymphoid hyperplasia from malignant B-cell lymphomas. Most normal B-cells are characterized by possession of one of the two immunoglobulin light chains (κ or λ) on their surfaces. Hyperplasias are characterized by mixtures of lymphocytes expressing κ or λ. Conversely, the vast majority of B-cell neoplasms have cells that express only one of the two light chains. This is often referred to as *light chain restriction* and by definition is evidence of monoclonality. Light chain restriction, however, may not be useful in poorly differentiated lymphomas that may not express light chains. Immunophenotyping is also quite valuable in distinguishing among the different types of small cell B-cell lymphomas. For example, both small cell lymphoma and mantle cell lymphoma are positive for CD5, whereas marginal cell lymphomas and small-cleaved cell lymphomas are usually negative for this antigen. Furthermore, small cell lymphoma, but not mantle cell lymphoma, usually expresses CD23. Thus, immunophenotyping may be used to distinguish among the small cell lymphoid neoplasms that show a high degree of morphologic overlap. For T-cell neoplasms, flow cytometry is capable of identifying cell populations with aberrant antigen expression. It is not useful for the diagnosis of Hodgkin's disease.

A major advantage of flow cytometry for immunophenotyping is that it possesses an explicitly high level of diagnostic sensitivity. Thus, it is able to detect a relatively small population of monoclonal neoplastic lymphocytes in a mixture that includes benign lymphoid elements. In addition, flow cytometry possesses a high level of diagnostic precision and usually is characterized by a rather rapid turnaround time.

Immunophenotyping also may be accomplished by immunocytochemistry, most commonly on cytospin preparations. Compared with flow cytometry, one major advantage of immunocytochemistry is that one is able to correlate directly the cytomorphology of the atypical lymphoid cells with the presence or absence of a specific cell surface antigen. In addition, fewer lymphoid cells are required for an adequate analysis.

Flow cytometry also has been used to determine the ploidy of a tumor cell population. Here, the cellular suspension is stained with propidium iodide. The latter stoichiometrically fluoresces in direct proportion to the deoxyribonucleic acid (DNA) content of a single nucleus. In this situation, cell cycle kinetics also may be used to determine the proportion of cells that are proliferating. This has been found most useful by some investigators in the evaluation of aspiration biopsies of malignant lymphomas and carcinoma of the breast.

Image Analysis

Image analysis is the use of standard microscopy of cellular samples to create digitized images of cells that then are evaluated by specific computer programs to measure different features of cells in the attempt to quantify objectively these attributes.

To date, the single measurement of greatest clinical utility is probably the determination of ploidy of neoplastic cells. For this, the Feulgen stain is by far the most widely used. The Feulgen preparation binds nuclear DNA in a stoichiometric fashion. Thus, the optical density of a nucleus is proportional to the amount of DNA present. When compared with a normal diploid control, the DNA content or ploidy of a specific nucleus can be determined. After an adequate number of cells have been so analyzed, the computer generates a histogram that demonstrates the modal DNA content. Generally, these ploidy data are more important prognostically than diagnostically. In many solid neoplasms, especially those in adults, an aneuploid DNA content is associated statistically with a worse prognosis than that associated with an equivalent diploid neoplasm. However, in certain neoplasms, particularly those in the pediatric population, it is the diploid pattern that may be associated with a poorer prognosis.

The image analysis procedure has had some clinical utility in patients with carcinoma of the breast. Cellular samples are stained for estrogen and progesterone receptors and then are analyzed to quantify nuclear staining. By so doing, calculation as to whether a tumor is positive or negative for a specific receptor is based on the staining intensity of the nuclei and the number that are stained. This again provides prognostic and therapeutic information.

In addition to nuclear calculations, the measurement of cytoplasmic and cell membrane constituents can also be evaluated after special staining. To date, this has shown little clinical utility for most quantifiable antigens, except for *Her-2-neu* in women with breast cancer and CD20 in patients with B-cell lymphomas.

Largely relegated today to investigative cytopathology, the measurement of specific cellular attributes has been extensively investigated by image analysis. Examples include quantification of nuclear area, characterization of chromatin texture, and evaluation of the irregularity of the nuclear outline.

Cytogenetics

In its broadest sense, cytogenetics is the study of genetic material and especially chromosomes of cells. The evaluation of chromosomes by karyotyping is the fundamental tool of the cytogeneticist. Karyotyping has evolved from an investigative procedure to one that may be used routinely in clinical laboratories. In the authors' experiences, karyotyping has had its greatest application with FNA biopsy and effusion fluids. This is related to the fact that certain human malignancies are associated with specific chromosomal ab-

TABLE 1-2

Specific Karyotypic Features of Neoplasms

Tumor	Abnormality
Follicular center cell lymphoma	t (14,18)
Burkitt's lymphoma	t (8,14)
Small cell lymphoma	t (11,14)
Anaplastic large cell lymphoma	t (2,5)
AML-M$_3$	t (15,17)
CML	t (9,22)
Alveolar rhabdomyosarcoma	t (2,13)
Ewing's sarcoma	t (11,22)
Intraabdominal small round cell tumor	t (11,22)
Synovial sarcoma	t (X, 18)
Myxoid liposarcoma	t (12,16)
Meningioma	trisomy 7

AML-M$_3$, Acute myelogenous leukemia-M$_3$ type; *CML,* chronic myelogenous leukemia.

normalities (Table 1-2). The detection of these pathognomonic karyotypic aberrations can be useful in confirming a specific primary diagnosis of various types of tumors and in recognizing recurrent and metastatic disease.

Basic karyotyping is performed on cells that undergo mitosis. Thus, the appropriate samples need to contain viable malignant cells that are actively dividing. Regardless of the specimen type, an aliquot needs to be placed in specific transport medium for preservation of the cells during their delivery to the cytogenetics laboratory. Cytologic preparations are quite suitable for karyotyping in that they often include a large proportion of individually dispersed cells. Different techniques may be used by different laboratories and/or for different types of suspected neoplasms. In some laboratories, the specimens are processed immediately with a direct procedure in which the cells are treated with colchicine. Colchicine is a microtubule toxin that blocks the activity of the mitotic spindle and thus arrests cells in the metaphase stage. The cells then are treated with a hypotonic solution that causes rupture of the cell membranes with the nucleus then releasing the chromosomes for only a short distance. The chromosomes are then fixed, often with a combination of methanol and glacial acetic acid. In other laboratories, cells are cultured before this process. Short-term cultures of 1 to 2 days may prove useful for improving the separation of lymphoproliferative disorders. Longer periods of culturing may be advantageous for solid neoplasms.

The classic morphology of chromosomes is grounded in the appearance of metaphase chromosomes. The latter are formed by two identical chromatid strands. Each chromosome has a centromere that forms a major constriction, dividing each chromosome into two arms that are generally of different lengths. Thus, chromosomes can be based on overall size, the position of the centromere, and the relative lengths of the longer and shorter arms.

The identification of chromosomes and various specific portions of each chromosome were markedly enhanced by the development of staining or banding techniques. The most widely used type of stain in the clinical laboratory is a Romanowsky stain, particularly the Giemsa stain. The re-

sulting patterns are referred to as *G bands,* which can be defined as an area of the chromosome that is either darker or lighter than the immediately adjacent segments. Typically, a short pretreatment with an enzyme such as trypsin precedes the application of the stain. This results in a permanent preparation that can be reviewed with conventional light microscopy and photographed.

After this preparation, analysis includes the determination of the number of chromosomes in a given cell, the identification of the number of each type of chromosome, and the examination of the banding pattern. In so doing, structural abnormalities may be identified. It is important to recognize that each metaphase may not allow determination of these features, and thus, a number of metaphases may need to be analyzed. Newer techniques used by some cytogenetic laboratories include synchronization of the cells before metaphase preparations. Another technique used to increase resolution is to use intercalating agents such as ethidium bromide, which increases the number of bands that may be detected.

All the previous information is predicated on the presence of well-preserved, viable, and mitotically active tumor cells. Techniques now have been developed that allow evaluation of chromosomes in nondividing or interphase nuclei.[8,9] Basically, this involves several sequential steps, including denaturization of the DNA, application of florescent-labeled specific probes, hybridization, and probe detection. The most widely used probes are directed against specific centromeres. This allows for enumeration of specific chromosomes. Other available probes may be directed against known genes involved in carcinogenesis and whole chromosome "painting" probes. Abati and colleagues demonstrated that equivalent nuclear signals could be obtained after several different types of fixation, including air-drying, methanol, 95% ethanol, and Carnoy's solution.[7] These authors found that poor nuclear staining followed formalin fixation, Diff-Quik and Pap stains.[7] Abati and colleagues also recommended that optimal results could be obtained through preparation of moderately cellular monolayers with cytospins and the enhancement of staining in some cases with a predigestion with proteinase K.[10]

Urine cytology plays an integral role in the diagnosis of primary and recurrent urothelial carcinoma of the urinary bladder. Unfortunately, it is also known for relatively low levels of diagnostic sensitivity. As recently reviewed by Bubendorf and colleagues, several groups have investigated the use of florescence in situ hybridization (FISH) to improve the detection of carcinoma in both spontaneously voided urine and bladder washing samples.[11] Using centromere-based probes to detect increased numbers of chromosomes and/or loss of specific genetic segments appears to increase both diagnostic specificity and sensitivity of urine cytology in the detection of urothelial neoplasia.

With the development of additional probes and improved technical aspects of the procedure, FISH may be used to detect reciprocal translocations characteristic of specific neoplasms. For example, aspiration biopsy of a spindle cell neoplasm—which demonstrates by FISH an X,18 reciprocal translocation—would be considered diagnostic of synovial sarcoma.[12]

Although most applications of FISH technology have been directed against the identification and detection of neoplastic cells, Rao and colleagues have used probes directed against the Y chromosome to detect male cells (spermatozoa and squamous epithelium) in cervicovaginal smears in cases of alleged sexual assault.[13] This technique proved to be much more sensitive for the detection of coital activity than the examination of routine Pap-stained specimens for spermatozoa.

Molecular Biology

During the last two decades, molecular biology has exploded on the medical scene, including numerous applications in pathology. Molecular biology may be defined as the analysis of DNA by hybridization and amplification techniques.[14] Probably the cornerstone of the foundation of molecular biology has been the development and application of the polymerase chain reaction (PCR). Before the introduction of PCR, hybridization testing of DNA and ribonucleic acid (RNA) sequences was performed directly on the target DNA after its extraction from cells. Thus, relatively small amounts of nucleic acid were available for analysis.

The beauty of the PCR is that it yields specific and rapid exponential amplification of nucleic acid sequences. This markedly increases the sensitivity of the detection of specific DNA and RNA sequences. The three basic steps used in the PCR are (1) denaturization, (2) hybridization of two synthetic oligonucleotides to complementary foci of the target nucleic acid that surround or flank the target nucleic acid to be amplified, and (3) extension for amplification. The initial denaturization is accomplished through heating of the isolated target DNA by elevation of the temperature within the system above 90° C. The single strands of DNA remain free in solution until the temperature is dropped—at which time the oligonucleotide primers anneal to the DNA. It is important to recognize a basic concept—that the primers are added in marked excess to the original target DNA and thus, the formation of hybrids between the target DNA and the added synthetic primers is markedly favored. The bottom line is that millions of copies of the target sequence of nucleic acid can be produced in only a few hours. A major advance was the identification of thermostable DNA polymerases, the prototype of which is Taq DNA polymerase.

With regard to cytology, probably the most widely used clinical molecular assay is the detection of human papillomavirus (HPV) using the hybrid capture test (Digene, Inc., Beltsville, Md.). With the hybrid capture assay, test DNA is harvested and denatured to form a single-strand solution. This solution is then exposed to a synthetic probe specific for HPV viral subtypes. Hybridization between the tests and probe nucleic acids occurs and then is captured by antibodies directed against the hybrid that are immobilized on the walls of the test wells. This is followed by the addition of another antibody directed against the hybrids, which is conjugated with alkaline phosphatase. Next, a substrate is added that emits light on breakdown of the alkaline phosphatase. Measurement of the amount of emitted light allows quantification of the amount of HPV DNA present in the original target sample. Digene provides two different hybrid capture tests—one for low-risk viruses and one for high-risk viruses. It appears as if the greatest use of this test will be for patients with a diagnosis of atypical squamous cells or glandular cells of undetermined significance.[15]

Both in situ hybridization and in situ PCR are instruments with the potential for numerous applications in diagnostic cytology because they combine the preservation of cytomorphology with specific nucleic acid data. In in situ hybridization the target nucleic acid (DNA or RNA) is fused with a known nucleic acid probe. The target DNA may include cells in cytologic smears. For visualization of the hybridization complex, probes are generally labeled with nonisotopic material such as digoxigenin or biotin. In addition to routine cytologic (or tissue) preparations, in situ hybridization requires nucleic acid denaturation, hybridization, detection, and often counterstain. In the experience of Abati and colleagues, cytospin preparations on charged slides are the specimen of choice.[10] PCR allows amplification of the desired nucleic acid sequence directly in intact cells—referred to as *in situ chain reaction.* Although the sensitivity of in situ PCR is much lower than when the nucleic acids are analyzed in solution, a marked increase in the target DNA for analysis is seen.

The PCR can be used, as discussed in Chapter 24, for the analysis of gene rearrangements of the immunoglobulin chain genes or the T-cell receptor genes to confirm the diagnosis of a B-cell or T-cell malignant lymphoproliferative disorder, respectively. In the authors' experiences, this is most commonly used for aspirates of lymphoid tissue in which a diagnosis of a T-cell lymphoma is suspected on the basis of clinical and cytomorphologic grounds or less often, when immunophenotyping fails to detect light chain restriction in a suspected B-cell neoplasm.

The PCR can also be used to amplify DNA in the search for specific reciprocal translocations that are considered pathognomonic for particular neoplasms. Examples include both lymphoreticular and nonlymphoreticular tumors such as Burkitt's lymphoma, follicular center cell lymphoma, mantle cell lymphoma, synovial sarcoma, and Ewing's sarcoma.

Loss of heterozygosity (LOH) may be defined as the loss of one allele in the DNA from a neoplasm as visualized in autoradiographs. Extracted targeted DNA is amplified via PCR and separated by electrophoresis. The markers used amplify segments that contain polymorphisms in the lengths of the alleles. Alleles of different sizes or configurations can be distinguished on electrophoretic gels based on their mobility. Patients who are heterozygous for this specific gene will manifest two distinct bands on the electrophoretic gel; these patients are often said to be informative for this specific allele. With LOH, the neoplasm typically manifests only one of the two bands on the gel. On the other hand, patients who are homozygous for the gene in their normal tissues manifest only one band on the gel and thus are considered to be noninformative, as LOH in the neoplasm cannot be detected by electrophoresis. Several applications of LOH technology have been described for cytopathology, particularly FNA biopsy. For example, Beaty and colleagues examined aspiration biopsies of known metastatic clear cell carcinomas of the kidney for LOH of the von Hippel-Lindau gene on the short arm of chromosome 3.[16] Approximately 75% of the informative cases showed the identical LOH in the primary and metastatic neoplasm. Abati and colleagues also have used a combination of microdissection and the PCR in FNA biopsies to aid in the distinction between benign and malignant aspirates of primary adrenal cortical proliferations.[17]

Both hyperplasia and adenomas lacked LOH for the markers studied, whereas 70% of the adrenocortical carcinomas examined showed LOH for at least one of the three tested markers.

Finally, one technique that may in the future have prominent impact on diagnostic cytology is the nucleic acid microarray.[14,18] This technique can be used to detect with extreme sensitivity a mutation in a specific gene or measure the levels of expression of thousands of genes in a single specimen.

References

1. Frable WJ. Thin-needle aspiration biopsy: a personal experience with 469 cases. Am J Clin Pathol 1976; 65:168-182.
2. Lever JV, Trott PA, Webb AJ. Fine needle aspiration cytology. J Clin Pathol 1985; 38:1-11.
3. Hajdu SI, Ehya H, Frable WJ, et al. The value and limitations of aspiration cytology in the diagnosis of primary tumors: a symposium. Acta Cytol 1989; 34:905-909.
4. Abati A, Fetsch P, Filie A. If cells could talk: the application of new techniques to cytopathology. Clin Lab Med 1998; 18:561-583.
5. Collins KA, Geisinger KR, Wagner PH, et al. The cytologic evaluation of lipid-laden alveolar macrophages as an indicator of aspiration pneumonia in young children. Arch Pathol Lab Med 1995; 119:228-231.
6. Bergman S, Graeme-Cook F, Pitman MB. The usefulness of the reticulin stain in the differential diagnosis of liver nodules on fine-needle aspiration biopsy cell block preparations. Mod Pathol 1997; 10:1258-1264.
7. Geisinger KR, Rainer RO, Field A. Lymph nodes. In: Geisinger KR, Silverman JF, editors. Fine needle aspiration cytology of superficial organs and body sites. New York: Churchill Livingstone; 1999. p.1-49.
8. Cajulis RS, Frias-Hidvegi D. Detection of numerical chromosomal abnormalities in malignant cells in body fluids by fluorescence in situ hybridization of interphase cell nuclei with chromosome-specific probes. Diagn Cytopathol 1992; 8:627-631.
9. Cajulis RS, Frias-Hidvegi D. Detection of numerical chromosomal abnormalities in malignant cells in fine needle aspirates by fluorescence in situ hybridization of interphase cell nuclei with chromosome-specific probes. Acta Cytol 1993; 37:391-396.
10. Abati A, Sanford JS, Fetsch P, et al. Fluorescence in situ hybridization (FISH): a user's guide to optimal preparation of cytologic specimens. Diagn Cytopathol 1995; 13:486-492.
11. Bubendorf L, Grilli B, Sauter G, et al. Multiprobe FISH for enhanced detection of bladder cancer in voided urine-specimens and bladder washings. Am J Clin Pathol 2001; 116:79-86.
12. Yang P, Hirose T, Hasegawat T, et al. Dual-colour fluorescence in situ hybridization analysis of synovial sarcoma. J Pathol 1998; 184:7-13.
13. Rao PN, Collins KA, Geisinger KR, et al. Identification of male epithelial cells in routine postcoital cervicovaginal smears using fluorescence in situ hybridization: application in sexual assault and molestation. Am J Clin Pathol 1995; 104:32-35.
14. Rimm DL. Molecular biology in cytopathology: current applications and future directions. Cancer Cytopathol 2000; 90:1-9.
15. Solomon D, Schiffman M, Tarone R. Comparison of three management strategies for patients with atypical squamous cells of undetermined significance: baseline results from a randomized trial. J Natl Cancer Inst 2001; 93: 293-299.
16. Beaty MW, Zhuang Z, Park WS, et al. Fine-needle aspiration of metastatic clear cell carcinoma of the kidney: employment of microdissection and the polymerase chain reaction as a potential diagnostic tool. Cancer Cytopathol 1997; 81:180-186.
17. Abati A, Sanjuan X, Wilker A, et al. Utilization of microdissection and the polymerase chain reaction for the diagnosis of adrenal cortical carcinoma in fine-needle aspiration cytology. Cancer Cytopathol 1999; 87:231-237.
18. Rimm DL. Impact of microarray technologies on cytopathology: overview of technologies and commentary on current and future implications for pathologists and cytopathologists. Acta Cytol 2001; 45:111-114.

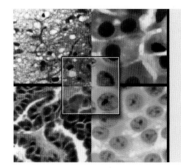

Fine-Needle Aspiration: Equipment, Basic and Clinical Techniques, and Results Reporting

CHAPTER
2

It would be difficult to think of a contemporary medical procedure that is less "high-tech" than fine-needle aspiration (FNA). Its initial clinical application antedated by decades the development of many modern diagnostic tests and devices.[1] At its simplest, only a needle without a syringe is required, as capillary action suffices to admit cells to the needle. The use of a syringe provides negative pressure to the needle tip, which extends the range of lesions that can be successfully sampled using this technique.

Although often a simple procedure, several technical improvements have occurred since its initial description. Modern needles are sterile, disposable and available in a wide range of diameters and lengths. The syringe holder that we use allows the operator to have one hand completely free during the procedure. This permits stabilization of target lesions leading to accurate puncture of even very small masses. The needle guide, invented by Dr. Sixten Franzen at Sweden's Karolinska Hospital, permits accurate, atraumatic aspiration of palpable masses in the prostate and perirectal or paravaginal masses.[2]

A successful marriage of low-tech and high-tech concepts occurs when modern radiographic techniques are used to guide a long, thin needle to a deep-seated, nonpalpable mass lesion. Long, flexible needles with either metal or plastic tips have been developed for use during endoscopy. These needles can be passed through the biopsy channel of either a gastrointestinal endoscope or a bronchoscope to sample pulmonary, mediastinal, or abdominal masses.[3] The current flowering of endoscopic ultrasound-guided FNA is the latest wave in cytology's advance.

Despite the use of radiologic or endoscopic techniques to extend the range of masses to which FNA can be applied, the basic technique remains quite simple. The same simplicity that makes FNA safe, rapid, inexpensive, and accurate can also be its most severe problem. This maneuver, although very powerful, is technically much less difficult to perform than many other common procedures such as bone marrow biopsy, central line placement, or tracheal intubation. Some pathologists fail to use FNA to its full advantage because they mistake the simple for the trivial and ignore its technical aspects.

A fear of those contemplating the use of FNA is that pathologists may be unable to interpret properly the material obtained. Certainly interpretation of cytologic preparations is very important, but in the authors' experience, more problems in FNA occur at the bedside than at the microscope. Accordingly, details of clinical aspiration are emphasized.

EQUIPMENT

Needles

Many advantages of tumor sampling by FNA are the direct result of the small diameter of the needles. These include an extremely low complication rate, excellent patient acceptance, no scars, and no need for anesthesia. In addition, the aspiration can be repeated as necessary for special studies, assessment of treatment effects, or obtaining additional tissue for a more complete or certain diagnosis. Nordenskjold and colleagues describe sequential aspiration of breast cancer patients for assessment of tumor cell thymidine labeling and the effects of treatment on the tumor.[4] Some of their patients accepted up to 40 FNA procedures.

Figure 2-1 shows a comparison of a 2-mm tissue core biopsy needle with the needles most often used for FNA. Most aspirations are performed with 23- to 27-gauge needles, which permit adequate sampling of a majority of masses. In the authors' experience the smallest needle that can adequately sample a given mass is preferred. For example, needles larger than 23 gauge cause increased bleeding rather than larger specimens. For this reason the diagnostic yield may be lower than that obtained with using smaller needles, and 23- or 25-gauge needles are used for most FNAs.

The appropriate needle length depends on the nature of the target lesion. Using 25-gauge needles, many lymph nodes can be reached with a ⅝-inch (1.6-cm) length. A 1.5-inch (3.8-cm) length can be used for many breast masses, whereas a patient with large breasts or palpable abdominal mass may require a 2-inch (5-cm) or 3.5-inch (8.8-cm) length. The authors use 1.5-inch, 25-gauge needle for the majority of aspirations.

This chapter is modified from Stanley MW, Löwhagen T. Fine needle aspiration of palpable masses. Butterworth-Heinemann: Boston; 1993.
Illustrations of sample preparation were staged for the purpose of photography. Optically opaque materials such as hand lotion were employed as surrogate specimens. During acquisition of actual patient materials, one should always observe the universal precautions that include gloves.

Needles with a plastic hub are preferred rather than a metal hub. This permits the operator to monitor the recovery of tissue, fluid, or blood as it appears in the hub. Diagnostic tissue fragments are often trapped in the needle hub. Using techniques to be discussed subsequently, an effort should be made to recover these fragments for microscopic examination. Thus, a clear view of the needle hub and its contents is helpful. A translucent colored hub is acceptable.

Syringes

Modern, sterile, disposable syringes made of clear plastic are excellent for use in FNA. Most clinicians use the 10-ml size, while others prefer the 20-ml size. Radiologists sometimes use a 50- or 60-ml size.

Table 2-1 summarizes the luminal pressure that can be generated by evacuating syringes of various sizes. The data were calculated by using the gas law to expand the dead space volume of the empty syringe to its maximum capacity. Using a standard Leur tip syringe fitted with a standard-size needle hub, the dead space volume is approximately 0.13 ml. When the initial pressure is 760 mm Hg, expanding this volume to the maximum final volume allowed by the syringe yields the luminal pressures shown. The final column in Table 2-1 shows the difference between the ambient pressure (760 mm Hg) and luminal pressure. Clearly, the differences among syringe sizes in the third column are trivial in terms of the *amount of suction* provided. Therefore, selection of a syringe size should be based on comfort, convenience, availability, and personal preference. Larger syringes do not give larger samples. Syringes with a lock device should not be used.

Syringe Holder

In most situations the metal syringe holder shown in Figure 2-2 is used. An exception is the aspiration without suction discussed later in this chapter (Zajdela technique). The metal syringe holder weighs only 190 g and is preferred over its plastic imitations. Such devices are usually available in two sizes that accommodate either a 10-ml or a 20-ml syringe.

Using the syringe holder permits both needle placement and application, as well as release of suction by the syringe to be accomplished with one hand. Suction is not applied until after the needle is within the mass and is released before it is withdrawn. Thus, suction in the syringe is sufficient to return the plunger to its neutral position at the conclusion of the aspiration. This action is automatic, requiring no additional effort by the physician performing the procedure. The other hand is completely free and available to locate and stabilize the target mass.

Quantity of Tissue

FNA often provides generous tissue sampling. The tissue obtained is frequently more abundant than that in well-accepted biopsy methods such as transbronchial biopsy, endoscopic bowel biopsy, or cutting needle core biopsy. Although qualitatively different, FNA specimens are often quantitatively superior to methods for biopsy of solid tissue fragments. FNA selectively removes tumor cells of carcinoma, melanoma, or lymphoma. Much of the connective tissue is left behind. The result is concentration of the diagnostic cells. Thus, FNA often gives better sampling than

TABLE 2-1		
Syringe Luminal Pressure for Different Syringe Volumes		
Syringe Volume (ml)	**Lumenal Pressure (mm Hg)**	**Ambient-Syringe Pressure Difference (mm Hg)**
3	30.4	730
5	18.2	742
10	9.1	751
12	7.6	752
20	4.5	756
50	1.8	758

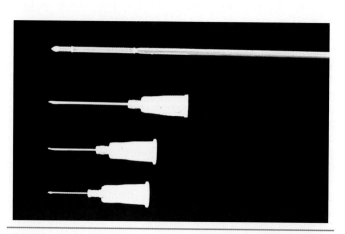

Figure 2-1 Needle used for fine-needle aspiration (FNA). A tissue core biopsy needle *(top)* is compared with fine needles of 23 (0.6 mm), 25 (0.5 mm), and 27 gauges (0.4 mm).

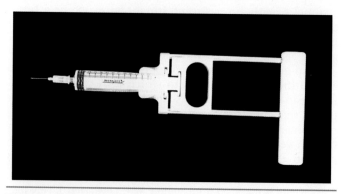

Figure 2-2 Metal pistol-grip syringe holder for FNA procedures. Illustrated here is the 10-ml size shown with a 12-ml syringe and a 25-gauge needle of 1.5-inch (38-mm) length.

biopsy methods that appear to remove larger pieces of tissue. In the latter instance, much of the tissue may be stroma rather than tumor cells.

BASIC TECHNIQUES IN FINE-NEEDLE ASPIRATION

The Aspiration Procedure

FNA can be adapted to many clinical settings and problems, but the basic procedure is constant. Although the total number of punctures performed on a given patient varies with the clinical situation, each aspiration takes about 5 to 10 seconds. Additional time is spent examining the lesion, preparing the skin, and processing the material obtained by FNA, but the actual aspiration event is brief. Important issues, including patient positioning, physical examination, and smear preparation, are discussed later in the chapter; this section concentrates on the basic process of performing the aspiration (Table 2-2).

The initial step is localization of the mass to be punctured. It is important to emphasize the need for delicacy and control. Large targets can be successfully punctured by any method, however unstudied. However, many masses that can be successfully studied by FNA are quite small and only a controlled approach will suffice.

For a right-handed clinician, two fingers of the left hand outline and immobilize the mass under study. With large tumors, the fingertips span only a portion of the mass. In smaller masses, two fingers often encompass the entire tumor. This approach also allows the aspirator to apply pressure to the mass so that even a mobile tumor becomes

a fixed target. In all cases the fingers are arched and extend from the hand, which is poised above a point near the palpable mass.

With the mass localized and stabilized, the previously assembled syringe holder with syringe and needle is now used. The needle is passed through the skin en route to the lesion. No suction has been applied at this point. The needle tip then enters the mass. Various aids to accomplishing this goal are described later in this chapter. For now, thinking of the needle as an extension of the right index finger and the mass as an extension of the palpating fingers of the left hand is helpful. Thus, the sometimes difficult task of hitting a small target resembles touching the tip of one index finger with the other. This concept creates the possibility of subtle nuances of touch and pressure between the needle and the mass. This delicacy and control are essential if small lesions are to be well sampled consistently.

The needle is advanced into the lesion, and suction is applied. Next, the process occurs that is most likely responsible for generous sampling with FNA, as the needle is moved back and forth through the mass in different directions by use of a "sewing-machine" motion. Suction is maintained throughout this process. By this method, the needle can cut loose many small pieces of tissue that are then aspirated because of the suction applied by the syringe. The actual motion causes the needle tip to describe a cone with its base in or near the mass and its apex at the point where the needle enters the skin, as shown in Figure 2-3.

In general, most aspirations are terminated when material begins to appear in the needle hub. This area is monitored for material during the aspiration procedure. In some instances, larger volumes of either cyst fluid or blood may be obtained.

The next step is designed to protect the specimen. All suction is released by allowing the syringe plunger to return gently to its resting position. Because the needle is still in the mass (or at least under the skin surface), the negative pressure within the syringe causes this to happen without any effort from the physician except for relaxing the fingers that have been pulling back on the plunger.

TABLE 2-2	
Summary of Steps in Basic Fine-Needle Aspiration	
Procedure Setup	**Suction Applied**
1. Locate, palpate, and stabilize the target lesion.	
2. Pass needle through the skin.	No
3. Advance needle into the lesion.	No
4. Apply suction.	Yes
5. Move needle repeatedly through the mass in various directions.	Yes
6. Release suction.	No
7. Remove needle from patient.	No
8. Detach needle from syringe.	
9. Fill syringe with air.	
10. Replace needle on syringe.	
11. Change grip on syringe holder.	
12. Touch needle tip to a microscope slide.	
13. Express specimen onto microscope slide.	
14. Prepare smears.	
15. Fix or dry smears.	
16. Reexamine the puncture site before leaving the patient's bedside.	

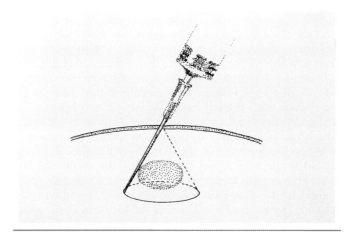

Figure 2-3 **The needle is moved back and forth through the mass in different directions.** Its tip describes a cone-shaped volume of sampled tissue with its base near the mass and its apex at the skin surface.

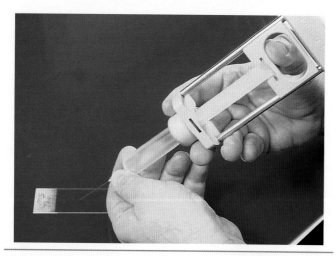

Figure 2-4   Syringe pistol grip used to carefully control the expression of aspirated material onto a glass microscope slide. The left hand holds the needle firmly on the syringe.

At this point in the procedure, most or all of the specimen is in the needle. A small amount may be in the needle hub. Except in the case of cyst fluids, bloody aspirations, or high-volume specimens such as an abscess or an area of necrosis, little or no material is in the syringe itself. The purpose of releasing suction before the needle is withdrawn is to leave the aspirated material largely in the needle. If it is withdrawn with suction still applied, the specimen is drawn quickly into the syringe, during which it breaks up into numerous small droplets. These are in turn deposited forcefully onto the walls of the syringe barrel where they are quickly desiccated and virtually impossible to recover intact. The vital importance of releasing suction before withdrawing the syringe was well illustrated by the study of Furnival and colleagues. By addition of this simple step to their aspiration protocol, these authors reduced the rate of unsatisfactory breast aspiration from 24.8% to 6% (total series = 237 cases).[5]

The needle is now withdrawn from the patient. With no suction applied to the syringe, the needle is detached from it. The syringe is now filled with air while the needle is detached. The needle with its specimen can now be replaced onto the syringe. The air in the syringe is used to expel the specimen onto a glass microscope slide. At this point, it is more efficient to use a different grip on the syringe pistol; it is held like a syringe being used for an injection (Figure 2-4). During this procedure the needle should be held on the syringe with the left hand. When it is not held to the syringe as the sample is expelled, the needle may fly forcefully from the syringe if the specimen is thick or clotted.

When the specimen is placed on the slide, the needle tip should be kept in actual contact with the surface of the slide, usually with the bevel at an angle of 45 degrees to 90 degrees to the slide's surface. Spraying the specimen onto the slide from a needle held above the slide causes the specimen to break up into droplets that are rapidly dried as they spread out on impact with the slide. Specimen desiccation is virtually nonexistent when the material is placed on the slide as a small droplet. Furthermore, if a moment or two is needed to care for the patient before attending to the spec-

imen, cytologic integrity is maintained by allowing the specimen to rest briefly in its tissue fluid. The aspirated material can be stored briefly either within the needle or as a small droplet on the glass slide.

Zajdela Technique

In many instances, capillary action without aspiration suffices to admit cells and tissue particles into a thin needle. This is the basis of the technique described by Zajdela.[6] In this method the mass is localized and stabilized with the fingers of the left hand as previously discussed. The right hand thumb, index finger, and middle finger hold the thin needle of appropriate length. After the needle is advanced into the lesion, it is moved about in a cone-shaped tissue volume similar to that discussed earlier and then withdrawn. A syringe filled with air is attached and used to expel the specimen onto a microscope slide for smear preparation.

This method is most useful for small lesions. The needle grip described above gives excellent control and an extraordinary degree of sensitivity to changes in the texture of tissues through which the needle passes. These benefits improve one's ability to puncture tiny masses. Zajdela and colleagues describe successful application of this method to study of small masses around the eye, including those in the lids.[6]

It has been suggested that adding aspiration—that is, performing FNA in the traditional manner—lowers the rate of inadequate sampling when benign breast masses are studied.[7] This probably reflects the fact that many of these masses consist largely of fibrofatty tissue and yield sparsely cellular samples under the best of circumstances. In the authors' experience, the Zajdela Method yields fewer cells than aspiration but provides sufficient material for diagnosis of most lesions. The needle can be concealed in the palm of the physician's hand and the patient is spared seeing the large syringe and syringe holder that some find alarming. Thus, patients are accepting of this technique.

Preparation of Samples

Glass Slides
An important consideration is slide labeling at the time of the procedure. Permanent labels with the laboratory's case accession number are affixed later. Labeling at the bedside should be rapid, convenient, and indelible. Most laboratories use two identifiers on each slide, such as the patient's name (or initials) and the site of the aspiration. Slides with one frosted end on both sides of the slide surface are preferred. A soft lead pencil is effective in labeling the frosted glass.

Slides are labeled at the bedside just before performing the aspiration to minimize any possibility of confusing material from different patients. In processing the smears after staining, it is important to apply a coverslip to the correct side of the slide and to ensure that the aspirated material is not wiped from the surface. By writing on the label and always applying smears to the same side as the label, no confusion over which side of the slide holds the specimen should occur. Scanty specimens may be difficult to identify by gross inspection of the slide so that some such method

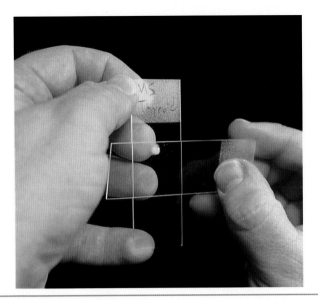

Figure 2-5 **One-step smear.** The end of the spreader slide is touched to the specimen slide at a 45-degree angle.

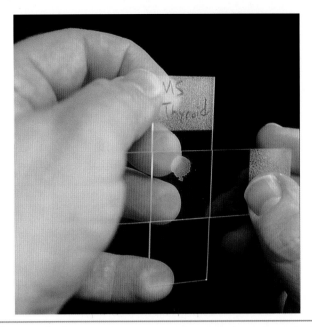

Figure 2-6 **One-step smear.** The top far edge of the spreader slide is lowered onto the specimen droplet. Gentle pressure is then used to flatten the material.

is important to ensure that occasional specimens are not lost when the slide is handled during processing.

Introduction to Smear Preparation

Although a variety of special studies can be applied to aspiration specimens, cellular material is most often spread on a glass slide to form a smear suitable for routine light microscopy. Cells should be spread over the slide surface. Some tissue fragments need to be spread apart with gentle pressure, and some remain intact. While accomplishing these goals, the pressure applied to the specimen must not be so great as to crush the cells. The end result should be a smear with well-preserved cells spread thinly enough to permit the transmission of light.

Selecting a smearing technique is dictated to some extent by the skills and preferences of the individual preparing the specimen. The physical properties of the specimen must also be considered; it is helpful to tailor the method to the specimen so that the best results are achieved. A small droplet of semisolid tissue for example, requires a different approach than that used for more fluid materials.

Many FNA slides have most or all of the specimen concentrated in a small area. These can be reviewed microscopically much more quickly than poorly made smears that do not concentrate tissue particles and cover most of the slide surface. In the authors' practice, most FNA smears do not require screening. This contributes to rapid turnaround time and improves laboratory efficiency.

Preparation of aspirated material is one of the most important parts of the entire process. Unless high-quality preparations are created, it does not matter how adroit the aspiration or how skilled the microscopist; the material is uninterpretable.

Two Slide-Pull Method

This is widely used and easy to learn. It is most useful with specimens of low volume. The specimen, or a small droplet-sized portion thereof, is placed near the center of the slide.

A second, clean, previously labeled slide is inverted over the first and gentle pressure is then applied, after which the two slides are pulled apart with a sliding motion. Both slides hold material, and both should be further processed. (The upper or spreader slide holds the specimen on its lower face and must be inverted before it is set aside for processing.)

If the specimen volume is too large, if excessive pressure is used in spreading the material, or if the droplet is placed too close to the end of the slide, the smear will have much of the material carried to the end of the slide where it forms a dense zone that is too thick for careful microscopic study.

One-Step Method

This produces high quality smears, especially with small-volume specimens. This technique is preferred to the two-slide pull because it allows precise control of the pressure applied to the specimen. Furthermore, it usually produces a smear that occupies a small area on the slide, thus facilitating rapid microscopic review.

In preparing to execute the maneuver, the slides are held as shown in Figure 2-5. The lower slide holds the specimen and is held in the left hand. Using the illustrated grip, the slide is securely supported, but its entire surface is virtually free and available for the smear. The upper slide is a spreader slide. When using this technique, the specimen is placed near the slide label. Thus, most of the slide's length is available for the smear.

The spreader slide is held at an angle so that its edge near the specimen is poised above the droplet and its other edge touches the lower slide in a hingelike fashion. It is then lowered onto the droplet as in Figure 2-6. Gentle pressure is applied to flatten but not crush the droplet. The spreader slide is then drawn along the length of the specimen slide by pulling it toward the preparer. The pressure applied to the lower slide must be constant and gentle.

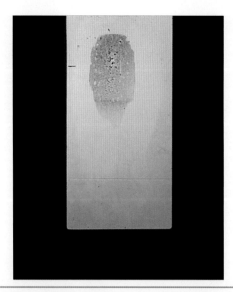

Figure 2-7 Typical smear produced by the one-step method. It occupies a small fraction of the total slide area and tissue particles are visible.

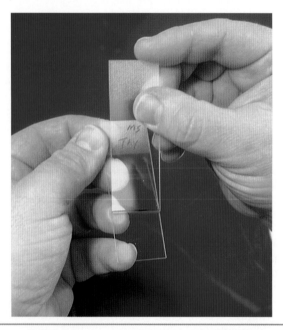

Figure 2-8 Two-step smear. Surface tension has distributed the entire specimen as a small line behind the end of the spreader slide. Tissue particles move with the fluid and are concentrated along this line.

During this procedure, the surfaces of the two slides are parallel. It is important that the spreader slide not be tilted to either side of parallel. If the edge away from the lower slide's label is tilting toward the lower slide, the pressure on the specimen is decreased, and the smear will be too thick. If the edge near the label is tilted down, the specimen will be scraped off of the lower slide onto the edge of the spreader slide where it forms a thick line from which diagnostic material is difficult to recover. Normally, little material is present on the spreader slide, so it is discarded. A typical smear prepared in this manner is shown in Figure 2-7. This preparation can be rapidly reviewed because it occu-

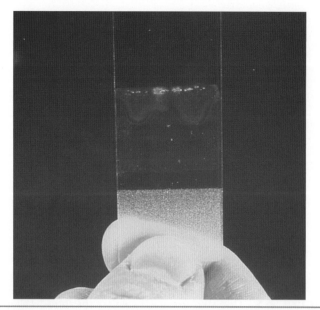

Figure 2-9 Two-step smear. The spreader slide has been pulled away from the specimen slide and retained for later use. The specimen slide is held vertically, with its label down. The tissue particles remain in a line in the middle of the slide while the fluid drains away toward the label end of the slide.

pies only a small area of the slide and contains visible tissue particles.

The Two-Step Method

The two-step method is tailored to liquid specimens within which cells and tissue particles are suspended. It is designed to handle a few drops of fluid at a time.

First, the fluid specimen is placed near the labeled end of the slide. Using the grip shown previously, the spreader slide is held vertically at a 45-degree angle to the specimen-bearing slide and its end is brought into contact with the lower slide in front of the specimen. It is then advanced toward the specimen slide's label until it just touches the specimen pool. Surface tension causes the liquid to spread out in a line behind the edge of the spreader slide (Figure 2-8). The tissue particles are carried with the fluid and are thus concentrated in a narrow band across the slide.

The spreader slide is then pulled away from the specimen slide label to about the middle of the lower slide. At this point, the two slides are tilted together as a unit so that the label ends point down. The spreader slide, which often bears some tissue at its distal end, is now quickly pulled away from the specimen slide. The spreader slide is retained in the right hand, while with the left hand, the specimen slide is held vertically. The larger tissue particles are now sedimented along the line where the spreader slide was placed, and much of the fluid drains toward the label of the specimen slide and away from the tissue (Figure 2-9).

The procedure from this point is much like the one-step method described previously. The same spreader slide (still with tissue fragments on its distal end) is turned perpendicular to the specimen slide and the line of tissue particles is smeared as before (Figure 2-10).

The tissue remaining on the distal end of the spreader slide must now be recovered. It can be placed either on the

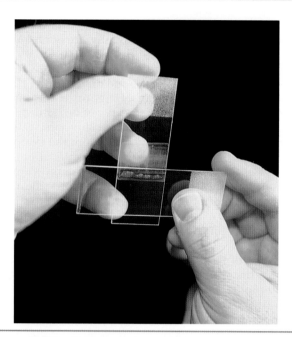

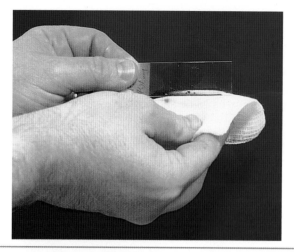

Figure 2-11 Modified two-step method. The particles have been allowed to sediment, the fluid is moved to the slide's edge by rotating the slide, and the gauze acts as a wick to remove the fluid.

Figure 2-10 Two-step smear. The line of particles shown in Figure 2-9 is now smeared with a spreader slide. At this point the method becomes much like the one-step smear process.

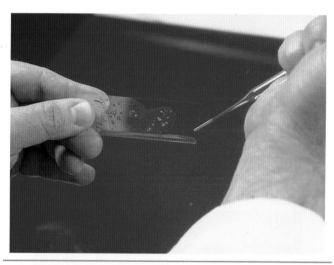

Figure 2-12 Modified two-step method. The excess fluid from the modified two-step smear method can be collected with a pipette and processed or saved for other studies.

smear that has just been made (if additional room is available on that slide), or it can be put on a new slide. The spreader slide is touched to the new slide near the label at a 45-degree angle with its line of fluid or tissue in the vertex of the angle. It is then lowered until it is parallel to the new specimen slide and drawn parallel to it much like with the two-slide pull.

The two-step method accomplishes two things. First, tissue particles are concentrated in a relatively small area of the slide for rapid viewing. Second, much of the fluid has been removed from the diagnostically important part of the specimen. This permits either rapid, thorough fixation or rapid drying of the slide, whichever is preferred. The high quality morphology of rapidly dried cells is lost if the cells are allowed to dry slowly in abundant fluid. The latter process causes the cells to appear exploded.

This technique is more complex, but it greatly increases the number of specimens that can be smeared in a few seconds at the bedside. This is important because all the alternatives to rapidly made smears involve either centrifugation or histology-based embedding. In either case, specimen preparation is much slower and requires more time from laboratory personnel. Because some of the chief advantages of FNA are its rapidity, simplicity, low cost, and lack of a need for highly skilled laboratory personnel, these alternative methods would reduce markedly its utility and attractiveness.

Modified Two-Step Method

This method has the same advantages as the two-step technique, but it is designed to handle a larger volume of blood or fluid—up to 0.5 ml per slide. In a few seconds, most of the tissue particles sediment. The slide can then be picked up and rotated gently. As the particles sediment over a large area of the slide, the fluid can be moved to the edge of the slide by this motion. Unless its volume is excessive, surface ten-

sion will keep the liquid on the slide. The slide is then tipped vertically, and the fluid is removed by bringing a piece of gauze to the edge of the slide. The gauze acts as a wick (Figure 2-11). Alternatively, this fluid can be removed with a small glass pipette and then processed by centrifugation for cytologic examination or special studies (Figure 2-12).

The particles on the slide must now be brought together and smeared. This is accomplished in the manner previously described for the two-step method.

Alternative to Rapid Preparation of Smears

Another method for specimen preparation rarely used in the authors' own practice is described here. The material obtained by aspiration can be expressed into a liquid fixative. Those that have been suggested include Saccomanno's fluid (2% Carbowax in 50% ethanol), 95% ethanol and 50% methanol. Once received in the laboratory, this fluid is processed by laboratory personnel using a centrifuge or made into a paraffin-embedded cell block. Liquid-based processing similar to that common in gynecologic cytology can also be employed, if the appropriate collection materials have been provided.

The advantage of this method is obvious; when non-pathologists perform aspirations, this technique relieves them of any need to be able to make smears. Furthermore,

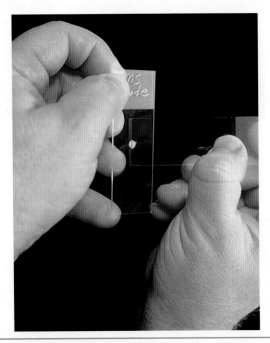

Figure 2-13 **Splitting sample.** In preparing to split a generous specimen, the edge of a spreader slide is used to partition a specimen pool as shown.

the specimen is preserved in a form suitable for transport to the laboratory, and laboratory personnel are not required to attend the procedure.

Disadvantages include the rising cost of FNA when processing is added and that turnaround time is longer than for direct smears. In the hospital setting, or in the clinic attached to the hospital, many smears can be stained, examined, and reported rapidly. For many clinicians, this is an important motivation for using FNA. From the cytopathologist's point of view, having only fixed material limits the staining possibilities. Specifically, Romanowsky stains (the group of staining methods applied to air-dried smears as in hematologic preparations) cannot be applied to fixed material. Some cytopathologists strongly prefer air-dried Romanowsky-stained smears in many settings.

Preparation of Several Smears from a Single Aspiration

It is often the case, especially with cancers, that a single aspiration provides more material than needed for one slide. Indeed, if too much material is placed on a single slide, it may be too thick for examination. In this instance the material is distributed among the original slide and one or more additional slides. Four or more good quality, cellular smears can be made from one puncture of a malignancy.

To begin, the entire specimen is expressed onto a specimen slide as described. The end of a spreader slide is then placed in the specimen pool at a 45-degree angle as shown in Figure 2-13. This is moved rapidly and smoothly to the edge of the specimen slide and carried off its edge. At this point the original specimen slide has a portion of its material still in place, and the spreader slide bears tissue on its distal end (Figure 2-14). The material on the specimen slide is smeared with the spreader slide as in the one-step method (Figure 2-15). The material on the end of the

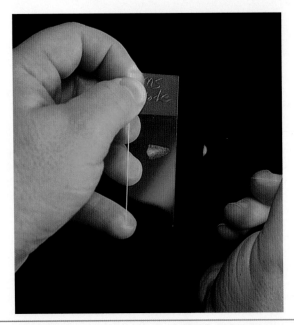

Figure 2-14 **Splitting sample.** The spreader slide has been moved off the edge of the specimen slide and now holds tissue on its distal end. The original specimen slide still has a portion of its original material.

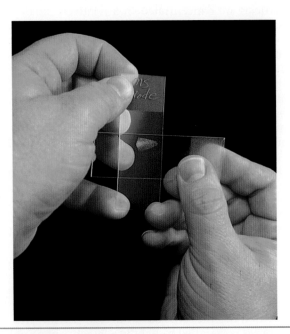

Figure 2-15 **Splitting sample.** The material that has been split, as shown in Figure 2-14, is smeared using the one-step method. Note that the spreader slide retains a portion of the aspirated material on its tip. This will be used to prepare a second smear. In this fashion, both fixed and dried slides can be prepared from a single aspirate.

spreader slide can now be placed onto a new slide and smeared.

If the specimen on the end of the spreader slide is sufficient, a small portion of it can be deposited on each of two or more slides by gently touching them with the specimen droplet. Each of the new specimen slides is then smeared by the one-step method. In this way, several smears have been rapidly prepared from one aspiration.

In a variation of this method, the edge or corner of a clean spreader slide is gently touched to an expressed specimen droplet, and a small amount will adhere. It can then be transferred by touching it to a new specimen slide. In this way, many small smears can be prepared. In the case of highly cellular material such as lymph node aspirations, these tiny smears may be thinner and better for microscopic examination than the thicker smears prepared from the entire specimen droplet.

These methods of splitting a specimen may also be applied to either the two-step or the modified two-step procedure. The spreader slide can be used to divide the line of tissue fragments produced early in these procedures. The remaining portion of the tissue particle line can then be smeared.

These methods can be mastered with practice and conducted in a few seconds. Just as the basic motions of the FNA procedure should be mastered before the patient is approached, so should the handling of aspirated material. Smear making can be practiced using droplets of lotion or liquid soap. The fluid-rich materials suitable for the two-step or modified two-step method can be simulated by material aspirated from an orange.

These techniques greatly increase the number of specimens that can be evaluated properly by FNA. The aspirated material is also of optimum quality when smears are well made, the tissue is concentrated, and the fluid or blood is largely removed. Unstained smears can be stored or transported as necessary.

Clotting of Aspiration Specimens

Extremely bloody specimens are always suboptimal, but many can be improved with the modified two-step smear technique. When clotting occurs, the material is unsuitable for cytologic examination and must be fixed (usually in formalin) and embedded for histologic study.

Some operators use heparinized syringes to reduce clotting. Those choosing this method should draw a small amount of heparin through the needle into the syringe. This should then be expelled as completely as possible. Tiny amounts are sufficient to impede clotting, but larger amounts may result in unwanted artifacts when cells are studied microscopically. Kung and colleagues state that heparin is rarely necessary. These authors discussed liver FNA, which often yields bloody material. They indicated that by handling the material quickly, clotting does not occur before smears are prepared.[8]

Embedded Cell Blocks (Histologic Preparation of Aspirated Material)

Occasional bloody specimens clot rapidly and completely. These are unsuitable for smears and cytologic interpretation. In other cases, histologic material is desirable in addition to cytologic preparations. In these instances, material is placed in a liquid fixative such as Bouin's or 10% neutral buffered formalin by expressing the needle's contents directly into fluid. This is then centrifuged, and the pellet is embedded for sectioning as any small tissue biopsy is handled. In other instances, FNA yields tissue particles of sufficient size, a few of which can be removed from a slide, fixed, and processed routinely.

Bloody specimens can be expressed onto a slide and intentionally set aside briefly to allow clotting. This material can then be placed in fixative solution. This method is often used, in addition to smear preparation, during radiographically directed aspirations when cell block material is desirable. Material obtained by rinsing the needle and syringe may also be suitable for preparation of cell blocks. This cell block method is especially useful in preparing large numbers of tissue sections for immunohistochemistry.

As FNA of palpable masses is easily repeated, and because most cases do not require histologic material for diagnosis, cell blocks are not prepared in all cases. On the other hand, when material is obtained with radiographic guidance or by endoscopic means, repeating the procedure is difficult and costly and causes delays in patient care. In these settings, cell blocks are prepared whenever sufficient material is available.

Additional Techniques

An effort should be made to recover all of the aspirated material. At times, some of this is lodged in the hub of the needle or in the distal part of the syringe. Tissue fragments in the needle hub are never recovered by repeated blasts of air from the syringe through the needle. These particles can be deposited on a slide by holding the needle in the hand and forcefully hitting the open end of the hub against the surface of the slide repeatedly. This maneuver has been executed several thousand times without incurring an accidental needle-stick injury. This technique should be practiced with sterile needles before applying it to needles with potentially infectious patient material. The needle can also be gripped with a hemostat to reduce the danger of an accidental needle stick. In another approach the needle is pushed through a rubber stopper in the end of a glass blood-drawing tube from which the vacuum has been released. This is then held horizontally with the open needle hub over a slide. The springlike quality of the needle allows it to be bent up away from the slide and snapped vigorously against the slide several times, releasing its contents.

Slides produced in any of these ways hold small fluid droplets or tissue particles. These can then be collected as in the modified two-step method so that they form a line to be smeared with another slide. The material in the hub is often the most diagnostic part of the specimen, the subsequently aspirated material having been contaminated with blood or fluid. Thus, recovery, smearing, and study of this portion of the specimen is important.

Tissue must also be recovered from the syringe. Small amounts of fluid or blood can be handled with the two-step or modified two-step smearing techniques. If clotting occurs, a cell block should be prepared. Volumes of nonclotting fluid greater than 0.5 ml are usually submitted to the cytology laboratory for centrifugation, after which the sedimented material is prepared by one of the smearing techniques previously described or as a fixed cell block for histologic study.

Small droplets or fragments often remain in the tip of the syringe. To recover this material the syringe without the needle is held as in Figure 2-4, and it is gently filled with air. The open end is placed on the glass slide and the plunger is rapidly, forcefully, and audibly pushed back to the empty position. This maneuver can be rapidly repeated several times so that all material can be recovered. It can then be collected and smeared as described for tissue that was recovered from the needle hub.

An alternative to this simple method involves rinsing of the syringe and needle with saline or fixative. This method is rarely used because the material obtained requires concentration by centrifugation or filtration.

After smears are prepared, some workers routinely rinse the needle and syringe with saline or fixative. This fluid is then centrifuged and examined for tumor cells. The authors prospectively studied 159 such needle rinse specimens obtained at FNA of 152 patients. Aspiration sites included the breast (70), lymph nodes (30), lung (15), soft tissue (14), salivary glands (12), thyroid (12), liver (5), and a single branchial cleft cyst. Malignancy was identified on smear material from 21 aspirates. In 16 of these (76%), the needle rinse material was also positive. No additional malignancies were detected by study of rinse material.[9]

It was concluded that routine preparation and study of needle rinse material contributes little to most FNA diagnoses. However, in all cases, efforts were made to recover material from the syringe tip and needle hub as previously described. In the absence of such methods, needle rinse material may be more useful. Furthermore, because many malignancies are represented in the rinse specimen, this method can be used to prepare additional slides if these are needed for special studies. This material can also be used to prepare histologic cell blocks.

Comments on Technical Assistance During Fine-Needle Aspiration

Those clinicians who perform aspirations often and are trained in the basic techniques of specimen preparation often perform the procedure well and send diagnostic material to the laboratory. However, a more common situation is that once obtained, the specimen is handed to a nurse or a resident physician who has no idea what to do with it. Thus, diagnostic material is converted to useless clots and crushed cells. Most clinicians who fail to enjoy the benefits of FNA experience more problems in specimen preparation than they do an inability to perform quality aspirations. Physicians wishing to perform FNA should take the time to master the entire procedure, including specimen preparation.

 ## ROUTINE AND RAPID STAINS

Unless intended for special studies or for cell block embedding as a histologic specimen, the aspirated material can only be handled in two ways. Once a smear is prepared, it can be either fixed or dried. The choice between these alternatives should be made before the procedure is carried out because either must be accomplished very rapidly once a smear has been prepared. Different stains are applied to these two types of slides so that they initiate very different sequences of events in the laboratory.

Preferences vary among different microscopists. Often a cytopathologist may prefer fixed slides for one kind of specimen and dried slides if other diagnostic possibilities are to be investigated. When someone other than the pathologist performs the aspiration, the laboratory should be consulted about preferred handling of the slides.

The relative merits of the two methods are discussed in the following sections. Because some processes are more easily diagnosed on one stain than the other and because surprises often occur in clinical medicine, these authors prefer preparing both dried and fixed slides in each case. It is often possible to split a single aspiration specimen into two or more slides, and one can usually prepare at least one dried and one fixed slide from each puncture. This technique is used routinely, and in the majority of cases, both smears contain diagnostic material.

Fixation of Smears

Fixatives are applied to a smear as a spray or by immersion of the slide into a liquid. The liquid fixatives include 95% ethanol, 100% ethanol, sequential application of methanol and ethanol, 100% methanol, Saccomanno's fixative, combined methanol/diethyl ether (Papanicolaou's original fixative), acetone, 80% isopropyl alcohol, combined acetone/methanol, and Esposti's fixative (95% ethanol with 5% glacial acetic acid). However, the most commonly used is 95% ethanol. This inexpensive, readily available liquid provides excellent cytologic detail. Its only disadvantages are the need to store and transport unstained slides in a container of liquid and to have this fluid and these containers at hand in the clinic.

The alternative to wet fixation is use of a commercially available spray fixative. These generally consist of various mixtures containing ethanol or isopropyl alcohol with carbowax (polyethylene glycol). The latter leaves a coating on the slide after the alcohol has evaporated and is said to prevent cell shrinkage. Such sprayed slides are dry within a few seconds and are then suitable for storage, mailing, or immediate processing. These coating fixatives must first be removed with a 10-minute soak in 95% ethanol before staining is performed. If this step is hastened, poor staining quality results.

After this initial step, the staining proceeds just as it would for wet-fixed smears. These commercial products can be purchased in small, easily carried bottles with a finger pump. Many clinicians find them convenient and easy to use. Furthermore, the manual pump eliminates the danger of cell damage by freezing, which can occur with pressurized cans of aerosol fixatives.

Aerosol spray fixatives are also in use. Many gynecologists are accustomed to using hair spray to fix cervical smears. This is inexpensive, readily available, and works fairly well. Aerosols expand isentropically when sprayed and thus are very cold. If the spray can is held closer to the smear surface rather than about 10 inches (25 cm) from it, the cells become rapidly frozen and severely damaged. The microscopic result resembles the air-drying artifact of fixed smears discussed in the following section and often renders the material unsuitable for cytologic examination.

Regardless of the fixative selected, it must be applied quickly because good results are obtained only if it is applied within a few seconds of making a smear. When cells dry, they swell, and their sizes appear altered. Furthermore, the distinct details of nuclear structure are no longer seen. Even in well-fixed smears, some drying artifact may occur at the smear edges. Marked drying renders Pap-stained slides unsuitable for interpretation.

Smear Drying

Alternatively, slides may be intentionally air-dried in preparation for a Romanowsky stain. This simple procedure consists of rapidly and completely drying a smear before any stain is applied. This is usually accomplished by setting the smear aside. For optimal results, drying should occur quickly. A slide can sometimes be held by the label and waved gently in the air for a few seconds. This hastens drying of a smear with excess blood or fluid.

One advantage of the drying technique when compared to wet or spray fixation is that drying eliminates one technical step; drying smears basically consists of doing nothing. Dried smears (stained appropriately) are preferable to smears that have been badly or slowly fixed and then Pap-stained. The former can be interpreted in the routine manner, whereas the latter is often difficult or impossible to interpret.

Stains Applied to Fixed Smears

The actions taken by the laboratory depend on whether a slide has been fixed or dried. Fixed material is usually stained by either the Papanicolaou method or the hematoxylin and eosin (H&E) method. Both employ one of the hematoxylins for nuclear staining. This dye colors the nucleic acids a dark purplish-blue color. The counterstaining is designed to show cytoplasmic characteristics. One hallmark of the Pap stain is the use of Orange-G, which stains cytoplasmic keratin a bright orange color. This is useful in identifying squamous differentiation.

Stains Applied to Air-Dried Smears

Any of several Romanowsky stains were originally developed for application to blood and bone marrow smears. Although numerous recipes exist, all are variable combinations of methylene blue and its breakdown products (Azure A, B, or C) with Eosin.[10] Most rely on methanol fixation. Cell drying results in cell swelling so that cells tend to appear larger in Romanowsky preparations.

An important chemical characteristic is the ability of Romanowsky stains to react metachromatically with a variety of tissue components. This is a shifting of the dye's absorption spectrum in the presence of negatively charged entities to give a reddish-purple color. Such reactions can be observed in nucleic acids (nuclear or nucleolar), various epithelial mucins, and extracellular matrix components. Some of these substances are stained poorly with the Pap or H&E stains.

Rapid-Staining Techniques

In many clinical situations, rapid results are desired. High-quality rapid-staining procedures are widely available and give excellent results. Many pathologists use an H&E stain adapted from the frozen section suite. These typically can be performed in 2 to 3 minutes. Rapid Pap stains give results comparable with those obtained by longer methods and can be completed in about 3 minutes.[11] When rapid Pap stains are performed outside the cytology laboratory (e.g., in the Radiology suite), xylene substitutes can be used. These often employ pleasant-smelling citrus terpenes and lack the irritating qualities of xylene.

Rapid Romanowsky Stains

Rapid Romanowsky stains are also available. The most common method is the commercially available Diff-Quik (DQ) method. Staining can be accomplished in 2 minutes or less. Cells left too long in solution II quickly darken and lose considerable microscopic detail. However, smears that are insufficiently stained can be returned to either staining solution until optimized.

Installing a permanent coverslip on Romanowsky-stained slides in the conventional manner requires that the slides dry completely before immersion in the appropriate solvent (xylene or its substitutes). To avoid this delay, these smears are often examined before they have been coverslipped. Only at high magnification does this present a somewhat blurred image. Because low and intermediate magnifications are sufficient for diagnosis of most FNA specimens, many can be examined immediately, while still wet, without sacrifice of diagnostic accuracy.

If high-power viewing is needed, the slide can be moistened with tap water and a coverslip applied immediately with water as a mounting medium. The resulting image is clear. This water mounting method permits rapid, high-quality examination (e.g., in the radiology suite) without the need to transport and handle the organic solvents and sticky mounting media used for permanent coverslip application. After initial rapid examination, the coverslip is removed and the slide should be dried thoroughly before application of a permanent coverslip. Examining the smear before permanent mounting by either of these methods can contribute to rapid diagnosis when this is needed. Ability to apply these stains is easily acquired and greatly facilitates rapid examination of FNA material.

One rapid method of Romanowsky staining that has been found unacceptable is the use of slide-staining machines that are often found in large volume routine hematology laboratories. These stains are often of poor quality, and their quality varies greatly from slide to slide.

Preparation of Slides for Immunocytochemical Stains

The majority of FNA specimens can be readily interpreted using routine stains applied to smears made at the bedside. These methods are inexpensive and give results quickly. A small number of cases require application of more advanced techniques.

Classification of malignant neoplasms has been greatly facilitated by modern immunocytochemical methods, which are readily adapted to cytologic material, including that obtained by FNA.[12] Important issues are optimum specimen preparation for maximum antigen preservation and minimum nonspecific background staining.

Many immunocytochemical stains can be applied to fixed smears. However, modern automated staining techniques require charged slides that are usually not used to

TABLE 2-3

Comparison of Papanicolaou and Romanowsky Stains as Applied to Aspiration Cytology

Cytologic Finding	Papanicolaou Stain	Romanowsky Stain
Nuclear detail	+	
Cytoplasmic keratin	+	
Cytoplasmic mucin		+
Cytoplasmic granules*		+
Extracellular mucin		+
Thyroid colloid		+
Extracellular matrix material†		
Close resemblance of cells from malignant lymphoma or other hematopoietic processes to those seen in standard hematologic preparations		

*Seen in some breast carcinomas and in approximately 20% of medullary thyroid carcinomas.
†Cartilage, osteoid, mesenchymal myxoid material, and the characteristic chondroid matrix of parotid pleomorphic adenoma.
Note: The plus sign (+) indicates that the stain is considered superior by the authors.

prepare direct smears at the time of FNA. Most workers prefer to use paraffin-embedded cell blocks discussed earlier. Multiple sections can be prepared for application of several primary antibodies. Most of the staining methods in common use were developed for formalin-fixed, paraffin-embedded tissue sections and are efficiently transferred to cytology cell blocks.

Comparison of Fixed (Papanicolaou-Stained) and Dried (Romanowsky-Stained) Cytologic Material

Highly reliable diagnosis occurs in some laboratories using mostly fixed smears and in other laboratories using mostly dried slides. Much of the difference amounts to personal preference based on training and experience. However, differences do exist; some of these are summarized in Table 2-3.

Cell Size

One fundamental difference is that of apparent cell size. Air drying results in an increase in cell size from flattening of the cells.[13] The increase in apparent nuclear area is approximately 20%.[14,15] This translates into a dried cell nuclear diameter of 110% of fixed cell nuclear diameter. Schulte also found that the coefficient of variation in measured nuclear size was less with dried than with fixed material.[15] Thus, dried slides may be more suitable for those wishing to perform morphometric studies or seeking to derive prognostic information from nuclear measurements as an expression of tumor grade.[16-21]

TABLE 2-4

Differences Between Aspiration Cytology and Exfoliative Cytology

Factor	Aspiration Cytology	Exfoliative Cytology
Smear findings		
High cellularity	Common	Uncommon
Tissue fragments	Common	Uncommon
Smear examination		
Pattern	Very important	Less important
Nuclear features	Less important	Very important
Use of high magnification	Occasionally	Frequently

Nuclear Detail

The most commonly cited advantage of fixed material is the exquisite nuclear detail available with this method. In traditional exfoliative cytology, it is precisely these details of nuclear morphology that form the basis for deciding that the cells in question are malignant. Chromatin details are less clear in air-dried material.

FNA, however, often gives a much larger number of tumor cells than are generally present in exfoliated material and also often yields tissue fragments. These tissue particles represent small biopsies and often reveal information about tumor architecture, stromal elements, extracellular tissue components, and the relations of tumor cells to one another. In this way, tissue particles and smear cellularity are the cytologist's equivalent of the histopathologist's concept of tissue architecture. Analysis of fine details of nuclear chromatin is replaced to a degree by other significant features, including smear pattern, cellularity, tissue fragment analysis, cell or nuclear size, degree of nuclear staining, and cell variability.

Accordingly, many FNA specimens are more effectively examined at a low or intermediate magnification similar to histologic sections. This is in contrast with the frequent need to use high magnification for detailed study of small numbers of cells in exfoliative cytology. Some of the contrasts between FNA and exfoliative cytology are summarized in Table 2-4.

Cytoplasmic Differentiation

The Pap stain was in part devised to reveal keratin as an indicator of squamous differentiation. Considering the common occurrence of squamous cell carcinomas and their metastases, this is an important use of this stain. The cytoplasmic keratin in squamous cell carcinomas avidly binds the Orange-G cytoplasmic counterstain of the Papanicolaou formulations. Aspirations from such tumors often have diagnostic cells scattered through large areas of blood, necrotic debris, and inflammatory cells. It is helpful to have the bright orange tumor cells stand out so clearly.

A variety of cytoplasmic granules and vacuoles have been described and are easily demonstrated using air-dried smears. Many of these are visualized poorly or not at all in fixed material. One example is the fine, red cytoplasmic granulation seen in 20% of medullary thyroid carcinomas.

Extracellular Materials

Extracellular mucin is much more easily identified in air-dried smears.[22,23] If present in small quantities, it may be nearly invisible on fixed preparations. Small droplets of intracellular mucin are well shown by the Romanowsky stains because they may be metachromatic.

In thyroid cytology, the presence, quantity, and quality of colloid is of great diagnostic significance. When abundant and free of blood, it can be identified grossly as a clear oily substance as the smear is prepared. If mixed with cyst fluid or blood, its presence may not be grossly appreciated. Microscopically, it is much more readily apparent in Romanowsky-stained than in Pap-stained smears.

When lesions of the thyroid or other organs are partially cystic, they often contain crystals. These dissolve away in the organic solvents used for either type of stain. In the dried material, a background of deeply stained colloid shows clear spaces, or windowpanes, that represent the negative image of the crystals. They are usually not seen in Pap-stained smears.

A variety of extracellular materials other than colloid and the epithelial mucins are of diagnostic importance. These include the characteristic chondroid matrix of pleomorphic adenomas, the basement membrane whorls of adenoid cystic carcinoma, and extracellular substances in a variety of mesenchymal neoplasms.

Another common situation is aspiration of the breast during pregnancy or lactation. The cytologic change of intense metabolic activity in these settings is a recognized cause of false-positive diagnoses. The cytology is actually rather characteristic, consisting of nuclear enlargement, mostly round nuclei, prominent nucleoli, and a tendency of the cells to be arranged in small acinar groups. Their abundant cytoplasm is fragile so that many of the cells appear as large, round, naked nuclei. The air-dried smear also shows a characteristic background. The secretory material and cytoplasmic fragments are present in the smear background as a blue-staining, frothy, or vacuolated material. This is very helpful in the secure identification of lactational or secretory changes. This background is much less apparent in fixed smears.

Hematopoietic Processes

Malignant lymphomas, leukemias, and benign lymphoproliferative processes are common and may pose formidable diagnostic problems. These may be addressed with a variety of special techniques, but the first step remains a careful evaluation of high-quality smears.

The foregoing discussion and examples are intended to suggest ways in which one stain or the other is preferable in different types of cases. The preferred method depends on the differential diagnostic considerations at hand, as well as the preference and experience of the cytopathologist. Thus, it is advisable to collect both air-dried and fixed material whenever feasible.

Liquid-Based Processing of Fine-Needle Aspiration Samples

One persistent cause of limitations in FNA utility is frequent preparation of poor-quality smears by various members of a clinical team. Elimination of this difficulty is a prime reason to recommend experienced pathologist or cy-

BOX 2-1

Cytomorphologic Alterations in Liquid-Based Preparations of Fine-Needle Aspiration Material

Cell clusters
Fragmentation and flattening of large cell clusters
Artifactual aggregation of lymphocytes

Overall preparation content
Decreased small mononuclear cells
Decreased myoepithelial cells
Decreased quantity of extracellular matrix materials

Individual cells
Rounded as any cells in fluid
Possibly smaller
Dissociation of small clusters

Nuclear alterations
Attenuation of chromatin detail
Nucleolar accentuation
Increased difficulty in identifying intranuclear inclusions

From Michael CW, McConnel J, Pecott J, et al. Comparison of ThinPrep and TriPath PREP liquid-based preparations in nongynecologic specimens: a pilot study. Diagn Cytopath 2001; 25(3):177-184; Kurtycz DF, Hoerl HD. Thin-layer technology: tempered enthusiasm. Diagn Cytopath 2000; 23(1):1-5; Michael CW, Hunter B. Interpretation of fine-needle aspirates processed by the ThinPrep technique: cytologic artifacts and diagnostic pitfalls. Diagn Cytopath 2000; 23(1):6-13.

totechnologist participation in specimen collection. Liquid-based processing (LBP) of cytologic specimens is a recently developed method that relies on expression of cellular material into a vial of fixative as a replacement for preparation of direct smears. Extensive literature and broad experience have led to nearly universal application of this method to cervicovaginal cytology. In that area, its benefits are largely a matter of consensus.

This method is appealing to those clinical teams for whom preparation of high-quality smears has remained an elusive skill or to whom laboratory participation at the time of FNA is not available. Comparisons between conventional cytologic material (CCM) and LBP have given variable results, some of which are more favorable[24-27] than others.[28-31] Some investigators have found LBP to be a viable alternative to CCM and have even indicated a slightly higher sensitivity for detection of malignancy by LBP.[24,25] However, others describe a greater yield using in CCM than LBP. For example, Salhadar and colleagues found 32 of 50 LBPs diagnostic as compared with 46 of 50 CCM.[30]

All studies of LBP describe a cleaner background in some cases than noted in CCM from the same specimen. However, morphologic differences between the two methods have been described[27,28] as summarized in Box 2-1. This was underscored by Dey and colleagues when they noted that experience is required for interpretation of this new type of preparation.[26]

At this writing, various investigators' opinions regarding application LBP to FNA range from enthusiastic endorsement to caution to statements that it is not warranted. Kurtycz and Hoerl underscored the idea that, "The patient is best served when the pathologist is directly involved with the initial sample acquisition," to the extent that "time and effort would be better spent on trying to educate select clinicians on how to obtain better samples than to totally convert to thin-layer methodologies."[28] Others have suggested that LBPs are simpler and less time-consuming than screening and interpretation of CCM.[26] This may be true for specimens such as body cavity fluids. However, many well-made direct FNA smears require very little screening and are less time-consuming than LBPs. This is especially true if rapid Romanowsky stains are applied to air-dried smears that will then be ready for microscopic examination in approximately 2 minutes.

Clearly, more work is forthcoming. However, at this time, it is possible to suggest several reasons for the current diversity of experience. Many of the published investigations are small, often describing less than 100 nongynecologic cytology cases, many of which often represent specimens other than FNAs. Many give aggregate results for a variety of FNA sites and combine these with other nongynecologic samples. The utility of LBP may differ among different types of material. Thus, variable case mix probably affects results of some studies. (Investigations that describe FNAs from a single body site are considered in the following section.)

Other methodologic considerations may contribute to the widely divergent outcomes of various studies. Some investigators express the entire contents of a dedicated FNA pass into the fixative vial, whereas others rely exclusively on needle rinses for the LBP sample. The diversity, quantity, and possibly the quality of CCM being compared with LBPs is also variable, with differing applications for smears, cell blocks, and cytocentrifuge material. This might also be a reason to evaluate the technology with studies confined to FNA, rather than examining aggregate evaluations of FNA and non-FNA specimens.

When LBPs are applied to breast FNA material, various authors have found that such components as stromal fragments, adipose tissue, all epithelial cells, single epithelial cells in benign lesions, myoepithelial cells, and cellular detail could be either increased or decreased when compared with conventional smears.[31-33] However, one large study found no difference in sensitivity and specificity for the diagnosis of malignancy when LBPs and conventional smears were compared.[34] In the experience of Perez-Reyes and colleagues, correlation between the results of the two methods occurred in only 62% of cases.[32] Furthermore, only four of 21 fibroadenomas (19%) were correctly interpreted using LBPs. This is reflected in these authors' finding that recovery of stroma was decreased by this method and that a greater tendency toward increased single epithelial cells was noted in benign lesions.[31] In addition to loss of stroma from fibroadenomas, these authors noted loss of mucin from colloid carcinomas and chondroid matrix material from metaplastic carcinoma.[32] It may prove very useful that two investigations have found LBPs suitable for immunohistochemical detection of estrogen and progesterone receptors.[35,36]

Application of LBP to thyroid FNA has also been described.[31,37-41] Some investigators find comparable diagnostic results when LBPs are contrasted with conventional smears.[39] Others have found decreased correlation with final diagnoses or lowered sensitivity when LBPs are used.[38,41] Frost and colleagues noted that 39% of 26 examples of chronic lymphocytic thyroiditis were not identified in LBPs, while only two of these same cases were inapparent using conventional smears.[38] Morphologic differences with LBPs have been described as improved nuclear detail, overall decreased cell preservation within tissue fragments, cytoplasmic damage with naked nuclei, decreased prominence of nuclear grooves and pseudoinclusions in papillary carcinoma, and loss of most colloid except particles of hard colloid.[41] Biscotti and colleagues also described loss of colloid. This finding is potentially important because the quantity of colloid in relation to the number of cells present is often the most important diagnostic picture in thyroid FNA. Because most cases represent benign colloid nodules, loss of the very common types of thin colloid could become a significant limiting factor in thyroid cytology based on LBPs. Clearly, additional evaluation is needed.

Comparing LBPs with conventional smears in salivary gland FNA, Al-Khafaji and Afify described better performance for the latter and noted morphologic differences that included loss or distortion of extracellular stromal elements, cellular shrinkage, and tissue particle fragmentation.[42] Examining sarcomas with LBP and conventional smears, Guiter and colleagues noted higher cellularity with conventional smear preparations. Furthermore, LBPs resulted in fewer thick tissue fragments, more single cells, and distortion of architectural patterns expected in sarcoma aspirates. Nuclear detail was better in LBPs, but loss of necrotic material could be a limiting factor for this method. Additional structural features such as the vascular pattern typical of myxoid liposarcoma, background myxoid material, and the matrix of low-grade chondrosarcomas were also lost.[43]

Results to date indicate that LBPs are suitable for immunocytochemistry.[43,44] Leung and Bedard described success with a wide range of antibodies. However, they achieved poor results when attempting to immunophenotype malignant lymphomas with this method.[44]

LBPs cannot be air-dried for Romanowsky staining. The experience and opinions of those who rely almost exclusively on fixed material for the practice of FNA cytology differs *a priori* from those who prefer air-dried smears or a combination of dried and fixed material. It is unlikely that these two groups will achieve agreement regarding the use of LBP for FNA. If LBPs continue to be favored over conventional smears by some groups, it is essential that the cytopathology community recognize the use of both this method and conventional smear preparations, as used by experienced individuals in different laboratories. At this time, strong evidence shows that the advent of this relatively new technology should not result in new definitions of the standard of care in cytopreparatory methodologies.

 ## WHO SHOULD PERFORM FINE-NEEDLE ASPIRATIONS?

Debate exists about who should perform FNAs, and no single best answer to this question is available. The primary responsibility for obtaining specimens by aspiration rests with different types of individuals in different institutions. A single individual often has the responsibility to see the patient, perform the aspiration, prepare the material obtained, microscopically examine the smears, and report the diagnosis. Another scenario often involves different people seeing the patient and performing the microscopy. In either system, the physician or physicians involved often need to consult their colleagues in the radiology suite or the microbiology or hematopathology laboratories.

The primary argument in favor of the separation of functions is that each physician is performing a limited role in which he or she has considerable expertise. Thus, the surgeon brings experience to the physical examination of mass lesions and to the performance of procedures directed at such lesions. These individuals are indeed qualified to implement FNA. However, good results depend on their having received training in aspiration with frequent performance of the technique and on having made provisions for proper handling of aspirated material by suitably schooled personnel.

When the clinician involved is not a surgeon but is an internist, gynecologist, or general clinician, the degree of expertise brought to the aspiration may be considerably less. These physicians may deal with patients in need of FNA less often and thus have little ongoing practice in the method. It has been shown that those performing aspirations on an occasional basis do not obtain the best results possible.[45,46]

FNA should be regarded as a first-line approach to the palpable mass and thus, an element of primary care. Many benign lesions do not require referral to a surgeon or other specialist.

There is ample support in the literature for the concept that the best results are obtained with the Swedish model in which the same individual performs the aspiration and interprets the material microscopically.[47-51] Hall and colleagues studied samples from 795 patients who underwent aspiration of thyroid nodules and found inadequate aspirations were obtained in 32.4% of cases by community clinicians, 15% of cases by medical center clinicians, and in only 6.4% of cases aspirated by a cytopathologist.[51]

Other advantages include the immediate correlation between the clinical impression of a mass and the gross appearance of the aspirated material. Many inadequate specimens can be recognized at once and the aspiration repeated immediately if the individual performing the procedure brings to the bedside expectations about the nature of the specimen to be produced. The constant review of specimens at the microscope in concert with clinical examination of patients is the only way to build this type of experience.

Furthermore, specimens can be accurately triaged by a cytopathologist at the time of the aspiration, based on differential diagnostic considerations, so that special studies are available on a timely basis without the need for frequent repeat aspirations. Either air-dried or fixed material may be strongly preferred by the microscopist depending on the diagnostic considerations at hand. If the person who is examining the material prepares the slides, either type of smear can be emphasized from the outset. Cell blocks can also be prepared as needed.

Some clinicians believe that a surgeon or other qualified clinician should obtain the specimen because of expertise in physical examination and assessment of masses. When a

pathologist performs aspirations, he or she usually reviews the cytologic material within a few minutes. No other physician has such complete and immediate feedback. The pathologist who performs several aspirations a day is probably the most skilled assessor of lumps and bumps.[52]

 ## FUNDAMENTAL RULES USED TO APPLY ASPIRATION CYTOLOGY

In their essay on the limitations of FNA, Hajdu and Melamed outline the ground rules for clinical application of this method.[53] Many of these were clearly defined in early descriptions of the technique by Martin and Ellis, Stewart, and Soderstrom.[54-56]

First, aspiration is always directed at a target lesion. This can either be a palpable mass or a tumor localized radiographically. FNA is not a screening test used to search for possible malignancy, even in a high-risk population.

The next two rules are really no different from the bases on which all biopsy pathology is practiced. A reasonable interpretation is possible only when the cytologic findings are placed in a clinical context. The minimum details needed include the age and gender of the patient and the exact site of the aspiration. A more detail description of the physical or radiographic findings and the information about the texture noted when a mass is penetrated by the needle further enhance diagnostic accuracy.

An important principle is that in a patient thought to have a malignancy, a negative report that does not provide a specific benign diagnosis leaves the clinical problem unsolved. The mass must be addressed either by repeat aspiration or by some other diagnostic maneuver. Only a specific benign diagnosis such as an infection that presents a reasonable alternative explanation for the clinical findings is acceptable.

 ## COMMUNICATION WITH PATIENTS BEFORE ASPIRATION

Patients come to the procedure with a range of possible expectations. To many, the idea of FNA is completely new. Patients often arrive at the clinic prepared for a complex, painful procedure that they think is implied by the word biopsy. The authors have encountered patients subjected to self-imposed overnight fasting who are prone to fainting. Patients such as these should be approached in a relaxed and friendly manner that will put them at ease.[57]

The medicolegal standard in North America demands that all patients be completely informed about medical procedures. This includes all pertinent information on the risks, benefits, and alternatives to a given procedure. The risks of aspiration are quite minimal.

 ## CLINICAL APPLICATION OF THE ASPIRATION PROCEDURE

The entire process should include several steps in addition to the puncture event itself. Ideally, it is nothing less than a synthesis of clinical, radiographic, laboratory, historical, tactile and cytologic findings to form a diagnosis that is as accurate and complete as possible. The various components of this process are summarized in Box 2-2. Although cumbersome to describe, the entire process usually requires about 10 minutes to complete. As previously mentioned, the needle is in the mass for approximately 5 to 10 seconds at each puncture. Thus, in one typical 10- to 15-minute appointment, the patient encounters the needle for only 5 to 40 seconds.

Learning about the Patient's Problem

The aspiration process begins by becoming familiar with the patient's problem. The referring physician often supplies this information. Its accuracy and completeness may vary from referral to referral. For example, the breast masses sent for aspiration by a surgeon are often much more highly selected than those from other physicians. This may place the physician performing the aspiration in the position of being the most experienced individual to examine the patient. Although this is a new role for most pathologists, after experience is obtained, it is a very appropriate role.

Another important factor is that masses change over time. This is certainly the case with cysts of many types. Rapid enlargement can contribute to the clinical suspicion that a mass is malignant. When a delay of several days or a few weeks separates the initial examination of benign lymphadenopathy from the aspiration appointment, the problem may resolve. Some of these patients will have received antibiotic therapy during the interval. Often, the indicated adenopathy is undetectable by even the most careful examination. These patients should not be aspirated because aspiration is always directed at a target lesion. It is made clear to the patient and referring physician that reevaluating the patient is necessary if adenopathy recurs.

Patient radiographs and laboratory studies are reviewed where appropriate. In the case of breast cytology, the mammograms can be helpful. A benign or inconclusive cytologic result does not obviate the need for further study of a patient with mammographic or clinical abnormalities indicative of possible malignancy.[58-60] Although not necessarily expert in diagnostic radiology, the physician performing the aspiration must always be aware of the radiographic findings and may often need to consult the radiologist. Other instances in which radiologic findings are very important include masses of the soft tissues, bones, and abdominal organ.

The next step in the FNA process is examination of the target lesion. Valuable information can be gained by careful physical examination. For example, the palpatory findings in the breast are different for diffuse fibrocystic change, fibroadenoma, and most breast carcinomas. The very firm, bosselated pleomorphic adenoma of the parotid differs from the soft, smooth, often cystic Warthin's tumor. The softness of a benign hyperplastic lymph node is different from the hard consistency of many nodes with Hodgkin's disease, tuberculosis, or metastatic carcinoma. The "rubbery" nodes of some malignant lymphomas present yet another sensation. The findings at physical examination need to be interpreted with other clinical features and with what is seen in the microscope.

Care must be taken to ensure that the area aspirated corresponds to that chosen by the referring physician or that the reason another area was selected is clearly documented. This is rarely a problem except in the case of extensive fibrocystic change of the breast. This chapter later illustrates some useful ways of describing puncture location.

Regardless of the quality or quantity of data supplied by the referring physician, it is useful to know what the patient thinks about the mass and elicit his or her description. For example, the patient who points with one finger to a breast mass is much more likely to have a significant lesion than the one who uses the palm of the hand or all of the fingertips together (usually in a circular motion) to indicate a large area of abnormality. However, patient descriptions may be incorrect. This is often encountered in the setting of a long-ignored, obviously malignant mass. Patients say that they noticed it only a few days ago or that it is getting smaller. In such instances the unequivocal diagnosis of malignancy provided by FNA is often the most rapid means by which the referring physician can break the psychologic wall of denial and thus help the patient begin dealing with the problem of malignancy.

Planning the Aspiration

Using strategies to be described in the next section, the lesion must be stabilized and held immobile, while still considering the comfort of the patient and the aspirator.

The number of punctures needed varies with the clinical situation. The cone-shaped biopsy volumes accessible to one needle pass can be expanded by multiple passes, as shown in Figure 2-16. In this way, even large areas of fibrocystic change in the breast can be sampled thoroughly. An effort is made to pass the needle through many portions of the palpable abnormality. Large primary malignant tumors

---

BOX 2-2

Stepwise Fine-Needle Aspiration Procedure

1. Question the patient or the referring physician about the history of the mass and other significant medical problems.
2. Review any relevant radiographs and laboratory studies, consulting specialists in these areas as necessary.
3. Examine the area to be aspirated.
4. Mentally plan the aspiration with respect to stabilization of the mass, needle size, and the number of punctures that might be necessary.
5. Plan the allocation of aspirated material to fixed slides, dried slides, cell blocks, and other studies.
6. Cleanse the skin with alcohol (briefly as for venipuncture).
7. Perform the aspiration with special attention to the tactile characteristics of the lesion when the needle enters it.
8. Apply pressure to the site after the aspiration.
9. Prepare the aspirated material.
10. Note the gross characteristics of the aspirated material.
11. Always inspect the puncture site before leaving the bedside.

are often aspirated two or more times to evaluate the spectrum of microscopic features. Conversely, metastases in patients with known malignancy or small primary tumors can often be adequately assessed as single pass, based on the knowledge that multiple smears can often be prepared from one aspiration. The gross inspection of aspirated material should also impart the impression of malignancy if the procedure is to be terminated after one puncture. This approach is useful in patients with disseminated malignancy for whom their disease or the procedure is a source of pain. When more than one puncture is planned, the patient should be informed of this before the initial aspiration. Having expected additional punctures canceled when the first yields adequate material is a pleasant and welcome surprise. Being asked to allow second or third punctures when only one was expected is always unwelcome.

Another factor that affects the number of punctures needed is the time elapsed during each aspiration. Some operators leave the needle in place only briefly, whereas others persist for up to 10 seconds. In most aspirations, the greatest pain derives from puncture of the skin. Deeper tissues are usually much less sensitive. Accordingly, aspirating for several seconds at each puncture reduces the total number of aspirations. The duration of the aspiration is to some extent governed by the nature and quantity of material recovered.

It is occasionally difficult to decide how many punctures suffice to exclude a diagnosis of malignancy. Some neoplasms are too small to be sampled confidently; others may be obscured by abnormal but benign tissue masses or cysts; still others may be very fibrous and yield few or no diagnostic cells. These considerations plus others give FNA a small, irreducible false-negative rate.

When special studies are likely to be necessary, planned allocation of the specimen to the various fixatives and media required can occur at this time. In a majority of cases, only good-quality smears are needed. Repeating the aspiration is done with no hesitation if the need for special studies becomes apparent after initial smear examination. The ability to do so is one of the benefits of FNA. The most common setting in which this occurs is the need for microbiologic culture of masses shown cytologically to be purulent or granulomatous.

The Aspiration

The actual aspiration procedure usually begins by cleansing the skin with alcohol, which is the preferred method. With this technique, aspiration site infections are virtually unheard of. A case could be made for more elaborate skin preparation for aspiration of immunosuppressed patients or for joint aspirations. The latter is common for rheumatologist but not common for the cytopathologist. Some use iodine-containing solutions and an elaborate preparation such as that commonly used for bone marrow aspiration or lumbar puncture.

Some patients are upset when they see the pistol-like syringe holder. The size of this instrument is in marked contrast with the delicacy of FNA as it will have been explained. For this reason, keeping this instrument out of the patient's field of vision is important. When this is not possible, the patient should be told that this instrument is for the clinician's convenience in securely holding such a small

needle, and the fact that nothing will touch him or her except the examiner's fingertips and the very thin needle should be emphasized. When moving the syringe pistol from a nearby table to the bedside, the patient usually does not observe it at all if the physician takes that moment to look at and speak to him or her.

The puncture is now executed. Issues of patient positioning are discussed later in this chapter as aspiration of particular body sites is considered. The range of motion and the size of the cone of sampled tissue varies with different anatomic sites. An aspiration volume used for large areas of thickening in the breast would clearly be inappropriate in the thyroid, for example. With very small nodules, the needle can go in and out but moves laterally rather slightly so that the cone is extremely narrow.

One should simultaneously maintain visual monitoring of the needle hub for return of material and of the patient's face for signs of distress. Even a patient who insists that no pain is experienced when he or she is in pain will be unconsciously betrayed by facial expressions. When the latter is noted, reassurance and a description of the procedure may help the patient relax. Better-quality material, a more rapid procedure, and a less traumatized patient results.

Just as physical examination provides clues to the possible nature of the lesion to be studied, the consistency of the mass as it is entered with the needle is also an important source of information. Most breast carcinomas are gritty and more firm than areas of fibrocystic change, which tend to be rubbery or doughy. Many malignant lymph nodes are much firmer than their benign counterparts. When masses are deeply located, the feeling of increased resistance as the lesion is punctured can be helpful in being sure that the needle has entered the mass.

At the conclusion of the aspiration, a gauze pad is pressed over the puncture site with mild pressure. In most instances, one can ask the patient to hold it in place. It is uncommon to have any bleeding after the time required to make smears of the aspirated material (usually less than one minute) has elapsed. If bleeding does persist, a few minutes of pressure are always sufficient to achieve hemostasis. Additional aspirations are then performed as needed. By these simple means, FNA can be safely performed even in patients with coagulopathies.

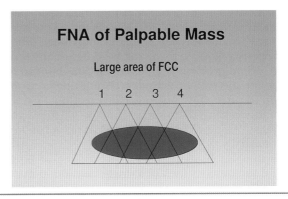

Figure 2-16 **Tissue sampling.** This diagram illustrates the way in which multiple, overlapping cone-shaped aspiration volumes can encompass the entirety of a large mass. This is especially applicable to large areas of fibrocystic change in the breast.

The aspirator is occasionally surprised to see a swelling, discolored area develop immediately after breast FNA. This problem can be related to numerous large irregular veins that are present throughout this organ. Surgeons describe occasional incidents of considerable blood loss after severing such a vein. Pressure suffices to limit the bleeding at the time of FNA. A small bruise will result.

Before Leaving the Patient

The final step in Box 2-2 is one to which considerable importance is attached. Before leaving the bedside, the puncture site should always be checked for bleeding or swelling, and an inquiry into the patient's comfort level should be made. Problems are extremely rare, but this small amount of additional time given to the patient is often appreciated. Care must be taken with the elderly, the weak, and those given to fainting. They must never be left unattended in a situation where a fall or other injury may occur.

Local Anesthesia for Transcutaneous Fine-Needle Aspiration

With rare exceptions, local anesthesia for FNA is not used with 23- or 25-gauge needles. Most patients agree that injection of anesthetic agents into the dermis is more painful than the aspiration itself. Certain anxious individuals, however, seem to derive some benefit from local cutaneous anesthesia.

Although most tissues deep to the dermis are not overly tender, aspiration of muscles is often painful. This usually occurs when thyroid or lymph node aspiration is approached incorrectly. The periosteum is also quite tender. Local anesthesia will not spare the patient these painful consequences of inept aspiration techniques.

Those using local anesthesia can apply it with a 30-gauge or 27-gauge needle. Anesthesia of the skin can be readily achieved, but it is not possible to deaden completely such masses as large areas of fibrocystic change within the breast. Four potential problems accompany the use of local anesthesia. The most serious is an allergic reaction to these agents. Rare individuals experience anaphylactic reactions with rapid cardiovascular collapse and death. The physician should always inquire about prior administration of local anesthetics. Most adults and many children have received these drugs previously for dental work and are free of allergic reactions. Those not possessing the experience and equipment to deal with severe reactions should probably not administer local anesthetic agents to individuals who have not previously received them and been free of any reaction.

The second problem is much less serious but can be distressing for the patient who expects anesthesia to remove the pain of cutaneous puncture. One occasionally discovers vials of these agents that simply do not work. Replacing this material with a new vial from a different manufacturer's lot number usually solves this problem.

The third problem relates to the volume of liquid injected. If too much is used in a single location, it may form a focus of soft tissue firmness that obscures the small lesion for which the patient needs FNA. This problem afflicts the neophyte who uses too much medication in an attempt to achieve a degree of anesthesia that is both impossible and unnecessary.

The last difficulty also occurs with overzealous injection of too large a volume of local anesthetic liquid. These fluids cause morphologic distortion of cells when included in the sample.

Two types of masses are often tender, even before FNA: granulomatous thyroiditis and some cases of fibrocystic breast disease. This symptom typifies the benign character of these lesions. The patient describes the pain, and palpation by the physician also causes pain. It is paradoxical that this pain is not increased by the needle puncture. Penetration of the skin causes brief sharp pain, but movement of the needle within the mass is not as unpleasant as palpation by the fingertips.

ASPIRATION OF SPECIFIC BODY SITES

Most aspirations are best performed with the patient in the supine position. This position is the most comfortable and relaxing position, and it eliminates the danger of an accidental fall. It also limits movement should the patient be startled by the puncture. However, if congestive heart failure is a problem, the patient should not be placed in a fully recumbent position, and the clinician should inquire about and observe the patient's breathing and comfort.

Although special situations are described subsequently, the goal is to provide good access to the target lesion with maximum comfort for the patient. If the procedure must be performed with the patient sitting on the bed or examining table, an assistant should be stationed behind the patient to provide support should fainting occur. It is an unavoidable fact of clinical medicine that some lesions simply cannot be adequately located in a supine patient.

Techniques for Thyroid Aspiration

General Approach

The basic anatomic relationships of the thyroid are summarized in Figure 2-17. Most of this organ's bulk lies along the posterolateral angle of the trachea in a gutter formed by the trachea medially and the sternocleidomastoid muscle laterally. Thus, although little tissue intervenes between the examining fingertips and the gland itself, deep palpation may be needed for adequate localization of all but the largest thyroid masses.

Most clinicians initially approach the thyroid by standing behind the patient and placing the fingertips of each hand in the anatomic gutters. This facilitates comparisons between the two lobes and helps locate small lesions, but it is not useful for the aspiration itself.

In many normal individuals, little or no thyroid tissue is palpable. The thyroid isthmus crosses the midline and is attached to tracheal rings two through four. Thus, when the patient swallows, the thyroid rises and falls with other neck structures. In this way, the gland substance passes under the fingertips and nodules become much more easily palpable. Many patients find such repetitive swallowing with the physician's fingertips on the neck difficult. This effort is often aided by encouraging the patient to take small sips of water to initiate swallowing.

After the mass is localized, note of its position should be made. The side on which a mass occurs is described, as is whether it is nearer the upper or lower pole. A few masses are in the midline. It is difficult to describe accurately the location of thyroid nodules in reference to external landmarks such as the sternal notch because distances between structures in the neck change depending on whether the cervical spine is in flexion or extension.

Figure 2-18 shows the preferred position for most thyroid aspirations. When a pillow is placed under the shoulders, the cervical spine is put in extension, which puts the soft tissue overlying the thyroid in a stretched attenuated position. This position also thrusts the larynx and upper trachea anteriorly and superiorly, bringing with them the thyroid. This positioning maximizes the ease with which small thyroid nodules can be located.

The needle should be angled slightly toward the midline and thus is directed toward the trachea and the vertebrae and away from the carotid sheath and its vascular contents. Furthermore, with the palpating fingertips between the trachea and the sternocleidomastoid muscle, the muscle is pushed laterally and out of the needle's path. Thyroid aspirations that contain abundant skeletal muscle have usually been obtained improperly.

When the needle is directed medially, the only structure likely to be inadvertently punctured is the trachea. When this happens, air enters the syringe so that suction is lost and the aspiration must be performed again. As a result, ciliated tracheal mucosal cells, macrophages, and mucus may occasionally be seen on the smears. In elderly patients, tracheal cartilage is often ossified and may contain fat and bone marrow. When marrow elements are aspirated unexpectedly, the immature granulocytes and large hyperchromatic megakaryocytes may be confused with cancer cells. This issue is discussed more completely in the discussion of contaminants in pulmonary samples. No adverse consequences are associated with tracheal puncture.

Cystic Thyroid Aspirations

Many thyroid nodules are variably cystic and thus may be evacuated by needle aspiration. Because vigorous needle motion may cause bleeding, some cysts may refill with blood almost immediately. Accordingly, the nodule is punctured with a single smooth motion, and a fluid return is anticipated while the needle is held stationary within the mass. If none appears, then progression to a gentle, low-amplitude needle motion is acceptable. Many thyroid lesions are highly vascular, and this type of motion suffices to obtain a specimen with minimal blood.

When cyst fluid is obtained, it should be processed by a concentration technique. After cyst evacuation, a careful repeat examination should be directed at the detection of any residual mass. If present, this mass should be aspirated.

Most thyroid cyst fluids represent benign lesions, but some degree of cystic degeneration is common in papillary carcinoma. One study found an incidence of cystic change of almost 17%.[61] Cystic change can also occur in follicular carcinomas.[62]

Clinical Goals

Nonfunctioning nodular goiter is common, affecting from 4% to 7% of the population.[63] Thyroid cancer, however, is uncommon, constituting 0.5% of all malignancies and 5% of patients referred for evaluation of a thyroid nodule.[64] Generally, FNA can accurately distinguish neoplastic from nonneoplastic lesions. The latter large group does not usually require surgery.

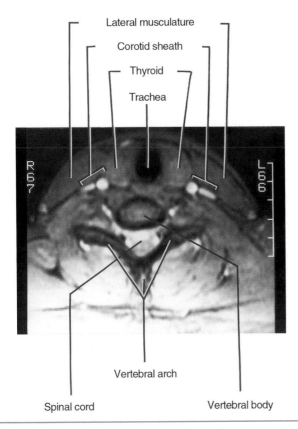

Lateral musculature

Corotid sheath

Thyroid

Trachea

Vertebral arch

Spinal cord   Vertebral body

Figure 2-17 **Thyroid anatomy.** This nuclear magnetic resonance scan of the neck shows the basic anatomic relationships of the thyroid.

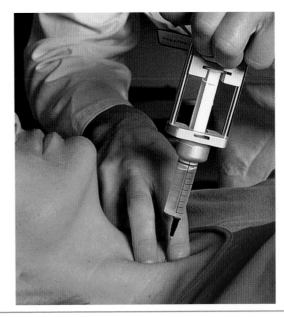

Figure 2-18 **The preferred position for most thyroid aspirations.** A pillow is placed beneath the patient's shoulders. This puts the cervical spine in extension, thereby thinning the soft tissues overlying the thyroid. Note that the needle is directed medially and the sternocleidomastoid muscle is displaced laterally as the two fingertips stabilize the mass.

Diagnostic Approaches to Breast Lesions

Surgical procedures excluded, four techniques commonly used to evaluate breast masses are physical examination, FNA cytology, mammography, and ultrasonography. In the case of palpable masses, one approach features FNA as soon as a lesion is detected. Other studies are then less urgent but are needed for evaluation of normal-appearing areas in the ipsilateral breast and opposite side. In the proper setting, guided aspiration of nonpalpable mammographic lesions can be undertaken.

In each case, the purposes are to diagnose malignancies preoperatively and identify and follow patients with benign disease. Because it is not possible to biopsy all diffusely lumpy breasts,[65] each of these diagnostic modalities is directed as skillfully as possible to detect breast cancer and identify women likely to harbor high-risk marker lesions.[66]

The diagnostic accuracy of each modality varies from series to series. From 8% to 38% of breast carcinomas are not detected by palpation alone. When mammography is added to the physical examination, up to 85% are detected preoperatively. By adding FNA, 93% to 100% are identified.[53,58,67] In the series of Kreuzer and Boquoi, concordance of the three methods indicated results that were correct more than 99% of the time.

Physical examination of the breast requires a great deal of experience to do well. Furthermore, results are plagued by some degree of subjectivism; not all observers agree about subtle findings. It is important that the patient's perception of masses, thickenings, or discomfort be elicited and taken seriously. Techniques for describing and recording the precise location of breast lesions are discussed in the section in this chapter on Evaluation of Breast Carcinoma.

Approach to Evaluation of Breast Cytology

False-negative diagnoses can occur as a result of poor technique or inaccurate targeting. Some breast carcinomas are extremely sclerotic and their dense fibrous stroma precludes aspiration of highly cellular material. This hypocellularity may be a diagnostic clue to infiltrating carcinoma of the lobular type and intraductal carcinoma.

The cytopathologist should not rely too heavily on the mammogram. The primary use of this test is identification of nonpalpable lesions. When a palpable mass is present, FNA can be the first-line diagnostic method. Mammography is then used to study nonpalpable disease in both breasts. Approximately 10% to 15% of palpable breast carcinomas are not visualized by mammography.

False-positive diagnoses may be related to cellular changes associated with pregnancy, lactation, or traumatic fat necrosis, and can be avoided if accurate clinical information is coupled with careful consideration of microscopic findings.

Histopathologists recognize a host of firm, stellate breast lesions that are benign but that can clinically, radiographically, and histologically mimic carcinoma. These are summarized in Box 2-3.[68-74] Keen and colleagues reviewed their experience with benign breast masses that clinically and mammographically appeared malignant. Their nine cases included examples of what was then called *indurative mastopathy, sclerosing papillary proliferation, infarcted papilloma, sclerosing adenosis,* and *fat necrosis.*[68]

Carcinoma must be diagnosed only when multiple cytologic criteria are met. Although suspicion of malignancy on clinical or mammographic grounds is sufficient to lead to an aspiration, neither is sufficient to result in an FNA diagnosis of carcinoma when it is not cytologically inescapable. Neither the radiologists' feeling that a given lesion may represent cancer nor the surgeon's being "sure it is cancer" constitutes a reason to diagnose carcinoma when the cytologic findings are not compelling.

Special Problems in Breast Aspiration

Cysts. A special situation is the handling of fluids aspirated from breast cysts. Less than 3% of cysts are associated with a malignancy.[58,75,76] Their significance is that they may conceal a malignancy from physical or radiographic examinations. Many surgeons aspirate cysts in the office and discard the fluid rather than submitting it for cytologic examination. With the typical pale yellow or light-green fluid in most cysts, this is an acceptable practice. If, however, the fluid is turbid or bloody, it should be centrifuged and examined microscopically. Fluids obtained from cysts that recur rapidly after drainage should also be examined microscopically.

Frable recommends the following steps in cyst evaluation:
1. Evacuate the cyst completely.
2. Carefully reexamine the patient for any residual mass in the area of the cyst. If any is found, it should be aspirated as any other breast mass.
3. Repeat the mammography to look for any suspicious areas that might have been obscured by the cyst.
4. Process the fluid and examine it microscopically, if indicated.[46]

Large, ill-defined breast thickenings. Many patients are referred for evaluation of breast lesions that are of low suspicion for malignancy. Historical and physical clues to the nature of benign fibrocystic change should be sought. These lesions are often areas of prominence or asymmetry in breasts that are diffusely lumpy or thickened. Focal thickenings or asymmetry between the two breasts may be reflected in the mammogram. These radiographs often confirm the abnormality but show no features suggestive of a malignant process. Such masses may be ill-defined on physical examination. Unless distinct, rounded cysts are present, the lesion may be difficult to delineate because its borders blend into the surrounding tissue.

Being numerous, not all of these cases can be reasonably approached surgically. However, a small number of such

---

BOX 2-3

Firm, Stellate Benign Breast Lesions that May Simulate Carcinoma Clinically, Mammographically, and Histologically

Sclerosing papillary proliferation
Radial scar
Fibromatosis
Fat necrosis
Elastosis in benign ductal proliferations
Granular cell tumor
Infarcted papilloma
Florid sclerosing adenosis (adenosis tumor)

thickenings obscure areas of malignancy. The addition of FNA to physical examination and mammography increases both the preoperative identification of cancer and the physician's confidence in nonsurgical follow-up of benign disease.

Adequate sampling is of paramount importance in these lesions but is difficult to define. A method of multiple, overlapping, cone-shaped aspiration volumes, as illustrated in Figure 2-16, is the best approach to larger thickenings in the breast. Generally, a minimum of three thorough aspirations is performed in such cases, but more may be needed in some instances. Although it is difficult to say how many aspirations are enough, it is usually clear that one is insufficient. Thorough, careful aspirations should always be performed, but the fact that this technique (like any other sampling method) has a small, seemingly irreducible false-negative rate remains. With this in mind, neither the quality of the procedure nor the thoroughness of patient follow-up can be allowed to diminish.

Small mobile lumps. Small mobile lumps make challenging targets for FNA. As discussed earlier, the techniques for stabilizing masses with the fingers of the left hand are useful in this situation. When the needle has entered the nodule, the fingertip can again be moved back and forth in an attempt to move the mass. If transfixed by the needle, the nodule is stationary and cannot be felt rolling under the fingertip. This technique can be applied to other small palpable lesions in many sites such as lymph nodes.

Deep-seated breast masses. Many breast masses are deeper than initial physical examination may suggest. The way in which this problem can be overcome is by feeling the lesion carefully with the needle tip. This usually suffices to ensure that the mass has been penetrated during the aspiration. In the patient with large breasts, one must also be careful to use a needle of sufficient length.

Multiple masses. Some patients are referred for evaluation of multiple areas of increased density that may involve both breasts. Each of these must be considered separately. Each may require more than one aspiration. Each lesion should be described, localized, and reported separately.

Complications of breast puncture. The patient with small breasts presents a special problem. The needle tip can come close to the chest wall soft tissues or even to the pleura. Pneumothorax caused by FNA is rare. One multi-institutional study described 74,000 breast aspirations performed with 21- to 23-gauge needles; 13 (0.18%) pneumothoraces occurred. None was severe, and none required chest tube placement for treatment.[77] In this series, pneumothorax caused sudden thoracic pain without dyspnea. To avoid this, breast lesions of this type should be entered with the needle oriented tangentially rather than perpendicular to the skin surface.

Painful aspiration of masses near the nipple. Retroareolar masses pose a problem because the skin of the nipple and areola is quite sensitive to pain. Because the retroareolar soft tissues are also sensitive, some pain is often unavoidable. The kindest thing that clinicians can do in this situation is to perform the aspiration skillfully and rapidly. To avoid the areolar skin, the retroareolar area can be entered tangentially. Another solution is to push the mass out from beneath the areolar area so that it can be aspirated through skin at some distance from this complex.

Aspiration of the male breast. Carcinoma is rare in the male breast but can be encountered. Aspiration of gyneco-

mastia is often very painful. Many men find the procedure difficult to tolerate. Again, skill and rapidity are important. Envisioning the area of gynecomastia as a thin, round, platelike area of tissue behind the areola, the clinician enters the skin tangentially some distance from the areola and then anticipates the firm feel as the needle enters the fibrous tissue. The needle is then moved back and forth and in and out in a much flattened version of the previously described cone-shaped tissue volume. Its motion is more like that of a fan-shaped distribution. This allows penetration of large areas of tissue in the medial to lateral and superior to inferior planes without close approach to the deep soft tissues and pleura.

Aspiration of breast carcinoma. Cytology can provide a firm, presurgical diagnosis of malignancy. This permits optimal counseling regarding treatment possibilities.

An indication for preoperative diagnosis of breast carcinoma by FNA is neoadjuvant chemotherapy. Cytotoxic agents are administered after diagnosis by FNA. Surgery is then performed. Tumor shrinkage may improve the resectability of larger lesions. Hormone receptor and DNA ploidy analyses need to be performed on aspirated material. Special specimen handling should be planned either at the time of the initial study or at the time of repeat FNA performed specifically to secure material for these studies.

When carcinomas are aspirated, they can often be felt as very firm. This perception is often described as gritty and is quite different from the rubbery or doughy feeling of benign breast lesions with dense fibrosis. An exception to this typical description is mucinous noma, which is very soft.[78,79] A similar situation occurs in medullary carcinoma because as its name implies, this tumor is fleshy in texture and is by definition well circumscribed.[79] (When diagnosed by rigorously applied criteria, medullary carcinoma is a very uncommon entity. In FNA material, it is impossible to distinguish from poorly differentiated infiltrating carcinoma that lacks the features of medullary carcinoma.)

As noted previously, many patients develop multiple breast abnormalities that may be studied by FNA. These may occur synchronously or at different times. It is imperative that the exact site, size, and clinical characteristics of the mass under study be described. The traditional description of the quadrant in which the lesion is found is not sufficient for this purpose. Two methods may be used. The first is to draw and label an illustration of the clinical findings. Although it is very helpful to receive such illustrations from the referring physician, they are very difficult to catalogue in the computerized archive that characterizes record keeping in the modern laboratory. A method of permanently recording this information uses a simple system of polar coordinates as illustrated in Figure 2-19. The data generated by this type of localization are very suitable for computerized reports.

The exact position of a mobile lesion may change depending on whether the patient is supine or sitting at the time of examination. The preferences is to perform most aspirations with the patient supine. Standardizing this practice minimizes any equivocation about the precise localization of a mobile breast mass. If, however, the lesion must be aspirated with the patient sitting, this should certainly be noted in the description of its localization.

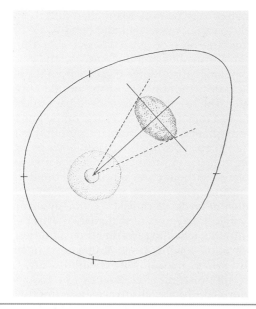

Figure 2-19 Localizing breast lesions. A system of polar coordinates can be used to accurately localize breast masses. The left breast lesion depicted here measures 2 × 3 cm, is located between 1 o'clock and 2 o'clock and is centered 6 cm from the nipple.

Techniques for Lymph Node Aspiration

Lymph nodes in the neck are commonly aspirated. Many of these are small and mobile. The ease with which they can be palpated may depend on the way in which the patient is examined. One may need to ask the patient to move the head in various ways to gain free access to small nodes. Final adjustments can be made when the physician moves the patient's head slightly with the right hand while palpating and stabilizing the target node with the fingers of the left hand.

Submandibular nodes may require bimanual palpation. The gloved fingers of the left hand push the node inferiorly by pressing in the sulcus between the floor of the mouth and the lower, inner border of the mandible. (It is much more comfortable for the patient if the gloved hand is moistened by running water before it is placed in the patient's mouth.) The lymph node can then be palpated subcutaneously with the fingers of the right hand in the usual fashion. One can then hold the node with the left hand between the index or middle finger (placed in the mouth) and the thumb on the skin surface beneath the mandible. In that way, one individual can perform the entire procedure, with the right hand being free for the syringe holder.

Nodes in the axilla or the supraclavicular fossa may lie close to the pleural surface, so some thought should be given to avoiding a possible pneumothorax. Nodes in the axilla can be very difficult to puncture accurately until considerable experience has been obtained. They are often mobile. If located high in the axilla, they must be pulled downward by the examining fingertips and stabilized by pressing them against the lateral chest wall. Palpation is facilitated by having the muscles that border the axilla in relaxation. These goals are facilitated by sitting beside the seated patient and asking him or her to rest the hand on the physician's shoulder. It is important to ensure, that should the patient be weak or should fainting occur, no fall or injury ensues. Thus, when executing this maneuver, an assistant should be positioned to help support the patient should this become necessary.

Aspiration of Salivary Glands

Technical aspects of parotid gland FNA are not significantly different from those of other subcutaneous masses such as lymph nodes. All but the largest submandibular masses may require bimanual palpation for localization and aspiration. This was described with submandibular lymph nodes. Intraoral masses that are covered by a smooth mucosa are often derived from minor salivary glands. Such lesions can occur in any part of the oral tissues and may be aspirated much as one would study subcutaneous masses. Topical anesthesia in the form of a spray can be easily applied to the mucosa.

Fear of complications, at first seemingly well founded, is unwarranted when carefully assessing the literature on this subject. The facial nerve and its branches divide within and course through the substance of the parotid. Some fear damage to this nerve either directly by the needle or as a result of compression by an enlarging hematoma. Although such a fear may be reasonable if one is using large, cutting-type core biopsy instruments, no instance of such damage has been reported by those using 23- or 25-gauge needles. The only local complication of salivary gland FNA seems to be the formation of small hematomas,[80] and this is not noted in most series.[46,81]

The other complication feared by some clinicians is local tumor recurrence. This is based on the fact that the most common salivary gland neoplasm is the benign mixed tumor (pleomorphic adenoma). Metastasizing cases of histologically benign mixed tumor are reportably rare. The real danger with this tumor is that if surgically violated by incision or by large cutting needle, it tends to multifocal local recurrence or implantation, which may be difficult to control with small surgical procedures. Thus, some clinicians forego all salivary gland aspiration. In fact, when small needles are used, there is no reported incident of such recurrence after FNA.[82,83]

Fine-Needle Aspiration of Skin Nodules

Although any palpable nodule can be aspirated, in North America the tendency is to use punch biopsy or excisional biopsy of cutaneous masses. If a malignancy (other than basal cell carcinoma) is strongly suspected on clinical grounds, some proceed to complete excision rather than use any type of biopsy.

Two dermal lesions are commonly studied. The first is the keratinous cyst, also known as *epidermal inclusion cyst* or *sebaceous cyst*. These firm, subcutaneous, dome-shaped dermal nodules may be up to several centimeters in greatest dimension. Their nature is usually suspected by the experienced clinician. Patients with a history of malignancy may be referred for evaluation of suspected metastatic disease. The caseous squamous debris that fills these cysts is immediately apparent when expelled from the needle. Also, the "rotten egg" odor of this material is characteristic. Thus, a diagnosis can often be rendered at the bedside before microscopic examination. In the clinical setting of known cancer, this finding can be reassuring. The rapidity with which it is achieved is always welcome.

Dermal recurrence of breast carcinoma is another setting in which cutaneous FNA can be very useful in providing rapid, reliable information by inexpensive means. Such lesions usually take the form of small (less than 5 mm), round or oval, firm, pale nodules. They may be much more apparent as the examining fingertips are moved lightly over the skin surface than they initially seem to be on visual inspection.

Palpable Masses of the Abdomen and Retroperitoneum

It is uncommon to see such patients before computed tomography (CT) or ultrasound studies have localized the mass and its potential extensions or metastases. Such studies often narrow the differential diagnostic possibilities that the cytopathologist must consider. Also, such lesions are usually aspirated by the radiologist with imaging guidance to ensure accurate needle placement.

When masses are readily palpable, however, little contraindication is evident to direct transcutaneous FNA at the bedside. Physicians familiar with the advantages of FNA may send the patient for this study before radiographic evaluation. This approach has been used for study of the palpably enlarged liver, which by CT scan shows a large burden of metastatic tumor in the form of numerous small masses. Such blind aspirations are often diagnostic and spare the patient other costly, painful studies. Palpation and percussion can localize the liver, and with the x-rays nearby, it is possible to be certain that no lung tissue overlies the selected area of aspiration. Longer needles than are often used may be required.

Some clinicians fear the consequences of entering the stomach, small intestine, or colon if abdominal aspiration is performed without radiographic guidance. In fact, penetration of bowel loops is quite common when radiologists direct needles into deep-seated lesions. In one study of 2500 transabdominal and transthoracic FNAs from Toronto General Hospital, the authors cited no instance of an infectious or hemorrhagic complication of bowel penetration.[52] They emphasized that the needles used are smaller than surgical suture material, which is commonly placed in the bowel wall with impunity.

 ## RESULTS REPORTING IN FINE NEEDLE ASPIRATION

The complete reporting method described here is for use by those who both perform the aspiration and interpret the microscopic findings. Those performing only part of this task issue only portions of such a report.

Medicolegal Considerations

In the section in this chapter on Breast FNA, potential malpractice issues were discussed that stem from the inevitable, small, but irreducible false-negative rate of FNA as it is applied to the large number of patients with apparently benign breast disease. It is an important principle of risk management that accurate documentation of the physician's actions provides the best defense during litigation.[84] The FNA report is the primary means of accomplishing this goal.

Potential problems arising from FNA can be categorized as false-positive diagnoses of malignancy, false-negative diagnoses of malignancy, and complications of the procedure. Many clinicians direct their energy to avoiding the potential complications of FNA that are extremely rare. The greatest source of liability arises not from patients injured by the procedure but from the diagnoses that are rendered.

False-negative diagnoses of malignancy represent a major source of potential liability for the FNA physician. Microscopy is one origin of this type of error but is probably not as common a problem as issues related to sampling or specimen preparation. Portions of this chapter are directed to minimizing errors by application of optimal techniques at each step of the FNA process. As noted earlier, more problems in FNA diagnosis occur at the bedside than at the microscope.

Components of the Fine-Needle Aspiration Report

These reports are modeled on the type of document generally used to report gross, microscopic and interpretive aspects of surgical biopsy specimens. Clinical, procedural, microscopic, interpretational, and follow-up issues should all be reflected in the final FNA report. This provides a complete assimilation of all available information and adequately documents performance of a high-quality, thorough procedure.

Demographic Section

The demographic section identifies the patient and referring physician. Note can also be made of other physicians or clinics in need of report copies. Dates should be given for the procedure itself, specimen receipt in the laboratory, and report generation. Some reimbursement plans mandate availability of results within a given time span. These dates document the process of specimen preparation and evaluation in the laboratory. Should delays be noted, this information can locate the problem within the laboratory itself or can be used to identify delays in specimen transport to the laboratory or in report generation.

Patient History

The history section of the report can be brief but should reflect signs, symptoms, chronology, and ancillary studies relevant to the lesion under study. This information is helpful in the cytopathologist's overall assessment of a case. It may highlight the need for additional studies if the cytologic diagnosis does not adequately explain key clinical findings. It can be used by those conducting reviews of procedures for appropriateness and cost-effectiveness. Finally, it can form an important database for clinical research.

Procedure

The procedure section of the report documents the thoroughness of the aspiration event. Its components describe performance of a procedure tailored to the clinical problem. It permits mention of special handling methods such as centrifugation of cyst fluid with smears prepared from the cell pellet. Gross findings of diagnostic significance can also be described, such as abundant colloid in a thyroid aspiration. If cyst fluid has been aspirated, one should document careful physical examination and reaspiration of any residual mass.

Microscopic Report

Microscopic descriptions should be brief; anyone needing to review these findings usually examines the glass slides. In many laboratories, microscopic descriptions are now omitted completely. If one elects to provide such a description, the key cellular features leading to the final diagnosis should be mentioned. Noncellular findings such as necrosis, inflammation, or thyroid colloid should also be noted.

This descriptive portion of the report is an excellent place for explanatory remarks. (Others place these comments in a separate section under the heading *Comments*.) For example, one may identify malignant cells but need to comment on an inability to further classify the neoplasm. Additional studies, recommendations for repeat aspiration, suggestion of surgical biopsy, or follow-up suggestions may be included here. One may also note the need to obtain slides of previous surgical or aspiration specimens for comparison with the material at hand.

One may also need to express inadequacy of the cytologic diagnosis in the light of clinical findings. The extent to which this is necessary often varies with the expertise of the referring physician. If the physical examination of a breast mass is highly suspicious for carcinoma but the cytology shows no malignancy, the surgeon may proceed appropriately to surgical biopsy. Others less skilled or experienced in breast examination and not realizing that FNA has a small false-negative rate may fail to obtain tissue surgically. If the cytopathologist is aware of the clinical findings, further evaluation can be recommended by surgical means or repeat FNA. Similar problems occur in other lesions for which provocative physical findings and false-negative cytology create a dissonance that demands resolution. The cytopathologist is in the unique position of using a detailed knowledge of the procedure's limitations (false-negative rate and difficulties in subclassification of uncommon tumors) to ensure correct application of the cytologic findings.

Diagnosis

Diagnoses are given in two parts: site (topography) and diagnosis (morphology). To the extent possible, the diagnostic terminology should reflect current practices in surgical pathology. The following are examples:

1. *Breast, right:* fibroadenoma
2. *Lymph node, cervical, right anterior:* metastatic squamous cell carcinoma
3. *Parotid gland, left:* pleomorphic adenoma
4. *Lymph node, inguinal, left:* malignant neoplasm (see description)

The historical method of reporting cytologic specimens as inadequate, benign, indeterminate, or malignant is now viewed by most as insufficient. Furthermore, the contemporary cytopathologist is often able to provide diagnoses of much greater specificity. In the uncommon instances in which diagnoses such as number 4 above are necessary, these should be accompanied by suggestion of means by which the disease process can be more fully classified.

References

1. Martin HE, Ellis EB. Biopsy by needle puncture and aspiration. Ann Surg 1930; 92:169-181.
2. Franzen S, Giertz G, Zajicek J. Cytological diagnosis of prostatic tumors by transrectal aspiration biopsy: a preliminary report. Br J Urol 1960; 32:193-201.
3. Shune D. Transbronchial needle aspiration: current status. Mayo Clin Proc 1989; 64:251-254.
4. Nordenskjold B, Löwhagen T, Westerberg H, et al. ³H-thymidine incorporation into mammary carcinoma cells obtained by needle aspiration before and during therapy. Acta Cytol 1976; 20:137-143.
5. Furnival CM, Hughes HE, Hocking MA, et al. Aspiration cytology in breast cancer: its relevance to diagnosis. Lancet 1975; 2:446-448.
6. Zajdela A, deMaüblanc MT, Schlienger P, et al. Cytologic diagnosis of periorbitalpalpable tumors using fine-needle sampling without aspiration. Diagn Cytopathol 1986; 2: 17-20.
7. Ciatto S, Catania S, Bravetti P, et al. Fine needle cytology of the breast: a controlled study of aspiration versus nonaspiration. Diagn Cytopathol 1991; 7:125-127.
8. Kung ITM, Chan S-K, Fung K-H. Fine-needle aspiration in hepatocellular carcinoma: combined clinical, cytologic and histologic approach. Cancer 1991; 67:673-680.
9. Henry-Stanley MJ, Stanley MW. Processing of needle rinse material from fine needle aspirations rarely detects malignancy not seen in smears. Diagn Cytopathol 1992; 8: 538-540.
10. Wittekind DH, Gehring T. On the nature of Romanowsky-Giemsa staining and the Romanowsky-Giemsa effect. I. Model experiments on the specificity of Azure B-Eosin Y stain as compared with other thiazine dye-Eosin Y combinations. Histochemical J 1985; 17:263-289.
11. Yang GC. Alvarez II. Ultrafast Papanicolaou stain: an alternative preparation for fine needle aspiration cytology. Acta Cytol 1995; 39:55-60.
12. Yazdi HM, Dardick I. Guides to clinical aspiration biopsy: diagnostic immunocytochemistry and electron microscopy. Igaku-Shoin: New York; 1992.
13. Schulte E: Air drying as a preparatory factor in cytology. Diagn Cytopathol 1986; 2:160-167.
14. Dziura DR, Bonfiglio TA. Needle cytology of the breast: a quantitative study of the cells of benign and malignant ductal neoplasia. Acta Cytol 1979; 23:332-334.
15. Schulte E, Wittekind C. The influence of the wet-fixed Papanicolaou and the air-dried Giemsa techniques on nuclear parameters in breast cancer cytology: a cytomorphometric study. Diagn Cytopathol 1987; 3:256-261.
16. Wallgren A, Zajicek J. The prognostic value of aspiration biopsy smear in mammary carcinoma. Acta Cytol 1976; 20:479-485.
17. Zajdela A, De LaRiva LS, Ghossein NA. The relation of prognosis to the nuclear diameter of breast cancer cells obtained by cytologic aspiration. Acta Cytol 1979; 23:75-80.
18. Cornelisse CJ, De Koning HR, Arentz PW, et al. Quantitative analysis of the nuclear area variation in benign and malignant breast cytology specimens. Acta Cytol 1981; 3:128-134.
19. Baak JPA, Kurver PHJ, Snoo-Nieuwlaat AJE, et al. Prognostic indicators in breast cancer-morphometric methods. Histopathology 1982; 6:327-339.
20. Fossa SD, Marton PF, Knudsen OS, et al. Nuclear Feulgen DNA content and nuclear size in human breast carcinoma. Hum Pathol 1982; 13:626-630.
21. Baak JPA, Van Dop H, Kurver PHJ, et al. The value of morphometry to classic prognosticators in breast cancer. Cancer 1985; 56:374-382.
22. Stanley MW, Tani EM, Skoog L. Mucinous breast carcinoma and mixed mucinous-infiltrating ductal carcinoma: a comparative cytologic study. Diagn Cytopathol 1989; 5:134-138.
23. Frable WJ: Thin-needle aspiration biopsy. Philadelphia: WB Saunders; 1983. pp.51-53.
24. Lee KR, Papillo JL, St. John T, et al. Evaluation of the ThinPrep processor for fine needle aspiration specimens. Acta Cytol 1996; 40(5):895-899.

25. Leung CS, Chiu B, Bell V. Comparison of ThinPrep and conventional preparations: nongynecologic cytology evaluation. Diagn Cytopath 1997; 16(4):368-371.

26. Dey P, Luthra UK, George J, Zuhairy F, et al. Comparison of ThinPrep and conventional preparations of fine needle aspiration cytology material. Acta Cytol 2000; 44(1):46-50.

27. Michael CW, McConnel J, Pecott J, et al. Comparison of ThinPrep and TriPath PREP liquid-based preparations in nongynecologic specimens: a pilot study. Diagn Cytopath 2001; 25(3):177-184.

28. Kurtycz DF, Hoerl HD. Thin-layer technology: tempered enthusiasm. Diagn Cytopath 2000; 23(1):1-5.

29. Michael CW, Hunter B. Interpretation of fine-needle aspirates processed by the ThinPrep technique: cytologic artifacts and diagnostic pitfalls. Diagn Cytopath 2000; 23(1): 6-13.

30. Salhadar A, Massarini-Wafai R, Wojcik EM. Routine use of ThinPrep method in fine-needle aspiration material as an adjunct to standard smears. Diagn Cytopath 2001; 25(2): 101-103.

31. Nasuti JF, Tam D, Gupta PK. Diagnostic value of liquid-based (ThinPrep) preparations in nongynecologic cases. Diagn Cytopath 2001; 24(2):137-141.

32. Perez-Reyes N, Mulford DK, Rutkowski MA, et al. Breast fine-needle aspiration: a comparison of thin-layer and conventional preparation. Am J Clin Pathol 1994; 102(3): 349-353.

33. Biscotti CV, Shorie JH, Gramlich TL, et al. ThinPrep vs. conventional smear cytologic preparations in analyzing fine-needle aspiration specimens from palpable breast masses. Diagn Cytopath 1999; 21(2):137-141.

34. Bedard YC, Pollett AF. Breast fine-needle aspiration: a comparison of ThinPrep and conventional smears. Am J Clin Pathol 1999; 111(4):523-527.

35. Tabbara SO, Sidawy MK, Frost AR, et al. The stability of estrogen and progesterone receptor expression on breast carcinoma cells stored as PreservCyt suspensions and as ThinPrep slides. Cancer 1998; 84(6):355-360.

36. Leung SW, Bedard YC. Estrogen and progesterone receptor contents in ThinPrep-processed fine-needle aspirates of breast. Am J Clin Pathol 1999; 112(1):50-56.

37. Biscotti CV, Hollow JA, Toddy SM, et al. ThinPrep versus conventional smear cytologic preparations in the analysis of thyroid fine-needle aspiration specimens. Am J Clin Pathol 1995; 104(2):150-153.

38. Frost AR, Sidawy MK, Ferfelli M, et al. Utility of thin-layer preparations in thyroid fine-needle aspiration: diagnostic accuracy, cytomorphology, and optimal sample preparation. Cancer 1998; 84(1):17-25.

39. Scurry JP, Duggan MA. Thin layer compared to direct smear in thyroid fine needle aspiration. Cytopath 2000; 11(2): 104-115.

40. Zhang Y, Fraser JL, Wang HH. Morphologic predictors of papillary carcinoma on fine-needle aspiration of thyroid with ThinPrep preparations. Diagn Cytopathol 2001; 24(6): 378-383.

41. Afify AM, Liu J, Al-Khafaji BM. Cytologic artifacts and pitfalls of thyroid fine-needle aspiration using ThinPrep: a comparative retrospective review. Cancer 2001; 93(3): 179-186.

42. Al-Khafaji BM, Afify AM. Salivary gland fine needle aspiration using the ThinPrep technique: diagnostic accuracy, cytologic artifacts and pitfalls. Acta Cytol 2001; 45(4): 567-574.

43. Guiter GE, Gatscha RM, Zakowski MF. ThinPrep vs. conventional smears in fine-needle aspirations of sarcomas: a morphological and immunocytochemical study. Diagn Cytopath 1999; 21(5):351-354.

44. Leung SW, Bedard YC. Immunocytochemical staining on ThinPrep processed smears. Mod Pathol 1996; 9(3): 304-306.

45. Borrows GH, Anderson TJ, Lamb JL, et al. Fine-needle aspiration of breast cancer: relationship of clinical factors to cytology results in 689 primary malignancies. Cancer 1986; 58:1492-1498.

46. Frable WJ: Fine-needle aspiration biopsy: a review. Hum Pathol 1983; 14:9-28.

47. Cohen MB, Miller TR, Gonzales JM, et al. Fine-needle aspiration biopsy: perceptions of physicians at an academic medical center. Arch Pathol Lab Med 1986; 110:813-817.

48. Zajicek J. Aspiration biopsy cytology. II. Cytology of infradiaphragmatic organs. New York: S Karger; 1974.

49. Zajdela A, Ghossein NA, Pilleron JP, et al: The value of aspiration cytology in the diagnosis of breast cancer: experience at the Foundation Curie. Cancer 1975; 35:499-506.

50. Franzen S, Zajicek J. Aspiration biopsy in the diagnosis of palpable lesions of the breast. Acta Radiol Ther Phys Biol 1968; 7:241:262.

51. Hall TL, Layfield LJ, Philippe A, et al. Source of diagnostic error in fine needle aspiration of the thyroid. Cancer 1989; 63:718-725.

52. Tao LC, Pierson FG, Delarne NC, et al. Percutaneous fine-needle aspiration biopsy. I. Its value to clinical practice. Cancer 1980; 45:1480-1485.

53. Hajdu SI, Melamed MR. Limitations of aspiration cytology in the diagnosis of primary neoplasms. Acta Cytol 1984; 28:337-345.

54. Martin HE, Ellis EB. Biopsy by needle puncture and aspiration. Ann Surg 1930; 92:169-181.

55. Stewart FW. The diagnosis of tumors by aspiration. Am J Pathol 1933; 9:801-815.

56. Soderstrom N. Fine needle aspiration biopsy. New York: Grune and Stratton; 1966.

57. Linsk JA, Franzen S. Fine-needle aspiration for the clinician. Philadelphia: JB Lippincott; 1986.

58. Bell DA, Hajdu SI, Urban JA, et al. Role of aspiration cytology in the diagnosis and management of mammary lesions in office practice. Cancer 1983; 51:1182-1189.

59. VanBogaert L-J, Mazy G. Reliability of the cyto-radioclinical triplet in breast pathology diagnosis. Acta Cytol 1977; 21:60-62.

60. Kreuzer G, Boquoi E. Aspiration biopsy cytology, mammography and clinical exploration: a modern set up in diagnosis of tumors of the breast. Acta Cytol 1976; 20:319-323.

61. Goellner JR, Johnson DA. Cytology of cystic papillary carcinoma of the thyroid. Acta Cytol 1982; 26:797-799.

62. Miller JM, Hamburger JI, Taylor CI. Is needle aspiration of the cystic thyroid nodule effective and safe treatment? In: Hamburger JI, Miller A, editors. Controversies in clinical thyroidology. Springer-Verlag: New York; 1981. pp.209-236.

63. Colacchio TA, LoGerfo P, Feird CR. Fine needle cytologic diagnosis of thyroid nodules: review and report of 300 cases. Am J Surg 1980; 140:568-571.

64. Ramacciotti CE, Pretorius HT, Chu EW, et al. Diagnostic accuracy and use of aspiration biopsy in the management of thyroid nodules. Arch Intern Med 1984; 144:1169-1173.

65. Hutter VP. Goodbye to fibrocystic disease. N Engl J Med 1985; 312:179-181.

66. Dupont WD, Page DL. Risk factors for breast cancer in women with proliferative breast disease. N Engl J Med 1985; 312:146-151.

67. Stanley MW. Fine needle aspiration: the ultimate opportunity for the pathologist to act as a clinical consultant: syllabus for American Society of Clinical Pathologists Course number 3404, Chicago: ASCP Press; 1990.

68. Keen ME, Murad TM, Cohen MI, et al. Benign breast lesions with malignant clinical and mammographic presentations. Hum Pathol 1985; 16:1147-1152.

69. Anderson JA, Gram JB. Radial scar in the female breast: a long-term follow-up study of 32 cases. Cancer 1984; 53: 2557-2560.

70. Hanna WM, Jambrosic J, Fish E. Aggressive fibromatosis of the breast. Arch Pathol Lab Med 1985; 109:260-263.

71. Flint A, Oberman HA. Infarction and squamous metaplasia of intraductal papilloma: a benign breast lesion that may simulate carcinoma. Hum Pathol 1984; 15:764-767.

72. Rickert RR, Ralisher L, Hutter RVP. Indurative mastopathy: a benign sclerosing lesion of breast with elastosis which may simulate carcinoma. Cancer 1981; 47:561-571.

73. Fenoglio C, Lattes R. Sclerosing papillary proliferations in the female breast: a benign lesion often mistaken for carcinoma. Cancer 1974; 33:681-700.

74. Strobel SL, Shah NT, Lucas JG, et al. Granular-cell tumor of the breast: a cytologic, immunohistochemical and ultrastructural study of two cases. Acta Cytol 1985; 29:598-601.

75. Kline TS, Joshi LP, Neal HS. Fine-needle aspiration of the breast: diagnosis and pitfalls: a review of 3545 cases. Cancer 1979; 44:1458-1464.

76. Strawbridge HTG, Bassett AA, Foldes I. Role of cytology in management of lesions of the breast. Surg Gynecol Obstet 1981; 152:1-7.

77. Catania S, Boccato P, Bono A, et al. Pneumothorax: a rare complication of fine needle aspiration of the breast. Acta Cytol 1989; 33:140.

78. Stanley MW, Tani EM, Skoog L. Mucinous breast carcinoma and mixed mucinous/infiltrating ductal carcinoma: a comparative cytologic study. Diagn Cytopathol 1989; 5:134-138.

79. Wargotz ES, Silverberg SG: Medullary carcinoma of the breast: a clinicopathologic study with appraisal of current diagnostic criteria. Hum Pathol 1988; 19:1340-1346.

80. Mavec P, Eneroth CM, Franzen S, et al. Aspiration biopsy of salivary gland tumors. I. Correlation of cytologic reports from 652 aspirations with clinical and histologic findings. Acta Otolaryngol 1964; 58:472-484.

81. O'Dwyer P, Farrar WB, James AG, et al. Needle aspiration biopsy of major salivary gland tumors. Cancer 1986; 57:554-557.

82. Engzell U, Esposti PL, Rubio C, et al. Investigation of tumor spread in connection with aspiration biopsy. Acta Radiol 1971; 10:385-398.

83. Eneroth CM, Zajicek J. Aspiration biopsy of salivary gland tumors. III. Morphologic studies on smears and histologic sections from 360 mixed tumors. Acta Cytol 1966; 10: 440-454.

84. Kline TJ, Kline TS. Communication and cytopathology. II. Malpractice. Diagn Cytopathol 1991; 7:227-228.

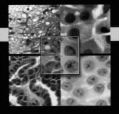

GYNECOLOGIC
CYTOLOGY

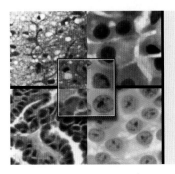

Normal Cytology of the Lower Female Genital Tract

The clinical and historical importance of gynecologic cytology as a cancer screening device cannot be overstated. The Papanicolaou (Pap) test is clearly the most effective, cost efficient, and minimally invasive cancer screening tool ever devised. Neither mammography nor occult blood testing for colorectal carcinoma can approach the success of Papanicolaou's method. Furthermore, the intellectual and cytomorphologic concepts of Pap test interpretation have formed the basis for the approach to most other cytodiagnostic investigations. Only when one encounters certain uncommon lesions accessible only by fine-needle aspiration (FNA) does the canon of diagnostic principles require alteration.

At this writing, much of the relevant literature antedates the Bethesda System 2001. To review studies from this period adequately, it is necessary to move occasionally between older and newer terminology. For example, the interpretation *atypical squamous cells of undetermined significance (ASCUS) favor low-grade squamous intraepithelial lesion (LGSIL)* is sometimes used. Failure to do so would render the result of numerous important studies uninterpretable because no comparable diagnostic category exists in the latest Bethesda System terminology.

 ## NORMAL CYTOLOGY OF THE VAGINA, CERVIX, AND ENDOCERVICAL CANAL

Vagina and Ectocervix

The vagina and external part of the uterine cervix (the portion visible from the vagina) are covered by a nonkeratinized stratified squamous epithelium. This is continuous over the fornices and recessed mucosal reflections between the portio and the vagina. The point at which this squamous mucosa meets the columnar mucosa of the endocervix is histologically described as the squamocolumnar junction. Physiologically, however, this intersection is dynamic and the actual point of mucosal convergence moves back and forth in response to a variety of stimuli. Hence, the term *transformation zone* has evolved. This transformation and the process by which it occurs (SM) are detailed in the subsequent discussion.

The stratified squamous epithelium consists of a variable number of cell layers. It rests on a basement membrane that is itself anchored to an underlying well-vascularized fibrous stroma. Table 3-1 and Figure 3-1 show this epithelium as having four histologic layers. The single layer of cells resting on the basement membrane is designated as the basal layer. These cells, together with the immediately superficial parabasal cells, are responsible for the proliferative activity that continuously replaces the entire epithelial thickness approximately every 7 days.[1-3] As assessed by the monoclonal antibody MIB-1, proliferative activity is decreased in atrophy and increased in SIL. The potential diagnostic implications of these observations are discussed more fully in Chapter 6, where the differential diagnosis of high-grade squamous intraepithelial lesion (HGSIL) with atrophy is considered.

Cells produced in the lower layers of the squamous epithelium migrate progressively toward the lumenal surface as they mature, where they are spontaneously exfoliated at the end of their life span. As these normal cells ascend, they mature (Figure 3-2, Table 3-2, and Box 3-1).[4] In short, the cells change from small and cyanophilic with scanty cytoplasm and open chromatin to large with abundant eosinophilic cytoplasm and small pyknotic nuclei. Open chromatin, cyanophilic (protein-poor) cytoplasm, and a high nuclear to cytoplasmic (N:C) ratio are all features of high metabolic activity in young cells. The opposite features characterize mature cells nearing senescence.

Distinction of parabasal cells from the cells of immature squamous metaplasia (SM) can be impossible, as noted subsequently, when the latter process is considered in detail. However, in a hormonal milieu that supports squamous cell maturation to the level of superficial cells and in the absence of significant inflammation, all three cell layers are not seen on a single smear. Thus, most mature smears show superficial and intermediate cells; any small immature cells of the type to be described below can be assumed to represent immature SM. In other hormonal settings, particularly the intermediate cell predominant patterns to be discussed during our consideration of hormonal cytology, such small immature cells may represent either SM or parabasal cells. In this setting the two cell types are indistinguishable. The nuclei of intermediate cells often show a thin horizontal groove; this is lost as maturation proceeds. In these types of cells, the pale, open chromatin sometimes allows visualization of the Barr body as a single small (≈ 1 μm) dark dot closely adherent to the inner surface of the nuclear membrane. The cytoplasm of intermediate cells may contain abundant glycogen. Sometimes, this has a pale golden color in Pap-stained preparations. At other times, it is clear, having been removed from the cells during processing through various solvents. When fully developed, the latter configuration results in the characteristic appearance of navicular (boat-shaped) cells; these are especially prominent during pregnancy (Figure 3-3).

Superficial cells are defined as having dark homogeneous nuclear staining without detectable chromatin substructure; their cytoplasm, through which light appears to pass easily, may be either cyanophilic or eosinophilic. These large, flat cells are polygonal and cover the mucosal surface just as cobblestones cover a street.

Endocervical Canal

Most of the canal is lined by a single layer of uniform columnar epithelial cells. Regeneration of this delicate layer is the role of poorly visualized reserve cells. Each mature cell features a tall column of pale to slightly basophilic mucin-filled cytoplasm. A round nucleus measuring approximately 50 μm² resides at the base of the cell. It is often rather pale with finely granular chromatin and may show a single small nucleolus. A Barr body may be visible. A curious nuclear modification is the nipplelike projection.[5] McCallum offered several clinical observations that suggest that formation of this structure may be related to the cell's exposure to increased levels of progesterone (progesterone-only contraceptives and possibly ovulation).

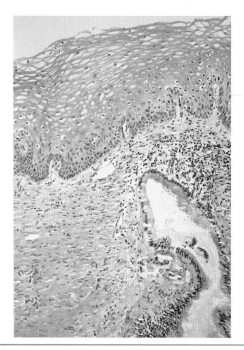

Figure 3-1 Normal squamous epithelium. This low-magnification image shows a multilayered squamous epithelium overlying cervical stroma with small, darkly staining chronic inflammatory cells and a single gland. Low-magnification evaluation makes the orderly maturation within the squamous epithelium apparent. The basal layer appears as a single, well-organized row of darkly staining small cells at the base of the epithelium. Immediately above that, the cells begin to mature as they acquire increased cytoplasm. This cytoplasm is eosinophilic because of cytokeratin protein deposition. The most mature cells at the upper levels of the epithelium have extremely small pyknotic nuclei and abundant eosinophilic cytoplasm. (Papanicolaou [Pap])

TABLE 3-1	
Layers of Normal Squamous Epithelium of the Vagina and Ectocervix	
Microanatomic Location	**Designation within the Epithelium**
Deepest single layer of cells	Basal cells
Lower one third (several layers)*	Parabasal cells
Middle one third (several layers)	Intermediate cells
Upper one third (several layers)†	Superficial cells

*The several cell layers immediately above the basal layer.
†The several cell layers closest to the lumenal surface.

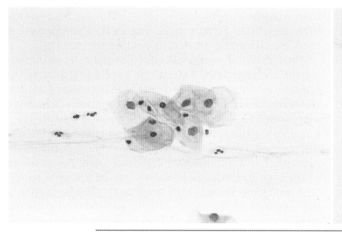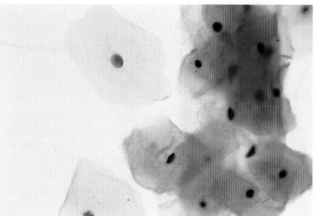

A   B

Figure 3-2 Normal squamous cells. **A,** This illustration shows a combination of intermediate cells and superficial cells. These mature squamous cells are large and flat and spread out to cover cervical surface with a hearty epithelium. Either cell type may show cyanophilic or eosinophilic cytoplasm. Intermediate cells are defined by nuclei that are pale, with stippled chromatin and smooth contours and an occasional small chromocenter **(B).** This higher-magnification image emphasizes these nuclear features. (Pap)

In smear material, these cells may lie singly, in flat sheets, or in three-dimensional clusters. When a sheet is viewed from the side, the columnar shape and lack of nuclear stratification that characterize this tissue is seen. When a flat sheet is viewed *en face,* the microscope can be focused through various planes to visualize either of two levels within this thin but still three-dimensional tissue fragment. The lower level contains the round uniform nuclei, each surrounded by a thin rim of cytoplasm. Each "respects" the others' boundaries, and no overlapping occurs, somewhat like eggs in a carton. If the sheet is viewed at its surface, the nuclei are no longer visible. Instead, a honeycomb pattern of closely apposed cell membranes is seen. The effects of atrophy on endocervical cells are considered in the section on Hormonal Cytology (Figure 3-4). In rare instances, mucus extruded from endocervical glands may form a long, thin basophilic spiral (Curschmann's spiral) identical to those seen more commonly in pulmonary samples.

The surface columnar epithelium is continuous with an identical tissue covering macroscopic lumenal folds of the endocervical lining and with the lining of numerous microscopic glands that extend below the surface. The gland openings may become overgrown and thus obstructed by squamous metaplastic epithelium. Furthermore, this metaplastic growth may extend into the glands for varying distances, replacing the normal columnar cells as it advances. When glands are obstructed, they become dilated and may lead to formation of submucosal cysts (Nabothian cysts). These often become sufficiently large as to be grossly visible in surgically resected material. These cysts are filled with secretory material, including a finely granular substance. The latter is occasionally detected in conventional Pap test smears as a granular background and should not be mistaken for the tumor diathesis pattern sometimes associated with invasive malignancies.

Columnar endocervical cells may show lumenal surface specialization in the form of a terminal plate and cilia, identical to those seen on tracheobronchial mucosal cells (Figure 3-5). It is important to note that ciliation alone does not constitute tubal metaplasia. The latter is a transformation of the simple columnar endocervical epithelium to a more complex ciliated epithelium identical to that of the fallopian tube. Careful evaluation of hysterectomy specimens indicated that this finding is virtually ubiquitous in the upper one third of the canal.[6]

Table 3-3 shows the cytomorphologic features of tubal metaplasia that have been described in detail[6-10] (Figure 3-6). Tissue fragments may show a smooth border, along which cilia may easily be detected. Problems arise when the cilia are not readily apparent and a cluster of small uniform cells with hyperchromatic nuclei and scanty cytoplasm is identified, or when rosettelike arrangements are noted. In this setting, a diagnosis of atypical glandular cells or adenocarcinoma in situ is likely to be rendered. In other instances, these small cells may be interpreted as HGSIL. Novotny and colleagues describe criteria useful in distinguishing these entities[9] (Table 3-4). These differential diagnostic considerations are also discussed in Chapter 8.

Occasionally, glandular cells or squamous metaplastic cells are encountered on a Pap test from a patient known to

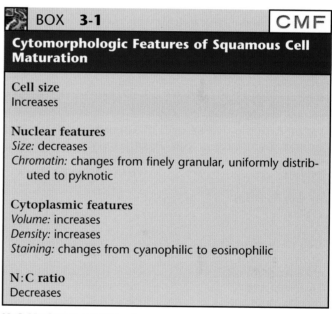

BOX 3-1 CMF

Cytomorphologic Features of Squamous Cell Maturation

Cell size
Increases

Nuclear features
Size: decreases
Chromatin: changes from finely granular, uniformly distributed to pyknotic

Cytoplasmic features
Volume: increases
Density: increases
Staining: changes from cyanophilic to eosinophilic

N:C ratio
Decreases

N:C, Nuclear to cytoplasmic.

TABLE 3-2

Maturation of Normal Squamous Epithelial Cells

Cell Type	Cell Area*	Nuclear Area*	N:C Ratio	Cytoplasmic Staining	Chromatin Pattern
Parabasal	Variable	50	Variable	Cyanophilic	Finely granular
Intermediate	1500	35	3% to 5%	Cyanophilic	Finely granular ± grooves
Superficial	1500	Variable (≤ 35)	2% to 3%	Cyanophilic or eosinophilic	Pyknotic

Summary

Immature Squamous Cells	Mature Squamous Cells
Small	Large
Cyanophilic	Cyanophilic or eosinophilic
Open chromatin	Dense chromatin
High N:C ratio	Low N:C ratio

Data are approximate, being rounded from the means of numerous measurements in Patten SF, Jr. Diagnostic cytopathology of uterine cervix. 2nd ed. Basel, Switzerland: S Karger AG; 1978.
N:C, Nuclear to cytoplasmic ratio (this is the ratio of these compartments' areas).
*All areas are in μm^2.

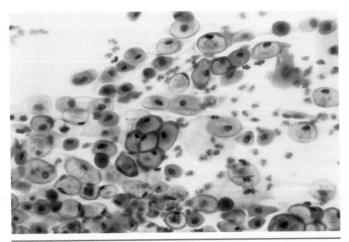

Figure 3-3   Glycogenated (navicular) squamous cells. In the center of this field are heavily glycogenated intermediate squamous cells known as *navicular cells*. Typical features are clear to lightly golden cytoplasm, thickened cell borders, and eccentric nuclei showing the features of benign intermediate or superficial cells. These bland nuclear features should prevent mistaking the clear cytoplasm for these cells for that of koilocytic atypia associated with papillomavirus infection (low-grade squamous intraepithelial lesion [LGSIL]). (Pap)

TABLE **3-3**   CMF

Cytomorphologic Features of Tubal Metaplasia in the Endocervical Canal

Feature	Description
Cell arrangements	
Commonly encountered	Clusters and sheets
Sometimes encountered	Rosettelike arrangements
Nuclear features	
Shape	Round to oval
Chromatin	Finely granular
Nucleoli	Inconspicuous
Cytoplasmic features	
Volume	Scanty
Staining	Cyanophilic
Cilia	Not always seen

TABLE **3-4**   CMF

Cytomorphologic Features of Tubal Metaplasia Contrasted with Those of in situ and Invasive Adenocarcinomas of the Uterine Cervix

Feature	Adenocarcinoma in Situ	Invasive Adenocarcinoma	Tubal Metaplasia
Background	Clean	Tumor diathesis possible	Clean
Cellularity	Variable, often high	Usually high	Variable, may be high
Cell arrangements:			
Crowded sheets	Numerous	Numerous	Few to numerous
Honeycomb sheets	Few	Few	Few to numerous
Feathered edges	Often present	Often present	Infrequent
Isolated strips	Few to numerous	Numerous	Absent or rare
Rosettes	Few to numerous	Numerous	Rare
Single cells	Few	Few to numerous	Few to numerous
Cytoplasmic features:			
Terminal bars/cilia	Absent	Absent	May be present
Cell shape	Columnar or cuboidal	Columnar or cuboidal	Columnar
Cytoplasm	Granular	Granular or vacuolated	Thin or dense
Nuclear features:			
Size	Enlarged	Enlarged	Enlarged
Anisonucleosis	Moderate	Moderate to marked	Slight to moderate
Shape	Elongated	Less elongated than AIS	Oval
Arrangement in groups	Stratified or palisaded	Stratified or palisaded	Evenly spaced
Chromatin:			
Granularity	Moderate to coarse	Moderate to coarse	Fine to moderate
Dispersion	Uniform	Less uniform than AIS	Uniform
Nucleoli	Very small or absent	Large and usually single	Very small or absent
Mitotic figures	Few to numerous	Numerous	Rare

From Novotny DM, Maygarden SJ, Johnson DE, et al. Tubal metaplasia: a frequent potential pitfall in the cytologic diagnosis of endocervical glandular dysplasia on cervical smears. Acta Cytol 1992; 36:1-10.
AIS, Adenocarcinoma in situ.

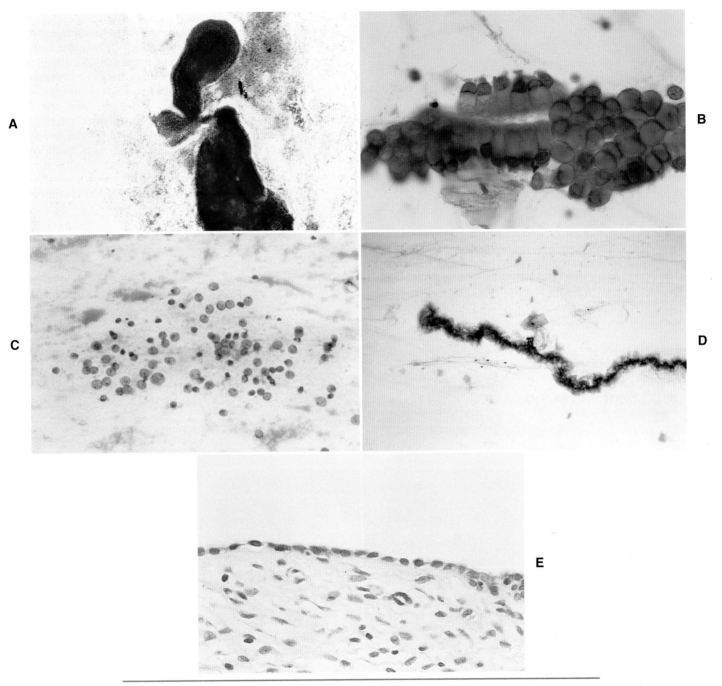

Figure 3-4 Normal endocervical cells. A, This low-magnification image shows a large, three-dimensional clublike fragment of endocervical glandular epithelium. The presence of such particles may suggest an endocervical polyp, but they are frequently seen in the absence of this lesion. (Pap) **B,** This high-magnification image shows endocervical cells both in transverse and *en face* projections. The transversely viewed cells show basally located nuclei beneath tall goblets of pale basophilic mucinous material. The luminal surface of this cell cluster shows a sharp border. At the edges of this tissue fragment the cell cluster has been twisted so that the endocervical cells are seen *en face* and their honeycomb-like lattice of membranes becomes apparent. **C,** Endocervical cells are fragile and are often damaged in the smearing process, so they lie as pale cytoplasmic remnants containing scattered, small, uniform nuclei. **D,** In some instances, mucus can be extruded from an endocervical gland to form a Curschmann's spiral similar to those more commonly encountered in respiratory material. **E,** This histologic preparation emphasizes the small, flat to cuboidal appearance exhibited by atrophic endocervical glandular cells. When present on a smear preparation, these small glandular cells can closely mimic endometrial cells. (**A-D,** Pap; **E,** Hematoxylin and eosin [H&E])

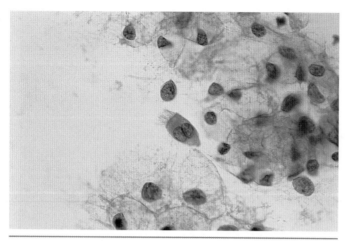

Figure 3-5 **Ciliated endocervical cells.** The presence of cilia and a terminal plate on columnar endocervical cells is common. This finding in isolation does not constitute tubal metaplasia, as it is illustrated in Figure 3-6. (Pap)

have had a hysterectomy. In the large published experience of Ramirez and colleagues, these are most often squamous metaplastic cells, with endocervical cells, glandular cells of nonspecific type, and mixtures of these cells occurring less often.[11] These investigators noted more frequent occurrence of glandular cells in patients who had undergone hysterectomy for treatment of a malignancy. However, it is not clear whether this may be an artifact of the authors' referral patient base. They postulate that some of these cells originate in vaginal adenosis that is not associated with in-utero diethylstilbestrol (DES) exposure. Other cases may be the result of supracervical hysterectomy. In some instances of vaginal hysterectomy, the fallopian tube remnants can shed glandular cells into the vaginal vault.

Squamous Metaplasia and Reserve Cell Hyperplasia

Glandular epithelia in many sites can participate in the process of SM whenever stress or injury requires a heartier covering than that afforded by a single layer of secretory

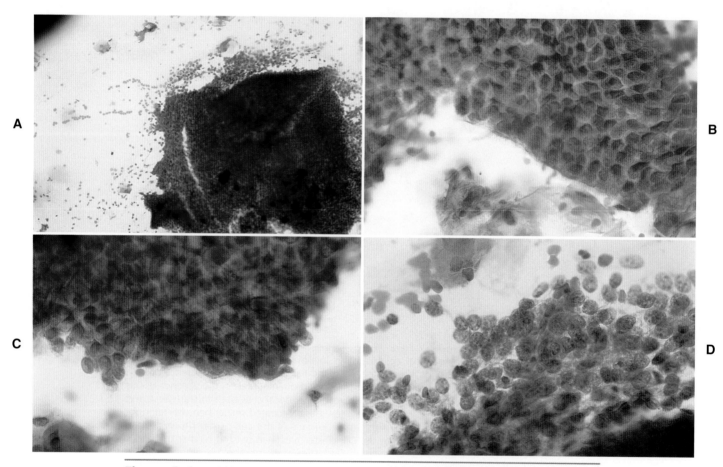

Figure 3-6 **Tubal metaplasia.** **A,** This low-magnification image shows a large tissue particle composed of densely packed small hyperchromatic cells. At this point, the differential diagnosis includes endometrial cells, a high-grade squamous intraepithelial lesion (HGSIL), atypical glandular cells of undetermined significance, adenocarcinoma in-situ, and tubal metaplasia (**B** and **C**). Each of these images shows a crowded cluster of small cells with hyperchromatic nuclei. The temptation to make a diagnosis of atypical glandular cells or HGSIL can be significant. However, careful examination with evaluation through multiple levels of focus shows that at least some portion of each particle is covered by columnar cells with sharp luminal borders and readily apparent cilia. These findings are diagnostic of tubal metaplasia. **D,** When tubal metaplastic cells are viewed in isolation or when the luminal border and cilia are not readily apparent, the danger of mistakenly diagnosing an HGSIL or an atypical glandular proliferation can be significant. (Pap)

cells. This process is considered in detail in connection with pulmonary epithelial abnormalities and neoplasia (see Chapters 15 and 16).

As noted previously, the squamocolumnar junction of the uterine cervix is a dynamic entity that moves continually through the transformation zone. As it moves proximally, SM is the process by which a glandular surface is exchanged for one covered by a stratified squamous epithelium. This process can be conceptually divided into three stages designated reserve cell hyperplasia, immature SM, and mature SM.

The dividing lines between these three stages are arbitrary. Histologically, reserve cell hyperplasia (RCH) appears as small immature cells with scanty cytoplasm that grow between the columnar endocervical cells and the underlying basement membrane. As these cells mature, they go through a series of alterations similar to those that characterize maturation in native squamous epithelia. The cells of RCH enlarge and begin to acquire more abundant eosinophilic cytoplasm. They may form several ill-defined layers in which cells have a syncytial relationship to one another. As maturation proceeds, cytoplasmic enlargement

continues, and the cells acquire histologically distinct cell borders; this point in the process is designated immature SM. Ultimately, this epithelium takes on the appearance of the more distally located squamous covering and is designated mature SM. The precise squamocolumnar junction will have advanced proximally to lie higher in the transformation zone. These histologic stages are illustrated in Figure 3-7.

Thus, SM is histologically divided into three stages. Cytologically, however, this maturational process goes through a smooth continuum. All gradations of cell size, nuclear maturity, and cytoplasmic volume can be appreciated. Another aspect of cytoplasmic maturation is readily apparent on Pap-stained preparations but not seen in histologic samples. In the latter, only one cytoplasmic counterstain, eosin, is available. This means that all cells show eosinophilic cytoplasm. In the more complex tinctorial repertory of the Pap stain, the cells' cytoplasm changes from cyanophilic to eosinophilic as maturation proceeds. Other cytoplasmic features of maturation are related to increasing deposition of keratin filaments. This leads to greater cytoplasmic density and sharp cell borders. These

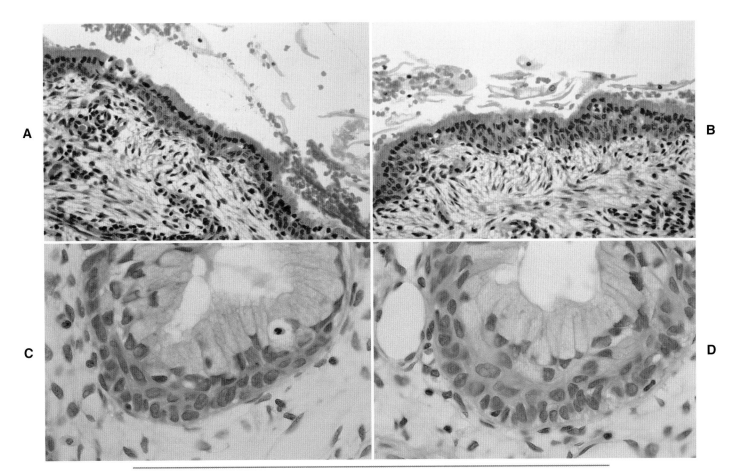

Figure 3-7 Developmental stages of squamous metaplasia (SM). **A** and **B**, These two images show reserve cell hyperplasia of the endocervical epithelium at low magnification. The residual layer of luminal columnar cells is underlain by one or two layers of small cells with scanty cytoplasm and no apparent cell borders **(A)**. As this process continues an increasing proliferation of these reserve cells occurs **(B)**. **C**, This higher-magnification image shows continued proliferation of basal cells beneath an intact layer of residual glandular cells. **D**, As this process continues, the reserve cells take on the features of immature squamous metaplastic cells as they acquire larger nuclei and more generous amounts of eosinophilic cytoplasm. Occasional intercellular borders can be identified. **(A&B,** Pap; **C&D,** H&E)

filaments are sometimes visualized at the light microscopic level as concentric cytoplasmic laminations.

The cytomorphology of these stages is illustrated in Figure 3-8. As discussed in Chapters 15 and 16 when RCH is considered in the context of bronchial SM, this most un-

differentiated portion of the process is rarely appreciated in cytologic samples. Most of the cell clusters illustrated as examples of RCH are morphologically indistinguishable from clusters of normal endometrial glandular cells (see the section on Endometrial Cells and Tissue Fragments).

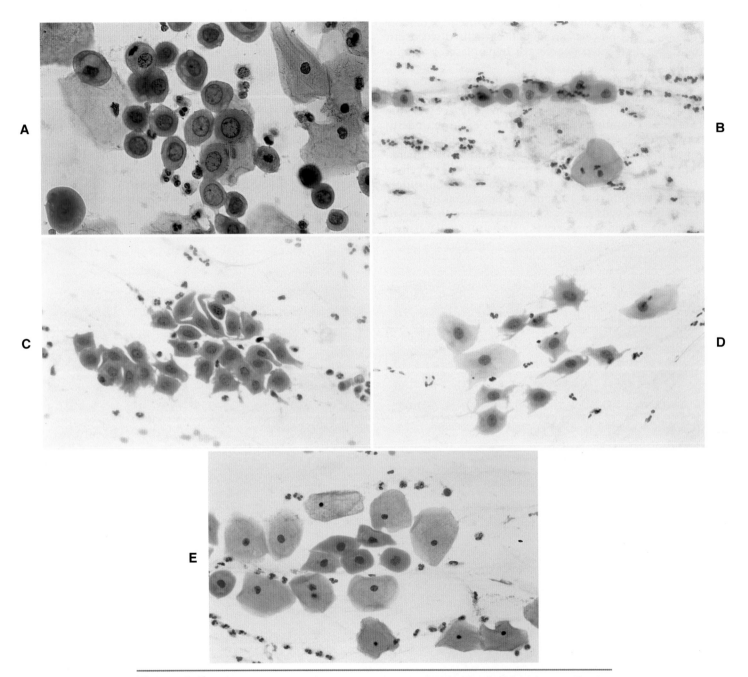

Figure 3-8   **Maturation of immature squamous metaplastic cells. A,** This high-magnification image shows immature squamous metaplastic cells in a background of intermediate and superficial cells. The metaplastic cells have a high nuclear to cytoplasmic (N:C) ratio and nuclei that are larger than those of intermediate cells. However, their chromatin is delicate, and their nuclear membranes are smooth. It is this high N:C ratio that occasionally causes these cells to be mistaken for those of HGSIL. The presence of small cytoplasmic vacuoles probably represents a response of these cells to background inflammation. **B** through **E,** This set of four images shows sequential maturation in immature squamous metaplastic cells. This is characterized by increasing cytoplasmic volume and decreasing N:C ratio. Intermediate and superficial cells are available for comparison with the metaplastic cells in **B** and **E. C,** This image shows the spider appearance of immature metaplastic cells as they are forced away from their basement membrane so that their previous surface attachments appear as cytoplasmic projections. Fully mature squamous metaplastic cells have an appearance indistinguishable from that of normal mature squamous cells. (Pap)

The importance of this process and its cytologic features cannot be overemphasized. When SILs are considered (see Chapter 6), it is noted that various grades of these preneoplastic abnormalities strongly resemble various stages of SM. It is as if development of a metaplastic epithelium is arrested at some stage in the process. Thus, a thorough understanding of the process and its cytology forms the basis for differential diagnostic thinking about SILs and their classification.

This is most important when immature SM is contrasted with HGSILs. For this reason the morphology of immature SM is summarized in Table 3-5. Two features are probably responsible for most of the differential diagnostic difficulties occasioned by this process. The cells of SM are small, as are those of a HGSIL, but their nuclei are slightly larger than those of intermediate cells (50 μm² vs. 35 μm²; see Tables 3-2, 3-3, and 3-5). These features combine to give them the appearance of small cells with scanty cytoplasm, nuclear enlargement, an elevated nucleocytoplasmic ratio, and the near total absence of nucleoli—hence, their resemblance to the cells of HGSIL. However, the cells of SM do not show hyperchromasia or irregularities of nuclear outline. Furthermore, the cells of HGSIL may be accompanied by those of LGSIL. As discussed more fully in Chapter 6, the latter are more readily recognized and their presence can afford considerable diagnostic relief.

Endometrial Cells and Tissue Fragments

Glandular and stromal cells of the endometrium may be either spontaneously shed or directly sampled. In the latter instance, this usually occurs when one of the newer devices designed to improve sampling the upper endocervical canal is employed. In some institutions, direct brushing or aspi-

ration of the endometrium has been used successfully, but these methods are not widely employed.[12-14]

Stromal cells may originate in the superficial endometrium (stratum functionalis) or in the deeper portions of this tissue (stratum basale) (Figure 3-9). Deep stromal cells are

TABLE 3-5		CMF
Cytomorphologic Features of Immature Squamous Metaplasia		
Feature	**Description**	
Cell arrangements	Some sheets	
	Single cells are common	
Cell size	300 to 500 μm²	
Nuclear size	50 μm²	
Nuclear outline	Smoothly round or oval	
N:C ratio (area)	Up to 16%*	
Chromatin	Finely granular	
	No hyperchromasia	
Nucleoli	Usually not present	
Cytoplasm	Dense	
	Cyanophilic	
	Sharp cell borders	
	May show concentric laminations	
	May show pointed projections (spider cells)	

*The high nucleocytoplasmic ratio of immature squamous metaplasia (SM) can cause confusion with the cells of a high grade squamous intraepithelial lesion (SIL). In contrast with the latter, however, the cells of SM lack nuclear hyperchromasia and any irregularities of nuclear contour.

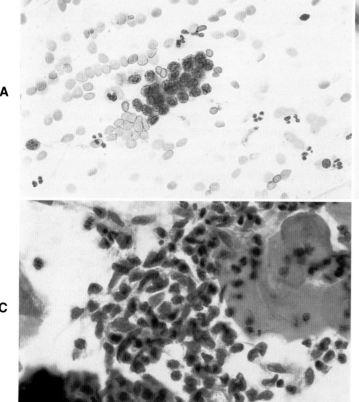

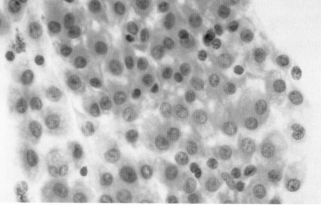

Figure 3-9 Normal endometrial cells. A, This cluster of well-preserved endometrial glandular cells shows small nuclei with stippled chromatin. In this excellent state of preservation, the nuclear features of these cells closely resemble those of intermediate cells. The hyperchromasia, wrinkling, and collapse that are often seen represent the effects of degeneration. **B,** This sheet of histiocyte-like cells represents endometrial stromal cells. Histiocytes lack this ability to form cohesive sheets but show similar vesicular nuclei and pale wispy cytoplasm. **C,** These deep endometrial stromal cells are typically shed on days 6 to 10. They lie in clusters or in loose aggregate and feature hyperchromatic, uniform spindle-shaped nuclei. (Pap)

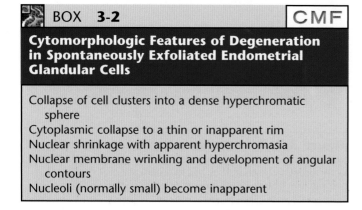

Figure 3-10   Endometrial exodus bodies. **A** and **B,** These two images show exodus bodies typical of endometrial shedding. **A,** The biphasic appearance with large glandular cells on the outside of a cell cluster and smaller stromal cells in the interior is typical. **B,** The tubular gland is associated with large numbers of histiocyte-like endometrial stromal cells. (Pap)

TABLE 3-6			CMF
Cytomorphologic Features of Endometrial Cells			
Cytologic Feature	**Endometrial Glandular Cells**	**Superficial Endometrial Stromal Cells***	**Deep Endometrial Stromal Cells**
Cell shape	Round or oval	Round or oval	Spindled
Cytoplasm	Scanty	Moderate	Scanty
	Cyanophilic	Ill-defined	Cyanophilic
	Variably vacuolated	Often vacuolated	Spindle shaped
Nuclear shape	Round or oval	Round oval or reniform	Spindle shaped, often with horizontal grooves
Nuclear size	40 μm^2	40 to 70 μm^2†	40 μm^2
Nucleoli	Small or absent	Small	Absent
Chromatin	Finely granular	Finely granular	Finely granular or coarse

*Superficial endometrial stromal cells are usually indistinguishable from histiocytes but may show a slightly greater tendency to appear cohesive and form loose sheets.
†The nuclei of superficial endometrial stromal cells enlarge progressively during the second half of the menstrual cycle.

BOX 3-2   CMF

Cytomorphologic Features of Degeneration in Spontaneously Exfoliated Endometrial Glandular Cells

Collapse of cell clusters into a dense hyperchromatic sphere
Cytoplasmic collapse to a thin or inapparent rim
Nuclear shrinkage with apparent hyperchromasia
Nuclear membrane wrinkling and development of angular contours
Nucleoli (normally small) become inapparent

---

typically shed on days 6 through 10 of the menstrual cycle. The cytomorphologic features of endometrial cells are summarized in Table 3-6. Subtle variations occur throughout the menstrual cycle, but these rarely intrude on the recognition and interpretation of endometrial cells.[15] At the time of late-cycle endometrial breakdown, exodus bodies may be nu-

merous and are usually associated with red blood cells (RBCs) and varying degree of acute inflammation. These darkly staining three-dimensional aggregates of small cells have a distinctly laminated appearance. A single layer of slightly larger, less hyperchromatic glandular cells surrounds a dense core of endometrial stromal cells (Figure 3-10).

The cytologic appearance of endometrial glandular cells depends on their state of preservation, as highlighted in Figure 3-9. Their most common presentation is as spontaneously exfoliated spherical cell clusters arriving at a cervical sampling device after varying periods of delay. In this situation, important aspects of their cytology are actually the result of degeneration, as summarized in Box 3-2. This appearance contrasts with that of well-preserved examples in which the nuclei closely resemble those of intermediate squamous cells, with the addition of an occasional small nucleolus.

Extremely well-preserved cells of both stroma and glands can be obtained, often in great quantity, when the lower uterine segment is brushed by various endocervical sampling devices.[16] (Figure 3-11). The most common presenta-

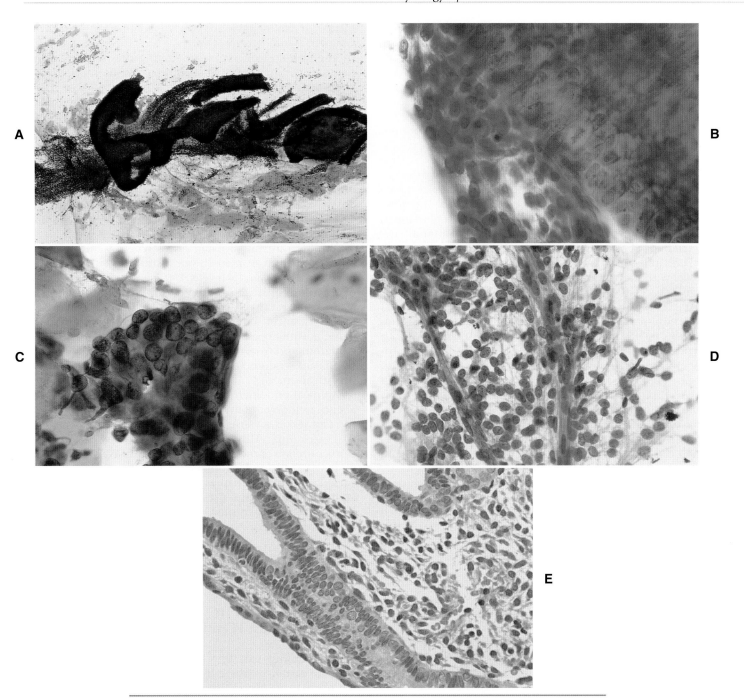

Figure 3-11 **Cytologic presentation of directly sampled endometrial tissue. A,** This low-magnification image shows a complex tissue fragment. Its biphasic nature is apparent as well-defined tubular structures alternate with a more diffuse proliferation of small blue cells. **B,** This high-magnification image shows the intersection of a gland (more eosinophilic) and a fragment of stromal tissue consisting of small basophilic cells. A mitotic figure is clearly visible in the glandular epithelium. This biphasic appearance is diagnostic of directly sampled endometrial tissue. **C,** When fragments of hyperchromatic stromal cells such as those seen in this image are encountered, the temptation to diagnose an HGSIL or an atypical glandular proliferation can be significant. **D,** This loose fragment of stromal tissue consists of small uniform hyperchromatic cells. However, it is interrupted by the presence of several easily recognized capillary-size blood vessels. The small blue cells of an in situ squamous or glandular carcinoma would represent an epithelium and hence, by definition, would not include blood vessels. **E,** This fragment of histologically obtained endometrium from the same patient whose smear was illustrated in images **A** to **D** recapitulates the cytologic features well. Here, tubular glands are set in a small blue cell stroma. The latter is interrupted by small capillaries. (**A-D,** Pap; **E,** H&E)

tion is as cohesive tissue fragments that are often larger than those usually encountered on Pap tests. The glands appear as long tubular structures composed of tightly packed, small uniform cells. These glands have very smooth borders and are sharply delineated from their surroundings. The stroma consists of even smaller hyperchromatic cells densely packed around the glands. Mitotic figures can occasionally be identified in either compartment. One interesting feature of the stroma is the common presence of easily identified capillaries.

When both glandular and stromal components are present, recognition of directly sampled endometrial tissue is usually straightforward. The similarity in the low-magnification biphasic appearance of endometrial tissue to that of phyllodes tumors of the breast as the latter are depicted by FNA and can be striking.

Difficulties may arise when fragments of stromal tissue occur without associated glands. These particles show tightly packed, small hyperchromatic cells that can be mistaken for an atypical glandular lesion (see Chapter 8) or HGSIL (see Chapter 6). The previously mentioned capillaries can be helpful in this differential diagnosis. Both atypical glandular lesions and HGSIL are exclusively intraepithelial processes. Because epithelia by definition do not contain blood vessels, their presence within the small blue cell proliferation effectively excludes these diagnoses from consideration. Thus, if a more ominous interpretation for these capillary-containing tissue fragments is entertained, the possibilities include neoplasms such as small cell carcinoma, endometrial stroma neoplasms, and adenoid cystic carcinoma. These differential diagnostic considerations are explored more fully in subsequent chapters.

Spontaneous shedding of endometrial cells is expected in each of the clinical situations listed in Box 3-3.[17-19] At this point, it is important to note that morphologically normal cells are being considered. Cells with atypia or cytologic ev-

idence of malignancy are considered in greater detail in Chapters 8 and 9, respectively.

The primary concern is identifying the minority of patients in whom abnormal shedding may be the herald of endometrial hyperplasia or adenocarcinoma. These conditions are quite uncommon before the age of 40, after which their prevalence rises with the passage of time. Thus, the patient's age affects the degree of concern aroused by the presence of endometrial cells in the second half of the menstrual cycle or after menopause. This is reflected in the Bethesda System 2001, which recommends reporting the presence of endometrial cells in patients age 40 or older. In postmenopausal women lacking the clinical conditions listed in Box 3-3, histologic investigation of the endometrium is usually warranted.

A more difficult problem arises when a smear from a postmenopausal woman shows histiocytes in the absence of endometrial glandular cells.[20,21] The ultimate significance of this finding is not entirely clear, but Nguyen and colleagues suggest that it is not a useful way of identifying the at-risk patients.[21] Interestingly, they note that, in a symptomatic postmenopausal woman, identification of histiocytes containing phagocytosed acute inflammatory cells suggests significant endometrial pathology and warrants further investigation.

Atypical endometrial cells may raise the possibility of adenocarcinoma. Many of these alterations are subtle, and the Pap test is an insensitive means of detecting endometrial carcinoma. (This fact is not clear to many patients who think of *cancer of the uterus* as a single disease.) Atypical endometrial cells and endometrial adenocarcinoma are discussed in detail in Chapters 8 and 9. Potentially significant atypia in endometrial glandular cells features cellular enlargement, increased nucleolar prominence, and irregularities of nuclear contour not associated with other features of degeneration. In contrast with the hyperchromasia of degeneration, the nuclei of many well-differentiated adenocarcinomas show pale staining.

 PHYSIOLOGIC ALTERATIONS RELATED TO PREGNANCY

Pap test findings can show alterations related to pregnancy. In some instances, these may be the harbinger of impending pregnancy loss. In others, they are sufficiently atypical to raise the possibility of malignancy.

Trophoblastic Cells

These placenta-derived cells may be of either the cytotrophoblastic or syncytiotrophoblastic (giant cell) type. Generally associated with pregnancy, trophoblastic cells can be seen for up to several months postpartum and are rarely associated with trophoblastic neoplasia in a nonpregnant woman. When encountered during pregnancy, they often signify that the patient is in danger of pregnancy loss, and their identification should instigate immediate notification of the clinical team.

Given the correct clinical situation, trophoblastic giant cells are readily recognized and rarely present diagnostic difficulties. Their closest mimics are the histiocytic giant

---

BOX   3-3

Spontaneous Exfoliation of Morphologically Normal Endometrial Cells

Clinical situations in which spontaneous exfoliation of morphologically normal endometrial cells may be expected are as follows:
- Second half of the menstrual cycle
- After giving birth
- After an abortion of any nature
- Dysfunctional uterine bleeding
- Endometriosis
- Endometritis
- Endometrial metaplasia of the cervix
- Endometrial polyps
- Use of an intrauterine device
- After endometrial inflammation
- Use of oral contraceptive agents
- Submucosal leiomyoma
- Endometrial hyperplasia or carcinoma

cells seen almost exclusively in postmenopausal patients and those who have received radiation therapy for a pelvic malignancy. These cell types are contrasted in Table 3-7.

Cells of the cytotrophoblast are smaller and more readily mistaken for SIL or squamous cell carcinoma. The cytologic features of these cells are summarized in Table 3-8.[22] Trophoblastic cells are illustrated in Figure 3-12.

Endocervical Decidual Change

Subepithelial stromal decidual change occurs in the endocervix in nearly one third of gravid uteri, and can be reflected in a Pap test from up to one third of those.[23] Cytologic features of these cells are summarized in Table 3-9. Based on these features, Schneider and Barnes suggested that the differential diagnosis may include reactive cellular changes (RCCs) (repair), SILs, and endocervical adenocarcinoma.[23] Subjectively, decidual cells are reminiscent of apocrine cells as seen in FNAs of the breast or nipple discharge material (Figure 3-13). Decidual change can persist after pregnancy and can be mimicked by alterations associated with oral contraceptive agents.

Hemosiderin and Hematoidin

The appearance of hemosiderin in cytologic preparations is described in detail during our consideration of diffuse pulmonary disorders (see Chapter 15). A wide variety of conditions can lead to hemorrhage, but most examples of both hematoidin cockleburrs and macrophages with cytoplasmic hemosiderin and are encountered in samples taken during the postpartum period[24,25] (Figure 3-14).

Arias-Stella Reaction

Classically described in the endometrium, the Arias-Stella reaction can occur in the cervix during pregnancy and is rarely associated with ectopic implantation in the cervix.[26,27] In the experience of Benoit and Kini, follow-up of 11 cases showed that this change resolves promptly after

---

TABLE 3-7

Comparison of Multinucleated Histiocytic Giant Cells with Syncytiotrophoblastic Giant Cells

Feature	Histiocytic Giant Cell	Trophoblastic Giant Cell
Clinical associations	Postmenopausal patient History of radiation therapy	Pregnancy Postpartum Threatened abortion Completed abortion Trophoblastic neoplasia
Relative size	Smaller	Larger
Cell shape	Round or oval	"Hand mirror"
Cytoplasmic features	Vacuolated Cyanophilic Ill-defined borders	Dense Cyanophilic or eosinophilic Sharp borders, often with a rim of condensation
Relative number of nuclei	Fewer	More
Nuclear features	50 μm^2 All identical Fine chromatin	50 μm^2 All identical Chromatin may be coarse

---

TABLE 3-8 — CMF

Cytomorphologic Features of Cytotrophoblastic Cells

Feature	Description
Cell arrangements	Single cells or small syncytial groups
Cytoplasmic features	Variable volume but may be scanty Small vacuoles are common
Nuclear features	One, two, or several nuclei per cell Finely granular chromatin Regular chromatin distribution Prominent nucleolus

---

TABLE 3-9 — CMF

Cytomorphologic Features of Decidual Cells

Feature	Description
Cell arrangements	Most cells in small clusters
Cytoplasm	Cyanophilic
Nuclear features	31 to 320 μm^{2*} (mean = 111) Finely granular chromatin May be multiple
Nucleolus	Prominent

*Data from Schneider V, Barnes LA. Ectopic decidual reaction of the uterine cervix: frequency and cytologic presentation. Acta Cytol 1981; 25:616-622.

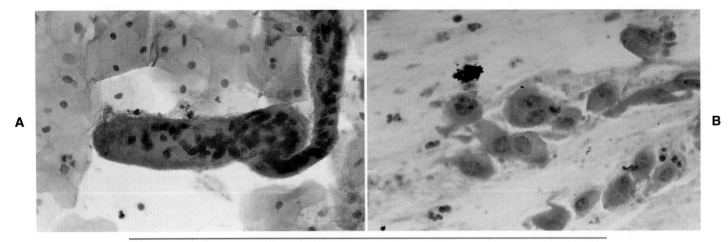

Figure 3-12 **Trophoblastic cells. A** and **B,** These images depict syncytial trophoblastic and cytotrophoblastic cells, respectively. The hand mirror shape and zonated cytoplasmic staining of the syncytial trophoblastic cell are characteristic. (Pap)

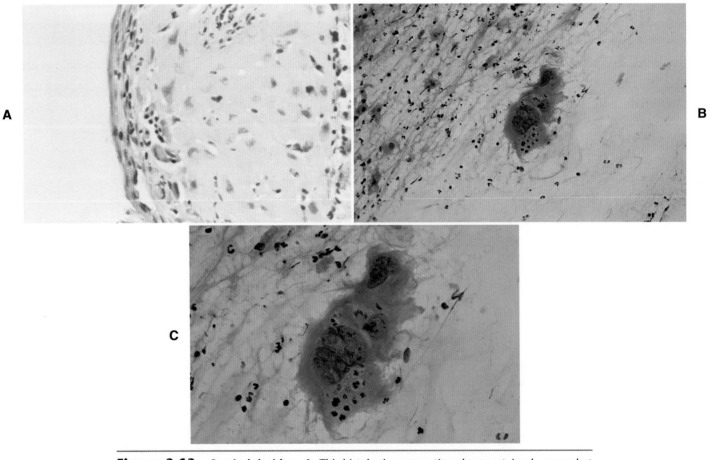

Figure 3-13 **Cervical decidua. A,** This histologic preparation shows retained, somewhat hyalinized decidua beneath an intact squamous mucosa. The decidual cells are large with pale-staining nuclei and abundant, lightly eosinophilic cytoplasm. **B** and **C,** The histologic features of decidual cells are recapitulated in its cytologic presentation. Although the cells are large with enlarged nuclei, they feature a low N:C ratio and evenly distributed chromatin. Nucleoli can be seen. (**A,** H&E; **B&C,** Pap)

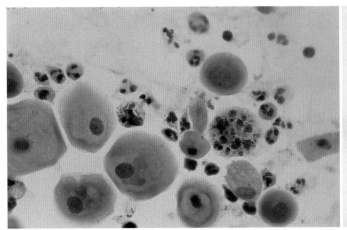

A

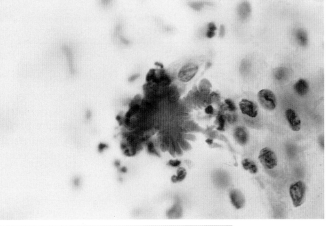

B

Figure 3-14　Hemosiderin and hematoidin. **A,** This smear from a postpartum patient shows a background of immature squamous cells and a few neutrophils. Also present is a macrophage with abundant, green-staining cytoplasmic hemosiderin pigment. **B,** This image also represents smear material from a postpartum patient. This complex branching eosinophilic structure represents a hematoidin cockleburr. Occasionally, some individuals mistake these for evidence of an infectious process. (Pap)

TABLE 3-10	
Arias-Stella Reaction in Endocervical Glandular Cells	
Feature	**Description**
Cell size	Enlarged vs. normal glandular cells
Cytoplasm	Vacuolated
Nucleocytoplasmic ratio	High
Nuclear features	Round to oval shape
	Rounded cytoplasmic pseudoinclusions
	Chromatin may appear degenerated

BOX 3-4

Guidelines for Specimen Collection and Suitability for Hormonal Assessment

Specimen collection guidelines
Smear taken from the lateral vaginal wall
Smear taken from the junction of the middle and upper one third of the vagina

Factors that make a smear unsuitable for hormonal assessment
Material not collected properly
Adequate clinical information not provided (age, menstrual status, obstetric condition, medications)
Inflammation
Evidence of an infection
Air-drying artifact

conclusion of the pregnancy.[26] The cytologic findings are summarized in Table 3-10.

 HORMONAL CYTOLOGY

The epithelia of the female genital tract are sensitive to estrogen, progesterone, androgens, and various additional steroid hormone derivatives and metabolites. The interactions among these molecules and an individual patient's cells are complex so that limited information about hormonal status can be obtained by examination of the cell sample. In general, estrogen promotes, and progesterone inhibits squamous cell maturation.

Guidelines for specimen collection and suitability for hormonal assessment are summarized in Box 3-4. In particular, it should be noted that collection from the cervix with targeting of the transformation zone is not suitable for hormonal assessment. Indeed, on this basis alone, many requests for hormonal evaluations of gynecologic specimens should not be honored.

Table 3-11 offers a generalized summary of smear patterns at various stages of life. One pattern of particular importance is that of intermediate cell predominance. Regardless of its cause, this pattern is the one most often associated with a shift in vaginal flora to coccobacilli and with cytolysis. These are more fully discussed when RCCs are considered in Chapter 4. The several clinical states with which this pattern may be associated are listed in Box 3-5. Another important picture is that of atrophy (Figure 3-15). Small squamous cells in dense clusters can closely mimic HGSIL, as discussed in Chapter 6. This problem can be particularly severe, if air-drying artifact is present, as is often the case in smears from postmenopausal patients. Also important in this regard are small, round, densely staining mucin droplets called *blue blobs*. These must be distinguished from the hyperchromatic nuclei of a HGSIL or even a squamous cell carcinoma.

TABLE 3-11

Hormonal Patterns at Different Stages of Life

Life Stage	Hormonal Pattern
Newborn	Sterile
	No inflammation
	Intermediate cells ± superficial cells
First 2 weeks of life	Acquire bacteria
	Neutrophils appear
	Atrophic cells
Childhood	Maturation and cyclic alterations occur months or years before menarche, due to cycles that are initially anovulatory.
Cycling woman, proliferative phase	Increasing squamous cell maturation
Cycling woman, postovulatory phase	Decreasing squamous cell maturation
Pregnancy	Resembles postovulatory pattern*
	Navicular cells may be numerous
Postpartum	Atrophy
Lactation	Atrophy persists but some maturation may appear slowly
Menopause	Atrophy or intermediate cell predominant pattern

*The appearance of parabasal cells suggests loss of hormonal support from either the corpus luteum or the placenta and may indicate intrauterine fetal demise, or impending loss of the pregnancy.

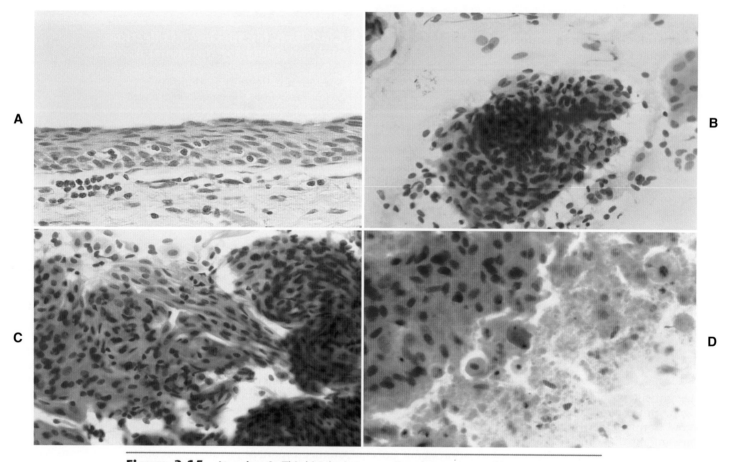

Figure 3-15 **Atrophy. A,** This histologic preparation shows an atrophic squamous epithelium. This covering is thin, consisting of only a few layers and lacks the complex progression of cell types illustrated in Figure 3-1. A distinct tendency toward spindling is seen near the surface. **B** and **C,** These Pap-stained tests from postmenopausal patients show clusters of atrophic squamous cells. **C,** Spindling similar to that noted in **A** is prominent. These immature cells are small with densely packed hyperchromatic nuclei and scanty cytoplasm. This can give rise to difficulties in recognizing an HGSIL in the background of atrophy. **D,** This high-power image from an atrophic smear shows darkly staining oval objects that are desiccated cervical mucus known as *blue blobs*. These have neither accompanying cytoplasm nor internal substructures suggestive of chromatin particles. Thus, these blue blobs should not be mistaken for the nuclei of dysplastic or malignant cells. (**A,** H&E; **B&C,** Pap)

BOX 3-5

Clinical States Associated with a Predominance of Intermediate Cells

Secondary amenorrhea
Castration
Secretory phase of the menstrual cycle
Pregnancy
Premenarche
Menopause
Long-term administration of exogenous estrogens

TABLE 3-12

Indices Used for Hormonal Assessment

Type of Index	Cell Type Ratio Compared
Maturation index*	Parabasal: intermediate: superficial (PIS)
Karyopyknotic index	Superficial: intermediate
Eosinophilic index	Eosinophilic: cyanophilic
Folded cell index	Folded cytoplasm: nonfolded cytoplasm
Crowded cell Index	Clusters of more than four cells: single cells

*The maturation index is the most commonly requested study.

Hormonal assessments are based on one or more indices generated by differential enumeration of various types of cells reflective of different maturational levels (parabasal, intermediate, and superficial cells). A count of 300 squamous cells is usually undertaken. The indices used are summarized in Table 3-12. In general, shifts from an estrogen-rich environment to one dominated by progesterone, such as that which occurs with each normal ovulation, induce squamous cells with greater cyanophilia, crowding within groups, and folding of cytoplasmic edges. As noted previously, these samples are more likely to show altered vaginal flora and cytolysis. The indices convey virtually nothing that is clinically useful in the vast majority of patients.

No single determination can reveal the onset of important events such as ovulation or conception, and even serial determinations are of limited value. Furthermore, hormonal cytology cannot be used to determine the point a woman has reached in her menstrual cycle.

The interactions in this physiologic system are so complex that only the most extreme morphologic patterns can be related to hormonal status. In particular, the concept that there exists some constellation of cellular findings that can be related in a stoichiometric fashion to estrogen levels is without foundation. In other words, an *estrogenic index* does not exist, since no set of cytologic findings varies dependably with estrogen levels. The idea that a woman's health can be optimized with administration of exogenous hormones guided by some type of cytologic hormone assessment now seems antiquated at best. The physician who has a standing order for hormonal assessment (usually a maturation index) on all or most Pap tests betrays considerable ignorance of this test. In current report terminology, hormonal assessments should be limited to a simple statement that the pattern is or is not consistent with the patient's age and history.

Hormonal assessments are based on squamous cell patterns. However, in some cases, endocervical cells also undergo atrophy (see Figure 3-4). This leaves the cells much smaller than previously described, with small, dark nuclei and scanty cytoplasm. In the most extreme examples, endocervical cells come to resemble endometrial cells. The practical implications of this observation for postmenopausal woman are obvious.

The hormonal pattern seen in patients using the long-term injectable contraceptive depot-medroxyprogesterone acetate is shifted markedly toward atrophy. Preliminary work suggests that these Pap tests are often obtained from individuals already at risk for SILs. Diagnostic difficulty occurs when small cells with high N:C ratios and some degree of nuclear hyperchromasia mimic a HGSIL.[28,29] It appears that false diagnoses of HGSIL and an increased rate of ASC diagnoses may occur in laboratories serving these patients. The magnitude of this problem and its possible solutions remain to be more fully explored.

Postmenopausal breast cancer patients being treated with tamoxifen show increased squamous cell maturation.[30] This finding is related to the fact that although tamoxifen is used as an antiestrogenic agent in these women, it also possesses some agonist activity. The degree to which the increased incidence of cervical polyps, endometrial polyps, and some gynecologic malignancies will ultimately alter gynecologic cytology is not yet clear.

Finally, smear patterns have been described in a large number of endocrinopathies. However, given the wide array of genetic, biochemical, and molecular evaluations now available, the importance of these observations is almost exclusively historical.

CYTOLOGY IN SEXUAL ASSAULT

Pap test cytology has been used in the evaluation of alleged sexual assault.[31,32] Traditionally, the process involves identification of spermatozoa on a smear. Costa and colleagues described a large series of such cases and found spermatozoa on 56% of smears from patients examined within 3 days of the alleged assault. They also indicated success in identifying cases missed by chemical means of semen detection.

As sperm degenerate, they lose the characteristic flagellum and appear as tiny oval- or teardrop-shaped structures. Thus, one is usually screening for the presence of sperm heads. These tiny oval or pointed structures are biphasic with lighter and darker poles. They can be present in low numbers and can be easily obscured by inflammatory cells. Specimen contamination and artifacts are relatively common; many individuals taking such samples work in the emergency department settings and may not be accustomed or even adequately trained in obtaining Pap test samples. Thus, this type of smear examination can be tedious.

The major cause of false-positive interpretations is misidentification of isolated nuclear lobes from degenerated neutrophils. These are the correct size for sperm heads but tend to be more uniformly round, rather than oval or teardrop shaped. Nuclear lobes have either coarse, "blocky" chromatin or when degenerated fully are uniformly pyknotic without chromatin details. Sperm heads are split into light and dark ends, with the latter corresponding to the acrosomal cap. This distinct biphasic appearance is not recapitulated by nuclear lobes.

Rao and colleagues used fluorescence in situ hybridization to identify Y chromosome–containing squamous cells on postcoital Pap tests. This method detected these cells on all cases with a coital history and was useful up to 3 weeks after coition. In contrast, cytologic detection of sperm was positive in only 41% of samples and never with a postcoital interval of greater than 2 weeks. The authors noted that this highly sensitive method can be applied to routine Pap tests, without the need for additional samples.

Regardless of the methodology employed, all clerical and laboratory personnel who participate in receiving, accessing, preparing, examining, or reporting these evaluations must be familiar with the requirements for integrity of a legal chain of custody. Failure to meet the necessary requirements at all stages or to provide adequate documentation negates the value of the sample and the test results in any evidentiary proceeding. Finally, those involved in this type of work must understand that some potential exists for receiving a subpoena for either a deposition or a court proceeding.

TRANSITIONAL CELL METAPLASIA OF THE UTERINE CERVIX

Transitional cell metaplasia (TCM) affects perimenopausal and postmenopausal women, and in studies of its histology, it is usually an incidental finding in resected or biopsied material.[33] It has been identified in hysterectomy material, curettings of the endometrium or endocervix, cervical biopsies, cervical conizations, and vaginal biopsies. TCM can occupy the surface, line endocervical glands, or rarely appear as isolated nests surrounded by cervical stroma.

Diagnostic difficulties may arise as TCM shows multiple layers of extremely small uniform cells that show little variation from one to another and essentially no maturation. Weir and Bell have contrasted TCM, HGSIL, atrophy, and tubal metaplasia.[34]

PAP TEST REPORT TERMINOLOGY: BETHESDA SYSTEM 2001

At this writing, the Bethesda System 2001 is the preferred diagnostic language for Pap test reporting in the United States. Other schemes have evolved in response to the different medical, cultural, and financial pressures operative in other locations.[35] It is unlikely that a universally acceptable terminology will be developed in the foreseeable future. The Bethesda System 2001 terminology is outlined in Box 3-6. Although many of the listed diagnoses are discussed in subsequent chapters, an overview of Pap test terminology is needed.

Chapter 6 explains the preparation-dependent variations in the cytologic appearance of cells representing SILs. The first entry in a the Bethesda System report is an indication of the type of preparation under review. Currently, these are classified as conventional material (smear) or as a liquid-based preparation (LBP). This forward-looking terminology allows for other specimen types that may be developed in the future.

In the most recent adjustment of the Bethesda System, *specimen adequacy* is defined as either satisfactory or unsatisfactory. Previous terms, including *less than satisfactory* and its successor *satisfactory but limited by,* have been eliminated in what seems to some a progressive limiting of laboratories' ability to call attention to the potential importance of diagnostic difficulties occasioned by technical problems. Specifying the presence or absence of an endocervical or transformation zone component is required. Problems such as obscuring blood, scant squamous cellularity, or excessive inflammation can be described in narrative appended to the specimen adequacy section of the report. However, technical problems occasionally increase diagnostic difficulty to the point that uncertainty exists in the pathologist's mind. Believing that it is unsafe to report such a Pap test as unsatisfactory, which precludes giving a diagnosis of any type, strict Bethesda System terminology forces a pathologist to declare the test satisfactory when it is less than satisfactory. (One's feeling of the inevitability of this phase might explain its existence in a former version of the Bethesda System.) The Bethesda System insistence that any Pap test with abnormal cells must be satisfactory seems oversimplified. It remains to be seen whether interpretations that may be compromised by technical factors will result in heightened medicolegal exposure, when the designation *satisfactory for evaluation* overshadows narrative verbiage. The current terminology seems superior to *satisfactory but limited by* which can be confusing. However, it is less clear and seems to offer the laboratory less protection than the original term *less than satisfactory.*

As discussed in Chapter 6, most SILs arise in the transformation zone. This is a circumferential zone in the endocervical canal in which the columnar epithelium can be reversibly converted to squamous epithelium by the process of SM. It is essential that this area be sampled to minimize the risk of a false-negative result from sampling. Thus, minimal acceptable evidence of sampling is identification of at least 10 endocervical cells or squamous metaplastic cells. Degenerated cells in mucus are likely to have been previously exfoliated, rather than directly sampled, and should not be considered adequate evidence of transformation zone sampling. In a hormonal setting that leads to atrophy (postmenopause, postpartum, or administration of progestational agents), it can be impossible to distinguish parabasal cells from squamous metaplastic cells so that it may be impossible to be sure that the transformation zone has been sampled. The laboratory can elect to describe this difficulty in the report.

As intuitively important as transformation zone sampling appears, its impact on actual SIL screening results is sometimes not great.[36-44] Pap tests with endocervical cells are more likely to show SIL cells, but women whose smears lack such cells do not show more SILs on follow-up. This suggests that even when this specimen adequacy indicator is not met, few false-negative Pap tests are detected by patient follow-up.

After applying minimal cellularity criteria, obscuring factors (blood or inflammatory cells) or air-drying may be evident. Many of these issues are encountered much less often with LBPs than with conventional smears. This is particularly true of air-drying artifact. Those who continue to work with conventional smears will wish to describe air-drying because it can sometimes place severe limitations on one's diagnostic certainty. Preliminary evidence suggests that slides that are only partially obscured (currently a narrative description under the term *satisfactory for diagnosis*) result in little increased risk of false-negative results.[42,43]

Unsatisfactory Pap tests are important because they leave the patient unscreened and can be associated with higher rates of SIL on follow-up than satisfactory samples. This may be because some of the factors that lead to an unsatisfactory Pap test are associated with high-risk behaviors as indicated by a Pap test with blood, severe inflammation, or evidence of sexually transmitted diseases.

The laboratory has sole responsibility for declaring a Pap test preparation to be unsatisfactory. The first reason for doing so is when the smear is unsuitable for examination because of inadequate identifying information or because it is received as a broken slide or as a leaking LBP container. In such cases, the sample is rejected *a priori* and never examined microscopically. The second reason is that after complete specimen processing and examination it is found unsuitable for evaluation for any epithelial abnormality. The latter can be the result of sparse cellularity, severe obscuring factors (inflammation or blood), and air-drying artifact.

Information reported in such cases can be a valuable source of education and quality improvement for the referring clinician or clinic. An unsatisfactory Pap test requires the most careful microscopic evaluation before it is concluded that no diagnosis is possible. Such tests can be time consuming.

Current Bethesda System criteria for an adequate number of squamous cells differ between a conventional smear and a LBP. A conventional smear should have between 8000 and 12,000 well-preserved and well-visualized squamous cells. This is an estimated minimal cell count range and does not suppose that any laboratory actually counts cells. Other types of cells and squamous cells that are obscured from view are not included in this tally. Even estimating cell numbers can be difficult if significant cell crowding or damage (cytolysis) occurs.

As the means to determine the number of squamous cells on a conventional Pap test slide is considered, it is important to note that most slides are obviously adequate and the issue of cell number estimation will not arise. However, a semiquantitative estimate of a slide's squamous cell number is recommended by the Bethesda System 2001 for those cases with a low or borderline squamous component. Be-

---

BOX 3-6

Bethesda System 2001 Diagnostic Terminology for Pap Tests

Specimen type
  Conventional smear
  Liquid-based preparation
  Other
Specimen adequacy
  Satisfactory for evaluation
  Unsatisfactory for evaluation
General categorization (optional)
  Negative for intraepithelial lesion
  Epithelial cell abnormality
Automated review
Ancillary testing
Interpretation/result
  Negative for intraepithelial lesion or malignancy
    Organisms
      Trichomonas vaginalis
      Fungal organisms morphologically consistent with
        Candida spp.
      Shift in bacterial flora suggestive of bacterial
        vaginosis
      Bacteria morphologically consistent with
        Actinomyces spp.
      Cellular changes consistent with herpes simplex
        virus
    Other nonneoplastic findings
      Reactive cellular changes associated with inflammation (includes typical repair)
      Radiation
      Intrauterine contraceptive device
      Glandular cells status post hysterectomy
      Atrophy
Other
  Endometrial cells in a woman ≥40 years of age

Epithelial cell abnormality
  Squamous cell
    Atypical squamous cells
      Of undetermined significance (ASC-US)
      Cannot exclude high-grade squamous intraepithelial lesion (ASC–H)
    Low-grade squamous intraepithelial lesion
      encompassing:
      Human papillomavirus cytopathic effect
      Mild dysplasia
      CIN 1
    High-grade squamous intraepithelial lesion
      encompassing:
      Moderate dysplasia/CIN 2
      Severe dysplasia/CIN 3/<15
  Invasive squamous cell carcinoma
  Glandular cell
    Atypical
      Endocervical cells
      Endometrial cells
      Glandular cells not otherwise specified
    Atypical
      Endocervical cells, favor neoplastic
      Endometrial cells, favor neoplastic
    Endocervical adenocarcinoma in situ
    Adenocarcinoma
      Endocervical
      Endometrial
      Extrauterine
      Not otherwise specified
  Other malignant neoplasm
Educational notes and suggestions

CIN, Carcinoma in situ; *CIS,* squamous cell carcinoma in situ.

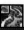 BOX 3-7

Inherent Smear Factors that Might Affect Apparent Cell Number on a Conventional Pap Test Smear

Relative cell crowding or cell dispersement
Cell (cytoplasmic) preservation
    Normal
    Cytolysis
Cell size
    Atrophic cytology
        Postmenopausal
        Postpartum
        Administration of progestational agents
    Cytology with prominent estrogen effect
Intervening elements in the visual field
    Mucus
    Endocervical cells
    Inflammatory cells

 BOX 3-8

Issues to Be Considered in Estimating Conventional Pap Test Squamous Cellularity by Comparison of Microscopic Fields with Standard Reference Images

Preparation of the images
It is probably not difficult.
Various magnifications may be required.
Cell number in a static image can be determined with great accuracy.
Even at a single magnification, a set of images is required to account for various field areas visualized with different manufacturers' optics.
Different image sets may be required to adjust for the inherent smear characteristics outlined in Box 3-7.
The agency responsible for standardization and field testing of reference images has not been determined.

Selection of images by the cytologist
What magnification is optimum?
Does the optimum magnification change based on either the factors in Box 3-6 or on a specific set of microscope optics?
Has the cytologist selected images that are matched to the optical characteristics of his or her individual microscope?
Unless all microscopes in the laboratory have identical optics, different cytologists may need to use different reference images.
It may be necessary to use several different images for a single smear.

Application of images in the field
Is 8000 to 12,000 estimated cells the best number?*
How accurate and reproducible are determinations of squamous cellularity based on reference images?†
If ×40 (final magnification) images are deemed useful, what fraction of screening cytotechnologists have ready access to ×4 objectives?
Does implementation of reference image methodology have any meaningful impact on the time that should be allotted to screen a slide to which it must be applied? How will this be documented and incorporated into management of workloads?
Does implementation of reference image methodology have different implications for laboratories with high rates of squamous intraepithelial lesions (SIL) and significant inflammation vs. those that evaluate specimens from mostly low-risk women with rare SILs and little inflammation?

*Outcome evaluation, efficiency of SIL detection, and false-negative fractions will need to be evaluated, as a function of this new approach to specimen adequacy determination.
†This question might be rigorously addressed by applying image analysis methods to smears.

cause the primary purpose of the Pap test is identification of squamous lesions, this effort is directed to these cells. Previous considerations regarding transformation zone sampling are not altered by this discussion. Furthermore, the presence of mucus and endocervical cells in any amount or number does nothing to ameliorate the sampling error represented by scant squamous cellularity. The estimated cell number supersedes previous Bethesda System recommendations that described acceptable smear cellularity in terms of the fraction of a slide's area occupied by squamous cells.[45-48] It is important to note that cell-by-cell counting has not been recommended, indicating that the cell number is to be estimated.

The method for estimated cell counting has not been fully developed at this writing. Some inherent smear characteristics might be expected to contribute to variations in apparent cell number (Box 3-7). Given these confounding visual factors, the difficulty and subjectivism involved in cell number estimation becomes clear. The proposed solution is comparison of the slide in question with reference images derived from smears showing various well-quantified levels of squamous cellularity.

At this writing, such images are not yet widely available and questions remain about their application (Box 3-8). It seems logical to expect that, when looking at a number of fields on a conventional smear with questionable cellularity, these fields are likely to differ considerably from one another. Thus, the cytologist may be in the position of testing several fields, perhaps against a number of different reference images and then mentally calculating a quasi-arithmetic sum of several subjective assessments. Based on the issues summarized in Boxes 3-7 and 3-8 and assuming that this method is accepted by the profession, the decisions used to select the correct template(s) for a given slide are summarized in Box 3-9. The reproducibility of this method remains to be investigated.

A similar semiquantitative approach is recommended for LBPs. Based in part on complete randomization of all cells in the liquid-filled test vial, a lower number of squamous cells is deemed adequate. An LBP slide should show a minimum of 5000 well-preserved, well-visualized squamous cells. Counts are based on 10 or more microscopic fields distributed along any diameters (lines that pass through the center of the preparation and extend to both edges).

Decisions that Might Be Used to Select a Reference Image for Evaluation of Squamous Cellularity on a Conventional Pap Test Smear*

Relative cell crowding
Cell preservation (normal vs. cytolysis)
Cell size (mature vs. atrophic)
Intervening materials (mucus or other cell types)
Select appropriate image for the desired magnification
Select appropriate image for a specific microscope's optics
Is more than one image required, based on field-to-field variability within the Pap test under evaluation?

*See Boxes 3-7 and 3-8.

In some instances, apparently inadequate cellularity is the result of technical or processing errors. To evaluate this possibility, the specimen vial can be retrieved and a second slide can be prepared. Even when additional slides are made, an adequate sample must show at least 5000 cells on a single slide; the cellularity of two or more preparations cannot be added to achieve this number. These determinations can be affected by same inherent cytologic factors described for conventional Pap tests (see Box 3-7). Evaluation of 10 or more fields represents a sample thought to predict the total number of cells present. It does not represent an evaluation of the entire slide.

When attempts are made to describe quantitatively the number of cells in a microscopic field, it is necessary to control for variations in field sizes among different microscopes. This, in turn, is a function of a given microscope's optical characteristics. The overall calculation of the average minimum number of cells required per microscopic field to predict a total of at least 5000 cells is as follows:

$$\text{Total cells required} = 5000$$
$$\text{Fields to be counted} \geq 10$$

The microscope field diameter in millimeters is determined by its inherent optical characteristics and calculated as follows:

$$\text{Field diameter} = \frac{\text{Eyepiece field number}}{\text{Objective magnification}}$$

These data are recorded by the microscope manufacturer on the eyepiece and objective, respectively. The area of this microscopic field can then be calculated as the area or any circle: $\pi(FD/2)^2$. Thus, the field diameter for a $\times 10$ objective viewed through eyepieces with a field number of 22 is as follows:

$$\frac{22}{10} = 2.2 \text{ mm}$$

and the area of the preparation encompassed by this single microscopic field is as follows:

$$\pi\left(\frac{2.2}{2}\right)^2 = 3.8 \text{ mm}^2$$

Given a 20-mm preparation diameter, the area of the slide occupied by the sample is as follows:

$$\pi\left(\frac{20}{2}\right)^2 = 314 \text{ mm}^2$$

and the total number of microscopic fields in the preparation using optics configured as above is as follows:

$$\frac{314}{3.8} = 83 \text{ Fields}$$

Because the field is circular, the number of completely nonoverlapping fields is something less than indicated by this simple calculation. The minimum average number of cells per microscopic field required to predict a total of 5000 is as follows:

$$\frac{5000}{83} = 60 \text{ Cells}$$

Thus, to achieve minimum adequate squamous cellularity, 10 or more individual fields along any diameters must each contain an average minimum of 60 cells. At this magnification, one diameter of a 20-mm slide preparation has a maximum of nine complete fields, as calculated by the following equation:

$$\frac{20\text{-mm Preparation}}{2.2\text{-mm Field diameter}} = 9.01 \text{ Fields per diameter}$$

Using this method, a preparation diameter of 13 mm encompasses a maximum of five complete fields. Thus, in any assessment it is necessary to examine fields along more than one diameter.

Using a given set of optics and a single type of preparation, calculations of this type can be easily tabulated for quick reference (Tables 3-13 and 3-14). Although a feeling of comfort in quantitation might accompany all this arithmetic, considerable subjectivism remains when this method is actually applied to a given LBP. This is especially true because only a small fraction of these cases require such an analysis, and many individuals may remain somewhat unpracticed in its application. Perhaps a system of reference images ultimately will be adopted in a manner similar to that discussed previously for conventional Pap tests. It is likely that field-to-field variability does not play the vexing role in LBP that it might for some conventional smears.

Statistical sampling issues not yet addressed may arise and require careful evaluation. For example, a cell number estimation based on 10 (or more) microscopic fields in an arrangement with 1600 available fields and a requirement of three or more cells per field may be very different from one requiring 143 or more cells in a preparation with 35 fields (see Tables 3-13 and 3-14). Studies designed to identify the most statistically robust but practical combinations of preparation type, microscope optics, and required number of counted fields should be undertaken. It is likely that a restricted range of statistically defensible but reasonable combinations will emerge.

As automation in cytology proceeds, it is quite possible that cell counting algorithms of this or some other type will be incorporated and that reliable data will be generated. For now, this method retains a degree of subjectivism.

The next section of the Bethesda System 2001 report is the general categorization of a Pap test into one of the following broad categories: negative for intraepithelial lesion or malignancy, positive for an epithelial cell abnormality, or showing some other significant finding. Important findings are then elaborated in the subsequent section listing interpretations and results in much more specific terms. Use of the general categorization portion of the report is optional.

TABLE **3-13**				
Average Number of Cells per Microscopic Field Required to Predict a Minimum Total of 5000 Cells				

Preparation diameter = 13 mm
Preparation area = 133 mm²

	EYEPIECE FIELD NUMBER 20		**EYEPIECE FIELD NUMBER 22**	
	×10 Objective	×40 Objective	×10 Objective	×40 Objective
Fields*	42	676	35	559
Cells required†	118	7	143	9

*This figure is the total number of microscopic fields encompassed by the entire preparation, given the specified preparation diameter and the specific microscope optical characteristics.
†This figure is the minimum average number of squamous cells per microscopic field required to predict a total of at least 5000 cells. As described in the text, 10 or more fields are examined.

TABLE **3-14**				
Average Number of Cells per Microscopic Field Required to Predict a Minimum Total of 5000 Cells				

Preparation diameter = 20 mm
Preparation area = 314 mm²

	EYEPIECE FIELD NUMBER 20		**EYEPIECE FIELD NUMBER 22**	
	×10 Objective	×40 Objective	×10 Objective	×40 Objective
Fields*	100	1600	83	1322
Cells required†	50	3	60	4

*This figure is the total number of microscopic fields encompassed by the entire preparation, given the specified preparation diameter and the specific microscope optical characteristics.
†This figure is the minimum average number of squamous cells per microscopic field required to predict a total of at least 5000 cells. Ten or more fields are examined, as described in the text.

The term *negative for intraepithelial lesion or malignancy* can be used as the interpretation/result portion of the report. A general categorization of *epithelial cell abnormality* or *other*, requires that additional information be given in the interpretation/results section of the report. An interpretation of negative can stand alone.

Before this more detailed interpretation, space is made for notations regarding automated slide review and a description of any ancillary testing that has been applied to the cell sample. Each of these should include a brief description of devices, methods, and results. These should be communicated in terms designed to be clearly understood by the clinician.

In the interpretation/results section of the report, each category in the general categorization (regardless of whether it is included as a separate report section) becomes a heading beneath which are listed a number of specific findings of varying clinical significance. When only organisms or other nonneoplastic findings are reported, it is important that this be superseded by the designation negative for intraepithelial lesion or malignancy. The latter may appear in either the general categorization or in the interpretation/results section, but must be included in the report. Specific entities in this category are discussed elsewhere in this chapter and in Chapter 4. In the Bethesda System 2001, the general categorization of *other* is limited in scope, describing inappropriate shedding of endometrial cell in a woman 40 years of age or older. The basis for this is that endometrial hyperplasia and carcinoma are very uncommon in younger women. However, inappropriate shedding of morphologically normal endometrial cells has been seen in young women, leading to a diagnosis of endometriosis. Some laboratories may wish to continue reporting the observation of endometrial cells in young women when these are detected in the second half of the menstrual cycle.

The final general categorization includes intraepithelial lesions and invasive malignancies. These are divided into squamous processes or glandular processes, and space is made for other types malignant neoplasms (hematopoietic, sarcoma, or malignant melanoma). Each of these is discussed in subsequent chapters.

The final section of the Bethesda System report allows one to communicate suggestions, or educational notes. These should be concise and consistent with published clinical follow-up guidelines from the appropriate professional organizations.

References

1. Payne S, Kernohan NM, Walker F. Proliferation in the normal cervix and in preinvasive cervical lesions. J Clin Pathol 1996; 49:667-671.
2. Bulten J, de Wilde PC, Schijf C, et al. Decreased expression of Ki-67 in atrophic cervical epithelium of post-menopausal women. J Pathol 2000; 190:545-553.
3. Mittal K. Utility of proliferation-associated marker MIB-1 in evaluating lesions of the uterine cervix. Adv Anat Pathol 1999; 6:177-185.

4. Patten SF, Jr. Diagnostic cytopathology of uterine cervix. 2nd ed. Basel, Switzerland: S Karger AG; 1978.

5. McCallum SM. New observations on the significance of nipplelike protrusions in the nuclei of endocervical cells. Acta Cytol 1988; 32:331-334.

6. Babkowski RC, Wilbur DC, Rutkowski MA, et al. The effects of endocervical canal topography, tubal metaplasia, and high canal sampling on the cytologic presentation of non-neoplastic endocervical cells. Am J Clin Pathol 1996; 105:403-410.

7. Selvaggi SM, Haefner HK. Microglandular endocervical hyperplasia and tubal metaplasia; pitfalls in the diagnosis of adenocarcinoma on cervical smears. Diagn Cytopathol 1997; 16:168-173.

8. Ducatman BS, Wang HH, Jonasson JG, et al. Tubal metaplasia: a cytologic study with comparison to other neoplastic and non-neoplastic conditions of the endocervix. Diagn Cytopathol 1993; 9:98-103.

9. Novotny DM, Maygarden SJ, Johnson DE, et al. Tubal metaplasia: a frequent potential pitfall in the cytologic diagnosis of endocervical glandular dysplasia on cervical smears. Acta Cytol 1992; 36:1-10.

10. Van Le L, Novotny D, Dotters DJ. Distinguishing tubal metaplasia from endocervical dysplasia on cervical Papanicolaou smears. Obstet Gynecol 1991; 78:974-976.

11. Ramirez NC, Sastry LK, Pisharodi LR. Benign glandular and squamous metaplastic-like cells seen in vaginal Pap smears of post hysterectomy patients: incidence and patient profile. Eur J Gynaecol Oncol 2000; 21:43-48.

12. Wu HH, Harshbarger KE, Berner HW, et al. Endometrial brush biopsy (Tao brush): histologic diagnosis of 200 cases with complementary cytology: an accurate sampling technique for the detection of endometrial abnormalities. Am J Clin Pathol 2000; 114:412-418.

13. Maksem JA. Performance characteristics of the Indiana University Medical Center endometrial sampler (Tao brush) in an outpatient office setting, first year's outcomes: recognizing histological patterns in cytology preparations of endometrial brushings. Diagn Cytopathol 2000; 22: 186-195.

14. Tajima M, Inamura M, Nakamura M, et al. The accuracy of endometrial cytology in the diagnosis of endometrial adenocarcinoma. Cytopathology 1998; 9:369-380.

15. Cosci-Porrazzi LO, Maiello FM, de Falco ML. The cytology of the normal cyclic endometrium. Diagn Cytopathol 1986; 1:198-203.

16. de Peralta-Venturino MN, Purslow MJ, et al. Endometrial cells of the "lower uterine segment" (LUS) in cervical smears obtained by endocervical brushings: a source of potential diagnostic pitfall. Diagn Cytopathol 1995; 12: 263-268.

17. Hanau CA, Begley N, Bibbo M. Cervical endometriosis: a potential pitfall in the evaluation of glandular cells in cervical smears. Diagn Cytopathol 1997; 16:274-280.

18. Mulvany NJ, Surtees V. Cervical/vaginal endometriosis with atypia: a cytohistopathologic study. Diagn Cytopathol 1999; 21:188-193.

19. Johnson TL, Kini SR. Endometrial metaplasia as a source of atypical glandular cells in cervicovaginal smears. Diagn Cytopathol 1996; 14:25-31.

20. Blumenfeld W, Holly EA, Mansur DL, et al. Histiocytes and the detection of endometrial adenocarcinoma. Acta Cytol 1985; 29:317-322.

21. Nguyen TN, Bourdeau JL, Ferenczy A, et al. Clinical significance of histiocytes in the detection of endometrial adenocarcinoma and hyperplasia. Diagn Cytopathol 1998; 19:89-93.

22. Frank TS, Bhat N, Noumoff JS, et al. Residual trophoblastic tissue as a source of highly atypical cells in the postpartum cervicovaginal smear. Acta Cytol 1991; 35:105-108.

23. Schneider V, Barnes LA. Ectopic decidual reaction of the uterine cervix: frequency and cytologic presentation. Acta Cytol 1981; 25:616-622.

24. Zaharopoulos P, Wong JY, Keagy N. Hematoidin crystals in cervicovaginal smears. Report of two cases. Acta Cytol 1985; 29:1029-1034.

25. Capaldo G, LeGolvan DP, Dramczyk JE. Hematoidin crystals in cervicovaginal smears. Review of 27 cases seen in one year. Acta Cytol 1983; 27:237-240.

26. Benoit JL, Kini SR. "Arias-Stella reaction"–like changes in endocervical glandular epithelium in cervical smears during pregnancy and postpartum states—a potential diagnostic pitfall. Diagn Cytopathol 1996; 14:349-355.

27. Mulvany NJ, Kahn A, Ostor A. Arias-Stella reaction associated with cervical pregnancy: report of a case with a cytologic presentation. Acta Cytol 1994; 38:218-222.

28. Valente PT, Schantz HD, Trabal JF. Cytologic changes in cervical smears associated with prolonged use of depot-medroxyprogesterone acetate. Cancer 1998; 84:328-334.

29. Volk EE, Jax JM, Kuntzman TJ. Cytologic findings in cervical smears in patients using intramuscular medroxyprogesterone acetate (Depo-provera) for contraception. Diagn Cytopathol 2000; 23:161-164.

30. Friedrich M, Mink D, Villena-Heinsen C, et al. Tamoxifen and proliferation of vaginal and cervical epithelium in postmenopausal women with breast cancer. Eur J Obstet, Gynecol, Reprod Biol 1998; 80:221-225.

31. Costa MJ, Tadros T, Tackett E, Naib Z. Vaginocervical cytology in victims of sexual assault. Diagn Cytopathol 1991; 7: 337-340.

32. Rao PN, Collins KA, GW, Geisinger KR, et al. Identification of male epithelial cells in routine postcoital cervicovaginal smears using fluorescence in-situ hybridization: application in sexual assualt and molestation. Am J Clin Pathol 1995; 104:32-35.

33. Weir MM, Bell DA, Young RH. Transitional cell metaplasia of the uterine cervix and vagina: an underrecognized lesion that may be confused with high-grade dysplasia. Am J Surg Pathol 1997; 21:510-517.

34. Weir MM, Bell DA. Transitional cell metaplasia of the cervix: a newly described entity in cervicovaginal smears. Diagn Cytopathol 1998; 18:222-226.

35. Schenck U, Herbert A, Solomon D. Terminology: IAC Task Force summary. Acta Cytol 1998; 42:5-15.

36. Birdsong GG. Pap smear adequacy: is our understanding satisfactory . . . or limited? Diagn Cytopathol 2001; 24: 79-81.

37. Mintzer MP, Curtis P, Resnick JC, et al. The effect of the quality of Papanicolaou smears on the detection of cytologic abnormalities. Cancer Cytopathol 1999; 87:113-117.

38. Vooijs PG, Elias A, Vander Graaf Y, et al. Relationship between the diagnosis of epithelial abnormalities and the composition of cervical smears. Acta Cytol 1985; 29: 323-328.

39. Kivlahan C, Ingram E. Papanicolaou smears without endocervical cells: are they adequate? Acta Cytol 1986; 30: 258-260.

40. Mitchell H. Longitudinal analysis of histologic high-grade disease after negative cervical cytology according to endocervical status. Cancer 2001; 93:237-240.

41. Mitchell H, Medley G. Longitudinal study of women with negative cervical smears according to endocervical status. Lancet 1991; 337:265-267.

42. Mitchell H, Medley G. Differences between Papanicolaou smears with correct and incorrect diagnoses. Cytopathology 1995; 6:368-375.

43. O'Sullivan JP, A'Hern RP, Chapman PA, et al. A case-control study of true-positive versus false-negative cervical smears in women with cervical intraepithelial neoplasia (CIN) III. Cytopathology 1998; 9:155-161.

44. Palefsky JM, Holly EA, Hogeboom CJ, et al. Anal cytology as a screening tool for anal squamous intraepithelial lesions. J AIDS Hum Retrovir 1997; 14:415-422.

45. Ransdell JS, Davey DD, Zaleski S. Clinicopathologic correlation of the unsatisfactory Papanicolaou smear. Cancer Cytopathol 1997; 81:139-143.

46. Gill GW. Pap smear cellular adequacy: What does 10% coverage look like: what does it mean? Acta Cytol 2000; 44:873.

47. Renshaw AA, Friedman MM, Rahemtulla A, et al. Accuracy and reproducibility of estimating the adequacy of the squamous component of cervicovaginal smears. Am J Clin Pathol 1999; 111:38-42.

48. Valente PT, Schantz HD, Trabal JF. The determination of Papanicolaou smear adequacy using a semiquantitative method to evaluate cellularity. Diagn Cytopathol 1991; 7:576-580.

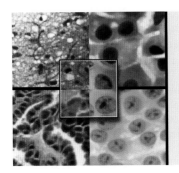

Negative for Intraepithelial Lesions and Malignancy

CHAPTER 4

Pap tests can exhibit a wide variety of nonneoplastic findings that connote no increased risk for future development of squamous intraepithelial lesions (SILs) or carcinoma. In some instances, these relate to infectious diseases that may be symptomatic and are amenable to specific therapy. Others are iatrogenic, and still others are associated with disease processes that primarily affect other tissues (pemphigus or Behçet's disease). Several alterations are important to recognize with confidence so that a false-positive interpretation of SIL or malignancy can be avoided. The working classification of these cytologic findings is summarized in Box 4-1.

Some of these entities have specific cytologic features that allow confident diagnosis, whereas others are less specific. Certain squamous cell alterations lie on a spectrum between cells that are within normal limits (WNL; see Chapter 3) and those that clearly indicate an SIL (see Chapter 6). When endocervical glandular cells are considered, some changes are clearly reactive in nature, whereas others may suggest a well-differentiated adenocarcinoma or adenocarcinoma in situ (AIS). Some of the most striking abnormalities are iatrogenic in nature. These can cause diagnostic difficulties if the patient's history is not clear to those in the cytology laboratory.

In addition to infections, this chapter concentrates on Pap test alterations that have traditionally been designated as *atypical*. The use of this term is quite restricted in the Bethesda System, where it appears only in connection with abnormal cells of undetermined significance (squamous or glandular). In practice, these interpretations raise the possibility of a preneoplastic condition. In contrast, the abnormalities discussed in this chapter have no such connotation. The term *atypia* is firmly entrenched in daily conversations and interpretations, and this is not likely to change in the near future. However, this chapter has adopted strict Bethesda System terminology (see Box 4-1). Thus, all of these alterations are initially classified as reactive cell changes (RCC) and then categorized as either infectious or reactive. In some instances, a more refined, often pathogenetically oriented interpretation is possible.

NONNEOPLASTIC FINDINGS: REACTIVE CELLULAR CHANGES

Nonspecific Inflammation Without Identifiable Infection or Specific Etiology

Inflammatory exudates are classified based on the types of immune effector cells involved. Virtually all Pap tests have at least occasional polymorphonuclear neutrophils (PMNs). When these cells are not prominent, the slide is sometimes said to be "clean." No established minimum number of PMNs is evident, nor is there density of infiltrate above which a patient is said to have clinically significant acute inflammation. The importance of the infiltrate depends entirely on any associated symptoms and other clinical findings. It is not assigned by the laboratory, which plays no role beyond the descriptive.

At the other end of the spectrum are those clearly unsatisfactory Pap tests that consist of mucus, PMNs, and little else. In other cases, abundant PMNs are accompanied by epithelial cells but obscure them from view, yielding a test that is unsatisfactory. The significance of PMNs is not always clear, even when the acute inflammation is striking. These cells may represent a response to bacterial vaginosis, candidiasis, or trichomoniasis. However, in most instances no morphologically apparent etiologic factors for acute inflammation are identified.

Eosinophils are rarely identified in Pap tests. These cells probably play a role in cervical ripening after the onset of labor during parturition.[1] When associated with invasive squamous cell carcinoma, some investigators have suggested that an eosinophilic infiltrate connotes a worsened prognosis.[2] For some patients, eosinophils probably represent an allergic response, particularly in the setting of recurring vaginal candidiasis.[3] The frequency with which eosinophils are present on Pap tests and thus, any diagnostic significance they may have is not known. In fixed smears the distinctive red granules are usually not seen, having been extracted during processing through organic solvents. They can be distinguished from neutrophils by their bilobed nuclei, rather than three nuclear lobes, but this exercise is not addressed with Pap tests in the manner sometimes employed in pulmonary cytology.

Small mature-appearing lymphocytes are often identified in the stroma of cervical biopsies, where a distinct distribution pattern of different immunologic subsets has been identified.[4] However, they are not often seen on Pap tests. Whether they are absent or simply rendered inconspicuous by their small size and dense hyperchromasia is not clear. When present in large numbers, lymphocytes usually indicate follicular cervicitis (FC) with formation of germinal centers in the cervical stroma. Sampling of a germinal center shows the features summarized in Box 4-2 and illus-

trated in Figure 4-1. Some investigators have found that this condition is associated with *Chlamydia trachomatis* more often than with other infectious agents.[5] As in other body sites, the lymphocytes' polymorphism is reassuring evidence of their benign nature. The cervix can be involved by malignant lymphoma, but this is rare and usually not considered in the evaluation of Pap tests.[6] Tingible body macrophages can be seen in any condition characterized by rapid cell turnover with release of nuclear debris from senescent cells. Thus, they are not pathognomonic of FC and can also be seen in small cell carcinoma or in high-grade malignant lymphoma. The benign nature of the lymphocytes is evidenced by their polymorphous morphologic features and not by the presence of tingible body cells. FC is discussed briefly in Chapter 6, when the differential diagnosis of small blue cells in high-grade SIL (HGSIL) is considered.

When histologic preparations are considered, chronic cervicitis more often shows a dense infiltrate of mature plasma cells than FC. As in the case of small lymphocytes, it is surprising that plasma cells are so uncommonly encountered on Pap tests; if present, they must usually be obscured by acute inflammatory cells. Rarely, the bulk of benign plasma cells may be so great as to clinically simulate cervical carcinoma.[7] Involvement of the uterine cervix by the malignant plasma cells of multiple myeloma is even less common, but presentation of this condition as a positive Pap test has been described.[8] Plasma cells can also be associated with cervical involvement by syphilis.[9]

General Reactive Patterns of Squamous Cells

Squamous cells can show reactive alterations in the absence of identifiable infectious agents. These changes have been traditionally termed *inflammatory atypia* and are now known as part of the RCCs associated with inflammation. Superficial, intermediate, and squamous metaplastic cells can all be affected.

When superficial or intermediate cells are involved, the differential diagnosis is between reactive cellular changes,

---

BOX 4-1

Classification of Nonneoplastic Findings

Reactive cellular changes (RCC)
  Nonspecific inflammation with no infection seen and no specific cause identified
    Acute
    Follicular
    Plasma cells
  General RCC patterns, squamous
    Reactive nuclear changes
    Keratosis and epidermalization
    Atrophic vaginitis
  General RCC patterns, glandular
    Reactive nuclear changes
    Microglandular hyperplasia
  General RCC patterns, other
    "Diathesis" pattern
    Repair and atypical repair
  Specific noninfectious RCC patterns
    Pemphigus
    Behçet's syndrome
    Folate deficiency
    Rheumatoid nodule (necrobiotic)
  Iatrogenic RCC patterns
    Intrauterine contraceptive devices

DES exposure
Suture granulomas
Radiation/chemotherapy
Induced folate deficiency
Rectovaginal fistula*
Tamoxifen therapy

Infections
  Infections, common nonviral
    Normal and altered bacterial flora
    Gonorrhea
    Chlamydia
    Candida and other fungi
    Actinomyces
    Leptothrix
    Trichomonas
  Infections, uncommon nonviral
    Enterobius
    Schistosomiasis
    Granuloma inguinale
    Entamoeba
    Syphilis
    Tuberculosis
  Infections, viral
    Herpesvirus
    Cytomegalovirus
    Adenovirus
    Human papillomavirus†

DES, Diethylstilbestrol.
*Rectovaginal fistula is included with the iatrogenic causes of reactive cellular changes because most examples are seen in the context of radiation therapy for a pelvic malignancy, including carcinoma of the uterine cervix.
†Human papillomavirus is included here for completeness but is discussed more fully when squamous intraepithelial lesions are considered in Chapter 6.

BOX 4-2   CMF

Cytomorphologic Features of Follicular Cervicitis

Numerous lymphocytes
Often appears as a streak in a localized area of a conventionally prepared smear
Much greater cell dispersal on liquid-based preparations can make this difficult to identify.
Lymphocytes vary in maturity, with a spectrum of the following:
  • Cell size
  • Nuclear size
  • Chromatin texture
  • Nucleolar number and prominence
  • Cytoplasmic volume
Tingible-body macrophages are usually seen*

*These can also be seen in high-grade malignancy of several types.

atypical squamous cells of undetermined significance (ASC-US), and low-grade SIL (LGSIL). The latter lesions are detailed in Chapters 5 and 6, respectively. All of these cells have a generous body of cytoplasm with minor alterations. As the cells become more significantly abnormal, their nuclei show increasing degrees of enlargement, hyperchromasia, irregularity of contour, and abnormality of chromatin distribution. The question then becomes: How large and how dark are cells designated as reactive, ASCUS, or LGSIL? Nuclei that stand out from surrounding cells and appear large and dark to the point of being conspicuous virtually always represent SIL. Diagnostic difficulty lies in the less severely abnormal range of cytologic alterations.

Normal intermediate cells and squamous cell RCCs associated with inflammation are summarized in Table 4-1 and illustrated in Figure 4-2. These cytologic alterations are contrasted with ASC in Chapter 5. Clearly, these distinctions are based on relatively minor morphologic alterations. Even the improvements in nomenclature embodied by the Bethesda System do not relieve these interpretations of considerable subjectivism. It has been suggested that even careful study of published Bethesda System example illustrations[11] does not improve interobserver agreement.[12] Classifying squamous cells at this level of abnormality is based primarily on mild nuclear enlargement with an attendant slight increase in nuclear to cytoplasmic (N:C) ratio.

The semiquantitative approach of expressing increased nuclear area as multiples of the normal nuclear size is congruent with the camera lucida measurements left to us by Patten.[10] The comparison of nuclear areas is operatively less cumbersome than comparing diameters. One can mentally pick up a nearby intermediate cell nucleus, imagine it superimposed on the nucleus of an abnormal cell, and determine how many could be fit over the nucleus in question. This approach is especially useful to those who are new to gynecologic cytology and is often used as a teaching tool.

Atypical squamous metaplasia (ASM) is a more difficult and potentially more dangerous problem. LGSIL usually has the appearance of intermediate cells with superimposed nuclear abnormalities. The type of HGSIL previously designated moderate dysplasia or cervical intraepithelial neoplasia grade II sheds cells that mimic immature squamous metaplasia with superimposed nuclear alterations (Figure 4-3). The cells of ASM often show one or more small nucleoli. Thus, troublesome alterations in ASM lead us to declare a smear abnormal (usually ASC–US) or to raise the diagnostic possibility of HGSIL (ASC–H). Again, the question becomes how big and how dark is the nucleus and how elevated is the N:C ratio before a confident interpretation of HGSIL can be rendered. It has been suggested that ASM suggestive of HGSIL should be aggressively investigated.[13] Atypical squamous metaplasia and its relationship to HGSIL is discussed more fully in the next chapter.

The normal cervical squamous epithelium is not keratinized. Mature superficial cells have eosinophilic cytoplasm, reflective of their high-protein content, but true orangeophilia indicates hypermaturity in the form of keratinization. Classically, such alterations have been described in association with uterine descensus or vaginal prolapse, but in most cases, no such predisposing condition is

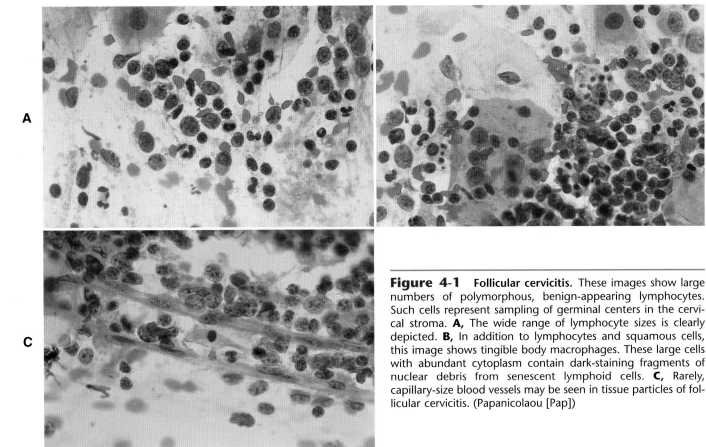

A **B** **C**

Figure 4-1 **Follicular cervicitis.** These images show large numbers of polymorphous, benign-appearing lymphocytes. Such cells represent sampling of germinal centers in the cervical stroma. **A,** The wide range of lymphocyte sizes is clearly depicted. **B,** In addition to lymphocytes and squamous cells, this image shows tingible body macrophages. These large cells with abundant cytoplasm contain dark-staining fragments of nuclear debris from senescent lymphoid cells. **C,** Rarely, capillary-size blood vessels may be seen in tissue particles of follicular cervicitis. (Papanicolaou [Pap])

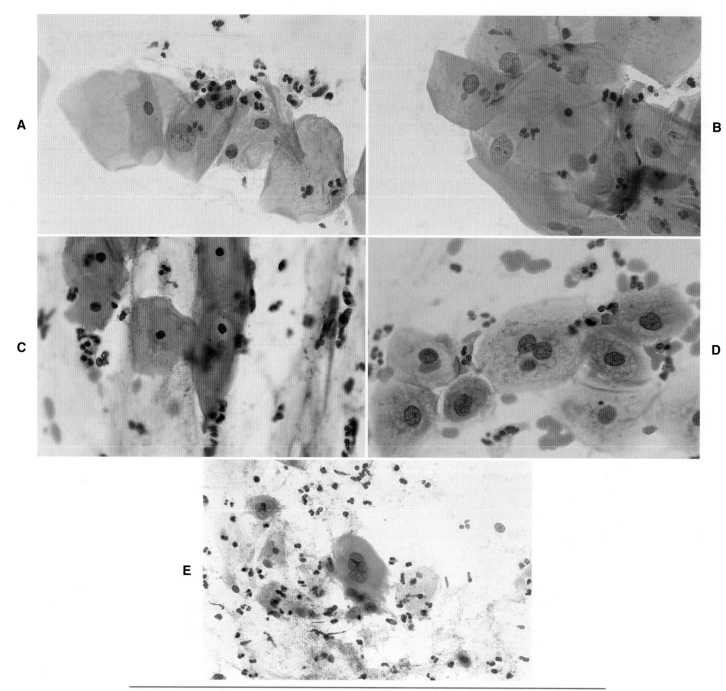

Figure 4-2 **Reactive cellular changes (RCCs) involving squamous cells. A** and **B,** In addition to normal intermediate cells, these images shows cells with mature cytoplasm and slight nuclear enlargement. No hyperchromasia is present, and the nuclear contours are smooth. These features help classify such minor abnormalities as RCCs. **C,** Small perinuclear halos are a common RCC in squamous cells. These are especially common in the setting of *Trichomonas vaginalis* infestation. These small halos with rather indistinct margins do not mimic the huge areas of cytoplasmic cavitation seen in human papillomavirus (HPV) cytopathic effect. **D,** Binucleation is another common reactive change in benign squamous cells. In the absence of other nuclear abnormalities or when associated with only mild nuclear enlargement, these alterations do not suggest HPV. **E,** Multinucleation is also a common RCC in benign squamous cells. At screening magnification, a cell such as this may appear provocative with marked nuclear enlargement. However, examination at this magnification shows that rather than one large hyperchromatic nucleus, this cell has several small nuclei that are identical to one another and show no evidence of either hyperchromasia or irregularities of nuclear contour. (Pap)

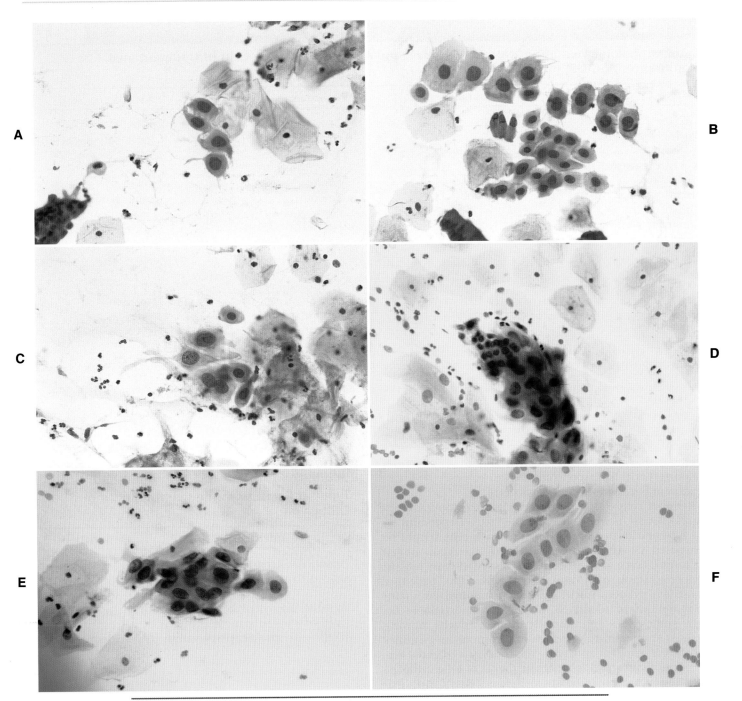

Figure 4-3 **Atypical squamous metaplasia. A** to **E,** Each of these images shows immature squamous metaplastic cells with varying degrees of nuclear enlargement. With this enlargement comes an increase in nuclear to cytoplasmic (N:C) ratio. However, hyperchromasia is minimal and each of these cells shows smooth nuclear contours. These features indicate that these cells represent a reactive cellular change rather than a high-grade squamous intraepithelial lesion (HGSIL). **F,** Air-drying artifact can cause striking nuclear enlargement. It also minimizes any hyperchromasia that may have been present. These features make air-dried examples of squamous metaplasia difficult to interpret. Some such cells may raise the possibility of an HGSIL. (Pap)

evident.[14] The terminology used to describe the various morphologic types of keratotic reactions is summarized in Table 4-2 and illustrated in Figure 4-4. The older term, *dyskeratosis,* is no longer in use. Its interpretation seems to have been too broad to be useful, as it has been applied to both the usually banal reactions in Table 4-2 and the potentially more significant lesions described below.

Anucleate hyperkeratotic cells can be introduced as contaminants from the vulva or distal vagina. The finding of simple changes such as those noted in Table 4-2 should be regarded as an RCC; none of these connote an increased likelihood of human papillomavirus (HPV) infection, SIL, or carcinoma. However, a banal-appearing keratotic reaction can overlie any of these more significant lesions,

TABLE 4-1

Cytomorphologic Features of Normal, Reactive, and Atypical Squamous Cells of Undetermined Significance (ASC-US) Intermediate Cells

Feature	Normal	Reactive	ASC-US
Cell size*	1500	1500	1500
Nuclear size*	35	Up to 2× normal (70)	Up to 3× normal (105)
Nuclear features:			
Hyperchromasia†	Absent	Minimal	Mild
Nuclear contour	Smooth	Smooth	Minimal irregularity
Chromatin texture	Finely granular	Finely granular	Finely granular
Chromatin clearing	Not seen	Not seen	Not seen
Multinucleation	Not seen	Common	May be seen
Nucleoli	Not seen	Not seen	Not seen
Cytoplasmic features:			
Polychromasia	Not seen	May be present	Not seen
Vacuolization	Not seen	May be present	Not seen
Perinuclear halos‡	Not seen	May be present	Not seen

*All sizes are given in μm² and are derived from Patten's average area measurement for intermediate squamous cells.[10]
†Well-fixed intermediated cell nuclei are *normochromatic* by definition. The term *hyperchromasia* means nuclear staining darker than that of intermediate cells in the same cytologic preparation.
‡These are small, concentric cytoplasmic clearings situated close to the nucleus and do not resemble the gaping cavitary cytoplasmic clearings associated with koilocytosis (see Chapter 6).

shielding the more deeply situated abnormal cells from sampling. For this reason, some suggest colposcopic investigation of persistent keratotic reactions.

Keratotic cells with additional nuclear or cytoplasmic abnormalities are not considered to be RCCs. Depending on the type and degree of abnormality, such cells should be designated ASC-US, SIL, or even keratinizing squamous cell carcinoma. (Each of these entities is discussed more fully in Chapters 5 through 7.) Parakeratotic cells of RCC have tiny completely pyknotic nuclei in which no residual chromatin structure can be identified. Small, dense, extremely orangeophilic cells with minimally shrunken nuclei showing retained chromatin substructure and contour irregularities may be the herald of an HGSIL. Abnormally configured keratotic cells with spindling, tadpole shapes or long cytoplasmic projections should be interpreted as signs of abnormal maturation. This is especially true, when these cytoplasmic derangements are associated with enlarged, hyperchromatic, or misshapen nuclei. Such forms are most often indicative of HPV effect but, as noted earlier, may be shed from more severe lesions.

The cytology of normal atrophy was discussed in Chapter 3. RCCs are relatively common in these preparations.[16,17] To some extent, these are the result of mild, diffuse air-drying that afflicts many Pap tests from these patients. Even when they are well-preserved, compact clusters of small atrophic cells with scant cytoplasm and the resultant nuclear crowding can arouse suspicion of a HGSIL, as discussed more fully in Chapter 6. Other examples show diffuse, mild-to-moderate nuclear enlargement without hyperchromasia or chromatin distribution abnormalities. Abati and colleagues have shown that this type of change is not a sign of ASC-US or SIL and that it is reversible with es-

TABLE 4-2

Types of Keratosis in the Cervical Squamous Epithelium

Cytologic Finding	Designation
Cytoplasmic keratohyalin granules	Prekeratinization
Anucleate mature squamous cells	Hyperkeratosis (orthokeratosis)
Miniature orangeophilic superficial cell with pyknotic nuclei	Parakeratosis
Keratohyalin granules plus keratosis	Epidermalization

trogen application (Figure 4-5). However, if karyomegaly is associated with hyperchromasia or irregularities of nuclear contour, the risk of ASC-US or SIL increases.[16]

Atrophic vaginitis may or may not show an acute inflammatory exudate. The cytologic features of this condition are summarized in Table 4-3 and illustrated in Figure 4-5. As highlighted in Table 4-3, a number of potential diagnostic errors can arise from this type of Pap test. The generalized nuclear enlargement of atrophy was discussed previously. The nature of blue blobs has been debated. However, a recent immunohistochemical and ultrastructural evaluation of these structures indicates that they may represent parabasal or intermediate squamous cells in an advanced state of degeneration.[18] Their only clinical significance is the small danger that they might be mistaken for SIL. Because of a combination of air-drying and degeneration, some parabasal cells show eosinophilic or

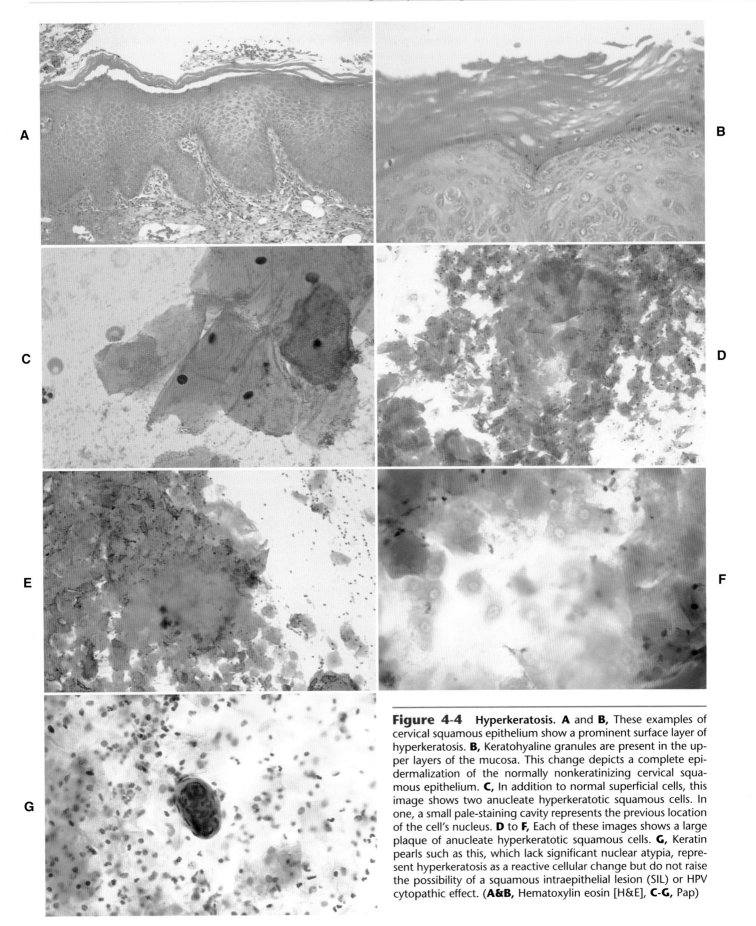

Figure 4-4   Hyperkeratosis. **A** and **B,** These examples of cervical squamous epithelium show a prominent surface layer of hyperkeratosis. **B,** Keratohyaline granules are present in the upper layers of the mucosa. This change depicts a complete epidermalization of the normally nonkeratinizing cervical squamous epithelium. **C,** In addition to normal superficial cells, this image shows two anucleate hyperkeratotic squamous cells. In one, a small pale-staining cavity represents the previous location of the cell's nucleus. **D** to **F,** Each of these images shows a large plaque of anucleate hyperkeratotic squamous cells. **G,** Keratin pearls such as this, which lack significant nuclear atypia, represent hyperkeratosis as a reactive cellular change but do not raise the possibility of a squamous intraepithelial lesion (SIL) or HPV cytopathic effect. (**A&B,** Hematoxylin eosin [H&E], **C-G,** Pap)

even orangeophilic staining and are sometimes confused with a keratotic reaction. Atrophic vaginitis represents profound atrophy, whereas parakeratosis represents a hypermature squamous epithelium. These two should not coexist, hence the term *pseudoparakeratotic parabasal cells.*

Reactive Patterns of Endocervical Columnar Cells

Mild, reactive alterations in endocervical glandular cells are described in Box 4-3 and illustrated in Figure 4-6. In mild forms, this change is characteristic and causes few diagnostic difficulties. The presence of nucleoli in cells with round,

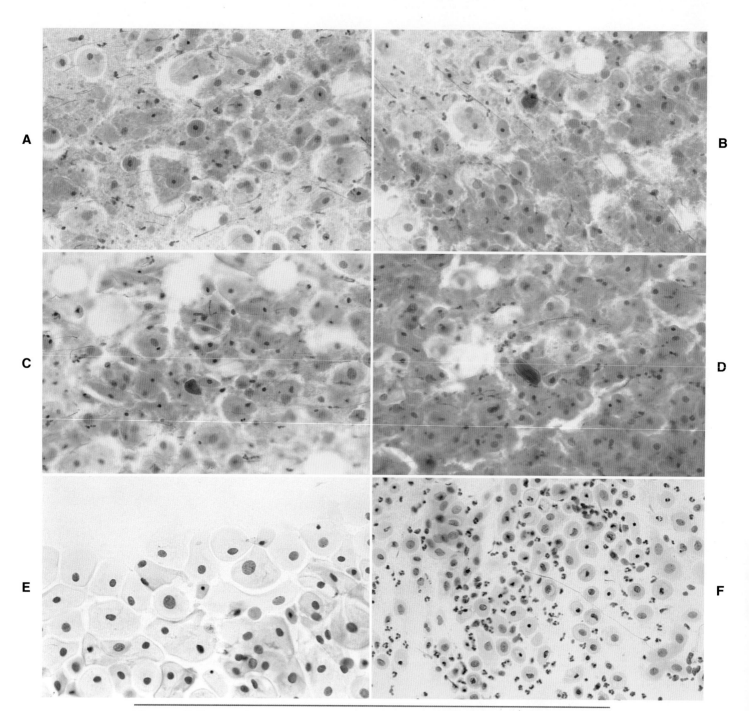

Figure 4-5   Atrophy. **A,** This atrophic smear shows a background of granular debris. This should not be mistaken for a tumor diathesis indicative of invasive malignancy. Near the center of the photograph is a small pseudoparakeratotic cell with dense orangeophilic cytoplasm and a completely pyknotic nucleus. This represents an advanced state of degeneration rather than parakeratosis. **B** to **D,** These images show atrophic smears. Near the center of each is a dark oval or irregularly shaped structure. Designated blue blobs, these fragments of acellular material should not be mistaken for the stripped nuclei of dysplastic or malignant cells. **E** to **F,** Each of these atrophic smears shows occasional cells with mild nuclear enlargement. This increase in nuclear size is not accompanied by hyperchromasia or by irregularities of nuclear contour. This degree of mild atypia is common in atrophic smears and should not lead to further evaluation of the patient. (Pap)

TABLE 4-3		CMF
Cytomorphologic Features of Atrophic Vaginitis		

Cytologic Finding	May Be Mistaken For . . .	Diagnostic Clue
Finely granular "dirty" background precipitate	May suggest a tumor diathesis	No other features of malignancy
Hyperchromatic blue blobs	Dysplastic nuclei	1. No apparent cytoplasm 2. Dense without a chromatin-like structure
Generalized nuclear enlargement	ASC-US or SIL	1. Smooth nuclear contour 2. Minimal hyperchromasia 3. Normal chromatin distribution
Pseudoparakeratotic parabasal cells Bare nuclei may be numerous	Parakeratosis	Does not occur in atrophy

ASCUS, Atypical squamous cells of undetermined significance; *SIL*, squamous intraepithelial lesion.

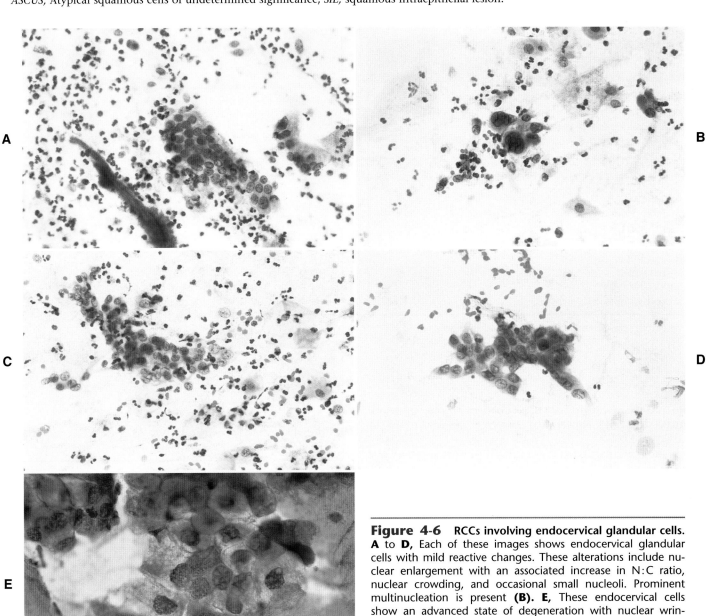

Figure 4-6 RCCs involving endocervical glandular cells. **A** to **D,** Each of these images shows endocervical glandular cells with mild reactive changes. These alterations include nuclear enlargement with an associated increase in N:C ratio, nuclear crowding, and occasional small nucleoli. Prominent multinucleation is present **(B). E,** These endocervical cells show an advanced state of degeneration with nuclear wrinkling and vacuolization. These alterations should not be interpreted as significant atypia. (Pap)

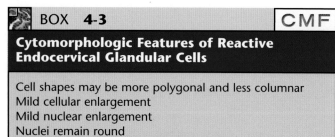

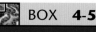

BOX 4-3 — CMF

Cytomorphologic Features of Reactive Endocervical Glandular Cells

Cell shapes may be more polygonal and less columnar
Mild cellular enlargement
Mild nuclear enlargement
Nuclei remain round
Chromatin becomes hypochromatic
No abnormalities of chromatin distribution
A single nucleolus of variable size
Cytoplasmic vacuoles

BOX 4-4

Histologic Findings in Microglandular Hyperplasia

Common patterns
Acute and chronic inflammation
Small closely packed rounded glands
Larger glands with or without intervening stroma
Squamous metaplasia

Uncommon variants
Solid growth
Reticular growth with edematous stroma*
Penetration up to several millimeters into the cervical stroma†
Nuclear hyperchromasia†
Hobnail cells†
Clear cells†
Occasional mitotic figures†

*This pattern can resemble endodermal sinus tumor.
†These features can resemble adenocarcinoma or clear cell carcinoma.

pale nuclei is reassuring. As these changes become more advanced, the cell's appearance converges on that of repair (see Box 4-1).

Microglandular hyperplasia (MGH) can occur at any age and is most often an incidental finding in histologic sections. The histology of MGH is highly variable, as summarized in Box 4-4.[19,20] Occasional examples may suggest carcinoma of various types, but the presence of areas with a more typical MGH pattern and the relatively low levels of atypia and mitotic activity usually lead to the correct interpretation. The long-cited association of this condition with oral contraceptives, hormonal replacement therapy, or pregnancy has been challenged.[21]

The cytology of MGH has been the subject of occasional reports,[22-24] as summarized in Box 4-5, and illustrated in Figure 4-7. Some examples show degenerative alterations and can be very difficult to interpret. Diagnoses of atypical glandular cells of undetermined significance, endocervical adenocarcinoma in situ, adenocarcinoma, or HGSIL is then shown by cone biopsy or hysterectomy to be in error.

BOX 4-5 — CMF

Cytomorphologic Features of Microglandular Hyperplasia

Most common features
Endocervical cells in flat sheets or small clusters
Nuclear enlargement
Nuclear overlapping and crowding
Oval nuclei
Finely granular chromatin
Small nucleoli
Abundant cytoplasm
Cytoplasmic vacuoles
Classic repair pattern in some cases

Degenerative features*
Cytoplasmic shrinkage
Cytoplasmic orangeophilia
Nuclear hyperchromasia
Nuclear pyknosis

From Valente PT, Schantz HD, Schultz M. Cytologic atypia associated with microglandular hyperplasia. Diagn Cytopathol 1994; 10:326-331.
*These features can lead to interpretations of atypical glandular cells, adenocarcinoma in situ, adenocarcinoma, or an HGSIL that is shown by subsequent histologic follow-up to be erroneous.

BOX 4-6 — CMF

Cytomorphologic Features of Repair

Cohesive flat sheets
Similar single cells are not present
Cells within a group maintain their polarity and may appear to be streaming in one direction
Enlarged cytoplasm
Cyanophilic cytoplasm
Cytoplasm may be vacuolated
Enlarged nuclei
Low N:C ratio
Smooth nuclear borders
Chromatin hypochromasia
Variably prominent nucleoli*
Mitotic figures may be seen
Neutrophils often infiltrate the cell sheet

N:C, Nuclear to cytoplasmic.
*Nucleoli may be single or multiple and vary in prominence from case to case.

Other General RCC Patterns

Repair is in this more general category because it represents a cluster of cytologic findings that can be superimposed on either glandular cells or immature squamous cells. As the cytologic alterations become more advanced, it may be difficult to determine the involved cells' origin. In evaluating repair cells identified after laser conization, Ueki and colleagues found that some were also of stromal origin.[25]

Most examples of repair are straightforward in cytologic samples and not likely to be confused with other reactive patterns or SIL[26] (Box 4-6 and Figure 4-8). As in the less ad-

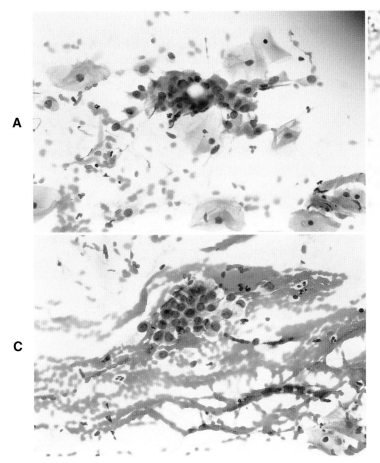

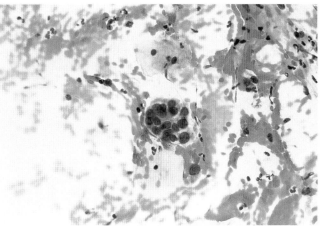

A

B

C

Figure 4-7 **Microglandular hyperplasia. A-C,** These endocervical cell clusters were derived from patients whose subsequent endocervical curettage specimens showed only microglandular hyperplasia. These cells have slightly enlarged nuclei with mild hyperchromasia and occasional small nucleoli. They also feature an increase in N:C ratio and tend to occur in small gland-like clusters. This latter architectural feature reflects the most common architectural pattern of microglandular hyperplasia in histologic samples. (Pap)

 BOX   4-7

Features of Atypical Repair that May Lead to a Classification of Atypical Squamous Cells of Undetermined Significance

Marked variability in nuclear size
Abnormalities of chromatin distribution
Marked variations in nucleolar size
Marked variations in nucleolar number

vanced endocervical reactive changes discussed previously, identification of cellular cohesion and prominent nucleoli in the face of nuclear pallor is reassuring. The primary differential diagnostic consideration is nonkeratinizing squamous cell carcinoma (see Chapter 7). The more advanced examples of repair were previously termed *atypical repair* (Box 4-7). This term does not appear in the Bethesda System 2001.

The pattern designated as *tumor diathesis* consists primarily of a granular protein and fibrin precipitate in the smear background, accompanied by varying amounts of lysed red blood cells (RBCs) and debris from damaged epithelial cells. As noted previously, such material is encountered less frequently in liquid-based Pap tests than in conventional smear preparations. This celebrated criterion for identification of invasive carcinomas of the uterine cervix is

absent in some invasive carcinomas, particularly those with invasion of less than 5 mm.[27] It is also absent from most invasive carcinomas with extensive keratinization. These issues are discussed more fully in Chapter 7. In the current context, it is important to note that a diathesis pattern can occur in benign conditions characterized by acute tissue destruction, including ulcerative lesions (herpesvirus), radiation damage, cervical stenosis, and pyometra. Thus, the presence or absence of this pattern may not assist in the differential diagnosis between repair and large cell nonkeratinizing squamous cell carcinoma.

Specific Noninfectious RCC Patterns

Pemphigus vulgaris (PV) is an autoimmune disorder characterized by blistering of the skin and mucosal sites, including the uterine cervix. All sites show identical histologic and immunofluorescence findings in biopsy material. Valente and colleagues noted an example of Pap test abnormality resulting from this condition that occurred despite disease that was otherwise well controlled by steroids. The patient had no symptoms referrable to the uterus or vagina.[28] Wright and colleagues identified similar cytologic abnormalities on a Pap test from a patient whose systemic PV had not yet been recognized.[29] Other patients present with vaginal discharge or bleeding; Dvoretsky and colleagues warned that PV may rarely coexist with carcinoma.[30]

Cytologically, the striking features of the abnormal cells in PV is their prominent nucleoli and nuclear pallor resembling those of repair. However, many of the cells are smaller than in the latter condition and are often described as parabasal in appearance. These features are summarized in Box 4-8 and illustrated in Figure 4-9. If frozen biopsy material is available or can be obtained, positive immunofluo-rescence for immunoglobulin G (IgG) and C3 can be confirmatory in clinically ambiguous cases.

Behçet's syndrome is characterized by a leukocytoclastic or lymphocytic vasculitis that causes ulcers in the skin, oral mucosa, eyes, colon, and genital tract. One case report in-

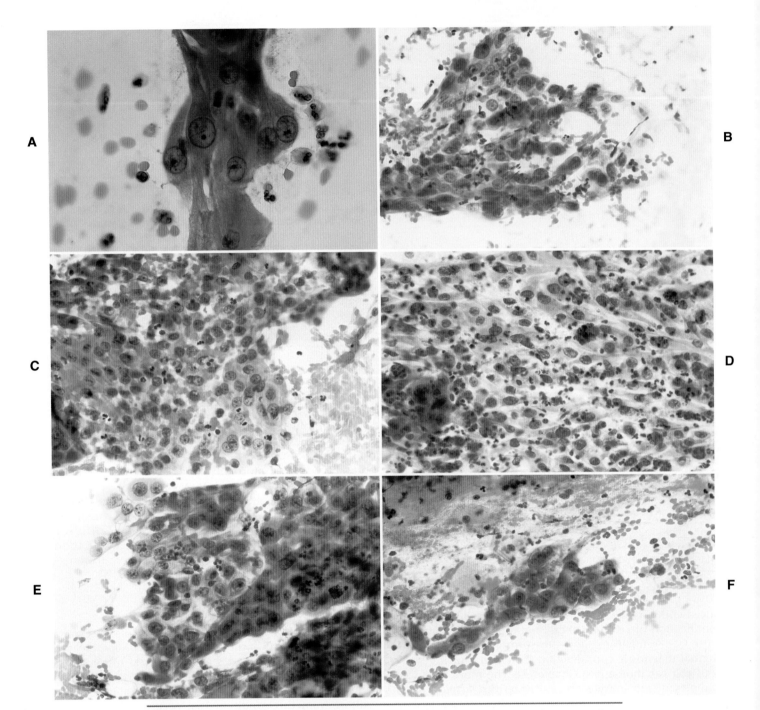

Figure 4-8   Repair. **A,** This high-magnification image shows the features of repair cytology. The nuclei are enlarged but pale, with even contours and prominent nucleoli. These cells are arranged in a flat, streaming sheet associated with inflammatory cells. No single cells with this nuclear morphology are apparent. **B to D,** These examples of repair also show a streaming arrangement of these cells within flat sheets. Infiltration by inflammatory cells is prominent. The nuclei are pale and nucleoli are easily identified. **E and F,** These examples of more advanced repair were previously termed *atypical repair*. These show greater degrees of nuclear hyperchromasia and nucleolar prominence. Mild irregularities of chromatin distribution are also apparent. An important key to the correct interpretation of these atypical cell clusters is that no single cells with similar morphology are identified. It is cells such as these that sometimes raise the differential diagnostic possibility of large cell nonkeratinizing squamous cell carcinoma. (Pap)

dicated that in addition to marked inflammation, a Pap test from a patient with active ulcerative disease showed atypical keratotic cells suspicious for squamous cell carcinoma.[31]

Folic acid deficiency leads to generalized cytologic alterations in numerous epithelia throughout the body. Mild deficits lead to megaloblastosis-like changes. Cells are enlarged, with enlarged nuclei showing extreme hypochromasia. More severe forms of folate deficiency are often induced by antineoplastic chemotherapy and are strongly radiomimetic, as discussed in the following section and in more detail during the discussion on diffuse diseases of the lung in Chapter 15.

The cervix is rarely involved by rheumatoid nodules. If sampled cytologically these show the same features noted elsewhere.

Iatrogenic RCC Patterns

The string from an intrauterine contraceptive device can lead to chronic irritation of the endometrium and the endocervix, with cytologic consequences listed in Box 4-9.[32-34] SIL is certainly not induced by the device, even in women who wear it for many years. The diagnosis of SIL is readily accomplished with follow-up Pap tests, but in some in-

stances it is necessary to use local vaginal treatment of inflammation to obtain a clean preparation that can be interpreted with confidence.

Vaginal adenosis after diethylstilbestrol (DES) exposure can be cytologically detected in women who have had a hysterectomy or when a directed upper vaginal wall sampling is obtained. Approximately one third of affected women do not have a history or in utero DES exposure. Adenosis also occurs as a secondary alteration following carbon dioxide laser vaporization or 5-fluorouracil treatment.[35] The cells of vaginal adenosis are cytologically indistinguishable from normal endocervical glandular cells, endometrial cells, or tubal cells; the endocervical type represents the majority of cases. The cytology of the closely related clear cell carcinoma is discussed in Chapter 10. It is noteworthy that although clear cell carcinoma of the cervix and endometrium continue to be recognized, the same tumor occurring as a primary vaginal mass has become very rare because gestational use of DES was discontinued decades ago.

Bardales and colleagues described foreign body reactions to suture material on Pap tests from six patients who had previously undergone hysterectomy.[36] Foreign body giant cells and histiocytes were assembled around linear fragments of suture material that were easily highlighted by visualization under polarized light (Figure 4-10).

Radiation and chemotherapy effects are described in detail during our consideration of pulmonary cytology. Similar alterations occur in gynecologic material. As mentioned previously, radiation change is mimicked by severe folate deficiency that in most instances is induced by antineoplastic chemotherapy. It is important to recall that radiation-induced cytologic alterations can persist for decades after therapy. The relationship between radiation for cervical carcinoma and subsequently identified SILs is discussed in Chapter 6.

Rectovaginal fistula is an uncommon complication of radiation therapy for pelvic malignancies, including carcinoma of the uterine cervix. It has numerous other causes and may be identified when fecal material is identified on a Pap test sample (Figure 4-11). An important component of

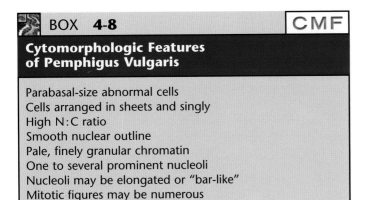

BOX 4-8 CMF

Cytomorphologic Features of Pemphigus Vulgaris

Parabasal-size abnormal cells
Cells arranged in sheets and singly
High N:C ratio
Smooth nuclear outline
Pale, finely granular chromatin
One to several prominent nucleoli
Nucleoli may be elongated or "bar-like"
Mitotic figures may be numerous

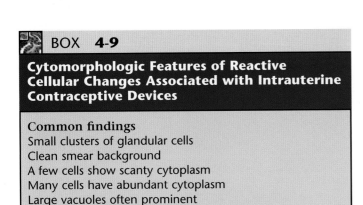

BOX 4-9

Cytomorphologic Features of Reactive Cellular Changes Associated with Intrauterine Contraceptive Devices

Common findings
Small clusters of glandular cells
Clean smear background
A few cells show scanty cytoplasm
Many cells have abundant cytoplasm
Large vacuoles often prominent
Vacuoles may displace the nucleus (signet ring cell appearance)
Neutrophils within the cell clusters or inside vacuoles
Degeneration may be seen
Some cells show a prominent nucleolus

Less common findings
Actinomyces
Psammoma body–like calcifications

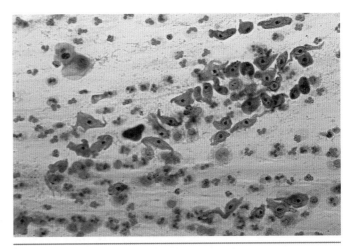

Figure 4-9 Pemphigus vulgaris. In a background of acute inflammatory cells, this illustration shows several cells with the cytoplasmic configuration of immature squamous metaplasia. Many of these feature striking nuclear clearing and a single large nucleolus. (Pap)

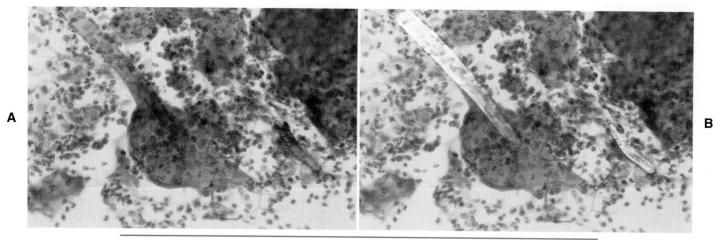

Figure 4-10 Suture granuloma on the Pap test of a patient who is status post-hysterectomy. **A** and **B,** These images show the same microscopic field: normal view **(A)** partially crossed polarizing filter view **(B).** A prominent inflammatory reaction includes foreign body giant cells that are attached to a narrow linear structure. When viewed under polarized light, this is readily visible and represents suture material that has incited a foreign body reaction. (Pap)

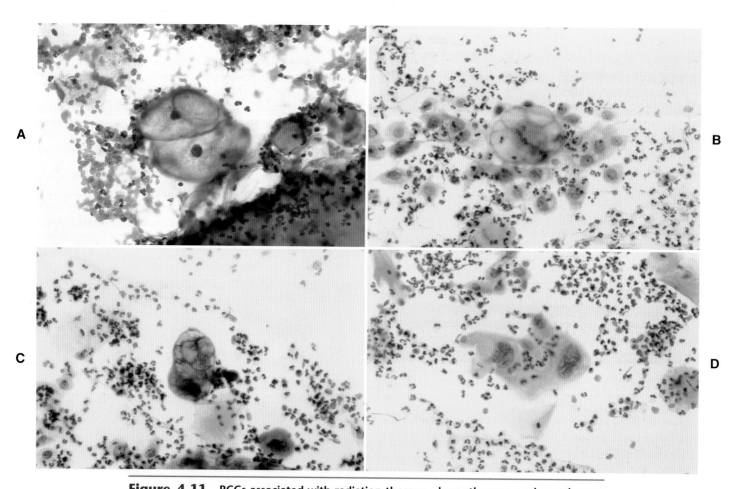

Figure 4-11 RCCs associated with radiation therapy, chemotherapy, and posttherapy rectovaginal fistula. **A** to **D,** These abnormal cells show reactive cellular changes after radiation therapy. They feature varying degrees of cellular enlargement, with increases in both the cytoplasmic and nuclear areas. This concomitant change results in maintenance of a low N:C ratio. Multinucleation, cytoplasmic vacuolization, strange cell shapes, and infiltration of the cytoplasm by neutrophils are also common features. **(A-D,** Pap)

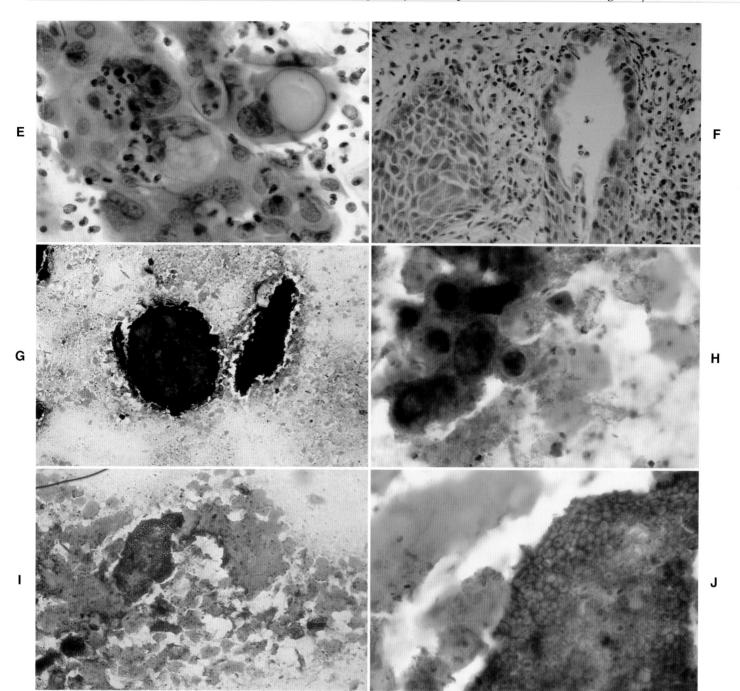

Figure 4-11, cont'd **E** and **F,** These images show chemotherapy and induced atypia in a Pap test and a corresponding cervical biopsy. The patient was a 21-year-old woman receiving intensive chemotherapy for Hodgkin's disease at the time of this examination. The changes are similar to those noted in the radiation-induced reactive cellular changes. The "soap bubble" vacuolization shown by some of these cells is typical. **G** and **H,** These images show amorphous acellular debris that litters the smear in an example of rectovaginal fistula associated with radiation therapy for a pelvic malignancy. **I** and **J.** This low- and high-magnification image pair shows vegetable matter on a Pap test from a patient with a rectovaginal fistula. The large, dark fragment features numerous cells with hyperchromatic nuclei. The keys to identifying these cells as vegetable in origin include their almost square or rectangular shape, their arrangement in regimented rows, and their separation by dense cell walls. (**E and G-J,** Pap; **F,** H&E)

TABLE **4-4**

Cytologic Comparison of 'Small Cells' in Tamoxifen Therapy with Endometrial Cells

Cytologic Feature	Small Cells	Endometrial Cells
Nuclear size	35-40 μm²	35-40 μm²*
Nuclear contour	Smooth	Wrinkled or grooved*
Cytoplasm	Absent	Scant
Cell arrangement	Loose	Tightly cohesive

Data from Opjorden SL, Caudill JL, Humphrey SK, et al. Small cells in cervical-vaginal smears of patients treated with tamoxifen. Cancer Cytopathol 2001; 93:23-28.
*The degree to which these features are present depends in part on the level of degenerative change exhibited by these cells.

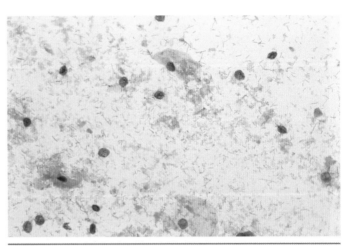

Figure 4-12 Cytolysis and Döderlein lactobacilli. This smear shows an intermediate cell predominant pattern with striking cytolysis. Most of the squamous cells have been reduced to wispy scraps of cyanophilic cytoplasmic debris and naked nuclei. Large numbers of uniform bacilli are prominent in this background. These represent the normal vaginal flora and comprise a large number of species. (Pap)

the latter can be vegetable cells. These are discussed in detail when we consider contaminants in pulmonary cytology preparations. Because they can show large hyperchromatic nuclei, they are occasionally mistaken for carcinoma cells. Other features that should lead to the correct interpretation include a square or rectangular cell shape, arrangement in regimented rows, and thick cell walls.

Breast cancer patients being treated with tamoxifen can experience a worsening of symptoms associated with the menopause. Increased estrogen effects are manifested by endometrial proliferative activity, and some individuals develop difficulties with postmenopausal bleeding, endometrial polyps, or endometrial adenocarcinoma. Abati and colleagues found that the presence of endometrial cells or histiocytes on the Pap test of a patient receiving tamoxifen suggests an increased risk for endometrial adenocarcinoma.[39]

The degree to which this therapy increases squamous cell maturation and atypia in Pap tests has been controversial.[37-39] However, most investigators indicate an increase in maturation. In a large study of bone marrow transplant recipients, it was suggested that squamous cell abnormalities are independent of both tamoxifen and high-dose chemotherapy (see Figure 4-11).[40]

Opjoreden and colleagues describe small cells on the Pap tests of tamoxifen-treated patients, most of whom were postmenopausal.[37] Careful review of control smears indicated that these cells were present with equal frequency in those with and without a history of tamoxifen therapy. However, these cells were much more readily detected when seen against the mature background squamous cells of the treated patients than when superimposed on the atrophic pattern typical of most untreated women. These investigators suggest that these small cells are parabasal or reserve cells similar to those described in Chapter 3. The major differential diagnostic distinction is endometrial cells, with which small cells are contrasted in Table 4-4. This distinction is important, since identification of endometrial cells on a Pap test of a postmenopausal woman often leads to an invasive investigation of suspected endometrial pathology.

Many of the tamoxifen studies published to date involve mostly older individuals who are at low risk for HPV and SIL. As a small subset of breast carcinoma patients who are

at high risk for HPV and SIL is identified, the effect on these conditions and on the possible development of invasive cervical carcinoma will require further investigation.

 NONNEOPLASTIC FINDINGS: ORGANISMS

Common Nonviral Infectious Agents

Although the normal vaginal flora have traditionally been referred to as the *Döderlein lactobacillus,* what appears on Pap tests to be a single type of bacterium is actually composed of numerous *Lactobacillus* spp. These readily identifiable rods are illustrated in Figure 4-12.

This group of organisms is probably responsible for the cytolysis observed in smears with an intermediate cell–predominant hormonal picture as described in Chapter 3. In this setting, the bacteria are numerous, and many squamous cells are severely damaged. Naked nuclei and fragments of cyanophilic cytoplasmic debris litter the smear.

Altered vaginal flora is the cytologic term given to a shift from these relatively large bacilli to a profusion of tiny coccobacillary forms. For practical purposes, these organisms resemble tiny basophilic dots at the magnification generally used for study of cytologic samples (rarely over ×400), and the usual, larger organisms are conspicuously absent. The abnormal organisms are present in enormous numbers and form a gray film or tinting of the background when conventional smear material is examined. Often, this film is separated from cell clusters by a thin clearing resulting from contraction at the time of fixation. These abnormal bacteria often coat squamous cells to form a clue cell (Figure 4-13). Previously such cells were felt to indicate the presence of *Gardnerella vaginalis* (formerly known as *Hemophilus vaginalis* or *Corynebacterium vaginalis*). However, it is now understood that the correlation between this morphologic picture and any particular type of organism is poor.[41,42]

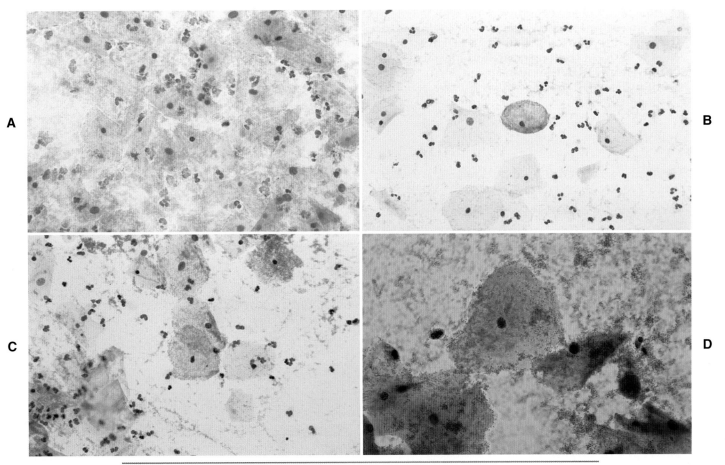

Figure 4-13 **Altered vaginal flora.** **A,** In contrast to the large rods that constitute the normal vaginal flora, this image shows altered flora. The background is tinted gray by large numbers of tiny coccobacillary forms. **B** to **D,** Each of these images shows a clue cell. These squamous cells are coated with large numbers of tiny coccobacillary bacteria. These are not diagnostic of any specific bacterial species. (Pap)

The relationships among the bacterial content of a Pap test, clinical symptoms of bacterial vaginosis, and culture results in both symptomatic and asymptomatic women are unclear. As a clinical entity, bacterial vaginosis features a malodorous discharge, vaginal pH greater than 4.5, and a fishy odor when an alkaline agent (10% potassium hydroxide) is added to the secretions. Clue cells and cytologically altered flora can be seen in patients with and without these signs. Thus, Pap test alterations correlate poorly with the clinical presence or absence of bacterial vaginosis. Mass and colleagues found that altered flora on a prenatal smear was associated with an increased risk of acute chorioamnionitis and preterm delivery.[43]

Gonococcus is occasionally encountered on Pap tests. However, this method has been found unsuitable in screening for this infection in asymptomatic women because of interobserver variability in identification of the diplococci and the prolonged screening time required for adequate microscopy.[44]

C. trachomatis is a venereally transmitted tiny intracellular bacterium that causes several diseases, including many cases of nongonococcal urethritis in both men and women. It was previously thought that squamous metaplastic cells with vacuoles containing tiny eosinophilic dots (so-called elementary particles) would permit cytologic identification of this organism. These inclusions probably represent mucinous or other vacuoles, the contents of which have undergone shrinkage during fixation. Correlation of this cytologic picture with microbiologic evidence of *C. trachomatis* infection is poor.[45] At this time, Pap test cytology has no role in diagnosis of this infection, and its presence or absence as determined by other laboratory methods should not alter other smear interpretations based on cytologic criteria.[46]

A number of fungi can be identified on Pap tests, including *Candida* spp., *Torulopsis glabrata,* and *Geotrichum.* All are morphologically similar with minor size differences. The yeast of *T. glabrata* are surrounded by a thin clear halo, and this organism does not form hyphae or the pseudohyphae typical of *Candida* spp.[47] The other yeast do form these elongated structures and lack halos. In most preparations the yeast are lightly eosinophilic (Figure 4-14). The Bethesda System reports fungi morphologically consistent with *Candida* spp., without further classification. Many women with fungi on a Pap test are asymptomatic.[48]

Fungi can be accompanied by significant cytologic alterations. The most alarming are large, thick plaques of keratotic squamous cells with varying degrees of nuclear abnormality. These may raise the possibility of a LGSIL and are often suggestive of HPV effect.

Infections by *Actinomyces* are associated with long-term, foreign-body residence within the uterus or vagina, particularly intrauterine contraceptive devices.[49] Extension of this infection leads to widespread pelvic inflammatory disease and may eventuate in tubo-ovarian abscess. Fluffy rounded masses of filamentous organisms show clublike peripheral knobs resulting from swollen filaments, and a background of marked acute inflammation is often evident (Figure 4-15). These masses have been described as resembling cotton balls or dust balls.

Leptothrix is a markedly elongated bacterial organism that is similar in width to the Döderlein bacilli. It has no clinical significance but is often present in combination with *Trichomonas vaginalis*[50] (Figure 4-16).

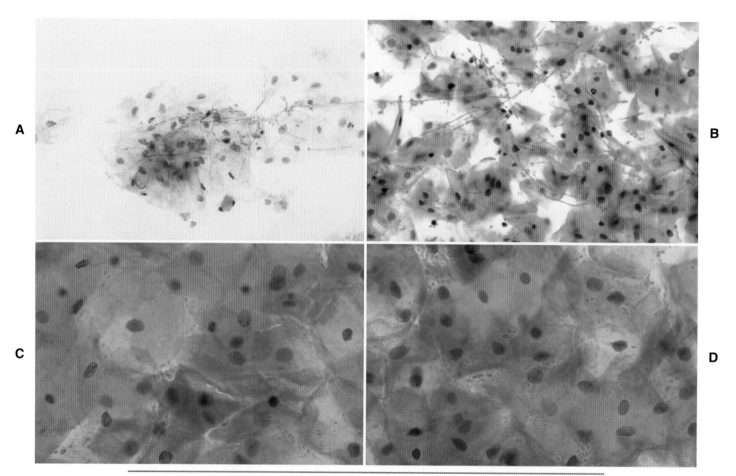

Figure 4-14   Yeast. **A** and **B**, These two images show the eosinophilic yeast and pseudohyphae of *Candida* spp. **C** and **D**, Small budding yeast without pseudohyphae are identified in these images. Each is surrounded by a small, clear halo indicative of *Torulopsis glabrata*. (Pap)

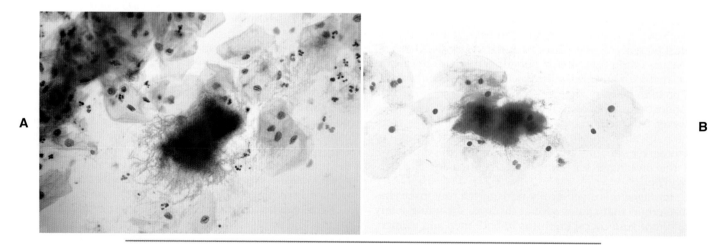

Figure 4-15   *Actinomyces.* **A** and **B**, These clusters of tiny filamentous organisms represent *Actinomyces* on Pap tests from patients wearing intrauterine contraceptive devices. (Pap)

Trichomoniasis results from venereally transmitted infestation with this protozoal organism. The prostate serves as a reservoir for this organism, where it is occasionally a cause of symptomatic, antibiotic resistant prostatitis, or urethritis.[51,52] In the latter instance, the organism is sometimes identified in the urine. Using immunohistochemical techniques, it also can be identified in other body sites.[53] *T. vaginalis* can be identified in Pap tests or visualized as motile organisms by microscopic examination of a fresh wet preparation in the clinic. Either test can be negative, even in the face of a symptomatic infestation.[54] When asymptomatic women are considered, false-positive identification of *T. vaginalis* can apparently occur.[55]

T. vaginalis are small triangular or sickle-shaped organisms that are pale gray with the Pap stain, and measure up to 30 μm in greatest dimension (Figure 4-17). Near one end is a small, slightly darker, sickle-shaped mass of nuclear material. The cytoplasm sometimes shows numerous tiny red granules. Careful attention to the size and shape of the organism, presence of red granules, and an eccentrically located nucleus increases the confidence of *T. vaginalis* identification and avoids false interpretation of debris or bits of cytoplasm as organisms. Paradoxically, this organism can be easier to find and classify on preparations that show air-drying artifact. Drying enlarges the cells and tends to accentuate the red granules and nucleus.

Intermediate and superficial cells tend to show exaggerated eosinophilia in the presence of *T. vaginalis*. In some instances, this is so pronounced that one can grossly appreci-

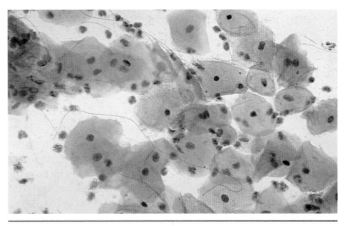

Figure 4-16   *Leptothrix.* These long, narrow filaments represent *Leptothrix.* This organism has no clinical significance but is often seen on in the presence of a *T. vaginalis* infestation. (Pap)

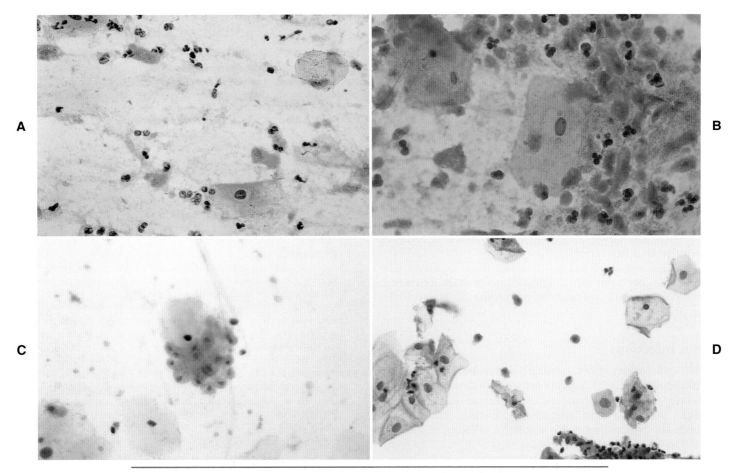

Figure 4-17   **Trichomoniasis. A,** Small, rectangular or triangular trichomonads are scattered through this image. Although cyanophilic, they show tiny red dots and a dark smudgy area of nuclear material. **B** and **C,** One occasionally encounters squamous cells that have been set upon by a herd of trichomonads. **D,** In liquid-based preparations, the organisms may appear more rounded than in conventional smears. Their nuclear material is visible, but the red dots may not be seen in the complete absence of air-drying typical of these preparations. (Pap)

ate the abnormal color of the slide even before beginning microscopy. Many cells show a perinuclear halo. As discussed previously in this chapter, these are small and in no way mimic the cytoplasmic cavitation seen in the koilocytes of HPV infections.

Uncommon Nonviral Infectious Agents

Enterobius vermicularis (pinworm) is a relatively common pediatric gastrointestinal infestation. Enormous quantities of 30 to 50 μm ova are shed and are so light, they become airborne and ingested by new hosts. Ova are sometimes present as a contaminant in Pap tests. They are oval with flattening along one side.[56,57]

The ova of various schistosomal species can be present on Pap tests from patients living in endemic areas, but most represent *Schistosoma haematobium*.[58,59] Ova are oval with a pointed terminal spine and measure up to 150 μm in length. Pelvic infestations usually center on the bladder, but the cervix or vagina and fallopian tubes can also be involved. Given the striking etiologic contribution of *S. haematobium* to carcinogenesis in squamous cell carcinoma of the urinary bladder, it is interesting to speculate about a causative role it might play in cervical carcinogenesis. Studies to date have been inconclusive.[60]

Cervical and vulvar involvement in granuloma inguinale have been described in Pap tests and vulvar scraping cytology, respectively.[61,62] Leiman and colleagues noted a combination of acute inflammation and epithelioid histiocytes and Donovan (the causative organism) bodies within cytoplasmic vacuoles of histiocytes.

Intestinal infestations with *Entamoeba histolytica* can be reflected in Pap tests. These large, histiocyte-like organisms have prominent nucleoli and their cytoplasm contains vacuoles and ingested RBCs. Immunohistochemical identification has been described.[63]

The necrotizing granulomatous inflammation of tuberculosis can be identified on Pap tests and is identical to that described in other sites, including lymph node aspirates.[64] Cervical tuberculosis has been identified using the polymerase chain reaction applied to previously fixed Pap test material.[65] The larvae of *Strongyloides stercoralis* have been identified in a Pap test.[66]

A single report of Loa loa first identified as a Pap test finding has been published. The authors provide a detailed review of parasitic infestations identified in gynecologic samples.[67]

Viral Infections

Viral cytopathic effect resulting from herpesvirus, cytomegalovirus (CMV), and adenovirus are described and illustrated during our consideration of diffuse diseases of the lungs. Similar cellular alterations are seen when these agents are detected on a Pap test.[68-71] CMV can be seen in patients with no history of immunosuppression.[69] The finding of herpes on a Pap test is potentially a medical emergency if the patient is pregnant and should always indicate immediate notification of the clinical team.

The major differential diagnostic problem occurs when multinucleated reactive cells are mistaken for herpetic cells. If the cells are degenerated, it may be impossible to make a confident determination of their nature. Reactive cells of-

ten show other alterations, as noted earlier. The presence of nucleoli is a strong indicator that viral cytopathic effect is not the cause of multinucleation. Of course, nucleoli must be distinguished from intranuclear viral inclusion bodies. The latter are usually larger and separated from a thickened or beaded nuclear membrane by a ring of clear karyoplasm. By contrast, nucleoli are set in a background of fine chromatin granules. Furthermore, the nuclei of reactive cells mold to one another less tightly than those seen in herpes.

References

1. Knudsen UM, Uldbjerg N, Rechberger T, et al. Eosinophils in human cervical ripening. Eur J Obstet, Gynecol, Reprod Biol 1997; 72:165-168.
2. van Driel WJ, Kievit-Tyson P, van den Broek LC, et al. Presence of an eosinophilic infiltrate in cervical squamous carcinoma results from a type-2 immune response. Gynecol Oncol 1999; 74:188-195.
3. Witkin SS, Jeremias J, Ledger WJ. Vaginal eosinophils and IgE antibodies to *Candida albicans* in women with recurrent vaginitis. J Med Vet Mycol 1989; 27:57-58.
4. Johansson EL, Rudin W, Wassen L, et al. Distribution of lymphocytes and adhesion molecules in human cervix and vagina. Immunology 1999; 96:272-277.
5. Hare MJ, Toone E, Taylor-Robinson D, et al. Follicular cervicitis: colposcopic appearances and association with Chlamydia trachomatis. Br J Obstet Gynaecol 1981; 88:174-180.
6. Mikhail MS, Runowicz CD, Kadish AS, et al. Colposcopic and cytologic detection of chronic lymphocytic leukemia. Gynecol Oncol 1989; 34:106-108.
7. Doherty MG, Van Dinh T, Payne D, et al. Chronic plasma cell cervicitis simulating a cervical malignancy: a case report. Obstet Gynecol 1993; 82:646-650.
8. Figueroa JM, Huffaker AK, Diehl EJ. Malignant plasma cells in cervical smear. Acta Cytol 1978; 22:43-45.
9. Iwasaka T, Ikeda N. Sugimori H. Secondary syphilis with extensive cervical lesion. Asia Oceania J Obstet Gynaecol 1987; 13:311-314.
10. Patten SF Jr. Diagnostic cytopathology of the uterine cervix. In: Wied GL, von Haam E, editors. Monographs in clinical cytology, vol 3, Basel Switzerland: S Karger AG; 1978.
11. Kurman RJ, Solomon D. The Bethesda System for reporting cervical/vaginal cytologic diagnoses: definitions, criteria, and explanatory notes for terminology and specimen Adequacy. New York: Spinger-Verlag; 1994.
12. Smith AE, Sherman ME, Scott DR, et al. Review of the Bethesda System atlas does not improve reproducibility or accuracy in the classification of atypical squamous cells of undetermined significance smears. Cancer 2000; 90: 201-206.
13. ChangChien CC, Lin H, Eng HL, et al. Clinical implication of atypical squamous cells of undetermined significance with or without favoring high-grade squamous intraepithelial lesion on cervical smears. Chang-Keng i Hsueh Tsa Chih 1999; 22:579-585.
14. Sorosky JI, Kaminski PF, Wheelock JB, et al. Clinical significance of hyperkeratosis and parakeratosis in otherwise negative Papanicolaou smears. Gynecol Oncol 1990; 39: 132-134.
15. Velasquez CTV. "Atypical parakeratosis" cells in cervical carcinoma cytology. Acta Cytol 1997; 41:614-616. (Letter).
16. Abati A, Jaffurs W, Wilder AM. Squamous atypia in the atrophic cervical vaginal smear: a new look at an old problem. Cancer 1998; 84:218-225.

17. Medley G, Surtees VM. Squamous atypia in the atrophic cervical vaginal smear: a plea for a more painstaking old style look versus a new look at the old problem. Cancer 1998; 84:200-201.

18. Abdulla M, Hombal S, Kanbour A, et al. Characterizing "blue blobs": immunohistochemical staining and ultrastructural study. Acta Cytol 2000; 44:547-550.

19. Leslie KO, Silverberg SG. Microglandular hyperplasia of the cervix: unusual clinical and pathological presentations and their differential diagnosis. Prog Surg Pathol 1984; 5: 95-114.

20. Young RH, Scully RE. Atypical forms of microglandular hyperplasia of the cervix simulating carcinoma. Am J Surg Pathol 1989; 13:50-56.

21. Greeley C, Schroeder S, Silverberg SG. Microglandular hyperplasia of the cervix: a true "pill" lesion? Int J Gynecol Pathol 1995; 14:50-54.

22. Valente PT, Schantz HD, Schultz M. Cytologic atypia associated with microglandular hyperplasia. Diagn Cytopathol 1994; 10:326-331.

23. Yahr LJ, Lee KR. Cytologic findings in microglandular hyperplasia of the cervix. Diagn Cytopathol 1991; 7:248-251.

24. Alvarez-Santin C, Sica A, Rodriquez M, et al. Microglandular hperplasia of the uterine cervix: cytologic diagnosis in cervical smears. Acta Cytol 1999; 43:110-113.

25. Ueki M, Ueda M, Kurokawa A, Morikawa M, et al. Cytologic study of the tissue repair cells of the uterine cervix: with special reference to their origin. Acta Cytol 1992; 36:310-318.

26. Yelverton CL, Bentley RC, Olenick S, et al. Epithelial repair of the uterine cervix: assessment of morphologic features and correlations with cytologic diagnosis. Int J Gynecol Pathol 1996; 15:338-344.

27. Rushing L, Cibas ES. Frequency of tumor diathesis in smears from women with squamous cell carcinoma of the cervix. Acta Cytol 1997; 41:781-785.

28. Valente PT, Ernst CS, Atkinson BF. Pemphigus vulgaris with subclinical involvement of the uterine cervix: report of a case with persistence of abnormal Papanicolaou smears posthysterectomy. Acta Cytol 1984; 28:681-683.

29. Wright C, Pipingas A, Grayson W, et al. Pemphigus vulgaris of the uterine cervix revisited: case report and review of the literature. Diagn Cytopath 2000; 22:304-307.

30. Dvoretsky PM, Bonfiglio TA, Patten SF Jr, et al. Pemphigus vulgaris and microinvasive squamous-cell carcinoma of the uterine cervix. Acta Cytol 1985; 29:403-410.

31. Wilbur DC, Maurer S, Smith NJ. Behçet's disease in a vaginal smear: report of a case with cytologic features and their distinction from squamous cell carcinoma. Acta Cytol 1993; 37:525-530.

32. Kaplan B, Orvieto R, Hirsch M, et al. The impact of intrauterine contraceptive devices on cytological findings from routine Pap smear testing. Eur J Contraception Reprod Health Care 1998; 3:75-77.

33. Fiorino AS. Intrauterine contraceptive device-associated actinomycotic abscess and *Actinomyces* detection on cervical smear. Obstet Gynecol 1996; 87:142-149.

34. Barter JF, Orr JW Jr, Holloway RW, et al. Psammoma bodies in a cervicovaginal smear associated with an intrauterine device. A case report. J Reprod Med 1987; 32:147-148.

35. Sedlacek TV, Riva JM, Magen AB, et al. Vaginal and vulvar adenosis: an unsuspected side effect of CO_2 laser vaporization. J Reprod Med 1990; 35:995.

36. Bardales RH, Valente PT, Stanley MW. Cytology of suture granulomas in post-hysterectomy vaginal smears. Diagn Cytopathol 1995; 13:336-338.

37. Opjorden SL, Caudill JL, Humphrey SK, et al. Small cells in cervical-vaginal smears of patients treated with tamoxifen. Cancer Cytopathol 2001; 93:23-28.

38. Gill BL, Simpson JF, Somlo G, et al. Effects of tamoxifen on the cytology of the uterine cervix in breast cancer patients. Diagn Cytopath 1998; 19:417-422.

39. Abadi MA, Barakat RR, Saigo PE. Effects of tamoxifen on cervicovaginal smears from patients with breast cancer. Acta Cytol 2000; 44:141-146.

40. Liu K, Marshall J, Shaw HS, Dodge RK, et al. Effects of chemotherapy and tamoxifen on cervical and vaginal smears in bone marrow transplant recipients. Acta Cytol 1999; 43:1027-1033.

41. Priestley CJ, Jones BM, Dhar J, et al. What is normal vaginal flora? Genitourin Med 1997; 73:23-28.

42. Greene JF 3rd, Kuehl TJ, Allen SR. The Papanicolaou smear: inadequate screening test for bacterial vaginosis during pregnancy. Am J Obstet Gynecol 2000; 182:1048-1049.

43. Mass SB, Brennan JP, Silverman N, et al. Association between a shift in vaginal flora on Papanicolaou smear and acute chorioamnionitis and preterm delivery. Diagn Cytopathol 1999; 21:7-9.

44. Genvert GI, Drusin LM, Seybolt JF, et al. Evaluation of the Papanicolaou-stained cytological smear as a screening technique for asymptomatic gonorrhoea. Br J Venereal Dis 1980; 56:400-403.

45. Caudill JL, Humphrey SK, Goellner JR. Cervicovaginal cytology and the diagnosis of Chlamydia trachomatis: a comparison with immunofluorescent results. Diagn Cytopathol 1994; 11:20-22.

46. Edelman M, Fox A, Alderman E, et al. Cervical Papanicolaou smear abnormalities and Chlamydia trachomatis in sexually active adolescent females. J Pediatr Adolesc Gynecol 2000; 13:65-69.

47. Boquet-Jimenez E, Alvarez San Cristobal A. Cytologic and microbiologic aspects of vaginal *Torulopsis*. Acta Cytol 1978; 22:331-334.

48. Shurbaji MS, Burja IT, Sawyer WL Jr. Clinical significance of identifying candida on cervicovaginal (Pap) smears. Diagn Cytopathol 1999; 21:14-17.

49. Christ ML, Haja J. Cytologic changes associated with vaginal pessary use: with special reference to the presence of Actinomyces. Acta Cytol 1978; 22:146-149.

50. Bibbo M, Harris MJ. Leptothrix. Acta Cytol 1972; 16:2-4.

51. Kuberski T. *Trichomonas vaginalis* associated with nongonococcal urethritis and prostatitis. Sexually Transmitted Diseases 1980; 7:135-136.

52. Gardner WA Jr, Culberson DE, Bennett BD. *Trichomonas vaginalis* in the prostate gland. Arch Pathol Lab Med 1986; 110:430-432.

53. O'Hara CM, Gardner WA Jr, Bennett BD. Immunoperoxidase staining of trichomonas vaginalis in cytologic material. Acta Cytol 1980; 24:448-451.

54. Wiese W, Patel SR, Patel SC, et al. A meta-analysis of the Papanicolaou smear and wet mount for the diagnosis of vaginal trichomoniasis. Am J Med 2000; 108:301-308.

55. Weinberger MW, Harger JH. Accuracy of the Papanicolaou smear in the diagnosis of asymptomatic infection with *Trichomonas vaginalis*. Obstet Gynecol 1993; 82:425-429.

56. Avram E, Yakovlevitz M, Schachter A. Cytologic detection of *Enterobius vermicularis* and *Strongyloides stercoralis* in routine cervicovaginal smears and urocytograms. Acta Cytol 1984; 28:468-470.

57. Bhambhani S, Milner A, Pant J, et al. Ova of *Taenia* and *Enterobius vermicularis* in cervicovaginal smears. Acta Cytol 1985; 29:913-914.

58. Berry A. Multispecies schistosomal infections of the female genital tract detected in cytology smears. Acta Cytol 1976; 20:361-365.

59. Mainguene C, Clement N, Gabriel S, et al. Urogenital schistosomiasis: an unusual discovery on cervical smears from a Caucasian female. Acta Cytol 1998; 42:1045-1046. (Letter).

60. Riffenburgh RH, Olson PE, Johnstone PA. Association of schistosomiasis with cervical cancer: detecting bias in clinical studies. East Afr Med J 1997; 74:14-16.

61. Leiman G, Markowitz S, Margolius KA. Cytologic detection of cervical granuloma inguinale. Diagn Cytopathol 1986; 2:138-143.

62. de Boer AL, de Boer F, Van der Merwe JV. Cytologic identification of Donovan bodies in granuloma inguinale. Acta Cytol 1984; 28:126-128.

63. Kobayashi TK, Koretoh O, Kamachi M, et al. Cytologic demonstration of Entamoeba histolytica using immunoperoxidase techniques. Report of two cases. Acta Cytol 1985; 29:414-418.

64. Angrish K, Verma K. Cytologic detection of tuberculosis of the uterine cervix. Acta Cytol 1981; 25:160-162.

65. Ferrara G, Cannone M, Guadagnino A, et al. Nested polymerase chain reaction on vaginal smears of tuberculous cervicitis: a case report. Acta Cytol 1999; 42:308-312.

66. Murty DA, Luthra UK, Sehgal K, et al. Cytologic detection of strongyloides stercoralis in a routine cervicovaginal smear: a case report. Acta Cytol 1994; 38:223-225.

67. Stelow EB, Pambuccian SE, Bardoles RH, et al. Loa loa presenting in a Pap test. Diagn Cytopathol (in press).

68. Hunt JL, Baloch Z, Judkins A, et al. Unique cytomegalovirus intracytoplasmic inclusions in ectocervical cells on a cervical/endocervical smear. Diagn Cytopathol 1998; 18:110-112.

69. Henry-Stanley MJ, Stanley MW, Burton LG, et al. Cytologic diagnosis of cytomegalovirus in cervical smears. Diagn Cytopathol 1993; 9:364-365.

70. Huang JC, Naylor B. Cytomegalovirus infection of the cervix detected by cytology and histology: a report of five cases. Cytopathology 1993; 4:237-241.

71. Laverty CR, Russell P, Black J, et al. Adenovirus infection of the cervix. Acta Cytol 1977; 21:114-117.

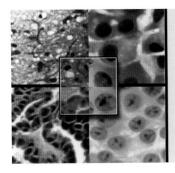

CHAPTER
5

Atypical Squamous Cells

In the Bethesda System, the term *atypical squamous cells (ASC)* is defined as an epithelial cell abnormality with "cellular changes that are more marked than those attributable to reactive changes but that quantitatively or qualitatively fall short of a definitive diagnosis of squamous intraepithelial lesion (SIL)."[1,2] This chapter examines the utility of nondefinitive diagnoses such as ASC, historical use of the term *atypia* in cervicovaginal cytology, cytologic features of ASC, frequency and clinical significance of an ASC interpretation, controversy surrounding ASC, and future of ASC. At the time of this writing, little data exist on the use of the 2002 Bethesda System term *ASC;* much of the data and discussion revolve around the previously used Bethesda System term *atypical squamous cells of undetermined significance (ASCUS)*.

 ## CYTOLOGIC ATYPIA

The cytologic diagnosis of atypia (regardless of specimen type) is a nondefinitive diagnosis, similar in nature to other nondefinitive diagnoses such as *suspicious, probably,* and *most likely.*[3-5] In Pap tests, the two nondefinitive diagnoses are ASC and atypical glandular cells (AGC), which are discussed in Chapter 8.[1,6,7] In contrast, definitive diagnoses include benign (e.g., no evidence of intraepithelial lesion or malignancy [NIL]) and SIL. As the previous definition of ASC implies, nondefinitive diagnoses are used in cervicovaginal cytology when specimens cannot be classified definitively into benign or pre-neoplastic/neoplastic categories. Reasons for the inability to classify specimens into definitive categories include the lack of specific cytologic features (e.g., absence of the well-defined features of SIL), the lack of a sufficient number of cytologic features (e.g., not enough cells with definitive features), and individual observer characteristics (e.g., experience).

Many practitioners believe that an atypical diagnosis such as ASC expresses a relatively high degree of uncertainty about outcome.[3,4] This conception has led to the belief that nondefinitive diagnoses are problematic because the perceived lack of certainty hinders the establishment of follow-up protocols or causes undue patient anxiety. Koss wrote that atypical cervicovaginal smear diagnoses gave little guidance to clinicians and most often resulted from

"timidity or inability."[8] Implicit in this view is the belief that a diagnosis is correct or incorrect (i.e., definitive diagnoses are correct and nondefinitive diagnoses are incorrect) and with enough knowledge or experience, pathologists could make correct diagnoses. Koss has stressed the need to limit atypical diagnoses in cervicovaginal cytology.[8]

The view that nondefinitive diagnoses are somehow inferior to definitive diagnoses is based on a fallacy and fails to take into account the probabilistic nature of all diagnoses.[3,5] This nature is apparent on examination of the follow-up of patients with specific diagnoses. For example, some women who have benign cervicovaginal diagnoses will have SIL on follow-up (i.e., a false-negative diagnosis), whereas some women who have SIL diagnoses will not have SIL on follow-up (i.e., a false-positive diagnosis). In actuality, a probability of disease or nondisease is inherent in every Bethesda System diagnosis, and consequently, no Bethesda System diagnosis is ever entirely definitive for disease or nondisease. Thus, the diagnoses of NIL, ASC, and SIL all carry a probability—albeit a different one for each diagnosis—for SIL being present.

Bayes' theorem uses the probabilities derived from laboratory tests such as Pap tests to calculate probabilities of disease in actual patients.[9] Thus, if Pap test diagnoses are viewed probabilistically, clinicians may act as Bayesian decision makers and use the probability of disease associated with a Bethesda System diagnosis with the pre-Pap test clinical probability of disease to determine the post-Pap test probability of disease. A means to calculate these probabilities involves likelihood ratios (LRs) that may be determined for specific diagnostic terms.[9-13] LRs generally range from 0 to infinity. The higher the LR, the more likely the target disease is present. A LR greater than 1.0 increases the post-test probability of disease compared with the pre-test probability of disease, and a LR less than 1.0 decreases the post-test probability of disease compared with the pre-test probability of disease. If the LR is 1.0 the post-test probability of disease remains the same as the pre-test probability of disease. Most clinicians act only in a quasi-Bayesian sense and do not calculate specific probabilities for each patient, although their thinking remains inherently probabilistic. Determining LRs for Pap test diagnoses illustrates the probabilistic meaning of these diagnoses.

TABLE 5-1

Likelihood Ratios for Three Fictitious Laboratories

| | LABORATORY 1 | | | LABORATORY 2 | | | LABORATORY 3 | | |
	%	SIL Follow-Up (%)	LR	%	SIL Follow-Up (%)	LR	%	SIL Follow-Up (%)	LR
NIL	89	2	0.21	92.2	1	0.18	90.8	3	0.3
ASC–US	7	50	10.3	5	40	11.7	0	—	—
Low-grade SIL	3	90	92.4	2	85	99.6	8	70	22.6
High-grade SIL	1	90	92.4	0.8	95	334	1.2	85	55.0

SIL, Squamous intraepithelial lesion; *NIL,* no evidence of intraepithelial lesion or malignancy; *ASC–US,* atypical squamous cells–undetermined significance.

TABLE 5-2

Diagnostic Schema Using Different Numbers of 'Atypical' Categories

Scheme 1	Scheme 2	Scheme 3	Scheme 4	Scheme 5
Benign	Benign	Benign	Benign	Benign
SIL	ASCUS (uncertain)	ASCUS-1 (probably benign)	ASCUS-1 (probably benign)	ASCUS-x
	SIL	ASCUS-2 (probably SIL)	ASCUS-2 (uncertain)	ASCUS-xi
		SIL	ASCUS-3 (probably SIL)	ASCUS-xj
			SIL	SIL

Example calculations of diagnostic LRs based on the probabilities for specific diagnoses for three fictitious laboratories are shown in Table 5-1. Laboratories 1 and 2 use the ASC category, and laboratory 3 does not. Patient follow-up and LRs for dysplasia for the diagnostic categories of ASC, low-grade SIL, and high-grade SIL for these laboratories also are shown. In laboratories 1 and 2 the LR for dysplasia for the ASC category is greater than 1.0, indicating that the post-test smear probability of a dysplasia is increased compared with the pre-test smear probability of a dysplasia. The percentage increase in post-test smear probability of a dysplasia given an ASC diagnosis is not as high as the percentage increase given a SIL diagnosis. Compared with laboratories 1 and 2, in laboratory 3—which does not use the ASC category—the probability of a dysplasia, given an NIL diagnosis, is higher, and the probability of a dysplasia, given a low-grade SIL or high-grade SIL diagnosis, is lower. In other words the probability of a false-negative diagnosis and a false-positive diagnosis is higher without the ASC category. Another laboratory that eschews the ASC diagnosis could have different results.

These calculations illustrate the probabilistic nature of all Pap test Bethesda System diagnoses. They do not show how, when, or why ASC or AGC diagnoses are made, and these questions have received little attention in the cytologic literature. Theoretically, for Pap tests a spectrum of nondefinitive diagnoses could be used (e.g., atypical, probably benign; atypical, uncertain; atypical, probably SIL), and each would have an LR for dysplasia. In theory, a number of *atypical* or ASC subclassification systems could be used (Table 5-2). One advantage of a multi-tier ASC subclassification system is that each subclass of ASC may be associated with a different probability of disease.[14,15] If these

probabilities are sufficiently different, these ASC subclasses may be clinically useful.[16] The more ASC subcategories used, the greater is the freedom to express shades of uncertainty.[14] One disadvantage of a multi-tier ASC subclassification system is that the subclasses may not be clinically useful and even may be clinically confusing. The appropriate number of ASC diagnostic categories is a matter of contention. The Bethesda Committee recommended subclassification of ASC and AGC diagnoses;[1] ASC subclassification follow-up is discussed on p. 96.

 ## HISTORY OF SQUAMOUS ATYPIA

Cervicovaginal nondefinitive diagnoses have been used since the original Pap classification system.[17-20] In this system, class II smears contained cells with benign atypia; class III smears contained cells suspicious for, but not diagnostic of, cancer; and class IV smears contained cells fairly conclusive of malignancy, although not entirely definitive.[18] Only classes I (benign) and V (malignant) were considered to be definitively diagnostic.[18] As the Pap classification system became outdated, smears were no longer placed into classes, although the concept of atypia remained.

One of the earlier uses of the term *atypia* was for koilocytotic atypia, described by Koss and Durfee (1956)[21] and Ayre (1949).[22] Originally, koilocytotic atypia was thought to be a risk factor for intraepithelial neoplasia and invasive neoplasia.[22] As it became known in the 1970s that koilocytotic atypia was a manifestation of human papillomavirus (HPV) infection and HPV infection itself was a risk factor for invasive neoplasia, the diagnostic term *HPV-change* gradually began to replace the term *koilocytotic atypia.*[23-27] In the Bethesda System, HPV change is incorporated into the diagnostic umbrella of low-grade SIL.[1] However, many pathologists still use the term *koilocytotic atypia,* even though atypia in this sense is *definitive* for HPV infection. This indicates that the concept of atypia still has several uses, is associated with different probabilities of disease, and does not necessarily reflect a high degree of uncertainty.

Large population-based studies of squamous atypia began appearing in the 1960s and 1970s. The earlier of these studies presented follow-up of women with class II Pap smears, which the authors referred to as *atypical.* For example, Hulka showed that 78.7% of women with a class II smear had a dysplasia or invasive cancer on histologic follow-up; however, on subsequent smear follow-up, the majority of women with a class II smear had a class I smear.[28] During these decades, simply following women with class II smears was not considered unusual, even though it was known that women with class II smears could have high-grade dysplasia.[28-31] Stafl and Mattingly showed that of patients with biopsy-diagnosed carcinoma in situ, 21.2% had a class II smear.[32]

Definitions of squamous atypia coupled with large population-based follow-up studies of atypical cervicovaginal smears began to appear in the mid-1970s. These studies are considered to have laid the groundwork for the current conception of ASC. In 1976, Melamed and Flehinger reported follow-up on women who had smears demonstrating squamous atypia that they defined as "minimal but significant abnormality of squamous epithelium not easily attributable to inflammation and thought possibly to represent early neoplastic changes but not suggesting any well defined precancerous lesion."[33] Melamed and Flehinger placed inflammatory atypia in the normal category. In their study population of 78,078 women, 1,973 (2.5%) had an atypical diagnosis, and the risk for these women of developing a more significant disease (dysplasia or cancer) was 9.4%; the probability of a woman with a normal smear to develop a more significant lesion was 1.3%.[33] Melamed and Flehinger did not provide photomicrographs illustrating squamous atypia.

In the *Compendium on Diagnostic Cytology,* Patten discussed and illustrated the concept of squamous atypia.[34] In his opinion of squamous atypia, the squamous cells exhibited cytologic features that fell short of dysplasia and yet were beyond those of reactive change; these features were mainly nuclear, such as nuclear enlargement (twice the nuclear size of an immature metaplastic squamous cell and three times the nuclear size of an intermediate squamous cell).[34-36] Patten thought that atypical squamous cells represented early manifestations of squamous intraepithelial neoplasia.[37] Patten advised that women who had smears with atypical squamous cells should remain under yearly surveillance.[38] Other authors such as Sandmire and colleagues,[39] Beyer-Boon and Verdonk,[40] Hasegawa and colleagues,[41] and Epstein[42] corroborated the data that women with atypical squamous cells are at increased risk to develop a more significant abnormality.

In addition to this early work documenting generic squamous atypia, several subtypes of squamous atypia also were introduced, in addition to koilocytotic atypia. These included atypical repair, atypia associated with atrophy, and atypical squamous metaplasia.

Classic repair involving squamous epithelium is not thought to be associated with an increased risk of neoplasia.[38,43] Several authors have disagreed with this hypothesis.[44] Geirsson and colleagues described the process of atypical epithelial repair, which they subdivided into the following three groups, each having a different incidence of neoplasia on follow-up[45]:

1. The atypical cells retained features of a specific cell line, either glandular or squamous, and the nuclei and nucleoli departed only slightly from normal.
2. The atypical cells did not possess morphologic features of a specific cell line. Most of the cells appeared to be related to immature squamous metaplasia. Marked deviation of nuclear and nucleolar structure was identified.
3. The atypical cells lost all morphologic features indicating the epithelium of origin, with significant nuclear and nucleolar alterations. The morphology depicted in illustrations suggested that these cells originated from squamous epithelium.[45]

The probability of cervical neoplasia associated with the subgroups of atypical repair was as follows: type I, 14%; type II, 22%; and type III, 62%.[36] Within each subgroup of atypical repair, predictability of the severity of the preneoplastic/neoplastic process could not be based on cytologic features. Although the term *atypical repair* was widely used in the pre-Bethesda System era, many cytologists did not use the three categories described by Geirsson and colleagues. Vooijs wrote that moderate atypia, often attributable to repair, should be followed by a repeat smear in 3 months.[46]

The concept of atypia associated with atrophy has long been recognized as a diagnostic conundrum.[8] In atrophy, parabasal cells predominate, and superficial cells are relatively nonexistent or sparse. Parabasal cells have higher nuclear-to-cytoplasmic ratios than intermediate squamous cells, and parabasal cell nuclei normally may be slightly hyperchromatic. The cytologic findings of SIL, particularly low-grade SIL, are not far removed, because SIL cells also have increased nuclear-to-cytoplasmic ratios and nuclear hyperchromasia.[47-50] Consequently, in some cases where a background of atrophy is present, occasional cells show slight nuclear enlargement, nuclear membrane irregularities, and hyperchromasia. Air-drying artifact, characteristic of atrophic smears, may further complicate interpretation. Women who had smears diagnosed as atrophy with squamous atypia were recommended to receive a short course of estrogen therapy followed by a repeat smear.[8,51] Atypical changes resulting from a benign cause theoretically would "resolve" after estrogen stimulation; atypical changes resulting from a pre-neoplastic process would persist and be detected more easily in a background of mature cells.[51]

Immature squamous metaplasia was known to be a pitfall for high-grade SIL in both cytology and surgical pathology.[52] The term *atypical squamous metaplasia* has had several different uses. In cytology, atypical metaplastic cells originally were described as metaplastic cells with nuclear atypia (e.g., nuclear hyperchromasia, membrane irregularity, irregular chromatic clumping, and so on) and increased nuclear-to-cytoplasmic ratios.[36] In the 1980s, it was reported that some patients with atypical squamous metaplasia had intraepithelial precancerous lesions, including cervical intraepithelial neoplasm (CIN) 2 or 3, on follow-up.[53,54] Crum and colleagues also introduced the term *atypical immature metaplasia* to reflect HPV infection in metaplastic cells, although this term has been controversial and not widely adopted.[55]

Thus, before the introduction of the Bethesda System, cytologists used the term *squamous atypia* to mean a number of different entities. The term has meant atypia secondary to reactive changes, subtypes of what is now called *SIL*, changes not diagnostic of either dysplasia or reactive change, or anything that was not considered "normal." Vooijs wrote that the causes of atypia included inflammation, regenerative reactions, deficiency states such as folic acid deficiency, and early neoplastic change.[56] The term *minimal dysplasia* also was used. This term generally meant that the cytologic features exceeded those of benign cellular changes but were not diagnostic of a mild dysplasia. Cytology textbooks, including that published by DeMay in 1995, continued to use the term *minimal dysplasia,* which DeMay included in the atypical squamous cells category.[57] DeMay wrote that these "minimally dysplastic lesions, however, rather than being of undetermined significance, when properly diagnosed, are of reasonably well-determined significance."[57] This statement continued to show the dialectic between expression of diagnostic certainty and the implied uncertainty associated with atypical diagnoses.

In summary, the Bethesda System terms for atypical squamous cells simply have replaced previous terms of *atypia* that had a similar risk of disease.

As mentioned in the introduction, in the earlier Bethesda classification systems, the term *ASCUS,* not *ASC,* was used. Initially, the 1988 Bethesda Committee did not qualify the term *ASCUS,* and this led to considerable confusion among cytologists and clinicians. After the second Bethesda Conference, the term *ASCUS* was defined to mean an epithelial cell abnormality having "cellular changes that are more marked than those attributable to reactive changes but that quantitatively or qualitatively fall short of a definitive diagnosis of squamous intraepithelial lesion."[1] The 1991 Bethesda Committee further wrote that "because the cellular changes in the ASCUS category may reflect an exuberant benign change or a potentially serious lesion, which cannot be unequivocally classified, they are interpreted as being of undetermined significance."[1] The 1991 Bethesda System criteria of ASCUS

are shown in Box 5-1, and 12 illustrations of ASCUS were shown in *The Bethesda System for Reporting Cervical/Vaginal Cytologic Diagnoses.*[1] No references were provided, although this conception of ASCUS was similar to Patten's conception of squamous atypia. A major benefit of the introduction of the term *ASCUS* was to codify the term *atypia* across laboratories.

Lesions classified as ASCUS were thought to lack sufficient features for a definitive benign or SIL diagnosis. This was a different view of atypia compared with some earlier, pre-Bethesda System views that tended to conceive of atypia as a pre–pre-neoplastic lesion (i.e., an early manifestation of dysplasia). The Bethesda view of squamous atypia was that a SIL may be present, although the criteria were not sufficient to make a SIL diagnosis. This concept was more risk-of-disease–centered than previously held concepts.

The 1991 Bethesda Committee recommended that ASCUS diagnoses be further qualified, if possible, into the categories of *favor reactive* and *favor SIL.*[1] This suggestion was affirmed by an International Academy of Cytology Task Force.[58] For those laboratories that further subclassified ASCUS using these terms, a third category of not otherwise specified (NOS) was sometimes added. Thus, this classification system was similar to the three-tier system discussed previously.

In *The Bethesda System for Reporting Cervical/Vaginal Cytologic Diagnoses,* explanatory notes and diagnostic problems associated with the ASCUS term were presented.[1] ASCUS was a diagnosis of exclusion for cytopathologic findings that were not sufficiently clear to permit a more specific diagnosis. Again without reference, the 1991 Bethesda Committee wrote that the laboratory ASCUS rate should not be greater than two to three times the SIL rate,[1] and Kurman, a member of the 1991 Bethesda Committee, and co-authors repeated this recommendation.[59] This statement influenced cytology laboratories to introduce the measure of an ASCUS:SIL ratio. In a College of American Pathologists Interlaboratory Comparison Program in Cervical Vaginal Cytology, Davey and colleagues reported that 97% of laboratories used the term *ASCUS* in 1997 and more than 80% of laboratories used the Bethesda System criteria for ASCUS.[60] The median laboratory ASCUS rate was 4.5%,[60] and in high-risk laboratories the ASCUS rate may be three times higher.[61] In 1996, Davey and colleagues reported that the mean ASCUS:SIL ratio was 2.3, with 80% of laboratories reporting ratios between 0.64 and 4.23.[60] The ASCUS:SIL ratio for individual cytopathologists also varied within laboratories.[62] Median laboratory ASCUS rates and ASCUS:SIL ratios increased from 1993 to 1996.[60] Using threshold analysis, Renshaw and colleagues reported variation in the sensitivity and specificity of observers using the ASCUS category.[63] The Bethesda Committee acknowledged that cytologists would use the term *ASCUS* differently.[1] Assuming a constant ASCUS rate and 50 million women per year having a Pap test, the total number of ASCUS diagnoses from 1990 to 2000 was 20 million.[64]

The 1991 Bethesda Committee wrote that *ASCUS* was not synonymous with the previously used terms of *atypia, benign atypia, inflammatory atypia,* or *reactive atypia,* which were classified as *reactive cellular changes.*[1] Sparsity of abnormal cells and artifacts such as air-drying contributed to making a diagnosis of ASCUS.[1]

BOX 5-1 | CMF

Bethesda System Cytomorphologic Features of Atypical Squamous Cells of Undetermined Significance

Nuclear enlargement is 2.5 to 3 times that of a normal intermediate squamous cell nucleus, with a slight increase in the nuclear-to-cytoplasmic ratio.

Variation in nuclear size and shape and binucleation may be observed.

Mild hyperchromasia may be present, but the chromatin remains evenly distributed without granularity.

Nuclear outlines usually are smooth and regular; very limited irregularity may be observed.

Several authors have pointed out that a woman cannot truly have an ASCUS lesion, and she will have either a SIL/cancer or a benign lesion on follow-up.[8,57] Thus, *ASCUS* exists only as a diagnostic term.

 ## DEFINITION OF ATYPICAL SQUAMOUS CELLS

The term *ASC* was created by the 2001 Bethesda Committee.[2] The definition of ASC essentially is the same as the definition of ASCUS. In the late 1980s and early 1990s, clinical management was closely linked to identifying all cases of SIL; all grades of SIL represented precursors that required colposcopy and treatment.[2] Thus, in the earlier Bethesda System classifications, ASCUS was a generic category that simply defined lesions that could not be classified as SIL. Currently, it is recognized that most low-grade SILs represent a self-limited HPV infection,[65] and the emphasis of clinical management is the detection and treatment of high-grade disease.[2] Thus, the 2001 Bethesda Committee emphasized the subcategorization of the term *ASC* to illustrate the difference between probabilities of low-grade and high-grade lesions.[2] The 2001 Bethesda Committee recommended eschewing the terms *favor reactive* and *favor SIL,* because all ASC was considered to be suggestive of SIL. The 2001 Bethesda Committee recommended that pathologists should "judiciously downgrade" a portion of cases previously interpreted as ASCUS.[2] ASC is not a diagnosis of exclusion.

It should be noted that the category of ASC (like the ASCUS category) is controversial,[66-68] and not all cytologists use this category. At the 2001 Bethesda workshop, a minority of participants argued for the elimination of ASC. One argument supporting this view is that the lesions currently diagnosed as ASC could be effectively classified into either the negative for intraepithelial lesion or malignancy (NIL) or SIL category. Raab showed that it could be cost effective to eliminate the ASC category if more than 70% of cases currently diagnosed as ASC were effectively reclassified.[69] Opposition to the elimination of ASC is based mainly on the belief that more errors (either false negatives or false positives) would occur.[69] The 2001 Bethesda Committee chose to maintain the use of an ASC category.

Subtypes of Atypical Squamous Cells

The 2001 Bethesda Committee recommended subclassifying ASC into two categories: atypical squamous cells-undetermined significance (ASC–US) and atypical squamous cells-cannot exclude high-grade SIL (ASC–H).[2] The category of ASC–US represents the majority of cases previously called *ASCUS;* the ASC–H category represents 5% to 10% of cases previously called ASCUS.[2,70-72] These two ASC categories were defined by studies showing different follow-up probabilities of disease. ASC–US cases are suggestive of low-grade SIL, although the qualifier of *undetermined significance* was retained to emphasize that some cases of ASC–US are associated with underlying CIN 2 or 3.[2] ASC–H cases are suggestive of high-grade SIL and its mimics.[2] In practice, all ASC cases may be subcategorized along morphologic lines, and ASC–H represents just one category. The other subcategories have been variably described and are discussed in the

following section to provide a framework for the making of ASC interpretations. (Thus, some of these subcategories generally are not used in day-to-day practice.) For each of these subcategories, the differential diagnosis includes benign entities (see Chapter 4) and neoplastic or pre-neoplastic entities (see Chapter 6). The criteria presented in the following section were described by the 1991 Bethesda Committee and subsequent publications by members of that Committee and additional researchers.

Subtypes of Atypical Squamous Cells–Undetermined Significance

Minimal Dysplasia or Changes Suggestive of Mild Dysplasia

The 1991 Bethesda Committee wrote that this subgroup is the most common of all the subtypes.[1] The cytologic differential diagnosis is benign (often reactive change) and mild dysplasia. The 1991 Bethesda System diagnostic criteria for ASCUS outlined in Box 5-1 essentially describe this entity. For comparison, the cytologic features of reactive change are presented in Box 5-2, and the cytologic features of low-grade SIL are shown in Box 5-3. This ASC–US subcategory is used if the cytologic features fall qualitatively short of low-grade SIL or if an insufficient number of cells indicative of a low-grade SIL are present. Hall and colleagues reported that the number of atypical cells present on the smear correlated with the probability of SIL on biopsy tissue.[73] The criteria in Box 5-1 are based on the qualitative diagnosis of this subcategory. In a case of this ASC–US subcategory, the squamous cell nuclei are slightly enlarged and possess smooth or slightly irregular nuclear membranes. DeMay reported that the average nuclear size of an atypical squamous cell nucleus was 100 μm^2, and the range of size was 70 μm^2 to 120 μm^2.[57] For comparison, Patten reported that the mean size of a mildly dysplastic cell nucleus was 165 μm^2, with a range of 120 μm^2 to 210 μm^2.[36] The chromatin is finely granular or mildly hyperchromatic. Thus, the nuclei have been interpreted as hypochromatic rather than hyperchromatic. Abu-Jawdeh and colleagues reported that coarse chromatin was the most important predictor of SIL in atypical squamous cell cases in which a SIL was found on follow-up.[74] Nucleoli are absent or inconspicuous, indicating that the cells should not be viewed as reactive in nature. The nuclear-to-cytoplasmic ratio is very slightly increased, although in contrast to a definitively mildly dysplastic cell, the nuclear-to-cytoplasmic ratio is lower. Thus, the nuclear-to-cytoplasmic ratio is generally less than 3:1. The cytoplasm is blue to pink to orange and essentially normal or reactive in appearance. In contrast, the cytoplasm of a mildly dysplastic cell has a slightly immature appearance. Figures 5-1 to 5-4 illustrate this ASC–US subtype. For comparison, Figures 5-5 and 5-6 show examples of low-grade SIL (CIN 1). If a large amount of acute inflammation is present, the changes may be reactive rather than possibly pre-neoplastic (i.e., an ASC–US diagnosis may not be warranted).

Changes Suggestive of Human Papillomavirus

This subcategory of ASC–US is perhaps the second most commonly used subcategory, and the differential diagnosis is between a low-grade SIL (secondary to HPV [last line of Box 5-2]) and reactive change due to a number of conditions, such as *Candida* infection or *Trichomonas vagi-*

BOX 5-2   CMF

Cytomorphologic Features of Reactive Changes with Inflammation

Nuclear enlargement is minimal (1.5 to 2 times the area of a normal intermediate squamous cell).

Occasional binucleation or multinucleation occurs.

Mild hyperchromasia may be present, but the chromatin structure and distribution remain uniformly finely granular.

Nuclear degeneration may result in karyopyknosis and karyorrhexis.

Nuclear outlines are smooth, rounded, and uniform.

Prominent single or multiple nucleoli are present.

The cytoplasm may show polychromasia, vacuolization, or perinuclear halos without peripheral thickening.

In typical repair the cells occur in flat, monolayer sheets with maintenance of nuclear polarity and typical mitotic figures; single cells with nuclear change are not seen.

BOX 5-3   CMF

Cytomorphologic Features of Low-Grade Squamous Intraepithelial Lesion

Cells occur singly or in sheets.

Nuclear abnormalities are generally confined to cells with mature or superficial-type cytoplasm.

Nuclear enlargement is at least three times the area of normal intermediate nuclei, resulting in an increased nuclear-to-cytoplasmic ratio.

Moderate variation is seen in nuclear size and shape.

Binucleation or multinucleation occurs.

Hyperchromasia is present, and the chromatin is uniformly distributed; alternatively, the chromatin may appear degenerated or smudged if associated with the cytopathic changes of human papillomavirus (HPV).

Nucleoli are rarely present or inconspicuous if present.

Nuclear membranes are either visible with slight irregularities or may be completely unapparent when the chromatin is smudged.

Distinct cell borders are present.

Cells that demonstrate a well-defined, optically clear perinuclear cavity and a peripheral dense rim of cytoplasm also must show the above nuclear abnormalities to be diagnostic of low-grade squamous intraepithelial lesion (SIL); perinuclear halos in the absence of nuclear abnormalities do not qualify for the diagnosis.

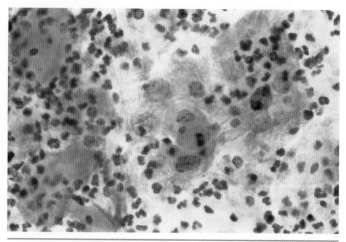

Figure 5-1 **Atypical squamous cells-undetermined significance (ASC–US) in a 35-year old woman.** Marked acute inflammation is admixed with intermediate squamous cells. The cells in the center show nuclear enlargement, slight nuclear hyperchromasia, and a slight increase in the nuclear-to-cytoplasmic ratio. The nuclear membranes also are slightly irregular in shape, although the nuclei are somewhat degenerated. The atypical squamous cells in this case may be representative of a cervical intraepithelial neoplasm (CIN 1), although reactive change cannot be completely excluded. (Papanicolaou [Pap])

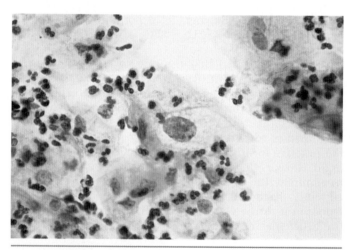

Figure 5-2 **ASC–US in a 24-year-old woman.** A single, large atypical squamous cell is seen in the center. This cell has a slightly enlarged nucleus, although the nucleus is not quite the size of most low-grade squamous intraepithelial lesion (SIL) nuclei. The nucleus also is somewhat hyperchromatic and shows mild irregularities in the nuclear membrane. Marked acute inflammation also is present. Similar to the Pap test seen in Figure 5-1, this cell may be representative of a low-grade SIL (CIN 1), although atypia from inflammatory change also cannot be completely excluded. (Pap)

nalis. Cytologic features of HPV are a well-defined, optically clear, perinuclear cavity; a peripheral rim of thickened cytoplasm; and nuclear atypia (e.g., hyperchromasia, irregular nuclear membranes, nuclear enlargement, nuclear pyknosis, etc.). Cells that display some but not all of these features may be classified as ASC–US. Thus, this ASC–US subcategory mainly is used for Pap tests containing cells with mild nuclear atypia and perinuclear clearing. The Bethesda Committee wrote that cytoplasmic vacuolization alone, without the nuclear atypia, is considered

a benign cellular change and should not be used as a feature of ASC–US.[1] Figures 5-7 through 5-10 show cytologic features of this ASC–US subgroup. For comparison, Figures 5-11 and 5-12 show examples of low-grade SIL (HPV). If only a few cells exhibit changes suggestive of HPV, an ASC–US diagnosis may be used rather than an outright low-grade SIL diagnosis. An example of this would be a case with rare cells showing changes suggestive of HPV in a background of marked acute inflammation and *Candida* organisms.

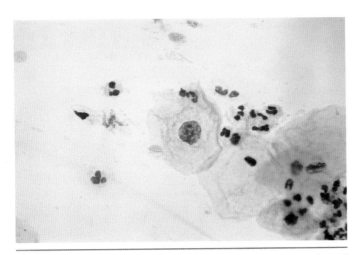

Figure 5-3 **ASC–US in a 42-year-old woman.** A single cell with an enlarged nucleus is seen in the center. Compared with the intermediate squamous cell nuclei seen at the edge, the nucleus is approximately three times the size. However, the nuclear-to-cytoplasmic ratio is not markedly increased, and the cytoplasm shows a slightly immature appearance. The differential diagnosis includes a low-grade SIL (CIN 1). (Pap)

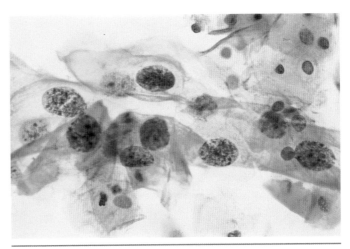

Figure 5-5 **Low-grade SIL in a 24-year-old woman.** In low-grade SIL, the cells occur singly and in sheets, and the nuclear enlargement is at least three times the area of a normal intermediate squamous cell nucleus. The nuclear-to-cytoplasmic ratio is increased, and moderate variation is seen in nuclear size and shape. Hyperchromasia is uniformly distributed, and the nuclear membranes show slight irregularities. In contrast to the cells depicted in Figures 5-1 through 5-4, the low-grade SIL cells shown here demonstrate greater nuclear enlargement, higher nuclear-to-cytoplasmic ratios, and more marked nuclear hyperchromasia. (Pap)

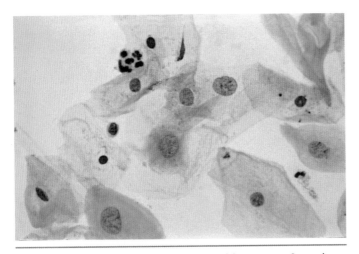

Figure 5-4 **ASC–US in a 20-year-old woman.** Several enlarged squamous cell nuclei are present. These nuclei are approximately three times the size of intermediate squamous cell nuclei and show slight hyperchromasia and irregular chromatin clumping. However, the hyperchromasia is not sufficient for a diagnosis of a low-grade SIL (CIN 1). A relative absence of inflammation is noted in this case, indicating that reactive change is less likely. (Pap)

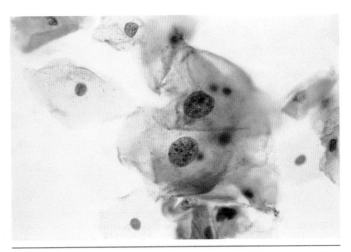

Figure 5-6 **Low-grade SIL in a 37-year-old woman.** Two low-grade SIL cells are seen in the center of the field. These cells show nuclear hyperchromasia and slight nuclear membrane irregularities. The nuclei are at least three times the size of intermediate squamous cell nuclei. (Pap)

Atypical Squamous Cells–Cannot Exclude High-Grade Squamous Intraepithelial Lesion

This subcategory of ASC, ASC–H, must be distinguished from benign squamous metaplasia and a high-grade SIL.[75-77] This category is also known as *atypical squamous metaplasia* and is similar to the atypical repair subgroup II described by Geirsson and colleagues.[45] For comparison, the cytologic features of a high-grade SIL are shown in Box 5-4. The cells of ASC–H show nuclear enlargement 1.5 to 2 times the size of a normal squamous metaplastic nucleus or 3 times the area of a normal intermediate squamous cell nucleus.[1] The normal metaplastic cell nucleus

measures 50 μm^2,[36] whereas an atypical metaplastic cell nucleus measures 60 μm^2 to 120 μm^2.[57] The ASC–H category is particularly problematic because the difference in size between a benign metaplastic cell and a high-grade SIL cell generally is slight.[78] Therefore, not a lot of wiggle room is present in an attempt to determine whether an atypical metaplastic cell is benign or pre-neoplastic. The nuclei of ASC–H may be hyperchromatic and have slightly irregular nuclear membranes. The nuclear membranes are more pronounced in a high-grade SIL. Unfortunately, in reactive conditions, benign metaplastic cells may have larger nuclei and greater nuclear membrane irregularity

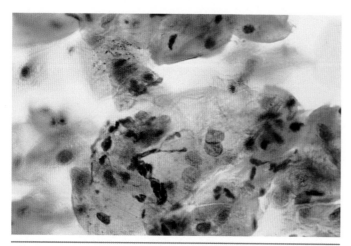

Figure 5-7 ASC–US in a 24-year-old woman. A binucleated cell is seen in the center of the field. This cell shows perinuclear cytoplasmic clearing, although the nuclear-to-cytoplasmic ratio is not markedly increased. The differential diagnosis includes a low-grade SIL, consistent with human papillomavirus (HPV) effect. Although binucleated, this cell does not show the nuclear hyperchromasia typically seen in HPV effect and the nuclear-to-cytoplasmic ratio is larger than expected in HPV effect. (Pap)

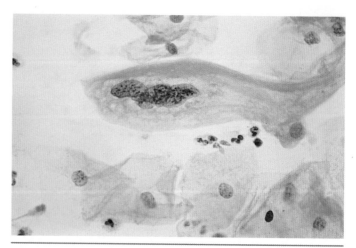

Figure 5-9 ASC–US in a 33-year-old woman. In this case, a single, multinucleated atypical squamous cell is seen. The nuclear-to-cytoplasmic ratio is not markedly increased, although slight cytoplasmic clearing is seen around the nuclei. The nuclei are hyperchromatic and overlapped. The differential diagnosis includes a low-grade SIL (HPV effect), although given the absence of more marked perinuclear halos, the low nuclear-to-cytoplasmic ratio, and the fact that this is the only cell present, a definitive diagnosis of low-grade SIL was not made. (Pap)

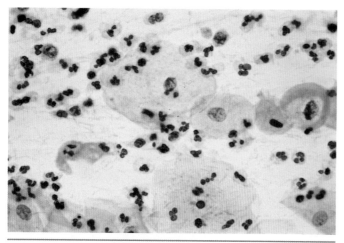

Figure 5-8 ASC–US in a 28-year-old woman. An ASC is seen in the right side of the field. This cell shows slight nuclear enlargement, slight nuclear degeneration, and perinuclear cytoplasmic clearing. In this case, only several cells on the entire Pap test show similar findings, and abundant acute inflammation is present. Thus, the differential diagnosis includes a low-grade SIL (HPV effect) and reactive change, which also may show cytoplasmic clearing. The nucleus does not show the hyperchromasia or the nuclear membrane irregularities typically seen in a low-grade SIL (HPV effect). (Pap)

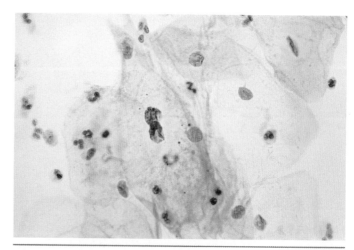

Figure 5-10 ASC–US in an 18-year-old woman. A binucleated squamous cell is seen. The nuclei are hyperchromatic and show overlapping and nuclear membrane irregularities. However, a lack of a cytoplasmic halo is noted, and acute inflammation is seen in the background. Thus, this cell may represent a low-grade SIL (HPV effect) or reactive change. (Pap)

and nuclear hyperchromasia. The cytoplasm of ASC–H cells usually is cyanophilic and occasionally vacuolated. Nucleoli are absent or inconspicuous. In usual squamous metaplasia, the nuclei are small and the cells have rounded outlines and slightly dense homogeneous cytoplasm. DeMay wrote that the nuclear abnormalities are subtle and difficult to distinguish from benign reactive changes on one hand and more advanced dysplasia on the other.[57] Figures 5-13 and 5-14 illustrate the ASC–H category. Figure 5-15 depicts an example of squamous metaplasia, and Figures 5-16 and 5-17 depict examples of high-grade SIL (CIN 3). Similar to the ASC–US subcategories, the diagnosis of ASC–H may be used when the cytologic criteria of a high-grade SIL are present, although the diagnostic cells are too few in number to make a definitive diagnosis.

Other Subtypes of Atypical Squamous Cells

Lesions that fall in these categories may be classified as either ASC–US or ASC–H and generally have not been well described by the Bethesda Committee.

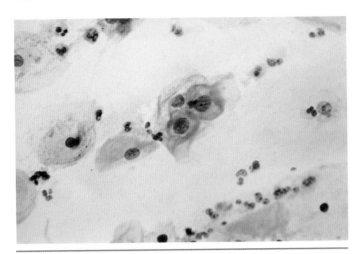

Figure 5-11 Low-grade SIL in a 24-year-old woman. Two cells demonstrate a well-defined, optically clear perinuclear cavity and a peripheral dense rim of cytoplasm. Nuclear abnormalities include nuclear enlargement, variation in nuclear size and shape, nuclear hyperchromasia that is uniformly distributed, and nuclear membranes with slight irregularities. These cells are classic examples of a low-grade SIL (HPV effect). (Pap)

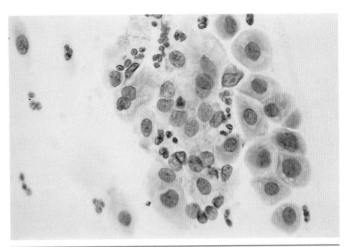

Figure 5-13 Atypical squamous cells–cannot exclude high-grade SIL (ASC–H) in a 29-year-old woman. A group of atypical squamous metaplastic cells is seen. These cells show variation in nuclear size, and the cells with the larger nuclei have relatively high nuclear-to-cytoplasmic ratios. The nuclei are slightly hyperchromatic and show nuclear membrane irregularities. The cytoplasm appears immature. The differential diagnosis includes benign squamous metaplasia and a high-grade SIL. The nuclei are slightly enlarged compared with the nuclei seen in benign squamous metaplasia, although the nuclear-to-cytoplasmic ratio is not quite as high as that seen in a high-grade SIL. (Pap)

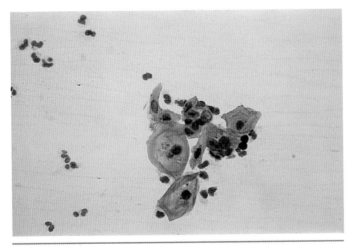

Figure 5-12 Low-grade SIL in a 33-year-old woman. A cluster of cells representative of a low-grade SIL (HPV effect) is present. These cells show perinuclear cavities with peripheral, irregular condensation of the cytoplasm. The nuclei are slightly enlarged and hyperchromatic. (Pap)

BOX 5-4   CMF

Cytomorphologic Features of High-Grade Squamous Intraepithelial Lesions

Cells usually occur singly, in sheets, or in syncytial-like aggregates.

Nuclear abnormalities occur predominantly in squamous cells with *immature,* lacy, and delicate or dense metaplastic cytoplasm; occasionally, the cytoplasm is *mature* and densely keratinized.

Nuclear enlargement is in the range of that seen in low-grade SIL, but the cytoplasmic area is decreased, leading to a marked increase in the nuclear-to-cytoplasmic ratios; the nuclear enlargement may be less than that in low-grade SIL.

High-grade SIL cell size is smaller than that in low-grade SIL.

Hyperchromasia is present, with finely or coarsely granular chromatin.

Nucleoli are generally absent.

Nuclear outlines are irregular.

Atypical Repair

This subcategory of ASC must be distinguished from typical repair and a high-grade SIL or invasive squamous cell carcinoma (SCC); it is used relatively infrequently, although actually may be another example of ASC-H (in addition to atypical squamous metaplasia). This ASC subcategory is similar to the type III atypical repair described by Geirsson and colleagues.[45] The findings of typical repair are presented at the bottom of Box 5-2. In benign repair the cells are seen in monolayer sheets and syncytia, and they contain prominent nucleoli. The chromatin pattern usually is pale, and nuclear membrane irregularities are absent. In those cases in which greater loss of nuclear polarity occurs, anisonucleosis, nuclear hyperchromasia, and irregular chromatin distribution are seen, and an ASC (atypical repair subtype) diagnosis may be rendered.[79] In this ASC subtype, large nucleoli and multiple nucleoli may be present. Greater nuclear membrane irregularities and nuclear rim thickening may be seen. Generally, if groups of atypical repair are admixed with a spectrum of reparative changes, a benign diagnosis is favored. Uniformity of atypical reparative changes favors the diagnosis of ASC. In most cases of atypical repair ASC, a background of acute inflammation is

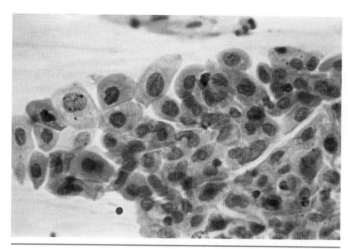

Figure 5-14 ASC–H in a 41-year-old woman. These atypical squamous metaplastic cells show an increased nuclear-to-cytoplasmic ratio, nuclear membrane irregularities, and variable nuclear hyperchromasia. Note that admixed with the atypical metaplastic cells are normal-appearing metaplastic cells with low nuclear-to-cytoplasmic ratios and relatively bland-appearing chromatin. Several of the larger atypical squamous cells show nuclear degeneration and smudging. The differential diagnosis includes a high-grade SIL and benign squamous metaplasia. (Pap)

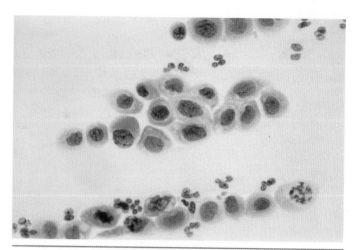

Figure 5-16 High-grade SIL in a 46-year-old woman. In a high-grade SIL, the cells occur singly, and the nuclear abnormalities predominate in immature squamous cells. These cells show lacy or delicate to dense cytoplasm. The nuclear enlargement is in the range of that seen in low-grade SIL, but the cytoplasmic area is decreased, leading to an increase in the nuclear-to-cytoplasmic ratio. The nuclei show hyperchromasia with coarsely granular chromatin. Nucleoli are absent, and the nuclear membranes are irregular. (Pap)

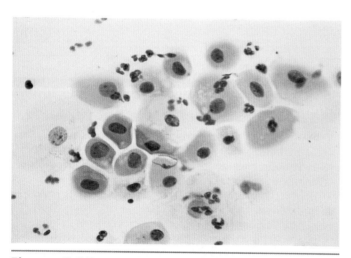

Figure 5-15 Squamous metaplasia in a 41-year-old woman. Benign squamous metaplastic cells are admixed with acute inflammatory cells. The squamous metaplastic cells show low nuclear-to-cytoplasmic ratios and nuclei that measure approximately 50 μm^2. Atypical squamous metaplastic nuclei are larger, ranging in size up to 120 μm^2. The nuclei in benign squamous metaplasia show nuclear hyperchromasia and nuclear membrane irregularities. However, in addition to the lack of marked hyperchromasia, no increase is noted in the nuclear-to-cytoplasmic ratio. (Pap)

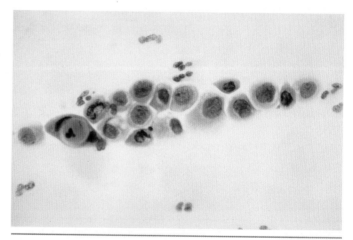

Figure 5-17 High-grade SIL in a 38-year-old woman. In this high-grade SIL, the cells show high nuclear-to-cytoplasmic ratios and nuclear hyperchromasia. Scattered cells show nuclear degeneration. The nuclear membranes are irregular, and the cytoplasm has a hard appearance. (Pap)

seen. Figures 5-18 and 5-19 show this ASC subtype; Figures 5-20 and 5-21 show reactive and reparative changes; and Figures 5-22 and 5-23 show high-grade SIL (CIN 3). In contrast to a high-grade SIL or invasive carcinoma, atypical repair ASC lacks single cells, tumor diathesis, and marked cytologic atypia.

Atypia with Atrophy
This subcategory of ASC is no different than the previously used category of atrophy with atypical squamous cells; it

must be distinguished from a benign atrophy and a SIL (either low- or high-grade) occurring in the setting of atrophy. The Bethesda System cytologic features of atrophy are shown in Box 5-5. Although the parabasal squamous cells seen in atrophy may demonstrate nuclear enlargement and hyperchromasia, the chromatin distribution and nuclear contours should remain uniform. Air-drying may cause artifactual nuclear enlargement in atrophic smears. Characteristic blue blobs also may be present.[80] The 1991 Bethesda Committee wrote that this subcategory should be considered if cells demonstrate (1) nuclear enlargement (at least two times the normal size of parabasal cells), (2) significant nuclear hyperchromasia, (3) irregularities in nu-

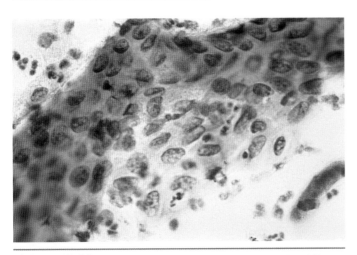

Figure 5-18 **ASC–H in a 44-year-old woman.** The differential diagnosis in this case is repair and a high-grade SIL. The cells show nuclear overlap and nuclear enlargement. Small nucleoli are present. Nuclear membrane thickening is seen, although the chromatin pattern is not markedly hyperchromatic. Nuclear membrane irregularities are pronounced. Inflammation is seen in the background. This is an example of atypical repair. (Pap)

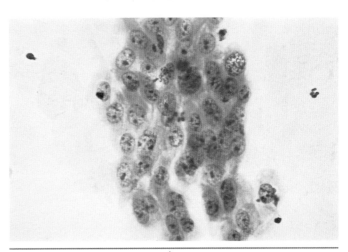

Figure 5-20 **Repair in a 33-year-old woman.** The cells predominantly lie in a flat sheet and show smooth nuclear outlines and single prominent nucleoli. Mild hyperchromasia is seen, although the chromatin structure and distribution remain finely granular. Occasional binucleation is seen. The nuclear enlargement is minimal. (Pap)

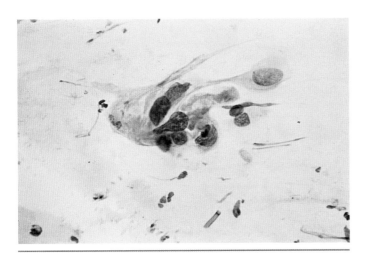

Figure 5-19 **ASC–H in a 32-year-old woman.** The cells show increased nuclear-to-cytoplasmic ratios and nuclear hyperchromasia. Anisonucleosis, nuclear polarity, and irregular chromatin distribution are seen. The differential diagnosis includes a reactive, reparative condition and a high-grade SIL. The nuclei are slightly air-dried, limiting definitive interpretation. (Pap)

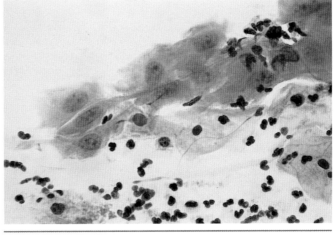

Figure 5-21 **Reparative change in a 37-year-old woman.** A flat sheet of cells showing cytoplasmic polychromasia is seen. The nuclei are centrally placed and generally show a prominent nucleolus. The nuclear membranes are round and smooth, and the chromatin is finely granular. Cytoplasmic extensions are seen along the edge of the cell, and acute inflammation is present in the background. (Pap)

clear chromatin distribution or contour, and (4) marked cellular pleomorphism in the form of tadpole or spindle cells.[1] Abati and colleagues reported that the most reliable cytologic features of pre-neoplastic atypia were nuclear hyperchromasia and irregular nuclear contours.[81] In this setting a short course of estrogen therapy (usually consisting of estrogen cream) followed by a repeat Pap test may be useful.[82] If a SIL is present, the dysplastic cells may be seen more clearly in a background of mature squamous cells. In some cases, atypia may persist, although no diagnostic abnormality may be present. Figures 5-24 and 5-25 show this ASC subcategory, and Figure 5-26 shows a Pap test from a woman after estrogen therapy—with Figure 5-25 demonstrating the Pap test from the same woman before estrogen

therapy. In this case, a maturation of the squamous epithelium is seen, and squamous atypia is no longer present.

Atypical Parakeratosis
This subcategory of ASC must be distinguished from benign parakeratosis (Koss having used the term *pseudoparakeratosis*),[8] HPV change (low-grade SIL),[83] and high-grade SIL (also known as *keratinizing dysplasia*).[84,85] Benign parakeratosis is a form of benign reactive change and is not a Bethesda System epithelial cell abnormality.[1] In parakeratosis, cells are seen in small clusters, and their nuclei are hyperchromatic, eccentrically placed, and generally small and degenerated. The nuclear-to-cytoplasmic ratio is low. The cytoplasm exhibits orangeophilia to cyanophilia, and an

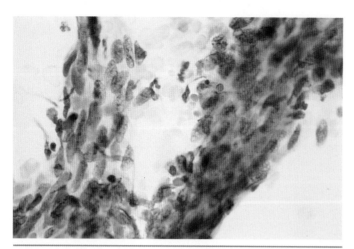

Figure 5-22   **High-grade SIL in a 45-year-old woman.** This high-grade SIL is an example of CIN 3 and shows tight clusters of pre-neoplastic cells with high nuclear-to-cytoplasmic ratios and nuclear overlap. The nuclei are hyperchromatic, and the chromatin is irregularly distributed. Many of the nuclei have a spindled appearance, and these cells most likely represent high-grade SIL in endocervical glands. (Pap)

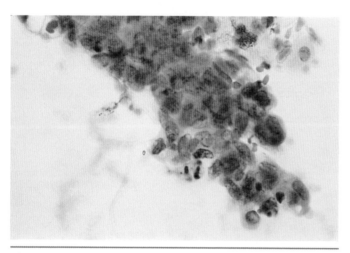

Figure 5-23   **High-grade SIL in a 44-year-old woman.** A three-dimensional group of cells showing high nuclear-to-cytoplasmic ratios and nuclear enlargement is seen. These cells are hyperchromatic and show marked nuclear membrane irregularities. An absence of nucleoli is evident, although slight polychromasia is observed. (Pap)

BOX   5-5   CMF

Bethesda System Cytomorphologic Features of Reactive Cellular Changes Associated with Atrophy with or without Inflammation

Generalized nuclear enlargement is seen in atrophic squamous cells or parabasal-like cells but without significant hyperchromasia.
Autolysis may result in naked nuclei.
Degenerated orangeophilic or eosinophilic parabasal-like cells with nuclear pyknosis resemble parakeratotic cells.
Abundant inflammatory exudate and basophilic granular background are present.
Basophilic amorphous material (blue blobs) may be seen.

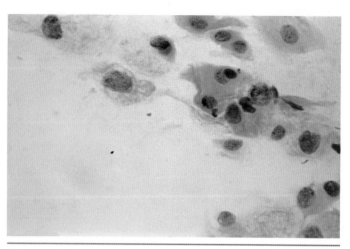

Figure 5-24   **ASC–US in a 68-year-old woman.** Several enlarged cells are seen in a background of atrophy. The majority of cells appear parabasal-like and lack significant hyperchromasia. A cell in the center portion of the field shows nuclear enlargement and slight nuclear hyperchromasia with nuclear membrane irregularities. This cell contains immature, lacy cytoplasm, and the nuclear-to-cytoplasmic ratio is enlarged. The differential diagnosis includes atrophy and a low-grade SIL. (Pap)

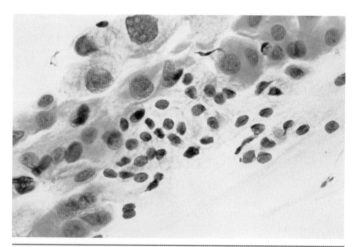

Figure 5-25   **ASC–US in a 58-year-old woman.** In this postmenopausal woman, numerous parabasal-like cells admixed with inflammation are visible in an atrophic background. Several of these cells have enlarged, hyperchromatic nuclei with increased nuclear-to-cytoplasmic ratios. The nuclei also show slight vacuolization and nuclear membrane irregularities. The differential diagnosis includes atrophy and a SIL, either low- or high-grade. (Pap)

inflammatory background usually is present. In the ASC subcategory of atypical parakeratosis, the cells may be seen in three-dimensional clusters and exhibit cellular pleomorphism, with cells having caudate or elongate shapes. In contrast to benign parakeratosis, the nuclei are larger, more hyperchromatic, and more irregular in shape. The nuclear-to-cytoplasmic ratio is increased. These changes previously have been referred to as *dyskaryosis*, a term that is equivalent to *dysplasia*. The cells of an atypical parakeratotic ASC lack the degree of atypia seen in the keratinizing form of high-grade SIL. Definitive features of HPV (low-grade SIL) also are absent. Figures 5-27 and 5-28 illustrate this ASC subtype, and Figure 5-29 depicts parakeratosis.

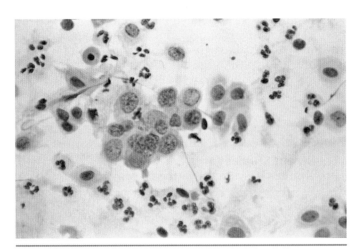

Figure 5-26 High-grade SIL in a 58-year-old woman. This Pap test is from the same woman as the Pap test depicted in Figure 5-25, although this Pap test was taken after estrogen therapy. A cluster of high-grade SIL cells is observed. These cells show high nuclear-to-cytoplasmic ratios, nuclear membrane irregularities, and nuclear hyperchromasia. (Pap)

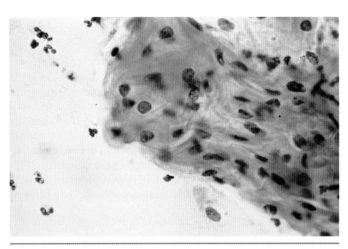

Figure 5-28 ASC–US in a 33-year-old woman. This cluster of cells represents atypical parakeratosis and shows nuclear enlargement, nuclear hyperchromasia, and nuclear membrane irregularities. The differential diagnosis includes a low-grade SIL (consistent with HPV effect) and benign parakeratosis. An absence of perinuclear clearing is present in this case. (Pap)

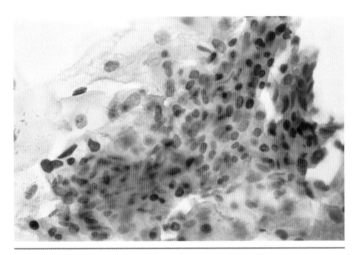

Figure 5-27 ASC–US in a 21-year-old woman. This example of ASC–US represents atypical parakeratosis. In normal parakeratosis the cells are seen in small clusters, and the nuclei are hyperchromatic, eccentrically placed, and generally small and degenerated. In this example, the cells are seen in a three-dimensional cluster and exhibit cellular pleomorphism, with cells having elongate or caudate shapes. The nuclei are larger and more hyperchromatic and exhibit nuclear membrane irregularities. The differential diagnosis includes a low-grade SIL and benign parakeratosis. (Pap)

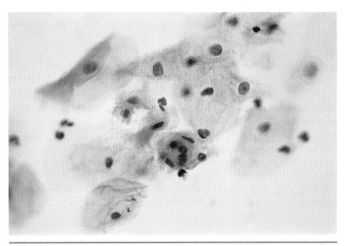

Figure 5-29 Parakeratosis in a 38-year-old woman. A small cluster of cells with hyperchromatic eccentrically placed nuclei is seen. These cells exhibit a degenerated appearance. The nuclear-to-cytoplasmic ratio is relatively low, and the cells appear orangeophilic. An absence of nuclear pleomorphism is evident, and the nuclear-to-cytoplasmic ratio is not markedly increased. (Pap)

Other Types of Atypical Squamous Cells

This category includes lesions that fall between reactive radiation atypia and radiation dysplasia,[86] reactive chemotherapeutic atypia and chemotherapeutic dysplasia,[87] and other benign and pre-neoplastic (or neoplastic) abnormalities (e.g., squamous atypia associated with pregnancy or vitamin deficiency).[88] In the spectrum of benign cellular changes secondary to radiation, squamous cells may exhibit an increased amount of cytoplasm, enlarged nuclei, cytoplasmic vacuolization, and nuclear degeneration (see

Chapter 4). In radiation dysplasia the cells exhibit the classic features of either high- or low-grade SIL (see Chapter 6 and Boxes 5-2 and 5-3). In smears from patients who have undergone radiation therapy, the cells may exhibit a slight increase in nuclear-to-cytoplasmic ratio, greater hyperchromasia, mild nuclear membrane irregularities, and unevenly distributed nuclear chromatin. These changes may be insufficient for a SIL diagnosis but may exceed the changes associated with radiation change alone and are classified as *ASC*. Similar problems may arise in patients undergoing chemotherapy. Figures 5-30 and 5-31 show ASC–US associated with women who have had radiation therapy, and Figure 5-32 shows an example of radiation change.

Follow-Up Studies of Women with an Interpretation of Atypical Squamous Cells

Follow-up studies of women who had a pre-Bethesda System diagnosis of squamous atypia are shown in Table 5-3.[53,54,89-107] These data are somewhat difficult to interpret because of the lack of uniformity of the term *atypia* in laboratory use. For example, some cases of class II (Pap) smears included cases of HPV change and/or dysplasia.[53,106] Nonetheless, these data show that women who had an atypical diagnosis were at increased risk for having or developing a SIL. The probability of having an invasive carcinoma was very small. Although a formal meta-analysis of these data has not been performed, the estimated mean percentage of women having an underlying SIL is about 40%, and approximately 10% of women had a high-grade SIL. Rare cases of invasive SCC after an atypical diagnosis also were reported.[89,99]

Since the introduction of the Bethesda System, a number of ASCUS follow-up studies have been published, and some

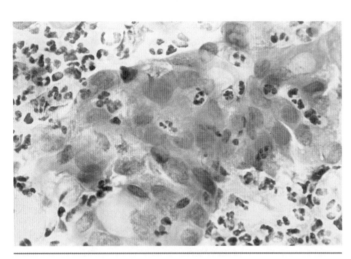

Figure 5-30 ASC–US in a 55-year-old woman status post–radiation therapy. A three-dimensional group of cells with marked acute inflammation is seen. These cells exhibit air-drying artifact and nuclear smudging. The nuclei are enlarged and show increased nuclear-to-cytoplasmic ratios. The nuclear membranes are irregular, and several of the cells show a nucleolus. The differential diagnosis includes radiation change and a low-grade SIL. (Pap)

TABLE 5-3

Follow-Up Studies for Women with a Pre-Bethesda System Diagnosis of Atypia

Reference	Number of Women	Women with SIL (%)	Women with High-Grade SIL (%)
107	104	19.2	9.6
104	86	69.8	46.5
102	429	31.0	14.0
105	110	44.5	25.5
89	46	52.2	37.0
90	214	85.0	61.2
103	97	56.7	8.2
53	236	24.5	4.7
91	406	18.7	7.6
92*	286	26.9	9.1
93	44	81.8	40.9
54	95	—	27.3
94	353	15.6	5.1
51	399	50.6	2.8
96	101	79.2	16.8
97	78	39.7	1.3
98	50	72.0	4.0
99	586	42.8	6.8
100†	31	48.0	16.0
101	336	—	25.3

*Does not include cases of human papillomavirus (HPV).
†Includes only pregnant women.

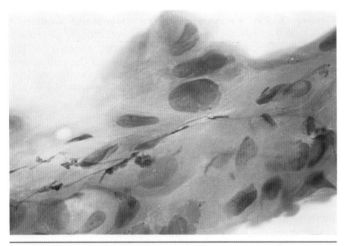

Figure 5-31 ASC–US in a 55-year-old woman status post–radiation therapy. A cluster of cells showing nuclear smudging and polychromasia is observed. Several of the cells show enlarged nuclei with irregular nuclear membranes. The nuclei do not appear markedly hyperchromatic, although the air-drying artifact limits definitive interpretation. The differential diagnosis includes radiation therapy and a low-grade SIL. (Pap)

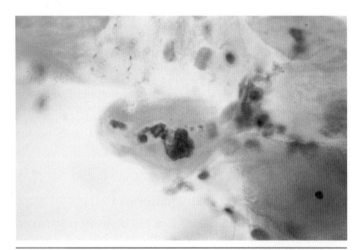

Figure 5-32 Radiation change in a 55-year-old woman status post–radiation therapy. A cell showing radiation change including nuclear smudging, multinucleation, nuclear membrane irregularities, increase in cytoplasmic area, and nuclear pyknosis is seen. (Pap)

of these data are shown in Table 5-4.[62,74,108-155] Similar to the follow-up data of the pre-Bethesda System diagnosis of squamous atypia, these data also are compromised by a lack of agreement of ASCUS use across laboratories. However, in summary, given an ASCUS diagnosis, the percentage of women who have or will develop a SIL is between 15% and 72%. The mean is approximately 50%. The number of women who had or would develop a high-grade SIL has between 1% and 18%, with a mean of approximately 10%. By performing a meta-analysis, Melnikow and colleagues reported that the probability of a high-grade SIL at 24 months was 7.1%.[156] For comparison, 50% to 70% of women who had low-grade SIL smears and 70% to 80% of women who had high-grade SIL smears had biopsy-proven follow-up of a SIL.[157-159] It is interesting to note that essentially the same percentage of women who had a pre-Bethesda System diagnosis of atypia had SIL follow-up as women who had an ASCUS diagnosis. It follows that the introduction of the term *ASCUS* resulted in uniformity of use (i.e., cytologists no longer using a spectrum of atypical diagnoses), but the percentage of women with SIL on follow-up did not change. Ghoussoub and Rimm reported that the type of follow-up (biopsy or repeat smear) influenced rates of SIL; these authors argued that patients with biopsy follow-up had a higher SIL rate, and most studies have not evaluated other parameters (e.g., past history, age, etc.).[160]

Table 5-5 divides studies measuring follow-up of ASCUS subclassification into the categories of favor reactive and favor SIL.* These data support the hypotheses that the diagnosis of ASCUS was heterogeneous (i.e., not all ASCUS diagnoses carrying the same risk of SIL) and that cytologists had some ability to stratify ASCUS cases according to probability of SIL. However, even if a reactive condition was favored, a woman still may have had a SIL, and favoring a SIL was no guarantee that a SIL was present. If a favor reactive diagnosis was made, the probability of a high-grade SIL was low (1% to 4%), and this was the rationale for the elimination of this subcategory in the 2002 Bethesda System.

*References 116, 122, 125, 129, 132, 135, 136, 140, 142, 153, and 162-164.

TABLE 5-4

Follow-Up Studies of Women with Atypical Squamous Cells of Undetermined Significance

Reference	Number of Women	Women with SIL (%)	Women with High-Grade SIL (%)	Reference	Number of Women	Women with SIL (%)	Women with High-Grade SIL (%)
124[a]	82	31.7	4.9	134	284	58.0	9.0
108[a,b]	295	14.0	6.0	126	52	46.2	13.5
109[a]	124	29.1	—	133	224	46.9	3.1
110[a]	63	49.0	14.0	124	223	16.0	2.6
111	31	61.3	3.2	146	203	24.1	8.4
112	271	25.1	11.4	99	452	23.7	12.8
113	159	60.4	9.4	151	995	—	7.3
141	171	16.4	9.9	81[d]	82	9.8	2.4
114	3850	27.0	4.0	128	560	36.3	16.8
115	122	54.9	12.3	148	227	30.0	5.3
116	124	46.0	4.8	129[e]	313	36.4	8.3
74	97	31.0	13.0	154	209	72.0	15.0
143	185	37.8	7.0	136	249	71.8	18.1
117	782	38.2	4.9	147	100	61.0	34.0
118	67	89.6	31.3	130[f]	20	30.0	5.0
144	62	27.4	8.1	116	476	26.9	9.0
119	181	30.9	6.1	153	65	30.8	18.5
120	118	44.9	11.0	138	105	71.4	27.6
140	83	34.9	3.6	139[g]	96	20.8	1.0
142	411	38.2	10.5	131	421	48.2	5.2
135	304	30.3	8.9	155	76	6.0	3.0
145[c]	46	34.8	10.9	132	186	36.6	12.9
121	181	13.3	5.0	150	178	38.2	29.8
122	296	13.5	5.1	149	360	22.2	5.3
123	39	38.5	17.9	152	137	36.4	6.1

[a]Abstract.
[b]Does not include cases of HPV.
[c]Patient population included only those of pediatric age.
[d]Patient population included only those with an initial atrophic smear pattern.
[e]Smears classified as "borderline."
[f]Patient population included only adolescents.
[g]Patient population included only women over age 55.

TABLE 5-5

Atypical Squamous Cells of Undetermined Significance Subclassification Follow-Up Studies

Reference	Number of Smears	PERCENTAGE OF WOMEN WITH FOLLOW-UP SIL OR CARCINOMA (%)			
		Favor Reactive	Not Otherwise Specified	Favor SIL	Favor High-Grade SIL
116	124	39.4	—	53.2	—
135	304	10.7	27.9	36.1	—
140	83	20.9	—	46.5	—
142	411	29.5	26.2	46.5	—
122*	296	—	—	—	60.0
125	452	7.0	21.4	33.1	55.6
163†	66	—	—	—	80.3
128	560	18.3	33.0	52.5	—
162	59	—	—	—	50.8
138	105	48.6	—	83.8	100
147	100	26.9	—	73.0	—
153	13	—	—	—	92.3
132	186	22.2	—	41.1	—
161	126	6.4	—	25.4	—
72	147	—	—	—	61.9

*Sheils and Wilbur used the category of atypical cells of immature metaplastic type instead of favor HGSIL.
†Schoolland and colleagues used the category "inconclusive, possibly high-grade epithelial abnormality."

The last column in Table 5-5 shows the follow-up data of the subclassification of the ASCUS subcategory of atypical squamous metaplasia. As stated previously, this category essentially has been renamed *ASC–H*. The estimated mean percentage of women who had this ASCUS subtype and had a high-grade SIL on follow-up was more than 50%. Using pre-Bethesda System data, Paavonen and colleagues reported that atypical squamous metaplasia had a three times more likely probability of progressing or being a dysplasia than generic squamous atypia.[54] Dressel and Wilbur showed that a SIL or a carcinoma were present in 37% of patients who had a diagnosis of atypical squamous metaplasia.[75] Hatem and Wilbur reviewed 17 cases of negative smears followed by a diagnosis of high-grade SIL.[76] Atypical squamous metaplastic cells were present in 65% of the cases. Thus, because this ASCUS subcategory was associated with a higher risk of a high-grade SIL than the generic ASCUS category, this category was split out (by the 2001 Bethesda Committee) and named *ASC–H*.

Follow-up studies of women with atypia associated with atrophy have shown a relatively low probability of a SIL.[51,137,150] Kaminski and colleagues reported that the probability of a SIL in women older than 50 and a single atypical smear was less than 5%.[51,165,166] Of 37 women who were put on estrogen replacement therapy, 84% had a normal second smear.[51] Of the remaining six patients with a diagnosis of persistent atypia, only one had evidence of HPV on follow-up. Rader and colleagues reported that the incidence of postmenopausal ASCUS was 1.8%; in this population the follow-up SIL rate was 15%, with 57% of women having a follow-up ASCUS diagnosis (with few patients in this study receiving estrogen cream).[139] Symmans and colleagues reported that only 17% of postmenopausal women with atypia had biopsy-proven SIL.[166] In contrast, pediatric patients who have an ASCUS diagnosis had the same risk of having or developing a SIL as the premenopausal adult population.[130,145]

Raab and colleagues showed that the follow-up for patients with an ASCUS diagnosis differed depending on the cytologist.[62] The probability of having or developing a SIL with an ASCUS diagnosis varied from 4.8% to 51.1%, depending on which cytopathologist made the ASCUS diagnosis.[62] This indicates that pathologists have different thresholds for using the ASCUS diagnosis, and the diagnosis of ASCUS confers a different risk of having or developing a SIL.

The more experienced cytologists tended to have moderate to high SIL follow-up probabilities (in the range of 30% to 40%). The less experienced cytologists may have been underusing ASCUS (hence a high SIL follow-up probability) or overusing ASCUS (hence a low SIL follow-up probability). Renshaw and colleagues reported that receiver operating curve analysis may help identify the sensitivity and specificity of ASCUS diagnoses for different cytologists; these data could then be used to alter individual thresholds for the diagnosis of ASCUS.[167]

Several studies have attempted to correlate an ASCUS diagnosis and risk of having a SIL with clinical factors.[51,62,137,165] As has been previously mentioned, the risk of having a SIL is lower in post-menopausal women.[51,62,137,165] Kobelin and colleagues reported that the risk of having a SIL is highest in women who had an ASCUS diagnosis and were under the age of 35;[168] Lousuebsakul and colleagues reported the highest incidence in women less than 25 years old.[131] The significance of this finding is uncertain, because the majority of women who develop invasive cervical cancer are over age 50. Raab and colleagues and Alameda and colleagues reported that the risk of having a SIL did not correlate with a previous diagnosis of SIL or ASCUS.[62,152]

Condel and colleagues examined the probability of a SIL in cases in which the cytotechnologist originally made an ASCUS diagnosis and the pathologists downgraded the diagnosis to benign.[169] Overall, the probability of a SIL was 8.8% and the probability of a high-grade SIL was 4.4%.[169] The probability of a follow-up SIL varied greatly by pathologist, with some pathologists having a probability of a SIL follow-up of 17% and others having a probability of a SIL follow-up of 0%.[169] These data may indicate that some pathologists downgrade too many ASCUS cases and other pathologists downgrade too few. The concept of setting thresholds is controversial, and a satisfactory numbers of "misses" have not been discussed.

Management of Women with Atypical Squamous Cells and Reporting Terminology

Throughout the 1990s, management protocols for women with ASC have varied and have depended on practitioner preference and perceived patient risk. In April 2002 the American Society for Colposcopy and Cervical Pathology (ASCCP) published guidelines on the management of women with cervical cytologic abnormalities, including ASC.[82] Performing immediate colposcopy, repeating the Pap test at specified intervals, HPV DNA testing for high-risk types, or combining a repeat Pap test with an adjunctive method are all acceptable methods used to manage a woman with ASC.[82] Each method has advantages and disadvantages.

An advantage of immediate colposcopy for women with ASC is that it immediately informs the clinician of the presence or absence of disease.[148] This strategy is advocated by some clinicians who believe that it is mandatory to detect and treat the subgroup of women who may have a high-grade SIL. Others question the reasoning behind this argument, given that the reported mean progression time of a carcinoma in situ to an invasive carcinoma is 10 years.[64,170-172] A meta-analysis of colposcopic performance showed that the mean sensitivity of disease detection was 96% and the mean specificity was 48%.[173] The disadvantages of immediate colposcopy include the increased cost, the discomfort that many women experience, and the potential for overdiagnosis and overtreatment. The ASCCP recommended that all women with ASC–H[153,162] and all immunosuppressed women with ASC–US be referred for immediate colposcopy.[82] It should be noted, however, that Holcomb and colleagues reported that human immunodeficiency virus (HIV) infection did not appear to increase the risk of a SIL in women who had an ASC diagnosis.[174] If immediate colposcopy is used to manage women with ASC–US, and CIN is found, these women should be managed according to the 2001 Consensus Guidelines for the Management of Women with Cervical Histological Abnormalities.[82] If CIN is not found, repeat Pap testing should be performed at 12 months.

A program of repeat Pap tests at specified intervals has been the most commonly used method (before HPV DNA testing) to manage women with ASC–US. An advantage of this method is the nonaggressive nature of this management strategy. The repeat Pap test may be taken at 4- to 6-month intervals until two consecutive NIL diagnoses have been obtained.[175-178] Then, a normal screening interval may be resumed. Most women who have a high-grade SIL will be identified on subsequent smears.[64,121] Ferris and colleagues reported that most women preferred a repeat Pap test rather than immediate colposcopy.[179] The threshold for referral of women for colposcopy on a repeat Pap test program is a diagnosis of ASC–US or higher.[70,180,181] Disadvantages for repeat Pap testing include a possible delay in the diagnosis of CIN 2 or 3, the relatively low sensitivity of the Pap test (resulting in false negatives), and the potential loss to follow-up.[82]

The ASCCP stated that HPV DNA testing for high-risk types is the preferred approach for the management of women with ASC–US;[82] HPV DNA testing is not recommended for women with ASC–H. The sensitivity of HPV DNA testing for the detection of histologically confirmed CIN 2 or higher in women with ASC ranges from 0.83 to 1.0,[82,182] and the negative predictive value of HPV DNA testing is greater than 98%. Between 31% and 60% of women with ASC will have high-risk types of HPV identified.[1,183,184] The proportion of women with high-risk HPV decreases with advancing age.[82] The concept of reflex HPV testing indicates that the HPV DNA test should be performed after an ASC–US diagnosis on either a liquid-based sample or a co-collected sample (with a conventional Pap smear). Reflex HPV DNA testing spares a woman from having to return for additional sample collection. Women who test positive for high-risk HPV DNA should be referred for colposcopic evaluation.[70,82,185-187] Women who test negative may receive a repeat Pap test in 12 months. Follow-up for women who test positive for high-risk HPV DNA but do not have a biopsy-confirmed CIN includes repeat Pap testing at 6 to 12 months and HPV DNA testing at 12 months.

The 2001 Bethesda Committee made recommendations regarding ancillary testing (e.g., HPV DNA testing) reporting terminology.[2] Methods of HPV DNA testing include hybrid capture, polymerase chain reaction, and in situ hybridization.[188,189] If HPV DNA testing is used, the results should be reported as positive or negative for HPV DNA of a certain type or class and the specific method of testing should be indicated. The HPV types included in the assay may be listed. If possible, the HPV test result and Pap test result should be reported simultaneously.

Different models used to report HPV DNA testing have been advocated. In the Bethesda System 2001 Workshop, the probabilistic model (reporting the HPV test result in conjunction with the ASC–US diagnosis and a statement of risk) was slightly favored over other models. However, some laboratories prefer other reporting models, and strengths and weaknesses of each model are evident. Several examples of reporting are provided as follows:

As a result only:

Interpretation: ASC–US with detection of high-risk HPV DNA

As a result associated with clinical management recommendations:

Interpretation: ASC–US with detection of high-risk HPV DNA

Recommendation: The ASCCP has recommended that this group of women undergo colposcopic examination. (Wright TC Jr, Cox JT, Massad LS, et al. JAMA 2002; 287:2120-2124.)

As a result plus a probabilistic statement of an underlying CIN 2 or 3 (probabilistic reporting model):

Interpretation: ASC–US with detection of high-risk HPV DNA

NOTE: These findings are associated with a 10% to 20% risk of underlying CIN 2 or higher lesion. (Solomon D et al. J Natl Cancer Inst 2001; 93:243-244.)

As a definitive interpretation that reflects both the cytomorphology and the HPV DNA status (interpretive reporting model):

Interpretation: Low-grade SIL

NOTE: The preliminary cytologic findings are ASC–US. High-risk DNA has been detected. In combination, these results are most consistent with a diagnosis of low-grade SIL.

Despite the ASCCP advocating the use of HPV DNA testing for women with ASC–US, some researchers have argued that the specificity of some methods of HPV DNA testing is too low.[179,190,191] Kaufman and Ferris and colleagues have concluded that HPV testing is of little use to the clinical practitioner.[192,193] The logic behind this conclusion is that if women receive appropriate follow-up examination, a SIL will be detected before it progresses to invasive carcinoma; knowing the HPV status may add little benefit if a pathologic diagnosis is needed before treatment is rendered.

Less aggressive management protocols have been advocated for women who have a diagnosis of ASC–US associated with atrophy.[51,137,165] The ASCCP reported that an acceptable management option is to provide a course of intravaginal estrogen cream followed by a repeat Pap test. This rationale is based on the follow-up studies showing that these women have a relatively low risk of having a SIL, and the majority of women who have a SIL have a low-grade SIL.

Several cost-effectiveness studies examining ASC–US management have been performed. Kim and colleagues reported that HPV DNA testing was more cost effective than other management strategies.[194] Raab and colleagues showed that repeat cervicovaginal smears were a more cost-effective strategy than aggressive strategies involving immediate colposcopy.[64] It should be noted, however, that with less aggressive follow-up strategies, more women would die of cervical cancer. However, the societal cost of the evaluation and treatment of women who had an ASC–US diagnosis would be markedly reduced. Raab and colleagues also demonstrated that with an effective means to triage women into different risk groups (e.g., HPV DNA testing), more aggressive treatment would be cost effective.[64] These results have been corroborated by Melnikow and colleagues and Cecchini and colleagues.[195,196]

In a study measuring clinical (gynecologist and family practitioner) perceptions of an ASC diagnosis, the estimated mean probability of a SIL given an ASC diagnosis was 34% and the mean probability of a high-grade SIL was 3%.[197] Of the clinicians, 33% thought that the probability of a high-grade SIL was 0%. These data indicate that clinicians have widely different views of the probability of a SIL in women who have an ASC diagnosis, and many clinicians underestimate the probability of a high-grade SIL.[197] Baldauf and colleagues reported that patient mismanagement may result in the development of invasive cancer in patients who receive regular cervicovaginal smears.[175,198]

Alternative methods used to manage women with ASC–US have been recommended, particularly outside the United States. These methods include cervicography or simply a repeat Pap test in 12 months. In Europe, less aggressive management methods are recommended. Eskridge and colleagues and August and colleagues recommended that follow-up for women who have an ASC–US diagnosis should consist of cervicography with repeat cervicovaginal smear instead of smear alone or colposcopy.[99,199]

New Cytology Technologies and Atypical Squamous Cells

Two liquid-based manufacturers (ThinPrep [Cytyc, Inc., Boxborough, Mass.] and SurePath [formerly Autocyte; TriPath Imaging, Inc., Burlington, N.C.]) have claimed that preparations using their technologies have less cellular overlapping and obscuring inflammation than conventional smears. Theoretically, one could conclude that fewer ASC diagnoses would be made with the liquid-based technologies because a percentage of ASC cases result from cellular overlapping and obscuring inflammation. A comparison of ASC rates using liquid-based preparations and conventional smears is shown in Table 5-6.[200-216] For ThinPrep, studies have shown either an increase or decrease in the ASC rate. In a meta-analysis of ThinPrep studies, Bernstein and colleagues reported that ThinPrep did not affect the ASC rate compared with the conventional Pap test.[217] An increased ASC rate after implementation of a liquid-based technology may be secondary to inexperience, and it has been hypothesized that the ASC rates would decrease over time after users became accustomed to differences in cellular detail. This has yet to be proved. In some of the ThinPrep studies that showed an increase in the ASC rate, other parameters such as the ASC/SIL ratio decreased. For example, Guidos and Selvaggi reported that the ASC/SIL ratio was reduced by 54% in the ThinPrep cohort compared with the conventional smear cohort.[202]

Authors recently have published follow-up SIL data for an ASC diagnosis using a liquid-based preparation and conventional smear. Weintraub and Morabia reported follow-up rates of a SIL and high-grade SIL in 43% and 22% of ThinPrep specimens and 76% and 44% of conventional specimens; these data indicate that an ASC diagnosis is associated with a higher risk of SIL on conventional smears compared with ThinPrep preparations.[205] It is interesting to note that the SIL follow-up rate after an ASC diagnosis reported by Weintraub and Morabia was higher than the rate reported by most other authors;[205] this suggests that this laboratory's threshold for ASC is different from other laboratories. Vassilakos and colleagues showed similar findings with Autocyte specimens (i.e., a decrease in an ASC diagnosis risk of SIL from 50% to 31% with use of the Autocyte preparation compared with the conventional smear).[207] These data emphasize the importance of multiple variables in any determination of the use of a liquid-based cytology.

The effect of automated rescreening/screening on ASC rates also has been addressed. O'Leary and colleagues showed limited use of PAPNET-assisted rescreening in 5,478 women; in this population, five additional ASCUS cases were identified at a cost of $5,825 per ASCUS diagnosis in 1997.[218] Automated rescreening presumably may be used to triage ASC cases. For example, Lerma and colleagues reported that in a review using PAPNET, 57 of 163 patients with an ASC diagnosis were classified correctly as negative.[219] Kok and colleagues also reported a decrease in ASC rates using PAPNET review.[220] Using the AutoPap System

(TriPath Imaging, Inc., Burlington, N.C.), 88% of ASC cases were ranked in the first three ranks, indicating that these cases would have been flagged for review.[221]

Interobserver Variability for Atypical Squamous Cells

Diagnostic reproducibility has been measured through (1) interobserver and intraobserver variability studies using preselected cases, (2) retrospective review of previously screened cases, and (3) studies measuring the use of ancillary techniques (e.g., HPV testing).[222-224] These studies have been performed over the past decades and thus encompass measurement of both pre-Bethesda System and post-Bethesda System classifications of squamous atypia.

Studies have reported diagnostic reproducibility in terms of percent agreement or the kappa statistic.[9] Crude agreement is the number of cases in which the diagnoses of one cytopathologist is in concordance with the diagnosis of a second cytologist. The kappa statistic is a more sophisticated measure of reproducibility that takes into account the agreement due to chance alone, whereas crude agreement does not. The kappa statistic is commonly reported on a -1.0 to 1.0 scale, with 1.0 representing perfect agreement and 0.0 representing chance agreement.[9] Positive kappa values show a level of agreement beyond chance agreement. Some have reported that kappa values less than 0.50 represent poor agreement; 0.50 to 0.80 represent good agreement, and 0.80 to 1.0 represent excellent agreement. In reproducibility studies it is important to evaluate the potential effect of interobserver disagreement. For example, if disagreement has no impact on clinical care, one could argue that the disagreement is meaningless. Some reproducibility studies have attempted to address this issue by scaling diagnoses (e.g., benign = 0; ASC = 1; and low-grade SIL = 2) and measuring interobserver agreement across different combined diagnoses (e.g., benign contrasted to a combined ASC and low-grade SIL category). Some researchers argue that differences in diagnosis by more than one category have no clinical significance.

In one of the largest pre-Bethesda reproducibility studies ever conducted, two American university laboratories exchanged 20,000 cases—10,000 from each laboratory.[225] These laboratories used the term *minimal dysplasia,* which is interpreted as an ASC–US subcategory. For the minimal dysplasia category used by the first laboratory, the exact agreement with the second laboratory was 9.2%. The second laboratory made a diagnosis of more than "two-steps," compared with the original diagnosis in 47.4% of cases. The second laboratory made a benign diagnosis in 40.1% of cases and a diagnosis of moderate or higher dysplasia in 7.3%. Although kappa statistics were not performed, studies such as this one led investigators to believe that interobserver agreement for the minimal dysplasia category was poor.

In a pre-Bethesda System study examining pre-selected cases, Klinkhamer and colleagues measured intraobserver variability in 19 Dutch observers, including 15 cytotechnologists.[226] Each observer screened 180 smears twice, with an interval of 6 months between screenings. Intraobserver variability differed considerably among different observers. In the grading of squamous or squamous metaplastic abnormalities, an average of 51.5% of the paired diagnoses from individual observers differed by one or more grades between the two screenings. Only 7% of paired observer diagnoses differed by two grades or more. Although this intraobserver disagreement may appear low, the study is

---

TABLE 5-6

Comparison of Atypical Squamous Cells of Undetermined Significance Rates with ThinPrep and AutoCyte against Conventional Smears

Reference	Technology	ASCUS (%)		Increase or (Decrease)	Increase or (Decrease) Per 10,000
		Conventional	Technology		
208	ThinPrep	2.3	2.9	26	61
200*	ThinPrep	3.1	2.4	(22.4)	(69)
201	ThinPrep	4.9	3.8	(23)	(116)
202†	ThinPrep	2.0	3.4	70	140
203	ThinPrep	12.5	6.9	(45)	(560)
204	ThinPrep	4.8	4.5	(4.8)	(23)
205	ThinPrep	1.5	2.4	60	90
211	ThinPrep	3.6	1.7	(53)	(192)
209	ThinPrep	1.5	1.1	(72)	(400)
212	ThinPrep	1.7	2.1	21	42
210	ThinPrep	3.2	2.6	(82)	(68)
213	ThinPrep	13.9	10.8	(23)	(310)
214	ThinPrep	6.3	9.5	34	325
206	AutoCyte	3.7	1.6	(57)	(110)
207	AutoCyte	3.5	1.9	(46)	(160)
215	AutoCyte	1.2	1.3	10	13
216	AutoCyte	3.8	5.5	47	175

*ASCUS neoplastic.
†ASCUS, low-grade SIL not excluded.

somewhat biased by the fact that only 12% of the study cases were originally diagnosed as *atypical squamous, squamous metaplastic cells present,* or *slight dysplasia.*

Because the Bethesda System contains fewer "risk" diagnostic categories compared with other classification systems (e.g., Pap class system), it is generally believed that its implementation has led to better interobserver agreement. The more recent reproducibility studies have focused on expert cytopathologists reviewing preselected cases. In a 1992 interobserver variability study by Sherman and colleagues in which Bethesda System categories were used, two cytopathologists examined 257 smears.[227] In 23.7% of cases, the cytopathologists disagreed by more than two categories. Of cases classified as *ASCUS* by cytopathologist 1, cytopathologist 2 made the diagnosis of benign, ASCUS, low-grade SIL, and high-grade SIL in 14.1%, 53.5%, 26.2%, and 6.1% of cases, respectively. Of cases classified as low-grade SIL by cytopathologist 1, cytopathologist 2 made the diagnosis of ASCUS 23.7% of cases.

More recent studies have supported these results. Young and colleagues circulated 20 slides to five expert cytopathologists in a 1994 study.[228] Of the cases, 16 were considered to be challenging, and exact agreement occurred in only seven cases. No unanimous agreement was made on an ASCUS diagnosis. In a study by Sherman and colleagues reexamining 200 cases originally diagnosed as ASCUS, five pathologists achieved perfect concordance in only 29% of cases.[229] In 9% of cases, none of the pathologists concurred, and in none of the cases did all the pathologists agree with the original ASCUS diagnosis. Sherman and colleagues showed that the detection of high-risk types of HPV DNA correlated strongly with the likelihood of a SIL diagnosis.[229]

In a more recently published Italian study examining an external quality assurance scheme, 110 slides were circulated to practicing cytopathologists. The overall kappa statistic for the pathologists in one laboratory for the diagnosis of ASCUS was 0.71.[230] The overall kappa statistic for the pathologists in this laboratory compared with the pathologists in other laboratories for the diagnosis of ASCUS was 0.33. Genest and colleagues reported that the intraobserver kappa for an ASCUS diagnosis was 0.51 and the interobserver kappa was 0.39.[125] These data indicate poor to average agreement—particularly between laboratories—for the ASCUS category. O'Sullivan and colleagues showed major differences between cytopathologists and nonspecialist pathologists in the grading of cervicovaginal smears; the cytopathologists were more consistent, compared with the nonspecialist pathologists in grading and diagnosing dysplasia.[231-233] Jones and colleagues showed that attendance at a training course and in-depth discussion improved some aspects of interobserver agreement.[234] However, Smith and colleagues reported that review of the *Bethesda System Atlas* did not improve diagnostic reproducibility.[235]

Using data from the Atypical Squamous Cells of Undetermined Significance–Low-Grade Squamous Intraepithelial Lesion Triage Study, Stoler and Schiffman reported moderate kappa values (κ = 0.46) for interpretation of ASCUS and low-grade SIL cases detected on monolayer preparations.[236] Interestingly, this interobserver variability was essentially equivalent to the variability of the interpretation of punch biopsy tissue specimens and loop electrosurgical excision procedure specimens.

 # SUMMARY

ASC is the most commonly used Bethesda System diagnosis for an epithelial cell abnormality. Compared with other Bethesda System epithelial abnormality diagnoses, an ASC–US diagnosis has a lower probability of having a SIL on follow-up. An ASC diagnosis expresses uncertainty that must be interpreted in context of the uncertainties associated with other Bethesda System epithelial abnormality diagnoses. Because of the introduction of the new terms *ASC–US* and *ASC–H* in 2001 and because of the relative novelty of HPV DNA testing for the management of women with ASC–US, data regarding the efficacy of these diagnostic categories and the use of HPV DNA testing are somewhat lacking. Thus, new studies on ASC diagnosis and management are currently being conducted and will affect how this diagnostic category is used.

References

1. Bethesda Committee. The Bethesda System for reporting cervical/vaginal diagnoses. New York: Springer-Verlag; 1994.
2. Solomon D, Davey D, Kurman R, et al. The 2001 Bethesda System terminology for reporting results of cervical cytology. JAMA 2002; 287:2114-2119.
3. Raab SS, Thomas PA, Lenel JC, et al. Pathology and probability: likelihood ratios and receiver operating characteristic curves in the interpretation of bronchial brush specimens. Am J Clin Pathol 1995; 103:588-593.
4. Schwartz WB, Wolfe HJ, Pauker SG. Pathology and probabilities: a new approach to interpreting and reporting biopsies. N Engl J Med 1981; 305:917-923.
5. Bryant GD, Norman GR. Expressions of probability: words and numbers (letter). N Engl J Med 1980; 302:411.
6. Bethesda Committee: The Bethesda System for reporting cervical/vaginal diagnoses. Acta Cytol 1993; 37:115-124.
7. The Bethesda Committee. Current issues: the 1991 Bethesda system for reporting cervical/vaginal diagnoses. Diagn Cytopathol 1993; 9:235-293.
8. Koss LG. Epidermoid carcinoma of the uterine cervix and related precancerous lesions. In: Koss LG, editor. Diagnostic vytology and its histologic basis. 4th ed. Philadelphia: JB Lippincott; 1992. pp.470-473.
9. Sackett DL, Haynes RB, Guyatt GH, et al, editors. Clinical epidemiology: a basic science for clinical medicine. 2nd ed. Boston: Little, Brown; 1991.
10. Giard RW, Hermans J. Interpretation of diagnostic cytology with likelihood ratios. Arch Pathol Lab Med 1990; 114:852-854.
11. Radack KL, Rouan G, Hedges J. The likelihood ratio: an improved measure for reporting and evaluating diagnostic test results. Arch Pathol Lab Med 1986; 110:689-693.
12. Raab SS, Oweity T, Hughes JH, et al. Effect of clinical history on diagnostic accuracy in the cytologic interpretation of bronchial brush specimens. Am J Clin Pathol 2000; 114:78-83.
13. Raab SS. Diagnostic accuracy in cytopathology. Diagn Cytopathol 1994; 10:68-75.
14. Renshaw AA, Genest DR, Cibas ES. Should atypical squamous cells of undetermined significance (ASCUS) be subcategorized? Accuracy analysis of Papanicolaou smears using receiver operating characteristic curves and implications for the ASCUS/squamous intraepithlelial lesion ratio. Am J Clin Pathol 2001; 116:692-695.

15. Pitman MB, Cibas ES, Powers CN, et al. Reducing or eliminating use of the category of atypical squamous cells of undetermined significance decreases the accuracy of the Papanicolaou smear. Cancer 2002; 96:128-134.

16. Raab SS. Subcategorization of Papanicolaou tests diagnosed as atypical squamous cells of undetermined significance. Am J Clin Pathol 2001; 116:631-634.

17. Papanicolaou GN. A survey of the actualities and potentialities of exfoliative cytology in cancer diagnosis. Ann Intern Med 1949; 31:661.

18. Solomon D. Nomenclature for cervicovaginal cytology. Tutor Cytol 1992; 40-43.

19. Reagan JW, Seidemann IL, Saracusa Y. The cellular morphology of carcinoma in situ and dysplasia or atypical hyperplasia of the uterine cervix. Cancer 1953; 6:224.

20. Ishizuka Y, Oota K, Masabuchi K, editors. Practical cytodiagnosis. Internatioanl Academy of Cytology: Chicago; 1972.

21. Koss LG, Durfee GR. Unusual patterns of squamous epithelium of the uterine cervix: cytologic and pathologic study of koilocytotic atypia. Ann NY Acad Sci 1956; 63:1245.

22. Ayre JE. The vaginal smear. "Precancer" cell studies using a modified technique. Am J Obstet Gynecol 1949; 58:1205.

23. Meisels A, Fortin R. Condylomatous lesions of the cervix and vagina. I. Cytologic patterns. Acta Cytol 1976; 20:505.

24. Purola E, Savia E. Cytology of gynecologic condyloma acuminatum. Acta Cytol 1977; 21:26-31.

25. Meisels A, Roy M, Fortier M, et al. Human papillomavirus of the cervix: the atypical condyloma. Acta Cytol 1981; 25:7-16.

26. Fu YS, Reagan JW, Richart RM. Definition of precursors. Gynecol Oncol 1981; 12:S220-231.

27. Crum CP, Fu YS, Levine RU, et al. Intraepithelial squamous lesions of the vulva: biologic and histologic criteria for the distinction of condyloma from vulvar intraepithelial neoplasia. Am J Obstet Gynecol 1982; 144:77-83.

28. Hulka BS. Cytologic and histologic outcome following an atypical cervical smear. Am J Obst Gynecol 1968; 101:190-199.

29. Bettinger HF, Reagan JW. Proceedings of the International Committee on Histologic Terminology for Lesions of the Uterine Cervix. In: Wied GL, editor. Proceedings of the First International Congress on Exfoliative Cytology. Philadelphia: Lippincott-Raven; 1962.

30. Stern E, Neely PM. Carcinoma and dysplasia of the cervix: a comparison of rates for new and returning populations. Acta Cytol 1963; 7:357.

31. Richart RM. The natural history of cervical intraepithelial neoplasia. Clin Obstet Gynecol 1968; 5:748.

32. Stafl A, Mattingly RF. Colposcopic diagnosis of cervical neoplasia. Obstet Gynecol 1973; 41:168-176.

33. Melamed MR, Flehinger BJ. Non-diagnostic squamous atypia in cervico-vaginal cytology as a risk factor for early neoplasia. Acta Cytol 1976; 20:108-110.

34. Patten SF Jr. Benign proliferative reactions of the uterine cervix. In: Wied GL, Koss LG, Reagan JW. Compendium on diagnostic cytology. Tutorials of cytology. Chicago: International Academy of Cytology; 1976. pp.53-60.

35. Patten SF Jr. Female genital tract: diseases of the uterine cervix. In: Keebler CM, Reagan JW, editors. A manual of cytotechnology. Chicago: American Society of Clinical Pathologists; 1975. pp.81-101.

36. Patten SF Jr. Diagnostic cytopathology of the uterine cervix. Monographs in clinical cytology. 2nd ed., vol. 3. New York: S Karger; 1978. pp.92-114.

37. Patten SF. Benign proliferative reactions and squamous atypia of the uterine cervix. Compendium on diagnostic cytology. Tutorials of cytology. 6th ed. Chicago: International Academy of Cytology; 1992. pp.77-81.

38. Patten SF. Benign proliferative reactions of the uterine cervix. In: Wied GL, Keebler CM, Koss LG, et al, editors. Compendium on diagnostic cytology. Tutorials of cytology. 6th ed. Chicago: International Academy of Cytology; 1988. pp.83-87.

39. Sandmire HF, Austin SD, Bechtel RC. Experience with 40,000 Papanicolaou smears. Obstet Gynecol 1976; 48:56-60.

40. Beyer-Boon ME, Verdonk GW. The identification of atypical reserve cells in smears of patients with premalignant and malignant changes in the squamous and glandular epithelium of the uterine cervix. Acta Cytol 1978; 22:305-311.

41. Hasegawa T, Tsutsui F, Kurihara S. Cytomorphologic study on the atypical cells following cryosurgery for the treatment of chronic cervicitis. Acta Cytol 1975; 19:533-537.

42. Epstein NA. The significance of cellular atypia in the diagnosis of malignancy in ulcers of the female genital tract. Acta Cytol 1972; 16:483-489.

43. Bibbo M, Keebler CM, Wied GL. The cytologic diagnosis of tissue repair in the female genital tract. Acta Cytol 1971; 15:133-137.

44. Sidawy MK, Tabbara SD. Reactive change and atypical squamous cells of undetermined significance in Papanicolaou smears: a cytohistologic correlation. Diagn Cytopathol 1994; 11:343-347.

45. Geirsson G, Woodworth FE, Patten SF, et al. Epithelial repair and regeneration in the uterine cervix I. An analysis of the cells. Acta Cytol 1977; 21:371-378.

46. Vooijs GP. Significance of cellular composition of smears for the reliability of cytological diagnoses. In: Goertler K, Feichter GE, Witte S, editors. New frontiers in cytology: modern aspects of research and practice. Berlin: Springer-Verlag; 1988. pp.412-420.

47. Buckley CH, Butler EB, Fox H. Cervical intraepithelial neoplasia. J Clin Pathol 1982; 35:1-13.

48. Koike N, Kasamatsu T. Efficacy of the cytobrush method in aged patients. Diagn Cytopathol 1994; 10:311-314.

49. Buckley CH, Herbert A. Johnson J, et al. Borderline nuclear changes in cervical smears: guidelines on their recognition and management. J Clin Pathol 1994; 47:481-492.

50. Ambros RA, Kurman RJ. Current concepts in the relationship of human papillomavirus infection to the pathogenesis and classification of precancerous squamous lesions of the uterine cervix. Semin Diagn Pathol 1990; 7:158-172.

51. Kaminski PF, Sorosky JI, Wheelock JB, et al. The significance of atypical cervical cytology in an older population. Obstet Gynecol 1989; 73:13-15.

52. Wright TC, Kurman RJ, Ferenczy A. Precancerous lesions of the cervix. In: Kurman RJ, editor: Blaustein's pathology of the female genital tract. New York: Springer-Verlag; 1994. pp.229-277.

53. Jones DED, Creasman WT, Dombroski RA, et al. Evaluation of the atypical Pap smear. Am J Obstet Gynecol 1987; 157:544-549.

54. Paavonen J, Kiviat NB, Wölner-Hanssen P, et al. Significance of mild cervical cytologic atypia in a sexually transmitted disease clinic population. Acta Cytol 1989; 33:831-838.

55. Crum CP, Egawa K, Fu YS, et al. Atypical immature metaplasia (AIM): a subset of human papillomavirus infection of the cervix. Cancer 1983; 51:2214-2219.

56. Vooijs GP. Benign proliferative reactions, intraepithelial neoplasia and invasive carcinoma of the uterine cervix. In: Bibbo M, editor. Comprehensive cytopathology, Philadelphia: WB Saunders; 1991. pp.153-230.

57. DeMay RM. The Pap smear. In: DeMay RM, editor: The art and science of cytopathology. Chicago: ASCP Press; 1995. pp.61-205.

58. Solomon D, Frable WJ, Vooijs GP, et al. ASCUS and AGUS criteria—International Academy of Cytology Task Force Summary: diagnostic cytology towards the 21st century: an international expert conference and tutorial. Acta Cytol 1998; 42:16-24.

59. Kurman RJ, Henson DE, Herbst AL, et al. Interim guidelines for management of abnormal cervical cytology: the 1992 National Cancer Workshop Institute. JAMA 1994; 271:1866-1869.

60. Davey DD, Woodhouse S, Styer P, Stastny J, Mody D. Atypical epithelial cells and specimen adequacy: current laboratory practices of participants in the College of American Pathologists interlaboratory comparison program in cervicovaginal cytology. Arch Pathol Lab Med 2000; 124:203-211.

61. Hudock J, Hanau CA, Hawthorne C, et al. Predictors of human papilloma virus in patients with keratinization. Diagn Cytopathol 1995; 12:28-31.

62. Raab SS, Bishop S, Zaleski S. Long-term outcome and relative risk in women with atypical squamous cells of undetermined significance. Am J Clin Pathol 1999; 112:57-62.

63. Renshaw AA, Lee KR, Granter SR. Use of statistical analysis of cytologic interpretation to determine the causes of interobserver disagreement and in quality improvement. Cancer 1997; 81:212-219.

64. Raab SS, Steiner AL, Hornberger J. The cost-effectiveness of treating women with a cervical vaginal smear diagnosis of atypical squamous cells of undetermined significance. Am J Obstet Gynecol 1998; 179:411-420.

65. Ho GY, Bierman R, Beardsley L, Chang CJ, Burk RD. Natural history of cervicovaginal papillomavirus infection in young women. N Engl J Med 1998; 338:423-428.

66. Frable WJ. ASCUS! ASCUS! Down the rabbit hole. Cancer Cytopathol 1999; 319-321.

67. Robb JA. The "ASCUS" swamp. Diagn Cytopathol 1994; 11:319-320.

68. Frable WJ. A rationale for the elimination of the use of ASCUS. Uncertainty in Gynecologic Cytology. Papanicolaou Society of Cytopathology Companion Meeting of the United States and Canadian Academy of Pathology Meeting, March 25, 2000.

69. Raab SS. Should the category of atypical squamous cells of undetermined significance (ASCUS) be eliminated? Mod Pathol 2000; 13:41 (abstract).

70. Solomon D, Schiffman M, Tarone R, for ALTS Group. Comparison of three management strategies for patients with atypical squamous cells of undetermined significance: baseline results from randomized trial. J Natl Cancer Inst 2001; 93:293-299.

71. Sherman ME, Solomon D, Schiffman M, for the ALTS Group. Qualification of ASCUS: a comparison of equivocal LSIL and equivocal HSIL cervical cytology in the ASCUS LSIL Triage Study. Am J Clin Pathol 2001; 116:386-394.

72. Quddus MR, Sung CJ, Steinhoff MM, et al. Atypical squamous metaplastic cells: reproducibility, outcome, and diagnostic features on ThinPrep Pap test. Cancer 2001; 93:16-22.

73. Hall S, Wu TC, Soudi N, et al. Low-grade squamous intraepithelial lesions: cytologic predictors of biopsy confirmation. Diagn Cytopathol 1994; 10:3-9.

74. Abu-Jawdeh GM, Trawinski G, Wang HH. Histocytological study of squamous atypia on Pap smears. Mod Pathol 1994; 7:920-924.

75. Dressel DM, Wilbur DC. Atypical immature squamous metaplastic cells in cervical smears: association with high-grade squamous intraepithelial lesions and carcinoma of the cervix. Acta Cytol 1992; 36:630.

76. Hatem F, Wilbur DC. High-grade squamous cervical lesions following negative Papanicolaou smears: false-negative cervical cytology or rapid progression. Diagn Cytopathol 1995; 12:135-141.

77. Wilbur DC, Bonfiglio TA. Editorial comment: atypical squamous cells in cervical smears—resolving a controversy. Diagn Cytopathol 1993: 9:429.

78. Gupta DK, Komaromy-Hiller G, Raab SS, et al. Interobserver and intraobserver variability in the cytologic diagnosis of normal and abnormal metaplastic squamous cells in Pap smears. Acta Cytol 2001; 45:697-703.

79. Crum CP, Cibas ES, Lee KR. Nondiagnostic squamous atypia. In: Crum CP, Cibas ES, Lee KR, editors. Pathology of early cervical neoplasia. New York: Churchill Livingstone; 1997. pp.139-175.

80. Ziabkowski TA, Naylor B. Cyanophilic bodies in cervicovaginal smears. Acta Cytol 1976; 20:340-342.

81. Abati A, Jaffurs W, Wilder AM. Squamous atypia in the atrophic cervical vaginal smear. Cancer Cytopathol 1998; 84:218-225.

82. Wright TC, Cox JT, Massad LS, et al. 2001 consensus guidelines for the management of women with cervical cytological abnormalities. JAMA 2002; 287:2120-2129.

83. Meisels A, Morin C. Human papillomavirus induced changes. In: Meisels A, Morin C, editors. Cytopathology of the uterine cervix. Chicago: American Society of Clinical Pathology, ASCP Press; 1990. pp.73-117.

84. Saito K, Saito A, Fu YS, et al. Topographic study of cervical condyloma and intraepithelial neoplasia. Cancer 1987; 59:2064-2070.

85. McLachlin CM, Shen L, Crum CP. High-grade cervical intraepithelial neoplasia: frequency and significance of co-existing condyloma. J Surg Pathol 1995; 1:165-172.

86. Koss LG, Melamed MR, Daniel WW. In situ epidermoid carcinoma of the cervix and vagina following radiotherapy for cervical cancer. Cancer 1961; 14:353-360.

87. Koss LG, Melamed MR, Mayer K. The effect of busulfan on human epithelia. Am J Clin Pathol 1965; 44:385-397.

88. Kitay DZ, Wentz WB. Cervical cytology in folic acid deficiency of pregnancy. Am J Obstet Gynecol 1969; 104:931-938.

89. Soutter WP, Wisdom S, Brough AK, et al. Should patients with mild atypia in a cervical smear be referred for colposcopy? Br J Obstet Gynecol 1986; 93:70-74.

90. Walker EM, Dodgson J, Duncan ID. Does mild atypia on a cervical smear warrant further investigation? Lancet (ii) 1986; 672-673.

91. Davis GL, Hernandez E, Davis JL, et al. Atypical squamous cells in Papanicolaou smears. Obstet Gynecol 1987; 69:43-46.

92. Noumoff JS. Atypia in cervical cytology as a risk factor for intraepithelial neoplasia. Am J Obstet Gynecol 1987; 156:628-631.

93. Tay SK, Jenkins D, Singer A. Management of squamous atypia (borderline nuclear abnormalities): repeat cytology or colposcopy? Aust NZJ Obstet Gynaecol 1987; 27:140-141.

94. Andrews S, Hernandez E, Miyazawa K. Paired Papanicolaou smears in the evaluation of atypical squamous cells. Obstet Gynecol 1989; 73:747-750.

95. Kaminski PE, Stevens CW, Wheelock JB. Squamous atypia on cytology: the influence of age. J Reprod Med 1989; 34:617-620.

96. Lindheim SR, Smith-Nguyen G. Aggressive evaluation for atypical squamous cells in Papanicolaou smears. J Reprod Med 1990; 35:971-973.

97. Lawley TB, Lee RB, Kapela R. The significance of moderate and severe inflammation on Class I Papanicolaou smear. Obstet Gynecol 1990: 76:997-999.

98. Borst M, Butterworth CE, Baker V, et al. Human papillomavirus screening for women with atypical Papanicolaou smears. J Reprod Med 1991; 36:95-99.

99. August N. Cervicography for evaluating the "atypical" Papanicolaou smear. J Reprod Med 1991; 36:89-94.

100. Kaminski PF, Lyon DS, Soroky KI, et al. Significance of atypical cervical cytology in pregnancy. Am J Perinatol 1992; 9:340-343.

101. Hirschowitz L, Raffle AE, Mackenzie EFD, et al. Long-term follow-up of women with borderline cervical smear test results: effects of age and viral infections on progression to high-grade dyskaryosis. BMJ 1992; 304:1209-1212.

102. Maier RC, Schultenover SJ. Evaluation of the atypical squamous cell Papanicolaou smear. Int J Gynecol Pathol 1986; 5:242-248.

103. Spitzer M, Krumholz BA, Chernys AE, et al. Comparative utility of repeat Papanicolaou smears, cervicography, and colposcopy in the evaluation of atypical Papanicolaou smears. Obstet Gynecol 1987; 69:731-735.

104. Kohan S, Noumoff J, Beckman EM, et al. Colposcopic screening of women with atypical Papanicolaou smears. J Reprod Med 1985; 30:383-387.

105. Reiter RC. Management of initial atypical cervical cytology: a randomized prospective study. Obstet Gynecol 1986; 68:237-240.

106. Morrison BW, Erickson ER, Doshi N, et al. The significance of atypical cervical smears. J Reprod Med 1988; 3:809-812.

107. Brown MS, Phillips GL Jr. Management of the mildly abnormal Pap smear: a conservative approach. Gynecol Oncol 1985; 22:149-153.

108. Sheils LA, Wilbur DC. The significance of atypical cells of squamous type (AS) on Papanicolaou smears: a five year follow-up study. Acta Cytol 1992; 36:580.

109. Howell LP, Davis RL. Follow-up of Papanicolaou smears diagnosed as atypical squamous cells of undetermined significance. Act Cytol 1993; 37:783.

110. Kaye KS, Dhurandhar NR. Atypical cells of undetermined significance: follow-up biopsy and Pap smear findings. Am J Clin Pathol 1993; 99:332.

111. Sidawy MK, Tabbara SO. Reactive change and atypical squamous cells of undetermined significance in Papanicolaou smears: a cytohistologic correlation. Diagn Cytopathol 1993; 9:423-429.

112. Taylor RR, Guerrieri JP, Nash JD, Henry MR, O'Connor DM. Atypical cervical cytology: colposcopic follow-up using the Bethesda System. J Reprod Med 1993; 38:443-447.

113. Slawson DC, Bennett JH, Herman JM. Follow-up Papanicolaou smear for cervical atypia: are we missing significant disease? A HARNET study. J Fam Pract 1993; 36:289-293.

114. Davey DD, Naryshkin S, Nielsen ML, et al. Atypical squamous cells of undetermined significance: interlaboratory comparison and quality assurance monitors. Diagn Cytopathol 1994; 11:390-396.

115. Slawson DC, Bennett JH, Simon LJ, et al. Should all women with cervical atypia be referred for colposcopy: a HARNET study. Harrisburg Area Research Network. J Fam Pract 1994; 38:387-392.

116. Widra EA, Dookhan D, Jordan A, et al. Evaluation of the atypical cytologic smear: validity of the 1991 Bethesda System. J Reprod Med 1994; 39:682-684.

117. Lonky NM, Navarre GL, Saunders S, et al. Low-grade Papanicolaou smears and the Bethesda System: a prospective cytohistopathologic analysis. Obstet Gynecol 1995; 85:716-720.

118. Shafi MI, Luesley DM. Management of low-grade lesions: follow-up or treat? Bail Clin Obstet Gynaecol 1995; 9:121-131.

119. Wright TC, Sun XW, Koulos J. Comparison of management algorithms for the evaluation of women with low-grade cytologic abnormalities. Obstet Gynecol 1995; 85:202-210.

120. Kaufman RH. Atypical squamous cells of undetermined significance and low-grade squamous intraepithelial lesion: diagnostic criteria and management. Am J Obstet Gynecol 1996; 175:1120-1128.

121. Alanen KW, Elit LM, Molinaro PA, et al. Assessment of cytologic follow-up as the recommended management for patients with atypical squamous cells of undetermined significance or low-grade squamous intraepithelial lesions. Cancer Cytopathol 1998; 84:5-10.

122. Sheils LA, Wilbur DC. Atypical squamous cells of undetermined significance: stratification of the risk of association with, or progression to, squamous intraepithelial lesions based on morphologic subcategorization. Acta Cytol 1997; 41:1065-1072.

123. Quitllet FA, Morta MC, Cañas A, et al. Cytologic atypia: clinical significance and follow-up recommendations. Acta Cytol 1997; 41:504-506.

124. Suh-Burgmann E, Darragh T, Smith-McCune K. Atypical squamous cells of undetermined significance: management patterns at an academic medical center. Am J Obstet Gynecol 1998; 178:991-995.

125. Genest DR, Cean B, Lee KR, et al. Qualifying the cytologic diagnosis of "atypical squamous cells of undetermined significance" affects the predictive value of a squamous intraepithelial lesion on subsequent biopsy. Arch Pathol Lab Med 1998; 122:338-341.

126. Auger M, Charbonneau M, Arseneau J. Atypical squamous cells of undetermined significance: a cytohistologic study of 52 cases. Acta Cytol 1997; 41:1671-1675.

127. Abati A, Jaffurs W, Wilder AM. Squamous atypia in the atrophic cervical vaginal smear: a new look at an old problem. Cancer 1998; 84:218-225.

128. Lachman MF, Cavallo-Calvanese C. Qualification of atypical squamous cells of undetermined significance in an independent laboratory: is it useful or significant? Am J Obstet Gynecol 1998; 179:421-429.

129. Heatley MK. Follow up of women with borderline cervical smears as defined by national guidelines. J Clin Pathol 1999; 52:787-788.

130. Edelman M, Fox AS, Alderman EM, et al. Cervical Papanicolaou smear abnormalities in inner city Bronx adolescents: prevalence, progression, and immune modifiers. Cancer Cytopathol 1999; 87:184-189.

131. Lousuebsakul V, Knutsen SMF, Gram IT, et al. Clinical impact of atypical squamous cells of undetermined significance: a cytohistologic comparison. Acta Cytol 2000; 44:23-30.

132. Vlahos NP, Dragisic KG, Wallach EE, et al. Clinical significance of the qualification of atypical squamous cells of undetermined significance: an analysis on the basis of histologic diagnoses. Am J Obstet Gynecol 2000; 182:885-890.

133. Yang M, Zachariah S. ASCUS on cervical cytologic smears: clinical significance. J Reprod Med 1997; 42:329-331.

134. Williams ML, Rimm DL, Pedigo MA, et al. Atypical squamous cells of undetermined significance: correlative histologic and follow-up studies from an academic medical center. Diag Cytopathol 1997; 16:1-7.

135. Collins LC, Wang HH, Abu-Jawdeh GM. Qualifiers of atypical squamous cells of undetermined significance help in patient management. Mod Pathol 1996; 9:677-681.

136. Dvorak KA, Finnemore M, Maksem JA. Histology correlation with atypical squamous cells of undetermined significance (ASCUS) and low-grade squamous intraepithelial lesion (LSIL) cytology diagnoses: an argument to ensure ASCUS follow-up that is as aggressive as that for LSIL. Diagn Cytopathol 1999; 21:292-295.

137. Cunnane MF, Rothblat IP. Atypical squamous cells in women over 50: histologic correlations. Acta Cytol 1993; 37:784.

138. Malik SN, Wilkinson EJ, Drew PA, Bennett BB, Hardt NS. Do qualifiers of ASCUS distinguish between low- and high-risk patients? Acta Cytol 1999; 43:376-380.

139. Rader AE, Rose PG, Rodriguez M, et al. Atypical squamous cells of undetermined significance in women over 55: comparison with the general population and implications for management. Acta Cytol 1999; 43:357-362.

140. Gonzalez D, Hernandez E, Anderson L, Heller P, Atkinson BF. Clinical significance of a cervical cytologic diagnosis of atypical squamous cells of undetermined significance: favoring a reactiave process or low-grade squamous intraepithelial lesion. J Reprod Med 1996; 41:719-723.

141. Goff BA, Muntz HG, Bell DA, et al. Human papillomavirus typing in patients with Papanicolaou smears showing squamous atypia. Gynecol Oncol 1993; 48:384-388.

142. Kline MJ, Davey DD. Atypical squamous cells of undetermined significance qualified: a follow-up study. Diagn Cytopathol 1996;14:380-384.

143. Delmore J, Williams CM, Nielsen ML, et al. Atypical squamous cells of undetermined significance: community incidence and management review. Kansas Med 1995; 96:133-134.

144. Selvaggi SM, Haefner HK. Reporting of atypical squamous cells of undetermined significance: is it significant? Diagn Cytopathol 1995; 13:352-356.

145. Rader AE, Labebnik R, Arora CD, et al. Atypical squamous cells of undetermined significance in the pediatric population: implications for management and comparison with the adult population. Acta Cytol 1997; 41:1073-1078.

146. Kobelin MH, Kobelin CG, Burke L, et al. Incidence and predictors of cervical dysplasia in patients with minimally abnormal Papanicolaou smears. Obstet Gynecol 1998; 92:356-359.

147. Ettler HC, Joseph MG, Downing PA, et al. Atypical squamous cells of undetermined significance: a cytohistological study in a colposcopy clinic. Diagn Cytopathol 1999; 21:211-216.

148. Nyirjesy I, Billingsley FS, Forman MR. Evaluation of atypical and low-grade cervical cytology in private practice. Obstet Gynecol 1998; 92:601-607.

149. Morin C, Bairati I, Bouchard C, et al. Cytologic predictors of cervical intraepithelial neoplasia in women with an ASCUS Pap smear. Acta Cytol 2000; 44:576-586.

150. al-Nafussi A, Rebello G, al-Yusif R, McGoogan E. The borderline cervical smear: colposcopic and biopsy outcome. J Clin Pathol 2000; 53:439-444.

151. Kinney WK, Manor MM, Hurley LB, et al. Where's the high-grade cervical neoplasia? The importance of minimally abnormal Papanicolaou diagnoses. Obstet Gynecol 1998; 91:973-976.

152. Alameda F, Fuste P, Conangla M, et al. ASCUS: Comparative follow-up results related to previous SIL diagnosis. Eur J Gynaecol Oncol 2000; 21:81-83.

153. Changchien CC, Lin H, Eng HL, et al. Clinical implication of atypical squamous cells of undetermined significance with or without favoring high-grade squamous intraepithelial lesion on cervical smears. Chang Keng I Hsueh Tsa Chih 1999; 22:579-585.

154. Holcomb K, Abulafia O, Matthews RP, et al. The significance of ASCUS cytology in HIV-positive women. Gynecol Oncol 1999; 75:118-121.

155. Giudice A, Rizzo M, Rossi RT, et al. Diagnosis and survey of abnormal/atypical squamous cells of undetermined significance: a retrospective study. Anticancer Res 2000; 20:1195-1199.

156. Melnikow J, Nuovo J, Willan AR, et al. Natural history of cervical squamous intraepithelial lesions: a meta-analysis. Obstet Gynecol 1998; 92:727-735.

157. Lee KR, Minter LJ, Crum CP. Division of low-grade SIL into subcategories on Papanicolaou smears does not predict biopsy follow-up. Mod Pathol 1996; 9:35.

158. Cox JT, Lorincz AT, Schiffman MH, et al. Human papillomavirus testing by hybrid capture appears to be useful in triaging women with a cytologic diagnosis of atypical squamous cells of undetermined significance. Am J Obstet Gynecol 1995; 172:946.

159. Hall S, Wu TC, Soudi N, Sherman ME. Low-grade squamous intraepithelial lesions: cytologic predictors of biopsy confirmation. Diagn Cytopathol 1994; 10:3-9.

160. Ghoussoub RA, Rimm DL. Degree of dysplasia following diagnosis of atypical squamous cells of undetermined significance is influenced by patient history and type of follow-up. Diagn Cytopathol 1997; 17:14-19.

161. Eltabbakh GH, Lipman JH, Mount SL, Morgan A. Significance of atypical squamous cells of undetermined significance on ThinPrep Papanicolaou smears. Gynecol Oncol 2000; 79:44-49.

162. Sherman ME, Tabbara SO, Scott DR, et al. "ASCUS, rule out HSIL": Cytologic features, histologic correlates, and human papillomavirus detection. Mod Pathol 1999; 12:335-342.

163. Schoolland M, Sterrett GF, Knowles SAS, Mitchell KM, Kurinczuk JJ. The "inconclusive-possible high-grade epithelial abnormality" category in Papanicolaou smear reporting. Cancer Cytopathol 1998; 84:208.

164. Quddus MR, Sung CJ, Steinhoff MM, et al. Atypical squamous metaplastic cells. Reproducibility, outcome, and diagnostic features on ThinPrep Pap test. Cancer Cytopathol 2001; 93:16-22.

165. Kaminski PF, Stevens CW Jr, Wheelock JB. Squamous atypia on cytology: the influence of age. J Reprod Med 1989; 34:617-620.

166. Symmans F, Mechanic L, MacConnell P, et al. Correlation of cervical cytology and human papillomavirus DNA detection in postmenopausal women. Int J Gynecol Pathol 1992; 11:204-209.

167. Renshaw AA, Dean BR, Cibas ES. Receiver operating characteristic curves for analysis of the results of cervicovaginal smears: a useful quality improvement tool. Arch Pathol Lab Med 1997; 121:968-975.

168. Kobelin MH, Kobelin CG, Burke L, Lavin P, Niloff JM, Kim YB. Incidence and predictors of cervical dysplasia in patients with minimally abnormal Papanicolaou smears. Obstet Gynecol 1998; 92:356-359.

169. Condel JL, Mahood LK, Grzybicki DM, Sturgis CD, Raab SS. Cases diagnosed as atypical by a cytotechnologist and downgraded to benign by a pathologist: a measure of laboratory quality. Am J Clin Pathol 2002; 117:520-522.

170. Richard RM. The natural history of cervical intraepithelial neoplasia. Clin Obstet Gynecol 1967; 10:748-784.

171. Fidler HK, Boyes DA, Worth AJ. Cervical cancer detection in British Columbia: a progress report. J Obstet Gynaecol Br Comm 1968; 75:392-404.

172. Kashgarian M, Dunn JE. The duration of intraepithelial and preclinical squamous cell carcinoma of the uterine cervix. Am J Epidemiol 1970; 92:211.

173. Mitchell MF, Schottenfeld D, Tortolero-Luna G, Cantor SB, Richards-Kortum R. Colposcopy for the diagnosis of squamous intraepithelial lesions: a meta-analysis. Obstet Gynecol 1998; 91:626-631.

174. Holcomb K, Abulafia O, Matthews RP, Chapman JE, Borges A, Lee YC, Buhl A. The significance of ASCUS cytology in HIV-positive women. Gynecol Oncol 1999; 75:118-121.

175. Baldauf JJ, Ritter J. Comparison of the risks of cytologic surveillance of women with atypical cells or low-grade abnormalities on cervical smear: review of the literature. Eur J Obstet Gynecol Reprod Biol 1998; 76:193-199.

176. Kurman RJ, Henson DE, Herbst AL, Noller KL, Schiffman MH. Interim guidelines for management of abnormal cervical cytology. JAMA 1994; 271:1866-1869.

177. American College of Obstetricians and Gynecologists. Cervical cytology: evaluation and management of abnormalities. Washington, DC: American College of Obstetricians and Gynecologists Technical Bulletin 183; 1993. pp.1-7.

178. Cox JT, Wilkinson EJ, Lonky N, et al. Management guidelines for the follow-up of atypical squamous cells of undetermined (ASCUS). J Lower Gen Tract Dis 2000; 4:99-105.

179. Ferris DG, Kiregel D, Cote L, et al. Women's triage and management preferences for cervical cytologic reports demonstrating atypical squamous cells of undetermined significance and low-grade squamous intraepithelial lesions. Arch Fam Med 1997; 6:348-353.

180. Cox T, Lorincz AT, Schiffman MH, Sherman ME, et al. Human papillomavirus testing by hybrid capture appears to be useful in triaging women with a cytologic diagnosis of atypical squamous cells of undetermined significance. Am J Obstet Gynecol 1995; 172:946-954.

181. Ferris DG, Wright TC Jr, Litaker MS, et al. Triage of women with ASCUS and LSIL on Pap smear reports. J Fam Pract 1998; 46:125-134.

182. Manos MM, Kinney WK, Hurley LB, et al. Identifying women with cervical neoplasia: using human papillomavirus DNA testing for equivocal Papanicolaou results. JAMA 1999; 281:1605-1610.

183. Wright TC Jr, Lorincz A, Ferris DG, et al. Reflex human papillomavirus deoxyribonucleic acid testing in women with abnormal Papanicolaou smears. Am J Obstet Gynecol 1998; 178:962-966.

184. Sherman ME, Schiffman M, Cox JT, et al. Effects of age and human papilloma virus load on colposcopy triage. J Natl Cancer Inst 2002; 94:102-107.

185. The Atypical Squamous Cells of Undetermined Significance/Low-grade Squamous Intraepithelial Lesions Triage Study (ALTS) Group. Human papillomavirus testing for triage of women with cytologic evidence of low-grade squamous intraepithelial lesions: baseline data from a randomized clinical trial. J Natl Cancer Inst 2000; 92:397-402.

186. Bergeron C, Jeannel D, Proveda JD, Cassonet P, Orth G. Human papillomavirus testing in women with mild cytologic atypia. Obstet Gynecol 2000; 95:821-827.

187. Manos MM, Kinney WK, Hurley LB, et al. Identifying women with cervical neoplasia: using human papillomavirus testing for equivocal Papanicolaou results. JAMA 1999; 281:1605-1610.

188. Nuovo GJ. Diagnosis of human papillomavirus using in situ hybridization and in situ polymerase chain reaction. Methods Mol Biol 2002; 179:113-136.

189. Nuovo GJ. Detection of human papillomavirus in Papanicolaou smears: correlation with pathologic findings and clinical outcome. Diagn Mol Pathol 1998; 7:158-163.

190. Sigurdsson K, Arnadottir T, Snorradottir M, et al. Human papillomavirus (HPV) in an Icelandic population: the role of HPV DNA testing based on hybrid capture and PCR assays among women with screen-detected abnormal Pap smears. Int J Cancer 1997; 72:446-452.

191. Crum CP, Genest DR, Krane JF, et al. Subclassifying atypical squamous cells in Thin-Prep cervical cytology correlates with detection of high-risk human papillomavirus DNA. Am J Clin Pathol 1999; 112:384-390.

192. Kaufman RH, Schreiber K. Carter T. Analysis of atypical squamous (glandular) cells of undetermined significance smears by neural network-directed review. Obstet Gynecol 1998; 91:556-560.

193. Ferris DG, Wright TC, Litaker MS, Richard RM, Lorincz AT, Sun XW, Woodward L. Comparison of two tests for detecting carcinogenic HPV in women with Papanicolaou smear reports of ASCUS and LSIL. J Fam Pract 1998; 46:136-141.

194. Kim JJ, Wright TC, Goldie SJ. Cost-effectiveness of alternative triage strategies for atypical squamous cells of undetermined significance. JAMA 2002; 287:2382-2390.

195. Melnikow J, Nuovo J. Paliescheskey M. Management choices for patients with "squamous atypia" on Papanicolaou smear: a toss up? Med Care 1996; 34:336-347.

196. Cecchini S, Iossa A, Bonardi R, Ciatto S, Cariaggi P. Comparing two modalities of management of women with cytology evidence of squamous or glandular atypia: early repeat cytology or colposcopy. Tumori 1997; 83:732-734.

197. Raab SS, Hart AR, D'Antonio JA, Grzybicki DM. Clinical perception of disease probability associated with Bethesda System diagnoses. Am J Clin Pathol 2001; 115:681-688.

198. Janerich DT, Hadjimichael O, Schwartz PE, et al. The screening histories of women with invasive cervical cancer in Connecticut. Am J Public Health 1995; 85:791.

199. Eskridge C, Begneaud WP, Landwehr C. Cervicography combined with repeat Papanicolaou test as triage for low-grade cytologic abnormalities. Obstet Gynecol 1998; 92:351-355.

200. Papillo JL, Zarka MA, St. John TL. Evaluation of the Thin-Prep Pap test in clinical practice: a seven-month, 16,314-case experience in Northern Vermont. Acta Cytol 1998; 42:203-208.

201. Dupree WB, et al. The promise and risk of new technology: The Lehigh Valley Hospital's experience with liquid-based cervical cytology. Cancer 1998; 84:202-207.

202. Guidos BJ, Selvaggi SM. Use of the Thin-Prep Pap test in clinical practice. Diagn Cytopathol 1999; 20:70-73.

203. Carpenter AB, Davey DD. Thin-Prep Pap test: performance and biopsy follow-up in a university hospital. Cancer 1999; 87:105-112.

204. Diaz-Rosario LA, Kabawat SE. Performance of a fluid-based, thin-layer Papanicolaou smear method in the clinical setting of an independent laboratory and an outpatient screening population in New England. Arch Pathol Lab Med 1999; 123:817-821.

205. Weintraub J, Morabia A. Efficacy of a liquid-based thin layer method for cervical cancer screening in a population with a low incidence of cervical cancer. Diagn Cytopathol 2000; 22:52-59.

206. Vassilakos P, Griffin S, Megevand E, Campana A. CytoRich liquid-based cervical cytologic test: screening results in a routine cytopathology service. Acta Cytol 1998; 42:198-202.

207. Vassilakos P, Schwartz D, de Marval F, et al. Biopsy-based comparison of liquid-based, thin-layer preparations to conventional Pap smears. J Reprod Med 2000; 45:11-16.

208. Bolick DR, Hellman DJ. Laboratory implementation and efficacy assessment of the Thin-Prep cervical cancer screening system. Acta Cytol 1998; 42:209-213.

209. Obwegeser JH, Brack S. Does liquid-based technology really improve detection of cervical neoplasia? A prospective, randomized trial comparing the ThinPrep Pap test with the conventional Pap test, including follow-up of HSIL cases. Acta Cytol 2001; 45:709-714.

210. Luthra UK, Chishti M, Dey P, et al. Performance of monolayered cervical smears in a gynecology outpatient setting in Kuwait. Acta Cytol 2002; 46:303-310.

211. Yeah GPS, Chan KW, Lauder I, Lam MB. Evaluation of the ThinPrep Papanicolaou test in clinical practice: 6-month study of 16,541 cases with histological correlation in 220 cases. Hong Kong Med J 1999; 5:233-239.

212. Monsonego J, Autillo-Touati A, Bergeron C, et al. Liquid-based cytology for primary cervical cancer screening: a multi-centre study. Br J Cancer 2001; 84:360-366.

213. Ring M, Bolger N, O'Donnell M, et al. Evaluation of liquid-based cytology in cervical screening of high-risk populations: a split study of colposcopy and genitourinary medicine populations. Cytopathology 2002; 13:152-159.

214. Biscotti CV, O'Brien DL, Gero MA, et al. Thin-Layer Pap test vs. conventional Pap smear. J Reprod Med 2002; 47:9-13.

215. Marino JF, Fremont-Smith M. Direct-to-vial experience with AutoCyte PREP in a small New England regional cytology practice. J Reprod Med 2001; 46:353-358.

216. Tench W. Preliminary assessment of the AutoCyte PREP. Direct-to-vial performance. J Reprod Med 2000; 45:912-916.

217. Bernstein SJ, Sanchez-Ramos L, Ndubisi B. Liquid-based cervical cytologic smear study and conventional Papanicolaou smears: a metaanalysis of prospective studies comparing cytologic diagnosis and sample adequacy. Am J Obstet Gynecol 2001; 185:308-317.

218. O'Leary TJ, Tellado M, Buckner S, Ali IS, Stevens A, Olllayos CW. PAPNET-assisted rescreening of cervical smears: cost and accuracy compared with a 100% manual rescreening strategy. JAMA 1998; 279:235-237.

219. Lerma E, Colomo L, Carreras A, Esteva E, Quilez M, Prat J. Rescreening of atypical cervicovaginal smears using PAPNET. Cancer 1998; 84:361-365.

220. Kok MR, Habers MA, Schreiner-Kok PG, Boon ME. New paradigm for ASCUS diagnosis using neural networks. Diagn Cytopathol 1998; 19:361-366.

221. Vassilakos P, Carrel S, Petignat P, Boulvain M, Campana A. Use of automated primary screening on liquid-based, thin-layer preparations. Acta Cytol 2002; 46:291-295.

222. Raab SS. Low-grade and ASCUS lesions of the cervix: diagnostic difficulties and reproducibility. Ann Pathol 1999; 19:S87-S89.

223. Llewellyn H. Observer variation, dysplasia grading, and HPV typing. Am J Clin Pathol 2002; 114(suppl 1):S21-S35.

224. Crum CP, Genest DR, Krane JF, et al. Subclassifying atypical squamous cells in Thin-Prep cervical cytology correlates with detection of high-risk human papillomavirus DNA. Am J Clin Pathol 1999; 112:384-390.

225. Yobs AR, Plott AE, Hicklin MD. Retrospective evaluation of gynecologic cytodiagnosis. II. Interlaboratory reproducibility as shown in rescreening large consecutive samples of reported cases. Acta Cytol 1987; 31:900-910.

226. Klinkhamer PJJM, Vooijs GP, de Haan AFJ. Intraobserver and interobserver variability in the diagnosis of epithelial abnormalities in cervical smears. Acta Cytol 1988; 32:794-800.

227. Sherman ME, Schiffman MH, Erozan YS, et al. The Bethesda System: a proposal for reporting abnormal cervical smears based on the reproducibility of cytopathologic diagnoses. Arch Pathol Lab Med 1992; 116:1155-1158.

228. Young NA, Naryshkin S, Atkinson BF, et al. Interobserver variabillity of cervical smears with squamous-cell abnormalities: a Philadelphia study. Diagn Cytopathol 1994; 11:352-357.

229. Sherman ME, Schiffman MH, Lorincz AT, et al. Toward objective quality assurance in cervical cytopathology: correlation of cytopathologic diagnoses with detection of high-risk human papillomavirus types. Am J Clin Pathol 1994; 102:182-187.

230. Confortini M, Biggeri A, Cariaggi MP, et al. Intralaboratory reproducibility in cervical cytology: results of the application of a 100-slide set. Acta Cytol 1993; 37:49-54.

231. O'Sullivan JP, Ismail SM, Barnes WSF, et al. Interobserver variation in the diagnosis and grading of dyskaryosis in cervical smears: specialist cytopathologists compared with non-specialists. J Clin Pathol 1994; 47:515-518.

232. O'Sullivan JP, Ismail SM, Barnes WS, et al. Inter- and intra-observer variation in the reporting of cervical smears: specialist cytopathologists versus histopathologists. Cytopathology 1996; 7:78-89.

233. O'Sullivan JP. Observer variation in gynaecological cytopathology. Cytopathology 1998; 9:6-14.

234. Jones S, Thomas GDH, Williamson P. Observer variation in the assessment of adequacy and neoplasia in cervical cytology. Acta Cytol 1996; 40:226-234.

235. Smith AE, Sherman ME, Scott DR, et al. Review of Bethesda System atlas does not improve reproducibility or accuracy in the classification of atypical squamous cells of undetermined significance smears. Cancer 2000; 90:201-206.

236. Stoler MH, Schiffman M. Interobserver reproducibility of cervical and histologic interpretations. JAMA 2001; 285:1500-1505.

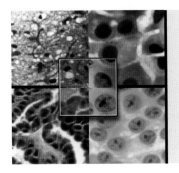

Squamous Intraepithelial Lesions

CHAPTER
6

 ## HUMAN PAPILLOMAVIRUS AND CERVICAL CARCINOGENESIS

Although both the incidence and mortality rates of carcinoma of the uterine cervix have declined in the United States, this cancer remains the second most common form of malignancy in women worldwide. For a number of decades, it has been recognized that squamous cell carcinoma of the cervix and its precursor lesions are related to several aspects of sexual behavior. Thus, it has long been suspected that carcinoma of the cervix may be the result of a sexually transmitted disease.[1] Although several putative infectious agents have been considered, it is now widely held that the vast majority of carcinomas are the consequence of infection by human papillomaviruses (HPV).[2-8] Similarly, HPV has been directly linked to the development of the precursor squamous intraepithelial lesions (SILs).[7-10] After a consideration of the epidemiologic, molecular biologic, and clinical factors that relate HPV infection to SIL and thus to invasive squamous cell carcinoma, the cytologic features and classification of the various SIL grades are discussed.

Epidemiologic Studies

The risk of developing carcinoma of the cervix is influenced strongly by two aspects of sexual activity, namely the age at the time of first intercourse and the number of lifetime sexual partners.[1] Younger onset ages correlate with increased risk as does multiple partners. Other statistically less powerful factors include lower socioeconomic status and the number of pregnancies. It is now believed that these factors should be considered covariables in the development of carcinoma in that they are all related to the sexual transmission of HPV.[1] Specifically, in several studies, when the effect of HPV infection is controlled for, these risk factors are not independently significant from a statistical view point. This is also true of SIL.

As the assays for detection of HPV have improved, this linkage of infection with SIL and carcinoma has grown stronger. In a large case control investigation, Schiffman and colleagues compared 500 women with SIL to 500 controls in Oregon.[9] The very sensitive polymerase chain reaction (PCR) was used to test for HPV and to subdivide them into three risk groups. Based on the evaluation of cervical biopsy tissue, 76% of the SILs contained HPV DNA. Although the authors did not provide exact numbers, they said that if cytologic evidence of HPV infection were included, the proportion of cases of SIL related to HPV infection would have increased. In contrast, only 18% of the controls without SIL were positive for HPV; the vast majority of these positive controls were in the low-risk group. The authors suggested that the proportion of cases associated with HPV could be excessively low as a result of inherent limitations in performing only a single HPV test to define the presence (or absence) of infection. The authors found increasing parity to be a potential risk factor for women with SIL independent of their HPV status. Parity was more strongly associated as a potential co-factor in women with low-grade SIL (LGSIL). Cigarette smoking was considered a possible co-factor for HPV-positive women with high-grade SIL (HGSIL). Koutsky and colleagues, in a large prospective cohort study, followed women who were cytologically negative and colposcopically normal for 2 years.[11] Of the women in the group, 30% were positive for HPV 16 DNA and developed an HGSIL.

Peng, in a case control study from China, demonstrated a strong association between HPV infection and invasive carcinoma of the cervix.[12] Another large case-control investigation that used PCR testing studied 436 women with carcinoma from Spain and Columbia.[13] The risk factor with the greatest association for invasive cancer was HPV infection. The largest investigation to date included 1035 women with cervical carcinoma from 22 countries including the United States.[5] This analysis also used PCR technology for HPV detection. Overall, HPV DNA was identified in 93% of the carcinomas. The proportion of positive carcinomas did not show significant geographic variation. With one exception, HPV 16 was the most prevalent, accounting for 50% of all positive neoplasms. The one exception was Indonesia, where HPV 18 was the most common. Overall, HPV 18 was identified in 24% of the carcinomas. This was followed by HPV 45 with 8% (a well-demonstrated clustering of HPV 45 infections was found in Western Africa) and HPV 31 in 5% of the malignancies. Overall, 20 different types of HPV DNA were detected in the cervical cancers. Bosch and colleagues also divided the neoplasms histologically.[5] HPV 16 was the most common in squamous cell carcinomas, whereas HPV

18 predominated in both adenocarcinomas and adenosquamous carcinomas. Bosch also pondered the occurrence of HPV-negative cervical carcinomas.[5] The greatest proportion of these cases occurred in Algeria. The authors suggested that these cancers might represent a distinct biological entity. On the other hand, it could be the result of false-negative DNA testing and/or the loss of HPV DNA during the development of the tumor.

The numerous HPV types have been divided into risk groups based on their association with specific forms of SIL and carcinoma of the cervix. Some authors divide them into two groups (high and low) and others into three groups (high, intermediate, and low risk). Lorincz and colleagues included HPV 6, 11, 42, 43, and 44 in their low-risk category.[14] These were almost always associated with LGSIL and almost never with either HGSIL or invasive cancer. The intermediate risk group included HPV 31, 33, 35, 51, and 52; although only uncommonly associated with invasive neoplasms, these viruses were associated with both LGSIL and HGSIL. HPV 16, 18, 45, and 56 were the high-risk group. They were associated with the vast majority of invasive squamous cell carcinomas (Table 6-1).

Lungu and colleagues evaluated cervical biopsies demonstrating SIL for HPV DNA using the PCR.[15] The authors demonstrated that one could not predict the HPV type from the histologic appearance of the LGSIL. Nearly double the proportion of cases of LGSIL was associated with intermediate and high-risk HPV compared with the proportion associated with low-risk viruses. More than one fifth of these specimens manifested two or more HPV types. Much tighter association was found between the histopathology and the HPV type in HGSIL. Nearly 90% of the cases were positive for either HPV 16, 18, or 33. Only 7% of the biopsies from these women contained multiple of virus types.

Using a Hybrid Capture assay, Hall and colleagues evaluated Pap test lavage specimens from 150 women who were referred to their institution with an abnormal cytologic diagnosis.[16] This assay divides the HPV into low- and high-risk groups. Forty of these women were considered to be free of disease (negative histology and cytology), whereas 69 had biopsy-proven SIL. A third group was considered to be equivocal for disease in that the Pap test cytology was ab-

normal but the biopsies were negative. Of the women with SIL or equivocal disease, 84% were positive for HPV DNA, whereas only 35% of the negative women were positive for HPV DNA. Overall, 92% of the HPV-positive women had high-risk viruses. The Hybrid Capture test allows quantification of the amount of HPV DNA, in addition to its simple detection.[16] The presence of biopsy proven SIL correlated well with large quantities of DNA. None of the women with HGSIL were infected only with the low-risk viruses (some had both high- and low-risk types).

It is traditionally considered that a large proportion of women who are positive for HPV DNA do not manifest any evidence of cervical disease. This is typically based on negative cytology findings in Pap tests. Moscicki and colleagues have demonstrated that in a population of young women (average age 18 years), the majority of subjects positive for HPV DNA have disease when examined by cytology, colposcopy, and biopsies.[17] One third had histologically proven cervical LGSIL; when the entire anogenital region was examined, 64% of the virus-positive women had disease.

Traditionally, it has also been taught that cervical adenocarcinomas are typically associated with HPV 18. It is also widely accepted that most cervical carcinomas are negative for *p53* mutations, as detected by immunohistochemistry. The study by Parker and colleagues found HPV DNA in 50% of a series of cervical adenocarcinomas.[18] Of these, 56% were positive for HPV 18, and the remainder were positive for HPV 16. In the series of Uchiyama and colleagues, 34% of the adenocarcinomas were HPV DNA positive.[19] Of the 11 positive cases, six were positive only for HPV 16, five for HPV 18, and 1 for both of these viral types. Both of these studies demonstrated a strong inverse relationship between the presence of HPV DNA and *p53* positivity in the tumor cells.[18,19]

Molecular Biologic Studies

The molecular biologic evidence of the involvement of HPV in cervical carcinogenesis is just as compelling as the epidemiologic data.[2-9,20] HPV are DNA tumor viruses in the family *Papovavirdae*.[3,4,6] These viruses are nonenveloped, have a icosahedral capsid, and measure approximately 50 nm in diameter. Inside the capsid is a circular double-stranded DNA molecule containing approximately 8000 base pairs. HPV are epitheliotropic viruses that are quite species specific and rather tissue specific; this latter quality is most likely related to postcellular transcription factors. Because the capsid proteins of HPV are highly conserved, especially *L1*, the different types cannot be readily differentiated serologically. Thus, DNA sequences are needed to distinguish the types. Currently, more than 80 types of HPV are recognized, with at least 25 that seek their homes in the anogenital epithelia. For a virus to be considered a new HPV type, at least 50% of its DNA has to be nonhomologous with known types.[21] Although HPV 16 and 18 are the two most common high-risk viruses, they are only distantly related phylogenetically.

Three major regions of the circular HPV genome are noted. One of theses is termed the *long controlling region (LCR)*, or the upstream regulatory region.[3-6] This portion of the genome does not code for proteins. Rather, it regulates replication and transcription of the virus. The LCR has binding sites for cellular transcription factors such as acti-

TABLE 6-1	
Human Papillomavirus Types Grouped by Differing Risk of Squamous Intraepithelial Lesions*	
Risk	**HPV Types**
Low*	6, 11, 42, 43, 44
Intermediate†	31, 33, 35, 51, 52
High‡	16, 18, 45, 56

From Lorincz AT, Reid R, Jenson AB, et al. Human papillomavirus infection of the cervix: relative risk associations of 15 common anogenital types. Am J Obstet Gynecol 1992; 79:328-337.
HPV, Human papillomavirus.
*Usually associated with low-grade squamous intraepithelial lesion.
†Associated with low or high-grade squamous intraepithelial lesion but rarely with invasive carcinoma.
‡Associated with the majority of invasive squamous cell carcinomas.

vator protein one and keratinocyte specific transcription factor-1 (KRF1). It is known that different forms of KRF1 are used by 16 and 18. Binding of these factors to the LCR regulates the activity of the open reading frames in the early regions of the genome.

The early region of the genome is so named because it is transcribed early in the life cycle of the virus. The early region has open reading frames that code for proteins involved in viral replication and in cellular transformation. The early region has six open reading frames (*E1-E7*, with no *E3*). Proteins coded for by both *E1* and *E2* are involved in episomal DNA replication.[6,22] The proteins encoded by *E1* bind to the LCR near the *E6* gene.[6] These proteins have both adenosine triphosphatase (ATPase) and helicase activities. The *E2* gene encodes two proteins of different lengths that assist in regulation following their binding to the LCR. The major role of the *E2* proteins may be in enhancing the attachment of the *E1* proteins to the LCR.

Although the *E4* gene is part of the early region, it encodes for proteins that resemble structural proteins that are coded relatively late in the viral life cycle.[23] These proteins are essential for maturation of HPV. The *E4* proteins, in some manner, interact with the cytokeratin skeleton of the cell; apparently, this permits the virions to leave the cell and thus be able to infect other cells. This creates the classic koilocytic morphology. Viral proteins also interfere with the mitotic spindle and cytokinesis. This explains the common finding of multinucleated cells in preinvasive lesions.[7] It has recently been demonstrated that condylomas related to high-risk viruses are more likely to have abnormally shaped mitotic figures than those related to the low-risk viruses.[24] The *E5* gene encodes for several peptides that are found within the membrane of the keratinocyte.[6] At least one function of these proteins is to enhance the interaction between epithelial growth factor receptor and their ligands. By promoting this interaction, they can enhance cellular growth. In some experimental systems, *E5* demonstrates weak transforming activity. It is often proposed that E5 proteins may in some way inhibit the host response to developing neoplasms. *E6* and *E7* encode proteins that are the major transforming products of HPV.[4,6,25,26]

The late region of the HPV genome contains two open reading frames that encode for capsid proteins.[6] The *L1* gene codes for a larger capsid protein that is highly conserved in nature. The *L2* protein is much smaller. The late region open reading frames are regulated by cellular transcription factors that are apparently not present in immature squamous epithelial cells. Thus, the late region genes are activated only in the intermediate and superficial squamous cells. Large quantities of the late region proteins are produced in LGSIL, whereas much smaller amounts are manufactured in HGSIL and cervical carcinomas.

Although many of the steps in the life cycle of HPV have been elucidated in the last decade, there are still many features that are relatively obscure.[3] It is thought that HPV enters the epithelium through small defects so they can reach the basal epithelial cells. It may be easier for HPV to infect cells in the transformation zone. One aspect of the cycle that is not well understood is the mechanism of lateral expansion of the infection and therefore the lesion.

Two major types of infection are latent and productive.[3,4,6] In the latent type, no clinical or morphologic (colposcopic, histologic, cytologic) signs are present indicating that the squamous epithelium has been infected. The only manner in which infection can be detected is by identification of HPV DNA using molecular techniques. The shedding of virus in quantities sufficient for detection apparently occurs transiently. During this phase, the DNA remains in the keratinocyte nucleus as a circular episome. The HPV DNA replicates only in conjunction with replication of human DNA. Approximately 20 to 100 copies of the virus per cell are present in a latent infection.

In the productive, or replicative, type of infection, viral replication occurs independent of the replication of host cellular DNA. The productive type of infection produces infective virions.[3,6] Most of the viral replication occurs in more mature intermediate and superficial epithelial cells. As the cells mature, the copies of viral DNA amplify into the thousands. Capsid proteins are produced concurrently with this amplification. The amplification appears to be related to cellular replication proteins, but this aspect is not well studied. Infection results in an increased mitotic activity and a prolonged life span of the squamous epithelial cells. However, these cells eventually do die and exfoliate after differentiation. Assembly of the virions occurs in the superficial cells, often resulting in koilocytic morphology, as the cells' cytoplasm comes to be filled with viral particles. The stimulus that actually converts a latent infection into a productive one remains unknown. It has been suggested that both host immunologic factors and the type of HPV may play a role. The process may be reversible.

The mechanism of malignant transformation of squamous epithelial cells by HPV has been well studied.[26] Persistent infection with a high-risk viral type is required for development of HGSIL. The *E6* and *E7* genes are intimately involved and required for malignant transformation. Both *E6* and *E7* are complimentary, resulting in a much higher efficiency of transformation. Both genes, especially *E6*, are probably needed for the maintenance of the malignant phenotype.

Occasional cervical carcinomas appear to contain only episomal HPV DNA both in primary neoplasms and metastases.[27] However, in the vast majority of these malignancies, the HPV DNA is integrated into the host DNA.[26,28] The circular DNA must be linearized before it can be integrated. Linearization usually occurs at *E2*.[7] Integration into the human DNA appears to occur at random sites. Characteristically, this integration results in an inactivation of the *E1* and *E2* genes. With in situ hybridization, the episomal and integrated forms of HPV DNA yield different reaction patterns in the squamous nuclei. With episomal DNA, a diffuse pattern is seen, whereas a dotlike or punctate pattern is present with integration. With in situ hybridization, HPV DNA can be detected in the nuclei of infected cells both in tissue and in cytologic samples.[29,30]

Normally, the expression of the *E2* gene results in a repression of the *E6* and *E7* genes.[26] Thus, integration allows the overexpression of *E6* and *E7* genes. This results in increased cellular proliferation and genetic instability. The small protein encoded by *E7* disrupts normal control mechanisms of cellular proliferation. The molecule *E2F* is a cellular proliferation-stimulating transcription factor that binds to and thus activates several human genes, inducing growth by shifting the cells from the G1 to the S phase of the cell cycle. A normal cellular mechanism to block *E2F* from binding and therefore stimulating growth is the pro-

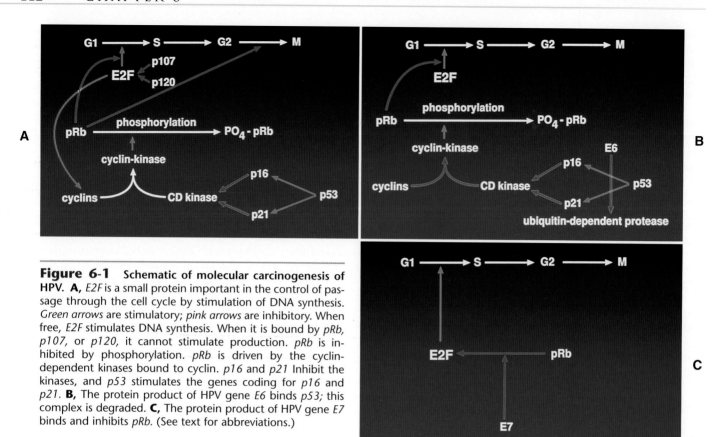

Figure 6-1 Schematic of molecular carcinogenesis of HPV. **A,** *E2F* is a small protein important in the control of passage through the cell cycle by stimulation of DNA synthesis. *Green arrows* are stimulatory; *pink arrows* are inhibitory. When free, *E2F* stimulates DNA synthesis. When it is bound by *pRb*, *p107*, or *p120*, it cannot stimulate production. *pRb* is inhibited by phosphorylation. *pRb* is driven by the cyclin-dependent kinases bound to cyclin. *p16* and *p21* Inhibit the kinases, and *p53* stimulates the genes coding for *p16* and *p21*. **B,** The protein product of HPV gene *E6* binds *p53;* this complex is degraded. **C,** The protein product of HPV gene *E7* binds and inhibits *pRb*. (See text for abbreviations.)

tein product of the retinoblastoma (RB) gene. In addition, it is thought that the retinoblastoma protein *(pRB)* may also in some manner reduce or inhibit transition from the G2 phase to the M phase of the cell cycle. In addition to growth regulation, *pRB* may also be used by some cells for normal differentiation.

The protein product of *E7*, which consists of 98 amino acids, acts primarily by binding to and thus inactivating *pRB*[26]—that is, when *E7* protein is bound to *pRB*, *pRB* cannot bind *E2F*. Thus, *E2F* is in its active state and can promote cellular growth. The passage from the G2 phase to the M phase is mediated at least in part by the proteins cyclin A and cyclin B. The cyclins are inactivated by the activity of cyclin dependent kinases. The *E7* protein binds to the kinases, inactivating these enzymes and thus increasing the quantities of cyclins.

To understand the transforming activity of the polypeptide coded for by the *E6* gene, it is essential to review briefly the activity of the tumor suppressor gene *p53*.[25,26] In normal cells, *p53* has only a small role. However, in cells that have damage to their DNA and that are capable of division, the *p53* gene is activated, resulting in increased levels of *p53* protein. The purpose of the *p53* gene and its product is to prevent the accumulation of potentially oncogenic mutations by cell cycle arrest or by inducing apoptosis. The *p53* peptide accomplishes cell cycle arrest by activating genes that code for cyclin-dependent kinase inhibitors (e.g., *p21*). By inhibiting the kinases, *p53* indirectly blocks the phosphorylation of the retinoblastoma protein. The end result is to reduce the amount of free *E2F*.

The polypeptide product of the *E6* gene is only slightly longer (158 amino acids) than the product of the *E7* gene.[26] *E6* polypeptide directly binds to the *p53* product. In so doing, *E6* inhibits *p53* activity and thus blocks the cell cycle arrest and apoptosis. This is because the *E6-p53* complex is rapidly degraded through the activity of the ubiquitin-dependent protease system. As with the *E7* peptide, the *E6* peptide in high-risk HPV manifests a high affinity for *p53*, whereas in low-risk groups a low affinity is apparent (Figure 6-1).

The laboratory test procedures for the detection of HPV DNA have been improved to the point that they can provide reliable and not massively cumbersome results for both clinical and epidemiologic studies.[31] The earliest test for HPV DNA involved Southern blot hybridization. This test is quite specific and rather sensitive and is considered by some to be the gold standard to which other tests are compared. Major disadvantages of this test include the fact that it is an extremely labor intensive and has a prolonged procedure that requires use of radioactive materials (and therefore is expensive). The first offshoots of this were filter in situ hybridization and dot blot methods. The filter in situ hybridization method is not sensitive and may also have a relatively low level of specificity. The dot blot tests, which are based on RNA-DNA hybridization, were an improvement.

One of the better currently available procedures is based on PCR. This should first use a general primer to detect the presence of HPV DNA, and then, if appropriate, use type-specific primers to determine the specific type of HPV DNA present.

The other major procedure, which has been widely used recently in epidemiologic and clinical investigations, is the Hybrid Capture assay (Digene Diagnostics, Inc., Gaithersburg, Md.).[9,31] This test, now in its second generation, permits a relatively quick evaluation of a specimen without the need for radioactive reagents. Furthermore, the assay permits positive specimens to be divided into those that contain low-risk and high-risk viruses. The amount of HPV DNA is quantitated on the basis of the amount of fluorescence. Schiffman and colleagues performed a large interlaboratory evaluation of the Hybrid Capture assay, comparing it with the results obtained using the polymerase chain reaction.[31] The authors demonstrated that the results of the Hybrid Capture test correlated well with the PCR standard and with the diagnoses of concurrently obtained cervical cytologic samples. More specifically, they demonstrated a strong correlation between the presence of high-risk HPV types and the presence of SIL. This was found for both the PCR-based reference and the Hybrid Capture test. DNA for high-risk HPV types can be detected in archived tissues a dozen years old with either hybrid capture or PCR.

Clinical Investigations

In addition to the previously discussed epidemiologic investigations, these HPV DNA assays can be used in more clinically relevant studies. For example, Elfgren and colleagues recently demonstrated that HPV DNA, using a PCR test, declined significantly after cone biopsy for SIL.[32] In this study of 23 women, four had postconization cytology that was positive for SIL or microinvasive carcinoma. Three of these women were positive for HPV DNA. Thus, one false-negative DNA result occurred. Eighteen other patients could be evaluated, and all were negative both cytologically and for HPV DNA. Interestingly, of the three women with positive HPV DNA tests after the cone biopsy, the HPV type changed in two of them; it remained the same type in the woman with microinvasive carcinoma. Male and female partners may not always harbor the same HPV type.[33]

According to Hatch and colleagues, for women with atypical squamous cells of undetermined significance (ASC–US), the most common form of management is to repeat the cytologic examination in a timely fashion.[34] If the abnormality persists or progresses, then the patient goes to colposcopy. Depending on the study cited, a wide variation is seen in the proportion of women who show SIL on colposcopically directed biopsies. Using the Hybrid Capture assay, Hatch and colleagues found that a positive result for a high-risk HPV type increased the likelihood of histologically discovering a HGSIL compared with a repeat cytologic examination alone.[34] Overall, they demonstrated an increased sensitivity for detecting clinically significant lesions by using both cytology and Hybrid Capture. Of special interest are the 44 women who had a cytologic diagnosis of ASC–US whose subsequent biopsies demonstrated SIL in 24 (55%). Of these, the majority were HGSIL. However, the Hybrid Capture assay was not perfect by any means; nine women who proved histologically to have HGSIL were negative for HPV DNA. Cox and colleagues have also evaluated the Hybrid Capture test by the means of triaging patients with a cytologic interpretation of ASC–US.[35] This study involved 217 women who were tested for HPV DNA by the

Hybrid Capture assay. The authors demonstrated a diagnostic sensitivity of the DNA assay for any level of SIL at 86%. For HGSIL, the sensitivity was 93%. The results of concurrently obtained cytologic examinations were not nearly as high. The authors concluded that diagnostic specificity for HGSIL could be greatly improved by referring only those women with an ASC–US diagnosis who also had high levels of HPV DNA of the high-risk type.

Concepts such as this led to the creation and institution of a huge study involving four university centers. This investigation is known as the *ASCUS-LGSIL Triage Study (ALTS)*.[36] A major goal was to determine the most effective clinical pathway to evaluate women with a cytologic diagnosis of ASC–US or LGSIL. At its inception, women with either diagnosis were randomized into one of three arms: immediate (within 3 weeks) colposcopy, follow-up cytology alone every 6 months, and HPV DNA testing (using the Hybrid Capture assay) to triage for colposcopy.[36,37] As discussed in more detail in Chapter 5, recommendations resulting from this work include referral to colposcopy for women with Pap test diagnoses of ASC–US and hybrid capture HPV assays positive for high-risk HPV types.

Additional Etiologic Factors

Although HPV appears to be the predominant carcinogenic effect in the uterine cervix, other factors also need to come in to play for the development of a large proportion of invasive carcinomas.[1] One of the most readily apparent features is immunosuppression. Notable causes of this suppression are renal transplantation and infection with human immunodeficiency virus (HIV). Both premalignant SIL and invasive tumors are increased overall in women who are immunosuppressed. Perhaps on the basis of immunosuppression, pregnancy may also confer a transient increased risk for the development of lesions secondary to HPV.

One of the more controversial potential factors is the use of oral contraceptives.[1] Several recent investigations have shown an association between long-term use of these agents and an increased risk for cervical disease. However, it is certainly not conclusive in that other studies have failed to manifest such a significant relationship. It is traditionally considered that postmenopausal women have a reduced risk of developing HPV-related cervical lesions. In light of this, the results of a recent study by Smith and colleagues prove interesting.[38] They evaluated the presence of HPV DNA in postmenopausal women who were receiving hormone replacement therapy. Over a 2-year period, the overall frequency of positivity for HPV DNA using a PCR-based test was 50%. Of these, HPV 16 was detected in 76%, and HPV 31 was found in 21%. It must be noted, however, that HPV DNA was also detected in a similar proportion of women who were not receiving exogenous steroids.[38]

Cigarette smoking has shown an independent role for the development of cervical disease independent of HPV infection in many studies.[1,39] Several investigations have demonstrated that the relative risk for developing cervical disease is correlated with both the duration of cigarette smoking and the number of cigarettes smoked. Thus, it appears as if cervical neoplasia may be related to cigarette smoking in a dose-dependent manner. Several studies have demonstrated the presence of components of tobacco smoke and their metabolites in cervical mucus.

For some time, the infectious agent that was most implicated in cervical carcinogenesis was herpes simplex virus (HSV).[1] Although HSV has been supplanted by HPV, it is thought by some that HSV may still play a role, possibly through mutagenesis, in the development of these neoplasms.

In has long been held that a high proportion of cases of mild dysplasia spontaneously regress, and a much smaller percentage of cases progress to invasive carcinoma. In an extensive review of four decades of literature, Ostor calculated regression, persistence, and progression rates for different levels of squamous dysplasia.[40] For patients with mild dysplasia, approximately 60% regress, and only 1% develop into an invasive carcinoma. On the other hand, only one third of severe dysplasias regress, and more than 12% develop into an invasive neoplasm. Ostor emphasized that based solely on histopathology, it was impossible to predict accurately which lesions would progress or regress.[40] One ancillary technique that may increase the ability to predict the fate of dysplastic lesions is the measurement of ploidy in the abnormal nuclei. Overall, dysplastic lesions that are either diploid or polyploid show a strong likelihood for a spontaneous involution, whereas those that are aneuploid are more apt to progress or at least persist. Histomorphologically, ploidy may be estimated by evaluation of chromosomal lag.[41] In many early invasive squamous carcinomas, a gain in the long arm of chromosome 3 has been demonstrated; this cytogenetic abnormality is not present in the majority of HGSIL. It has been hypothesized that a progressive imbalance between proliferation and programmed cell death may play a role in the evolution of squamous dysplasias.[42] Allelic imbalances, especially at the short arm of chromosome 3, occurs in a relatively low proportion of LGSIL lesions. It appears as if allelic reduction is more heterogeneous in LGSIL than in HGSIL, suggesting that the latter is genetically more homogeneous (fewer different abnormal clones). It has been suggested that women who are infected with HPV are more likely to experience early spontaneous abortions than those who are not infected.[44]

Sherman and colleagues have recently reviewed the potential for a prophylactic HPV vaccine.[45] The latent HPV proteins have been the major antigens used in attempts to generate a vaccine. Some vaccines have been developed using viruslike particles; the latter are hollow capsid structures lacking HPV DNA and can be produced by molecular techniques. In the proper conformation, the *L1* protein induces type-specific neutralizing antibodies of the immunoglobulin G (IgG) type (work is in progress on immunoglobulin A [IgA] antibody induction). The *L2* protein, although capable of stimulating low levels of antibodies, does not contribute significantly. The vaccine does not require an adjuvant. Humoral reactions appear to be sufficient to prevent infection. Sherman proposed that a widespread vaccine program is a number of years away.[45]

Work is also in progress to develop an agent that not only prevents HPV infection but also destroys an established infection. This is being attempted through the stimulation of the cell-mediated immune response. One experimental cocktail includes HPV proteins *L1*, *L2*, *E2*, and *E7*.

 # CYTOLOGY OF HUMAN PAPILLOMAVIRUS AND SQUAMOUS INTRAEPITHELIAL LESIONS

Introduction and Terminology

The Pap test's tremendous success in preventing cervical carcinoma lies in its ability to detect preinvasive epithelial alterations. Underlying this is the idea that most invasive carcinomas arise from carcinomas in situ that have in turn arisen from lesser degrees of abnormality. However, it is clear that some tumors do not pass through this sequence or do so very quickly. Furthermore, some appear to arise *de novo* from apparently normal epithelium. Assertions of this type leave unaddressed the possibility of false-negative antecedent biopsies resulting from sampling or interpretation.

Low-grade intraepithelial lesions may be associated with low-risk HPV types and have a low risk of progression. Some such lesions may be biologically indolent and almost a separate disease process than the high-grade lesions with their high-risk HPV types. This would imply that at least a substantial fraction of high-grade lesions are high-grade *ab initio* and do not develop by progression of a low-grade lesion. However, at least some LGSILs harbor high-risk virus types and pose a risk for progression to HGSIL.

Histologically, *dysplasia* is defined as a delay in maturation of basal-layer cells along with acquisition of various degrees of morphologic derangement. An assessment of the degree of abnormality has great clinical importance. Over the years, a number of grading schemes have been employed. In general, the trend over several decades has been toward fewer subdivisions, until, in the current classification, only two grades remain. Table 6-2 summarizes the relationships among various grading schemes.

Dysplasia remains a useful term in histopathology and seems firmly entrenched in the colloquialisms of cytopathology, but the concept of intraepithelial neoplasia (or lesions) is in keeping with our ideas about preinvasive alterations in other body sites. The grades of dysplasia are meant to connote an increasing delay in maturation associated with increasingly abnormal cellular morphology. As described in Chapter 3, the normal cervical squamous epithelium is divided into a basal layer of cells, several strata of parabasal cells, layers of intermediate cells, and a lumenal

TABLE 6-2

Grading Schemes for Preinvasive Abnormalities of the Uterine Cervical Squamous Epithelium

Traditional Dysplasia Classification	Cervical Intraepithelial Neoplasia (CIN)	Intraepithelial System Classification*
Mild dysplasia	CIN 1	LGSIL
Moderate dysplasia	CIN 2	HGSIL
Severe dysplasia	CIN 3	HGSIL
Carcinoma in situ	CIN 3	HGSIL

LGSIL, Low-grade squamous intraepithelial lesion; *HGSIL,* high-grade squamous intraepithelial lesion.
*This system is currently applied only to cytologic preparations and has not been widely adopted for histologic material.

surface of superficial cells. In the normal state, basal cell maturation begins immediately in the first layer of parabasal cells. This gives the basal layer a very well-demarcated appearance, as the cells above it begin to acquire increasingly abundant cytoplasm and progressive nuclear pyknosis.

A delay in maturation of basal cells indicates that these small dark cells remain so as they ascend for some distance into the upper layers of the epithelium. When this involves the lower one third of the epithelium and maturation begins above that point, it is *mild dysplasia*. If the maturational delay continues into the middle one third of the epithelium, the process is termed *moderate dysplasia*. The basal cells do not retain normal cytologic features. In the traditional scheme, the histologic distinction between severe dysplasia and carcinoma in situ was based on a thin layer of surface maturation. It is difficult to distinguish true matu-

ration from a slight surface flattening that often occurs in carcinoma in situ, so that reproducible distinction between these two categories was never achieved. In cytologic preparations, striking morphologic abnormalities accompany the maturational delay. These cytologic abnormalities are reflected in altered cellular polarity within the epithelium and by the presence of mitotic figures in layers above the basal layer. Figure 6-2 summarizes the histologic findings in cervical intraepithelial neoplasia (CIN) 1, 2, and 3.

The Bethesda System's two-tier classification is appealing for its improved reproducibility and its direct correlation with clinical significance. Furthermore, its clinical relevance underscores recognition of high- and low-risk HPV types and their relevance to lesion progression. A similar dichotomy exists in the ploidy of SILs. Those that are diploid or polyploid are more likely to regress, whereas those that

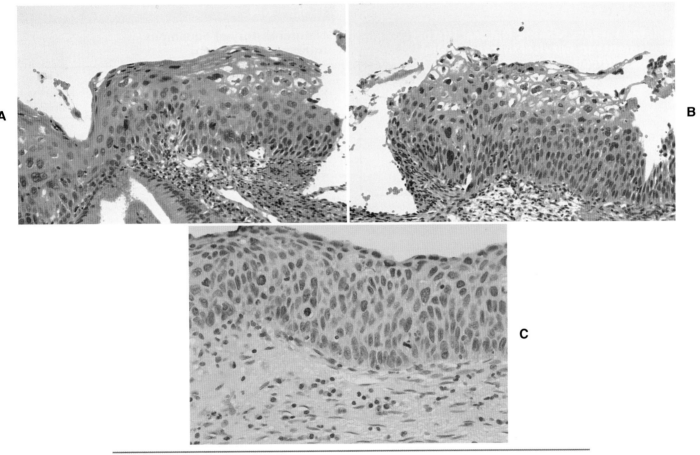

Figure 6-2 **Histopathology of cervical intraepithelial neoplasia in the squamous epithelium of the uterine cervix. A,** This metaplastic squamous epithelium overlies a gland-bearing area of the endocervix. The squamous epithelium shows a slight arrest of maturation with small, dark, somewhat vertically polarized cells occupying the lower one third of the epithelium, representing cervical intraepithelial neoplasia (CIN) I. Above this, the epithelium shows koilocytes with large hyperchromatic nuclei and prominent cytoplasmic vacuolization. This and the next illustration show the way in which koilocytic cells representing HPV infection occupy the upper layers of the epithelium, while dysplastic cells extend upward from the basal layer. This explains the now-archaic designation of koilocytic change as inverted atypia. **B,** This example of CIN 2 shows small hyperchromatic, vertically polarized and slightly spindled basal layer-like cells occupying the lower one half to two thirds of the squamous epithelium. Surface koilocytes are noted in a manner similar to that described in Figure 6-1, *A.* **C,** This example of CIN 3 (squamous cell carcinoma in situ) shows a transepidermal arrest of maturation. This is manifested by small, dark, vertically polarized cells with little cytoplasm that extend completely through the epithelial thickness. The surface shows neither normal maturation nor koilocytic change. (Hematoxylin eosin [H&E])

TABLE 6-3

Risk of Progression to Invasive Carcinoma for Various Grades of Intraepithelial Neoplasia

		WOMEN DEVELOPING INVASIVE CARCINOMA (%)		
Reference Number	Number of Patients	CIN 1	CIN 2	CIN 3
49*	43	14		86
50†	62	2	7	82
51	70,236	1.0	5.0	42.3

CIN, Cervical intraepithelial neoplasia.
*A two-tired (low grade vs. high grade) system was used in this study.
†These authors studied women with carcinoma and smears previously considered negative. The diagnoses reflected in these data are review interpretations. Clearly, such a sample is highly skewed toward the aggressive lesions.

BOX 6-1

Variable Factors Making Natural History Assessments in Cervical Intraepithelial Lesions Difficult

Length of follow-up
Diagnostic criteria
Diagnostic reproducibility
Methods of clinical follow-up
Associated risk factors or conditions
Accurate identification of the most severe disease present
Interim interventions*

*It is possible that inflammation and regeneration engendered by a biopsy can alter the natural history of a preneoplastic lesion.

TABLE 6-4

Natural History of Squamous Intraepithelial Lesions

Initial Diagnosis	Regress	Persist	Progress to Carcinoma in Situ	Progress to Carcinoma
CIN 1	57	32	11	1
CIN 2	43	35	22	5
CIN 3	32	56	–	12

Data from Ostor AG: Natural history of cervical intraepithelial neoplasia: a critical review. Int J. Gynecol Pathol 1993; 12: 176-192.
CIN, Cervical intraepithelial neoplasia.

are aneuploid tend to persist or progress.[46-48] However, the ultimate utility of Bethesda System terminology lies in the fact that it is predictive of patient outcome, in terms of risk for development of invasive carcinoma.

Table 6-3 summarizes three investigations that indicate the low risk for invasive carcinoma that is associated with LGSIL.[49-51] The term *SIL* has not been uniformly adopted for use in histopathology. Hence, this designation is used in discussion of cytology, and use of CIN terminology is retained for discussions of histopathology. SIL lesions can regress, persist, or progress. A number of factors make it difficult to derive accurate risk assessments, as summarized in Box 6-1. This is especially true for patients with a potentially serious condition who do not wish to undergo prolonged follow-up without treatment. As summarized in Table 6-4, Ostor evaluated rates of persistence, progression, and regression. These too are difficult to investigate for the previously cited reasons.[52] Regression after conclusion of a pregnancy seems more clearly established. This could be due to either regeneration following the trauma of delivery or the altered immune status after parturition. It is also important to note that even though a lesion may no longer be detectable by cytology or colposcopy, the patient remains at high risk for recurrent dysplasias and invasive carcinoma. Appropriate surveillance is important.

The data in Tables 6-3 and 6-4 are highly variable, and to a great extent, this reflects the difficulties cited in Box 6-1. However, the trend is clear: LGSIL rarely progresses, whereas HGSIL does so more commonly. Thus, the dichotomous division of SIL into high and low grade reflects the virology, ploidy, and clinical outcome. As molecular biologic investigations continue, it will be interesting to see whether this division extends to even finer levels.

Anatomic and Pathologic Considerations

The point at which the ectocervical squamous mucosa meets columnar cell mucinous epithelium of the endocervix is the squamocolumnar junction. This point is not static and moves proximally through the transformation zone as inflammation, infection, or other irritations necessitate that the distal canal be lined by a heartier squamous epithelium. It can then recede when conditions normalize. Histologically, one does not commonly see the abrupt transition between epithelia connoted by the term *junction*. Instead, the mature squamous mucosa is separated from the columnar cell surface by a zone of squamous metaplasia of variable width. Thus, the concept of a zone rather than a junction seems clear.

The surface of the endocervical canal is complex, with folds or clefts, and glands that extend below the surface. A dysplastic growth can follow these natural contours to yield a complex histologic appearance. Distinctions between carcinoma in situ, microinvasive carcinoma, and frankly invasive carcinoma are considered in Chapter 7. Abdul-Karim and colleagues described the linear (surface) extent and depth of dysplasias as a function of grade.[53] Their data are summarized in Table 6-5 and have obvious implications for

TABLE 6-5

Relationship of Dysplasia Grade with Linear Extent and Depth of Dysplastic Lesions*

Grade of Dysplasia	Average Linear Extent	Average Depth Below Surface
CIN 1	4.1	0.42
CIN 2	5.8	0.93
CIN 3	7.6	1.35

From Abdul-Karim FW, Fu YS, Reagan JW, et al. Morphometric study of intraepithelial neoplasia of the uterine cervix. Obstet Gynecol 1982; 60:210-214.
*All measurements are in mm.

the size and depth of conization procedures needed to remove dysplastic tissue.

After arising in the transformation zone, dysplasias undermine and then replace the endocervical epithelium. Extension to the ectocervix is less common. This process most often occurs on the anterior cervical lip. Lesions that show more than one grade of dysplasia are very common. When this occurs, the higher-grade process is usually situated proximal (e.g., higher) in the endocervical canal than the lower-grade lesion. This is one explanation for negative or low-grade colposcopic examination and biopsies in the face of cytology with clear evidence of HGSIL.

One additional issue related to the distribution of squamous dysplasia is important. Most lesions are localized and can be eradicated. This is in contrast with adenocarcinoma in situ. This glandular lesion is usually situated beyond the range of the colposcope, a fact of little consequence, since it grows as multiple foci that are microscopic in extent. Confidently eradicating these lesions is a complex issue.

The sequence of HPV/dysplasia/carcinoma in situ/invasive carcinoma is probably the route through which most squamous cell carcinomas of the uterine cervix arise. In most instances, the progression happens over a period of several years. This has been reflected by the traditionally cited average ages for cytologic detection of dysplasia (early 30s), carcinoma in situ (early 40s), and invasive carcinoma (early 50s).[54] However, a few tumors appear to arise directly from normal epithelium or have a fast transition through precursor stages.

Low-Grade Squamous Intraepithelial Lesion, Including Human Papillomavirus

Normal squamous epithelial cells and the process of squamous metaplasia were described in Chapter 3. The histologic components of dysplasia are summarized in Table 6-6. In LGSIL, these alterations are mild and by definition are seen only in the deepest one third of the epithelium (see Figure 6-2). However, in addition to parabasal cell layers that show this degree of maturational delay, the surface layers may show HPV cytopathic effect. The Bethesda System combines the cytologic picture that reflects CIN 1 with changes of HPV cytopathic effect with the designation LGSIL. The cytologies of these entities are discussed separately in this chapter, as they were classically described. Then, the chapter will return to the discussion on unification of these findings under the rubric LGSIL. Overlapping cytodiagnostic criteria, virtually

identical clinical implications, and a strong tendency toward association with low-risk HPV types justify this unification. Furthermore, the therapeutic implications of both diagnoses are currently identical.

The cells of LGSIL that do not show HPV effect resemble normal superficial or intermediate cells in size and cytoplasmic staining. This cytoplasmic configuration is an important criterion in distinguishing LGSIL from HGSIL. Superimposed on this picture are nuclear abnormalities summarized in Table 6-7.[55] These alterations are illustrated in Figure 6-3. Normal squamous cells, those with benign reactive alterations and ASC–US, were contrasted in Chapter 4, and this comparison is now expanded to include LGSIL without HPV cytopathic effect (Table 6-8). All of these cell types show essentially the same cytoplasmic volume, configuration, and tinctorial properties. Distinction among them is based on differences in nuclear morphology and the attendant feature of nuclear to cytoplasmic (N:C) ratio. Despite the rather clear-cut–sounding criteria of the Bethesda System, cutoff points for passing from reactive cellular changes (RCC) to ASC–US and from ASC–US to LGSIL remain somewhat subjective.

A paradox surrounds the diagnosis of LGSIL. In the absence of confounding technical problems, the cytologic diagnosis of LGSIL is usually straightforward. The cells are large with large hyperchromatic nuclei and often stand out clearly at screening magnification. If the nuclear alterations are fully developed and RCC is not a consideration, interpretation is subject to little or no equivocation. In some cases, difficulty occurs in achieving unanimity in distinguishing LGSIL from HGSIL.[56] In histologic preparations, on the other hand, subtle alterations with minimal nuclear atypia and little appreciable increase in mitotic activity can lead to great subjectivism and poor reproducibility in the diagnosis of CIN 1 among pathologists. This problem is greatly exacerbated by tangential sections of small biopsies. Such difficulties also can extend to other levels of CIN.[57-59] When evaluating cervical biopsies that seem equivocal for low-grade dysplasia, it is the authors' practice to review any available Pap test cytologic sample that led to colposcopy and biopsy.

Most vulvar and vaginal condylomata are exophytic and clearly visible. In contrast, most condylomata of the uterine cervix are flat (condyloma planum) and invisible until turned white by application of dilute acetic acid. (Acetowhite patches are a common target for cervical biopsy.)

HPV cytopathic effect results in cellular alterations termed *koilocytosis*. In histologic samples, the affected cells occupy the upper levels of the squamous epithelium, rather than spreading upward from the basement membrane, as is the case for dysplasias. Hence, the now outmoded term *inverted atypia* was used before the relationship of these cells to HPV infection was clarified. The cytologic characteristics of koilocytes and less diagnostic associated changes are summarized in Box 6-2. Cytoplasmic cavitation, thickened cell borders, and the listed nuclear abnormalities are required for this diagnosis. The nuclei of HPV lesions are abnormal by definition so that terms such as *atypical condyloma* have no place in the current diagnostic lexicon. The features of koilocytosis are illustrated in Figure 6-4.

As noted in Chapter 4, small perinuclear halos are a common reactive change, especially with *Trichomonas* infesta-

---

TABLE 6-6

Histologic Features of Dysplasia

Normal Squamous Epithelium	Dysplastic Squamous Epithelium
Distinct basal cell layer	Loss of a distinct basal cell layer
Orderly maturation from base to surface	Cellular disorganization
Horizontal polarity of nuclei at levels above the basal layer	Vertical polarity
Orderly cytoplasmic maturation:	Delayed maturation:
• Increased cell size	• Cells remain small
• Increasing cytoplasmic volume	• Cytoplasmic volume remains small
• Decreasing nucleocytoplasmic ratio	• Nucleocytoplasmic ratio remains high
Progressive development of nuclear pyknosis	Retain nuclear features of immaturity
Mitotic activity confined to the basal layer	Mitotic figures above the basal layer
All mitotic figures are normal	Some mitotic figures may be abnormal

---

TABLE 6-7

Bethesda System Cytomorphologic Features for Low-Grade Squamous Intraepithelial Lesion Not Showing Human Papillomavirus Effect

Cytomorphologic Feature	Finding in LGSIL Without HPV Effect
Cell arrangements	Single cells and sheets of cells
Cytoplasmic features	Resemble superficial or intermediate cells:
	• Eosinophilic or cyanophilic
	• Abundant
	• Well-defined polygonal cell borders
Nuclear features	Less severe than in HGSIL:
	• Nuclear enlargement up to ×3*
	• Resultant increase in N:C ratio
	• Moderate variation in size and shape
	• Slight irregularities in nuclear outline
	• Hyperchromasia†
	• Uniformly distributed chromatin
	• Finely granular chromatin
	• Nucleoli are usually not seen
	• Well-defined nuclear membrane

From Kurman RJ, Solomon D. The Bethesda System for reporting cervical/vaginal cytologic diagnoses: definitions, criteria, and explanatory notes for terminology and specimen adequacy. New York: Springer-Verlag; 1994.

HGSIL, High-grade squamous intraepithelial lesion; *LGSIL,* low-grade squamous intraepithelial lesion; *HPV,* human papillomavirus; *N:C,* nuclear to cytoplasmic ratio.

*In the Bethesda System, nuclear sizes are described in terms of their apparent areas, and are given as multiples of the normal intermediate cells' nuclear area of 35 μm². In LGSIL with features of cervical intraepithelial neoplasia (CIN) 1, the average N:C ratio is 15%, rather than the 2% to 3% in normal intermediate cells.

†Well-fixed intermediated cell nuclei are *normochromatic* by definition. The term *hyperchromasia* means nuclear staining darker than that of intermediate cells in the same cytologic preparation.

tions. These have less distinct borders and do not achieve the voluminous cavitary, or "cookie-cutter," appearance of koilocytosis. Glycogenation is also common and can result in substantial cytoplasmic clearing with thickened cell borders. This is especially true for navicular cells associated with pregnancy. For this reason, nuclear abnormalities are another *sine qua non* of koilocytosis. Cells showing HPV cytopathic effect have enlarged hyperchromatic nuclei that are often wrinkled, or "raisinlike." Their chromatin is often smudgy without the fine granularity of LGSIL cells with features of CIN 1 (see Table 6-7). Substantial nuclear abnormalities are also required for diagnosis of condyloma in histologic preparations. Failure to insist on this criterion leads some to overdiagnose HPV infections in cervical biopsy samples. These low-grade findings do not constitute a medical emergency, and conservatism is order because of the adverse social implications of glibly diagnosing a sexually transmitted disease.

HPV may lead to striking keratosis. This is often shed as large, thick, orangeophilic plaques. Close examination shows either polygonal cells or spindle cells with the latter representing a flattening of the epithelial surface. The nuclei of these cells may be enlarged and hyperchromatic. In some instances, a clear diagnosis of LGSIL is possible. This is especially true when such plaques are associated with koilocytes elsewhere in the preparation. In the absence of both koilocytes and nuclei fully diagnostic of LGSIL, these plaques should be interpreted as ASC–US. If the suggestion of LGSIL is strong, a comment to that effect may be added to the report. Finally, multinucleation is a common reactive alteration in both squamous and glandular cells of the cervix. Although true koilocytes often show multinucleation, this finding alone is insignificant unless coupled with the other more important diagnostic features of HPV effect.

The separation of LGSIL with classic features of CIN 1 from cases with fully developed HPV cytopathic effect facilitates a discussion of both ends of the LGSIL spectrum. However, this construct is highly artificial. Many cytologic samples show a morphologic range, and cells with both types of features occur together. It is also possible to have samples with straightforward CIN 1 cells and incompletely developed koilocytes. Such findings still constitute LGSIL. In the experience of Sherman and colleagues, experienced pathologists are no better than chance alone in distinguishing these two entities in a given cytologic sample, affirming the unified concept of LGSIL.[59]

The only differential diagnostic considerations for LGSIL involve intermediate or superficial-type cells with lesser de-

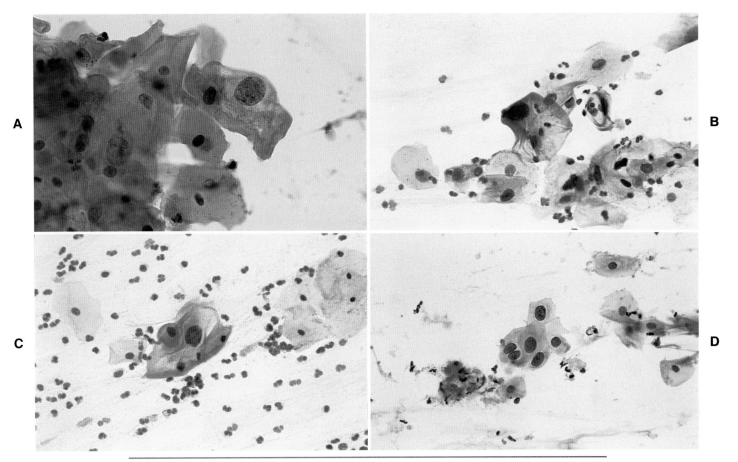

Figure 6-3 Low-grade squamous intraepithelial lesion (LGSIL); human papillomavirus (HPV) viral cytopathic effect not shown. These cytologic alterations are known in classical cytology as *mild dysplasia,* and in histopathology they should be reflected in CIN 1. **A** to **D,** Each of these images show cells that have the cytoplasmic configuration and staining qualities of intermediate or superficial cells. However, their nuclei are strikingly abnormal. Compared with normal intermediate cell nuclei elsewhere in these images, these cells of LGSIL show nuclei that are markedly enlarged and hyperchromatic with varying degrees of chromatin granularity or even smudging. (Papanicolaou [Pap])   *Continued*

grees of nuclear atypia. Such cells should either be considered a benign cellular change (see Chapter 3) or ASCUS (see Chapter 5). The current version of the Bethesda System (2001) does not employ the term *ASCUS favor LGSIL.* However, individual practitioners are free to add descriptive comments that they feel more fully convey a diagnostic impression to the treating physician.

High-Grade Squamous Intraepithelial Lesion

As noted in Table 6-2, this Bethesda System category includes cytologic findings previously termed *moderate dysplasia, severe dysplasia, carcinoma in situ, CIN 2,* and *CIN 3.* The cells are smaller than those of LGSIL and generally resemble some stage in the process of squamous metaplasia, as it was described and illustrated in Chapter 3—hence, the now antiquated term *metaplastic dysplasia.* Many histopathologists still use a three-tiered system, so that different types of HGSIL are referred to as showing features of CIN 2 or features of CIN 3. It is the authors' belief that although this diagnostic distinction has no significant clinical, prognostic, or therapeutic implications, it facilitates description of the

full range of cytomorphology now subsumed under the rubric of HGSIL (Figures 6-5 and 6-6).

The Bethesda System criteria for HGSIL are summarized in Table 6-9. These cells encompass a wide range of cell sizes, N:C ratios, and degrees of nuclear abnormality. Resembling a stage in the process of squamous metaplasia, they are always smaller than the cells of LGSIL, with less cytoplasm, a higher N:C ratio, and much more conspicuous nuclear abnormalities. At the extreme, some HGSILs yield only small, isolated cells that are few in number; there can be widely scattered and easily missed at the time of initial screening. Many HGSILs are accompanied by cells more typical of LGSIL or condyloma. These do not alter the diagnosis, and pathologists should report only the highest grade lesion identified.

The cell arrangements in HGSIL include single cells, sheets, loosely streaming collections of cells similar to those often seen in squamous metaplasia, and syncytial clusters. The latter vary widely in size and are seen much more frequently in conventional smears than in liquid-based preparations. A syncytium contains variable numbers of closely packed intensely hyperchromatic nuclei that

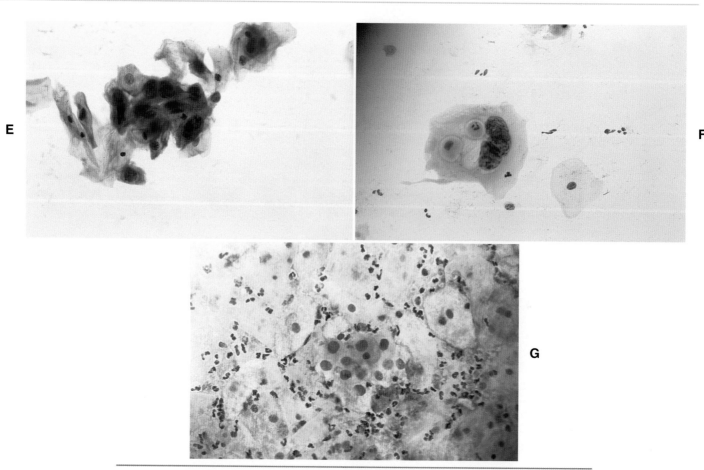

Figure 6-3, cont'd **E,** Similar abnormal nuclei are present in some of these cells in this thick cluster. However, such nuclei, although enlarged and hyperchromatic, can be easily missed at screening magnification, as they are obscured within the three dimensions of this cell cluster. When viewed at the microscope, they stand out as the focus is varied. **F,** This extremely large cell shows the features of LGSIL noted in Figures 6-2, A-D. When compared with the adjacent normal intermediate cell, this abnormal cell is shown to be extremely large. As noted in Table 6-2, this is a common finding in smears that elsewhere manifest clear-cut evidence of HPV viral cytopathic effect. The term *giant superficial cells* has been applied to this type of LGSIL cell. **G,** This conventional smear preparation suffers from cell crowding, acute inflammation, and a striking degree of air-drying artifact. In this setting the major diagnostic criteria for LGSIL, including nuclear size and hyperchromasia, are lost. The diagnostic reproducibility is greatly hampered. Some observers considered this normal, whereas others described abnormal squamous cells of uncertain significance. (Pap)

mold to one another, as little cytoplasm separates adjacent cells. No cell borders can be perceived so that the cluster appears as a disorganized collection of nuclei. Mitotic figures and apoptotic bodies can often be seen within the larger clusters.

The nuclei in HGSIL, especially those with features of CIN 3, are often smaller than those of LGSIL. The cells are made even smaller and given a high N:C ratio because they have little cytoplasm. Irregularities of nuclear contour may be striking, and this is especially true when newer liquid-based preparatory methods are used. Chromatin may be either finely or coarsely granular but is usually distributed uniformly. Nucleoli are not typical of HGSIL but may be seen when the process grows inward by following the intact, pre-existing basement membrane of endocervical glands.

The small dark cells of HGSIL with features of CIN 3 are often associated with small orangeophilic cells that super-

ficially resemble the cells of parakeratosis. Closer inspection shows that these cells and their nuclei often have irregular shapes and nuclei that are larger than the tiny pyknotic bodies that define parakeratosis. Furthermore, the nuclei, although extremely hyperchromatic, are not completely smooth as expected in parakeratosis. Rather, they retain some coarse chromatin structure with areas of clearing and are often irregular in shape. It is possible that some of these cells represent differentiation of dysplastic cells. However, this would seem to be at odds with the extremely immature nature of the HGSIL cells. These cells are suggested to be degenerating dysplastic cells, the abnormal nuclei of which have begun to collapse. Their orangeophilia is also degenerative in nature, much like that seen in pseudoparakeratotic parabasal cells that are common among the atrophic cells from postmenopausal patients.

TABLE 6-8

Cytomorphologic Features of Normal Cells, Reactive Cells, Atypical Squamous Cells of Undetermined Significance, and Low-Grade Squamous Intraepithelial Lesions

Feature	Normal	Reactive	ASC–US	LGSIL
Cell size*	1500	1500	1500	1500
Nuclear size*	35	up to ×2 normal (70)	up to ×3 normal (105)	≥ ×3 normal (≥105)
Nuclear features				
Hyperchromasia†	Absent	Minimal	Mild	Present and obvious†
Nuclear contour	Smooth	Smooth	Minimal irregularity	Mild irregularity
Chromatin texture	Finely granular	Finely granular	Finely granular	Finely granular
Chromatin clearing	Not seen	Not seen	Not seen	Not seen
Multinucleation	Not seen	Common	May be seen	May be seen
Nucleoli	Not seen	Not seen	Not seen	Rarely seen
Cytoplasmic features				
Polychromasia	Not seen	May be present	Not seen	Not seen
Vacuolization	Not seen	May be present	Not seen	Not seen
Perinuclear Halos‡	Not seen	May be present	Not seen	Not seen‡

ASC–US, Atypical squamous cells of undetermined significance; *LGSIL*, low-grade squamous intraepithelial lesion.
*All sizes are given in μm² and are derived from Dr. Patten's average area measurement for intermediate squamous cells.[10]
†Well-fixed intermediated cell nuclei are "normochromatic" by definition. The term hyperchromasia means nuclear staining darker than that of intermediate cells in the same cytologic preparation.
‡These are small concentric cytoplasmic clearings situated close to the nucleus, and do not resemble the gaping cavitary cytoplasmic clearing associated with koilocytes (see Chapter 4).

BOX 6-2

Human Papillomavirus–Associated Alterations in Cytologic Samples

Required for identification of koilocytosis*
Large punched-out appearing clear cytoplasmic cavity occupies most of the cell volume
Thickened cell border and peripheral cytoplasm
Nuclear abnormalities:
• Enlargement
• Hyperchromasia
• Irregularities of contour

Additional abnormalities that may be seen†
Keratosis:
• May contain abnormal nuclei (enlarged, hyperchromatic, smudged)
• May show a prominent spindle cell configuration
• Often shed in large, thick plaques
Multinucleation
Smudging of chromatin may be striking
Cytomegaly with "giant superficial cells"
Anucleate ("ghost") cells

*These cytomorphologic features constitute the definition of koilocytosis. All must be present to warrant a diagnosis of low-grade squamous intraepithelial lesion showing human papillomavirus (HPV) cytopathic effect.
†Whether singly or in combination, these findings do not fulfill the definition of koilocytosis and are not diagnostic of HPV cytopathic effect.

Once the abnormal cells have been identified (e.g., not missed in screening), two major problems attend the accurate diagnosis of HGSIL, as summarized in Table 6-10.

HGSIL is distinguished from squamous metaplasia by nuclear enlargement, hyperchromasia, and membrane irregularities, together with a marked elevation in N:C ratio. In histologic preparations, mitotic figures can be found in the upper levels of dysplastic squamous epithelium, and some may be abnormal as evidenced by asymmetric or multipolar metaphases. Abnormal mitotic figures have been significantly associated with aneuploidy, polyploidy, and high-risk HPV types.[60-62]

Patten described the cytology of three types of carcinoma in situ, based on cell size, nuclear size, and N:C ratio.[63] The large cell type of carcinoma in situ is virtually indistinguishable from CIN 2 by these means. The smallest cells of HGSIL with features of CIN 3 can be difficult to distinguish from very immature forms of squamous metaplasia. Using Patten's camera lucida cell measurements, the cells he called *small cell* and *intermediate cell carcinomas in situ* are contrasted with those of immature squamous metaplasia in Table 6-11.[63] These data are rounded averages derived from his more detailed descriptions. With this in mind, it is obvious that considerable overlap is possible and that distinction of HGSIL with features of CIN 3 from immature squamous metaplasia can be difficult.

If careful application of cytologic criteria cannot resolve this diagnostic dilemma, a diagnosis of *ASC, favor HGSIL* (ASC–H) would be appropriate. Sherman and colleagues indicated that many such samples herald a true HGSIL.[64] Prospective evaluation of this diagnostic category will undoubtedly be facilitated by its recent elevation to the status of an official entry in the Bethesda System diagnostic terminology.

Atypical immature metaplasia (AIM) is poorly defined and of unclear clinical significance. Histologically, it is operatively defined as an *immature squamous metaplasia* with

less atypia than seen in carcinoma in situ. As summarized in Box 6-3, its features were outlined by Crum and colleagues.[65] Based on finding a wide range of Ki-67 indices and variable HPV status in 27 microdissected examples of AIM, Geng and colleagues suggested that this entity represents a heterogenous group of lesions.[66] However, noting a

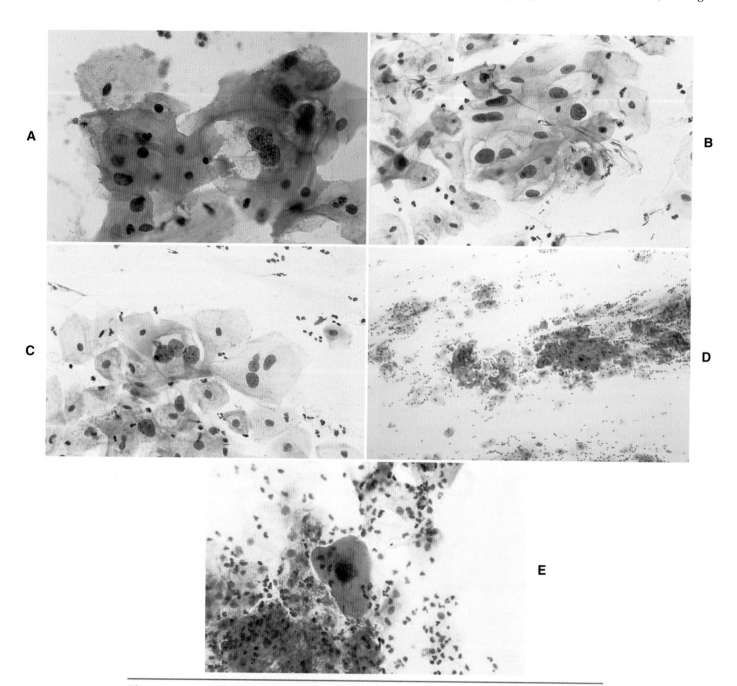

Figure 6-4 HPV cytopathic effect. **A** to **C,** Classic koilocytic change is illustrated in these images. The cells have the cytoplasmic configuration and volume of intermediate or superficial cells. However, this is altered by large cavitary cytoplasmic clearing with sharp borders. This clearing pushes the remaining cytoplasm outward so that the cells have very thick rims with sharp borders. The nuclear features in these examples are similar to those in LGSIL without HPV cytopathic effect. In other examples, varying degrees of nuclear smudging are evident. **D,** This image of a conventional smear shows koilocytes at low magnification. Even at this screening lens view, the cytoplasmic clearing is apparent (×100). **E,** This extremely large keratotic and somewhat misshapen squamous cell does not show classic koilocytic morphology. However, this degree of cytomegaly, keratosis, and nuclear abnormality are diagnostic of LGSIL and suggestive of HPV cytopathic effect. (Pap)

high rate of concurrent or subsequently developing HGSIL in association with AIM, these investigators called for close clinical follow-up for these patients, especially in the face of positive HPV testing or a high Ki-67 labeling index. However, it has also been suggested that most cases of AIM share the cytologic features of LGSIL.[65] At this time, the histologic diagnosis of AIM is regarded as problematic, and it is not recognized as a distinct cytodiagnostic entity. Using current terminology, it is likely that most such cases would be called *ASC–H.*

The small cells of normal atrophic squamous epithelium can occur singly or in sheets and clusters. Within aggregates, their nuclei can appear crowded because the cells have little cytoplasm. Mild air-drying is a common condi-

tion that can lead to nuclear enlargement. Other examples show diffuse mild-to-moderate nuclear enlargement without hyperchromasia or chromatin distribution abnormalities. Abati and colleagues have shown that this change is not a sign of ASC or SIL and that it is reversible with estrogen application. On the other hand, if karyomegaly is associated with hyperchromasia or irregularities of nuclear contour, the risk of ASC or SIL increases.[67] However, Jonanovic and colleagues describe pseudokoilocytosis as another type of postmenopausal squamous atypia. In their evaluation of 30 cervical biopsies from women over age 50 and older, they found no evidence of HPV by PCR. They suggested that most of these troublesome, but nondysplastic atypias differ from true koilocytosis in the following

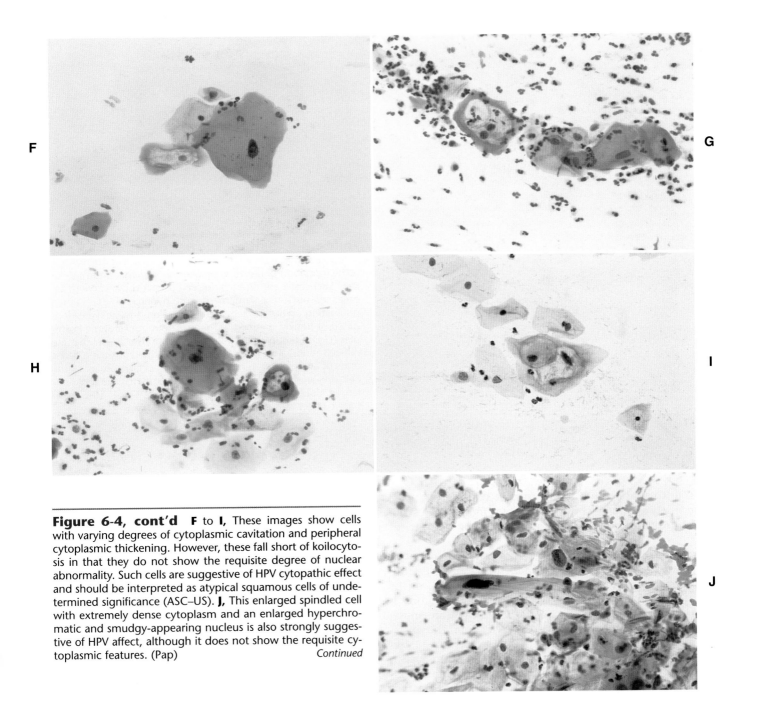

Figure 6-4, cont'd   **F** to **I,** These images show cells with varying degrees of cytoplasmic cavitation and peripheral cytoplasmic thickening. However, these fall short of koilocytosis in that they do not show the requisite degree of nuclear abnormality. Such cells are suggestive of HPV cytopathic effect and should be interpreted as atypical squamous cells of undetermined significance (ASC–US). **J,** This enlarged spindled cell with extremely dense cytoplasm and an enlarged hyperchromatic and smudgy-appearing nucleus is also strongly suggestive of HPV affect, although it does not show the requisite cytoplasmic features. (Pap) *Continued*

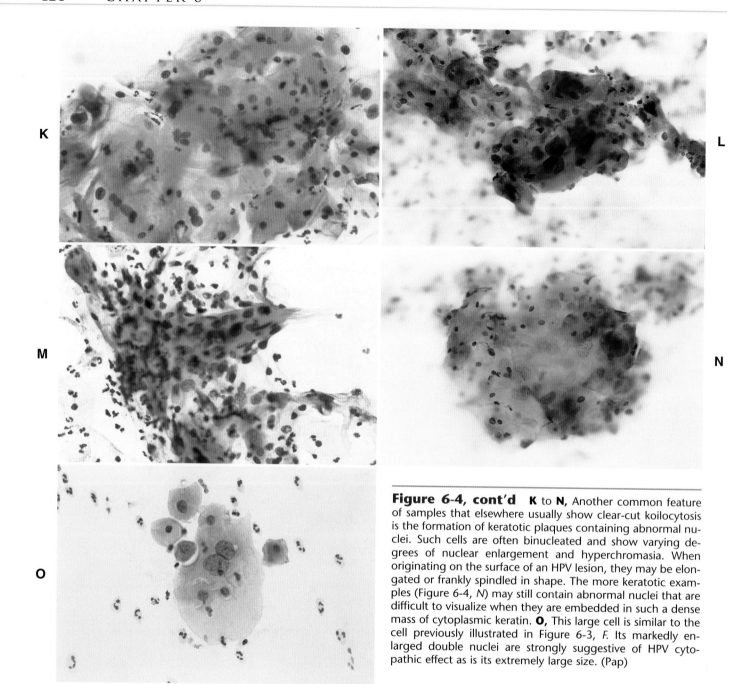

Figure 6-4, cont'd **K** to **N,** Another common feature of samples that elsewhere usually show clear-cut koilocytosis is the formation of keratotic plaques containing abnormal nuclei. Such cells are often binucleated and show varying degrees of nuclear enlargement and hyperchromasia. When originating on the surface of an HPV lesion, they may be elongated or frankly spindled in shape. The more keratotic examples (Figure 6-4, *N*) may still contain abnormal nuclei that are difficult to visualize when they are embedded in such a dense mass of cytoplasmic keratin. **O,** This large cell is similar to the cell previously illustrated in Figure 6-3, *F.* Its markedly enlarged double nuclei are strongly suggestive of HPV cytopathic effect as is its extremely large size. (Pap)

ways: less variation in nuclear size and staining intensity, more finely granular chromatin, more uniformly distributed chromatin, and greater uniformity of perinuclear halos.[68]

In those cases in which the question of HGSIL in a postmenopausal patient cannot be confidently resolved by routine methods, a small amount of topical estrogen can be used to stimulate maturation of the cervical epithelium. If a repeat Pap test shows dysplastic cells, they are much more clearly delineated once removed from the background of small dark atrophic cells. The problem of a false-negative repeat resulting from sampling error has not been satisfactorily investigated in this setting. Ejersbo and colleagues described an alternative to the method of repeat after estrogen administration. They applied a Ki-67 immunostain to previously Pap-stained samples and found that a negative result was a reliable indicator of atrophy and not HGSIL.[69]

A number of essentially normal types of glandular cells present as small clusters with dark staining and occasionally require distinction from HGSIL. These include tubal metaplasia, exfoliated endometrial cells, directly sampled lower uterine segment endometrial cells, and damaged or atrophic endocervical cells (see Chapter 3).

Transitional cell metaplasia (TCM) was also described in Chapter 3. Weir and Bell have contrasted TCM, HGSIL, atrophy, and tubal metaplasia.[70] Key points in the differential diagnosis between this normal, but uncommon finding and HGSIL are summarized in Table 6-12. Importantly, TCM lacks the marked hyperchromasia, coarse chromatin, nu-

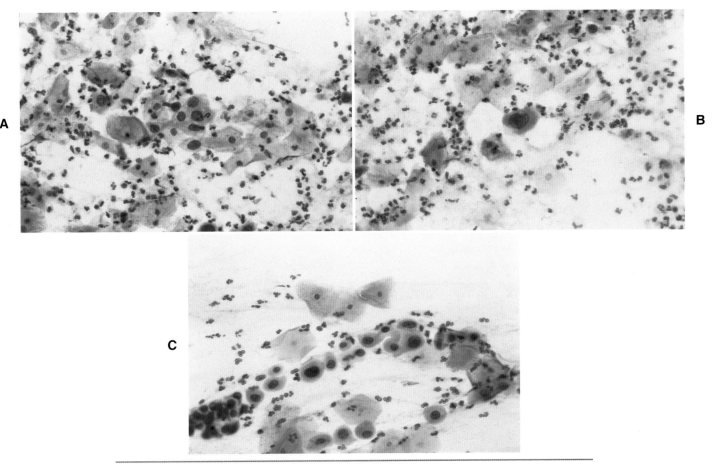

Figure 6-5 High-grade squamous intraepithelial lesion (HGSIL) of the type previously designated *moderate dysplasia.* (The histological correlate of this cytologic finding is CIN 2.) **A** and **B,** The abnormal cells in the center of this image show cytoplasm that has the configuration and staining quality of immature squamous metaplastic cells. Thus, the cells are smaller than the surrounding intermediate and superficial cells. However, their nuclei are strikingly enlarged and hyperchromatic. **C,** These abnormal cells also resemble immature squamous metaplastic cells with superimposed marked nuclear abnormalities. However, these cells show less cytoplasm and a higher nuclear to cytoplasmic (N:C) ratio than those illustrated in Figures 6-4, *A* and *B.* Although still representing HGSIL, these are cells that in the previous classifications would have been considered intermediate between moderate dysplasia and severe dysplasia/carcinoma in situ. Histologically, such cells may correspond to either lesion. (Pap)

clear contour irregularities, and high N:C ratios of HGSIL. Nuclear grooves can be found in either condition but are much more common in TCM.

Keratinizing Squamous Intraepithelial Lesions

LGSIL with HPV effect can show strikingly atypical keratinized cells that on an individual basis may mimic those of invasive keratinizing squamous cell carcinoma. Hence, the older term pleomorphic dysplasia. The diathesis pattern that sometimes accompanies invasive carcinomas is usually absent in tumors with marked keratinization. Furthermore, intermediate stages of keratinizing dysplasia have not been defined in cytologic terms, and no recognized entity can be considered keratinizing carcinoma in situ. Should all examples keratinizing dysplasia carry a disclaimer, such as *cannot exclude invasive carcinoma*? In the author's practice, they do not. Atypical keratosis as a part of HPV cytopathic effect is much more common than floridly keratinized car-

cinoma. The latter diagnosis must rest on clinical or histologic findings.

Squamous Intraepithelial Lesions in Special Clinical Circumstances

By definition, abnormal cells should not be interpreted as postradiation dysplasia during the first 6 months after treatment for cervical carcinoma. After that time, cells showing classical features of an intraepithelial lesion have long been held as a warning sign of recurrent carcinoma, especially if detected within the first three years following therapy.[71] However, most of this literature antedates current practices in radiation therapy and the significance of cytologic abnormalities following radiation has not been adequately reevaluated in the new era. All such findings should prompt careful clinical evaluation.

SIL has also been noted after chemotherapy and immunosuppression[72-74] and in patients infected with HIV.[75-79]

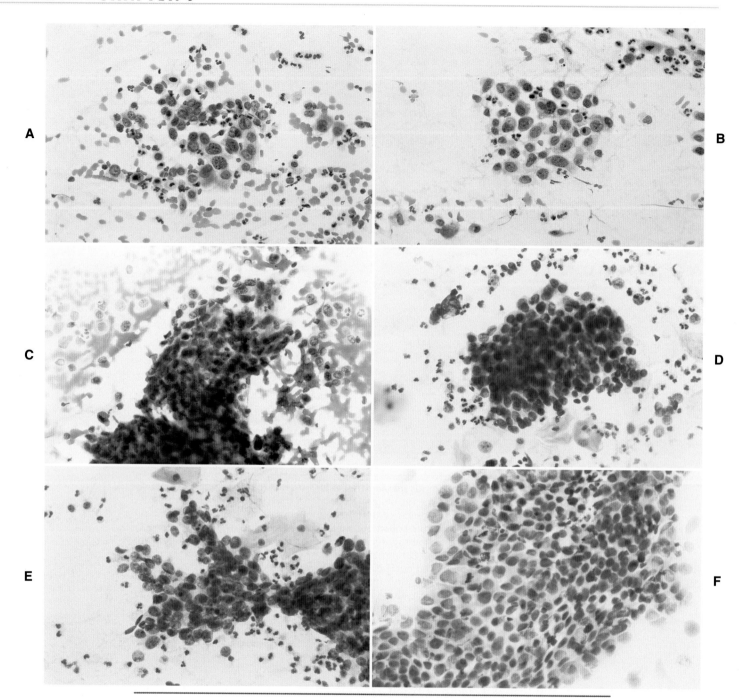

Figure 6-6 HGSIL with features of severe dysplasia/carcinoma in situ. The histologic correlate of this cytologic picture is CIN 3. **A** and **B,** These images show loose clusters of small cells. These have the size and cytoplasmic configuration of immature squamous metaplastic cells or parabasal cells. However, their nuclei are enlarged to the extent that each cell has a high N:C ratio. When individual cells are examined closely, the nuclei range from minimally to moderately hyperchromatic and the chromatin can be either finely granular or more coarsely stippled. **C** and **D,** These tightly cohesive three-dimensional cell clusters show small hyperchromatic nuclei with no apparent cytoplasmic borders. This syncytial pattern is seen in many examples of HGSIL. They are much more common in conventional smears than in liquid-based preparations. Only at the edge of such cell clusters can one appreciate the nuclear hyperchromasia and coarse chromatin pattern of individual nuclei. **E,** This syncytial group of HGSIL cells shows features similar to those in Figures 6-6, *C* and *D.* Near the center of the photograph, small, round, intensely hyperchromatic fragments of nuclear material represent individual cell apoptosis. **F,** Air-drying artifact renders this syncytial cluster of HGSIL cells as large and pale. However, careful examination of this cluster shows mitotic figures and apoptotic bodies indicating the rapid cell proliferation typical of HGSIL cell clusters. (Pap)

Table 6-13 compares the rate of dysplasia in various patient groups with and without HIV infections.[79] Another study found a similar increase in SIL among women with HIV. However, after multivariate analysis, these investigators found clinical acquired immune deficiency syndrome (AIDS), as opposed to HIV seroconversion without clinical AIDS, and morphologically demonstrated HPV infection to be the only independent variables capable of predicting the presence of an SIL. In the work of Davis and colleagues, CD4 lymphocyte counts and viral load measurements cor-

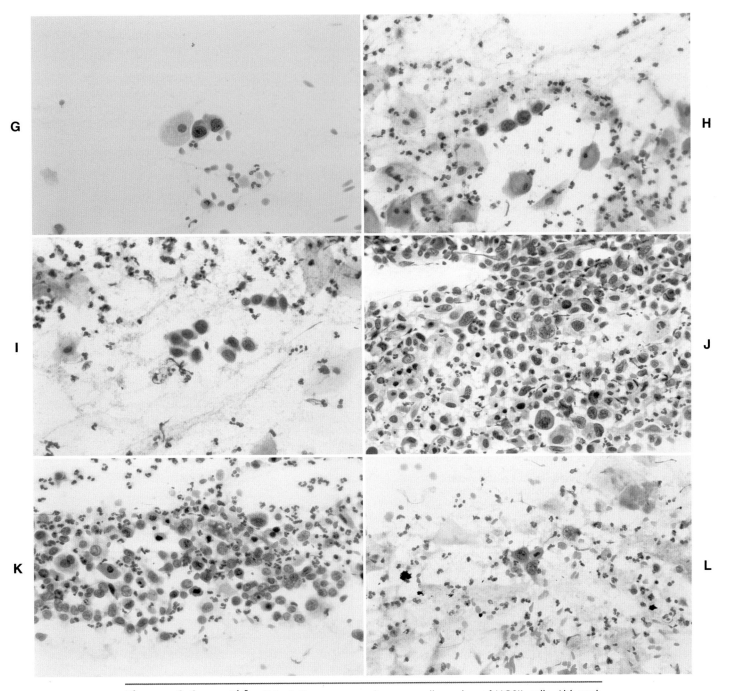

Figure 6-6, cont'd **G** to **I**, Some smears show a small number of HGSIL cells. Although they still feature high N:C ratio, nuclear hyperchromasia and varying degrees of chromatin clumping, they can be difficult to identify at screening magnification. **J** to **L**, Each of these images shows cells typical of HGSIL. Scattered among these cells are small, intensely eosinophilic cells with hyperchromatic nuclei. These cells are distinguished from the cells of reactive parakeratosis in that their nuclei are large, sometimes irregular in shape and are not completely pyknotic as one expects in parakeratosis. Instead, these nuclei are somewhat open and retain an identifiable chromatin structure. This picture is caused by degeneration of HGSIL cells. When cells such as these are seen in the absence of cells with more clear-cut features of HGSIL, they should be regarded as a possible herald of this lesion and interpreted as ASC with a note that HGSIL cannot be excluded (ASC–H). (Pap)

TABLE 6-9

Bethesda System Cytomorphologic Features for High-Grade Squamous Intraepithelial Lesion

Cytomorphologic Feature	Finding in HGSIL
Cell arrangements	Single cells, sheets, syncytial clusters
Cell size	Smaller than LGSIL
Cytoplasmic features	Resemble a stage of immature squamous metaplasia: • Moderate or scant in amount • Cyanophilic* • Delicate and lacy or • Dense with concentric laminations • May be vacuolated
Nuclear features	Nuclear enlargement of ×2-3 Resultant marked increase in N:C ratio Moderate variation in size and shape Irregularities in nuclear outline may be marked† Hyperchromasia is variable; some are hypochromatic† Uniformly distributed chromatin Finely or coarsely granular chromatin Nucleoli are usually not seen

From Kurman RJ, Solomon D. The Bethesda System for reporting cervical/vaginal cytologic diagnoses: definitions, criteria, and explanatory notes for terminology and specimen adequacy. New York: Springer-Verlag; 1994.
N:C, Nuclear to cytoplasmic ratio; HGSIL, high-grade squamous intraepithelial lesion; LGSIL, low-grade squamous intraepithelial lesion.
*Problems related to high-grade lesions with keratinized cytoplasm are discussed separately. Furthermore, some high-grade squamous intraepithelial lesion (HGSIL) cells show a degenerative orangeophilia.
†These may be especially prominent in liquid-based preparations.

TABLE 6-10

Differential Diagnostic Problems in High-Grade Squamous Intraepithelial Lesion

HGSIL Pattern	Differential Diagnosis
Small single cells	Immature squamous metaplasia Atypical immature squamous metaplasia
Syncytial cell clusters	Atrophy Tubal metaplasia Exfoliated endometrial cells Directly sampled lower uterine segment endometrial cells Endocervical cells Transitional cell metaplasia

HGSIL, High-grade squamous intraepithelial lesion.

BOX 6-3

Histologic Features of Atypical Immature Metaplasia

Uniform basal cell population
Minimal nuclear crowding
Basal cells with variable hyperchromasia
Basal cells with uniform chromatin distribution
Preserved cellular polarity within the epithelium
Enlarged or multiple nuclei confined to suprabasilar areas
Absence of abnormal mitotic figures

From Crum CP, Egawa K, Fu YS, et al. Atypical immature metaplasia (AIM): a subset of human papillomavirus infection of the cervix. Cancer 1983; 51(12):2214-2219.

BOX 6-4

High-Grade Squamous Intraepithelial Lesion Cells in Liquid-Based Preparations: Contrasts with Conventional Smears

Few abnormal cells may be present
High-grade squamous intraepithelial lesion cells may appear smaller
Chromatin clumping can be less apparent
Hyperchromasia is less striking; some lesions yield hypochromasia
Syncytial groups are not commonly seen

---

related with the presence of SIL, and CD4 counts emerged from multivariate analysis as an independent risk factor for SIL or invasive squamous cell carcinoma.[76] In the experience of Stratton and colleagues, pregnancy does little to alter the incidence of SIL in HIV positive women.[77]

Liquid-Based Preparations

Liquid-based preparation of Pap test cytology samples is now a widespread practice. The current version of the Bethesda System suggests reports that have a specimen-type designation where the type of processing may be specified. At the time of this writing, the categories are conventional, liquid based, and the forward-looking "other." Many laboratories enjoy these usually artifact-free preparations, whereas clinicians and patients benefit from improved detection rates. Both benefits result from a decrease in preparatory ar-

tifacts such as air-drying. Cytologic interpretation in most conditions is little altered from conventional material. However, significant differences in the appearance of HGSIL cells can cause difficulties. These are summarized in Box 6-4. Despite these differences, irregularities of nuclear contour may be more striking than in conventional preparations, and the abnormal cells show a high N:C ratio.

TABLE 6-11

High-Grade Squamous Intraepithelial Lesion (Patten's Small Cell Carcinoma In Situ) Contrasted with Immature Squamous Metaplasia

Type of Lesion	Average Size	Average Nuclear Size	Average N:C Ratio
HGSIL (small cell carcinoma in situ)	100 μm²	70 μm²	70%
HGSIL (intermediate cell carcinoma in situ)	200 μm²	100 μm²	50%
Immature squamous metaplasia	300 μm²	50 μm²	17%

N:C, Nuclear to cytoplasmic ratio; *HGSIL,* high-grade squamous intraepithelial lesion.

TABLE 6-12

Differential Diagnosis of Transitional Cell Metaplasia and High-Grade Squamous Intraepithelial Lesion

Feature	Transitional Cell Metaplasia	HGSIL
Architecture	Sheets, multilayered, streaming	Syncytia, multilayered, nuclear overlap
Nucleoli	Small	Chromocenters only
Nuclear shape	Oval, spindled, tapered	Round, oval
Chromatin	Powdery	Hyperchromatic; fine or coarse
N:C ratio	Low	High
Grooves	Present	Rare
Contour	Wrinkled, regular	Irregular
Size*	×1.5-2.5	×1.5-2.0
Halos	Present	Absent

Data from Weir MM, Bell DA. Transitional cell metaplasia of the cervix: a newly described entity in cervicovaginal smears. Diagn Cytopathol 1998; 18:222-226.
N:C, Nuclear to cytoplasmic ratio; *HGSIL,* high-grade squamous intraepithelial lesion.
*Size comparison with an intermediate squamous cell nucleus

TABLE 6-13

Incidence of Biopsy Proven Squamous Intraepithelial Lesion as a Function of Human Immunodeficiency Virus Status

Patient Profile	Number Studied	Percentage with Dysplasia or Carcinoma
HIV positive	111	41
HIV-negative intravenous drug users	76	9
HIV-negative general clinic population	526	4

From Schafer A, Friedmann W, Mielke M, et al. The increased frequency of cervical dysplasia-neoplasia in women infected with the human immunodeficiency virus is related to the degree of immunosuppression. Am J Obstet Gynecol 1991; 164:593-599.
HIV, Human immunodeficiency virus.

Careful evaluation of these two features is essential to accurate diagnosis of HGSIL (Figure 6-7). The 2001 Bethesda System designation *ASC–H* is appropriate for those cases in which small cells of immature squamous metaplasia cannot be distinguished from those of a HGSIL.

 ## SCREENING

The goal of cervical cancer screening is obviously not detection of established malignancies. Rather, preventing development of these often lethal tumors is accomplished by detecting and eradicating a potentially premalignant process. It seems fitting to consider issues related to screening as a part of the discussion of SILs. Criteria of the World Health Organization (WHO) for a screening program are summarized in Table 6-14.[80]

Cervical cancer screening based on Pap tests is the most effective cancer prevention strategy ever devised. It has lowered the death rate from cervical cancer by 70%.[81,82] However, the United States continues to experience 13,000 cases annually and 4100 deaths from cervical carcinoma. Schneider and colleagues outline the evidence that a screening program may be failing and summarize reasons for such shortcomings[82,83] (Box 6-5).

Janerich and colleagues reviewed the screening history of 481 women diagnosed with invasive cervical carcinoma over a 5-year period in Connecticut.[84] Their results are similar to those in other studies.[85-87] Some of the Connecticut data are summarized in Table 6-15. The 20-year age difference between women who were and were not receiving screening suggests that this important test may not be a regular part of older women's health care. Furthermore, older individuals have a tendency to present with higher stage

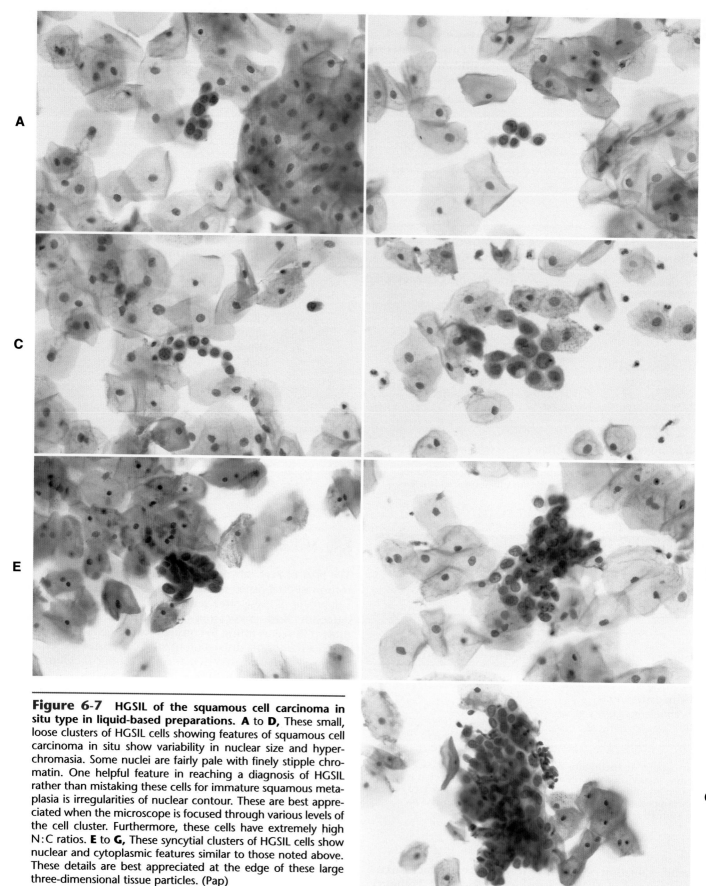

Figure 6-7 HGSIL of the squamous cell carcinoma in situ type in liquid-based preparations. **A** to **D,** These small, loose clusters of HGSIL cells showing features of squamous cell carcinoma in situ show variability in nuclear size and hyperchromasia. Some nuclei are fairly pale with finely stipple chromatin. One helpful feature in reaching a diagnosis of HGSIL rather than mistaking these cells for immature squamous metaplasia is irregularities of nuclear contour. These are best appreciated when the microscope is focused through various levels of the cell cluster. Furthermore, these cells have extremely high N:C ratios. **E** to **G,** These syncytial clusters of HGSIL cells show nuclear and cytoplasmic features similar to those noted above. These details are best appreciated at the edge of these large three-dimensional tissue particles. (Pap)

carcinomas than younger women. The most important observation from this table is that 57.8% of new cervical cancer patients have either never been screened or have not been screened for several years. When those who were screened but did not receive adequate follow-up for detected abnormalities are added, cancer prevention is discovered to have been possible for 68.6%. Schneider and colleagues highlighted population groups that are often underscreened[82] (Box 6-6) and suggested innovative approaches for reaching these groups.[88,89]

Nearly one fourth of new cervical cancer patients in this study had previous normal Pap tests. (It is important to note that this statement is based on review of available slides. A lack of such review with attendant heavy reliance on medical records is a weakness of many studies of this type.) To what extent this reflects sampling error at the time of specimen collection is not completely clear. However, Gay and colleagues found that 63% of negative conventional smears taken within 1 year of a diagnosis of carcinoma or carcinoma in situ were negative, resulting from unsuccessful lesion sampling.[90]

The remaining data in the work of Janerich and colleagues showed that 6.9% of new cervical carcinoma cases were associated with previous abnormal Pap tests that had been mistakenly interpreted as within normal limits. These false-negative results resulting from interpretive errors are much less common than false-negative results resulting from apparent sampling errors. (Setting aside the issues of rapidly progressive tumors and those that do not pass through recognizable precursor stages, these are cases with a negative test in a patient who develops carcinoma.) Numerous studies of false-negative interpretation have

---

TABLE 6-14

World Health Organization Guidelines for a Screening Medical Test

Test Feature	Guidelines
Characteristics of the disease	Must be an important public health problem
	Must have a recognizable early stage
	Natural history must be known
Effect of treatment	Treatment of abnormalities detected by screening must be effective
Characteristics of the test	A suitable test must be available
	The test must be acceptable to large numbers of at-risk patients
	The test's harm must be less than its benefit
	Must be economically beneficial, based on cost-benefit analysis

Modified from Schneider V, Henry MR, Jimenez-Ayala M, et al. Cervical cancer screening, screening errors and reporting. Acta Cytol 2001; 45:493-498.

BOX 6-5

Screening Program Failures

Signs of failure
Failure to reach women at risk
Low coverage rate*
Long screening interval
Inadequate follow-up of abnormal smears
High false-negative rates

Reasons for failure
Lack of patient participation in programs
Poor-quality smears
Inaccurate smear interpretation
Inadequate follow-up or treatment
Inherent tumor biology†

From Schneider V, Henry MR, Jimenex-Ayala M, et al. Cervical cancer screening, screening errors and reporting. Acta Cytol 2001; 45:493-498.
*Percent of the at-risk population being screened.
†As noted in the text, a minority of cervical carcinomas arise *de novo*, without detectable preinvasive (dysplastic) stages. Others may pass through recognizable noninvasive phases but seem to do so with a rapidity that allows them to elude standard screening practices.

TABLE 6-15

Screening Histories of Women Newly Diagnosed with Invasive Cervical Carcinoma (N = 481)

Screening History	%	Mean Age ± SD
Never screened	28.5	64.5 ± 14.4
Previous smear correctly interpreted and not requiring follow-up:		
Excessive screening interval (>5yr)	23.5	49.7 ± 13.0
Long screening interval (3-5 yr)	5.8	47.9 ± 16.1
Short screening interval (<3 yr)	24.5	43.2 ± 12.3
Previous smear incorrectly interpreted as normal*	6.9	45.5 ± 16.4
Incomplete follow-up after a smearing requiring investigation	10.8	46.6 ± 12.7

From Janerich DT, Hadjimichael O, Schwartz PE, et al. The screening histories of women with invasive cervical cancer, Connecticut. Am J Public Health 1995; 85:791-794.
SD, Standard deviation.
*When reevaluated by the investigators, these are smears felt to show an abnormality that would require follow-up.

BOX 6-6

Population Groups that Are Often Underscreened

Indigenous peoples
Recent immigrants
Minorities
Inner city residents
Rural poor

Schneider V, Henry MR, Jimenez-Ayala M, et al. Cervical cancer screening, screening errors and reporting. Acta Cytol 2001; 45:493-498.

TABLE 6-16

False-Negative Rate Due to Screening Errors

Reference	All SILs and Carcinomas (%)	HGSIL and Carcinoma (%)
91	14.4	7.1
92	10.6	10.1

From Gay JD, Donaldson LD, Goellner JR. False negative results in cervical cytologic studies. Acta Cytol 1985; 29:1043-1046; Wilbur DC, Prey MU, Miller WM, et al. The AutoPap system for primary screening in cervical cytology: comparing the results of a prospective, intended-use study with routine manual practice. Acta Cytol 1998; 42:214-220.
SIL, Squamous intraepithelial lesion; *HGSIL*, high-grade squamous intraepithelial lesion.

 BOX 6-7

Factors that May Make a Smear More Likely to Receive a False-Negative Interpretation

Few abnormal cells present
Abnormal cells present on only part of a conventional smear
Abnormal cells singly rather than in groups
HGSIL cells that are small
HGSIL cells that lack nuclear hyperchromasia

From Mitchell H, Medley G. Differences between Papanicolaou smears with correct and incorrect diagnoses. Cytopathology 1995; 6:368-375; Smith PA, Turnbull LS. Small cell and "pale" dyskaryosis. Cytopathology 1997; 8:3-8.
HGSIL, High-grade squamous intraepithelial lesion.

been published, but variations in methodology often make comparisons impossible. Two studies that report comparable data are summarized in Table 6-16.[91,92]

Mitchell and Medley described factors that may make a Pap test more likely to receive a false-negative diagnosis[93,94] (Box 6-7). Most of these are not surprising. Small pale cells of a HGSIL can be difficult to locate and even more difficult to interpret, once they have been identified.

It is clear that there exists a subset of HGSIL that is very difficult to interpret correctly. Bergeron and colleagues reviewed Pap tests taken from 585 women within 3 years of biopsy-proven squamous cell carcinoma in situ.[95] Of these, 132 were originally classified as negative, representing 87 patients (14.8%). When reviewed, 27 of these (20%) showed HGSIL, 10 showed LGSIL, 10 were considered to show ASCUS, and seven were unsatisfactory. In addition, 78 (59%) were considered negative on review.

However, in looking at the problem of false-negative HGSILs, the overall issue must be put into proper perspective. Most Pap tests are normal. A given false-negative rate is a percentage of an already small fraction of all cases. Thus, a 5% false-negative rate in a low-risk population with a 1% HGSIL rate means that one in 2000 is a false-negative HGSIL. This tiny 0.05% error rate would be something of which this profession could be proud, were it not for the fact that each error has a potential for terrible impact in a woman's life.

In the work of Gay and colleagues laboratory errors were almost equally divided between screening and interpretive errors.[90] Davey provided a detailed discussion of the problems that arise as we try to agree on a definition of a false-negative result.[96] She discussed the variables involved and highlighted the range of definitions that have led to publication of false-negative rates ranging from 10% to more than 70%. Her operative definition is one that these authors would adopt:

> "A test riginally reported as negative or normal, which is found to have sufficient numbers of carcinoma or dysplastic (SIL) cells on review. The abnormal cells should be verifiable by more than one experienced cytologist in a blind fashion, and it is ideal if the lesion is confirmed by biopsy or other confirmatory test."[96]

Even this seemingly straightforward definition has some difficulties. It should be clear from the foregoing that the number of abnormal cells on a Pap test is an important factor in determining the probability that it will result in a false-negative interpretation. This problem affects quality control measures but is even more severe when cytopathologists are reviewed as a result of a medicolegal proceeding.

It is important that this definition stresses reproducibility in recognition of previously missed abnormal cells. The abnormality must not be equivocal. A corollary of this concept is that it is usually unreasonable to consider as false-negative diagnoses of ASC or atypical glandular cells of undetermined significance (AGUS). The lack of reproducibility at this level of cytologic abnormality is great. These authors have seen medicolegal proceedings that have turned on the idea that treatment would have differed significantly if a test had been interpreted as ASC-US rather than as negative. In most instances, this cytologic distinction is too subjective to form the basis for allegations of malpractice, regardless of the clinician's insistence that this distinction would have been of great clinical import.

Describing a false-negative rate as a simple percentage of cases requires analyzing a large fraction of the total caseload. Furthermore, it ignores the enormous range in disease prevalence among different laboratories or even among different clinics sending material to a given laboratory. Hence, the concept of a false-negative fraction (FNF) as defined in the following way[97-99]:

$$FNF = \frac{\text{Estimated false-negative results}}{(\text{True-positive results} + \text{Estimated false-negative results}) \times 100}$$

This calculation begins with information about a laboratory's historic false-negative rate, as determined by ongoing quality control measures, such as rescreen of tests interpreted as negative. Then, by employing this estimated false-negative rate in both parts of the fraction, it is independent of disease prevalence. This permits interlaboratory comparisons in a way that would be meaningless using a simple false-negative rate.

Naryshkin summarized previously published FNF.[98] A range from 1.6% to 27.7% is probably reflective of variations in the method used to determine the estimated false-negative rate. Another factor is the diligence of slide review. In some settings, rescreening is delegated to a pathologist, who often performs only a cursory examination of the

BOX 6-8

Quality Control Strategies for Reducing the Number of False-Negative Smears

100% rescreen
Rescreen 10% of randomly selected negative smears
Rescreen 10% of smears, targeting a high risk population
Rapid rescreen of most or all cases
Automated rescreening

TABLE 6-17

Interobserver Agreement in Pap Test Diagnosis and Interpretation of Histologic Material

Cytologic Diagnosis	Kappa Statistic
All liquid-based Pap tests	0.59
Negative vs. atypical squamous cells	0.56
Atypical squamous cells vs. LGSIL	0.64
LGSIL vs. HGSIL	0.51
Histologic Diagnosis	**Kappa Statistic**
Cervical biopsy	0.56
LEEP conization	0.58

Data from Stoler MH, Schiffman M. Interobserver reproducibility of cervical cytologic and histologic preparations: Realistic estimates from the ASCUS-LSIL triage study. J Am Med Assoc 2001; 285:1500-1505.
HGSIL, High-grade squamous intraepithelial lesion; *LGSIL,* low-grade squamous intraepithelial lesion.

TABLE 6-18

Initial Pap Test Findings in Patients Ultimately Shown to Have a High-Grade Squamous Intraepithelial Lesion

Cytologic Diagnosis	PERCENTAGE OF HISTOLOGIC HGSIL PRESENTING WITH THIS CYTOLOGIC DIAGNOSIS	
	Patients <40 Years Old	Patients >40 Years Old
ASC	43.6	44.3
AGC	8.3	16.3
LGSIL	20.2	9.4
HGSIL	29.7	30.0

Data from Kinney WK, Manor MM, Hurley LB, et al. Where's the high grade cervical neoplasia? The importance of minimally abnormal Papanicolaou diagnoses. Obstet Gynecol 1998; 91:379-386.
HGSIL, High-grade squamous intraepithelial lesion; *ASC,* atypical squamous cell; *AGC,* atypical glandular cell; *LGSIL,* low-grade squamous intraepithelial lesion.

slide. This does not constitute appropriate rescreening and is complicated by the fact that pathologists have a higher screening error rate than experienced cytotechnologists. Rescreening for quality control purposes should be conducted in a manner that recapitulates the laboratory's day-to-day operations as closely as possible. The slow, exaggerated rescreening that often takes place under testing or investigative circumstances might exaggerate the error rate, and will try to measure a type of performance other than that actually taking place. This reaches its peak when slides are reviewed for medicolegal purposes and one is monetarily compensated for lavishing enormous amounts of time on a single Pap test. One can look at the slide until cells that could never be detected by a technologist screening under normal laboratory circumstances are identified. Review of slides in this manner bears no relationship to actual practice. As a quality control methodology, it is misleading. As an expert witness's behavior, it is probably unethical.

Box 6-8 summarizes strategies for reducing the number of false-negative results. The most common method is either random or targeted rescreen of 10% of negatives. This technique is laborious and has the capacity to find only 10% of abnormal false-negative results. In many laboratories, the rate of significant abnormalities is so low that few screening errors are identified by this method. An alternative method has been mandatory in the United Kingdom since 1995. This involves a rapid (60 seconds) rescreen of all negative slides.[100-102] Dudding indicated that considerable differences were noted in competence among various individuals involved in rapid rescreening. However, his interesting experiment with Americans not accustomed to the method indicates that up to 50% of LGSIL and 60% of HGSIL can be identified by this method. It is ironic that after a decade of mounting evidence showing that this method is superior to the 10% rescreen, the United States will require an act of Congress before making the switch. The ultimate utility of automated screening for quality control is not yet clear.[103]

Regardless of the quality control method in use, false-negative results cannot be completely eliminated at this time. Naryshkin suggests that an FNF of 5% may be the *irreducible sustainable floor.*[98] Considerably higher values will occur under some circumstances, particularly if analyses are conducted over short-term intervals. Despite its imperfections, and the need for careful quality control, the Pap test remains the most effective cancer screening tool ever devised. Its continued success will require access to regular screening at appropriate intervals for all at-risk women. This will be facilitated by educational efforts directed by this profession to the public, physicians, and legislators. While celebrating the success of cervical cancer screening, professionals must work to dispel the widely held expectation of complete diagnostic success with a 0% false-negative rate.

At the heart of these issues is the fact that cervical cytology and even histopathology remain somewhat subjective diagnostic exercises. This is exemplified by the moderate levels of intraobserver agreement that are revealed when Kappa statistics are examined,[104] as summarized in Table 6-17. Furthermore, diagnostic uncertainty, when coupled with sampling issues ultimately mean that only a minority of histologically proven HGSILs present as such at the time of initial Pap testing[105] (Table 6-18).

The ALTS trial was described during discussion of atypical squamous cells. Data from early phases of the investigation indicate that as much as 8.8% of atypical squamous cells cases and 14.1% of LGSIL Pap tests can be reclassified as HGSIL at the time of central review. Using this information with the number of each diagnosis rendered annually in the United States, it is estimated that as many as 352,000 cases of HGSIL present as either atypical squamous cells or LGSIL annually.

In the United States, the Bethesda System, now in its third incarnation, will be the officially sanctioned cervical cytology terminology for the foreseeable future (see Chapter 3). Schenck and colleagues emphasized that no terminology universally acceptable to the entire world is likely to emerge but that comparisons are possible.[106] The most important aspects of any terminology are that it is used clearly and that it is understood by the clinical recipients of these reports.

 ## EVOLVING TREATMENT RECOMMENDATIONS

Current consensus guidelines for evaluation and follow-up of women whose Pap tests show atypical squamous cells were discussed in Chapter 5. Currently, there is a tendency to emphasize detection of HGSILs and to play down the importance of LGSILs. The latter often regress spontaneously, but if all are evaluated by colposcopy, the annual cost to the United States health care system would be approximately $1 billion. This conservative approach is seen by many to lessen the patients' testing, treatment, anxiety, and potential complications.

Unlike the case for atypical squamous cells, HPV testing has no role to play in evaluation of LGSIL. Because the majority are positive, this additional information plays no role in patient triage or follow-up.

References

1. Franco EL. Epidemiology of anogenital warts and cancer. Obstet Gynecol Clin North Am 1996; 23:597-623.
2. Van Ramst N, Van Ranst M, Kaplan JB, Buck RD. Phylogenetic classification of human papillomaviruses: correlation with clinical manifestations. J Gen Virol 1992; 73:2653-2660.
3. Laimins LA. The biology of human papillomaviruses: from warts to cancer. Infect Agents Dis 1993; 2:74-86.
4. Zur Hausen H, de Villiers E-M. Human papillomaviruses. Annu Rev Microbiol 1994; 48:427-447.
5. Bosch FX, Manos MM, Munoz N, et al. Prevalence of human papillomavirus in cervical cancer: a worldwide perspective. J Natl Cancer Inst 1995; 87:796-802.
6. Turek LP, Smith EM. The genetic program of genital human papillomaviruses in infection and cancer. Obstet Gynecol Clin North Am 1996; 23:735-758.
7. Richart RM, Masood S, Syrjanen KJ, et al. Human papillomavirus: International Academy of Cytology task force summary—diagnostic cytology towards the 21st century: an International expert conference and tutorial. Acta Cytol 1998; 42:50-58.
8. Stoler MH. Human papillomaviruses and cervical neoplasia: a model for carcinogenesis. Int J Gynecol Pathol 2000; 19:16-28.
9. Schiffman MH, Bauer HN, Hoover RN, et al. Epidemiologic evidence showing that human papillomavirus infection causes most cervical intraepithelial neoplasia. J Natl Cancer Inst 1993; 85:958-964.
10. Schiffman M, et al. Why, how, and when the cytologic diagnosis of ASCUS should be eliminated. J Lower Gen Tr Dis 1998; 2:165-169.
11. Koutsky LA, Holmes KK, Critchlow CW, et al. A cohort study of the risk of cervical intraepithelial neoplasia grade 2 or 3 in relation to papillomavirus infection. N Engl J Med 1992; 327:1272-1278.
12. Peng HQ, Liu SL, Mann V, et al. Human papillomavirus types 16 and 33, herpes simplex virus type 2 and other risk factors for cervical cancer in Sichuan Provice, China. Int J Cancer 1991; 47:711-716.
13. Bosch FX, Munoz N, de Sanjose S, et al. Risk factors for cervical cancer in Columbia and Spain. Int J Cancer 1992; 52:750-758.
14. Lorincz AT, Reid R, Jenson AB, et al. Human papillomavirus infection of the cervix: relative risk associations of 15 common anogenital types. Am J Obstet Gynecol 1992; 79:328-337.
15. Lungu O, Sun XW, Felix J, et al. Relationship of human papillomavirus type to grade of cervical intraepithelial neoplasia. JAMA 1992; 267:2493-2496.
16. Hall S, Lorincz A, Shah F, et al. Human papillomavirus DNA detection in cervical specimens by hybrid capture: correlation with cytologic and histologic diagnosis of squamous intraepithelial lesions of the cervix. Gynecol Oncol 1996; 62:353-359.
17. Moscicki AB, Palefsky JM, Gonzales J, et al. Colposcopic and histologic findings and HPV DNA test variability in young women positive for HPV DNA. J Infect Dis 1992; 166:951-957.
18. Parker MF, Arroyo GF, Geradts J, et al. Molecular characterization of adenocarcinoma of the cervix. Gynecol Oncol 1997; 64:242-251.
19. Uchiyama M, Iwasaka T, Matsuo N, et al. Correlation between human papillomavirus positivity and *p53* gene overexpression in adenocarcinoma of the uterine cervix. Gynecol Oncol 1997; 65:23-29.
20. Nindl I, Greinke C, Zahm DM, et al. Human papillomavirus distribution in cervical tissues of different morphology as determined by Hybrid Capture assay and PCR. Int J Gynecol Pathol 1997; 16:197-204.
21. Astori G, Arzise A, Pipan C, et al. Characterization of a putative new HPV genomic sequence from a cervical lesion using *L1* consensus primers and restriction fragment length polymorphism. Virus Res 1997; 50:57-63.
22. Bernard BA, Bailly C, Lenoir MC, et al. The human papillomavirus type 18 *E2* gene product is a repressor of the HPV 18 regulatory region in human keratinocytes. J Virol 1989; 63:4317-4324.
23. Palefsky JM, Winkler B, Rabanus JP, et al. Characterization of in vivo expression of the human papillomavirus type 16 *E4* protein in cervical biopsy tissues. J Clin Invest 1991; 87:2132-2141.
24. Mittal K, Demopoulos RI, Tata M. A comparison of proliferative activity and atypical mitoses in cervical condylomas with various HPV types. Int J Gynecol Pathol 1998; 17:24-28.
25. Kessis TD, Slebos RJ, Nelson, et al. Human papillomavirus 16 *E6* expression disrupts the *p53*-mediated cellular response to DNA damage. Proc Nat Acad Sci 1993; 90:3988-3992.
26. Vousden KH. Regulation of the cell cycle by viral oncoproteins. Semin Cancer Biol 1995; 6:109-116.
27. Matsukura T, Koi S, Sugase M, et al. Both episomal and integrated forms of human papillomavirus type 16 are involved in invasive cervical cancers. Virology 1989; 172:63-72.

28. Kalantari M, Karlsen F, Kristensen G, et al. Disruption of the E1 and E2 reading frames of HPV16 in cervical carcinoma is associated with poor prognosis. Int J Gynecol Pathol 1998; 17:146-153.

29. Autillo-Touati A, Joannes M, d'Ercole C, et al. HPV typing by in situ hybridization on cervical cytologic smears with ASCUS. Acta Cytol 1998; 42:631-638.

30. McGoogan E, Seagar AL, Cubie HA, et al. Detection of high-risk human papillomavirus nucleic acid in archival cervical smears. Acta Cytol 1998; 42:1079-1083.

31. Schiffman MH, Kiviat NB, Burk RD, et al. Accuracy and interlaboratory reliability of human papillomavirus DNA testing by hybrid capture. J Clin Microbiol 1995; 33: 545-550.

32. Elfgren K, Bistoletti P, Dillner L, et al. Conization for cervical intraepithelial neoplasia is followed by disappearance of human papillomavirus deoxyribonucleic acid and a decline in serum and cervical mucus antibodies against human papillomavirus antigens. Am J Obstet Gynecol 1996; 174:937-942.

33. Gomousa-Michael M, Deligeorgi-Politi H, Condi-Paphiti A, et al. Human papillomavirus identification and typing of both sexual partners. Acta Cytol 1997; 41:244-250.

34. Hatch KD, Schneider A, Abdel-Nour W. An evaluation of human papillomavirus testing for intermediate and high-risk types as triage before colposcopy. Am J Obstet Gynecol 1995; 172:1150-1157.

35. Cox JT, Lorincz AT, Schiffman MH, et al. Human papillomavirus testing by Hybrid Capture appears to be useful in triaging women with a cytologic diagnosis of atypical squamous cells of undetermined significance. Am J Obstet Gynecol 1995; 172:946-954.

36. Schiffman M, Adrianza ME. ASCUS-LSIL Triage Study: design, methods and characteristics of trial participants. Acta Cytol 2000; 44:726-742.

37. The ALTS Group: Human papillomavirus testing for triage of women with cytologic evidence of low-grade squamous intraepithelial lesions: baseline date from a randomized trial. JNCI 2000; 92:397-402.

38. Smith EM, Johnson SR, Figueres EJ, et al. The frequency of human papillomavirus detection in postmenopausal women on hormone replacement therapy. Gynecol Oncol 1997; 65:441-446.

39. Cerqueira EM, Santoro CL, Donozo NF, et al. Genetic damage in exfoliated cells of the uterine cervix: asssociation and interaction between cigarette smoking and progression to malignant transformation. Acta Cytol 1998; 42:639-649.

40. Ostor AG. Natural history of cervical intraepithelial neoplasia: a critical review. Int J Gynecol Pathol 1993; 12: 186-192.

41. Burger MP, van Leeuwen AM, Hollema H, et al. Human papillomavirus type influences the extent of chromosomal lag during mitosis in cervical intraepithelial neoplasia grade III. Int J Gynecol Pathol 1997; 16:10-14.

42. Harmsel B, Kuijpers J, Smedts F, et al. Progressing imbalance between proliferation and apoptosis with increasing severity of cervical intraepithelial neoplasia. Int J Gynecol Pathol 1997; 16:205-211.

43. Luft F, Gerbert J, Schneider A, et al. Frequent allelic imbalance of tumor suppressor gene loci in cervical dysplasia. Intern J Gynecol Pathol 1999; 18:374-380.

44. Hermonat PL, Han L, Wendel PJ, et al. Human papillomavirus is more prevalent in first trimester spontaneously aborted products of conception compared to elective specimens. Virus Genes 1997; 14:13-17.

45. Sherman ME, Schiffman MH, Strickler H, et al. Prospects for a prophylactic HPV vaccine: rationale and future implications for cervical cancer screening. Diagn Cytopathol 1998; 18:5-9.

46. Fu YS, Reagan JW, Richart RM, et al. Definition of cervical cancer precursors. In: Grundman E, editors. Cancer campaign: cancer of the uterine cervix (vol 8). Gustav Fisher Verlag: Stuttgart; 1985. p.67.

47. Bibbo M, Dytch HE, Alenghat E, et al. DNA ploidy profiles as prognostic indicators in CIN lesions. Am J Clin Pathol 1989; 92:261-265.

48. Fu YS, Reagan JW, Richart RM: Definition of precursors. Gynecol Oncol 1981; 12:S220-S231.

49. Stanbridge CM, Sluleman BA, Persad RV, et al. A cervical smear review in women developing cervical carcinoma with particular reference to age, false negative cytology and the histologic type of the carcinoma. Int J Gynecol Cancer 1992; 2:92-100.

50. Robertson JH. Woodend B, Elliott H. Cytological changes preceding cervical cancer. J Clin Pathol 1994; 47:278-279.

51. Narod SA, Jain TM, Wall C, et al. Dysplasia and the natural history of cervical cancer: early results of the Toronto cohort study. Eur J Cancer 1991; 27:1411-1416.

52. Ostor AG: Natural history of cervical intraepithelial neoplasia: a critical review. Int J. Gynecol Pathol 1993; 12: 176-192.

53. Abdul-Karim FW, Fu YS, Reagan JW, et al. Morphometric study of intraepithelial neoplasia of the uterine cervix. Obstet Gynecol 1982; 60:210-214.

54. Patten SF. Diagnostic cytology of the uterine cervix. Baltimore: Williams and Wilkins; 1978.

55. Kurman RJ, Solomon D. The Bethesda System for reporting cervical/vaginal cytologic diagnoses: definitions, criteria, and explanatory notes for terminology and specimen adequacy. New York: Springer-Verlag; 1994.

56. Woodhouse SL, Stastny JF, Styer PE, et al. Interobserver variability in subclassification of squamous intraepithelial lesions: results of the College of American Pathologists Interlaboratory Comparison Program in Cervicovaginal Cytology. Arch Pathol Lab Med 1999; 123(11): 1079-1084.

57. de Vet HC, Knipschild PG, Schouten HJ, et al. Interobserver variation in histopathological grading of cervical dysplasia. J Clin Epidemiol 1990; 43(12):1395-1398.

58. de Vet HC, Knipschild PG, Schouten HJ, et al. Sources of interobserver variation in histopathological grading of cervical dysplasia. J Clin Epidemiol 1992; 45(7):785-790.

59. Sherman ME, Schiffman MH, Erozan YS, et al. The Bethesda System: a proposal for reporting abnormal cervical smears based on the reproducibility of cytopathologic diagnoses. Arch Pathol Lab Med 1992; 116(11): 1155-1158.

60. Reid R, Fu YS, Herschman RB, et al. Genital warts and cervical cancer (VI): the relationship between aneuploid and polypoid cervical lesions. Am J Obstet Gynecol 1984; 150:189-199.

61. Pieters WJLM, Koudstaal J, Ploem-Zaayer JJ, et al. The three-group metaphase as a morphologic indicator of high ploidy cells in cervical intraepithelial neoplasia. Anal Quant Cytol Histol 1992; 14:227-232.

62. Bergeron C, Ferenczy A, Shah KV, et al. Multicentric human papillomavirus infections of the female genital tract: correlation of viral types with abnormal mitotic figures, colposcopic presentation, and location. Obstet Gynecol 1987; 69:736-742.

63. Patten SF Jr. Diagnostic cytopathology of the uterine cervix. In: Wied GL, von Haam E, editors. Monographs in clinical cytology (vol 3). Basel, Switzerland: S Karger AG; 1978.

64. Sherman ME, Tabbara SO, Scott DR, et al. *ASCUS, rule out HSIL*: cytologic features, histologic correlates, and human papillomavirus detection. Mod Pathol 1999; 12(4): 335-342.

65. Crum CP, Egawa K, Fu YS, et al. Atypical immature metaplasia (AIM): a subset of human papilloma virus infection of the cervix. Cancer 1983; 51(12):2214-2219.

66. Geng L, Connolly DC, Isacson C, et al. Atypical immature metaplasia (AIM) of the cervix: is it related to high-grade squamous intraepithelial lesion (HSIL)? Hum Pathol 1999; 30:345-350.

67. Abati A, Jaffurs W, Wilder AM. Squamous atypia in the atrophic cervical vaginal smear: a new look at an old problem. Cancer 1998; 84:218-225.

68. Jovanovic AS, McLachlin CM, Shen L, et al. Postmenopausal squamous atypia: a spectrum including "pseudo-koilocytosis." Mod Pathol 1995; 8(4):408-412.

69. Ejersbo D, Jensen HA, Holund B. Efficacy of Ki-67 antigen staining in Papanicolaou (Pap) smears in postmenopausal women with atypia: an audit. Cytopathology 1999; 10(6):369-374.

70. Weir MM, Bell DA. Transitional cell metaplasia of the cervix: a newly described entity in cervicovaginal smears. Diagn Cytopathol 1998; 18:222-226.

71. Wentz WB, Reagan JW. Clinical significance of postradiation dysplasia. Am J Obstet Gynecol 1970; 106:812-817.

72. Koss LG, Melamed MR, Mayer K. The effect of busulfan on human epithelia. Am J Clin Pathol 1965; 44:385-397.

73. Ringrose CAD. Carcinoma in situ of the cervix after amethopterin therapy. Am J Obstet Gynecol 1974; 119:1132-1133.

74. Kay S, Frable JW, Hume D. Cervical dysplasia and cancer developing in women on immunosuppression therapy for renal homotransplantation. Cancer 1970; 26:1048-1052.

75. Pugliese A, Saini A, Andronico L, et al. Sexually transmitted infections and cervicovaginal dysplasia in a cohort of human immunodeficiency virus-positive women in Turin. Cancer Detect Prev 2001; 25(1):32-39.

76. Davis AT, Chakraborty H, Flowers L, et al. Cervical dysplasia in women infected with the human immunodeficiency virus (HIV): a correlation with HIV viral load and CD4+ count. Gynecol Oncol 2001; 80(3):350-354.

77. Stratton P, Gupta P, Riester K, et al. Cervical dysplasia on cervicovaginal Papanicolaou smear among HIV-1–infected pregnant and nonpregnant women: Women and Infants Transmission Study. J Acquir Immune Defic Syndr 1999; 20(3):300-307.

78. Hocke C, Leroy V, Morlat P, et al. Cervical dysplasia and human immunodeficiency virus infection in women: prevalence and associated factors: Groupe d'Epidemiologie Clinique du SIDA en Aquitaine (GESCA). Eur J Obstet, Gynecol, Reprod Biol 1998; 81(1):69-76.

79. Schafer A, Friedmann W, Mielke M, et al. The increased frequency of cervical dysplasia-neoplasia in women infected with the human immunodeficiency virus is related to the degree of immunosuppression. Am J Obstet Gynecol 1991; 164:593-599.

80. Wilson JM, Jungner YG. Principles and practice of screening for disease. Geneva: World Health Organization; 1968.

81. Anderson GH, Boyes DA, Benedet JL, et al. Organisation and results of the cervical cytology screening programme in British Columbia, 1955-1985. Br Med J 1988; 296:975-978.

82. Schneider V, Henry MR, Jimenez-Ayala M, et al. Cervical cancer screening, screening errors and reporting. Acta Cytol 2001; 45:493-498.

83. Miller AB. Failures of cervical cancer screening. Am J Public Health 1995; 85:761-762.

84. Janerich DT, Hadjimichael O, Schwartz PE, et al. The screening histories of women with invasive cervical cancer, Connecticut. Am J Public Health 1995; 85:791-794.

85. Cervical cancer control: Rhode Island. MMWR 1989; 659-662.

86. Nasca PC, Ellish N, Caputo TA, et al. An epidemiologic study of Pap screening histories in women with invasive carcinoma of the uterine cervix. NY State J Med 1991; 91:152-156.

87. Kinney W, Sung HY, Kearney KA, et al. Missed opportunities for cervical cancer screening of HMO members developing invasive cervical cancer. Gynecol Oncol 1998; 71:428-430.

88. Hislop TG, Clarke HF, Deschamps M, et al. Cervical cytology screening: How can we improve rates among First Nations in women in urban British Columbia? Can Fam Physician 1996; 42:1701-1708.

89. Burack RC, Gimotty PA, George J, et al. How reminders given to patients and physicians affect Pap smear use in a health maintenance organization: results of a randomized controlled trial. Cancer 1998; 82:2391-2400.

90. Gay JD, Donaldson LD, Goellner JR. False negative results in cervical cytologic studies. Acta Cytol 1985; 29:1043-1046.

91. Wilbur DC, Prey MU, Miller WM, et al. The AutoPap system for primary screening in cervical cytology: comparing the results of a prospective, intended-use study with routine manual practice. Acta Cytol 1998; 42:214-220.

92. Bishop JW, Kaufman RH, Taylor DA. Multicenter comparison of manual and automated screening of AutoCyte gynecologic preparations. Acta Cytol 1999; 43:34-38.

93. Mitchell H, Medley G. Differences between Papanicolaou smears with correct and incorrect diagnoses. Cytopathology 1995; 6:368-375.

94. Smith PA, Turnbull LS. Small cell and "pale" dyskaryosis. Cytopathology 1997; 8:3-8.

95. Bergeron C, Debaque H, Ayivi J, et al. Cervical smear histories of 585 women with biopsy-proven carcinoma in situ. Acta Cytol 1997; 41:1676-1680.

96. Davey DD. Quality and liability issues with the Papanicolaou smear. Arch Pathol Lab Med 1997; 121:267-269.

97. Krieger P, Naryshkin S. Random rescreening of cytologic smears: a practical and effective component of quality assurance programs in both large and small cytology laboratories. Acta Cytol 1994; 38:291-298.

98. Naryshkin S. The false-negative fraction for Papanicolaou smears: how often are "abnormal" smears not detected by a "standard" screening cytologist? Arch Pathol Lab Med 1997; 121:270-272.

99. Dolinar J, Ollayos CW, Tellado M, et al. The false-negative fraction: a statistical method to measure the efficacy of cervical smear screening laboratories. Mil Med 1999; 164(6):140-411.

100. Baker A, Melcher D, Smith R. Role of rescreening of cervical smears in internal quality control. J Clin Pathol 1995; 48:1002-1004.

101. Johnson SJ, Hair T, Gibson L, et al. An assessment of partial rescreening as an internal quality control method for cervical smears. Cytopathology 1995; 6:376-387.

102. Dudding N. Rapid rescreen: a viable alterative to 1:10? Diagn Cytopathol 2001; 24:219-221.

103. Sawaya GF, Grimes DA. New technologies in cervical cytology screening: a word of caution. Obstet Gynecol 1999; 94:307-310.

104. Stoler MH, Schiffman M. Interobserver reproducibility of cervical cytologic and histologic preparations: realistic estimates from the ASCUS-LSIL triage study. J Am Med Assoc 2001; 285:1500-1505.

105. Kinney WK, Manor MM, Hurley LB, et al. Where's the high grade cervical neoplasia? The importance of minimally abnormal Papanicolaou diagnoses. Obstet Gynecol 1998; 91:379-386.

106. Schenck U, Herbert A, Solomon D: Terminology: IAC Task Force summary. Acta Cytol 1998; 42:5-15.

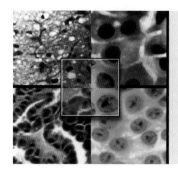

Invasive Squamous Cell Carcinoma

CHAPTER
7

The powerful late twentieth-century impetus to diagnose malignancy by cytologic means was propelled by the striking success of cervical cancer screening using the method of Papanicolaou. (Similar methods were independently devised by Aurel Babé's working in Romania.) At the close of the last century, the United States had enjoyed a 70% decline in deaths from this lethal cancer. Unfortunately, approximately 13,000 new cases continued to be detected annually, leading to more than 4100 deaths per year. The success of cytologic screening is put into perspective by the observation that most of these deaths occur in women who have either never received cytologic screening or who have not been studied during the several years immediately preceding their presentation with invasive carcinoma.[1]

As emphasized in Chapter 10, a wide range of malignancies can arise in the uterine cervix. In numerical terms, however, squamous cell carcinoma is overwhelmingly the most important. The astounding success of cytologic screening hinges on the following two characteristics of this malignancy: (1) most cases of invasive carcinoma are preceded by a predictable series of noninvasive, nonlethal precursor lesions—that is, the squamous intraepithelial lesions discussed in the previous chapter; (2) progression of the lesion through these stages happens slowly in the majority of cases. This explains the enormous success of cervical cancer screening despite the often-cited limitations in the sensitivity of a single test—that is, frequent false-negative results occur for a variety of reasons, but most women do not experience the consequences of the test's limitations because they receive multiple evaluations in the face of a disease that progresses slowly. At odds with this description of the most common circumstance is the minority of carcinomas that seem to develop explosively, possibly without passing through a set of detectable preneoplastic, noninvasive lesions.

MICROINVASIVE SQUAMOUS CELL CARCINOMA

As with many malignancies, tumor stage is one of the most important prognostic factors in squamous cell carcinoma of the uterine cervix. Tumors with minimal invasion detected by histologic examination are designated microinvasive carcinomas. Such carcinomas have an excellent prognosis with an extremely low incidence of lymph node metastases. One consequence of this is that microinvasive carcinomas can be treated by cervical conization in a manner that allows most younger women to retain their fertility. By definition, such tumors are clinically undetectable and diagnosed solely on the basis of cytologic screening and subsequent histologic findings. Box 7-1 summarizes the current International Federation of Gynecology and Obstetrics (FIGO) definition of microinvasive squamous cell carcinoma.

The epithelium from which a microinvasive carcinoma originates may show carcinoma in situ or dysplasia. Rarely, it may be normal.[2] The invasive component is often multifocal. The cells of microinvasive carcinoma show considerably more conspicuous squamous differentiation than the small immature cells of the overlying squamous cell carcinoma in situ. In the earliest histologically demonstrable examples, a field of small blue carcinoma in situ cells is interrupted where it rests on and begins to penetrate the basement membrane. The invasive cells stand out because they are much larger with abundant eosinophilic cytoplasm and prominent nucleoli. Frank keratinization of individual cells may be seen. At the point where the basement membrane has been breeched, the epithelium takes on an irregular contour, as the microinvasive cell nest extends into the subjacent stroma. Another histologic correlate of invasion is alteration of the surrounding stroma. It may assume an edematous or desmoplastic appearance that is often paler than the normal, more maturely collagenized fibrous stroma adjacent to nearby abnormal but noninvasive epithelium. A mixture of acute and chronic inflammatory cells is usually present. For unknown reasons, eosinophils are prominent in some patients. Adjacent areas of multifocal microinvasion may remain distinct or may show a tendency to become confluent, thus forming larger areas of invasive, albeit shallow, disease. The prognostic significance of confluent microinvasion is controversial at this time.[3-5]

In histologic preparations the presence of lymphatic or capillary vascular space involvement can be difficult to assess accurately and must be distinguished from the stromal retraction artifacts that are common in paraffin sections. The frequency of this morphologic finding depends on the depth of tumor invasion, number of levels examined, and criteria for identification of vascular spaces. The latter include the use of immunohistochemical methods to identify the endothelial cells that most unequivocally localize these spaces. In most analyses, the depth of tumor invasion correlates with the presence of lymph node metastases to a greater extent than vascular invasion (Table 7-1). The latter finding acquires importance primarily in tumors showing more than 3.0 mm of invasion.[6-9]

Given the previously cited cytologic alterations attending the histologic sections of microinvasion, it seems reasonable to suggest that Pap test findings should allow distinctions between carcinoma in situ, microinvasive carcinoma, and frankly invasive carcinoma. Criteria for these distinctions have been described[10-12] but are difficult to apply consistently. One reason for this is that the histologic definition of microinvasion became more conservative after the initial cytologic criteria had been advanced. Recognition of invasion in cytologic preparations is significantly more straightforward using the older definition of up to 5-mm invasion but much more difficult with minimally invasive disease. Nguyen was able to suggest invasion based on assessment of cytologic samples from 88% of tumors as deep as 3 mm but in only 14% of those invading only up to 1 mm.[11]

The cytologic findings in these three entities vary along a continuous spectrum, and it is not possible to draw clear distinctions. It is also not necessary. Diagnoses such as *high-grade squamous intraepithelial neoplasia with features suggestive of invasion* or *invasion cannot be excluded* are operatively preferable to attempts at more detailed classification in cytologic samples. Not only is the accuracy of such subclassification limited, but the patient's treatment and prognosis also depends on tumor type, size, and depth of invasion and on other staging information that can only be obtained by detailed histologic evaluation of excised tissue in concert with other clinical evaluations. In this regard the Bethesda System makes no mention of microinvasive squamous cell carcinoma as a diagnostic entity. Thus, this diagnosis and its numerical niceties are histologically and clinically important but are largely irrelevant to Pap test interpretation.

INVASIVE SQUAMOUS CELL CARCINOMA

A proportion of early carcinomas that have been detected by cytologic means may not be grossly apparent either in vivo or at the surgical pathology cutting bench. More advanced examples show varying degrees of necrosis, ulceration, protrusion, and endophytic growth. A large polypoid exophytic tumor may present as a mass in the upper vagina with relatively little invasive growth. In advanced cases, destruction of the entire cervix with or without fistula formation may occur.

Table 7-2 shows squamous cell carcinomas of the uterine cervix that are classified as keratinizing, large cell nonkeratinizing, or small cell. The third entity can be further divided into small cell squamous cell carcinomas and small cell neuroendocrine tumors. The latter are identical to those arising in many other epithelia, particularly the bronchi, and are discussed in the next chapter with other uncommon tumors of the cervix. Evidence of squamous differentiation in small cell carcinoma may be difficult to demonstrate. When studied at the ultrastructural level, these tumors may show various combinations of squamous, glandular and neuroendocrine differentiation, blurring distinctions between the hypothetically different types of what, at the light microscopic level presents as a small cell carcinoma.[13]

The prognostic significance of this tumor classification is limited, as is assignment of Broders-type grading. Considering stage 1B tumors, Zaino and colleagues found that grade and tumor type were much less predictive of lymph node metastases and patient outcome than the depth of invasion (measured in mm), and the presence or absence of vascular space involvement.[14] Another confounding factor is the limited reproducibility of tumor classification among different pathologists. Opinions and subjective impressions regarding the amount of keratin required to designate a carcinoma as keratinizing are variable, poorly reproducible, and subject to sampling errors. One proposed simplification considers any carcinoma with even single cell keratinization as a keratinizing carcinoma.[15] In this scheme, keratinizing tumors emerge as more aggressive than nonkera-

---

BOX 7-1

Definition of Microinvasive Squamous Cell Carcinoma of the Uterine Cervix (Stage 1A1*)

Invasion less than 3 mm†
Surface extent less than 7 mm†
No evidence of vascular space invasion

---

*Carcinomas with invasion between 3.1 and 5 mm are designated *stage 1A2.* Stage 1B tumors exceed these numeric criteria or present with clinically apparent disease.
†Measurements of the depth of invasion are taken from the invasive carcinoma's point of origin. This may be the surface epithelium or the lining of a subsurface gland, the columnar lining of which has been replaced by abnormal squamous epithelium. Tangential sectioning in histologic sections may introduce ambiguity into these measurements.

TABLE 7-1

Correlation of the Depth of Microinvasive Squamous Cell Carcinoma with the Incidence of Lymph Node Metastases

Depth of Invasion	Patients with Lymph Node Metastases (%)
<1.0 mm	0.4
0.1 to 3.0 mm	1.2
3.1 to 5.0 mm	6.8

From Fu YS, Berek JS. Minimal cervical cancer: definition and histology. Recent Results Cancer Res 1988; 106:47-56; Benson WL, Norris HJ. A critical review of the frequency of lymph node metastasis and death from microinvasive carcinoma of the cervix. Obstet Gynecol 1977; 49:632-638.

tinizing carcinomas. This may seem paradoxical because keratin production is usually considered to be the hallmark of a well-differentiated squamous cell carcinoma. However, one conceptual approach notes that the normal cervical epithelium is not keratinized. Thus, overt production of keratin represents aberrant differentiation that further removes the neoplastic cells from their nonneoplastic counterparts.

Histologic Variants of Squamous Cell Carcinoma

Box 7-2 summarizes the variants of squamous cell carcinoma that are recognized in the uterine cervix. Spindle cell squamous carcinoma is rare in the uterine cervix and may be mistaken for a sarcoma, malignant melanoma, or metastatic deposit from a neoplasm originating in another site.[16] As is the case with most spindle cell carcinomas, these tumors tend to be of high nuclear grade and show numerous mitotic figures. If immunohistochemical evidence of epithelial differentiation is not forthcoming with stains for cytokeratins, ultrastructural demonstration of tonofilaments and desmosomes may be required for accurate diag-

nosis. Clinical and radiographic exclusion of tumors in other body sites and a negative immunoprofile for malignant melanoma are probably the most important diagnostic imperatives.

Squamous cell carcinomas that are largely papillary may be entirely exophytic or may have an underlying invasive component. Adequate excision is required for proper classification.[17] Clinically, these carcinomas mimic condyloma or verrucous carcinoma. However, true papillary squamous cell carcinomas show a much greater degree of nuclear atypia than encountered in either of these other lesions.

Verrucous carcinoma of the uterine cervix is a rare entity.[18] Clinically, it is usually thought to represent a condyloma. This erroneous impression is strengthened both clinically and in superficial biopsies by prominent surface keratinization. By definition, this tumor does not show the nuclear features usually associated with malignancy. Its accurate recognition depends on histologic sampling that is sufficiently generous to show the characteristic pushing stromal infiltration by blunt ingrowths from the surface epithelium. Local recurrences are much more common than metastases. However, radiation therapy can turn a locally aggressive verrucous carcinoma into a much more cytologically anaplastic carcinoma with increased metastatic potential. Initial control is best achieved by adequate excision. Many tumors for which this is not achieved recur.

Lymphoepithelioma-like carcinoma shows syncytial tumor cell growth with dense lymphocytic infiltration in a manner similar to its counterpart in the nasopharynx and other sites.[19] Few examples have been reported during the contemporary therapeutic era so that earlier suggestions of a prognosis better than that of typical squamous cell carcinoma are difficult to evaluate.[20]

Mixed carcinomas occur rarely in the cervix. Vuong and colleagues described a squamous cell carcinoma in situ associated with an invasive adenoid cystic carcinoma.[21] Given the relative frequency of the former, the significance of this pairing is difficult to assess.

Cytology of Invasive Squamous Cell Carcinoma

The cytologic basis for classifying squamous lesions of the uterine cervix originates with the concept that a continuum of increasingly severe nuclear abnormalities is associated with disease progression. Hence, the central axiom of classical cytology is that *a cell's biologic potential can be read in the details of its nuclear morphology.* These details include the following: progressive increases in nucleocytoplasmic ratio,

TABLE 7-2	
Classification and Histologic Features of Invasive Squamous Cell Carcinomas of the Uterine Cervix	
Carcinoma Type	**Histologic Features**
Keratinizing carcinoma	Large cells
	Eosinophilic cytoplasm
	Large hyperchromatic nuclei*
	Coarse chromatin clumping
	Whorls of keratinized or parakeratotic cells
	Necrosis is common
	Cytoplasmic differentiation features intercellular bridges and keratohyaline granules
Large cell nonkeratinizing carcinoma	Large cells
	Eosinophilic cytoplasm
	Coarse chromatin clumping
	Prominent nucleoli
	Keratin whorls are not present
	Intercellular bridges are difficult to identify
Small cell carcinoma	Small cells
	Scanty cytoplasm
	Little evidence of squamous differentiation
	Keratin whorls not present
	Individual cell keratinization not present
	Hyperchromatic nuclei
	Densely clumped chromatin
	Small nucleoli
	Numerous mitotic figures
	Necrosis may be prominent

*Some nuclei are so densely hyperchromatic and show so little chromatin structure as to be termed *India ink spots.*

BOX 7-2

Histologic Variants of Squamous Cell Carcinoma in the Uterine Cervix

Spindle cell (sarcomatoid) carcinoma
Papillary carcinoma
Verrucous carcinoma
Lymphoepithelioma-like carcinoma
Mixed carcinomas

TABLE 7-3   CMF

Cytomorphologic Features of Progression from Carcinoma in Situ to Invasive Squamous Cell Carcinoma

Type of Carcinoma	Chromatin	Chromatin Particle Size	Chromatin Clearing	Nucleoli
Carcinoma in situ	Finely or coarsely granular	Uniform	None	None
Microinvasive carcinoma	Coarsely granular	Uniform	Minor	Small
Invasive carcinoma*	Coarsely granular	Nonuniform	Definite interparticle spaces	Larger

*In many cases, each of these cytomorphologic features is manifested by a minority of the tumor cells. Careful assessment of many cells with a mental addition of accumulated abnormal findings is often required for an accurate diagnosis.

TABLE 7-4

Cytomorphologic Comparison of Various Types of Squamous Cell Carcinoma of the Uterine Cervix

Type of Carcinoma	Cell Size*	Nuclear Size*	Nucleocytoplasmic Ratio (%)
Keratinizing carcinoma	300	75	30
Nonkeratinizing carcinoma	250	90	35
Small cell carcinoma	170	70	40

From Patten SF. Diagnostic cytology of the uterine cervix. Baltimore: Williams and Wilkins; 1978.
*All measurements are in μm² and are rounded from those published by Patten based on his camera lucida drawings.

chromatin clumping, abnormalities of chromatin distribution with areas of clearing, irregularities of nuclear membrane contour, and nucleolar prominence. These are summarized in Table 7-3.[22] Practical difficulties with the cytologic diagnosis of microinvasive carcinoma have been cited previously.

As an aside, it is useful to take this opportunity to reflect on the intellectual edifice that has been erected on this axiom and then strengthened by the success of cervical cancer screening programs. Assessment of a lesion's biologic potential for invasion and metastasis by careful evaluation of nuclear morphology forms the basis for the traditional cytomorphologic criteria of malignancy. The use of these criteria is then extended by making these findings the measure by which malignancy is distinguished from reactive and regenerative cellular alterations in other body sites. This intellectual construct is useful when squamous cell carcinoma of the uterine cervix, its precursors, and its mimics are considered among various reactive processes. However, the flood of new experience and understanding that accompanied the flowering of fine-needle aspiration (FNA) and endoscopy in the late twentieth century has shown that this model is not applicable to cytologic evaluation of numerous other human neoplasms. Examples include the following: some carcinomas of the breast or pancreas are cytologically bland and do not meet the traditional nuclear criteria of malignancy; the nuclei of adenoid cystic carcinoma and basal cell adenoma of salivary gland origin are indistinguishable, and neither shows malignant features; reactive type-II pneumocytes seen in a variety of pulmonary conditions show many of the features usually ascribed to malignant cells. Thus, care must be exercised in trying to apply concepts valid for exfoliative cytology of the uterine cervix and other sites (sputum, urine, and so on) to directly sampled lesions (FNAs, bronchoalveolar lavage, and so on).

The nosologic niceties previously discussed are not reflected in contemporary Bethesda System cytodiagnostic

TABLE 7-5   CMF

Cytomorphologic Features of Invasive Squamous Cell Carcinoma of the Uterine Cervix

Feature	Description
Cell arrangements	Syncytial groups and single cells*
Average cell size	300 μm²†
Cytoplasmic eosinophilia	Present in up to 25% of cells‡
Average nuclear size	75 μm²†
Chromatin clumping	Coarse
Chromatin distribution	Irregular with clearing between clumps
Chromatin particle size	Variable
Densely hyperchromatic (opaque) nuclei	Present in up to 20% of cells†
Macronucleoli	Present in up to 25% of cells†

*The presence of single cells with malignant nuclear features is often a key to recognizing invasive carcinoma.
†Measurements are from Patten's camera lucida drawings.
‡This contrasts with the uniformly cyanophilic cytoplasm typical of high-grade squamous intraepithelial lesion cells.

terminology; all types of invasive squamous cell carcinoma are represented by a single diagnosis in Bethesda System. However, the lessons learned from histologic subclassification of these neoplasms leads to appreciating the variations encountered in cytologic samples. Table 7-4 summarizes some of the cytologic differences among the various types of squamous cell carcinoma. The cytologic findings in invasive squamous cell carcinoma are summarized in Figures 7-1 to 7-4.

Much has been made of the importance of a tumor diathesis background in the cytologic diagnosis of invasive carcinoma. This pattern is evidence of tissue destruction and consists of lysed blood, fragments of cellular debris,

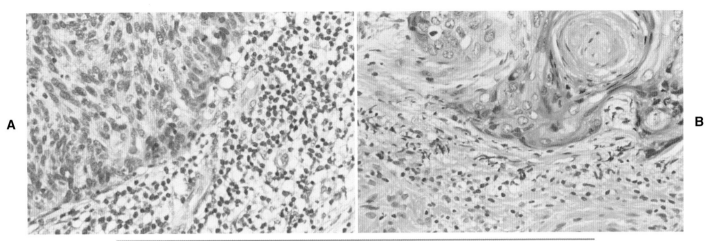

Figure 7-1 **Histology of infiltrating squamous cell carcinoma of the uterine cervix.** **A,** This large cell nonkeratinizing squamous cell carcinoma shows a pushing border where it infiltrates the highly inflamed stroma. **B,** This keratinizing squamous cell carcinoma infiltrates in a much more irregular or ragged fashion. (Papanicolaou [Pap])

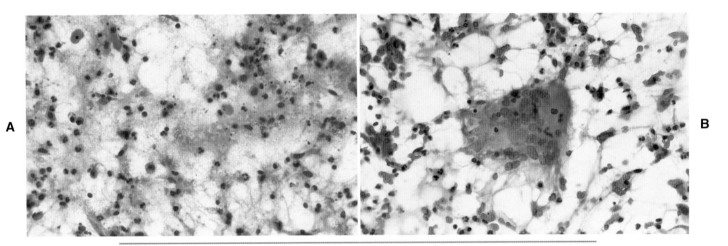

Figure 7-2 **Patterns of inflammation associated with infiltrating squamous cell carcinomas.** **A,** This background of proteinaceous granular precipitate, fragments of damaged cells, and inflammatory cells constitutes a tumor diathesis. This pattern represents tissue destruction by an invasive carcinoma. **B,** This multinucleated foreign body giant cell is set against a tumor diathesis background. It may represent a part of the stromal reaction to tissue damage associated with invasive malignancy. Alternatively, such cells may appear in response to keratin produced by tumor cells. This material incites a foreign body reaction wherever it gains access to stromal tissue. (Pap)

and a protein precipitate. In conventional smears, it may be spread diffusely over the slide, or it may be focal. The precipitate may be either eosinophilic or cyanophilic. This background may be seen in other conditions associated with tissue destruction, including cervical stenosis or pyometra. Other causes of tissue destruction including ulceration resulting from herpesvirus or acute radiation injury also litter the smear with similar material. (Clinically, cervicovaginal cytologic samples should not be collected during acute radiation injury.) In the experience of Rushing and Cibas, only half of smears from 28 invasive cervical carcinoma cases showed this background.[23] In cases with invasion to a depth of less than 5 mm, a diathesis was a particularly unreliable indicator of malignancy. Thus, a tumor diathesis is neither sufficient nor essential for the cytologic

diagnosis of invasive cervical carcinoma. This background is also not present in most cervicovaginal cytologic samples prepared by liquid-based methods.

The cytologic findings in invasive squamous cell carcinoma are summarized in Table 7-5. Key features associated with invasion may be illustrated by a minority of cells and include variably sized, irregularly distributed chromatin clumps separated by areas of clear karyoplasm, nucleoli, and shedding of single cells with these malignant nuclear features. The degree to which a given sample exhibits various combinations of these findings allows carcinoma to be distinguished from a high-grade squamous intraepithelial lesion (HGSIL).

Large cell nonkeratinizing carcinomas may shed cells with nuclear pallor. The differential diagnosis for these tu-

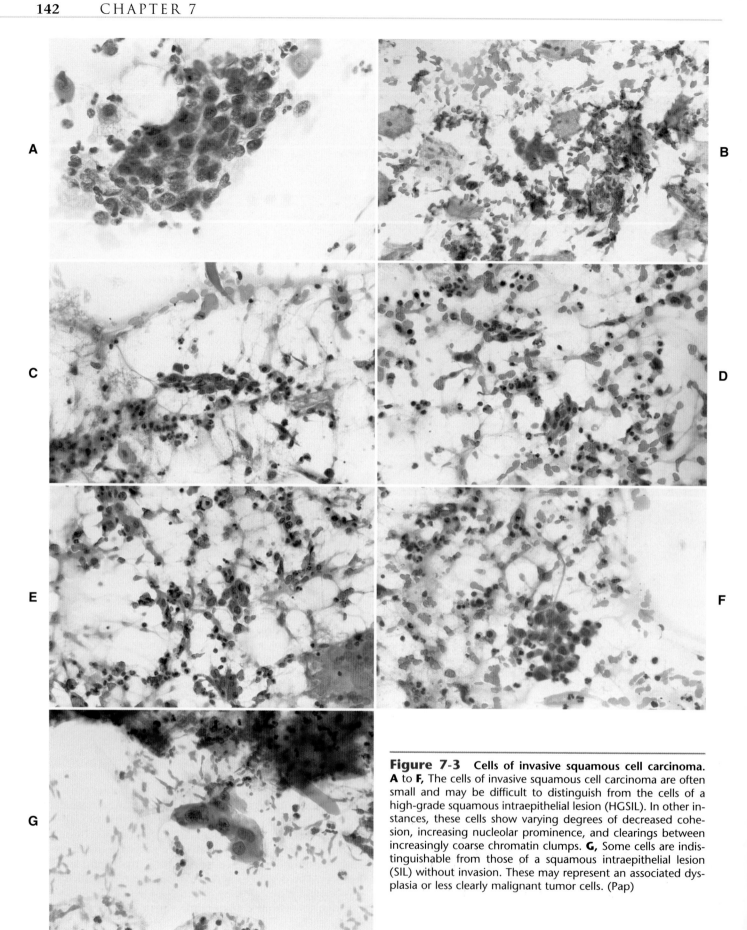

Figure 7-3   Cells of invasive squamous cell carcinoma. **A** to **F,** The cells of invasive squamous cell carcinoma are often small and may be difficult to distinguish from the cells of a high-grade squamous intraepithelial lesion (HGSIL). In other instances, these cells show varying degrees of decreased cohesion, increasing nucleolar prominence, and clearings between increasingly coarse chromatin clumps. **G,** Some cells are indistinguishable from those of a squamous intraepithelial lesion (SIL) without invasion. These may represent an associated dysplasia or less clearly malignant tumor cells. (Pap)

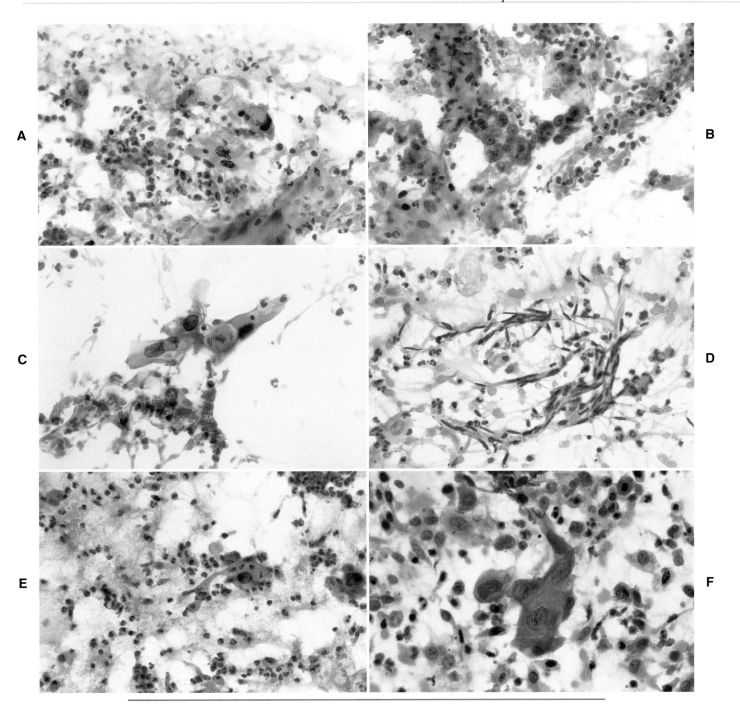

Figure 7-4 **Keratinizing squamous cell carcinoma A,** Tumor diathesis is usually lacking in keratinizing carcinomas. The presence of extensive keratin can impart a low nuclear to cytoplasmic (N : C) ratio to many of the tumor cells, making them difficult to recognize as malignant. Furthermore, the nuclei of many tumor cells are homogeneously dark ("India ink spots") and lack the nucleoli and chromatin clumping typical of nonkeratinizing carcinoma cell. The keratotic cells seen in this illustration have brightly orangeophilic cytoplasm and intensely hyperchromatic nuclei. Although associated with carcinoma in this instance, cells of this type can be seen in low-grade squamous intraepithelial lesions (LGSIL) with no evidence of invasion. **B,** In addition to keratinized cells, this image also shows a cluster of small hyperchromatic cells that are more clearly malignant. Careful observation shows small nucleoli and areas of chromatin clearing in some of these small cells. **C,** The clear background and abnormal keratinizing cells in this image are most suggestive of LGSIL. However, they were associated with an infiltrating carcinoma. **D,** Keratinized cells may be spindled, as in these examples of what some have called *fiber cells.* **E,** Other keratinized cells may take on bizarre shapes. This is evidence of abnormal maturation but can also be seen in noninvasive lesions. In this instance a tumor diathesis background helps point toward the correct diagnosis of invasive carcinoma. **F,** Some keratinizing lesions shed cells with more clear-cut features of malignancy. (Pap)

mors is repair or atypical repair, the cytology of which is described in Chapter 4. Mitotic figures can be seen in either condition. The finding of atypical cells in flat, streaming cohesive sheets is characteristic of repair. This streaming arrangement contrasts with the haphazard arrangement of cells in the syncytia typical of carcinoma. Another hallmark of repair is that cells similar to those in the sheets are not found singly, indicating maintenance of cellular cohesion. In carcinoma, however, single abnormal cells are an important hallmark of malignancy. The chromatin of repair cells is pale, uniform, and finely granular. This contrasts with the irregularly distributed chromatin clumping of most carcinomas. Thus, as is so often the case in cytology, a correct diagnosis is based on mental addition of several features identified by study of numerous cells or cell groups.

The diagnosis of keratinizing carcinoma and its distinction from noninvasive lesions with prominent keratinization is difficult in cytologic samples. Because of the appearance of maturation embodied in surface keratin production, an entity that might be designated as keratinizing carcinoma in situ has not been described. The marked atypia that can be seen with some condylomas can mimic that of keratinizing carcinoma. The traditional observation that keratinizing carcinomas do not show a tumor diathesis background heightens the diagnostic difficulty. Nucleoli are absent from most cells with advanced cytoplasmic keratinization. In the past, it was suggested that all keratinizing lesions with nuclear atypia (keratinizing dysplasia) be reported with a warning that invasive carcinoma could not be excluded. Given the frequency with which human papillomavirus (HPV) lesions with abnormal keratinized cells are encountered, this currently seems outmoded and excessive.

Subclassification of small cell carcinomas into squamous, glandular, neuroendocrine, and mixed is probably not possible in cytologic samples. Recognition of the small cell carcinomas depends on identification of small hyperchromatic cells with scanty cytoplasm. Such cells may be mistaken for endometrial cells or a HGSIL. Necrosis, individual cell necrosis (apoptotic bodies), and mitotic figures are keys to the correct diagnosis.

Hoerl and colleagues indicate the difficulty of this diagnosis in liquid-based preparations.[24] Nuclear pallor, lack of background necrosis, absence of smearing artifact, and inapparent nuclear molding contributed to diagnostic difficulties. These investigators conclude that in liquid-based preparations, it is difficult or impossible to distinguish small cell neuroendocrine carcinoma from small cell squamous cell carcinoma. This is not surprising, as the same difficulty has been noted in conventional smear material. (Much has been made of nuclear molding. However, this is in large part an artifact of cellular degeneration and cell damage during preparation of conventional smears. It is not surprising that this diagnostic criterion is less useful in liquid-based preparations. Similar preparation-dependent cytomorphologic features are discussed during consideration of neuroendocrine carcinomas of the lung.) The observation that these small cell malignancies closely mimic endometrioid adenocarcinomas is more alarming.[24]

Few examples of verrucous carcinoma,[25] papillary squamous cell carcinoma,[17,26] and lymphoepithelioma-like carcinoma[27,28] of the uterine cervix have been described in cytologic samples. Verrucous carcinoma lacks cytologic features of malignancy, and is likely to be misinterpreted as a benign keratotic lesion in most cases. Polymerase chain reaction (PCR) analysis has shown that most papillary squamous cell carcinomas are HPV-related. They are distinguished from verrucous carcinoma, in part by showing cytologic atypia not found in the latter neoplasm.

References

1. Jemal A, Thomas A, Murray T, et al. Cancer statistics, 2002. CA Cancer J Clin 2002; 52:25-47.
2. Ng ABP, Reagan JW. Microinvasive carcinoma of the uterine cervix. Am J Clin Pathol 1969; 52:511-519.
3. Rubio CA, Soderberg G, Einhorn N. Histological and follow-up studies in cases of microinvasive carcinoma of the uterine cervix. Acta Pathol Microbiol Scand 1974; 82[A]: 397-410.
4. Savage EW. Microinvasive carcinoma of the cervix. Am J Obstet Gynecol 1972; 113:708-717.
5. Roche WD, Norris HJ. Microinvasive carcinoma of the cervix: the significance of lymphatic invasion and confluent patterns of growth. Cancer 1975; 36:180-186.
6. Sedlis A, Sol S, Tsukada Y, et al. Microinvasive carcinoma of the uterine cervix: a clinical-pathologic study. Am J Obstet Gynecol 1979; 133:64-74.
7. Fu YS, Berek JS. Minimal cervical cancer: definition and histology. Recent Results Cancer Res 1988; 106:47-56.
8. Benson WL, Norris HJ. A critical review of the frequency of lymph node metastasis and death from microinvasive carcinoma of the cervix. Obstet Gynecol 1977; 49:632-638.
9. van Nagell JR Jr, Greenwell N, Powell DF, et al. Microinvasive carcinoma of the cervix. Am J Obstet Gynecol 1983; 145:981-991.
10. Ng ABP, Reagan JW, Linder EA. The cellular manifestations of microinvasive squamous cell carcinoma of the cervix. Acta Cytol 1972; 16:5-13.
11. Nguyen GK. Exfoliative cytology of microinvasive squamous cell carcinoma of the uterine cervix: a retrospective study of 42 cases. Acta Cytol 1984; 28:457-460.
12. Sugimori H, Iwasaka T, Yoshimura T, et al. Cytology of microinvasive squamous cell carcinoma of the uterine cervix. Acta Cytol 1987; 31:412-416.
13. Gersell DJ, Mazoujian G, Mutch DG, et al. Small-cell undifferentiated carcinoma of the cervix. Am J Surg Pathol 1988; 12:684-698.
14. Zaino RJ, Ward S, Delgado G, et al. Histopathologic predictors of the behavior or surgically treated stage 1B squamous cell carcinoma of the cervix: a gynecologic oncology group study. Cancer 1992; 69:1750-1758.
15. Stock RJ, Zaino R, Bundy BN, et al. Evaluation and comparison of histopathologic grading systems of epithelial carcinoma of the uterine cervix: Gynecologic Oncology Group studies. Int J Gynecol Pathol 1994; 13:99-108.
16. Steeper TA, Piscioli F, Rosai J. Squamous cell carcinoma with sarcoma-like stroma of the female genital tract: Clinicopathologic study of four cases. Cancer 1983; 52: 890-898.
17. Randall ME, Andersen WA, Mills SE, et al. Papillary squamous cell carcinoma of the uterine cervix: a clinicopathologic study of nine cases. Int J Gynecol Pathol 1986; 5:1-10.
18. Tiltman AJ, Atad J. Verrucous carcinoma of the cervix with endometrial involvement. Int J Gynecol Pathol 1982; 1:221-226.
19. Weinberg E, Hoisington S, Eastman AY, et al. Uterine cervical lymphoepithelioma-like carcinoma: absence of Epstein-Barr virus genomes. Am J Clin Pathol 1993; 99:195-199.
20. Husami K, Sugano H, Sakamoto G, et al. Circumscribed carcinoma of the uterine cervix, with marked lymphocytic infiltration. Cancer 1977; 39:2503-2507.

21. Vuong PN, Neveux Y, Schoonaert MG, et al. Adenoid cystic (cylindromatous) carcinoma associated with squamous cell carcinoma of the cervix uteri: cytologic presentation of a case with histologic and ultrastructural correlations. Acta Cytol 1996; 40:289-294.

22. Patten SF. Diagnostic cytology of the uterine cervix. Baltimore: Williams and Wilkins; 1978.

23. Rushing L, Cibas ES. Frequency of tumor diathesis in smears from women with squamous cell carcinoma of the cervix. Acta Cytol 1997; 41:781-785.

24. Hoerl HD, Schink J, Hartenbach E, et al. Exfoliative cytology of primary poorly differentiated (small-cell) neuroendocrine carcinoma of the uterine cervix in ThinPrep material: a case report. Diagn Cytopathol 2000; 23:14-18.

25. Szczepulska E, Nasierowska-Guttmejer A, Bidzinski M. Cervical verrucous carcinoma involving endometrium: case report. Eur J Gynaecol Oncol 1999; 20:35-37.

26. Randall ME, Andersen WA, Mills Mills SE, et al. Papillary squamous cell carcinoma of the uterine cervix: a clinicopathologic study of nine cases. Int J Gynecol Pathol 1986; 5:1-10.

27. Brinck U, Jakob C, Bau O, et al. Papillary squamous cell carcinoma of the uterine cervix: report of three cases and a review of its classification. Int J Gynecol Pathol 2000; 19: 231-235.

28. Reich O, Pickel H, Purstner P. Exfoliative cytology of a lymphoepithelioma-like carcinoma in a cervical smear: a case report. Acta Cytol 1999; 43:285-288.

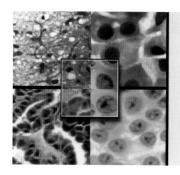

Atypical Glandular Cells of Undetermined Significance

CHAPTER
8

In 1988 the Bethesda System introduced the diagnostic category of atypical glandular cells of undetermined significance (AGUS) to denote atypical cytologic changes in endocervical or endometrial cells that exceed the expected spectrum of reactive alterations yet fall short of adenocarcinoma.[1] The diagnostic terminology was intended for use in pre-neoplastic and reactive glandular lesions. Due to the great deal of difficulty with this morphologic interpretation and the lack of diagnostic reproducibility, AGUS has been used for mostly reactive lesions.[2] The literature relates the incidence of AGUS to be between 0.2% to 1.8%.[3-8] The reported rates of clinically significant lesions (i.e., dysplasia or malignancy) on follow-up range from 17% to 80%.[4-6,8-12]

The diagnostic application of the terms *AGUS*, or simply *atypical glandular cells (AGC)*, is considered tenuous by many because of the overlapping cytomorphology present within the spectrum of reactive-to-malignant glandular cells. The intrinsic problems encountered with the category of AGC are derived from the following facts:

- Although some women in the AGC category (previously referred to in the last Bethesda System terminology as *AGUS*) on the Papanicolaou (Pap) test had benign/reactive pathology, a meaningful subset of patients had demonstrable lesions of potentially high-grade squamous, endocervical, or endometrial morphology. Thus, AGC represents a potential triple threat.
- Atypical/dysplastic/neoplastic squamous cells mimic AGC.
- Reactive glandular cells can appear very similar to neoplastic glandular cells. Although endocervical cells are usually the only glandular cells that the cytopathologist is called upon to evaluate in a normal Pap test (i.e., unless a woman is within 12 days of her last menstrual period and then endometrial cells may be seen in varying proportions), abnormal Pap tests may contain glandular cells from outside the cervix (i.e., endometrial cells in women over the age of 40).
- The morphologic distinction of different populations of glandular cells, whether normal or abnormal, can be exceedingly difficult on the Pap test.

With the previously stated concerns as the reality of the situation, the most recent rendition of the Bethesda System (May 2001) and the American Society for Colposcopy and Cervical Cytology have recommended terminology and clinical management guidelines that yield a detailed and comprehensive decision-making tree based on cytologic criteria and follow-up statistics for the previous diagnostic terminology of AGUS. Despite considerable morphologic overlap, the current recommendations of the Bethesda System 2001 allow for specific classification when deemed possible, as well as grouping under the more amorphous terminology of *AGC of undetermined etiology*.[13,14]

Keeping in mind that the concept of AGC remains a work in progress, this chapter outlines the current recommendations, cytologic criteria, clinical correlates, and management triage of AGC.

 ## HISTORICAL PERSPECTIVE: CHANGES IN TERMINOLOGY

Although many women previously assigned the diagnosis of AGUS on a Pap test have had benign/reactive lesions, histologically, high-grade epithelial lesions—particularly squamous type—have been found in about 14% to 17.4% of cases in a community-based population.[3,15] The terminology of AGUS was born and modified at the 1989 and 1991 Bethesda System Workshops, following in the footsteps of its squamous counterpart (ASCUS), atypical squamous cells of undetermined significance.[1,16] The AGUS terminology was used to replace the previously ill-defined category of glandular cell atypia.

The glandular cell diagnostic components of the 1991 Bethesda System updates were as follows[17]:

1. Endometrial cells, cytologically benign, in a postmenopausal woman (inclusive of endometrial glandular cells and stromal cells)
2. Atypical glandular cells of undetermined significance
3. Atypical endometrial cells of undetermined significance
4. Atypical endocervical cells, favor reactive
5. Atypical endocervical cells, probably neoplastic
6. Endocervical adenocarcinoma
7. Endometrial adenocarcinoma
8. Extrauterine adenocarcinoma

As stated previously, the diagnosis of AGUS was applied to Pap tests with cytologic changes in endocervical or

TABLE 8-1

Follow-Up Data on the Diagnostic Category of Atypical Glandular Cells of Undetermined Significance: 13 Studies Published Since 1992

Study Reference Number*	AGUS Rate (%)	SIL (%)	AIS (%)	EMH (%)	CA (%)
3	0.5	54.3	0	NA	4.3
4	0.46	39.7	7.9	3.2	3.2
5	0.2	9.1	3.9	NA	NA
9	1.8	43.7	3.3	NA	4.0
11	0.63	27	1.9	1.1	6.0
12	0.17	22	NA	NA	8.2
15	0.5	15.4	3.6	NA	<1
19	NA	39.6	5.8	NA	5.8
20	0.11	19.2	1.9	9.6	1.9
21	0.27	21.2	1.2	11.8	9.4
Taylor and colleagues (1993)†	0.18	37	NA	NA	NA
Veljovich and colleagues (1998)‡	0.53	22.6	2.5	2.5	4.0
Chhieng and colleagues (2000)§	0.5	19.5	0	0	5.3

AGUS, Atypical glandular cells of undetermined significance; *SIL*, squamous intraepithelial lesion; *AIS*, adenocarcinoma in situ; *EMH*, Endometrial hyperplasia; *CA*, carcinoma.
*See the References of this chapter.
†Taylor RR, Guerrieri LP, Nash JD, et al. Atypical cervical cytology: colposcopic follow-up using the Bethesda System. J Reprod Med 1993; 38:443-447.
‡Veljovich DS, Stoler MH, Anderson WA, et al. Atypical glandular cells of undetermined significance: a five-year retrospective histopathologic study. Am J Obstet Gynecol 1998; 179:382-390.
§Chhieng DC, Elgert PA, Cangiarella JC, et al. Clinical significance of atypical glandular cells of undetermined significance: a follow-up study from an academic medical center. Acta Cytol 2000; 44:557-566.

endometrial cells that exceeded the usual spectrum of reactive changes but that lacked sufficient features for a diagnosis of adenocarcinoma.[1,16] This terminology and classification gave pathologists an important framework from which to study glandular lesions of the cervix. Subsequent studies tested these cytologic criteria for the glandular diagnostic categories and yielded important pathologic and clinical data within the ensuing 10 years.

With Bethesda 2001 the cytologic criteria have remained the same, and the diagnostic terminology categories have expanded with the exception of AGUS, favor reactive, which has been removed as a diagnostic category. If the glandular cells are truly thought to be reactive, they are now considered part of the general categorization of *negative for squamous intraepithelial lesion (SIL)* and in the subcategorization of *benign reactive cellular changes*. Reactive endocervical cells are considered to be part of the spectrum of a normal Pap test. However, if the changes in the endocervical or other glandular cells cannot be deemed confidently as benign/reactive, or frankly malignant, they are designated as AGC of undetermined etiology, atypical endocervical cells (AEC), or atypical endometrial cells. This step was taken to reduce the false sense of benignity conveyed to many with this terminology, as a significant majority of cases were associated with clinically important lesions in 5% to 39% of cases.[18]

Recently published clinicopathologic studies have shown that the 1991 Bethesda System category of AGUS carries a high risk for the women categorized as such. In this population, SIL rates have been reported to be as high as approximately 40%[4,19]; endocervical adenocarcinoma in

situ (AIS) rates have been as high as approximately 6% to 8%[4,19]; endometrial hyperplasia rates have approximated 10% to 12%[20,21]; and carcinoma rates in general have been reported as high as up to 9%[21] (Table 8-1). In postmenopausal women diagnosed with AGUS, carcinomas most frequently detected on follow-up are endometrial or extrauterine in origin.[22] This assortment of possible pathologic correlates highlights the aforementioned issue of cytologic overlap within the AGUS and AGC categories. A lesion designated as AGC on a Pap test may be endocervical, squamous, endometrial, or even extrauterine in origin and the proposed clinical management rubric has been designed to take this into account.[14]

A diagnosis of AGUS in the postmenopausal population portends a clinically significant lesion in 32.7% of patients. A majority of these lesions are adenocarcinomas (53%) or high-grade squamous intraepithelial lesions (HGSIL) (26%).[23] Conversely, in the pregnant and postpartum population a diagnosis of AGUS was associated with a biopsy rate of SIL of 29%.[24]

Since the 1991 Bethesda Conference the cytologic criteria for endocervical AIS have been found to be predictive and reproducible.[25] Thus, in the current proposed terminology the specific category exists for *endocervical AIS*, whereas in the 1991 system, cells with this morphology would have been put into the *AGUS, probably neoplastic* category.[18]

Although not considered to be atypical, the presence of benign glandular cells (squamous metaplastic, endocervical, or benign glandular cells not otherwise classifiable) in a woman after a hysterectomy warrants reporting. This falls under the category of *other nonneoplastic findings*. Studies have shown essentially no risk of de novo or recurrence of malignancy in patients with these findings regardless of the prior history.[26-28] Vaginal endometriosis, uterine tube prolapse, fistula, glandular metaplasia (associated with previous treatment for neoplasia), and vaginal adenosis (not associated with exposure to diethylstilbestrol) are common causes of this phenomenon.[26,28]

Although the Pap test is not considered to be an accurate screening tool for the detection of endometrial adenocarcinoma, a small percentage of cases may be detected through this testing mode, heralded by the presence of shed or exfoliated endometrial glandular cells. However, these are most often found in asymptomatic women who do not present with the usual symptoms of abnormal bleeding that would lead one to suspect endometrial carcinoma.[29-31] The presence of endometrial cells in patients using hormone replacement therapy and chemopreventive agents (such as tamoxifen) remains under study.[32,33]

With the previous Bethesda System terminology, normal-appearing endometrial cells out of phase (after day 12 of the last menstrual period) were reportable. These cells are rarely associated with meaningful endometrial pathology in premenopausal women and thus are not to be reported in the current Bethesda System terminology.[34-37] The current terminology proposes that endometrial cells in all women over age 40 should be reported. Endometrial cells in the Pap test of a woman over age 40 may signal a possible hyperplastic or neoplastic condition of the endometrium and thus should be reported. This falls under the *general categorization* category of *other*. This may be followed by an educational note explaining that endometrial cells in a woman over age 40 may be associated with a normal endometrium, hormonal therapy, or endometrial/uterine pathology. Clinical correlation and tissue sampling may be recommended.[37]

 ## PROPOSED 2001 TERMINOLOGY

An abbreviated proposed 2001 terminology as set forth by the National Cancer Institutes (NCI) Bethesda 2001 Conference for AGC is as follows (Box 8-1):

II. General Categorization
  A. Negative for intraepithelial lesion or malignancy
  B. Epithelial cell abnormality (specify as squamous or glandular as appropriate)
  C. Other; *see interpretation/diagnosis*
VIII. Glandular Cell Abnormalities (attempt to subclassify, if possible)
  A. Atypical glandular cells
    1. Atypical endocervical cells
    2. Atypical endometrial cells
    3. Atypical glandular cells of undetermined etiology
  B. Atypical glandular/endocervical cells, favor neoplastic
  C. Endocervical adenocarcinoma in situ
  D. Adenocarcinoma
    1. Endocervical
    2. Endometrial
    3. Extrauterine
    4. Not otherwise specified

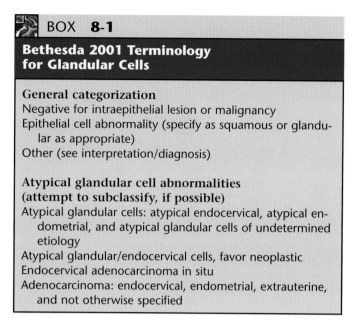

BOX 8-1

Bethesda 2001 Terminology for Glandular Cells

General categorization
Negative for intraepithelial lesion or malignancy
Epithelial cell abnormality (specify as squamous or glandular as appropriate)
Other (see interpretation/diagnosis)

Atypical glandular cell abnormalities (attempt to subclassify, if possible)
Atypical glandular cells: atypical endocervical, atypical endometrial, and atypical glandular cells of undetermined etiology
Atypical glandular/endocervical cells, favor neoplastic
Endocervical adenocarcinoma in situ
Adenocarcinoma: endocervical, endometrial, extrauterine, and not otherwise specified

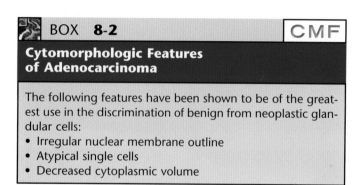

BOX 8-2   **CMF**

Cytomorphologic Features of Adenocarcinoma

The following features have been shown to be of the greatest use in the discrimination of benign from neoplastic glandular cells:
- Irregular nuclear membrane outline
- Atypical single cells
- Decreased cytoplasmic volume

 ## CYTOLOGIC CRITERIA: ATYPICAL GLANDULAR CELLS

The Bethesda terminology proposed in 2001 attempts to use cytologic criteria to assign AGC to the appropriate cell of origin. The category of AGC can be used in cases that exhibit some but not all of the criteria for AIS or one of the *probably neoplastic* designations. The cytologic features that have been shown to be of the greatest use in discerning benign from neoplastic glandular cells are irregular nuclear membrane outline, atypical single cells, and decreased cytoplasmic volume.[38] With this in mind the following are the cytologic criteria for the spectrum of benign/reactive to malignant glandular cells. Examples of the normal glandular components of the Pap test that must be discriminated from AGC are illustrated in Figures 8-1 to 8-13. The cytologic criteria for each of these cell types is discussed in greater detail in Chapter 3 and 4 (Box 8-2 and Table 8-2).

Reactive Atypical Endocervical Cells

Uniform nuclear enlargement with prominent nucleoli and hyperchromasia in the absence of feathering, rosettes, and chromatin irregularities represent features of reactive endocervical cells.[15,18] These cells now fall under the cate-

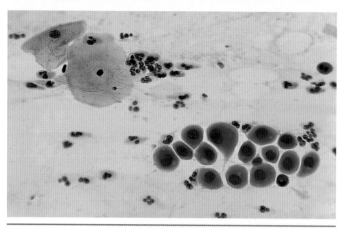

Figure 8-1 Squamous metaplasia. Normal mature eosinophilic superficial cell in one corner with sheet of basophilic squamous metaplastic cells opposite. The metaplastic cells appear to fit together as if pieces in a cobblestone type puzzle. The nuclei approximate the size of adjacent neutrophils and are basophilic without prominent nucleoli in this instance. Cytoplasm varies from dense to focally vacuolated. (Papanicolaou [Pap])

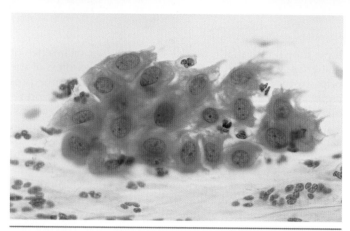

Figure 8-2 Squamous metaplasia. Sheet of cyanophilic squamous metaplastic cells with delicate, lacy cytoplasm and interlacing cytoplasmic processes. Cells have slightly increased nuclear volume with smooth nuclear contours, open chromatin pattern, and small, eosinophilic chromocenters. (Pap)

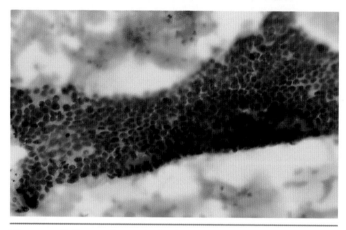

Figure 8-3 Endocervical cells. Flat sheet of normal endocervical cells. Cells are in a honeycombed pattern with nuclei arranged next to one another. Cytoplasm does not appear abundant as the cells are viewed from above rather than tangentially. Nuclei appear slightly hyperchromatic with some cells having visible chromocenters. Cytoplasm is lightly basophilic. Cell sheet appears "rolled over" in the central portion of the slide. (Pap)

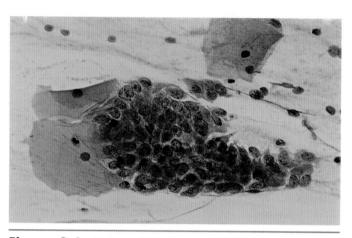

Figure 8-4 Endocervical cells. Curved sheet of endocervical cells in a monolayered honeycomb. Nuclei have a finely stippled chromatin pattern with small basophilic chromocenters. Basophilic cytoplasm is elongated/columnar and lacy. Straight edge of columnar cytoplasm is evident in the three detached cells. Intermediate squamous cells are adjacent. (Pap)

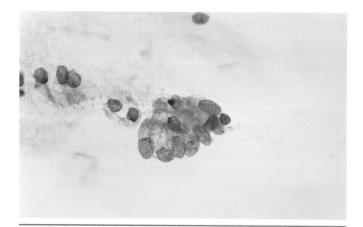

Figure 8-5 Endocervical cells. Strip of endocervical cells with vacuolated, columnar, cyanophilic cytoplasm and basally oriented nuclei. The nuclei exhibit an open chromatin pattern with small, eosinophilic chromocenters. The usually oval nuclear contours appear irregular in areas by overlying vacuoles or folding. (Pap)

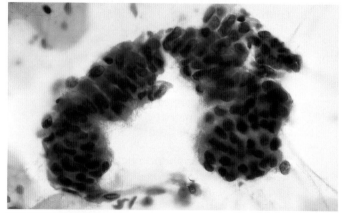

Figure 8-6 Tubal metaplasia. Ciliated columnar endocervical cells appear in sheets and strips with rounded, intermediately placed, mildly hyperchromatic nuclei and abundant eosinophilic cilia present on the luminal surface. The nuclei appear stratified. (Pap) (From Kurman RJ, Solomon D. The Bethesda System for Reporting Cervical/Vaginal Cytologic Diagnoses. New York: Springer-Verlag; 1994.)

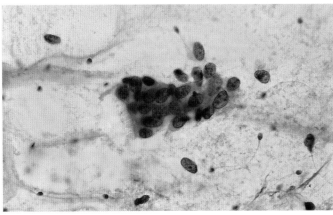

Figure 8-7 **Tubal metaplasia.** Ciliated columnar endocervical cells in a small vertical sheet. Abundant eosinophilic cilia noted coming from the luminally placed terminal bar. The round nuclei appear hyperchromatic with stippled chromatin and visible basophilic chromocenters. Nuclei are stratified, and the columnar cytoplasm is cyanophilic. (Pap) (From Kurman RJ, Solomon D. The Bethesda System for Reporting Cervical/Vaginal Diagnoses. New York: Springer-Verlag; 1994.)

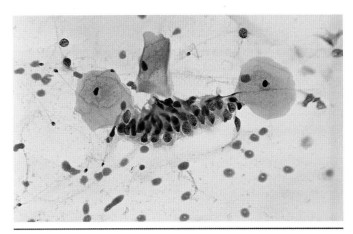

Figure 8-8 **Tubal metaplasia.** Ciliated columnar endocervical cells in a strip with obvious cyanophilic staining luminal cilia. The cells have stratified round to oval nuclei, which appear hyperchromatic, and the cytoplasm is cyanophilic. The nuclei are centrally placed within the cytoplasm. Adjacent superficial squamous cells are present. (Pap)

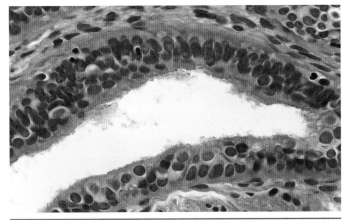
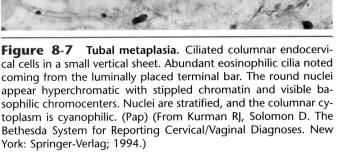

Figure 8-9 **Histologic section: tubal metaplasia.** Ciliated columnar endocervical cells in a gland with luminal cilia. Some of the cells are vacuolated. Nuclei are round to oval, hyperchromatic and stratified. Eosinophilic nucleoli are present in some of the cells. (Hematoxylin and eosin [H&E])

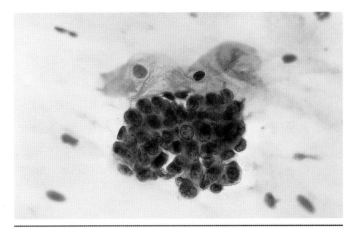

Figure 8-10 **Endometrial cells.** Rounded, cohesive cluster of shed endometrial cells. The small cells have a paucity of amphophilic cytoplasm with round nuclei and a finely stippled, mildly hyperchromatic chromatin pattern. Adjacent squamous cells are present for size comparison. (Pap) (From Kurman RJ, Solomon D. The Bethesda System for Reporting Cervical/Vaginal Diagnoses. New York: Springer-Verlag; 1994.)

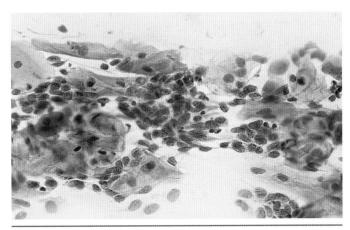

Figure 8-11 **Endometrial stromal cells.** Discohesive, spindled/elongated endometrial stromal cells. The cells are composed of elongated and in some instances, carrot-shaped, nuclei with wisps of amphophilic cytoplasm. The nuclei appear mildly hyperchromatic with finely stippled chromatin. Squamous cells and a few neutrophils are present for size comparisons. (Pap)

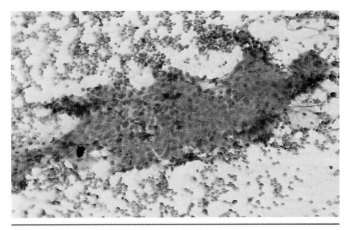

Figure 8-12 **Lower uterine segment.** Sheet of endometrial cells from the lower uterine segment obtained from a brush sample. Round normochromatic nuclei appear as a monolayer with little, if any, intervening cytoplasm. (Pap)

TABLE 8-2   CMF
Cytomorphologic Features of Endocervical Cells for Conventional Pap Tests

	Probably Reactive	Atypical, Probably Neoplastic	Adenocarcinoma in Situ
Cell arrangements	Sheets and strips May be honeycombed	Sheets, strips, and rosettes	Sheets, strips, and rosettes
Nuclear overlap	Minimal	Present	Present; marked crowding
Increased nuclear size	Increase up to three to five times normal	Present	Present Irregular contours Pleomorphism
Nuclear feathering	Absent	Present	Present Marked
Cytoplasmic volume	Normal	Diminished	Diminished
Nucleoli	Present	Inconspicuous	Inconspicuous
Hyperchromasia	Mild	Present	Present
Variation in nuclear size and shape	Mild	Present	Present May be marked
Chromatin	Variable	Finely to moderately granular	Coarsely granular Evenly distributed

From Kurman RJ, Solomon D. The Bethesda System 1991 for reporting cervical/vaginal cytological diagnosis. Diagn Cytopathol 1993; 9:235-246.

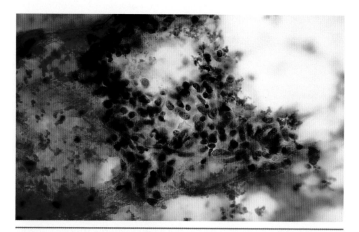

Figure 8-13 **Endometriosis.** Bloody smear with mixture of endometrial stromal and epithelial cells. The stromal and epithelial cells are tightly packed with hyperchromatic, rounded, and elongated nuclei with wispy intervening cytoplasm. (Pap)

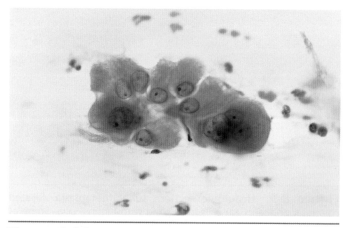

Figure 8-14 **Reactive endocervical cells.** These columnar endocervical cells show enlarged hypochromatic nuclei, with prominent eosinophilic nucleoli, a slight degree of variation in nuclear size, and focal multinucleation is present. Smooth nuclear borders are maintained for the most part. Cytoplasm is wispy and cyanophilic. (Pap)

gory of *negative for intraepithelial lesion, benign reactive cellular changes* (Figures 8-14 to 8-17), which is described as follows:
- Cells are present in flat sheets and strips with a small amount of nuclear overlap.
- Nuclear enlargement may be present with nuclei three to five times the size of a normal endocervical cell nucleus.
- Nuclear size and shape may be mildly variable.
- Mild degree of hyperchromasia may be apparent.
- Nucleoli are usually visible (may have macronucleoli).
- Cytoplasm is abundant.
- Distinct cell borders are evident.

Reactive Atypical Endocervical Cells in Liquid-Based Preparations

The following are the minor differences in appearances noted on reactive/reparative endocervical cells in liquid-based preparations[39] (Figures 8-18 and 8-19):
- Single atypical cells may be noted.

- Sheets of cells may round up in solution and appear more tightly arranged and less pulled out or flattened.

Atypical Endocervical Cells, Probably Neoplastic

Characteristics of atypical endocervical cells that are probably neoplastic are as follows[17,18] (Figures 8-20 to 8-25):
- Cells present in sheets, thin strips, and rosettes
- Honeycomb pattern lost in sheets
- Increased nuclear-to-cytoplasmic (N:C) ratio*
- Ill-defined cell borders
- Nuclear crowding and overlap prominent
- Distinct hyperchromasia with chromatin pattern that is moderately to finely granular
- Indistinct nucleoli

---

*Items identify the best distinguishing features for neoplastic outcome.[38]

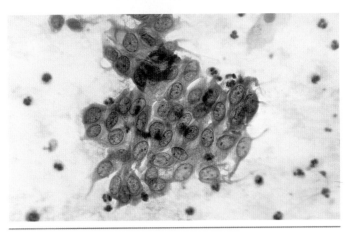

Figure 8-15 Rectovaginal fistula. These reactive/reparative endocervical cells are arranged in a flat sheet with the long axis of the nuclei arranged in parallel. The nuclei show a uniform enlargement with distinct chromatin clearing and eosinophilic or basophilic chromocenters. Nuclear contours are oval, and the nuclear membrane is smooth. Columnar cytoplasm is fluffy and amphophilic. Neutrophils are present for size comparison. (Pap)

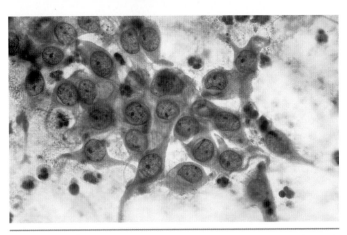

Figure 8-16 Rectovaginal fistula. These reactive endocervical cells are arranged in a flat sheet and show diffuse nuclear enlargement with a mild increase in the N:C ratio. The nuclei have a round to oval shape, show a finely stippled chromatin pattern and obvious basophilic nucleoli, which in some of the cells are quite prominent. Neutrophils are present for size comparison. (Pap) (From Kurman RJ, Solomon D. The Bethesda System for Reporting Cervical/Vaginal Diagnoses. New York: Springer-Verlag; 1994.)

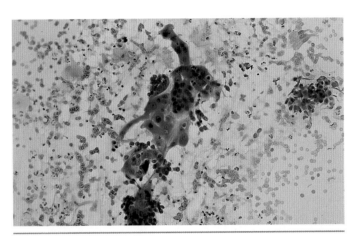

Figure 8-17 Reactive endocervical cells. Normal endocervical cells are next to reactive endocervical cells infiltrated by neutrophils. The smear has a bloody and mildly inflammatory background. The central and peripherally placed reactive endocervical cells are adjacent to a group of centrally placed reactive squamous metaplastic cells. The metaplastic cells have dense, abundant cytoplasm and round nuclei with prominent nucleoli.

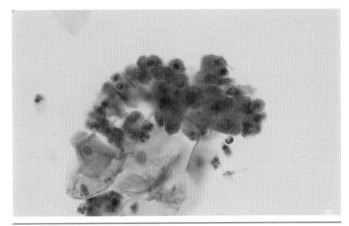

Figure 8-18 Reactive endocervical cells from ThinPrep. These endocervical cells have enlarged nuclei with visible eosinophilic nucleoli. Although the N:C ratio appears to be slightly increased, the nuclei are normochromatic, and the cells remain in an architecturally intact monolayer. (Pap)

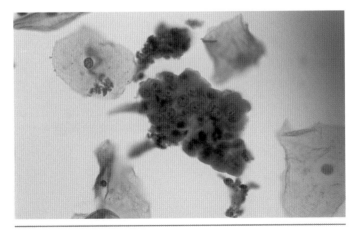

Figure 8-19 Reactive endocervical cells from ThinPrep. These endocervical cells have enlarged nuclei with large eosinophilic nucleoli and focal chromatin clumping. The cells remain in an architecturally intact monolayer. (Pap)

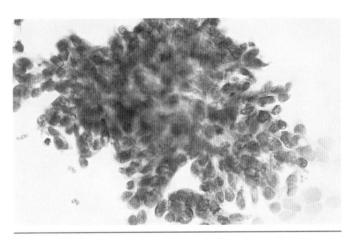

Figure 8-20 Atypical endocervical cells, probably neoplastic. Three-dimensional cluster of atypical endocervical cells. These cells have high N:C ratios, thickened nuclear membranes, and hyperchromasia. Occasional nuclear palisading is seen. On follow-up, this patient had an invasive endocervical adenocarcinoma, well differentiated. (Pap)

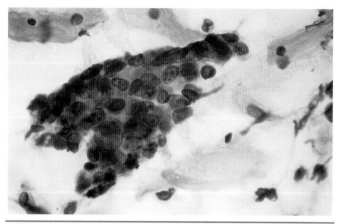

Figure 8-21 **Atypical endocervical cells, probably neoplastic.** A three-dimensional cluster of atypical glandular cells is present. The cells are hyperchromatic and show enlarged nuclei with a slight increase in N:C ratios. On follow-up, this patient had AIS. (Pap)

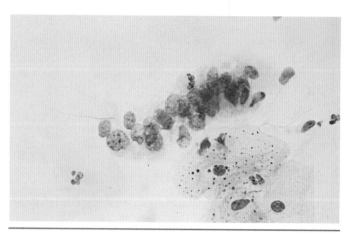

Figure 8-22 **Atypical endocervical cells, probably neoplastic.** A row of atypical endocervical cells is observed. These cells show high N:C ratios and nuclear hyperchromasia. Palisading is present. On follow-up, this patient had a HGSIL. (Pap)

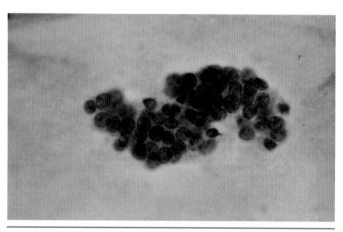

Figure 8-23 **Atypical endocervical cells, probably neoplastic.** A three-dimensional cluster of atypical endocervical cells. These cells show high N:C ratios, nuclear hyperchromasia, and nuclear overlap. Cellular dissociation is not seen. On follow-up, this patient had HGSIL. (Pap)

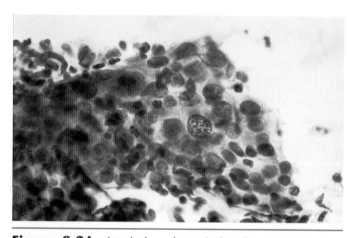

Figure 8-24 **Atypical endocervical cells, probably neoplastic.** A three-dimensional group of atypical endocervical cells is present. These cells are admixed with inflammation. Scattered nuclei are enlarged and hyperchromatic. Irregular chromatin patterns are seen. On follow-up, this patient had a low-grade SIL (LGSIL). (Pap)

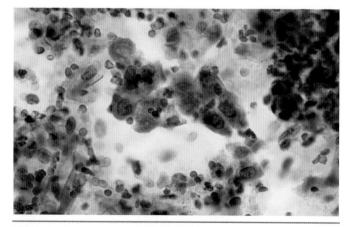

Figure 8-25 **Atypical endocervical cells, probably neoplastic.** A two-dimensional group of atypical endocervical cells is present. These cells exhibit metaplastic cytoplasm and enlarged nuclei. On follow-up, this patient had a LGSIL. (Pap)

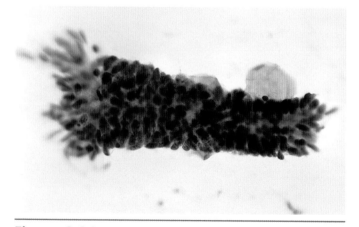

Figure 8-26 **AIS.** Two-dimensional sheet of neoplastic endocervical cells exhibiting elongated hyperchromatic nuclei with extensive nuclear overlapping and coarsely granular chromatin. The cells have a uniform increase in the N:C ratios with significant nuclear pleomorphism present and irregular nuclear contours. The nuclei exhibit peripheral pseudostratification. (Pap)

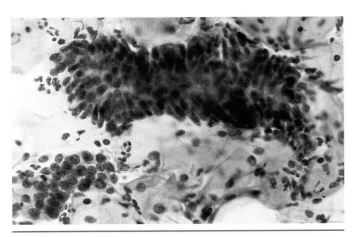

Figure 8-27 AIS. Two-dimensional sheet of neoplastic endocervical cells exhibiting elongated hyperchromatic nuclei with extensive nuclear overlapping and coarsely granular chromatin with obvious nucleoli. Peripheral nuclear pseudostratification is prominent. Mild nuclear pleomorphism is noted. A uniform increase in the N:C ratios is noted. (Pap)

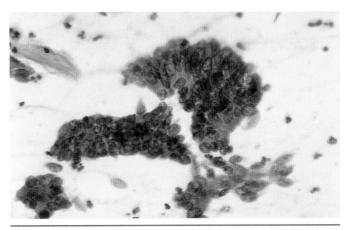

Figure 8-28 AIS. Several sheets of neoplastic endocervical cells. Although one of the sheets appears two-dimensional the other is largely a monolayer with extreme nuclear crowding. The columnar morphology of the cells is evident. Marked nuclear enlargement and pleomorphism is noted. The nuclei are hyperchromatic, and some of the cells have irregular nuclear outlines. Rare single cells are present in the background. A smaller third strip of similar appearing cells is also present. Neutrophils are present for size comparison. (Pap)

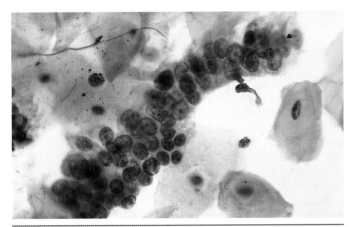

Figure 8-29 AIS. Strips of enlarged, atypical columnar endocervical cells with round or oval hyperchromatic nuclei and extensive nuclear pseudostratification. The nuclei exhibit hyperchromasia. Chromatin clumping, prominent nucleoli, and anisonucleosis are present. (Pap)

- Mitotic figures may be present
- Nuclei are enlarged, elongated and stratified in the majority of the cases
- Nuclear palisading, a prominent feature, with nuclei projecting in a stratified manner along the edges of the cell strips and clusters
- Variation in nuclear size and shape* (See note, p. 152.)

Endocervical Adenocarcinoma In Situ (Common Type)

Previously, (Bethesda 1988 and 1991) no diagnostic category exsisted for AIS, but rather the cases thought to be AIS were placed into the *atypical endocervical cells, probably neoplastic* category. Cases of AIS that are underdiagnosed on Pap tests exhibit several cytologic patterns—one in which the cells resemble reactive endocervical cells and the other in which the cells are small and mimic endometrial cells or endocervical cells from high in the canal and/or tubal metaplasia[18,40-42] (Figures 8-26 to 8-33).

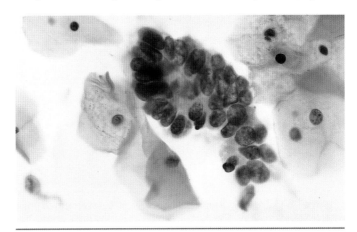

Figure 8-30 AIS. Atypical endocervical cells arranged in a strip and in a rosette. The nuclei exhibit pseudostratification, hyperchromasia, anisonucleosis, irregular nuclear contours, increased N:C ratios, and significant enlargement. Squamous cells are present. (Pap)

The following criteria have been shown to be statistically significant and favored the diagnosis of AIS: the absence of endometrial stromal cells and endometrial-like tubules, coarse chromatin, extreme nuclear crowding (with a lack of honeycombing), mitotic figures, and feathering.[42]

In a study of 70 histologically confirmed cases of endocervical adenocarcinoma, the mean patient age was 37 (range of 22 to 70). Most cases were asymptomatic with only 3% of patients presenting with abnormal bleeding. During colposcopy, 95% of patients had a normal appearing cervix, whereas 5% appeared suspicious. Within this group, nine cases revealed the cytologic features of the endometrioid subtype, and 15 cases revealed cytologic features of the intestinal subtype, as described in the following text.[40] Cytologically, rosettes and epithelial strips with pseudostratification were reported to be present in at least 90% of diagnostic cases.[40] AIS is reported to have a coexistent HGSIL in more than half the cases.[43] Cytologic features are as follow:
- Pattern similar to atypical endocervical cells, probably neoplastic, but more marked

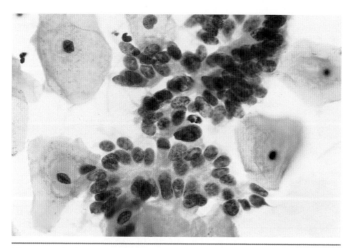

Figure 8-31   AIS. Atypical endocervical cells arranged in a strip and rosette. The nuclei exhibit pseudostratification, hyperchromasia, obvious pleomorphism, irregular nuclear contours, increased N:C ratios, and significant enlargement. Squamous cells are present. (Pap)

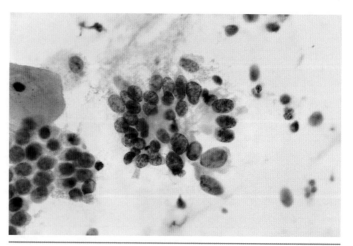

Figure 8-33   AIS. Atypical endocervical cells arranged in two rosettes. The nuclei exhibit pseudostratification, hyperchromasia, obvious pleomorphism, irregular nuclear contours, increased N:C ratios, and significant enlargement. (Pap)

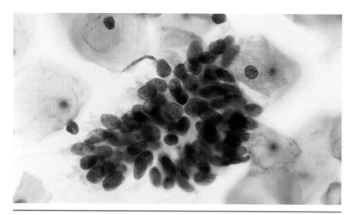

Figure 8-32   AIS. Atypical endocervical cells arranged in a rosettelike formation. The nuclei exhibit pseudostratification, hyperchromasia, obvious pleomorphism, irregular nuclear contours, increased N:C ratios, and significant enlargement. Squamous cells are present. (Pap)

- Elongated hyperchromatic nuclei with extensive nuclear overlap
- Nucleoli not prominent
- Increased N:C ratios and decreased cytoplasmic volume*
- Visible variation in nuclear size with obvious pleomorphism
- Irregular nuclear contours*
- Evenly disbursed, coarsely granular chromatin; parachromatin clearing
- Honeycomb pattern lost with columnar cells present in two dimensional sheets and rosettes with pseudostratified nuclei (feathering), which may be the most significant architectural feature
- Single atypical cells*
- Mitoses
- Apoptotic bodies possibly present
- Inflammatory background

---

*Items identify the best distinguishing features for neoplastic outcome.[38]

- Possible nuclear enlargement (75µm²)
- Nuclei one to three times the size of a normal endocervical cell nucleus

Endocervical Adenocarcinoma in Situ: Endometrioid Subtype

Recent studies evaluating cases diagnosed as *endocervical adenocarcinoma, endometrioid subtype* revealed that the cytologic presentation of this subtype of AIS as groups of crowded small cells leads to underdiagnosis.[40-43] The following list outlines the cytologic features:
- Thick, chunky strips of cells with marked nuclear pseudostratification
- Rosettes with characteristic markedly crowded nuclei
- Little to no cytoplasm present
- Three-dimensional balls of glandular cells resembling abnormal endometrial cells
- Absent intracytoplasmic mucin

Endocervical Adenocarcinoma in Situ: Intestinal Subtype

The intestinal subtype of endocervical AIS is characterized by the following[40,44]:
- Sheets of neoplastic glandular cells (may be honeycombed) with abundant opaque cytoplasm with large secretory granules
- Large cells with round nuclei resembling columnar cells desquamated from the colonic mucosa
- Pattern is never seen alone; may be in conjunction with endometrioid pattern or with conventional pattern

Endocervical Adenocarcinoma in Situ: Liquid-Based Preparations

Although AIS appears similar in conventional and liquid-based preparations, the following features have been noted on liquid-based material[18] (Figures 8-34 to 8-36):
- Apparent increase in the density and three-dimensional quality to the crowded groups

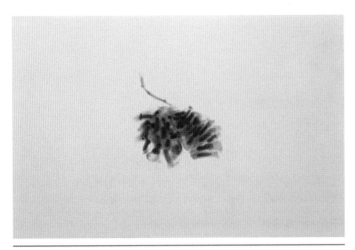

Figure 8-34 **AIS on ThinPrep.** These strips of atypical columnar cells show stratified nuclei with hyperchromatic chromatin and prominent eosinophilic nucleoli. Some cytoplasmic vacuolization is evident. (Pap)

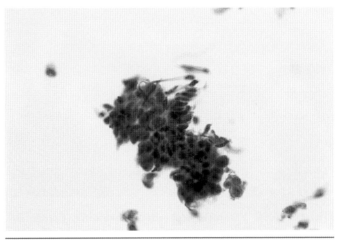

Figure 8-36 **AIS on ThinPrep.** This group of cells is arranged in a three-dimensional aggregate with a strip present at the end. The nuclei are palisading, crowded, and hyperchromatic. The nuclei are oval or rounded. Eosinophilic nucleoli are prominent. (Pap)

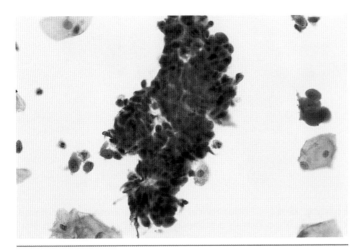

Figure 8-35 **AIS on ThinPrep.** This group of cells is arranged in a three-dimensional aggregate with strips and a rosette present at the end. The nuclei are palisading, crowded, and hyperchromatic. The nuclei are oval or rounded. (Pap)

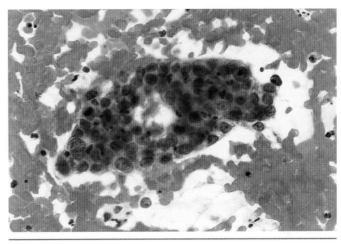

Figure 8-37 **Endocervical adenocarcinoma.** Two-dimensional sheet of atypical cells with increased N:C ratios, round nuclei, prominent eosinophilic macronucleoli, parachromatin clearing, and a cuboidal shape. Rare single cells present in the bloody background. (Pap)

- Hyperchromasia may appear more marked
- Increased difficulty in visualizing individual nuclei
- May have abnormal honeycomb-like arrangement
- Architectural features may be more elusive than in conventional smears
- Decreased feathering (nuclear protrusions) with sharper, smoother, contoured edges of the cell groups
- Strips with pseudostratified nuclei (feathering) may be the most conspicuous architectural feature

Endocervical Adenocarcinoma

Considerable morphologic overlap is evident between AIS and endocervical adenocarcinoma (Figures 8-37 to 8-43).[17]

Although well-differentiated invasive endocervical adenocarcinoma may not have a tumor diathesis and parachromatin clearing, the presence of a tumor diathesis, macronucleoli, and parachromatin clearing suggest an invasive carcinoma.[17] In a study of 40 such cases, syncytia of glandular cells, crowded sheets, and papillary groupings, when seen in conjunction with AIS, were suggestive of microinvasion. Also associated with microinvasion were cellular pleomorphism, frequent cellular dissociation, irregular chromatin and macronucleoli, with or without a tumor diathesis, as noted in the following list[45]:

- Single cells, two-dimensional sheets and clusters
- Enlarged nuclei with prominent, sometimes macronucleoli
- Irregular chromatin and parachromatin clearing
- Possible necrotic tumor diathesis
- Cells may be rounded or maintain a columnar shape with eosinophilic or cyanophilic cytoplasm
- Possible accompanying abnormal squamous cells as part of neoplasia

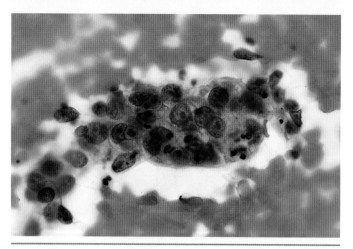

Figure 8-38 Endocervical adenocarcinoma. Two-dimensional aggregate of cells with vacuolated cytoplasm, round nuclei, eosinophilic macronucleoli with extensive parachromatin clearing, and clumping. Malignant cells are admixed with neutrophils. The background is bloody. (Pap)

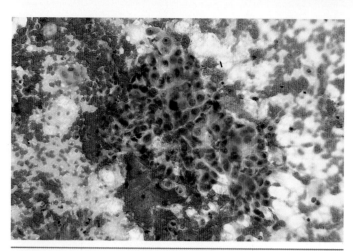

Figure 8-39 Endocervical adenocarcinoma. Two-dimensional sheet of cells with amphophilic cytoplasm, round nuclei, macronucleoli with parachromatin clearing, and clumping. The background is bloody and inflammatory. (Pap)

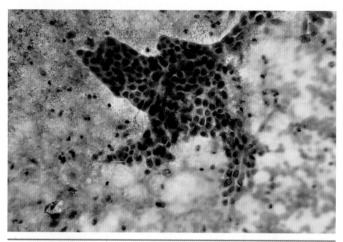

Figure 8-40 Endocervical adenocarcinoma. Two-dimensional sheet of cells with smooth borders, amphophilic cytoplasm, round nuclei, and variable nucleoli with chromatin clumping. The background is bloody and inflammatory. This may represent an admixed squamous component. (Pap)

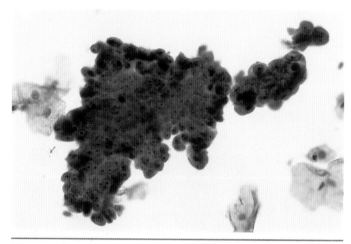

Figure 8-41 Endocervical adenocarcinoma on ThinPrep. This preparation reveals a monolayer of cells exhibiting high N:C ratios with eosinophilic macronucleoli, and chromatin clearing. A three-dimensional cluster of cells is adjacent revealing similar morphologic features. (Pap)

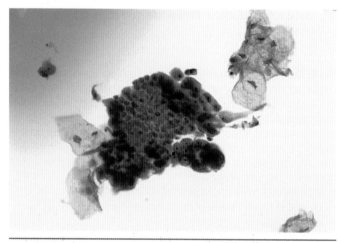

Figure 8-42 Normal endocervical cells adjacent to endocervical adenocarcinoma on ThinPrep. A sheet of normal, benign endocervical cells is adjacent to a cluster and a sheet of atypical cells with high N:C ratios and eosinophilic macronucleoli. The cytoplasmic features of the sheet of cells and the adjacent groups of cells are similar. Note the contrasting nuclear features. (Pap)

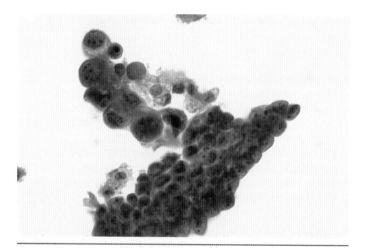

Figure 8-43 Atypical endocervical cells adjacent to endocervical adenocarcinoma on ThinPrep. A sheet of atypical endocervical cells is adjacent to a cluster of larger atypical cells with high N:C ratios and eosinophilic macronucleoli. The cells in the sheet have higher N:C ratios than those in the cluster, which have abundant vacuolated cytoplasm. Atypical nuclear features are similar in the sheet and cluster but are more pronounced in the cluster. (Pap)

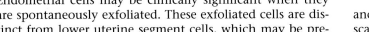

Benign Endometrial Cells

Endometrial cells may be clinically significant when they are spontaneously exfoliated. These exfoliated cells are distinct from lower uterine segment cells, which may be present due to vigorous sampling from the endocervical brush or ectropion[17] (see Figures 8-10 to 8-13). These cells are only mentioned in the reports of women over age 40.[37,46] Exfoliated endometrial stromal cells and histiocytes do not carry pathologic significance.[30,47,48]

Epithelial Cells

Lower uterine segment cells: nonshed. Lower uterine segment cells may be present in sheets that have penetrating glands. Nuclei are small and round and are about the size of an intermediate cell nucleus.

Endometrial cells: benign, shed. Cells occur in small clusters and may be present as single cells. They may or may not have small, visible nucleoli, but they can have ill-defined cell margins. Basophilic cytoplasm is scant and may be vacuolated.

Stromal Cells

Deep. Deep stromal cells are round or spindle shaped and have small oval nuclei. Basophilic cytoplasm is also scant in these cells.

Superficial. With decidual changes, superficial stromal cells may have abundant eosinophilic cytoplasm. It also may be difficult to distinguish from histiocytes and endometrial epithelial cells.

Atypical Endometrial Cells

Because atypical endometrial cells may signal a neoplastic, hyperplastic, or pre-neoplastic condition of the endometrium, they should always be mentioned in the report regardless of the patient's age[17,49] (Figures 8-44 to 8-47). When compared with the *benign, shed* endometrial morphology, the only two different features for the diagnosis of atypical endometrial cells are the presence of *slight nuclear enlargement and mild hyperchromasia.*

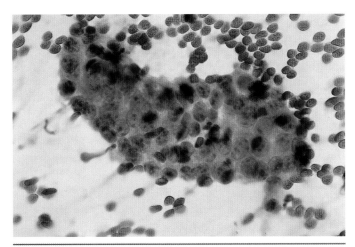

Figure 8-44 **Atypical endometrial cells.** The cells are in a tight cluster with enlarged nuclei, indistinct cytoplasmic borders, scant cytoplasm, mild hyperchromasia, and obvious nucleoli. (Pap)

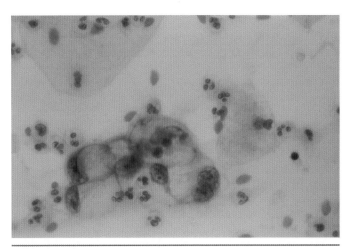

Figure 8-46 **Atypical endometrial cells.** This cluster of cells shows marked cytoplasmic enlargement and vacuolization with peripherally placed, compressed nuclei. The nuclei have prominent eosinophilic nucleoli. (Pap)

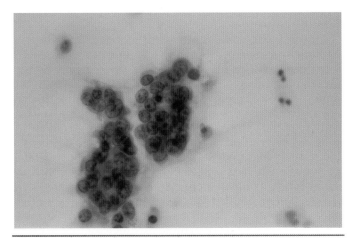

Figure 8-45 **Atypical endometrial cells.** The cells are in two clusters and have enlarged nuclei, indistinct cytoplasmic borders, scant cytoplasm, mild hyperchromasia, and obvious nucleoli. (Pap)

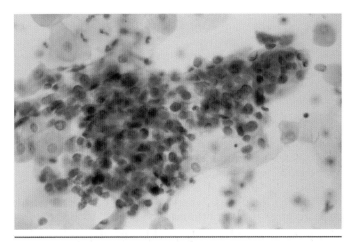

Figure 8-47 **Atypical endometrial cells.** The cells are in loose sheets and have enlarged nuclei, indistinct cytoplasmic borders, scant cytoplasm, mild hyperchromasia, and nucleoli. (Pap)

In addition, other characteristics of atypical endometrial cells are as follows:

- Cells in small clusters/balls
- Slight enlargement of nucleus
- Mild hyperchromasia
- Small nucleoli
- Cytoplasmic borders indistinct
- Scant cytoplasm (as compared with endocervical cells) that may be vacuolated

 ## DIFFERENTIAL DIAGNOSIS OF ATYPICAL GLANDULAR CELLS

Benign/Reactive Changes

Benign/reactive endocervical cells with cytologic features that by definition are atypical, yet are not pre-neoplastic, may be seen in a variety of conditions. Infections and reparative processes are notorious. The background changes on the Pap test are clues as to the reactive nature of the lesion. However, reactive changes in endocervical cells can also accompany neoplastic lesions. Microglandular hyperplasia and Arias-Stella changes of the endocervical glands can also give rise to atypical but reactive changes in the endocervical cells.[17]

Ciliated endocervical cells, commonly referred to as *tubal metaplasia* (but more appropriately termed *tubal differentiation*) are distinguished by their columnar shape, basally placed oval hyperchromatic nuclei, and their long eosinophilic cilia[25] (see Figures 8-6 to 8-9). At times, these cells can be reminiscent of AIS or even invasive adenocarcinoma of the endocervix (see Figures 8-26 to 8-43). Tubal differentiation cells are usually present in clusters and may appear pseudostratified. The best distinguishing feature is the presence of cilia on these benign cells. The nuclei of these ciliated cells are round to oval, and show more finely granular evenly dispersed chromatin than the cells of AIS. Also feathering and pseudorosette formation are not present in groups of these ciliated endocervical cells.[17]

Glandular Versus Squamous Lesions

Of cases diagnosed as AGUS, 14% to 80% on follow up will have a clinically significant lesion* (Figure 8-48). Three recent publications have reported this number to be at about 25%.[12,15,20] The majority of these high-grade lesions are squamous in type. As would be expected, older patients (≥50) diagnosed as AGUS have a higher probability of having a glandular lesion as opposed to a squamous lesion.[50] Although a significant degree of cytologic overlap exists between glandular and squamous lesions, particularly HGSIL involving endocervical glands, a recent study has identified cytologic features in the areas of cell shape, cytoplasm, and architecture, which are helpful in this distinction.[15] Smears in which the abnormal cells are polygonal or ovoid are more likely squamous, whereas in glandular lesions the cells are more likely columnar or cuboidal. Vacuolated cy-

*References 3, 5-7, 10-12, 15, 19, and 20.

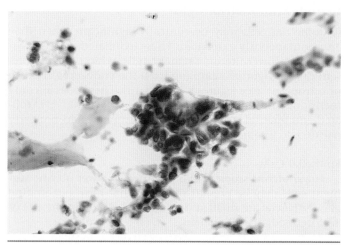

Figure 8-48 **HGSIL-simulating glandular lesion.** This represents a HGSIL within endocervical glands, simulating a glandular lesion. The cells appear in strips of varying width. They have dark, irregular nuclei and exhibit significant nuclear piling up and high N:C ratios. The cytoplasm is dense. (Pap)

toplasm was not seen in squamous lesions. Dense cytoplasm, although present in all squamous lesions (e.g., HGSIL) in this study, was present also in some of the glandular lesions. The architectural features of feathering, rosettes, and palisades were absent in squamous lesions (e.g., HGSIL), but were a prominent feature in some of the cases of AIS.[15] The distinguishing features suggesting a HGSIL are as follows:

- Cells are arranged as sheets or fragments.
- Atypical single cells rare.
- Cell shape is polygonal or oval.
- Dense cytoplasm is present.
- Ovoid, enlarged central hyperchromatic nuclei with chromatin irregularities are present.
- Fragments have a smooth edge along one aspect with cells with elongated nuclei and small amounts of cytoplasm.
- The long axes of the nuclei are arranged parallel to the edge of the cellular sheet rather than perpendicular (as in feathering).
- Rare cellular fragments with features suggestive of feathering may be present.

Clearly, glandular and squamous lesions may coexist in the same specimen because they are frequent coinhabitants of the cervix.[44] This may be indicated cytologically by features of both squamous and glandular differentiation in the same sample (i.e., groups of atypical cells with smooth, flattened edges and areas with rosettes and feathering). The use of these criteria to separate squamous versus glandular lesions has been shown to have good cytohistologic correlation.[15] With that said, several cases with purely glandular cytology on Pap tests yielded biopsy-proven HGSIL without any glandular component at all.[15]

The aforementioned study reviewed 137 smears originally diagnosed as AGUS and the subsequent biopsies. When an expert panel of pathologists reviewed these cases, the diagnosis of AGUS was only maintained on 44 of these original 137 cases, although the proportions of follow-up diagnoses were similar[15] (Table 8-3).

TABLE 8-3

Histologic Results and Detection of Carcinoma-Associated Human Papillomavirus DNA in Atypical Glandular Cells of Undetermined Significance Pap Tests

Original Cytology Diagnosis of AGUS (n = 137); Histologic Diagnosis	Number of Cases (%)	Number of Individuals with HPV (%)	Review Cytology Diagnosis of AGUS (n = 44); Histologic Diagnosis	Number of Individuals with HPV (%)
Negative/nondiagnostic histology	109 (80.1)	18 (16.5)	34 (79.1)	8 (18.2)
Low-grade squamous intraepithelial lesion (LGSIL)	9 (6.6)	5 (55.6)	2 (4.7)	1 (50%)
High-grade squamous intraepithelial lesion (HGSIL)	12 (8.8)	11 (91.7)	2 (4.7)	2 (100)
HGSIL + adenocarcinoma in situ (AIS)	2 (1.5)	2 (100)	1 (2.3)	1 (100)
AIS	3 (2.2)	3 (100)	3 (7.0)	3 (100)
Endometrial carcinoma	1 (0.07)	0	1 (2.3)	0
TOTAL*	136 (100)	39 (28.7)	43 (100)	15 (34.1)

From Ronnett BM, Manos MM, Ransley JE, et al. Atypical glandular cells of undetermined significance (AGUS): cytopathologic features, histopathologic results, and human papillomavirus DNA detection. Hum Pathol 1999; 30:816-825.
*One case had insufficient tissue for diagnosis on follow-up histology.

Glandular Lesions

". . . The majority of significant AGUS lesions are squamous dysplasias, and from 40% to 68% of squamous dysplasias are high-grade lesions. . . ."[51]

The diagnostic meaning of the Bethesda category of AGUS/AGC has been questioned, as has the ability to diagnose glandular lesions by Pap tests. Using the Bethesda System criteria, the category of AGUS seems to diagnose mostly cases of HGSIL which are, by definition, not glandular.

The sensitivity of glandular lesion diagnosis by the Pap test is highest for endocervical adenocarcinoma and lowest for endometrial carcinoma. Only a small percentage of women with AIS and most women with invasive adenocarcinoma will be diagnosed as having disease on a Pap test. Sampling, screening, and interpretative errors have been implicated as contributing to the lower detection rate of AIS on Pap tests.[41,52]

Endometrial adenocarcinoma is rarely diagnosed on Pap tests. It is estimated that of women with endometrial adenocarcinoma, only about one third shed abnormal cells that may be detected through the Pap test.[51,53-57]

Among women with endometrial carcinoma, a Pap test performed in the 2-year period immediately preceding the diagnosis found evidence of possible disease in only 28% of cases.[53] As the definitive cytologic criteria for endometrial carcinoma in the Pap test milieu require further elucidation, the proposed terminology stops at atypical endometrial cells and does not further elaborate on neoplastic probability unless the criteria fulfill that of endometrial adenocarcinoma. A recent study evaluated the clinical implications of *AGUS, favor endometrial origin*.[49] The patients ranged in age from 29 to 88, with a mean age of 53 years; 55% of the patients were postmenopausal. Follow-up revealed clinically significant uterine lesions in 31%, including endometrial adenocarcinoma (13%), endometrial hyperplasia (11%), and significant squamous lesions (high-grade or carcinoma) (7%).[49] The remaining patients had benign or normal pathology results. Thus, one third of the women with a diagnosis of *AGUS, favor endometrial origin* will have a significant uterine lesion on biopsy, with a majority of these lesions being endometrial in origin.[49]

AGUS/AGC is a poorly reproducible cytologic interpretation.[2,7,58] When four expert cytopathologists reviewed 100 cases originally diagnosed as AGUS, in no case did all of the cytopathologists use the same diagnosis. In this group, little agreement was reached on which cytologic criteria were important in separating clinically significant and benign lesions, with 46% having benign follow-up and 54% having a clinically significant lesion on follow-up.[2] The authors concluded that the AGUS category is poorly understood, that poor interobserver diagnostic agreement exists, and that no agreement exists on diagnostic cytologic criteria.[2]

Another study evaluating this phenomenon found that when an expert panel of five pathologists reviewed 135 cases originally diagnosed as AGUS, the AGUS designation was retained by three or more of the five reviewers in only 29% of conventional Pap tests. The interobserver variability in designating a smear as AGUS was marked. The best agreement was reached for lesions designated as high-grade squamous or glandular in type.[58]

The current Bethesda System approach to the interpretation of atypical glandular cells recommends that the sign-out terminology for AGC should be as specific as possible, as determined by the cytologic features of the abnormalities. The cytologic features of both atypical endocervical cells and atypical endometrial cells have been defined by the 1991 Bethesda Conference, and it is believed that by strictly using defined morphologic guidelines, most cases can be placed into either the endocervical or endometrial categories. Thus, if the glandular cell type can be identified, neoplasia is favored, or the diagnosis of a particular type of carcinoma can be made with certainty, it should be noted as such in the diagnostic line. However, the system recognizes that the morphology can be ambiguous, thus, the categorization of simply AGC of undetermined significance. The criteria for an unqualified AGC of undetermined significance are less well-defined and reproducible and will invariably include *reactive, benign* cases. Thus, laboratories should be cognizant of AGC rates to ensure that they are not placing reactive, benign Pap tests into this category. AGC rates for typical cytology laboratories should be below 1% for conventional and liquid-based preparations.[18] The current Bethesda System guidelines have placed the category of *AGUS, favor reactive* into the *negative, benign/reactive* cellular changes category. Whether this will cause an actual decrease in the AGC/AGUS rate or these cases will be relegated to the *AGC,* the *unqualified* category is yet to be seen (Box 8-3).

Preliminary studies show that the follow-up for AGC diagnosed on liquid-based preparations seems to yield a higher degree of pathologic abnormalities.[59-61] The clinical management approach—which includes colposcopy and cervical, endocervical, and endometrial sampling—will undoubtedly assist in this learning curve.[14]

Human Papillomavirus Detection

HPV DNA hybrid capture techniques (Digene, Gaithersburg, Md.) for carcinoma-associated HPV have been shown to be useful for the triaging of ASCUS into high-risk and low-risk categories.[62,63] As many of the cases originally diagnosed as AGUS eventually are proven to be SILs, particularly HGSIL, HPV hybrid capture studies may prove useful in lesions diagnosed as AGC/AGUS.[15] A recent study evalu-

ated this approach using the HPV hybrid capture II microplate method for HPV 16, 18, 31, 33, 35, 39, 45, 51, 52, 56, and 58 (see Table 8-3). Although 16% to 18% of AGUS cases revealed HPV positivity with HPV hybrid capture, what appears most captivating are the figures for the true glandular and squamous lesions—in which HPV was detected in 50% to 100% of various biopsy confirmed lesions (see Table 8-3). These figures suggest the rationale for a more aggressive follow-up course in women diagnosed with AGUS/AGC with detectable HPV found by hybrid capture. In this study, HPV DNA testing was deemed more sensitive than a repeat Pap test (94.1% vs 62.5%) in identifying patients with a histologically confirmed high-grade lesion (e.g., HGSIL, AIS), although this difference did not reach statistical significance. These authors recommend a triage approach using a combination of review of cytologic diagnosis and HPV testing to yield the best results. If all of the women in the study who had positive HPV results and abnormal cytologic reviews were referred to colposcopy, all HGSILs would have been detected. These data also suggest that a negative HPV DNA test gives good reassurance that a high-grade lesion is not present. A negative HPV DNA test, however, is not useful in ruling out an endometrial lesion.[15]

MANAGEMENT OF ATYPICAL GLANDULAR CELLS

The array of possible pathologic associations with the category AGUS has broadened the current management guidelines for AGC with a comprehensive management approach that includes the sampling of endocervix, ectocervix, and endometrium, particularly in women over the age of 35[14] (see Table 8-1). In women over age 35 the majority of cancers in this spectrum are endometrial in origin.[3,22] Previous practice guidelines have recommended colposcopy, endocervical cell sampling, and sometimes endometrial sampling or curettage.[64-66] Clinical practices have, however, been at variance with these guidelines.[67]

The recommendation for initial management of a woman diagnosed with AGC (all subcategories) is as follows:

- *All women with atypical glandular or endocervical cells should have colposcopy and endocervical sampling.*[14] This initial management should not vary based on the qualification of the atypia or on the presence of accompanying squamous abnormalities on the Pap test. Managing AGC of any type by a repeat Pap test is unacceptable.[14]
- *All women with atypical endometrial cells should initially have endometrial sampling. If the endometrial sampling is negative, then these women should have colposcopy and endocervical sampling.*
- *In cases in which an increase risk is deemed by the qualifiers favor neoplasia, favor AIS, or AIS, the patient should have a cervical excisional procedure following colposcopy.* For this, a cold cone or electrosurgical microneedle excision is favored over a loop electrosurgical excision procedure for evaluation and treatment because of the increased potential for burn artifact at the excision margins with the latter procedure.[14] The exception to this recommendation would be for women that are found to have invasive carcinoma on biopsy or endocervical sampling done during colposcopic examination, as they require definitive therapy.[14]

BOX 8-3

Approach to the General Categorization of Atypical Glandular Cells

When the cytopathologist is unable to determine the cell type with certainty, the cells should be classified as follows:
- Atypical glandular cells, unqualified
- Atypical glandular cells, favor neoplasia

When the cytopathologist has deemed the atypical cells to be of endocervical etiology, the cells should be classified as follows:
- Atypical endocervical cells, unqualified
- Atypical endocervical cells, favor neoplasia
- Atypical endocervical cells, probably adenocarcinoma in situ
- Adenocarcinoma in situ

When the cytopathologist has deemed the atypical cells to be of endometrial origin, the cells should be classified as follows:
- Atypical endometrial cells

When the atypical cells in any of the above categories are accompanied by squamous abnormalities, the cells should be classified as follows:
- Atypical glandular cells (from any of the approved diagnostic categories), with squamous abnormality (specify the abnormality)

When the atypical glandular cells are from an origin other than the cervix or endometrium (e.g., ovary, fallopian tube), the cells should be classified as follows:
- Atypical glandular cells suggestive of (state origin other than cervix or endometrium)

Women over age 35 have an increased risk for endometrial neoplasia. Along with that, the recognition of atypical endometrial cells noted on cervical cytology and unexplained vaginal bleeding at any age are all factors that increase the risk for endometrial neoplasia.[14]

- *Direct endometrial sampling (e.g., endometrial pipelle or dilatation and curettage) should be performed in women of any age, when their cytology has been diagnosed as atypical endometrial cells; women with AGC with unexplained vaginal bleeding; and women over age 35 with any glandular cell abnormality detected on Pap test. Additionally, endo-* metrial sampling should also be done on postmenopausal women who have endometrial cells in their Pap tests and who are not on hormonal replacement therapy.[14]

- *When the atypical cells are deemed to be of glandular, other than cervical or endometrial, origin, it is recommended that appropriate procedures for evaluating the possible site of origin should be performed, in addition to the initial colposcopy and endocervical sampling conducted on diagnosis of AGC.*

Initial management and follow-up guidelines are outlined in Tables 8-4 and 8-5.

TABLE 8-4

Initial Management and Follow-Up Guidelines for Atypical Glandular Cells

Initial Diagnosis	Initial Workup	Follow-Up
- AGC, NOS - Atypical endocervical cells, NOS	Negative colposcopy Negative biopsy Negative endocervical sampling	Repeat Pap test every 4-6 months until the patient has had three or four normal Pap tests.
- AGC, favor neoplasia - Atypical endocervical cells, favor neoplasia - Atypical endocervical cells, probably AIS - AIS - Other neoplasm (if negative on more specific workup)	Negative colposcopy Negative biopsy Negative endocervical sampling	Perform cervical excisional procedure. Some may prefer to have the Pap test reviewed before a cervical excision procedure is begun.

From American Society for Colposcopy and Cervical Cytology. Draft guidelines: ASCPP Consensus Conference on Cytological Abnormalities and Cervical Cancer Precursors, accessed September 6-9, 2001 [http://consensus.asccp.org].
AGC, Atypical glandular cells; *NOS,* not otherwise specified; *AIS,* adenocarcinoma in situ.

TABLE 8-5

Follow-Up Management Guidelines for Atypical Glandular Cells for Women Negative on Initial Examination

Initial Diagnosis	Initial Workup	Follow-Up
Initial colposcopy, biopsy, and ECC negative and initial Pap test: - AGC, NOS - Atypical endocervical cells - NOS	Negative follow-up for three or four Pap tests	Return patient to routine screening at 4- to 6-month intervals.
Initial colposcopy, biopsy, ECC negative and initial Pap test: - AGC, NOS - Atypical endocervical cells - NOS	Follow-up Pap test equivocal or LGSIL or ASCUS	Repeat colposcopy and indicated procedure.
Initial colposcopy, biopsy, and ECC negative and initial Pap test: - AGC, NOS - Atypical endocervical cells, NOS	Follow-up Pap test HGSIL or AGUS	Consider referral to expert in the evaluation of abnormal Pap tests or: - Repeat colposcopy and indicated procedures; review with pathologist.
Initial colposcopy, biopsy, and ECC negative and initial Pap test: - Repeat ACG - AGC, favor neoplasia - Atypical endocervical cells, suggestive of AIS - AIS - Other	Negative endometrial sampling Negative excisional cervical procedure	Consider referral to expert in the evaluation of abnormal Pap tests or: - Pelvic ultrasound - Abdominopelvic CT - Hysteroscopy in women over age 35 - Review of slides with pathologist.

ECC, Endocervical cells; *AGC,* atypical glandular cell; *NOS,* not otherwise specified; *LGSIL,* low-grade squamous intraepithelial lesion; *ASCUS/AGUS,* atypical squamous cells of undetermined significance; *HGSIL,* high-grade squamous intraepithelial lesion; *AIS,* adenocarcinoma in situ; *CT,* computed tomography.

References

1. National Cancer Institute Workshop. The 1988 Bethesda System for reporting cervical/vaginal cytological diagnosis. JAMA 1989; 262:931-934.
2. Raab SS, Geisinger KR, Silverman JF, et al. Interobserver variability of a Papanicolaou smear diagnosis of atypical-glandular cells of undetermined significance. Am J Clin Pathol 1998; 110(5):653-659.
3. Valdini A, Vaccaro C, Pochinsky M, et al. Incidence and evaluation of an AGUS Papanicolaou smear in primary care. J Am Board Fam Pract 2001; 14:172-177.
4. Goff BA, Atanosoff P, Brown E, et al. Endocervical glandular atypia in Papanicolaou smears. Obstet Gynecol 1992; 79:101-104
5. Kennedy AW, Salmieri SS, Wierth SL, et al. Results of the clinical evaluation of atypical glandular cells of undetermined significance (AGUS) detected on cervical cytology screening. Gynecol Oncol 1996; 63:14-18.
6. Lee KR, Manna EA, St John T. Atypical endocervical glandular cells: accuracy of cytologic diagnosis. Diagn Cytopathol 1995; 13:202-208.
7. Raab SS, Snider TE, Potts SA: Atypical glandular cells of undetermined significance: diagnostic accuracy and interobserver variability using select cytologic criteria. Am J Clin Pathol 1997; 107:299-307.
8. Chhieng DC, Elgert P, Cangiarella JF, Cohen JM: Variation in the incidence of AGUS between different patient populations. Acta Cytol 2001; 45:287-293.
9. Nasu I, Meurer W, Fu YS. Endocervical glandular atypia and adenocarcinoma: a correlation of cytology and histology. Int J Gynecol Pathol 1993; 12:208-218.
10. Bose S, Kannan V, Kline TS. Abnormal endocervical cells. Really abnormal? Really endocervical? Am J Clin Pathol 1994; 101:708-713.
11. Eddy GL, Strumpf KB, Wojtowycz MA, et al. Biopsy findings in five hundred thirty-one patients with atypical glandular cells of uncertain significance as defined by the Bethesda system. Am J Obstet Gynecol 1997; 177:1188-1195.
12. Duska LR, Flynn CF, Chen A, et al. Clinical evaluation of atypical glandular cells of undetermined significance on cervical cytology. Obstet Gynecol 1998; 91:278-282.
13. NCI Bethesda System. 2001 terminology, accessed May 2001 [http://bethesda2001.cancer.gov/terminology.html].
14. American Society for Colposcopy and Cervical Cytology: Draft guidelines: ASCCP Consensus Conference on Cytological Abnormalities and Cervical Cancer Precursors, accessed Sept 6-9, 2001; [http://consensus.asccp.org.]
15. Ronnett BM, Manos MM, Ransley JE, et al. Atypical glandular cells of undetermined significance (AGUS): cytopathologic features, histopathologic results, and human papillomavirus DNA detection. Hum Pathol 1999; 30:816-825.
16. Bethesda System. The Bethesda System 1991 for reporting cervical/vaginal cytological diagnosis. Diagn Cytopathol 1993; 9:235-246.
17. Kurman RJ, Solomon D. The Bethesda System for reporting cervical/vaginal cytologic diagnoses. New York: Springer Verlag; 1994.
18. Wilbur D, Chhieng D, Cox JT, et al. Draft recommendations: atypical glandular cells of undetermined significance: draft recommendations (Bethesda 2001 Workshop). Bethesda, Md: National Cancer Institute; 2001.
19. Jones B, Novis D. Cervical biopsy-cytology correlation: a College of American Pathologists Q-Probes study of 22,439 correlations in 348 laboratories. Arch Pathol Lab Med 1996; 20:523-531.
20. Soofer SB, Sidawy MK. Atypical glandular cells of undetermined significance: clinically significant lesions and means of patient follow up. Cancer (Cancer Cytopathol) 2000; 90:207-214.
21. Zweizig S, Noller K, Real EF, et al. Neoplasia associated with atypical glandular cells of undetermined significance on cervical cytology. Gyncecol Oncol 1997; 65:314-8.
22. Obenson K, Abrero F, Grafton W. Cytohistologic correlation between AGUS and biopsy-detected lesions in postmenopausal women. Acta Cytol 2000; 44:1;41-45.
23. Chhieng D, Elgert P, Cohen JM, Cangiarella JF: Clinical significance of AGUS in postmenopausal women. Cancer 2001; 93:1-7.
24. Chhieng D, Elgert P, Cangiarella JF, Cohen JM: Significance of AGUS Pap smears in pregnant and postpartum women. Acta Cytol 2001; 45:294-299.
25. Solomon D, Frable WJ, Vooijs GP, et al. ASCUS and AGUS criteria: IAC task force summary. Acta Cytol 1998; 42:16-24.
26. Tambouret NC, Pitman MB, Bell DA. Benign glandular cells in posthysterectomy vaginal smears. Acta Cytol 1998; 42:1403-1408.
27. Ponder TB, Easley KO, Davila RM. Glandular cells in vaginal smears from posthysterectomy vaginal smears. Acta Cytol 1997; 41:1701-1704.
28. Ramirez NC, Sastry LK, Pisharodi LR. Benign glandular and squamous metaplastic-like cells seen in vaginal Pap smears of post hysterectomy patients: incidence and patient profile. Eur J Gynecol Oncol 2000; 21:43-48.
29. Cherkis RC, Patten SF, Andrews TJ, et al. Significance of normal endometrial cells detected by cervical cytology. Obstet Gynecol 1998; 71:242-244.
30. Zucker PK, Kadson EJ, Feldstein ML. The validity of Pap smear parameters as predictors of endometrial pathology in menopausal women. Cancer 1985; 56:2256-2263.
31. Gomez-Fernandez CR, Ganjei-Azar P, Capote-Dishaw J, et al. Reporting normal endometrial cells in Pap smears: an outcome appraisal. Gynecol Oncol 1999; 74:381-384.
32. Abadi MA, Barakat RR, Saigo PE. Effects of tamoxifen on cervical smears from patients with breast cancer. Acta Cytol 2000; 44:141-146.
33. Sarode VR, Radar AE, Rose PG. Significance of cytologically normal endometrial cells in cervical smears from postmenopausal women. Acta Cytol 2001; 45:153-156.
34. Ng ABP, Reagan JW, Hawliczek S, et al. Significance of endometrial cells in the detection of endometrial carcinoma and its precursors. Acta Cytol 1974; 18:356-361.
35. Gondos B, King EB. Significance of endometrial cells in cervicovaginal smears. Ann Clin Lab Sci 1977; 7:486-490.
36. Gray J, Nguyen G-K. Cytologic detection of endometrial pathology by Pap smears. Diagn Cytopathol 1999; 20:181-182.
37. Moriarty A, Cibas E, Gill G, et al. Draft recommendations: endometrial cells (Bethesda 2001 Workshop). Bethesda, Md: National Cancer Institute; 2001.
38. Raab SS, Isacson C, Layfield LJ, et al. Atypical glandular cells of undetermined significance: cytologic criteria to separate clinically significant from benign lesions. Am J Clin Pathol 1995; 104:574-582.
39. Young N, Bibbo M, Buckner SB, Colgan T, Rosenthal D, Wilkinson E. Draft recommendations: benign cellular changes and infections (Bethesda 2001 Workshop). Bethesda, Md: National Cancer Institute; 2001.
40. Ayer B, Pacey F, Greenberg M, et al. The cytologic diagnosis of adenocarcinoma in situ of the cervix uteri and related lesions I: adenocarcinoma in situ. Acta Cytol 1987; 31(4):397-411.
41. Lee KR, Minter LJ, Granter SR. Papanicolaou smear sensitivity for adenocarcinoma in situ of the cervix: a study of 34 cases. Am J Clin Pathol 1997; 107:30-35.

42. Lee KR, Genest DR, Minter LJ, et al. Adenocarcinoma in situ in cervical smears with a small cell (endometrioid) pattern: distinction from cells directly sampled from the upper endocervical canal or lower segment of the endometrium. Am J Clin Pathol 1998; 109:738-742.

43. Lee KR. Adenocarcinoma in situ with a small cell (endometrioid) pattern in cervical smears: a test of the distinction from benign mimics using specific criteria. Cancer (Cancer Cytopathol) 1999; 87:254-258.

44. Jaworski RC. Endocervical glandular dysplasia, adenocarcinoma in situ, and early invasive (microinvasive) adenocarcinoma of the uterine cervix. Semin Diagn Pathol 1990; 7:190-204.

45. Ayer B, Pacey F, Greenberg M. The cytologic diagnosis of adenocarcinoma in situ of the cervix uteri and related lesions II: microinvasive adenocarcinoma. Acta Cytol 1988; 32(3):318-324.

46. De Peralta-Venturino MN, Perslow MJ, et al. Endometrial cells of the "lower uterine segment" (LUS) in cervical smears obtained by endocervical brushings: a source of potential diagnostic pitfall. Diagn Cytopathol 1995; 12:263-271.

47. Chang A, Sandweiss L, Bose S. Cytologically benign endometrial cells in the Papanicolaou smears of postmenopausal women. Gyncol Oncol 2001; 80:37-43.

48. Nguyen TN, Bourdeau J-L, Ferenczy A, et al. Clinical significance of histiocytes in the detection of endometrial adenocarcinoma and hyperplasia. Diagn Cytopathol 1998; 19:89-93.

49. Chhieng DC, Elgert P, Cohen JM, et al. Clinical implications of atypical glandular cells of undetermined significance, favor endometrial origin. Cancer Cytopathol 2001; 93:351-356.

50. Koonings PP, Price JH. Evaluation of atypical glandular cells of undetermined significance: is age important? Am J Obstet Gynecol 2001; 184:1457-1461.

51. Raab SS. Can glandular lesions be diagnosed in Pap smear cytology? Diagn Cytol 2000; 23(92):127-133.

52. Boon ME, Guilloud JCD, Kok LT, et al. Efficacy of screening for cervical squamous and adenocarcinoma: the Dutch experience. Cancer 1987; 59:862-866.

53. Mitchell H, Giles G, Medley G. Accuracy and survival benefit of cytological prediction of endometrial carcinoma on routine cervical smears. Int J Gynecol Pathol 1993; 12:34-40.

54. Salamao DR, Raab SS. Atypical glandular cells of undetermined significance, favor endometrial origin: diagnostic criteria to separate benign from malignant lesions. Acta Cytol 1998; 42:1212.

55. Larson DM, Johnson KK, Reyes CN, et al. Prognostic significance of malignant cervical cytology in patients with endometrial cancer. Obstet Gynecol 1994; 84:399-403.

56. Demirkiran F, Arvas M, Erkun E, et al. The prognostic significance of cervico-vaginal cytology in endometrial cancer. Eur J Gynaecol Oncol 1995; 6:403-409.

57. Schneider ML, Wortmann M, Wegel A. Influence of histologic and cytologic grade and the clinical and postsurgical stage on the rate of endometrial adenocarcinoma detection by cervical cytology. Acta Cytol 1986; 30:616-622.

58. Lee KR, Darragh TM, Joste NE, et al. Atypical glandular cells of undetermined significance (AGUS): interobserver reproducibility in cervical smears and corresponding thin-layer preparations. Am J Clin Path 2002; 117:96-102.

59. Roberts JM, Thurloe JK, Bowditch RC, et al. Comparison of ThinPrep and Pap smears in relation to prediction of adenocarcinoma in situ. Acta Cytol 1999; 43:74-80.

60. Ashfaq R, Gibbons D, Vela C, et al. ThinPrep Pap test: accuracy for glandular disease. Acta Cytol 1999; 43:81-85.

61. Eltabbakh GH, Lipman JN, Mount SL, et al. Significance of atypical glandular cells of undetermined significance on ThinPrep Papanicolaou smears. Gynecol Oncol 2000; 78:245-250.

62. Atypical Squamous Cells of Undetermined Significance/Low-Grade Squamous Intraepithelial Lesions Triage Study Group (ALTS). Human papillomavirus testing triage of women with cytologic evidence of low-grade squamous intraepithelial lesions: baseline data from a randomized trial. J Natl Cancer Inst 2000; 92:397-402.

63. Manos MM, Kinney WK, Hurley LB, et al. Identifying women with cervical neoplasia: using human papillomavirus testing for equivocal Papanicolaou results. JAMA 1999; 281:1605-1610.

64. American College of Obstetricians and Gynecologists. Cervical cytology: evaluation and management of abnormalities. ACOG Techn Bull 183. Washington, DC: American College of Obstetricians and Gynecologists; 1993.

65. Cox JT. ASCCP Practice guideline: management of glandular abnormalities in the cervical smear. J Lower Genital Tract Dis 1997; 1:41-46.

66. Partridge E. NCCN practice guidelines for cervical screening. Oncology 1999; 13:550-574.

67. Chin AB, Bristow RE, Korst LM, et al. The significance of atypical glandular cells on routine cervical cytologic testing in a community-based population. Am J Obstet Gynecol 2000; 182:1278-1282.

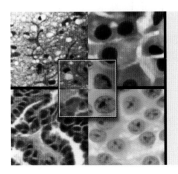

Invasive Glandular Malignancies of the Gynecologic Tract

This chapter focuses on the invasive glandular malignancies that may be seen in cervicovaginal preparations. The Bethesda System recommends that these malignancies be classified as *endocervical adenocarcinoma, endometrial adenocarcinoma,* and *extrauterine adenocarcinoma* (Box 9-1).[1] The pre-neoplastic and benign mimics of these entities are presented, with additional discussion of these nonmalignant entities in Chapters 3, 4, and 6.

 ## ENDOMETRIAL ADENOCARCINOMA

History

In the United States, endometrial carcinoma is the most common gynecologic malignancy, with 36,100 newly diagnosed cases and 6,500 cancer related deaths in 2000.[2] Approximately 80% of all endometrial malignancies are adenocarcinomas; the cytologic detection of other endometrial carcinomas and sarcomas is discussed in Chapter 10. The majority (74%) of endometrial adenocarcinomas are confined to the uterine corpus and consequently may be cured with excision.[3] Endometrial carcinoma is still the seventh leading cancer-related cause of death in women.[2] Approximately 75% of cases occur in postmenopausal women[4] (generally in women in their sixth or seventh decades of life), although 25% occur in women less than 50 years of age[3] and 5% occur in women less than 40 years of age. Symptoms of endometrial carcinoma include abnormal vaginal discharge (90%), abnormal bleeding (80%), and leukorrhea (10%).[3]

The pathogenesis of adenocarcinoma is thought to occur along two independent pathways, and Kurman and colleagues refer to these types as *types I* and *II* (Table 9-1).[1] Apparently, the majority of adenocarcinomas (type I) develop as a result of unopposed estrogen stimulation with various levels of hyperplasia serving as intermediate morphologic stages.[5,6] The women who develop these adenocarcinomas tend to be younger than women with type II adenocarcinomas, and their adenocarcinomas tend to be low grade.[7,8] The second group of adenocarcinomas (type II) develop de novo, without unopposed estrogen stimulation[9,10] Well-studied risk factors for the development of adenocarcinoma are shown in Box 9-2. Other putative risk factors include gonadal dysgenesis,[11] tamoxifen exposure,[12] and pelvic radiation.[13]

Different histologic classifications of hyperplasia have been proposed.[4] One of the more widely adopted classification systems is the system of Kurman and Norris.[14] In this system, hyperplasias are classified according to glandular architecture (i.e., simple or complex) and cytologic atypia (i.e., not atypical or atypical).[14] Tavassoli and Kraus reported that patients who had atypical hyperplasia had the highest risk (in the range of 25%) of developing adenocarcinoma.[15] Patients with endometrial hyperplasia without atypia were at a lower risk (1.6%).[14] Thus, atypical hyperplasia is a definite precursor of endometrial adenocarcinoma (type I), whereas hyperplasia without atypia may not be.

The prognosis of women with endometrial adenocarcinoma depends on the tumor stage (Table 9-2),[16] histologic and nuclear tumor grade, and depth of myometrial tumor invasion. After staging, 74% of patients are stage I, 13% are stage II, 9% are stage III, and 3% are stage IV.[3] Five-year survival by stage is as follows: stage I, 89%; stage II, 80%; stage III, 30%; and stage IV, 9%.[3] Tumor grading is based on the International Federation of Gynecology and Obstetrics (FIGO) system, which takes into account the growth pattern (i.e., amount of glandular versus solid growth) and nuclear atypia.[17] Approximately 50% of adenocarcinomas are grade I, 35% are grade II, and 15% are grade III.[4]

The most common histologic type of uterine adenocarcinoma morphologically recapitulates normal endometrium and hence is classified as the endometrioid type. Variants of the endometrioid type include adenoacanthoma, adenosquamous carcinoma, secretory carcinoma, villoglandular carcinoma, and ciliated carcinoma.[18] Nonendometrioid types include mucinous adenocarcinoma, serous adenocarcinoma, and clear cell carcinoma.[18] Kurman and colleagues have argued that clear cell carcinoma is not a distinct clinicopathologic entity, high-grade clear cell carcinomas are actually serous adenocarcinomas, and low-grade clear cell carcinomas are actually endometrioid adenocarcinomas.[1] This chapter treats clear cell adenocarcinoma as a distinct entity but acknowledges the overlap with other adenocarcinoma subtypes. Different endometrioid subtypes may occur together, and nonendometrioid subtypes may occur in conjunction with endometrioid subtypes. Extension of endometrial adenocarcinoma to the

BOX 9-1

Bethesda Categories of Glandular Malignancy

Endocervical adenocarcinoma
Endometrial adenocarcinoma
Extrauterine adenocarcinoma
Other

TABLE 9-1

Characteristics of Endometrial Adenocarcinoma

| Characteristic | ADENOCARCINOMA TYPE | |
	Type I	Type II
Age	Younger, pre- or peri- menopausal	Older, post- menopausal
Pre-existing hyperplasia	Yes	No
High estrogen	Yes	No
Histologic grade	Low	High
Myometrial invasion	Minimal	Deep

From Kurman R, Zaino R, Norris H. Endometrial carcinoma. In: Kurman RJ, editor. Blaustein's pathology of the female genital tract. New York: Springer-Verlag; 1994. p.441.

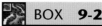 **BOX 9-2**

Risk Factors for Endometrial Adenocarcinoma

Obesity
Diabetes
Hypertension
Longstanding unopposed estrogen use
Functioning granulosa cell tumors or thecomas
Infertility
Dysfunctional bleeding
Failure of ovulation (e.g., Stein-Leventhal syndrome)
Atypical endometrial hyperplasia
Low parity

From Kurman R, Zaino R, Norris H. Endometrial carcinoma. In: Kurman RJ, editor. Blaustein's pathology of the female genital tract. New York: Springer-Verlag; 1994. p.440.

TABLE 9-2

Endometrial Carcinoma Staging

Stage	Description
IA	Confined to corpus and limited to the endometrium
IB	Confined to the corpus with invasion to less than one half the myometrium
IC	Confined to the corpus with invasion to more than one half the myometrium
IIA	Involves corpus and shows endocervical glandular involvement only
IIB	Involves corpus and shows cervical stromal invasion
IIIA	Extends outside the uterus, but not outside the pelvis; tumor invades the serosa, adnexa, and/or positive peritoneal cytology
IIIB	Extends outside the uterus but not outside the pelvis; vaginal involvement
IIIC	Extends outside the uterus but not outside the pelvis; metastases to pelvic and/or paraaortic lymph nodes
IVA	Tumor invasion of bladder and/or bowel mucosa
IVB	Distant metastases including intra-abdominal and/or inguinal lymph nodes

cervix occurs in more than 10% of cases with consequent upstaging.[19]

Sensitivity of Detection

Although the conventional Pap smear may be used to detect endometrial carcinoma, this specimen is not useful for endometrial cancer screening.[20] Kurman and colleagues wrote that cytological screening for endometrial carcinoma was not cost-effective, even though cost data supporting this conclusion are unsubstantiated.[1] The low opinion of conventional smears for endometrial cancer screening largely reflects its reported relatively low sensitivity for the detection of endometrial cancer.

Endometrial cancer detection depends on patient, sampling, interpretive, and screening factors. Detection correlates with shedding of neoplastic cells from the primary location into the cervix and vagina and not all adenocarcinomas readily shed tumor cells. Some authors have reported very low sensitivity rates; for example, Mitchell and colleagues reported that among women with endometrial carcinoma, a cervical smear performed in the 2 years preceding the diagnosis predicted the presence of disease in only 28% of the cases.[21] Burk and colleagues reported that the positive rate for endometrial cancer detection on cervical smears was 18%[20]; other authors have reported similar findings.[22-27]

However, higher sensitivities of adenocarcinoma detection have been presented by other authors. Schneider and colleagues reported a false-negative rate of 40%, which related largely to low-grade carcinomas.[28] Reagan reported that the sensitivity of endometrial adenocarcinoma detection was higher than 80% and depended on the sampling

method (i.e., cervical sampling was the least sensitive method).[29] Berg and Durfee presented similar data.[30] Koss wrote that with vaginal pool material, the positive rate ranged from 64% to 75%.[31-33] Many clinicians do not specifically sample the vaginal pool to increase diagnostic sensitivity. Koss has advocated that a vaginal smear should be part of every examination in women older than age 50 and in younger women who have signs and/or symptoms suggestive of endometrial disease.[37]

Demirkiran and colleagues reported that the overall sensitivity of the conventional smear for endometrial cancer detection was 46%; however, sensitivity depended on tumor stage and grade.[34] Of women with FIGO stage I carcinomas, 19% had positive cytology, whereas 60% of women with stage II carcinomas had positive cytology.[34] Fukuda and colleagues reported that malignant and suspicious cervical smears statistically correlated with grade, stage, depth of myometrial involvement, and metastases.[35] Tumor detection also depends on the portion of the endometrial cavity involved by neoplasm and whether the cervix is involved.[36]

Sensitivity of cancer detection also depends on what counts for a positive cytologic diagnosis. If nondefinitive diagnoses such as atypical glandular cells (AGC) or endometrial cells in a postmenopausal woman are considered to indicate disease, then the sensitivity is higher.

In summary, although a meta-analysis of endometrial cancer cytology detection studies has not been performed, the sensitivity of detection on cervical smears is probably in the range of 25% to 60%, with most papers reporting a sensitivity higher than 50%. The lower-grade tumors shed no or few cells and because most endometrioid adenocarcinomas are low grade, many of these adenocarcinomas go undetected. For comparison, Fahey and colleagues reported that the sensitivity of the detection of pre-neoplastic squamous lesions of the cervix ranged from 11% to 99%, with studies demonstrating a sensitivity of approximately 50%.[38] Thus, the sensitivity of endometrial cancer detection on cervical smears may not be much different than the sensitivity of squamous dysplasia detection. However, because of the different biologic potentials of cervical dysplasia and endometrial carcinoma, missing endometrial lesions is of greater immediate clinical significance, and therefore screening with conventional cytology cannot be relied on as the sole means for endometrial carcinoma detection. Fortunately, clinical signs and symptoms, as mentioned earlier, are the main clinical guide for endometrial cancer detection. Detecting endometrial carcinoma through conventional cytology is an added, albeit small, bonus.

The sensitivity of endometrial hyperplasia detection on cervicovaginal samples is low. The conventional opinion is that endometrial hyperplasia cannot be definitively diagnosed, and that, at most, endometrial hyperplasia may be diagnosed as *atypical glandular cells (AGC), favor endometrial origin*. Ng reported that endometrial cells are seen in vaginal smears in 5% of cases of hyperplasia.[39] These endometrial cells generally have a completely benign appearance. In endocervical samples, benign endometrial cells are seen in 25% of patients who have hyperplasia and atypia and 10% of patients who have hyperplasia and no atypia.[39]

Similar to conventional smears, liquid-based Pap tests do not directly sample the endometrial vault. Thus, these preparations also are probably not suitable for endometrial cancer screening, although this statement has not been proven. However, also like conventional smears, liquid-based preparations have been shown to detect endometrial disease.[40]

In contrast to their low sensitivity, Pap tests are believed to be highly specific in that they generally do not falsely diagnose endometrial adenocarcinoma. Although the specificity is well over 99.99%,[41,42] false-positive diagnoses do occur. For example, Mitchell and colleagues reported that 25% of women with cytologic diagnoses of adenocarcinoma did not have malignancy on histologic follow-up.[21] Gray and Nguyen reported that one in six women with a diagnosis of malignant endometrial cells had a benign diagnosis on follow-up.[41]

Direct sampling of the endometrial vault increases the sensitivity of adenocarcinoma detection. Although a num-

TABLE 9-3

Endometrial Sampling Methods

Method	Reference*
Endometrial aspiration cannula	Jordan and colleagues (1956)[a]
Endometrial brush	Johnsson and Stormby (1968)[b]
Endometrial jet irrigation	50
Endometrial sponge biopsy	Chatfield and Bremner (1972)[c]
Isaacs' endometrial sampler	51
Endometrial aspiration pistol	Vassilakos and colleagues (1975)[d]
Medhosa cannula	Jimenez-Ayala and colleagues (1975)[e]
Endometrial Mi-Mark cannula	45
Endometrial masubuchi aspirator	52
Endocyte sampler	48
Endometrial Pistolet sampler	44
Endo-pap sampler	47
Endosearch sampler	46
Uterobrush	53
Abradul endometrial cell sampler	55
Endometrial brush biopsy (MedScand Cytobrush)	Maksem and Knesel (1996)[f]

*For numbers, refer to reference list.
[a]Jordan MJ, Bader GM, Namgzie AS. Comparative accuracy of preoperative cytologic and histologic diagnosis in endometrial lesions. Obstet Gynecol 1956; 7:646-653.
[b]Johnsson JE, Stormby NG. Cytological brush technique in malignant disease of the endometrium. Acta Obstet Gynecol Scand 1968; 47:38-51.
[c]Chatfield WR, Bremner AD. Intrauterine sponge biopsy: a new technique to screen for early intrauterine malignancy. Obstet Gynecol 1972; 39:323-328.
[d]Vassilakos P, Wyss R, Wenger D, et al. Endometrial cytohistology by aspiration technique and by Gravlee Jet Washer: a comparative study. Obstet Gynecol 1975; 45:320-324.
[e]Jimenez-Ayala M, Vilaplana E, Becerro de Bengoa C, et al. Endometrial and endocervical brushing techniques with a Medhosa cannula. Acta Cytol 1975; 19:557-563.
[f]Maksem JA, Knesel E. Liquid fixation of endometrial brush cytology ensures a well-preserved, representative cell sample with frequent tissue correlation. Diagn Cytopathol 1996; 14:367-373.

ber of sampling methods (e.g., endometrial aspiration, jet wash, endometrial lavage, endometrial brushing, suction curettage, tampon smear, and brushing with confocal microscopy) have been introduced over the years (Table 9-3). many of these methods no longer are in use.[43-55]

The sensitivity for endometrial adenocarcinoma detection using direct endometrial sampling in part depends on whether tissue fragments are obtained. In some centers, tissue fragments are processed as cell blocks and treated as histologic specimens.[37] If tissue fragments are not present, the sensitivity for a cancer diagnosis is approximately 90%, and the sensitivity for a hyperplasia diagnosis is 50%.[29,56,57] Some investigators have decried that these high sensitivities are only obtained with considerable experience, which presumably most centers lack.[37] Nonetheless, recently published papers investigating direct endometrial sampling, such as using the Tao brush, have shown considerable success. For example, Smith and colleagues reported that the sensitivity of detecting hyperplasia/carcinoma using the Tao brush was 57%; all the false-negative cases were focal hyperplasias, and adenocarcinomas were not missed.[58] Wu and colleagues reported that the sensitivity and specificity for hyperplasia and adenocarcinoma detection were 100%, although the sample size of patients with hyperplasia or adenocarcinoma was small.[59]

If tissue fragments are present, the sensitivity for adenocarcinoma detection is greater than 95% and the sensitivity for hyperplasia detection is greater than 90%.[29,57]

Currently, none of these methods have been widely adopted, and therefore the use of these methods for endometrial cancer screening is largely unknown.[60] These methods probably are useful for screening for cancer, but not for precursor lesions.[61] Paradoxically, using direct endometrial sampling for screening, Sato and colleagues reported that fewer high-risk women were detected to have endometrial cancer than a control group of women[62]; this may indicate that the currently accepted risk factors for endometrial cancer need to be reexamined. The acceptance of these cytologic sampling techniques by clinicians and patients depends on the acceptability and replacement/ conjunctive use of these techniques with currently used histologic methods; this largely lies outside the scope of cytology laboratories.

Cytologic Features of Endometrioid Type Neoplasia (Hyperplasia and Endometrioid Adenocarcinoma)

In indirect endometrial samples (cervical and vaginal), for the most part the neoplastic cells are shed spontaneously, whereas in direct samples (endometrial) the endometrial cells are abraded. Sampling and shedding lead to different morphologic patterns. For this reason, the cytologic findings in these two specimen types are presented separately. The Bethesda Committee provided a cytologic description of adenocarcinomas on indirect samples; direct samples were not discussed.

Cervical and Vaginal (Indirect) Sampling

The differences between the cytologic literature (particularly in the 1970s and early 1980s) and the Bethesda Committee descriptions of endometrial disease are telling. Some cytology textbooks and much of the literature are replete with cytologic descriptions of endometrial hyperplasia and adenocarcinoma. From these studies, one could conclude that the diagnosis of hyperplasias and adenocarcinomas, if not straightforward, is at least possible. However, other authors have treated the concept of actually making these diagnoses with disdain.[37] The Bethesda Committee seems to have adopted this latter viewpoint.[1]

As outlined previously, endometrial neoplasia and preneoplasia may be classified histologically into the categories of hyperplasia without atypia, atypical hyperplasia, and adenocarcinoma. In the Bethesda System, the categories of endometrial cell abnormalities are as follows: (1) endometrial cells in a postmenopausal women; (2) *AGC, endometrial origin*; and (3) endometrial adenocarcinoma.[1] Clearly, a one-to-one correlation between these histologic and cytologic categories does not exist, although both systems describe a spectrum of change from atypical to carcinoma. The lack of correlation is most evident when the histologic category of atypical hyperplasia is compared with the cytologic category of *AGC, endometrial origin*.[63] The *AGC, endometrial origin* category is viewed as a risk diagnosis for adenocarcinoma rather than a cytologic description of atypical endometrial hyperplasia. In fact, the majority of women who have *AGC, endometrial origin* do not have an atypical endometrial hyperplasia.[64,65]

A summary of the early cytologic endometrial neoplasia literature follows with the authors' comments regarding how the early cytologic classification systems mesh with the Bethesda System categories for endometrial cell abnormalities.[66] The authors believe that the majority of hyperplasias and some endometrial adenocarcinomas cannot be diagnosed definitively using indirect cytologic sampling methods. Thus, these authors concur with the Bethesda Committee's general approach to the diagnoses of endometrial neoplasia.[66] However, the framework provided by the early cytologic descriptions are key to understanding the cytologic manifestations of endometrial malignancy. As many authors agree, the cytologic features of the endometrial cells in benign conditions, atypical hyperplasia, and well-differentiated adenocarcinoma exhibit considerable overlap.[67]

One last point regarding indirect endocervical sampling should be made. Authors such as Koss have argued that the cytologic findings in vaginal, cervical, and endocervical smears may be quite different.[37] Vaginal and cervical smears tend to show few endometrial cells (the fewest cells are seen in cervical smears), and cells in both these smear types are degenerated (the cells are more degenerated in vaginal smears).[37] Endocervical samples show the greatest number of nondegenerated endometrial cells.

Hyperplasia without atypia. Based on retrospective review, Ng and colleagues reported that hyperplasia without atypia was characterized by the observation of only five[1] endometrial cell groups, on the average, per smear (Table 9-4).[67] The endometrial cell nuclei were slightly enlarged compared with the normal group, and the cytoplasm generally lacked vacuoles and was scant.[67-72] Skaarland, however, reported that nuclear size alone could not be used to separate hyperplasia without atypia from malignancy.[73] Ishii and Fujii reported that all hyperplasias and adenocarcinomas had papillary clusters, although the clusters became more complex as lesions progressed from hyperplasia without atypia to hyperplasia with atypia to adenocarcinoma.[74] In hyperplasia without atypia, the nuclear chromatin was finely granular and not irregularly distributed (Figure 9-1).[67] Koss wrote that the only difference between benign endometrial cells and endometrial cells in hyperplasia without atypia was a slight increase in nuclear hyperchromasia and nucleolar prominence.[37] For most practicing cytologists, these changes are so subtle that distinction from normal endometrial cells is virtually impossible. Thus, these cell groups probably are flagged as *normal in appearance* in postmenopausal women or in cycling women if the endometrial cells occur after day 12. Only in unusual circumstances would a diagnosis of *AGC, endometrial cell origin* be made.

Hyperplasia with atypia. Ng and colleagues reported that in atypical hyperplasia, more endometrial cell clusters (average of 12) were present.[67] The endometrial cell nuclei were enlarged and, in most cases, exceeded the size range of normal endometrial cell nuclei (40 μm^2) (see Table 9-4).[67-70]

Similar to the glandular cell nuclei in hyperplasia without atypia, nuclei were round with finely granular chromatin.[70] The cells remained in tight clusters, and the cytoplasm was mostly basophilic.[67] Kashimura and colleagues reported that anisokaryosis, internuclear distance, and stratification of nuclei were features helpful in separating hyperplasia with atypia from hyperplasia without atypia (Figure 9-2).[75] Endometrial stromal cells were seen in slightly more than 25% of cases.[67] A tumor diathesis always was absent.[67] In some cases of atypical hyperplasia, one may be able to recognize the subtle increase in nuclear size and render an atypical *(AGC, endometrial origin)* diagnosis. In other cases, the nuclear size may be worrisome enough for a diagnosis of endometrial adenocarcinoma to be made.

Endometrioid type adenocarcinoma. The Bethesda System criteria for endometrioid type adenocarcinoma are shown in Box 9-3.[66] The cytologic features depend on the degree of differentiation, and the more poorly differentiated endometrioid adenocarcinomas may have few recognizable endometrial cell features. In general, compared with endometrial hyperplasias, endometrial adenocarcinomas shed more cells that are larger in size and contain a larger nucleus (Figure 9-3). The malignant cells are usually present in small clusters, although cellular dissociation may be evident, in contrast with the hyperplasias where the observation of single endometrial cells is highly unusual. The number of cells is variable, and Ng and colleagues reported that a mean of 18 cell groups per smear was seen in grade I adenocarcinomas. The number of shed malignant cells depends on several factors, including the surface area of the endometrium involved by tumor and the degree of differentiation.[76] Many clinicians do not specifically sample the vaginal pool to increase diagnostic sensitivity. Koss has advocated that a vaginal smear should be part of every examination in women older than age 50 and in younger women who have signs and/or symptoms suggestive of endometrial disease.[37] Smears from women who have high-stage (but still low-grade) adenocarcinomas with spread to the cervix may show more numerous cell clusters; these malignant cell groups may be arranged in sheets or even rosettes (a more common feature in endocervical adenocarcinomas).[77] Cellular degeneration may be a prominent finding, limiting

TABLE 9-4   CMF

Comparison of Cytomorphologic Features of Endometrial Neoplasia

Criterion	Hyperplasia	Atypical Hyperplasia	Adenocarcinoma, Well-Differentiated
Number of cells	Few	Moderate	Many
Nuclear size (um²)	42-49	53	57-60
Irregular chromatin	(+)	(+)	(+++)
Nuclear hyperchromasia	(++)	(++)	(+++)
Micronucleoli	(+/−)	(+)	(+++)
Multiple nucleoli	(−)	(−)	(+)
Uniform chromatin	(+++)	(++)	(+)
Diathesis	(−)	(−)	(+++)

From Ng ABP, Reagan JW, Cechner RL. The precursors of endometrial cancer: a study of their cellular manifestations. Acta Cytol 1973; 17:439-448.

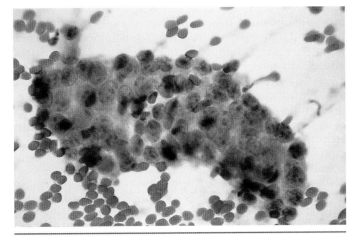

Figure 9-1 **Endometrial hyperplasia without atypia in a cervical specimen.** A pseudopapillary cluster containing cells with slight nuclear hyperchromasia is present. The cells exhibit slight nuclear overlapping. (Papanicolaou [Pap])

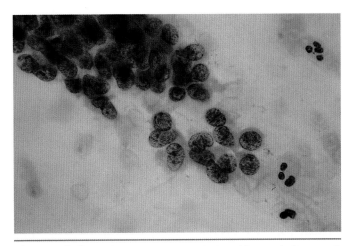

Figure 9-2 **Endometrial hyperplasia with atypia in a vaginal specimen.** The nuclei exhibit piling and anisonucleosis. Cellular dissociation is not evident. Nuclear membrane irregularities are present. (Pap)

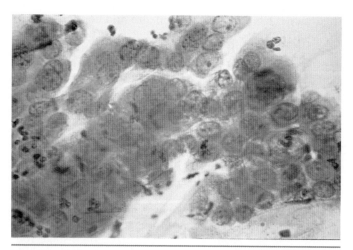

Figure 9-3 Endometrioid type adenocarcinoma, well-differentiated, in a vaginal specimen. Large clusters with slight cellular dissociation are observed. Nucleoli are seen and the cells exhibit increased nuclear to cytoplasmic (N:C) ratios. (Pap)

BOX **9-3** CMF

Bethesda System Cytomorphologic Features of Endometrial Adenocarcinoma

1. Cells typically occur singly or in small, loose clusters
2. In well-differentiated tumors, nuclei may be increased only slightly in size and become larger with the increasing grade of tumor
3. Variation in nuclear size and loss of nuclear polarity are evident
4. Particularly in higher-grade tumors, nuclei display moderate hyperchromasia, irregular chromatin distribution, and parachromatin clearing
5. Small to prominent nucleoli are present; nucleoli become larger with the increasing grade of tumor
6. Cytoplasm is scant, cyanophilic, and often vacuolated
7. A watery, finely granular tumor diathesis is variably present

definitive classification.[78] Degenerated single malignant cells often are inconspicuous and small (Figure 9-4), measuring about the size of parabasal cells (i.e., 10 μm^2 to 20 μm^2 in diameter)[37] and thus are easily overlooked. Larger cell clusters (predominantly three-dimensional) may have a papillary appearance with the groups containing more than 20 cells, although most cell groups contain fewer than 12 cells.[77]

Psammoma bodies may accompany the neoplastic endometrial cell clusters (Figure 9-5), although psammoma bodies may be seen in other malignancies and benign conditions.[78-92] Ng and colleagues reported that psammoma bodies were seen in one of every 125 cases of endometrial adenocarcinoma.[78] Kern reported that benign psammoma bodies were seen in approximately one of every 78,000 cervicovaginal smears, although the presence of a psammoma body usually bespoke a malignant process.[92]

Because many endometrial adenocarcinomas occur in an older patient population, the smear background is often at least partially atrophic. Older women with endometrial adenocarcinoma secondary to unopposed estrogen however may show increased squamous maturation.[93] Stoll reported that 35% of postmenopausal women show full squamous maturation.[94] Berg and Durfee reported that postmenopausal women who have increased squamous maturation have a 15 times greater probability of having an endometrial cancer than women who have an atrophic smear pattern.[30] Thus, some authors have recommended that postmenopausal women who have increased squamous maturation need to undergo a thorough clinical examination to rule out endometrial carcinoma.[95] Koss recommended that cytopathologists also need to search for endometrial adenocarcinoma in postmenopausal women with abnormal bleeding or with a vaginal smear with benign-appearing endometrial cells and/or necrosis.[37] Gronroos and colleagues reported that obese and/or diabetic postmenopausal women who had cytolytic or karyopyknotic smears had higher than normal levels of serum estrogen and were at increased risk for endometrial adenocarcinoma.[96]

In vaginal smears, the malignant cells of endometrial adenocarcinoma, even the well-differentiated ones, often are accompanied with blood, debris, neutrophils, and macrophages.[37]

The cytoplasm of FIGO grade I endometrioid adenocarcinomas often is scant and may be vacuolated (Figure 9-6), with some cells containing degenerated debris or neutrophils.[30] Engulfed neutrophils are not pathognomonic because engulfed neutrophils may be seen within reactive endocervical cell (mucus-containing) cytoplasm. In low-grade endometrial adenocarcinomas, the malignant cells may be seen singly and in loose clusters (Figure 9-7) and not in tight aggregates.[97] Single cancer cells are oval to spherical and only slightly enlarged.[97] The single cells often are degenerated with poorly defined membranes and easily confused with histiocytes or neutrophils.[98] The cytoplasm stains basophilic to gray. The nucleus of a well-preserved FIGO grade I endometrioid adenocarcinoma is not quite twice the size of an intermediate squamous cell nucleus (60 μm^2 compared with 35 μm^2).[57]

The malignant cells may be columnar, round, or oval in shape. Ng reported that well-differentiated endometrioid adenocarcinomas have more palely staining chromatin compared with either benign endometrial cells or hyperplastic endometrial cells.[67] However, the chromatin pattern in well-differentiated endometrioid adenocarcinomas is more irregularly clumped than the chromatin pattern in nonmalignant conditions. The number and size of nucleoli correlate with the degree of tumor differentiation; a single, small nucleolus typically is seen in well-differentiated endometrioid adenocarcinomas (Figure 9-8).[99] The diagnosis of endometrial adenocarcinoma should be rendered with caution if a nucleolus is not observed. A watery tumor diathesis may accompany smears of well-differentiated endometrial adenocarcinoma (Figure 9-9), even if the neoplastic cell clusters are few in number.[98] It is basophilic and finely granular (not necrotic) and corresponds to the watery vaginal discharge seen clinically. The granular material consists of necrotic fragments of nuclear material.[98,100]

A valid question is whether pathologists are able cytologically to diagnose well-differentiated endometrioid adenocarcinoma (and separate this malignancy from other lesions such as atypical hyperplasia). Little has been pub-

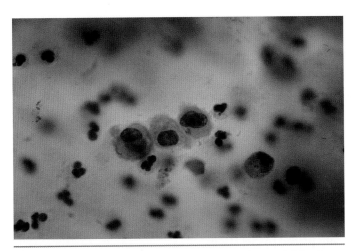

Figure 9-4 **Degenerated cells of an endometrioid adeno-carcinoma in a vaginal specimen.** The malignant cells are about the size of parabasal cells and show hyperchromatic nuclei. Numerous inflammatory cells are present. (Pap)

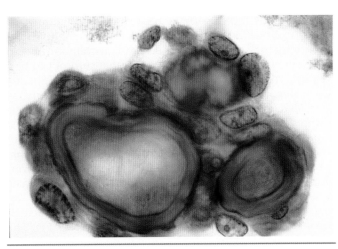

Figure 9-5 **Psammoma bodies accompanying an en-dometrioid adenocarcinoma in a vaginal specimen.** The malig-nant cells contain prominent nucleoli and coarse chromatin. (Pap)

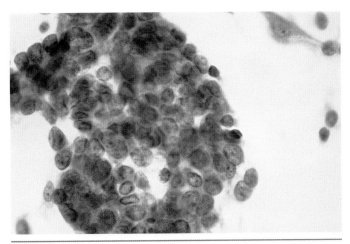

Figure 9-6 **Well-differentiated endometrioid adenocarci-noma in a cervical specimen.** The neoplastic cells show nuclear overlapping and small nucleoli. Variation in nuclear size and slight cellular dissociation are seen. (Pap)

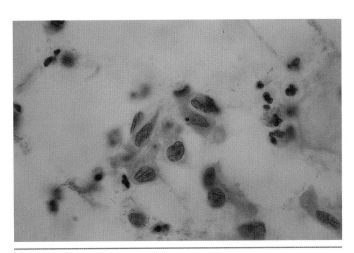

Figure 9-7 **Well-differentiated endometrioid adenocarci-noma in a vaginal specimen.** The malignant cells show wispy cy-toplasm, oval nuclei, and nuclear grooves. (Pap)

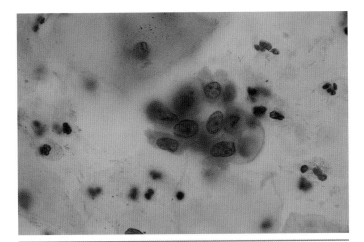

Figure 9-8 **Well-differentiated endometrioid adenocarci-noma in a cervical specimen.** The neoplastic nuclei contain a sin-gle, small nucleolus. The cytoplasm is moderate in amount and has a basophilic appearance. (Pap)

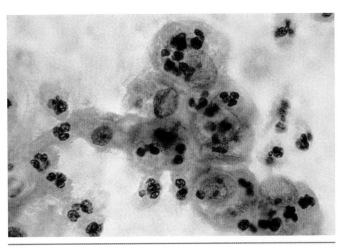

Figure 9-9 **Watery tumor diathesis accompanying a well-differentiated endometrioid adenocarcinoma in a vaginal specimen.** The diathesis is basophilic and finely granular; large necrotic chunks are absent. Several of the malignant cells have en-gulfed neutrophils. (Pap)

lished on this topic, perhaps because seeing endometrial cells suspicious for adenocarcinoma or even definitive cells of endometrial adenocarcinoma is an uncommon event. Some cytologists tend to classify cases that turn out to be a well-differentiated endometrial adenocarcinoma in the AGC category. Others use the adenocarcinoma category.

In FIGO grade II and III adenocarcinomas, the cytologic features of malignancy are more easily recognized. Most importantly, the nuclear area increases as the grade increases, and the nuclei show more hyperchromasia (Figure 9-10). However, compared with the hyperchromasia in cervical squamous malignancies, the nuclear hyperchromasia is less in high-grade endometrial adenocarcinomas. In high-grade endometrioid adenocarcinomas, the nucleoli become more prominent and numerous (Figure 9-11). The interchromatic regions also become more prominent as the carcinoma becomes more poorly differentiated.[97] The cells in high-grade adenocarcinomas are larger than in low-grade adenocarcinomas.[101] In grade II and III endometrioid adenocarcinomas the cells may form tight three-dimensional balls, compared with the loose clusters seen in grade I endometrioid adenocarcinomas.[97] Cytoplasmic vacuoles may indent the nucleus, creating a signet ring cell appearance (Figure 9-12). Necrotic, instead of watery, tumor diathesis may accompany high-grade endometrioid adenocarcinomas. In some high-grade adenocarcinomas, large sheets of malignant cells may be shed (Figure 9-13). These cell groups may mimic a squamous cell carcinoma in situ, although adenocarcinoma cells have less dense cytoplasm, less coarse chromatin, and more prominent nucleoli.

In vaginal smears (but generally not in cervical smears), histiocytes and stromal endometrial cells may accompany cells of endometrioid adenocarcinoma. The histiocytes have finely vacuolated cytoplasm and elongated, eccentrically placed nuclei (Figure 9-14). The presence of these cells in a postmenopausal woman requires careful examination to rule out an endometrioid adenocarcinoma.

As the cells of an endometrial carcinoma may be shed infrequently, a suspicious (e.g., AGC) or malignant diagnosis

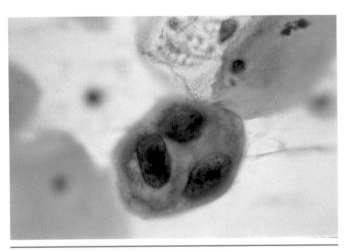

Figure 9-10 Moderately differentiated endometrioid adenocarcinoma in an endocervical specimen. The nuclei are hyperchromatic and large, and nucleoli are seen. The cytoplasm is vacuolated and basophilic. (Pap)

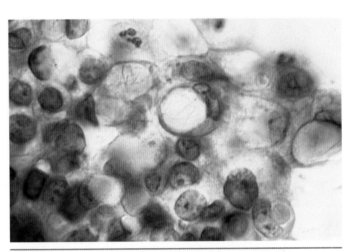

Figure 9-12 Slightly degenerated poorly differentiated endometrioid adenocarcinoma in a vaginal specimen. Numerous cytoplasmic vacuoles give some of the cells a signet ring appearance. The nuclei vary considerably in size. (Pap)

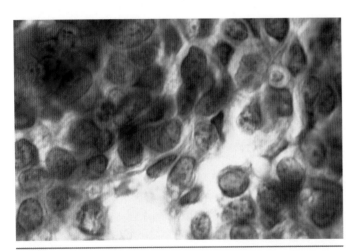

Figure 9-11 Poorly differentiated endometrioid adenocarcinoma in a cervical specimen. Prominent and multiple nucleoli are seen. The chromatin pattern is relatively open, and nuclear membrane irregularities are pronounced. (Pap)

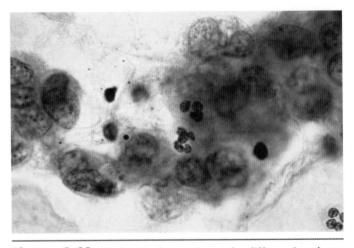

Figure 9-13 A large sheet of poorly differentiated endometrioid adenocarcinoma in a vaginal specimen. The malignant cells show extensive nuclear overlapping and slight cellular dissociation. Note the necrotic tumor diathesis in the background. (Pap)

may be followed by negative smears. Koss reported that this was more often the case if cervical instead of vaginal smears were obtained.[37] Thus, long-term follow-up and good clinical communication is mandatory if cells on a vaginal smear are worrisome for an endometrial malignancy.

Endometrial (Direct) Sampling

Direct samples of endometrial neoplasia usually are highly cellular. If gross tissue fragments are present, these may be processed as a histologic specimen.[102] Otherwise, the specimen may be smeared or concentrated on a slide.

Hyperplasia without atypia. Koss reported that the identification of endometrial hyperplasia without atypia is virtually impossible on direct endometrial samples.[37] This is particularly true for pre- and perimenopausal women, where hyperplasia without atypia may be indistinguishable from proliferative phase endometrium. In postmenopausal women, hyperplasia without atypia may be suggested, simply because proliferative phase endometrium is a less common event.[61,103] The endometrial

cells of a hyperplasia usually are present in variably sized aggregates. Unlike indirect samples, the cells of a hyperplasia may occur singly. Koss reported that in hyperplasia without atypia, slight nucleolar prominence may be seen (Figure 9-15).[104]

Hyperplasia with atypia. In atypical hyperplasia, greater nuclear and nucleolar abnormalities and large cohesive cellular sheets may be seen.[104] In tissue fragments, the glands, although crowded, lack a back-to-back architecture. Not unexpectedly, difficulties arise in separating atypical hyperplasia from well-differentiated adenocarcinoma. Meisels and Jolicoeur reported that the cytologic features most important in diagnosing hyperplasia were cellular overlapping, presence of nucleoli, anisokaryosis, chromatin granularity, and presence of stromal cells (Figure 9-16)[103]; from this study, it is unclear if atypical and nonatypical hyperplasias could be separated from each other. Coscia-Porrazzi reported that the greater the chromatin clumping and anisokaryosis (Figure 9-17), the more likely a lesion was an atypical hyperplasia.[105]

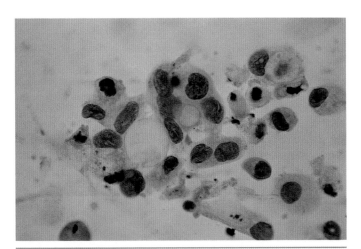

Figure 9-14 **Histiocytes in association with a moderately differentiated endometrioid adenocarcinoma in a cervical specimen.** It is difficult to determine whether some of the degenerated cells are malignant glandular cells or histiocytes. (Pap)

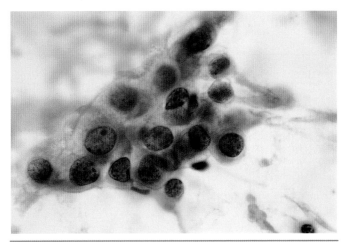

Figure 9-16 Direct sample of endometrial hyperplasia with atypia. The cells show nuclear overlapping and granular chromatin. Several of the cells show prominent nucleoli. (Pap)

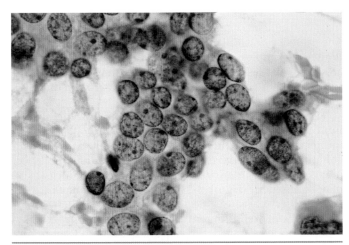

Figure 9-15 Direct sample of endometrial hyperplasia without atypia. The specimen is cellular, and large groups of cells are seen. The endometrial cell nuclei are hyperchromatic and show little variation in nuclear size. (Pap)

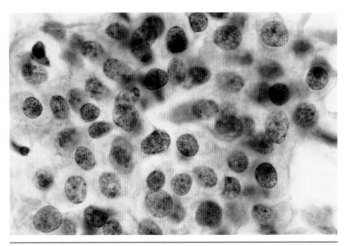

Figure 9-17 Direct sample of endometrial hyperplasia with atypia. The nuclei are hyperchromatic, and the chromatin is slightly coarse. Variation in nuclear size also is present. Single neoplastic cells are not seen. (Pap)

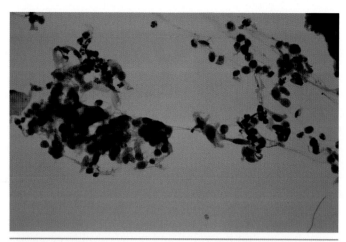

Figure 9-18   Direct sample of a well-differentiated endometrioid adenocarcinoma. This low-power view shows large, variably sized fragments of neoplastic cells. Nuclear overlapping is seen. (Pap)

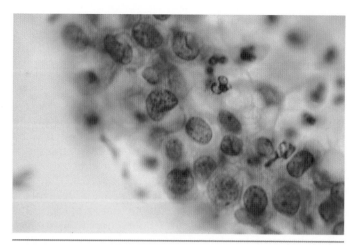

Figure 9-20   Direct sample of a moderately differentiated endometrioid adenocarcinoma. A fragment of moderately differentiated tumor with nuclear overlapping and variability in nuclear size is present. (Pap)

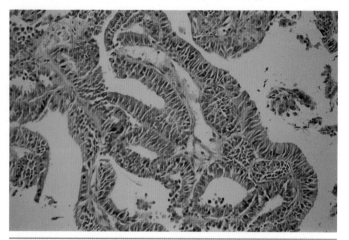

Figure 9-19   Direct sample of an endometrioid adenocarcinoma (cell block). This tumor is moderately differentiated and shows back-to-back glands and moderate variation in nuclear size. Some laboratories prefer cell block preparations over smears. (Pap)

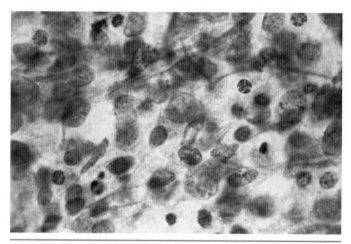

Figure 9-21   Direct sample of a poorly differentiated endometrioid adenocarcinoma. This high-power view shows cells with high N:C ratios and nuclear hyperchromasia. Nucleoli are seen, and nuclear streaking is present. (Pap)

Endometrioid adenocarcinoma. The appearance of the malignant cells of an endometrioid adenocarcinoma depends on several factors such as tumor grade and sampling. For the most part, the malignant cells are observed singly and in small or large groups (Figure 9-18). The groups tend to be larger in direct samples compared with indirect samples. Microtissue fragments may be present on cytologic smears or cell block preparations (Figure 9-19); these fragments vary in size and shape and consist of malignant cells in whole or partial glands admixed with stroma. The glands appear crowded and show lack of cellular polarity (Figure 9-20). In poorly differentiated adenocarcinomas, the neoplastic cells may form sheets without easily recognizable gland formation. Extensive cellular overlapping is common. Strips of malignant endometrial cells may be seen, although cellular strips are seen more commonly with endocervical adenocarcinomas. In well-differentiated endometrioid adenocarcinomas, fragments of hyperplastic endometrial cells may be admixed with malignant cell fragments. Foam cells

may surround malignant glands in microtissue fragments. The presence of cellular balls is not as apparent in direct endometrial samples. In addition, fewer degenerative features are seen in direct samples. In cancers that do not extensively involve the endometrial cavity, a tumor diathesis may be absent.

The single malignant cells in direct samples generally exhibit the same cytologic features as previously discussed in indirect samples. The malignant cells appear cuboidal, columnar (an unusual feature in indirect endometrial specimens), round, or oval. Variation in cellular and nuclear size may be apparent (Figure 9-21). The cytoplasm may be difficult to observe because of cellular crowding (Figure 9-22); in single cells of well-differentiated adenocarcinomas, the cytoplasm appears frayed and delicately stained. Psammoma bodies occasionally are present.

The neoplastic cell nuclei show granular chromatin, and nucleoli are seen. Similar to indirect samples, the nucleoli are larger and more numerous in the more poorly differen-

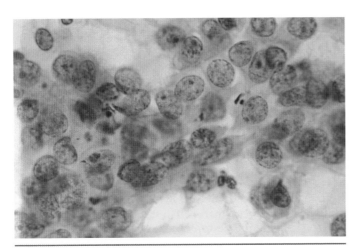

Figure 9-22 Direct sample of a poorly differentiated endometrioid adenocarcinoma. The nucleoli are enlarged and inflammatory cells are admixed with the tumor cells. Three-dimensional groups of tumor cells are present. (Pap)

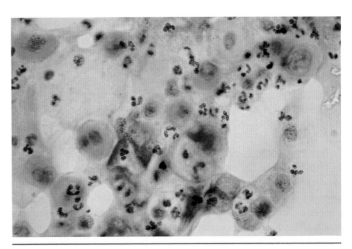

Figure 9-23 High-power view of degenerated squamous metaplastic cells and malignant glandular cells from an endometrioid adenocarcinoma in a vaginal smear. Despite the degeneration, the squamous metaplastic cells maintain their hard-appearing cytoplasm. The malignant glandular cells have foamy cytoplasm. Tumor diathesis is admixed. (Pap)

tiated adenocarcinomas. Mitotic figures usually are present; this cytologic feature is unusual in indirect samples, mainly because of limited sampling.

False-Positive and False-Negative Specimens

In indirect samples, the causes of a false-positive diagnosis (Box 9-4) of an endometrioid adenocarcinoma include benign endometrial and endocervical conditions.

False-positive diagnoses related to endometrial disease include reactive and inflammatory endometrial conditions (e.g., chronic endometritis or tuberculous endometritis) and Arias-Stella reaction.[106-109] endometrial polyps (sometimes with infarct),[41,110] radiation effect,[111] lower uterine segment cells,[112-114] endometrial hyperplasia, trophoblastic cells,[115] menstrual phase endometrium, atypical endometrium overlying stromal breakdown,[116] and uterine material shed because of intrauterine contraceptive devices.[117,118] In these conditions, the endometrial cell nuclei may appear larger and more hyperchromatic, and the nuclear membranes may be more irregular in contour. In addition, nucleolar prominence in reactive conditions may simulate the changes seen in endometrial adenocarcinoma. The benign endometrial cells in these processes usually are quite cohesive and thus single cells rarely are seen. Syncytial trophoblastic cells are multinucleated, and the nuclei lack significant atypia; in endometrial adenocarcinomas the malignant cells usually contain a single nucleus and the nuclear atypia is greater.[119]

Ng and colleagues wrote that the most common cause of a false-positive diagnosis was reactive endocervical, metaplastic, or parabasal cells.[120] In these cervical conditions, the benign cells usually maintain a low nuclear to cytoplasmic (N:C) ratio, and the cytoplasm is vacuolated. Mitoses may be more readily apparent in endocervical conditions than in endometrial adenocarcinoma, and in repair, inflammatory cells are admixed with monolayer sheets of glandular cells. In reactive glandular conditions the nuclear chromatin is pale, and a tumor diathesis is absent. Other conditions such as microglandular hyperplasia,[121] tubal metapla-

BOX 9-4

Causes of a False-Positive Diagnosis of Endometrial Adenocarcinoma

Endocervical repair
Intrauterine device
Endometrial inflammation
Radiation effect
Arias-Stella reaction
Endometrial hyperplasia
Lower uterine segment cells
Endometrial polyp
Endometriosis
Trophoblastic cells
Degenerated squamous metaplastic cells
Stripped nuclei in atrophic smears
Microglandular hyperplasia
Artifacts (collection, fixation, staining)

sia,[122] or endometriosis[123,124] also may mimic an endometrial adenocarcinoma.

Squamous metaplastic cells undergoing degeneration may be confused with malignant endometrial cells (Figure 9-23). When these cells degenerate, cytoplasmic vacuoles, similar to the vacuoles in endometrial adenocarcinoma, may form. Portions of the cytoplasm however, should remain dense and cyanophilic, unlike the frayed cytoplasm of endometrial adenocarcinoma. In addition, nucleoli should not be evident in squamous metaplastic cells.

Artifactual changes in endocervical or endometrial cells also may lead to a false-positive diagnosis.[42] Artifactual changes may result from improper collection, fixation, or staining and may result in nuclear and/or cellular enlargement, nuclear hyperchromasia, and cytoplasmic vacuolation. In some atrophic smears, nuclear stripping results in single atypical nuclei that may be mistaken for malignancy (Figure 9-24). In some cases an endometrial malignancy has been mistakenly diagnosed on insufficient material.[42] Caution should be made when definitively diagnosing an endometrial adenocarcinoma in women less than 40 years of age.

In direct endometrial samples, many of the same pitfalls occur. Koss claimed that polyps may be a particular cause for concern.[37]

Endocervical, extrauterine (e.g., nonendometrioid ovarian or fallopian tube), and metastatic adenocarcinomas, squamous cell carcinoma, and some sarcomas may be confused with an endometrioid adenocarcinoma. For adenocarcinomas, separation of the site of origin may not be possible, and it should be remembered that any adenocarcinoma subtype may occur anywhere in the gynecologic tract. Site of tumor origin depends mainly on determining where the bulk of the tumor lies. It so happens that most endometrial adenocarcinomas are endometrioid type and most endocervical adenocarcinomas are mucinous type, and this is why (and not unreasonably so) the Bethesda

System proposed different criteria for adenocarcinomas arising in these different locations. Thus, determination of the site of origin of an adenocarcinoma is based more on probabilities and less on specific or defining cytologic features.

As compared with most endocervical (mucinous) adenocarcinomas, most endometrial (endometrioid) adenocarcinomas shed fewer cells (or have fewer cells abraded), have cells of smaller size, have smaller nuclei, have smaller and fewer nucleoli, have less granular chromatin, and have a more watery and less necrotic tumor diathesis (Table 9-5).[57] These differences result partly from the differences in cell type and partly from the differences in how the cells were obtained (endometrial-shed; endocervical-abraded). Malignant endocervical cells are columnar in shape, whereas malignant endometrial cells are round to oval. The cells of an endocervical adenocarcinoma form strips, rosettes, and sheets; the cells of an endometrial adenocarcinoma form balls, loose clusters, and acini. Malignant endocervical cells have granular, eosinophilic cytoplasm, and malignant endometrial cells have finely vacuolated, cyanophilic cytoplasm. When cells having an endometrial appearance are seen in large groups, these cells may have been abraded, rather than sloughed, which may suggest endocervical involvement by an endometrial adenocarcinoma or a primary cervical neoplasm with endometrioid differentation.[125] As cervical cytology may lead to an incorrect site of origin classification, Costa and colleagues recommended a uniform clinical response (i.e., endocervical and endometrial sampling) for all cervical smears diagnosed as adenocarcinoma.[126]

When seen in cervical or vaginal smears, most extrauterine tumors are poorly differentiated and lack an associated tumor diathesis. In comparison, most poorly differentiated endometrial adenocarcinomas are associated with tumor diathesis.[78]

Squamous cell carcinoma, particularly the nonkeratinizing variant, also may mimic endometrial adenocarcinoma. In contrast with endometrial adenocarcinoma, squamous cell carcinoma samples are more cellular; rarely contain papillary groups; contain cells with denser cytoplasm, more hyperchromatic nuclei, more granular chromatin, and fewer macronucleoli; and show more tumor diathesis.[127]

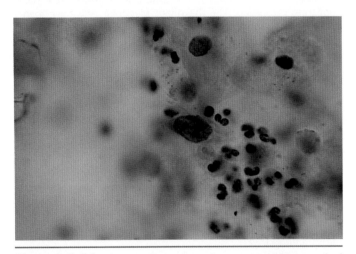

Figure 9-24 **Stripped nucleus in an atrophic cervical smear.** This nucleus is a mimic for an endometrioid adenocarcinoma. Although hyperchromatic, this nucleus has a degenerated appearance, and a prominent nucleolus is not seen. One should be cautious of making a malignant diagnosis if cytoplasm is not seen with the atypical nucleus. (Pap)

TABLE 9-5		
Comparison of Endometrial and Endocervical Adenocarcinoma in Pap Tests		
Cytologic Feature	**Endometrial Adenocarcinoma**	**Endocervical Adenocarcinoma**
Number of cells	Few	Many
Nuclear area (μm^2)	60	90
Cell size	Smaller	Larger
Cell forms	Round to oval	Columnar
Cell arrangements	Balls, loose clusters	Strips, sheets, rosettes
Cytoplasmic tincture	Cyanophilic	Eosinophilic
Cytoplasmic granularity	Less granular	Granular
Cytoplasmic vacuoles	Vacuolated	Less vacuolated
Nuclear hyperchromasia	Less	More
Chromatin granularity	Fine	Coarse
Number of nucleoli	Fewer	More
Size of nucleoli	Smaller	Larger

From Reagan JW, Ng ABP. The cells of uterine adenocarcinoma. In: Wied GL, editor. Monographs in Clinical Cytology. 2nd rev. ed. New York: S, Karger. 1973; pp.96-112.

Most squamous cell carcinomas arise in the cervix, although pure squamous cell carcinoma rarely may arise in the endometrium.

The most common cause of a false-negative diagnosis is sampling.[126] Screening errors may occur when the malignant cells are few in number or are mixed with obscuring blood or inflammation. Interpretive errors generally occur when the adenocarcinoma is well differentiated and the malignant endometrial cells are mistaken for benign endometrial cells or are simply overlooked.

Cytologic Features of Other Endometrial Adenocarcinoma Subtypes

Little data have been published on the cytologic descriptions of some of the subtypes of endometrial adenocarcinoma (the nonpure endometrioid subtype). The importance of these descriptions is more academic than practical because the main role of cytology is to alert the clinician that malignancy is present rather than to subclassify the endometrial adenocarcinoma. Recognizing the subtypes may be important for distinguishing the particular pitfalls, which mimic the less common adenocarcinoma variants. These subtypes may be more easily recognizable in direct endometrial samples (because more cells are obtained), although the cytologic features are quite similar in both indirect and direct endometrial samples.

Endometrioid Adenocarcinoma with Squamous Differentiation

Endometrioid adenocarcinomas may be associated with benign squamous metaplasia (adenoacanthoma) or malignant squamous differentiation (adenosquamous carcinoma). However, some authorities prefer to refer to all of these entities as endometrial adenocarcinoma with squamous differentiation because prognosis is related to the grade of the glandular component. In both conditions, malignant glandular cells, as described above, should be present. The malignant glandular component usually is well or moderately differentiated. In adenoacanthoma, the benign squamous

cells may form balls, and the cytoplasm is abundant (Figure 9-25). In some cases, the metaplastic squamous cells cannot be distinguished from cervical metaplastic squamous cells. However, Reagan described the benign squamous cell cytoplasm as *oxyphilic* and reported that this cytoplasmic character is seen exclusively in benign endometrial squamous cells.[97] Buschmann and colleagues coined the term keratin bodies for these clusters.[128] If keratin bodies are observed in vaginal smears, the findings are suspicious for an endometrial primary; if keratin bodies are observed in cervical smears, the findings are more suspicious for an endocervical primary.[37] Becker reported that pseudokeratin bodies may be seen in nonmalignant conditions such as vaginitis.[129]

In endometrial adenosquamous cell carcinoma, the malignant squamous component may be keratinizing, nonkeratinizing, or small cell type.[49] Reagan reported that the most commonly seen malignant squamous component had a large cell keratinizing appearance.[97] In these malignant squamous cells the cytoplasm is abundant, the chromatin is moderately granular (Figure 9-26), and macronucleoli may be observed. In this subtype, the malignant squamous cells are rounded, whereas in many cervical squamous cell carcinomas the malignant squamous cells have more irregular shapes.[37] The malignant glandular and squamous components may be seen in the same aggregates, but more often, this is not the case. The glandular component usually predominates.

Serous Adenocarcinoma

Endometrial serous adenocarcinoma is a high-grade variant, and cytologic preparations show an anaplastic carcinoma. Wright and colleagues described the cervical smears of the serous adenocarcinoma variant to be more cellular and consistently to show tumor diathesis.[130] True papillae, irregularly shaped cell clusters, tight cell balls, and stripped malignant cell nuclei also tended to be present (Figure 9-27).[130] Kuebler and colleagues reported that the smears of serous adenocarcinoma were unlikely to contain histiocytes and the neoplastic cells rarely contained phagocytosed mater-

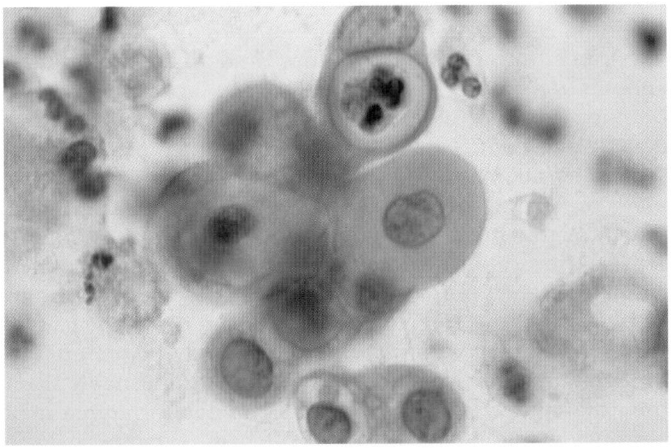

Figure 9-25 Benign squamous metaplastic cells in an adenoacanthoma in a cervical smear. The squamous metaplastic cells are present in balls and have relatively low N:C ratios. The squamous cells show an absence of nuclear atypia. (Pap)

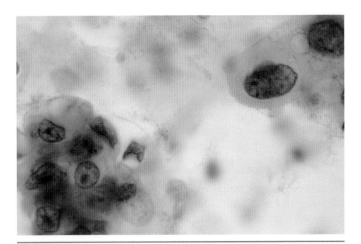

Figure 9-26 Endometrioid adenosquamous carcinoma in a cervical smear. Clusters of malignant glandular cells are admixed with malignant squamous cells *(upper right)*. Note the hard orangeophilic appearance of the malignant squamous cell cytoplasm. The malignant glandular cells have prominent nucleoli and are seen in a three-dimensional cluster. (Pap)

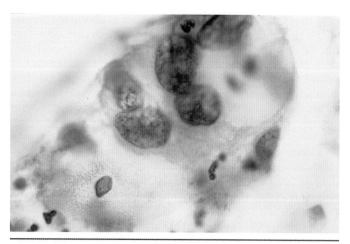

Figure 9-27 **Endometrial serous adenocarcinoma in an endocervical smear.** Identification of this entity requires observation of papillae (papillae are not seen here) and anaplastic cytologic features. Note the marked anisonucleosis, nuclear hyperchromasia, and prominent nucleoli, which are all anaplastic cytologic features. (Pap)

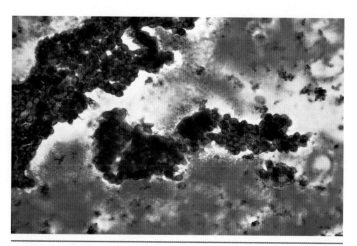

Figure 9-29 **Endometrial villoglandular adenocarcinoma in a cervical specimen.** This high-power view shows the malignant cells lining a fibrovascular core. Moderate cellular dissociation is present. In contrast to a serous adenocarcinoma, the malignant cells shown here display only moderate cellular atypia. (Pap)

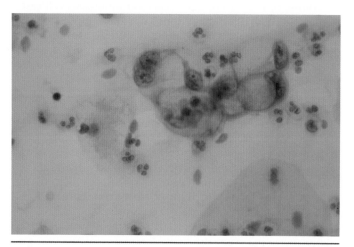

Figure 9-28 **Clear cell adenocarcinoma in a vaginal specimen.** The poorly differentiated malignant cells have frayed and finely vacuolated cytoplasm. In this case, the chromatin is finely granular, and a prominent nucleolus is observed. The cytoplasmic vacuoles may indent the nucleus, yielding a signet ring appearance. (Pap)

ial.[131] Psammoma bodies are more likely to be seen in serous adenocarcinoma than in other adenocarcinoma subtypes. Eddy and colleagues reported that if smears were diagnosed as frank adenocarcinoma rather than AGC, these smears were more likely to contain high-risk subtypes (e.g., serous adenocarcinoma or clear cell adenocarcinoma).[36]

Secretory Adenocarcinoma

Endometrial secretory adenocarcinoma is a very rare low-grade adenocarcinoma. Kusuyama and colleagues reported that the malignant cells in secretory adenocarcinoma tended to be shed in large clusters.[132] In the larger clusters, the cytoplasm had a clear or vacuolated appearance and nuclear polarity was lost.[132] Only minor degrees of nuclear atypia were seen and the differential diagnosis included Arias-Stella reaction, histiocytes, and secretory endometrium.

Clear Cell Adenocarcinoma

As mentioned on p. 167, clear cell adenocarcinomas are a heterogeneous group of malignancies and therefore may have a spectrum of appearances. Common to all clear cell adenocarcinomas is the appearance of the cytoplasm, which is vacuolated. Reagan described the cytoplasm as frayed and delicately stained (Figure 9-28).[97] In degenerated samples, this cytoplasmic quality usually is lost. The nuclei vary in their degree of atypia but generally exhibit finely granular chromatin.[133] Nucleoli are irregularly shaped[133] and prominent.[134] Ohwada and colleagues described clear cell carcinomas as having a "mirrorball" pattern.[135] In the more poorly differentiated tumors, single cells and large tumor clusters are seen. A tumor diathesis usually is present.

Mucinous Adenocarcinoma

Most endometrial mucinous adenocarcinomas are well to moderately differentiated. Endometrial mucinous adenocarcinomas appear similar to the more common endocervical mucinous adenocarcinomas, and distinction of an endometrial source is impossible based purely on cytomorphology. In addition, endometrial mucinous adenocarcinomas may be confused with endometrial mucinous metaplasia.[136] The neoplastic cells have vacuolated cytoplasm that may contain slightly eosinophilic material, consistent with mucin. A mucin stain could be used to confirm the nature of this intracellular material. Intracellular phagocytosed material rarely is present. In some cases, the mucin vacuoles may be so large as to give the cells a signet ring appearance. Large collections of extracellular mucin may be present, although these mucin collections are indistinguishable from the usual endocervical cell mucin. The nuclear atypia may be considerable.[137]

Ciliated Cell Adenocarcinoma

Endometrial ciliated cell adenocarcinoma has been described on endometrial brush cytology.[54] The malignant cells appear well to moderately differentiated and have cilia on their apical surfaces.[54] The presence of cilia on cytologic specimens almost always entails a benign process, and this malignancy represents an exceedingly rare exception.

Villoglandular Adenocarcinoma

Endometrial villoglandular adenocarcinoma is a well-differentiated malignancy; accordingly the malignant cells may be difficult to separate from nonmalignant processes. The cells may be seen in large sheets or papillae; papillary structures covered with cells exhibiting slight atypia should raise the possibility of a villoglandular adenocarcinoma rather than a serous adenocarcinoma in which the cells have larger and more irregular nuclei with much more prominent nucleoli (Figure 9-29).

Mixed Müllerian Carcinoma

Mixed müllerian carcinomas, which also contain a malignant glandular component, are described in Chapter 10.

ENDOCERVICAL ADENOCARCINOMA

Endocervical adenocarcinomas arise in the glandular epithelium, which lines the endocervical canal and which may extend out onto the cervix. Endocervical adenocarcinoma is increasing in frequency compared with cervical squamous cell carcinoma. Before the 1970s, only 5% of invasive cervical/endocervical cancers were adenocarcinomas (95% were squamous cell carcinomas).[138,139] After the 1970s, cancer registries and clinical series indicated that from 17% to 27% of cervical/endocervical malignancies were adenocarcinomas.[140-143] Some studies have shown no appreciable increase in frequency of endocervical adenocarcinoma in the last two decades,[144,145] although other studies report the opposite.[146] The mean age of presentation is between 47 and 53,[140,147-149] although the incidence of women less than 35 years of age with invasive endocervical adenocarcinoma is increasing.[144,145] The most common symptom of endocervical adenocarcinoma is abnormal vaginal bleeding (75%). Infrequently, presenting symptoms are pelvic pain or vaginal discharge.[140,150] In 15% of patients, no gross cervical lesions are seen.[151]

In all likelihood, invasive endocervical adenocarcinomas arise from a subcolumnar reserve cell in the transformation zone.[152] Endocervical adenocarcinoma in situ is thought to be the precursor lesion and is discussed in Chapter 8. Risk factors for the development of endocervical adenocarcinoma are shown in Box 9-5. The risk factors for endocervical adenocarcinoma include the same risk factors as for cervical squamous cell carcinoma[142,144,153] In more than 50% of cases, endocervical adenocarcinoma is found in association with cervical intraepithelial neoplasia.[154-156] More than 70% of invasive endocervical adenocarcinomas are associated with human papillomavirus (HPV), particularly HPV 18.[157-159] Although early studies showed that women who used oral contraceptives were at increased risk,[145,160] recent investigations have not supported this finding.[141,142] Some women may have a general predisposition to develop both endocervical (particularly the minimal deviation type) and ovarian mucinous tumors.[161]

The prognosis of women who have endocervical adenocarcinoma depends on the tumor stage (Table 9-6),[16] tumor size, lymph node status, histologic subtype, and tumor

---

BOX 9-5

Risk Factors for Endocervical Adenocarcinoma

Human papillomavirus
Squamous intraepithelial lesions
Genetic predisposition
Hypertension
Multiple sexual partners
Young age of first intercourse
Increased sexual activity
Tobacco use
Nulliparity
Diabetes
Obesity

TABLE 9-6

Endocervical Adenocarcinomas Staging System

Stage	Description
IA	Invasive carcinoma confined to the uterus and diagnosed only by microscopy
IB	Invasive carcinoma confined to the uterus and clinically visible
IIA	Tumor invades beyond the uterus but not to the pelvic wall or to lower third of vagina; without parametrial invasion
IIB	Tumor invades beyond the uterus but not to the pelvic wall or to lower third of vagina; with parametrial invasion
IIIA	Tumor involves lower third of vagina; no extension to pelvic wall
IIIB	Tumor extends to the pelvic wall and/or causes hydronephrosis or nonfunctioning kidney
IVA	Tumor invades the mucosa of the bladder or rectum and/or extends beyond the true pelvis
IVB	Distant metastasis

---

grade.[162] In North America, 80% of patients are stage I or II.[138,150] In a recent Norwegian study, Alfsen and colleagues reported that the distribution by FIGO stage was as follows: stage I, 62%; stage II, 21%; stage III, 12%; and stage IV, 5%.[146] Five-year survival rates for stage I, stage II, stage III, and stage IV endocervical adenocarcinomas are 75.9%, 62.9%, 29.2%, and 0%, respectively.[149,163-166] Chen and colleagues reported that the 5-year survival rates for stages I or II cervical adenocarcinoma were lower than for stages I or II squamous cell carcinoma when radiotherapy was the primary treatment; otherwise, survival rates were similar.[163] Tumor grading is based on the FIGO system that takes into account the growth pattern (i.e., amount of glandular versus solid growth) and nuclear atypia.[167]

As with endometrial adenocarcinomas, endocervical adenocarcinomas are a heterogeneous group of malignancies exhibiting several histologic patterns. These subtypes are often found together, and some authors prefer to classify the adenocarcinoma according to the most prevalent histologic pattern. If additional histologic subtypes comprise more than 10% of the total tumor pattern, some authors recommend that these subtypes be separately listed.[167] Generally, the most common subtype is mucinous adenocarcinoma,[150,164,165] although other authors have reported that endometrioid adenocarcinoma is more common.[168,169] Together, these two subtypes comprise up to 90% of all endocervical adenocarcinomas.[146,168,169] Lee and Flynn reported that the histogenesis of the mucinous and endometrioid type was the same, although the endometrioid type arose higher in the endocervical canal.[170] The more rare adenocarcinoma subtypes include clear cell adenocarcinoma (10%),[165] serous adenocarcinoma, mesonephric adenocarcinoma, villoglandular adenocarcinoma, adenoid cystic carcinoma, and adenoid basal carcinoma. Adenosquamous carcinomas and mucoepidermoid carcinomas (carcinomas without recognizable gland formation but with focal mucin positivity) are discussed in Chapter 7.

Some authors use the term *microinvasive endocervical adenocarcinoma* to refer to those adenocarcinomas that have invaded to less than 5 mm in depth.[171] Zaino argued that the term microinvasive endocervical adenocarcinoma is poorly defined and not reproducible.[172] Thus, for the purposes of this text, this entity has not been recognized. Regardless of one's viewpoint, some investigators described the cytologic features of this entity to be indistinguishable from the more typical invasive endocervical adenocarcinoma.[57,152,173-176]

Sensitivity and Specificity

Angel and colleagues reported that only a minority of patients with invasive endocervical adenocarcinoma were detected through cytologic screening.[177] Hurt and colleagues reported that of 43 patients with invasive endocervical adenocarcinoma who had undergone screening, 18 (41.9%) had a normal smear.[150] Boddington and colleagues found the false-negative rate for invasive endocervical adenocarcinoma to be 26.7%; in six of 13 patients with negative smears, retrospective review showed that malignant cells were present.[178] Sampling error also may play a role in the cytologic underdiagnosis of invasive endocervical adenocarcinoma because some of these neoplasms rise very high in the endocervical canal. Kristensen and colleagues presented similar sensitivity data with 30% of women with en-

docervical adenocarcinoma having negative smears.[179] Benoit and colleagues showed that only 25 of 84 (29.8%) women had negative screening examinations within 3 years of the malignant diagnosis.[180]

Other authors have reported that the majority of invasive endocervical adenocarcinomas are detected through cervicovaginal smear cytology. Reagan and Ng reported that the diagnostic accuracy was 97%, Korhonen and colleagues 86%, Saigo and colleagues 91%, and Ayer at al 95.7%.[57,176,181]

Sensitivity of cancer detection also depends on what counts for a positive cytologic diagnosis. If nondefinitive diagnoses such as AGC are considered to indicate disease, then the sensitivity is higher.

In summary, the sensitivity of invasive endocervical adenocarcinoma detection ranges from approximately 40% to more than 90%, with most studies reporting sensitivities greater than 70%. Thus, the sensitivity of invasive endocervical adenocarcinoma detection is higher than the sensitivity of adenocarcinoma in situ or squamous intraepithelial lesion detection.[38] False-negative diagnoses are mainly a result of sampling,[183] although interpretive and screening errors also play a role. The transformation zone recedes with age, making sampling more difficult.[154] Invasive endocervical adenocarcinoma also may be focal and deep, limiting the ability to sample.[184]

The specificity of cervicovaginal smears in not falsely diagnosing invasive endocervical adenocarcinoma is high and probably more than 99.9%. Causes of false-positive diagnoses are discussed in the following section.

Cytologic Features of Invasive Mucinous Endocervical Adenocarcinoma

Although not specifically stated, the Bethesda System cytologic features of invasive endocervical adenocarcinoma appear to describe the mucinous variant. The cytologic features of the other variants are described subsequently. The Bethesda System criteria for invasive endocervical adenocarcinoma are shown in Box 9-6. The cytologic features of invasive mucinous endocervical adenocarcinoma overlap with the cytologic features of adenocarcinoma in situ. Separating invasive and in situ adenocarcinoma is difficult, and perhaps, only the more poorly differentiated invasive endocervical adenocarcinomas may be diagnosed definitively.

In surgical pathology practice, four subtypes of invasive mucinous endocervical adenocarcinoma are described.[167] The first three subtypes are the endocervical, intestinal, and signet ring forms. The fourth subtype, minimal deviation adenocarcinoma, is discussed separately. In the endocervical subtype, the malignant glands are composed of mucin-containing columnar cells resembling endocervical mucosa. These cancers usually are well to moderately differentiated.[185] In the intestinal subtype the malignant glands are composed of cells resembling colonic mucosa. These malignancies usually are moderately differentiated. In the signet ring subtype, single poorly differentiated malignant cells invade the stroma. This subtype rarely occurs as a pure form and more often is mixed with the other two subtypes. Similar to endometrial adenocarcinomas, endocervical mucinous adenocarcinomas are graded on architectural features and nuclear grade.[150,168] These three subtypes rarely are

---

BOX 9-6 CMF

Bethesda System Cytomorphologic Features of Endocervical Adenocarcinoma

1. Cytologic criteria include those outlined for atypical endocervical cells, probably neoplastic (see Table 8-2)
2. Single cell, two-dimensional sheets, or clusters may be seen
3. Enlarged nuclei demonstrate irregular chromatin distribution and parachromatin clearing
4. Macronucleoli may be present
5. A necrotic tumor diathesis may be present
6. Columnar cell shape may be retained with eosinophilic or cyanophilic cytoplasm
7. Abnormal squamous cells may be present, representing either a coexisting squamous lesion or the squamous component of an adenocarcinom

described separately in the cytology literature, although their differences have important bearings on their cytologic appearance. The 1991 Bethesda Committee criteria not only failed to describe the various nonmucinous subtypes of invasive endocervical adenocarcinoma but also failed to describe the various mucinous subtypes.

Endocervical smears differ in the cellularity of the malignant cell population depending on if the invasive malignant foci are sampled directly or if the malignant cells are spontaneously shed. Most invasive endocervical adenocarcinomas may be reached with the currently employed sampling devices, although sampling still depends on clinical skill and some patient factors such as the presence or absence of cervical stenosis. If the lesions are sampled directly, the malignant endocervical component is highly cellular. Otherwise, the number of malignant cells is low and depends on several factors such as the histologic grade. Malignant cell degeneration is more likely in cases in which the malignant cell component is shed rather than abraded. Vaginal pool specimens tend to not contain many malignant cells, regardless of whether the tumor cells are shed or abraded.

If directly sampled, the malignant cells usually are seen singly and in clusters (Figure 9-30). The number of single cells depends on tumor differentiation, with greater cellular dissociation in the more poorly differentiated mucinous adenocarcinomas. Thus, if a signet ring cell component is present, a greater proportion of single malignant cells is observed. In the intestinal and endocervical mucinous adenocarcinomas, rosettes, large sheets, and strips are present (Figure 9-31)[173]; these findings are similar to those seen in adenocarcinoma in situ.[174,175,186,187] Cell balls are associated with directly sampled, more poorly differentiated endocervical adenocarcinomas; this cytologic feature is more commonly seen in endometrial adenocarcinomas. In addition, syncytial aggregates may be seen, although this is a more common feature of adenocarcinoma in situ. Ayer and colleagues have suggested that the presence of papillary-like groups is suggestive of an invasive adenocarcinoma, rather than an adenocarcinoma in situ.[188] In well-differentiated

adenocarcinomas the sheets may appear quite orderly, and the group architecture is not the defining feature of malignancy (Figure 9-32).

In both in situ and invasive adenocarcinoma, the cell groups may exhibit *feathering*, which refers to protrusion of the malignant cell nuclei from the edges of the groups (Figure 9-33). These large nuclei may be bare or encircled with only scant cytoplasm; Lee and colleagues reported that feathering is not seen in benign endocervical conditions.[175]

Except for well-differentiated mucinous adenocarcinomas (see the section entitled Minimal Deviation Adenocarcinoma), abundant extracellular mucin is not present. This is true for even the endocervical subtype; the mucin that accompanies malignant cells is most likely produced by benign endocervical mucosa. As a rule the intestinal subtype is not associated with extracellular mucin.

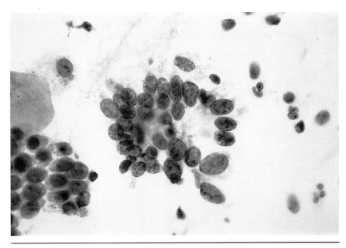

Figure 9-31 **Endocervical mucinous adenocarcinoma in an endocervical specimen.** At this high power, rosettes, strips, and single cells are observed. The malignant single cells possess cytoplasm with an elongated appearance. Marked variation in nuclear size is present. (Pap)

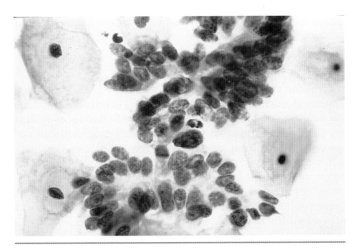

Figure 9-30 **Endocervical mucinous adenocarcinoma in a cervical specimen.** This tumor was directly sampled and shows malignant cells arranged in clusters, pseudorosettes, and strips. The chromatin is granular and dark and this smear resembles that of an adenocarcinoma in situ. (Pap)

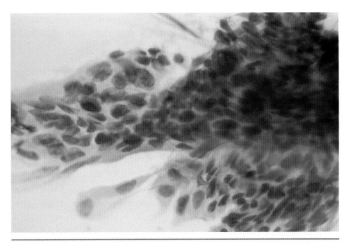

Figure 9-32 **Endocervical mucinous adenocarcinoma in a cervical specimen.** This malignancy is well differentiated, and the malignant cells appear quite orderly. Only moderate cellular atypia is present. Note the absence of an inflammatory component. (Pap)

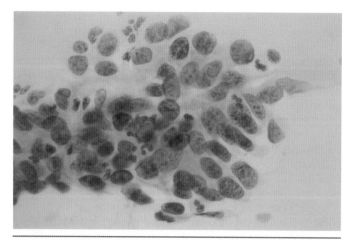

Figure 9-33 **Endocervical mucinous adenocarcinoma in an endocervical specimen.** In this malignant cell group, the cells display feathering, or extension of the nuclei beyond the edges of the group. This feature may be seen in both endocervical adenocarcinoma in situ and invasive adenocarcinoma. The nuclear chromatin is dark and rosettes also are present. (Pap)

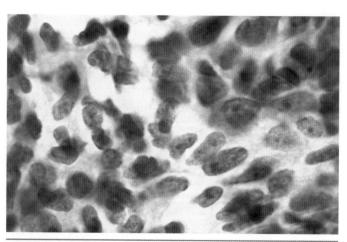

Figure 9-35 **Endocervical mucinous adenocarcinoma in an endocervical specimen.** At this high power, the malignant cells show columnar shapes and an eccentrically placed nucleolus. This tumor is an example of the endocervical variant. (Pap)

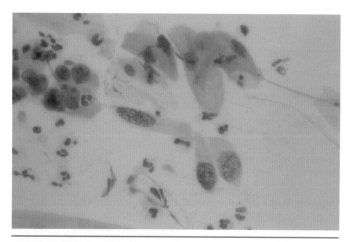

Figure 9-34 **Endocervical mucinous adenocarcinoma in a cervical specimen.** At this high power, the malignant cells are admixed with a necrotic tumor diathesis. In contrast to the diathesis seen with most endometrial adenocarcinomas, the diathesis seen here consists of degenerated tumor cell debris and neutrophils (rather than a watery diathesis). Single tumor cells with elongated hyperchromatic nuclei are present. (Pap)

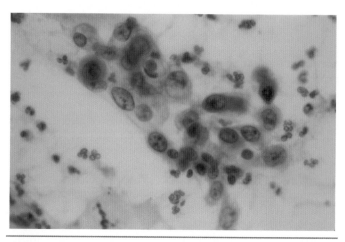

Figure 9-36 **Endocervical mucinous adenocarcinoma in an endocervical specimen.** Fine cytoplasmic vacuoles are seen in this example of the intestinal variant. It is rare to see large cytoplasmic vacuoles in the intestinal variant. The cells have an elongated shape with irregularly clumped nuclear chromatin and prominent nucleoli. (Pap)

The amount of tumor diathesis depends on the degree of differentiation. Tumor diathesis is not a feature of adenocarcinoma in situ, so if even a small amount of tumor diathesis is present, an invasive carcinoma may be suggested. Endocervical adenocarcinoma tumor diathesis consists of necrotic cellular debris and neutrophils (Figure 9-34); it does not have the watery quality so characteristic of endometrial adenocarcinoma tumor diathesis. Psammoma bodies rarely accompany pure invasive mucinous endocervical adenocarcinomas.

The malignant cells of both the intestinal and endocervical subtypes are roughly equal in size and larger than benign endocervical cells. In well- and moderately differentiated mucinous adenocarcinomas, the malignant cells have a tall columnar configuration with eccentric nuclei (Figure 9-35).[173] In cellular groups, the nuclei may appear pali-

saded. The cytoplasm has a granular quality, and the cytoplasmic borders may be indistinct.[173,189] Intracellular mucin vacuoles may be observed in the endocervical subtype and are rare in the intestinal subtype. In well-differentiated endocervical intestinal adenocarcinomas, multiple fine vacuoles are observed (Figure 9-36). In the signet ring form, larger cytoplasmic vacuoles indenting the nucleus are common (Figure 9-37). The cytoplasm is eosinophilic[190] to cyanophilic in the endocervical and intestinal subtypes and is cyanophilic in the signet ring subtype.

In endocervical mucinous adenocarcinomas the N:C ratio is increased, and the nuclei appear crowded. The nuclear features are the key to the cytologic recognition of malignancy; the cytoplasmic features are of secondary importance. The size of the nuclei of the mucinous adenocarcinoma subtype depends on the degree of tumor differentiation (Figure

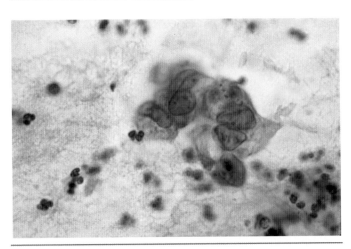

Figure 9-37 **Endocervical mucinous adenocarcinoma in an endocervical specimen.** At this high power, a signet ring cell is seen. This cell displays prominent cytoplasmic vacuoles that indent the nucleus. The signet ring form most commonly is seen in association with the other variants. Nuclear membrane irregularities are pronounced. (Pap)

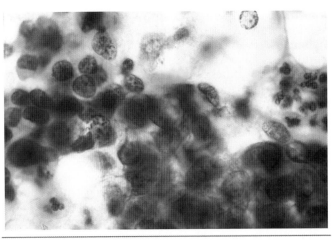

Figure 9-39 **Endocervical mucinous adenocarcinoma in a cervical specimen.** This high-grade malignancy shows cells with large hyperchromatic nuclei. In several cells, the nuclear chromatin appears hypochromatic. Considerable variability in nuclear size is evident. (Pap)

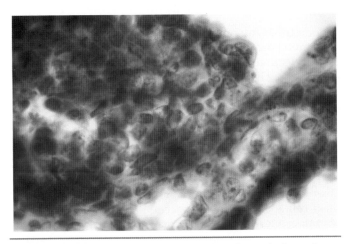

Figure 9-38 **Poorly differentiated endocervical mucinous adenocarcinoma in an endocervical specimen.** The malignant cells have a high N:C ratio and irregular nuclear outlines. These large nuclei are indicative of poor differentiation. Extensive nuclear overlap and prominent nucleoli are seen. (Pap)

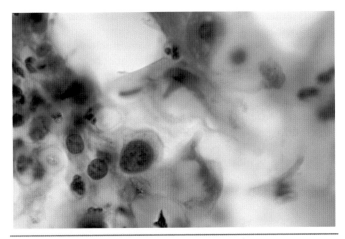

Figure 9-40 **Endocervical mucinous adenocarcinoma in an endocervical specimen.** A moderately dysplastic squamous cell is seen in the background of this moderately differentiated adenocarcinoma. The dysplastic squamous cell appears metaplastic. (Pap)

9-38).[174,191] Reagan and colleagues reported that the malignant nuclei range in size from 73 μm^2 to 165 μm^2; in contrast benign endocervical nuclei vary from 50 μm^2 to 60 μm^2. Thus, in the well-differentiated subtypes, the nuclei are in the size range of the nuclei in reactive endocervical conditions. Pacey and Ng reported that in 25% of cases, the malignant nuclei are smaller than the nuclei of normal endocervical nuclei[192]; this small nuclear size has not been the authors' experience.

Malignant nuclei are hyperchromatic even in well-differentiated adenocarcinomas. The chromatin is coarse, although some authors report the opposite.[192] In high-grade mucinous adenocarcinomas, the chromatin may appear finer (the opposite is the case in many endometrial adenocarcinomas) and less hyperchromatic (Figure 9-39). The nuclei generally are oval and nuclear membrane irregularities are usually apparent. Nucleoli are not characteristic of well-differentiated mucinous adenocarcinomas but are observed in moderately to poorly differentiated adenocarcinomas.[182] The nucleoli remain round but may be enlarged and multiple in the poorly differentiated mucinous adenocarcinomas. Mitoses may be seen but usually are not numerous except in the poorly differentiated tumors. Squamous intraepithelial neoplasia may be seen in the background of invasive endocervical mucinous adenocarcinoma subtypes (Figure 9-40).

Liquid-based preparations of invasive endocervical mucinous adenocarcinoma show the same cytologic features as described above in direct smears.[193] Van Aspert van Erp reported that the detection of endocervical glandular neoplasia was reproducible using video observation.[194]

Minimal Deviation Adenocarcinoma (Adenoma Malignum)

Minimal deviation adenocarcinoma is a special variant of endocervical mucinous adenocarcinoma, although recent classification systems have been expanded to include endometrioid and clear cell variants.[151,195-197] This malignancy is extremely well differentiated and difficult to classify as malignant, even on histologic specimens.[195] Surgical pathologists have written that these adenocarcinomas lack the cytologic features of malignancy but architecturally exhibit atypical glands that vary in size, shape, and location.[167] Minimal deviation adenocarcinomas account for 1% to 3% of all endocervical adenocarcinomas.[197] They are strongly associated with Peutz-Jeghers syndrome.[198] Some series have presented data indicating that women with minimal deviation adenocarcinoma have worse survival,[199,200] whereas other series have presented data indicating a prognosis equal to that of women with ordinary well-differentiated mucinous adenocarcinoma.[195,197]

Clinically, a copious watery or mucinous vaginal discharge may be apparent. Cytologically, abundant extracellular mucin may be observed.[201] In the mucinous variety, numerous loose sheets of bland-appearing endocervical vacuolated cells may be seen.[187,202-204] Glandular openings in the honeycomb sheets of cells may be appreciated, and within the groups the malignant cells do not exhibit well-developed stratification.[205] Single, columnar cells with lacy cytoplasm may also be present.[201] The nuclei are only slightly enlarged, but the chromatin is dark, although fine to granular.[152] Nucleoli are small or inconspicuous, although Kudo and colleagues described macronucleoli. Szyfelbein and colleagues reported that mitoses may be quite numerous.[152,201] Although the cytologic findings may be likened to repair, in most smears the most important finding is the marked increase in the number of bland-appearing endocervical glandular groups. Despite these excellent cytologic descriptions, minimal deviation adenocarcinoma cannot be diagnosed outright on cytologic preparations, and at best an AGC diagnosis may be rendered.[205]

False-Positive Diagnoses of Endocervical Mucinous Adenocarcinoma

Causes of false-positive diagnoses include reactive and inflammatory endocervical conditions,[206] microglandular hyperplasia,[122,207-209] tubal metaplasia,[122,209,210] endocervical polyps,[206] brushing artifact,[211] degenerated endometrial cells, exogenous hormone effect, Arias-Stella reac-

tion,[106,119,212] cervical endometriosis,[123] lower uterine segment endometrium,[112] and radiation or chemotherapy effect[213,214] (Box 9-7). In all these conditions the glandular cells may be enlarged and exhibit well-developed nuclear changes. In some of these conditions, feathering has been reported. The presence of marked atypia and numerous single cells usually signifies an adenocarcinoma, although a definitive diagnosis hardly is possible in all cases.

Other malignancies such as squamous cell carcinoma or squamous dysplasia in endocervical glands may be confused with an invasive endocervical adenocarcinoma. In all these squamous lesions, atypical nuclei are seen. The presence of rosettes, feathering, and cytoplasmic fragility are more indicative of an adenocarcinoma.[215] The cytologic separation of squamous from glandular origin may not be possible, and it should be remembered that squamous and glandular neoplasia often occur in combination.

The cytologic features useful in separating endocervical mucinous adenocarcinoma from endometrial endometrioid adenocarcinoma are shown in Table 9-5.

Cytologic Features of Invasive Endocervical (Nonmucinous) Adenocarcinoma Subtypes

Endometrioid Adenocarcinoma

This subtype of endocervical adenocarcinoma is cytologically indistinguishable from the endometrioid adenocarcinoma arising in the endometrium. Extensively degenerated endometrioid adenocarcinomas are more likely to be from the endometrium. Clinically, endometrial primaries usually present with uterine enlargement with secondary endocervical involvement. Endocervical primaries present with cervical/endocervical enlargement without enlargement of the uterine corpus.

Clear Cell Adenocarcinoma

Clear cell adenocarcinomas account for approximately 4% of endocervical adenocarcinoma.[216,217] Clear cell adenocarcinomas arising in young women more often are linked to DES exposure, whereas those arising in post-menopausal women tend to develop in the absence of DES exposure.[218] Three histologic patterns of tumor growth are recognized: solid, tubulocystic, and papillary.[191]

Cytologically, many clear cell adenocarcinomas may resemble other poorly differentiated adenocarcinomas.[210] Endocervical clear cell adenocarcinomas appear identical to those arising in the endometrium or vagina. The nuclei are enlarged, variably hyperchromatic, and often stripped.[192] Nucleoli are typically prominent. The cytoplasmic characteristics, the major histologically defining feature of this adenocarcinoma type, may be absent as a result of degeneration of cytologic specimens. In nondegenerated specimens the cytoplasm may be wispy, abundant, and cyanophilic (Figure 9-41). In low-grade clear cell adenocarcinomas, the malignant cells may have bland chromatin.[219]

The differential diagnosis includes Arias-Stella reaction, repair, and microglandular hyperplasia. In all these benign conditions the nuclear atypia is lacking.

Serous Adenocarcinoma

Primary serous adenocarcinomas of the endocervix are exceedingly rare high-grade malignancies. Cytologically, they resemble serous adenocarcinomas arising in the ovary or

---

BOX 9-7

Causes of a False-Positive Diagnosis of Endocervical Adenocarcinoma

Endocervical repair
Radiation and/or chemotherapy effect
Arias-Stella reaction
Endometrial hyperplasia
Lower uterine segment cells
Endocervical polyp
Endometriosis
Tubal metaplasia
Chemotherapy effect
Degenerated squamous metaplastic cells
Stripped nuclei in atrophic smears
Microglandular hyperplasia
Artifacts (collection, fixation, staining)

endometrium. Pseudopapillary fragments, balls, and sheets of moderately pleomorphic cells are present[222] (Figure 9-42). Tumor diathesis tends to be abundant in primary endocervical serous adenocarcinoma and is less commonly observed in endometrial or ovarian primaries.[220] Psammoma bodies may be present.[81]

Mesonephric Carcinoma

Mesonephric carcinomas are exceedingly rare malignancies that arise in the deep lateral cervical wall; the location of mesonephric duct remnants.[221] For the histologic diagnosis, involvement of the endocervical mucosa should not be present.[267] Consequently, an exfoliative cytologic specimen of a mesonephric carcinoma would be highly unusual. The authors are unaware of any published reports.

Villoglandular Adenocarcinoma

Villoglandular adenocarcinoma is a well-differentiated malignancy that occurs in young women and has been associated with oral contraceptive use.[222-224] Patients have an excellent prognosis.[223,224] Histologically, these malignancies are characterized by papillae lined by bland cells having endocervical, intestinal, or endometrioid features.

Cervical smears usually are highly cellular, with malignant cells seen in papillary clusters, cohesive sheets, rosettes, and tissue fragments,[225] in which nuclear palisading, pseudostratification, and crowding are evident. The nuclei are small and hyperchromatic and contain inconspicuous nucleoli. Feathering, cell balls, and single malignant cells are reported to be absent.[226] The differential diagnosis includes inflammatory conditions, cells from the lower uterine segment, papillary adenofibroma, and müllerian papilloma.[222,227] Squamous cell carcinoma in situ also may be a mimic.[225] Chang and colleagues reported that no cases of villoglandular adenocarcinoma were definitively diagnosed as malignant on cervicovaginal smears.[226]

Adenosquamous Carcinoma, Glassy Cell Carcinoma, and Mucoepidermoid Carcinomas

These malignancies are described in greater detail in Chapter 7.

Adenoid Cystic Carcinoma

Although adenoid cystic carcinomas account for less than 1% of all cervical adenocarcinomas,[185,228,229] stage for stage, they are more lethal than other endocervical adenocarcinoma variants.[230] These carcinomas occur in postmenopausal women and may by associated with ovarian mucinous tumors. Morphologically, these neoplasma are similar to those arising in the salivary gland, breast, skin, and airways.[231,232] Bittencourt and colleagues described that smears of adenoid cystic carcinoma contained sheets of uniform cells surrounding spaces containing hyaline deposits (Figure 9-43).[233] Ravinsky and colleagues reported that the cells exhibited a cribriform pattern and that dysplastic squamous cells were seen.[234]

Adenoid Basal Carcinoma

Adenoid basal carcinomas account for less than 1% of all cervical adenocarcinomas, generally occur in postmenopausal women,[228,229] and usually are not aggressive. Histologically, adenoid basal carcinomas resemble basal cell

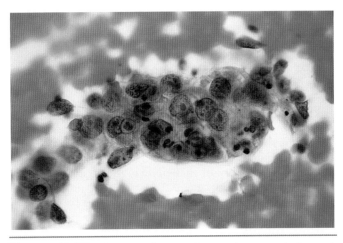

Figure 9-42 **Serous adenocarcinoma in a cervical specimen.** The malignant cells are in a large cluster admixed with acute inflammation. The cells exhibit variability in size and shape. (Pap)

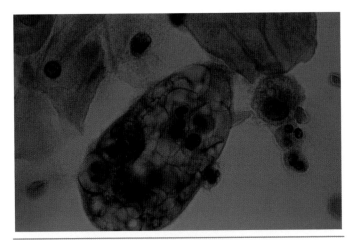

Figure 9-41 **Clear cell adenocarcinoma in a cervical specimen.** This poorly differentiated malignancy shows a large cell cluster and a single cell. Numerous cytoplasmic vacuoles are present. In this case, the neoplastic nuclei are not much larger than the benign intermediate squamous cell nuclei. (Pap)

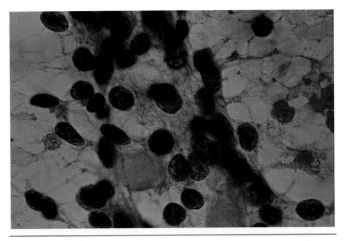

Figure 9-43 **Adenoid cystic adenocarcinoma in an endocervical specimen.** Note the cytologic similarities to the salivary gland counterpart. The malignant cells are seen in clusters surrounding hyaline deposits. The cells contain a small amount of cytoplasm and the nuclei are relatively monomorphic and hyperchromatic. (Pap)

carcinomas of the skin. The cytologic diagnosis of adenoid basal carcinoma is quite difficult, particularly in the separation of adenoid basal carcinoma from benign conditions.[235] In cervicovaginal smears a predominance of small, uniform cell clusters with hyperchromatic nuclei are seen.[236] Peripheral palisading may be evident.[235] The more conventional invasive adenocarcinoma features such as rosettes, feathering, and columnar cells are lacking.

CYTOLOGIC FEATURES OF EXTRAUTERINE ADENOCARCINOMA

Extrauterine neoplasms, which may be detected on cervicovaginal smears include adenocarcinomas arising in the fallopian tube, ovary, peritoneum; adenocarcinomas that secondarily invade the gynecologic tract; vaginal adenocarcinomas; and metastatic adenocarcinomas. Ng and colleagues reported that of every 100,000 smears screened, 11 extrauterine cancers were detected.[78] Approximately seven uterine cancers are detected per every one extrauterine cancer detected.[78] Excluding vaginal adenocarcinomas, 42% of extrauterine cancers detected were from the ovary, 8% from the fallopian tube, and 50% from nongynecologic sources.[78] The most common nongynecologic source is the gastrointestinal tract followed by breast,[237-240] with adenocarcinomas from the pancreas, lung, urethra, kidney and other sites seen less often.[78,241-243]

Recognizing that a Pap test contains a malignancy that is extrauterine has important clinical ramifications. First, if the woman has no history of malignancy, the diagnosis initiates and guides the clinical evaluation. Second, if the woman has a history of malignancy, the recognition may help document tumor stage.[244] Factors that influence the presence of extrauterine adenocarcinomas in Pap tests include the location and extent of spread of the primary malignancy, patency of the fallopian tube, tumor type, and degree of tumor differentiation. In most cases, the cytologic appearance of the extrauterine malignant cells lack defining features for the site of origin to be determined.

Regardless of the site of origin, Ng and colleagues and others have reported that most extrauterine malignancies detected in Pap tests were poorly differentiated and contained obviously numerous malignant cells with large, hyperchromatic nuclei.[78,245,246] Gupta and Balsara wrote that in 64% of Pap tests in which an extrauterine adenocarcinoma was present, the diagnosis of metastasis was made (other diagnoses such as AGC were made on most of the other smears).[244] Ng and colleagues reported that false-positive diagnoses of extrauterine cancer are rare.[39]

Ovarian and Tubal Adenocarcinomas

Ovarian, fallopian tube, and peritoneal adenocarcinomas that may be detected in cervicovaginal smears usually are high-grade malignancies.[78,87,88,245-265] Ng and colleagues reported that a feature helpful in distinguishing ovarian or fallopian tube adenocarcinomas from uterine adenocarcinomas was the absence of diathesis.[78] Tumor diathesis was absent in 80% of smears of ovarian and fallopian tube adenocarcinomas, whereas it was present in 85% and 93% of smears of endocervical and endometrial adenocarcinomas, respectively.[78] The Bethesda System used this criterion as a feature of extrauterine adenocarcinoma (Box 9-8).[1] The presence of a very poorly differentiated adenocarcinoma, especially with papillary features, not associated with tumor diathesis is even more supportive of an ovarian or fallopian tube adenocarcinoma (Figure 9-44).[39] If diathesis is present with an extrauterine malignancy, it usually is watery rather than necrotic.[39] Psammoma bodies may be suggestive of extrauterine origin,[88,253] but psammoma bodies also may be seen in uterine adenocarcinomas.

Direct sampling of the endometrium also may be used to detect primary ovarian or fallopian tube adenocarcinomas.[261,265,266]

Adenocarcinomas Secondarily Invading the Gynecologic Tract

Adenocarcinomas arising in the rectum or urinary tract may secondarily involve the gynecologic tract. Invasive rectal adenocarcinomas may result in the formation of a rectovaginal fistula; Angeles and Saigo reported that 30% of rectovaginal fistulas were secondary to malignancy.[267] In contrast with ovarian and fallopian tube tumors seen on cervicovaginal smears, rectal adenocarcinomas invading the gynecologic tract are often associated with necrotic tumor diathesis. The malignant cells usually are columnar and contain an eccentrically placed nucleus (Figure 9-45). The chromatin is hyperchromatic and coarse. Separating rectal adenocarcinomas from endocervical adenocarcino-

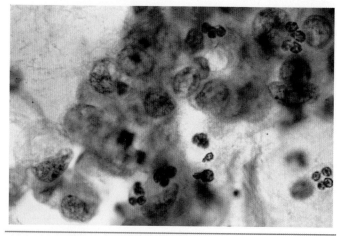

Figure 9-44   Ovarian serous adenocarcinoma in a vaginal specimen. The malignant cells appear markedly anaplastic, and tumor diathesis is absent. The cells are present in a large group having a three-dimensional appearance. (Pap)

BOX 9-8

Bethesda System Criterion for Extrauterine Adenocarcinoma

When cells diagnostic of adenocarcinoma occur in association with a clean background or with morphology unusual for tumors of the uterus/cervix, an extrauterine neoplasm should be considered.

mas of the intestinal subtype and from endometrioid adenocarcinomas on cytologic grounds is impossible. However, if malignant cells having an intestinal appearance are seen predominantly on the vaginal (rather than cervical) portion of a smear (if performed separately) and are well preserved, a rectal origin may be suspected. Also, if feces are evident, this points to a primary rectal tumor.

Vaginal Adenocarcinoma

Primary adenocarcinoma of the vagina accounts for approximately 1% of invasive gynecologic tract malignancies.[268] A significant proportion of these adenocarcinomas are clear cell adenocarcinomas, which are related to in utero DES. Melnick and colleagues estimated that the risk that a clear cell adenocarcinoma will develop in an exposed female from birth through age 34 years was 1:1000.[269] In 1990 and 1991, 53 new cases of vaginal clear cell adenocarcinoma were reported.[270] The sensitivity of detection of clear cell adenocarcinoma is high. Taft and colleagues reported that in 11 patients, the cervicovaginal smear served as the primary means of detection.[271] In addition, in 43 of 55 patients who had prior positive biopsy tissue diagnoses, the smears were positive or suspicious for adenocarcinoma.[271] Hanselaar and colleagues reported that vaginal smears were *always* positive, whereas cervical smears were positive in 85% of the cases.[272]

Clear cell adenocarcinomas of the vagina arise in regions of vaginal adenosis where the normal squamous epithelium is replaced by mucus-producing endocervical type epithelium. Adenocarcinomas arising in adenosis may involve the cervix in 40% of cases. Bibbo and colleagues recommended that for women who are at risk to develop adenosis or adenocarcinoma, four separate scrape smears from the four quadrants of the proximal vagina should be obtained.[273] Clear cell adenocarcinomas may recur more than 15 years after initial diagnosis, and continued close vaginal smear follow-up is mandatory.[274]

The cytologic features of vaginal clear cell adenocarcinoma are similar to the features in endometrial and cervical clear cell adenocarcinomas, although the cells may be better preserved in the vaginal primaries (Figure 9-46). The smears may be cellular, and in ulcerated tumors, neutrophils may be admixed with the malignant cells.[271] Vaginal adenocarcinomas may have different degrees of differentiation, and in some smears the cells may have a bland appearance. Clusters of mucus-secreting cells from regions of adenosis may be admixed with malignant cell clusters, and definitive diagnosis of adenocarcinoma may not be possible. Taft and colleagues indicated that poorly differentiated clear cell adenocarcinomas may be confused with squamous cell carcinomas.[271]

Metastatic Adenocarcinoma

Case reports of metastatic adenocarcinomas to the gynecologic tract abound. Adenocarcinomas may metastasize through the lymphatic spaces, hematogenously, or by spread through the peritoneal space. Adenocarcinomas from the upper gynecologic tract may spread by seeding the lower tract.[275,276] In many cases of metastatic disease, the tumor remains confined to the vascular or lymphatic spaces,[277] and Pap tests are then negative. In other cases, cervical erosion may occur, allowing the malignant cells to be present on Pap tests. In most cases, clinical signs and symptoms of metastatic disease are present, and only 6% of women who have metastatic disease are asymptomatic.[278]

Song reported that in metastatic malignancies, the tumor cells tend to predominate in the vaginal, rather than the cervical portion of the smear.[257] If ulceration has not occurred, the smears lack tumor diathesis and few cells are seen.[279] Most metastatic adenocarcinomas, although classifiable as malignant, cannot be definitively identified by site of origin on cytologic grounds alone. Some exceptions exist. For example, in metastatic lobular adenocarcinomas, the cells may be small and bland, rather than poorly differentiated (Figure 9-47).[280] Metastatic breast cancer cells may resemble histiocytes. Kashimura and colleagues described that cervicovaginal smears of metastatic gastric carcinoma tended to contain fewer malignant cells and that these cells exhibited coarser chromatin and discrete vacuoles compared with primary endocervical adenocarcinomas.[279]

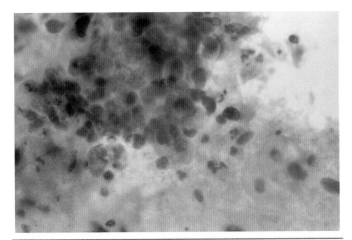

Figure 9-45 **Rectal adenocarcinoma in a vaginal specimen.** The malignant cells are seen in a cluster and have large, slightly degenerated, elongated nuclei. Extensive tumor necrosis is present in the background. (Pap)

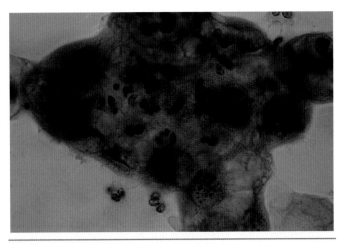

Figure 9-46 **Clear cell adenocarcinoma in a vaginal specimen.** The malignant cells are well preserved and present in a large cluster. The malignant cells have anaplastic nuclei and wispy, finely vacuolated cytoplasm. (Pap)

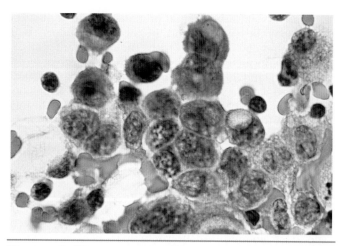

Figure 9-47 **Lobular carcinoma of the breast metastatic to the vagina in a vaginal specimen.** The malignant cells have high N:C ratios and coarse chromatin. Rare cells have large cytoplasmic vacuoles. Nuclear molding is seen. (Pap)

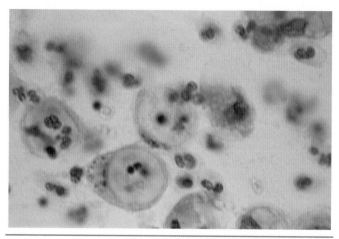

Figure 9-48 **Metastatic gastric adenocarcinoma in a cervical specimen.** The tumor shows signet ring forms with engulfed neutrophils. Abundant necrosis is present. (Pap)

Matsuura and colleagues reported that sheetlike arrangements of malignant cells was unusual in metastatic gastric adenocarcinoma.[281] McGill and colleagues reported that some gastric adenocarcinomas may present with a signet ring cell appearance (Figure 9-48)[282]; cervicovaginal smears, with a pure signet ring cell appearance from a uterine primary, are highly unusual.

References

1. Kurman R, Zaino R, Norris H. Endometrial carcinoma. In: Kurman RJ, editor. Blaustein's pathology of the female genital tract. New York: Springer-Verlag; 1994. pp.439-485.
2. Greenlee RT, Murray T, Wingo PA. Cancer statistics. Ca Cancer J Clin 2000; 50:7-33.
3. Young RC. Gynecologic malignancies. In: Fauci AS, Braunwald E, Isselbacher KJ, et al., editors. Harrison's principles of internal medicine. New York: McGraw-Hill; 1998. pp.605-611.
4. Rosai J. Female reproductive system. In: Rosai J, editor: Ackerman's surgical pathology. St. Louis: Mosby; 1996. pp.1319-1564.
5. Gusberg SB, Hall RE. Precursors of corpus cancer. III. The appearance of cancer of the endometrium in estrogenically conditioned patients. Obstet Gynecol 1961; 17:397-412.
6. Kaufman RH, Abbott JP, Wall JA. The endometrium before and after wedge resection of the ovaries in the Stein-Leventhal syndrome. Am J Obstet Gynecol 1959; 77:1271-1285.
7. Bokhman JV. Two pathogenetic types of endometrial carcinoma. Gynecol Oncol 1983; 15:10-17.
8. Smith M, McCartney AJ. Occult, high-risk endometrial cancer. Gynecol Oncol 1985; 22:154-161.
9. Beckner ME, Mori T, Silverberg SG. Endometrial carcinoma. Nontumor factors in prognosis. Int J Gynecol Pathol 1985; 4:131-145.
10. Deligdisch L, Cohen CJ. Histologic correlates and virulence implications of endometrial carcinoma associated with adenomatous hyperplasia. Cancer 1985; 56:1452-1455.
11. McCarty JKS, Barton TK, Peete JCH, et al. Gonadal dysgenesis with adenocarcinoma of the endometrium. An electron microscopic and steroid receptor analyses with a review of the literature. Cancer 1978; 42:512-520.
12. Fisher B, Costantino JP, Redmond CK, et al. Endometrial cancer in tamoxifen-treated breast cancer patients. Findings from the National Surgical Adjuvant Breast and Bowel Project (NSABP) B-14. J Natl Cancer Inst 1994; 86:527-537.
13. Rodriguez J, Hart WR. Endometrial cancers occurring 10 or more years after pelvic irradiation for carcinoma. Int J Gynecol Pathol 1982; 1:135-144.
14. Kurman R, Kaminsky P, Norris H. The behavior of endometrial hyperplasia. A long-term study of "untreated" hyperplasia in 170 patients. Cancer 1985; 56:403-412.
15. Tavassoli F, Kraus FT. Endometrial lesions in uteri resected for atypical endometrial hyperplasia. Am J Clin Pathol 1978; 70:770-779.
16. Benedet JL, Bender H, Jones H, et al. FIGO staging classifications and clinical practice guidelines in the management of gynecologic cancers. Int J Gynecol Obstet 2000; 70:209-262.
17. Zaino RJ, Kurman RJ, Diana KL, et al. The utility of the revised International Federation of Gynecology and Obstetrics histologic grading of endometrial adenocarcinoma using a defined nuclear grading system. A Gynecologic Oncology Group study. Cancer 1995; 75:81-86.
18. Scully RE, Poulson H, Sobin LH. International histological classification and histologic typing of female genital tract tumors. Berlin: Springer-Verlag; 1994.
19. Frauenhoffer EE, Zaino RJ, Wolff TV, et al. Value of endocervical curettage in the staging of endometrial carcinoma. Int J Gynecol Pathol 1987; 6:195-202.
20. Burk JR, Lehman HF, Wolf FS. Inadequacy of Papanicolaou smears in the detection of endometrial cancer. N Engl J Med 1974; 291:191-192.
21. Mitchell H, Giles G, Medley G. Accuracy and survival benefit of cytological prediction of endometrial carcinoma on routine cervical smears. Int J Gynecol Pathol 1993; 12:34-40.
22. Sjolin KE. Cytologic findings and their significance in gynecology: clinico-pathologic and cytologic correlation. Acta Obstet Gynecol Scand 1970; 49:7-12.
23. Christopherson WM, Mendez WM, Parker JE, et al. Carcinoma of the endometrium: a study of changing rates over a 15-year period. Cancer 1971; 27:1005-1008.
24. Nahhas WA, Lung CJ, Rudolph JH. Carcinoma of the corpus uteri: a 10-year review of 225 patients. Obstet Gynecol 1971; 38:564-570.
25. Frick HCI, Munnell EW, Richart RM, et al. Carcinoma of the endometrium. Am J Obstet Gynecol 1973; 115:663-676.

26. Lederer H, Lambourne A. The results of screening by cervical cytology and of histological examination of gynaecological operation specimens. J Obstet Gynaecol Br Commonw 1973; 80:67-71.

27. vandenBosch T, Vandendael A, Wranz P, et al. Cervical cytology in menopausal women at high risk for endometrial disease. Eur J Cancer Prev 1998; 7:149-152.

28. Schneider ML, Wortmann M, Weigel A. Influence of the histologic and cytologic grade and the clinical and post-surgical stage on the rate of endometrial carcinoma detection by cervical cytology. Acta Cytol 1986; 30:616-622.

29. Reagan JW, Ng ABP. The cells of endometrial cancer. In: Wied GL, Keebler CM, Koss LG, et al, editors. Compendium on diagnostic cytology. 7th ed. Chicago: Tutorials of Cytology; 1992. p.126.

30. Berg JW, Durfee GR. The cytological presentation of endometrial carcinoma. Cancer 1958; 11:158-172.

31. Koss LG, Durfee GR. Cytologic diagnosis of endometrial carcinoma. Result of ten years of experience. Acta Cytol 1962; 6:519-531.

32. Reagan JW. Cytologic aspects of endometrial neoplasia. Acta Cytol 1980; 24:488-489.

33. Vuopala S. Diagnostic accuracy and clinical applicability of cytological and histological methods for investigating endometrial carcinoma. Acta Obstet Gynecol Scand 1977; 70 (Suppl):1-72.

34. Demirkiran F, Arvas M, Erkun E, et al. The prognostic significance of cervico-vaginal cytology in endometrial cancer. Eur J Gynaecol Oncol 1995; 16:403-409.

35. Fukuda K, Mori M, Uchiyama M, et al. Preoperative cervical cytology in endometrial carcinoma and its clinicopathologic relevance. Gynecol Oncol 1999; 72:273-277.

36. Eddy GL, Wojtowycz MA, Piraino PS, et al. Papanicolaou smears by the Bethesda System in endometrial malignancy: utility and prognostic importance. Obstet Gynecol 1997; 90:999-1003.

37. Koss LG. Proliferative disorders and carcinoma of the endometrium. In: Koss LG, editor. Diagnostic cytology and its histologic bases. Philadelphia: J.B. Lippincott; 1992. pp.535-586.

38. Fahey MT, Irwig L, Macaskill P. Meta-analysis of Pap test accuracy. Am J Epidemiol 1995; 141:680-689.

39. Ng ABP. Endometrial hyperplasia and carcinoma and extrauterine cancer. In: Bibbo M, editor. Comprehensive cytopathology. Philadelphia: W.B. Saunders; 1997. pp.251-277.

40. Guidos BJ, Selvaggi SM. Detection of endometrial adenocarcinoma with the ThinPrep (R) Pap test-trade mark. Diagn Cytopathol 2000; 23:260-265.

41. Gray JA, Nguyen GK. Cytologic detection of endometrial pathology by Pap smears. Diagn Cytopathol 1999; 20:181-182.

42. Tajima M, Inamura M, Nakamura M, Sudo Y, Yamagishi K. The accuracy of endometrial cytology in the diagnosis of endometrial adenocarcinoma. Cytopathology 1998; 9:369-380.

43. Tao LC. Direct intrauterine sampling: the IUMC Endometrial Sampler. Diagn Cytopathol 1997; 17:153-159.

44. Vuopala S, Klemi PJ, Maenpaa J, et al. Endobrush sampling for endometrial cancer. Acta Obstet Gynecol Scand 1989; 68:345-350.

45. Milan AR, Markley RL, Fisher RS, et al. Endometrial cytology: using the Milan-Markley technic. Obstet Gynecol 1976; 48:111-116.

46. Ueda M, Ueki M, Kumaga K, et al. Clinical evaluation of the Endosearch sampler in endometrial cytology: a preliminary report. J Med 1994; 25:305-318.

47. Palermo VG. Interpretation of endometrium obtained by the Endo-Pap sampler and a clinical study of its use. Diagn Cytopathol 1985; 1:5-12.

48. Yazigi R, Sanchez J, Duarte I, et al. Cytologic detection of endometrial carcinoma by the endocyte technique. Gynecol Oncol 1983; 16:346-351.

49. Schachter A, Beckerman A, Bahary C, et al. The value of cytology in the diagnosis of endometrial pathology. Acta Cytol 1980; 24:149-152.

50. Gravlee LCJ. Jet-irrigation method for the diagnosis of endometrial adenocarcinoma: its principle and accuracy. Obstet Gynecol 1969; 34:168-172.

51. Isaacs JH, Wilhoite RW. Aspiration cytology of the endometrium: office and hospital sampling procedures. Am J Obstet Gynecol 1974; 118:679-687.

52. Inoue Y, Ikeda M, Kimura K, et al. Accuracy of endometrial aspiration in the diagnosis of endometrial cancer. Acta Cytol 1983; 27:477-481.

53. Sato S, Yaegashi N, Shikano K, et al. Endometrial cytodiagnosis with the Uterobrush and Endocyte. Acta Cytol 1996; 40:907-910.

54. Maksem JA. Ciliated cell adenocarcinoma of the endometrium diagnosed by endometrial brush cytology and confirmed by hysterectomy: a case report detailing a highly efficient cytology collection and processing technique. Diagn Cytopathol 1997; 16:78-82.

55. Boon ME, Luzzatto R, Brucker N, et al. Diagnostic efficacy of endometrial cytology with the Abradul cell sampler supplemented by laser scanning confocal microscopy. Acta Cytol 1996; 40:277-282.

56. Skaarland E. New concept in diagnostic endometrial cytology: diagnostic criteria based on composition and architecture of large tissue fragments in smears. J Clin Pathol 1986; 39:36-43.

57. Reagan JW, Ng ABP. The cells of uterine adenocarcinoma. In: Wied GL, editor. Monographs in clinical cytology. 2nd ed. New York: S, Karger AG; 1973. pp.96-112.

58. Smith RA, Breitkopf DM, Wong JY, et al. Comparison of endometrial cytology to endometrial histology in the detection of hyperplasia and carcinoma. Obstet Gynecol 2000; 95:S28.

59. Wu HH, Harshbarger KE, Berner HW, et al. Endometrial brush biopsy (Tao brush): histologic diagnosis of 200 cases with complementary cytology: an accurate sampling technique for the detection of endometrial abnormalities. Am J Clin Pathol 2000; 114:412-418.

60. Porrazzi LC, Quarto F, Maiello FM, et al. The value of endometrial cytology by scraping in 1,798 cases: screening in asymptomatic women and diagnosis in symptomatic ones. Diagn Cytopathol 1987; 3:112-120.

61. Mencaglia L. Endometrial cytology: six years of experience. Diagn Cytopathol 1987; 3:185-190.

62. Sato S, Matsunaga G, Konno R, et al. Mass screening for cancer of the endometrium in Miyagi Prefecture, Japan. Acta Cytol 1998; 42:295-298.

63. Raab SS. Can glandular lesions be diagnosed on Pap smears? Diagn Cytopathol 2000; 23:127-133.

64. Raab SS, Snider TE, Potts SA, et al. Atypical glandular cells of undetermined significance. Diagnostic accuracy and interobserver variability using select cytologic criteria. Am J Clin Pathol 1997; 107:299-307.

65. Salomão DR, Hughes JH, Raab SS. Atypical glandular cells of undetermined significance, favor endometrial origin: criteria for separating low-grade endometrial carcinoma from benign endometrial lesions. Acta Cytol 2002; 46:458-464.

66. Kurman R, Solomon D. The Bethesda System for reporting cervical/vaginal diagnoses. New York: Springer-Verlag, 1994.

67. Ng ABP, Reagan JW, Cechner RL. The precursors of endometrial cancer: a study of their cellular manifestations. Acta Cytol 1973; 17:439-448.

68. Boschann HW. Cytometry on normal and abnormal endometrial cells. Acta Cytol 1958; 2:520-522.

69. deBrux JA, Froment-Dupre J. Cytology of endometrial hyperplasia. Acta Cytol 1958; 2:613-617.

70. Bibbo M, Bartels PH, Bahr GF, et al. Data bank for endometrial cells. Operation of the TICAS file project. Acta Cytol 1970; 14:574-582.

71. Arrighi AA. Cytology of endometrial hyperplasia. Acta Cytol 1958; 2:613.

72. Ferreira CA. Cytology of endometrial hyperplasia. Acta Cytol 1958; 2:617.

73. Skaarland E. Nuclear size and shape of epithelial cells from the endometrium: lack of value as a criterion for differentiation between normal, hyperplastic, and malignant conditions. J Clin Pathol 1985; 38:502-506.

74. Ishii Y, Fujii M. Criteria for differential diagnosis of complex hyperplasia or beyond in endometrial cytology. Acta Cytol 1997; 41:1095-1102.

75. Kashimura M, Baba S, Shinohara M, et al. Cytologic findings in endometrial hyperplasia. Acta Cytol 1988; 32:335-340.

76. Lozowski MS, Mishriki Y, Solitare GB. Factors determining the degree of endometrial exfoliation and their diagnostic implications in endometrial adenocarcinoma. Acta Cytol 1986; 30:623-627.

77. Akin MR, Nguyen GK. Cytologic manifestations of advanced endometrial adenocarcinomas in cervical-vaginal smears. Diagn Cytopathol 1999; 20:108-110.

78. Ng ABP, Reagan JW, Hawkiczek S, et al. Significance of endometrial cells in the detection of endometrial carcinoma and its precursors. Acta Cytol 1974; 18:356-361.

79. Benson PA. Psammoma bodies found in cervico-vaginal smears, case report. Acta Cytol 1973; 17:64-66.

80. Differding JT. Psammoma bodies in a vaginal smear. Acta Cytol 1967; 11:199-201.

81. Seltzer V, Spitzer M. Psammoma bodies in papillary adenocarcinoma of the endocervix. Int J Gynecol Pathol 1988; 2:216-221.

82. Mussett R, Nuovo V. Une observation de tumeur vegetante de l'ovaire reconnue et traitee relativement precocement, grace a la methode des frottis vaginaux. Bull Assoc Gynec Obstet 1950; 2:408.

83. Navratil E. Mittels des zelltestes nach papanicolaou festgestelltes primares adenokarzinom des ovars und adenokarzinom der tube. Krebsarzt 1951; 6:66-72.

84. Fujimoto I, Masubuchi S, Miwa H, et al. Psammoma bodies found in cervicovaginal and/or endometrial smears. Acta Cytol 1982; 26:317-322.

85. Valicenti JJF, Priester SK. Psammoma bodies of benign endometrial origin in cervicovaginal cytology. Acta Cytol 1977; 21:550-552.

86. Jenkins DM, Goulden R. Psammoma bodies in cervical cytology smears. Acta Cytol 1977; 21:112-113.

87. Luzzatto R, Sisson G, Luzzatto L, et al. Psammoma bodies and cells from in situ fallopian tube carcinoma in endometrial smears: a case report. Acta Cytol 1996; 40:295-298.

88. Takashina T, Ono M, Kanda Y, et al. Cervicovaginal and endometrial cytology in ovarian cancer. Acta Cytol 1988; 32:159-162.

89. Karpas CM, Bridge MF. Endometrial adenocarcinoma with psammomatous bodies. Am J Obstet Gynecol 1963; 87:935-941.

90. Kirkland N, Hardy N. Psammoma bodies found in cervicovaginal smears: a case report. Acta Cytol 1979; 23:131-133.

91. Spjut HJ, Kaufman RH, Carrig SS. Psammoma bodies in the cervicovaginal smear. Acta Cytol 1964; 8:352-355.

92. Kern SB. Prevalence of psammoma bodies in Papanicolaou-stained cervicovaginal smears. Acta Cytol 1991; 35:81-88.

93. Cassano PA, Saigo PE, Hajdu SI. Comparison of cytohormonal status of postmenopausal women with cancer to age-matched controls. Acta Cytol 1986; 30:93-98.

94. Stoll P. Vaginal smears in menopause. Acta Cytol 1960; 4:148-150.

95. Efstratiades M, Tamvakopoulou E, Papatheodorou B, Batrinos M. Postmenopausal vaginal cytohormonal pattern in 597 healthy women and 301 patients with genital cancer. Acta Cytol 1982; 26:126-130.

96. Gronroos M, Tyrkko J, Siiteri PK, et al. Cytolysis and karyopyknosis in postmenopausal vaginal smears as markers of endometrial cancer, diabetes and obesity: studies based on a ten-year follow-up. Acta Cytol 1986; 30:628-632.

97. Reagan JW. Can screening for endometrial cancer be justified? Acta Cytol 1980; 24:87-89.

98. Berry AV, Livni NM, Epstein N. Some observations on cell morphology in the cytodiagnosis of endometrial carcinoma. Acta Cytol 1969; 13:530-533.

99. Long MR, Doko F, Taylor JHC. Nucleoli and nucleolar ribonucleic acid in nonmalignant and malignant human endometria. Am J Obstet Gynecol 1958; 75:1002-1014.

100. Anderson WAD. Pathology. 5th ed. St. Louis: Mosby; 1966. p.74.

101. Papanicolaou GN. Atlas of exfoliative cytology. Cambridge: Harvard University Press; 1954.

102. Yang GC, Wan LS, Papellas J, Waisman J. Compact cell blocks: use for body fluids, fine needle aspirations and endometrial brush biopsies. Act Cytol 1998; 42:703-706.

103. Meisels A, Jolicoeur C. Criteria for the cytologic assessment of hyperplasias in endometrial samples obtained by the Endopap Endometrial Sampler. Acta Cytol 1985; 29:297-302.

104. Koss LG, Schreiber K, Oberlander SG, et al. Detection of endometrial carcinoma and hyperplasia in asymptomatic women. Obstet Gynecol 1984; 64:1-11.

105. Coscia-Porrazzi LO. Cytologic criteria of hyperplastic lesions in endometrial samples obtained by the endocyte sampler. Diagn Cytopathol 1988; 4:283-287.

106. Shrago SS. The Arias Stella reaction. A case report of a cytologic presentation. Acta Cytol 1977; 21:310-313.

107. Kobayashi TK, Fujimoto T, Okamoto H, et al. Cytologic evaluation of atypical cells in cervicovaginal smears from women with tubal pregnancies. Acta Cytol 1983; 27:28-32.

108. Murad TM, Terhart K, Flint A. Atypical cells in pregnancy and postpartum smears. Acta Cytol 1981; 25:623-630.

109. Benoit JL, Kini SR. Arias-Stella reaction-like changes in endocervical glandular epithelium in cervical smears during pregnancy and postpartum states: a potential diagnostic pitfall. Diagn Cytopathol 1996; 14:349-355.

110. Chhieng DC, Elgert PA, Cangiarella JF, et al. Cytology of polypoid adenomyomas: a report of two cases. Diagn Cytopathol 2000; 22:176-180.

111. Kim HS, Underwood D. Adenocarcinomas in the cervicovaginal Papanicolaou smear: analysis of a 12-year experience. Diagn Cytopathol 1991; 7:119-124.

112. Babkowski RC, Wilbur DC, Rutkowski MA, et al. The effects of endocervical canal topography, tubal metaplasia, and high canal sampling on the cytologic presentation of non-neoplastic endocervical cells. Am J Clin Pathol 1996; 105:403-410.

113. Heaton RB, Harris TF, Larson DM, et al. Glandular cells derived from direct sampling of the lower uterine segment in patients status post-cervical cone biopsy: a diagnostic dilemma. Am J Clin Pathol 1996; 106:511-516.

114. dePeralta-Venturino MN, Purslow MJ, Kini SR. Endometrial cells of the "lower uterine segment" (LUS) in cervical smears obtained by endocervical brushings: a source of potential diagnostic pitfall. Diagn Cytopathol 1995; 12:263-268.

115. Frank TS, Bhat N, Noumoff JS, et al. Residual trophoblastic tissue as a source of highly atypical cells in the postpartum cervicovaginal smear. Acta Cytol 1991; 35:105-108.

116. Ehrmann RL. Atypical endometrial cells and stromal breakdown of two case reports. Acta Cytol 1975; 19:463-469.

117. Gupta PK, Burroughs F, Luff RD, et al. Epithelial atypias associated with intrauterine contraceptive devices (IUD). Acta Cytol 1978; 22:286-291.

118. vonLudinghausen M, Anastasiadis P. Anatomic basis of endometrial cytology. Acta Cytol 1984; 28:555-562.

119. Mulvany NJ, Khan A, Ostor A. Arias-Stella reaction associated with cervical pregnancy. Report of a case with a cytologic presentation. Acta Cytol 1994; 38:218-222.

120. Ng ABP, Reagan JW. Normal benign and neoplastic processes simulating adenocarcinoma of uterus. In: Wied GL, Keebler CM, Koss LG, et al, editors. Compendium on diagnostic cytology. 6th ed. Chicago: Tutorials of Cytology; 1990. p.176.

121. Shidham VB, Dayer AM, Basir Z, et al. Cervical cytology and immunohistochemical features in endometrial adenocarcinoma simulating microglandular hyperplasia: a case report. Acta Cytol 2000; 44:661-666.

122. Ducatman BS, Wang HH, Jonasson JG, et al. Tubal metaplasia: a cytologic study with comparison to other neoplastic and non-neoplastic conditions of the endocervix. Diagn Cytopathol 1993; 9:98-105.

123. Mulvany NJ, Surtees V. Cervical/vaginal endometriosis with atypia: a cytohistopathologic study. Diagn Cytopathol 1999; 21:188-193.

124. Hanau CA, Begley N, Bibbo M. Cervical endometriosis: a potential pitfall in the evaluation of glandular cells in cervical smears. Diagn Cytopathol 1997; 16:274-280.

125. Zuna RE, Erroll M. Utility of the cervical cytologic smear in assessing endocervical involvement by endometrial carcinoma. Acta Cytol 1996; 40:878-884.

126. Costa MJ, Kenny MB, Naib ZM. Cervicovaginal cytology in uterine adenocarcinoma and adenosquamous carcinoma. Comparison of cytologic and histologic findings. Acta Cytol 1991; 35:127-134.

127. Patten JSF. Diagnostic cytology of the uterine cervix. 2nd ed. New York: S, Karger AG; 1978.

128. Buschmann C, Hergenrader M, Porter D. Keratin bodies: a clue in the cytological detection of endometrial adenoacanthoma. Report of two cases. Acta Cytol 1974; 18:297-299.

129. Becker SN. Keratin bodies and pseudokeratin bodies endometrial adenoacanthoma versus "ligeneous" vaginitis. Acta Cytol 1976; 20:486-488.

130. Wright CA, Leiman G, Burgess SM. The cytomorphology of papillary serous carcinoma of the endometrium in cervical smears. Cancer 1999; 87:12-18.

131. Kuebler DL, Nikrui N, Bell DA. Cytologic features of endometrial papillary serous carcinoma. Acta Cytol 1989; 33:120-126.

132. Kusuyama Y, Yoshida M, Imai H, et al. Secretory carcinoma of the endometrium. Acta Cytol 1988; 33:127-130.

133. Vooijs PG, Ng AB, Wentz WB. The detection of vaginal adenosis and clear cell carcinoma. Acta Cytol 1973; 17:59-63.

134. Wolinska WH, Melamed MR. Clear cell endometrial adenocarcinoma in a young woman: report of a case detected by cytology. Gynecol Oncol 1979; 8:119-120.

135. Ohwada M, Suzuki M, Ohno T, et al. Appearance of primary endometrial and ovarian clear cell adenocarcinoma 17 months postpartum: a case report. Acta Cytol 1998; 42:765-768.

136. Galvera-Davidson H, Fernandez A, Navarro J, et al. Mucinous metaplasia to neoplastic lesions in endometrial samples with cytohistologic correlation. Diagn Cytopathol 1989; 5:150-153.

137. Yoshida M, Kusuyama Y, Imai H, et al. A case of mucinous adenocarcinoma of the endometrium. J Jpn Soc Clin Cytol 1987; 26:1154-1157.

138. Helper TK, Dockerty MB, Randall LM. Primary adenocarcinoma of the cervix. Am J Obstet Gynecol 1952; 63:800-808.

139. Mikuta JJ, Celebre JA. Adenocarcinoma of the cervix. Obstet Gynecol 1969; 33:753-756.

140. Leminen A, Paavonen J, Forss M, et al. Adenocarcinoma of the uterine cervix. Cancer 1990; 65:53-59.

141. Hopkins MP, Morley GW. A comparison of adenocarcinoma and squamous cell carcinoma of the cervix. Obstet Gynecol 1991; 77:912-917.

142. Horowitz IR, Jacobson LP, Zucker PK, et al. Epidemiology of adenocarcinoma of the cervix. Gynecol Oncol 1988; 31:25-31.

143. Anderson GH, Benedet JL, LeRiche JC, et al. Invasive cancer of the cervix in British Columbia: a review of the demography and screening histories of 437 cases seen from 1985-1988. Obstet Gynecol 1992; 80:1-4.

144. Parazzini F, LaVecchia C. Epidemiology of adenocarcinoma of the cervix. Gynecol Oncol 1990; 39:40-46.

145. Peters RK, Chao A, Mack TM, et al. Increased frequency of adenocarcinoma of the uterine cervix in young women in Los Angeles county. J Natl Cancer Inst 1986; 76:423-428.

146. Alfsen GC, Thoresen SO, Kristensen GB, et al. Histopathologic subtyping of cervical adenocarcinoma reveals increasing incidence rates of endometrioid tumors in all age groups: a population based study with review of all nonsquamous cervical carcinomas in Norway from 1966 to 1970, 1976 to 1980, and 1986 to 1990. Cancer 2000; 89:1291-1299.

147. Brinton LA, Tashima KT, Lehman HF, et al. Epidemiology of cervical cancer by cell type. Cancer Res 1987; 47:1706-1711.

148. Ireland D, Hardiman P, Monaghan JM. Adenocarcinoma of the uterine cervix: a study of 73 cases. Obstet Gynecol 1985; 65:82-85.

149. Anton-Culver H, Bloss JD, Bringman D, et al. Comparison of adenocarcinoma and squamous cell carcinoma of the uterine cervix: a population based epidemiologic study. Am J Obstet Gynecol 1992; 186:1507-1514.

150. Hurt GW, Silverberg SG, Frable WJ, et al. Adenocarcinoma of the cervix: histopathologic and clinical features. Am J Obstet Gynecol 1977; 129:304-315.

151. Teshima S, Shimosato Y, Kishi K, et al. Early stage adenocarcinoma of the uterine cervix. Histopathologic analysis with consideration of histogenesis. Cancer 1985; 56:167-172.

152. Kudo R, Sagae S, Hayakawa O, et al. Morphology of adenocarcinoma in situ and microinvasive adenocarcinoma of the uterine cervix: a cytologic and ultrastructural study. Acta Cytol 1991; 35:109-116.

153. Brand E, Berek JS, Hacker NF. Controversies in the management of cervical adenocarcinoma. Obstet Gynecol 1988; 71:261-269.

154. Fu YS, Berek JS, Hilborne LH. Diagnostic problems of in situ and invasive adenocarcinomas of the uterine cervix. Appl Pathol 1987; 5:47-56.

155. Maier RC, Norris HJ. Coexistence of cervical intraepithelial neoplasia with primary adenocarcinoma of the endocervix. Obstet Gynecol 1980; 56:361-364.

156. Qizilbash AH. In situ and microinvasive adenocarcinoma of the uterine cervix. J Clin Pathol 1975; 64:155-170.

157. Wilczynski SP, Bergen S, Walker J, et al. Human papillomavirus and cervical cancer: analysis of histopathological features associated with different viral types. Hum Pathol 1988; 19:697-704.

158. Tase T, Okagaki T, Clark BA, et al. Human papillomavirus types and localization in adenocarcinoma and adenosquamous carcinoma of the uterine cervix: a study by in situ hybridization. Cancer Res 1988; 48:993-998.

159. Griffin NR, Dockey D, Lewis FA, et al. Demonstration of low frequency of human papilloma virus DNA in cervical adenocarcinoma and adenocarcinoma in situ by polymerase chain reaction and in situ hybridization. Int J Gynecol Pathol 1991; 10:36-43.

160. Jones MW, Silverberg SG. Cervical adenocarcinoma in young women: possible relationship to microglandular hyperplasia and use of oral contraceptives. Obstet Gynecol 1989; 73:984-989.

161. Kaminski PF, Norris HJ. Coexistence of ovarian neoplasms and endocervical adenocarcinoma. Obstet Gynecol 1984; 64:553-556.

162. Chen RJ, Chang DY, Yen ML, et al. Prognostic factors of primary adenocarcinoma of the uterine cervix. Gynecol Oncol 1998; 69:157-164.

163. Chen RJ, Lin YH, Chen CA, et al. Influence of histologic type and age on survival rates for invsive cervical carcinoma in Taiwan. Gynecol Oncol 1999; 73:184-190.

164. Kleine W, Rau K, Schwoeorer D, et al. Prognosis of the adenocarcinoma of the cervix uteri: a comparative study. Gynecol Oncol 1989; 35:145-149.

165. Saigo PE, Cain JM, Kim WS, et al. Prognostic factors in adenocarcinoma of the uterine cervix. Cancer 1986; 57:1584-1593.

166. Kilgore LC, Soong SJ, Gore H, et al. Analysis of prognostic features in adenocarcinoma of the cervix. Gynecol Oncol 1988; 31:137-153.

167. Wright TC, Kurman RJ, Ferenczy A. Carcinoma and other tumors of the cervix. In: Kurman RJ, editor. Blaustein's pathology of the female genital tract. New York: Springer-Verlag; 1994. pp.229-326.

168. Berek JS, Hacker NF, Fu YS, et al. Adenocarcinoma of the uterine cervix: histologic variables associated with lymph node metastases and survival. Obstet Gynecol 1985; 65:46-52.

169. Raju KS, Kjorstad KE, Abeler V. Prognostic factors in the treatment of stage 1B adenocarcinoma of the cervix. Int J Gynecol Cancer 1991; 1:69-74.

170. Lee KR, Flynn CE. Early invasive adenocarcinoma of the cervix. Cancer 2000; 89:1048-1055.

171. Koss LG. Adenocarcinoma and related tumors of the uterine cervix. In: Koss LG, editor. Diagnostic cytology and its histologic bases. Philadelphia: J.B. Lippincott; 1992. pp.513-534.

172. Zaino RJ. Glandular lesions of the uterine cervix. Mod Pathol 2000; 13:261-274.

173. Nguyen GK, Jeannot AB. Exfoliative cytology of in situ and microinvasive adenocarcinoma of the uterine cervix. Acta Cytol 1983; 28:461-467.

174. Betsill WLJ, Clark AH. Early endocervical glandular neoplasia. I. Histomorphology and cytomorphology. Acta Cytol 1986; 30:115-126.

175. Lee KR, Manna EA, Jones MA. Comparative cytologic features of adenocarcinoma in situ of the uterine cervix. Acta Cytol 1991; 35:117-126.

176. Saigo PE, Wolinska WH, Kim WS, et al. The role of cytology in the diagnosis and follow-up of patients with cervical adenocarcinoma. Acta Cytol 1985; 29:785-794.

177. Angel C, duBeshter B, Lin YL. Clinical presentation and management of stage I cervical adenocarcinoma: a 25-year experience. Gynecol Oncol 1992; 44:71-78.

178. Boddington MM, Spriggs AI, Cowdrell RH. Adenocarcinoma of the uterine cervix: cytological evidence of a long preclinical evolution. Br J Obstet Gynaecol 1976; 83:900-903.

179. Kristensen GB, Skyggebjerg KD, Holund B, et al. Analysis of cervical smears obtained within three years of the diagnosis of invasive cervical cancer. Acta Cytol 1991; 35:47-50.

180. Benoit AG, Krepart GV, Lotocki RJ. Results of prior cytologic screening in patients with a diagnosis of stage I carcinoma of athe cervix. Am J Obstet Gynecol 1984; 148:690-694.

181. Korhonen MO. Adenocarcinoma of the uterine cervix. Acta Pathol Microbiol Immunol Scand 1978; 264:1-51.

182. Ayer B, Pacey F, Greenberg M. The cytologic diagnosis of invasive adenocarcinoma of the cervix uteri. Cytopathology 1991; 2:181-191.

183. Gay JD, Donaldson LD, Goellner JR. False-negative results in cervical cytologic studies. Acta Cytol 1985; 29:1043-1046.

184. Jaworski RC, Pacey NF, Greenberg ML, et al. The histologic diagnosis of adenocarcinoma in situ and related lesions of the cervix uteri: adenocarcinoma in situ. Cancer 1988; 61:1171-1181.

185. Abell MR, Gosling JRG. Gland cell carcinoma (adenocarcinoma) of the uterine cervix. Am J Obstet Gynecol 1962; 83:729.

186. Crum CP, Cibas ES, Lee KR. Glandular precursors, adenocarcinomas, and their mimics. In: Crum CP, Cibas ES, Lee KR, editors. Pathology of early cervical neoplasia. New York: Churchill Livingstone; 1997. pp.177-240.

187. Nguyen GK, Daya D. Cervical adenocarcinoma and related lesions: cytodiagnostic criteria and pitfalls. Pathol Annu 1993; 28:53-75.

188. Ayer B, Pacey F, Greenberg M. The cytologic diagnosis of adenocarcinoma in situ of the cervix uteri and related lesions. II. Microinvasive adenocarcinoma. Acta Cytol 1988; 32:318-324.

189. Bousfield L, Pacey R, Young Q, et al. Expanded cytologic criteria for the diagnosis of adenocarcinoma in situ of the cervix and related lesions. Acta Cytol 1980; 24:283-296.

190. van Aspert van Erp AJ, Grootenboer van't Hof AE, et al. Endocervical columnar cell intraepithelial neoplasia (ECCIN). III. Interobserver variability in feature use. Anal Cell Pathol 1996; 10:115-135.

191. Clark AH, Betsill WLJ. Early endocervical glandular neoplasia. II. Morphometric analysis of the cells. Acta Cytol 1986; 30:127-134.

192. Pacey NF, Ng ABP. Glandular neoplasms of the uterine cervix. In: Bibbo M, editor. Comprehensive cytopathology. Philadelphia: W.B. Saunders; 1997. p.231-250.

193. Johnson JE, Rahemtulla A. Endocervical glandular neoplasia and its mimics in ThinPrep Pap tests: a descriptive study. Acta Cytol 1999; 43:369-375.

194. van Aspert van Erp AJ, Grootenboer van't Hof BE, et al. Identifying cytologic characteristics and grading endocervical columnar cell abnormalities: a study aided by high-definition television. Acta Cytol 1997; 41:1659-1670.

195. Silverberg SG, Hurt WG. Minimal deviation adenocarcinoma (adenoma malignum) of the cervix: a reappraisal. Am J Obstet Gynecol 1975; 121:971-975.

196. Young RH, Scully RE. Minimal deviation endometrioid adenocarcinoma of the uterine cervix: a report of five cases of a distinctive neoplasm that may be misinterpreted as benign. Am J Surg Pathol 1993; 17:660-665.

197. Kaminski PF, Maier RC. Clear cell adenocarcinoma of the cervix unrelated to diethylstilbestrol exposure. Obstet Gynecol 1983; 62:720-727.

198. McGowan L, Young RH, Scully RE. Peutz-Jeghers syndrome with adenoma malignum of the cervix: a report of two cases. Gynecol Oncol 1980; 10:125-133.

199. Kaku T, Enjoji M. Extremely well-differentiated adenocarcinoma (adenoma malignum) of the cervix. Int J Gynecol Pathol 1983; 2:28-41.

200. Gilks CB, Young RH, Aguirre P, et al. Adenoma malignum (minimal deviation adenocarcinoma) of the uterine cervix: a clinicopathological and immunohistochemical analysis of 26 cases. Am J Surg Pathol 1989; 13:717-729.

201. Szyfelbein WM, Young RH, Scully RE. Adenoma malignum of the cervix: cytologic findings. Acta Cytol 1984; 28:691-698.

202. Ishii K, Katsuyama T, Ota H, et al. Cytologic and cytochemical features of adenoma malignum of the uterine cervix. Cancer 1999; 87:245-253.

203. Fukazawa I, Iwasaki H, Endo N. A case report of adenoma malignum of the uterine cervix. Acta Cytol 1992; 36:780.

204. Sato S, Ito K, Konno R, et al. Adenoma malignum: report of a case with cytologic and colposcopic findings and immunohistochemical staining with antimucin monoclonal antibody HIK-1083. Acta Cytol 2000; 44:389-392.

205. Granter SR, Lee KR. Cytologic findings in minimal deviation adenocarcinoma (adenoma malignum) of the cervix: a report of seven cases. Am J Clin Pathol 1996; 105:327-333.

206. Ghorab Z, Mahmood S, Schinella R. Endocervical reactive atypia: a histologic-cytologic study. Diagn Cytopathol 2000; 22:342-346.

207. Yahr LJ, Lee KR. Cytologic findings in microglandular hyperplasia of the cervix. Diagn Cytopathol 1991; 7:248-251.

208. Valente PT, Schantz HD, Schultz M. Cytologic atypia associated with microglandular hyperplasia. Diagn Cytopathol 1994; 10:326-331.

209. Selvaggi SM, Haefner HK. Microglandular endocervical hyperplasia and tubal metaplasia: pitfalls in the diagnosis of adenocarcinoma on cervical smears. Diagn Cytopathol 1997; 16:168-173.

210. Pacey F, Ayer B, Greenberg M. The cytologic diagnosis of adenocarcinoma in situ of the cervix uteri and related lesions. III. Pitfalls in diagnosis. Acta Cytol 1988; 32:325-330.

211. Fiorella RM, Casafrancisco D, Yokota S, Kragel PF. Artifactual endocervical atypia induced by endocervical brush collection. Diagn Cytopathol 1994; 11:79-83.

212. Pisharodi LR, Jovanoska S. Spectrum of cytologic changes in pregnancy: a review of 100 abnormal cervical smears, with emphasis on diagnostic pitfalls. Acta Cytol 1995; 39:905-908.

213. Murad TM, August C. Radiation-induced atypia: a review. Diagn Cytopathol 1985; 1:137-152.

214. Shield PW. Chronic radiation effects: a correlative study of smears and biopsies from the cervix and vagina. Diagn Cytopathol 1995; 13:107-119.

215. Siziopikou KP, Wang HH, Abu-Jawdeh G. Cytologic features of neoplastic lesions in endocervical glands. Diagn Cytopathol 1997; 17:1-7.

216. Noller KL, Decker GG, Dockerty MB, et al. Mesonephric (clear cell) carcinoma of the vagina and cervix: a retrospective analysis. Obstet Gynecol 1974; 43:640-644.

217. Herbst AL, Cole P, Norusis MJ, et al. Epidemiologic aspects and factors related to survival in 384 registry cases of clear cell adenocarcinoma of the vagina and cervix. Am J Obstet Gynecol 1979; 135:876-886.

218. Kaminski PF, Norris HJ. Minimal deviation carcinoma (adenoma malignum) of the cervix. Int J Gynecol Pathol 1983; 2:141-152.

219. Young QA, Pacey NF. The cytologic diagnosis of clear cell adenocarcinoma of athe cervix uteri. Acta Cytol 1978;22:3-6.

220. Zhou C, Matisic JP, Clement PB, et al. Cytologic features of papillary serous adenocarcinoma of the uterine cervix. Cancer 1997; 81:98-104.

221. Lang G, Dallenbach-Hellweg G. The histogenetic origin of cervical mesonephric hyperplasia and mesonephric adenocarcinoma of the uterine cervix studied with immunohistochemical methods. Int J Gynecol Pathol 1990; 9:145-157.

222. Young RH, Scully RE. Villoglandular papillary adenocarcinoma of the uterine cervix: a clinicopathologic analysis of 13 cases. Cancer 1989; 63:1773-1779.

223. Jones MW, Silverberg SG, Kurman RJ. Well-differentiated villoglandular adenocarcinoma of the uterine cervix: a clinicopathological study of 24 cases. Int J Gynecol Pathol 1992; 12:1-7.

224. Hopson L, Jones MA, Boyce CR, et al. Papillary villoglandular carcinoma of the cervix. Gynecol Oncol 1990; 39:221-224.

225. Ballo MS, Silverberg SG, Sidawy MK. Cytologic features of well-differentiated villoglandular adenocarcinoma of the cervix. Acta Cytol 1996; 40:536-540.

226. Chang WC, Matisic JP, Zhou C, et al. Cytologic features of villoglandular adenocarcinoma of the uterine cervix: comparison with typical endocervical adenocarcinoma with a villoglandular component and papillary serous carcinoma. Cancer 1999; 87:5-11.

227. Young RH, Clement PB. Pseudoneoplastic glandular lesions of the uterine cervix. Semin Diagn Pathol 1991; 8:234-249.

228. Dinh TV, Woodruff JD. Adenoid cystic and adenoid basal carcinomas of the cervix. Obstet Gynecol 1985; 65:705-709.

229. Ferry JA, Scully RE. Adenoid cystic carcinoma and adenoid basal carcinoma of the uterine cervix: a study of 28 cases. Am J Surg Pathol 1988; 12:134-144.

230. Prempree T, Willasanta U, Tang CK. Management of adenoic cystic carcinoma of the uterine cervix (cylindroma). Cancer 1980; 46:1631-1635.

231. Grafton WD, Kamm RC, Cowley LH. Cytologic characteristics of adenoid cystic carcinoma of the cervix uteri. Acta Cytol 1976; 20:164-166.

232. Dayton V, Henry M, Stanley MW, et al. Adenoid cystic carcinoma of the uterine cervix. Cytologic features. Acta Cytol 1990; 34:125-128.

233. Bittencourt AL, Guimaraes JP, Barbosa HS, et al. Adenocystic carcinoma of the uterine cervix: report of six cases and review of the literature. Acta Med Port 1979; 1:697-706.

234. Ravinsky E, Safneck JR, Chantziantoniou N. Cytologic features of primary adenoid cystic carcinoma of the uterine cervix. A case report. Acta Cytol 1996; 40:1304-1308.

235. Peterson LS, Neumann AA. Cytologic features of adenoid basal carcinoma of the uterine cervix. A case report. Acta Cytol 1995; 39:563-568.

236. Powers CN, Stastny JF, Frable WJ. Adenoid basal carcinoma of the cervix: a potential pitfall in cervicovaginal cytology. Diagn Cytopathol 1996; 14:172-177.

237. Lemoine NR, Hall PA. Epithelial tumors metastatic to the uterine cervix: a study of 33 cases and review of the literature. Cancer 1986; 57:2002-2005.

238. Way S. Carcinoma metastatic in the cervix. Gynecol Oncol 1980; 9:298-302.

239. Kumar NB, Hart WR. Metastases to the uterine corpus from extragenital cancer. A clinicopathologic study of 63 cases. Cancer 1982; 50:2163-2169.

240. Mazur MT, Hsueh S, Gersell DJ. Metastases to the female genital tract. Analysis of 325 cases. Cancer 1984; 53:1978-1984.

241. Vinette-Leduc D, Yazdi HM, Payn G, Villeneuve N. Metastatic salivary duct carcinoma to the uterus: report of a case diagnosed by cervical smear. Diagn Cytopathol 1999; 21:271-275.

242. Parsons L, Taymor MD. Carcinoma of the breast metastatic to the peritoneum as a source of positive vaginal smears. Am J Obstet Gynecol 1953; 66:194-196.

243. Queiroz C, Bacchi CE, Oliveira C, et al. Cytologic diagnosis of vaginal metastasis from renal cell carcinoma: a case report. Acta Cytol 1999; 43:1098-1100.

244. Gupta D, Balsara G. Extrauterine malignancies: role of Pap smears in diagnosis and management. Acta Cytol 1999; 43:806-813.

245. Figge DC, de Alvarez RD. Diagnosis of ovarian carcinoma by vaginal cytology. Obstet Gynecol 1956; 8:655-663.

246. Rubin DK, Frost JK. The cytologic detection of ovarian cancer. Acta Cytol 1963; 7:191-195.

247. Takashina T, Ito E, Kudo R. Cytologic diagnosis of primary tubal cancer. Acta Cytol 1985; 29:367-372.

248. Wachtel E. Cytology of ovarian carcinoma. In: Transactions of the Sixth Annual Meeting of the Inter-Society Cytology Council. 1959. pp.69-75.

249. Fidler HK, Lock DR. Carcinoma of the fallopian tube detected by cervical smears. Am J Obstet Gynecol 1954; 67:1103-1111.

250. Dance EF, Fullmer CD. Extrauterine carcinoma cells observed in cervico-vaginal smears. Acta Cytol 1970; 14:187-191.

251. Garret R. Extrauterine tumor cells in vaginal and cervical smears. Obstet Gynecol 1959; 14:21-27.

252. Masukawa T. Intestinal, endometrial, and ovarian carcinoma detection and diagnosis by vaginal-cervical smears. Marquette Med Rev 1968; 34:Winter.

253. Masukawa T, Wada Y, Mattingly RF, et al. Cytologic detection of minute ovarian, endometrial and breast carcinomas, with emphasis on clinical-pathological approaches. Acta Cytol 1973; 17:316-319.

254. McGarvey RN. Cytologic diagnosis of ovarian cancer; report of case, review of literature. Obstet Gynecol 1955; 5:257-261.

255. Graham RM, VanNiekerk WA. Vaginal cytology in cancer of the ovary. Acta Cytol 1962; 6:496-499.

256. Sedlis A. Primary carcinoma of the fallopian tube. Obstet Gynecol Survey 1961; 16:209-226.

257. Song YS. Significance of positive vaginal smears in extrauterine carcinomas. Am J Obstet Gynecol 1957; 73:341-348.

258. Maher CF, Haran MV, McLaughlin J. Abnormal cervical ctyology leading to the diagnosis of a primary serous adenocarcinoma of the peritoneum. Aust NZJ Obstet Gynaecol 1996; 36:100-101.

259. Pairwuti S. Results of Pap smear examinations in women with abnormal ovaries. J Med Assoc Thai 1991; 74:248-252.

260. Minato H, Shimizu M, Hirokawa M, et al. Adenocarcinoma in situ of the fallopian tube: a case report. Acta Cytol 1998; 42:1455-1457.

261. Hirai Y, Chen JT, Hamada T, et al. Clinical and cytologic aspects of primary fallopian tube carcinoma. A report of ten cases. Acta Cytol 1987; 31:834-840.

262. Benson PA. Cytologic diagnosis in primary carcinoma of fallopian tube. Case report and review. Acta Cytol 1974; 18:429-434.

263. Hopfel-Kreiner I, Mikuz G. Accidental cytological findings in routine vaginal smear in primary carcinoma of the fallopian tube. Pathol Res Pract 1978; 163:163-167.

264. Fox CH. Adnexal malignancy detected by cervical cytology. Am J Obstet Gynecol 1978; 132:148-150.

265. Takashina N, Hirai Y, Yamauchi K, et al. Clinical usefulness of endometrial aspiration cytology and CA-125 in the detection of fallopian tube carcinoma. Acta Cytol 1997; 41:1445-1450.

266. Jobo T, Arai M, Iwaya H, Kato Y, et al. Usefulness of endometrial aspiration cytology for the preoperative diagnosis of ovarian carcinoma. Acta Cytol 1999; 43:104-109.

267. Angeles MA, Saigo PE. Cytologic findings in rectovaginal fistulae. Acta Cytol 1994; 38:373-376.

268. Clark AH, Betsill WLJ. A morphometric study of primary adenocarcinoma of the vagina. Acta Cytol 1986; 30:323-333.

269. Melnick S, Cole P, Anderson D, et al. Rates and risks of diethylstilbestrol-related clear-cell adenocarcinoma of the vagina and cervix: an update. N Engl J Med 1987; 316:514-516.

270. Trimble E, Rubinstein LV, Menck HR, et al. Vaginal clear cell adenocarcinoma in the United States. Gynecol Oncol 1996; 61:113-115.

271. Taft PD, Robboy SJ, Herbst AL, et al. Cytology of clear-cell adenocarcinoma of genital tract in young females: review of 95 cases from the registry. Acta Cytol 1974; 18:279-290.

272. Hanselaar AG, Boss EA, Massuger LF, Bernheim JL. Cytologic examination to detect clear cell adenocarcinoma of the vagina or cervix. Gynecol Oncol 1999; 75:338-344.

273. Bibbo M, Ali I, Al-Naqeeb M, et al. Cytologic findings in female and male offspring of DES treated mothers. Acta Cytol 1975; 19:568-572.

274. Fishman DA, Williams S, Small JW, et al. Late recurrences of vaginal clear cell adenocarcinoma. Gynecol Oncol 1996; 62:128-132.

275. Jimenez-Ayala M, Martinez-Cabruja R, Casado ML, et al. Serous surface papillary carcinoma of the ovary metastatic to a cervical polyp: a case report. Acta Cytol 1996; 40:765-769.

276. Korhonen M, Stenback F. Adenocarcinoma metastatic to the uterine cervix. Gynecol Obstet Invest 1984; 17:57-65.

277. Imachi M, Tsukamoto N, Amagase H, et al. Metastatic adenocarcinoma to the uterine cervix from gastric cancer: a clinicopathologic analysis of 16 cases. Cancer 1993; 71:3472-3477.

278. Nguyen GK. Cytopathologic aspects of a metastatic malignant mixed müllerian tumor of the uterus: report of a case with trans-abdominal fine needle aspiration biopsy. Acta Cytol 1982; 26:521-526.

279. Kashimura M, Kashimura Y, Matsuyama T, et al. Adenocarcinoma of the uterine cervix metastatic from primary stomach cancer: cytologic findings in six cases. Acta Cytol 1983; 27:54-58.

280. Mallow DW, Humphrey PA, Soper JT, et al. Metastatic lobular carcinoma of the breast diagnosed in cervicovaginal samples: a case report. Acta Cytol 1997; 41:549-555.

281. Matsuura Y, Saito R, Kawagoe T, Toki N, Sugihara K, Kashimura M. Cytologic analysis of primary stomach adenocarcinoma metastatic to the uterine cervix. Acta Cytol 1997; 41:291-294.

282. McGill F, Adachi A, Karimi N, et al. Abnormal cervical cytology leading to the diagnosis of gastric cancer. Gynecol Oncol 1990; 36:101-105.

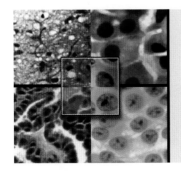

Unusual Malignancies of the Gynecologic Tract

CHAPTER
10

This chapter focuses on the nonglandular and non-squamous malignancies that may be detected on the Papanicolaou (Pap) test. These malignancies include primary neuroendocrine carcinomas, sarcomas, mixed epithelial-mesenchymal malignancies, malignant melanoma, trophoblastic tumors, lymphoma/leukemia, germ cell malignancies, and metastatic nonglandular malignancies.

 NEUROENDOCRINE CARCINOMAS

The following three types of neuroendocrine carcinoma have been described histologically: (1) small undifferentiated neuroendocrine carcinomas, (2) intermediately differentiated neuroendocrine carcinomas (e.g., atypical carcinoid tumors), and (3) cervical adenocarcinomas with neuroendocrine differentiation that are similar to intestinal carcinoid tumors. The first two neuroendocrine carcinomas usually are classified together as small cell carcinomas.[1] Although the cellular origin of these malignancies is unknown, they presumably arise from cells of argyrophil lineage.[1,2] If the Pap test shows neuroendocrine carcinoma, the site of origin is almost invariably the cervix or endocervix, although neuroendocrine carcinoma may arise in other gynecologic tract sites such as the ovary.

Small Cell Carcinomas

Small cell carcinomas are aggressive malignancies that comprise from 0.5% to 5% of all cervical neoplasms.[1,3,4] These malignancies may occur in both the young and elderly adult with a mean age of occurrence between 36 and 42 years.[1,3-7] As with most cervical squamous cell carcinomas and adenocarcinomas, the majority of women are asymptomatic, although bleeding may be observed.[4,8,9] Rarely, neuroendocrine hormonal symptoms may be present.[7] Compared with nonkeratinizing squamous cell carcinomas, small cell carcinomas are more commonly associated with human papillomavirus (HPV) type 18 and less commonly associated with HPV 16.[10,11] The scattered reports of these malignancies have indicated that detection occurs more often by histology than by cytology.[6,7]

Survival of women who have cervical small cell carcinoma mainly depends on tumor stage.[5-7,12] However, compared with cervical carcinoid-like tumors and stage-matched, poorly differentiated squamous cell carcinomas with small cell features, small cell carcinomas have a worse prognosis.[5,7] In other words, they are intrinsically highly aggressive cancers.

The cytologic findings of small cell carcinoma of the cervix are similar to those seen in the lung[7,13-16] (Box 10-1). The malignant cells, which may be seen in clusters and singly, possess high nuclear to cytoplasmic (N:C) ratios (Figure 10-1). The defining cytologic features are nuclear and the malignant cells show finely granular (salt and pepper) chromatin, nuclear molding, nuclear crush artifact, and a small or inconspicuous nucleolus (Figure 10-2). Similar to pulmonary small cell carcinomas, cervical small cell carcinomas may have a non–small cell component (large cell or mixed adenocarcinoma or squamous cell carcinoma). Squamous dysplastic cells may be admixed.

Ancillary studies may be helpful but are often not practical, especially for the cytologic diagnosis. Smears may be destained and then restained with the Grimelius stain (to demonstrate argyrophilia) or immunohistochemical stains such as synaptophysin and neuron-specific enolase.[17] The Grimelius stain is not sensitive and may display high background staining. Small cell carcinomas also may show little neuroendocrine immunohistochemical reactivity. In addition, conventional adenocarcinomas and squamous cell carcinomas may display neuroendocrine reactivity.[7,9] Electron microscopy may be used in some cases to demonstrate neuroendocrine granules.[18]

The differential diagnosis includes a squamous intraepithelial lesion (SIL) of small cell type, glandular neoplasia, malignant lymphoma, endometrial stromal sarcoma, metastatic carcinoma (e.g., breast origin), malignant melanoma, rhabdomyosarcoma, and primitive neuroectodermal tumor.[17] SILs show more nuclear hyperchromasia and coarser chromatin, and invasive squamous cell carcinomas may display a prominent nucleolus. The cytoplasm of glandular neoplasias has a wispy, foamy appearance, and although neoplastic glandular nuclei may be stripped, an absence of nuclear molding and crush artifact is evident. The possibil-

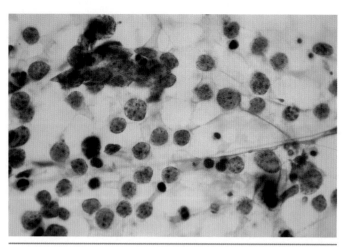

Figure 10-1 Small cell carcinoma on a Pap test of a 37-year-old woman. The neoplastic cells appear dissociated and have high nuclear to cytoplasmic (N:C) ratios and a salt-and-pepper nuclear chromatin pattern. The nucleoli are inconspicuous, and necrotic debris is present.

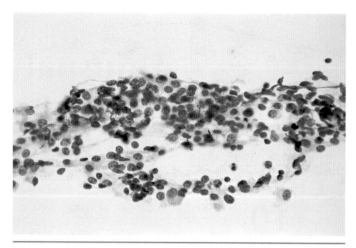

Figure 10-3 Carcinoid-like tumor on a Pap test of a 39-year-old woman. The neoplastic cells are seen in a loose cluster. The cells are dissociated, and single-stripped nuclei are present. The nuclei are round and are less atypical than the nuclei of a small cell carcinoma.

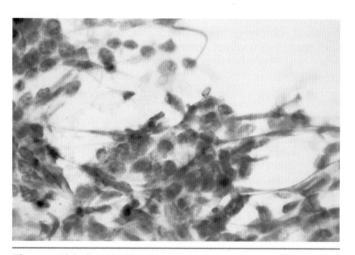

Figure 10-2 Small cell carcinoma on a Pap test of a 40-year-old woman. The neoplastic cells are seen in clusters and show nuclear molding and crush artifact.

BOX 10-1 CMF

Cytomorphologic Features of Small Cell Carcinoma

Cellular smears with cells in clusters or singly
High N:C ratios
Salt-and-pepper chromatin
Nuclear molding and crush artifact
Inconspicuous nucleolus
Non–small cell component may be present
Necrosis
Lack of lymphoglandular bodies

N:C, Nuclear to cytoplasmic.

BOX 10-2 CMF

Cytomorphologic Features of Carcinoid-Like Tumor

Cellular smears with monotonous cells in clusters or singly
Finely granular chromatin pattern
High N:C ratios
Lack of marked cytologic atypia
Nuclear molding
Lack of necrosis

ity of a metastatic small cell carcinoma from another site always should be considered.

Carcinoid-Like Tumor

Malignancies originally described as carcinoid tumors of the cervix are now thought to be adenocarcinomas with neuroendocrine differentiation.[1] In some foci, these malignancies histologically resemble intestinal carcinoids.[19-24] In other foci, these tumors show glandular features including mucin production. Wright and colleagues reported that these tumors are not associated with the carcinoid syndrome,[1] and it is unclear if pure carcinoid tumors exist.[25] Well-differentiated neuroendocrine carcinomas also may arise in the uterine corpus, ovary, or vagina. True carcinoid tumors from nongynecologic sites may metastasize to the gynecologic tract.

Cytologically, carcinoid-like tumors are characterized by a monotonous population of small cells with high N:C ra-

tios (Box 10-2). The malignant cells are often seen singly, although small cell clusters also may be present (Figure 10-3). The nuclei are round, and the chromatin pattern is finely granular; nucleoli are inconspicuous or absent. Necrosis generally is lacking except in cases in which mucosal ulceration has occurred. Glandular features, including cytoplasmic vacuoles and three-dimensional balls, are generally seen, and the mitotic rate may be brisk.

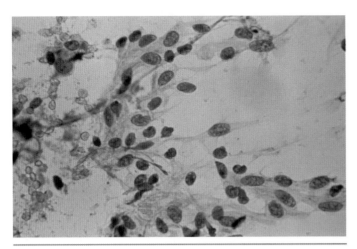

Figure 10-4   Leiomyosarcoma on a Pap test of a 58-year-old woman. In this well-differentiated leiomyosarcoma, the malignant cells are in loose clusters and are seen singly. The cells have elongated nuclei with even chromatin patterns.

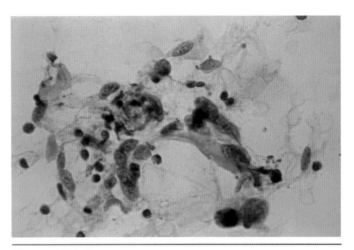

Figure 10-5   Leiomyosarcoma on a Pap test of a 81-year-old woman. The malignant cells are present in a loose cluster and have basophilic, poorly defined cytoplasmic boundaries. Variability in nuclear size is apparent. Necrotic debris and degenerated cells are present.

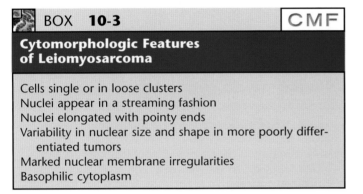

BOX **10-3**	CMF
Cytomorphologic Features of Leiomyosarcoma	

Cells single or in loose clusters
Nuclei appear in a streaming fashion
Nuclei elongated with pointy ends
Variability in nuclear size and shape in more poorly differentiated tumors
Marked nuclear membrane irregularities
Basophilic cytoplasm

 ## SARCOMAS

The sarcomas that have been reported on Pap tests include leiomyosarcoma, stromal sarcoma, rhabdomyosarcoma and fibrosarcoma. Sarcomas may arise from the ovary, fallopian tube, uterine corpus or cervix, or vagina.

Leiomyosarcoma

Leiomyosarcoma is the most common primary sarcoma of the gynecologic tract with the most common site of origin being the uterine myometrium. Leiomyosarcomas account for 1.3% of uterine malignancies, and the mean age of presentation is 52.[26-28] Signs and symptoms include an abdominal or pelvic mass, vaginal bleeding and/or lower abdominal pain.[27,29] Patient prognosis mainly depends on tumor stage,[30] and the overall 5-year survival rate is 15% to 25%.[26,28,31] It is extremely rare for a leiomyosarcoma to arise in the cervix or vagina.[32]

Histologically, the diagnostic separation of a leiomyosarcoma from a leiomyoma depends on cellularity, nuclear atypia, and the number of mitoses.[31] Leiomyosarcomas are graded histologically, and several histologic subtypes are recognized (e.g., epithelioid leiomyosarcoma, myxoid leiomyosarcoma).

Myometrial leiomyosarcomas rarely are diagnosed on cervicovaginal specimens because in most cases, they are not directly sampled (most are intramural), and leiomyosarcomas are not prone to shed cells even if they are in continuity with the endometrial cavity. Hajdu and Hajdu reported that of 38 patients with a leiomyosarcoma, only six had malignant cells on their Pap tests.[33] In some instances, myometrial leiomyosarcomas may extend into the endocervical canal and may be directly sampled. The leiomyosarcomas that are sampled tend to be of higher histologic grade.[34]

On the Pap test, the malignant cells of a conventional leiomyosarcoma, similar to the cells of many sarcomas, are spindle shaped (Box 10-3). These cells may be observed in small, loose clusters but are often seen singly. The cells may be arranged in interlacing fascicles or in a streaming fashion (Figure 10-4). Considerable variability in cell and nuclear size and shape from both case to case and microscopic field to field may be observed. Tumor cell cytoplasm is poorly delineated and basophilic (Figure 10-5). Cytoplasmic borders are absent in the loose cell clusters. The neoplastic nuclei are elongated and tend to have pointy ends (Figure 10-6). In the more poorly differentiated examples, multinucleation and bizarre nuclear forms are common. Nuclear membrane irregularities abound, and the nuclear chromatin is coarse but evenly dispersed. One or several prominent nucleoli often are easily recognizable. A tumor diathesis may be necrotic or finely granular.

Epithelioid leiomyosarcomas may resemble poorly differentiated carcinomas because the tumor cells have polygonal contours and better defined cytoplasmic boundaries compared with the nonepithelioid variants. Furthermore, the cells in epithelioid leiomyosarcomas may form three-dimensional clusters. A Pap test of myxoid leiomyosarcoma may show a large amount of myxoid material in which the neoplastic spindle cells may be sparse.

The differential diagnosis of leiomyosarcoma includes other sarcomas (e.g., malignant fibrous histiocytoma or fibrosarcoma), mixed müllerian tumors, and sarcomatoid carcinomas. A submucosal benign uterine leiomyoma may ulcerate and shed atypical cells (most likely as a result of reparative change), and these cells may be worrisome for a leiomyosarcoma.

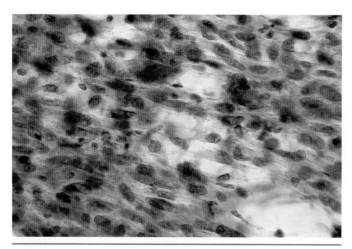

Figure 10-6 Leiomyosarcoma on a Pap test of a 59-year-old woman. The malignant cells have elongated nuclei and irregular nuclear membranes. The chromatin pattern is coarsely clumped. The cytoplasm is scant and the cytoplasmic borders are poorly defined. This large fragment of cells most likely is a result of direct sampling.

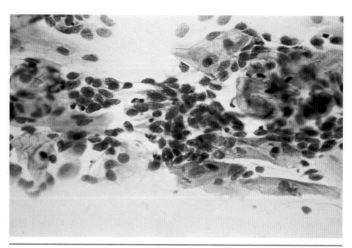

Figure 10-7 Low-grade endometrial stromal sarcoma on a Pap test of a 62-year-old woman. The neoplastic cells are seen in loose clusters, and the cytoplasm trails from the edges of the cells. The cytoplasm is basophilic, and the cells have high N:C ratios. These neoplastic stromal cells resemble normal stromal cells.

Endometrial Stromal Tumors

Endometrial stromal tumors may be subclassified as endometrial stromal nodule, low-grade endometrial stromal sarcoma, and high-grade endometrial stromal sarcoma. Endometrial stromal nodules are benign, whereas endometrial stromal sarcomas are capable of metastasizing. These neoplasms most often arise in the endometrium, but rarely have been reported to arise in extrauterine sites such as foci of endometriosis.

Endometrial stromal nodules make up less than 25% of all endometrial stromal tumors. The mean age at diagnosis is 47 years.[35] The main symptoms of an endometrial stromal nodule are bleeding and menorrhagia.[35] Histologically, the neoplastic cells resemble normal proliferative phase stromal cells, and the cells do not invade the myometrium.[35,36]

Endometrial stromal sarcomas comprise less than 10% of all uterine sarcomas; of these, 67% are low grade.[26] More than 50% are detected in premenopausal women.[37,38] The main clinical symptoms are abdominal pain, vaginal bleeding, and menorrhagia. Histologically, the individual neoplastic cells of a low-grade endometrial stromal sarcoma morphologically resemble the stromal cells of proliferative phase endometrium, but they invade the myometrium.[38,39] The neoplastic cells of a high-grade endometrial stromal sarcoma appear much more atypical. Survival is most strongly associated with tumor stage, and women with a stage I low-grade endometrial stromal sarcoma have a 5-year survival of greater than 80%.[37,38] Women who have a stage I high-grade endometrial stromal sarcoma have a 5-year survival of more than 50%.[37,40] Unusual variants of stromal tumors include uterine neoplasm resembling an ovarian sex cord tumor and combined smooth muscle-stromal tumor.[41,42]

The majority of endometrial stromal nodules and low-grade endometrial stromal sarcomas are not detected on Pap tests because the cells are not sufficiently atypical.[43,44] Some high-grade endometrial stromal sarcomas may be detected on a Pap test, particularly when these malignancies ulcerate the endometrial surface and shed cells.[44,45]

> **BOX 10-4**   **CMF**
>
> **Cytolomorphologic Features of Endometrial Stromal Sarcoma**
>
> Cellular differentiation depends on tumor grade
> Smears with few cells in loose clusters or single
> Low-grade tumors have a monomorphic appearance with cells that have an oval nucleus, high N:C ratios, and minimal nuclear atypia. The cytoplasm trails from the cell, lending a cometlike appearance
> High-grade tumors are pleomorphic with cells having bizarre nuclear forms, brisk mitotic rate, and nucleoli

In cytologic specimens the tumor cells of low-grade endometrial stromal sarcomas (and endometrial stromal nodules) resemble normal proliferative endometrial stromal cells in loosely cohesive clusters (Figure 10-7). The tumor cells are described as having a cometlike appearance, with the cytoplasm trailing from one edge of the nucleus (Box 10-4).[46,47] In the cell clusters, the cytoplasmic borders are poorly defined and the cytoplasm has a basophilic tincture. The cells mostly have a monomorphic appearance with round to slightly oval nuclei possessing mildly irregular nuclear borders. The N:C ratios are high. The chromatin is hyperchromatic and a small nucleolus may be observed. In a low-grade endometrial stromal sarcoma the cytologic atypia is minimal. However, if a large number of endometrial stromal cells with mildly atypical nuclei is present, a low-grade endometrial stromal sarcoma may be suspected.

The cytologic features of a high-grade endometrial stromal sarcoma usually are more reminiscent of other poorly differentiated sarcomas. Although some of the cells may be cytologically similar to normal endometrial stromal cells,[44] other cells may have a bizarre appearance with hyperchromatic and irregularly shaped nuclei and discernible nucleoli (Figure 10-8).[46,47] Mitotic figures may be identified easily.[43-45] Tumor diathesis may be present.[47]

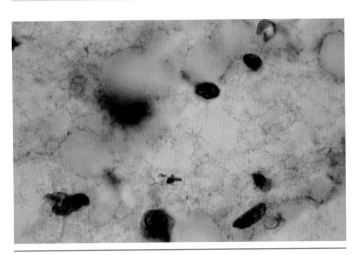

Figure 10-8 High-grade endometrial stromal sarcoma on a Pap test of a 55-year-old woman. The neoplastic cells are pleomorphic and are seen singly. Bizarre, hyperchromatic nuclei are present. The findings are similar to those of other high-grade sarcomas.

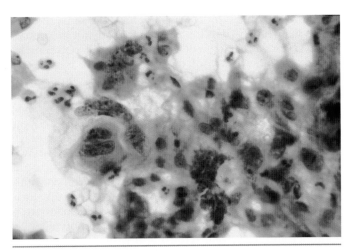

Figure 10-9 Rhabdomyosarcoma on a Pap test of a 6-year-old girl. The malignant cells are seen singly and are round to oval. The N:C ratios are high, and multinucleated forms are present.

BOX 10-5 CMF

Cytomorphologic Features of Rhabdomyosarcoma

Features similar to other small blue cell malignancies
Single cells and rare cell clusters
High N:C ratios
Nuclei eccentrically placed and round to oval
Chromatin may be hyperchromatic
Nuclear crush artifact may be seen
Eosinophilic cytoplasm with rare cells showing cross striations

---

Rhabdomyosarcoma

Embryonal rhabdomyosarcoma is the most common vaginal neoplasm in infants and children. The most common presentation is in a child less than 2 years of age with 90% occurring in children less than 5 years of age.[48,49] Rarely, rhabdomyosarcomas occur in the gynecologic tract of adults. In children, most embryonal rhabdomyosarcomas have a gross grapelike appearance, are of the subtype termed sarcoma botryoides, and may protrude from the vagina.[50] With chemotherapy and surgery the overall 3-year survival probably is more than 85%.[51]

Embryonal rhabdomyosarcomas usually are diagnosed on clinical findings and biopsy; consequently, a Pap test in a young child for a primary diagnosis of embryonal rhabdomyosarcoma generally is never performed. Histologically, the malignant cells lie below the epithelium, and unless mucosal ulceration is present, it would be highly unlikely for these malignant cells to be sampled on a smear.

Cytologically, embryonal rhabdomyosarcomas look similar to other small blue cell malignancies (Box 10-5). Pap tests show single round to spindle cells, occasional multinucleated cells, and rare loosely cohesive clusters. The neoplastic cell cytoplasm is eosinophilic, and cytoplasmic cross striations, a feature of skeletal muscle differentiation, rarely are seen (Figure 10-9). In an embryonal rhabdomyosarcoma, the malignant cell nuclei are eccentrically placed, round to oval, and may display a prominent nucleolus. The chromatin pattern tends to be open. If necessary, immunocytochemistry (i.e., reactivity for desmin, muscle specific actin, and myogenin) or electron microscopy may aid in confirming the diagnosis. Cells having a skeletal muscle appearance also may be seen in mixed müllerian tumors but are seen in a totally different clinical context.

Other Primary Sarcomas

Other pure sarcomas that have been described in the gynecologic tract include chondrosarcoma, liposarcoma, osteosarcoma, paraganglioma, malignant fibrous histiocytoma, alveolar soft part sarcoma, malignant rhabdoid tumor, angiosarcoma, and primitive neuroectodermal tumor. Of these rare primary gynecologic malignancies, alveolar soft part sarcoma has been described in Pap test specimens.[52] Alveolar soft part sarcomas are characterized by anaplastic mesenchymal cells having an epithelioid appearance; these cells contain abundant eosinophilic, granular cytoplasm and a large nucleus with a prominent nucleolus.[52]

 # MIXED EPITHELIAL-MESENCHYMAL MALIGNANCIES

The mixed epithelial-mesenchymal malignancies include mixed müllerian tumor, adenosarcoma, and carcinofibroma. Mixed müllerian tumors are composed of both malignant epithelial and mesenchymal components. Adenosarcomas are composed of benign epithelial elements and malignant mesenchymal elements. Carcinofibromas consist of malignant epithelial components and benign mesenchymal components.

Mixed Müllerian Tumors

Mixed müllerian tumors occur in the ovary, fallopian tube, endometrium, and cervix; an endometrial origin is the most common. The median age of clinical presentation is 65 years.[28,36,53] Symptoms include vaginal bleeding, lower abdominal pain, and a palpable mass lesion.[54,55] Women who develop these tumors generally have the same risk factors as women who develop endometrial adenocarcinomas; however, for women who develop mixed müllerian tumors, the association with prior radiation exposure is greater.[56] Primary ovarian mixed müllerian tumors comprise less than 1% of all primary ovarian malignancies, and patients usually present with abdominal enlargement and pelvic pain. For low-stage uterine mixed müllerian tumors, 5-year survival rates range from 40% to 50%.[57-59] For high-stage treated uterine mixed müllerian tumors, 5-year survival rates range from 25% to 30%.[57,58]

Histologically, the epithelial component of mixed müllerian tumors is an adenocarcinoma, squamous cell carcinoma, or a mixture of both carcinomas. The adenocarcinomatous component may consist of any subtype (e.g., endometrioid, clear cell, serous) and is more often poorly differentiated but occasionally well differentiated.[36,60,61] If the sarcomatous element is composed of elements normally found in the uterus (e.g., leiomyosarcoma or stromal sarcoma), the sarcomatous component is referred to as *homologous*. If the sarcomatous component is composed of elements not normally found in the uterus (e.g., rhabdomyosarcoma, osteosarcoma, or chondrosarcoma), the sarcomatous component is referred to as *heterologous*. Heterologous mixed müllerian tumors are more common. The nature of the sarcomatous element (i.e., heterologous or homologous) has no bearing on patient survival.[57,61]

Despite the name *mixed müllerian*, Silverberg and colleagues and others have argued that these malignancies most likely are of epithelial origin and the sarcomatous elements represent mesenchymal differentiation in an otherwise poorly differentiated carcinoma.[61,62]

The sensitivity of the Pap test for tumor detection depends on sampling method and tumor extent.[43,53,63-66] On Pap tests, Barwick and colleagues reported that only 27% of patients with an endometrial mixed müllerian tumors had the diagnosis made on the smear.[67] Costa and colleagues reported a sensitivity of detection of 61%,[65] and other authors have reported a similar sensitivity of detection.[43] With direct

endometrial sampling, sensitivity may approach 100%. Similar to endometrial adenocarcinomas, the malignant cells of mixed müllerian tumors are more frequently seen on the vaginal rather than the cervical smear.[68] The malignancy invariably is not detected on Pap tests in patients with ovarian mixed müllerian tumors, unless it is widely metastatic.

The Pap test is often bloody, and a tumor diathesis may be present (Box 10-6). If the malignancy has not extended into the cervix, the diathesis may be watery. On indirect samples, the carcinomatous component is seen more often than the sarcomatous component,[55] although both components may be present (Figure 10-10).[43,69] On direct samples, both components usually are evident.[63,70,71] When the carcinomatous component is an adenocarcinoma, the malignant cells appear similar to the cells seen in smears of pure endometrial adenocarcinoma (usually the endometrioid type is present). When the carcinomatous component is squamous, the Pap test may be indistinguishable from a smear of an invasive cervical squamous cell carcinoma. If the carcinomatous component is poorly differentiated, it may not be possible to classify the malignant cells as epithelial.[65]

On the Pap test, the sarcomatous component may be difficult to identify. Most commonly, malignant single spindle

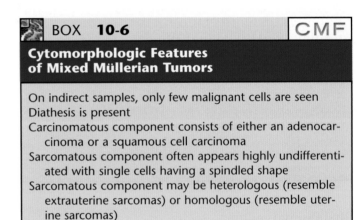

BOX   10-6   CMF

Cytomorphologic Features of Mixed Müllerian Tumors

On indirect samples, only few malignant cells are seen
Diathesis is present
Carcinomatous component consists of either an adenocarcinoma or a squamous cell carcinoma
Sarcomatous component often appears highly undifferentiated with single cells having a spindled shape
Sarcomatous component may be heterologous (resemble extrauterine sarcomas) or homologous (resemble uterine sarcomas)

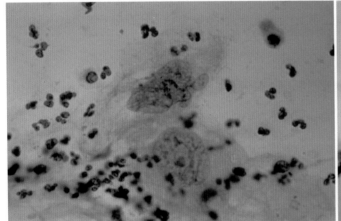

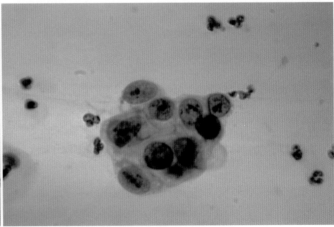

A   B

Figure 10-10   Mixed müllerian tumor on a Pap test of a 67-year-old woman. **A,** Two large multilobated malignant cells are admixed with acute inflammation. The cells have indistinct cytoplasmic boundaries. These cells represent the sarcomatous component of a mixed müllerian tumor. **B,** This photomicrograph is from the same patient as the photomicrograph shown in **A.** This group of cells represents an adenocarcinomatous component of a mixed müllerian tumor. The cells are seen in a small cluster with malignant nuclei along the edge. Nuclear overlap is present, and the nuclei have high N:C ratios. The cytoplasm is foamy, and the nuclear membranes are irregular in shape.

cells are seen.[63] These cells most often appear as undifferentiated mesenchymal cells and cannot be identified definitively as homologous or heterologous (Figure 10-11). The malignant spindle cells have an eccentrically placed nucleus, ill-defined cytoplasmic boundaries and eosinophilic or basophilic cytoplasm[71] (Figure 10-12). The chromatin is hyperchromatic and coarse. Multinucleation is common. In heterologous mixed müllerian tumors, skeletal muscle, chondroid, or osteoid differentiation may be appreciated.[69] A rhabdomyosarcoma component may display cytoplasmic cross striations; the malignant cells of a chondrosarcoma show bluish cytoplasm and round nuclei. The malignant cells of an osteosarcoma may be admixed with osteoid, which consists of strands of eosinophilic matrix. All of these events are extremely unusual.

On the Pap test, the differential diagnosis of mixed müllerian tumors includes pure sarcomas and sarcomatoid carcinomas.

Adenosarcomas

Adenosarcomas most often arise in the endometrium but also may occur in the cervix, ovary, fallopian tube, and paraovarian tissues.[26,72,73] The median age of presentation is 57 years, and the clinical symptoms include vaginal bleeding, pelvic pain, and an abdominal mass.[26] Adenosarcomas are not as aggressive as mixed müllerian tumors because only 25% of patients with adenosarcoma die of their tumor.[74,75]

Histologically, the glandular epithelial component most often is inactive but may be proliferative. The sarcomatous element is homologous in 75% to 80% of cases and heterologous in the remainder.[75,76] The cytologic features of the mesenchymal cells of adenosarcomas are similar to the features of the mesenchymal cells of mixed müllerian tumors, although a malignant epithelial component is lacking in adenosarcomas (Figure 10-13).

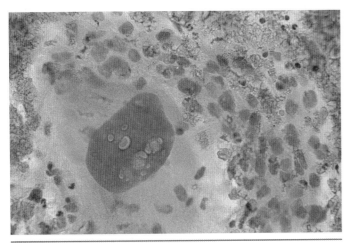

Figure 10-11 **Mixed müllerian tumor on a Pap test of an 80-year-old woman.** The sarcomatous component is homologous, and a large malignant sarcomatous cell is seen. The cytoplasm is abundant, and the nucleus is hyperchromatic and shows marked membrane irregularities. A carcinomatous component consists of a sheet of malignant cells.

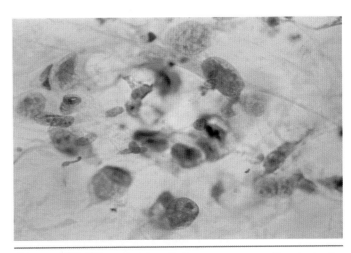

Figure 10-12 **Mixed müllerian tumor on a Pap test of a 66-year-old woman.** The sarcomatous component consists of single cells with eccentrically placed nuclei and eosinophilic cytoplasm.

A 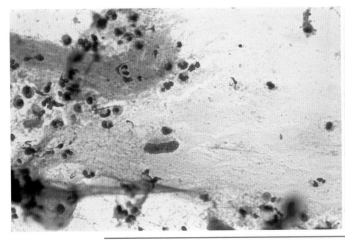 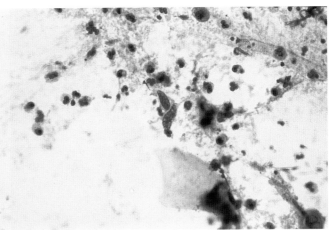 B

Figure 10-13 **Adenosarcoma on a Pap test of a 58-year-old woman. A,** The smear shows abundant necrosis and scattered single malignant cells. These cells have enlarged nuclei and high N:C ratios. **B,** Scattered large malignant cells are present in a background of necrosis. These cells have abundant cytoplasm and enlarged nuclei with pronounced nuclear membrane irregularities.

Carcinofibroma

Carcinofibromas are the least common of the mixed epithelial-mesenchymal malignancies. Direct endometrial sampling has shown a malignant glandular component and scattered nonepithelial cells without significant atypia.[77] The malignant epithelial cells appear identical to the carcinomas previously described.

MALIGNANT MELANOMA

Up to 5% of all malignant melanomas in women occur in the gynecologic tract.[78] Malignant melanomas more commonly occur on the vulva but also may arise in the vagina, particularly the distal one third,[79] cervix,[80-82] or ovary. Chung and colleagues reported that approximately 3% of vaginal malignancies are malignant melanomas.[83] The incidence of cervical malignant melanoma is very low. The mean age at diagnosis is 57 years with clinical symptoms including bleeding

and a mass.[83] The five-year survival rate is between 10% and 20%.[79,83] Metastatic malignant melanoma to the gynecologic tract is more common than a primary malignant melanoma, and most patients have a history of this malignancy before the secondary occurrence.[81,84-86] However, identification of a primary extragynecologic tract site may be made after the malignancy is identified in the gynecologic tract.[86] Melanoma metastatic to the endometrium has been detected on the Pap test and direct endometrial samples.[87]

The cytologic appearance of melanoma is myriad (Box 10-7). The most common Pap test appearance is the presence of mostly single cells with occasional cell clusters.[80,82,88-95] The single tumor cells most often have a plump, epithelioid appearance with basophilic cytoplasm and fine, lacy intracytoplasmic vacuoles (Figure 10-14). The cytoplasmic borders may be poorly delineated or sharp (Figure 10-15) when the cytoplasm has a metaplastic appearance. Intracytoplasmic melanin pigment may or may not be present.[82,86,96-98] Extracellular melanin or melanin in macrophages also may be noted. In some instances, the malignant cells may have a spindled appearance[88] (Figure 10-16). Bizarre giant cells may be seen[93,99] Malignant melanoma nuclei are large, round to oval, and peripherally located; multinucleation is fairly common. Intranuclear pseudoinclusions may be present.[84] The nuclei may be hyperchromatic or hypochromatic. Prominent nucleoli com-

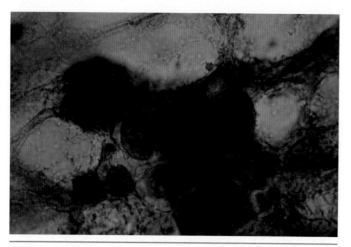

Figure 10-14 Malignant melanoma on a Pap test of a 72-year-old woman. The cells are seen in a cluster and have scant cytoplasm. The N:C ratios are high, and the chromatin pattern is coarse.

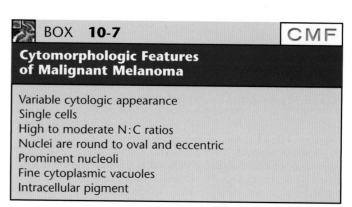

BOX   **10-7**   CMF

Cytomorphologic Features of Malignant Melanoma

Variable cytologic appearance
Single cells
High to moderate N:C ratios
Nuclei are round to oval and eccentric
Prominent nucleoli
Fine cytoplasmic vacuoles
Intracellular pigment

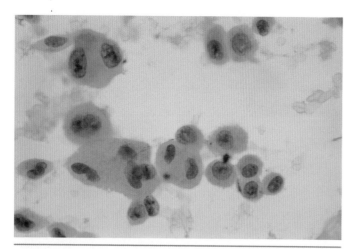

Figure 10-15 Malignant melanoma on a Pap test of a 45-year-old woman. Single cells with an occasional intranuclear cytoplasmic pseudo-inclusion are seen. The nuclei are large, and multinucleated neoplastic cells are present.

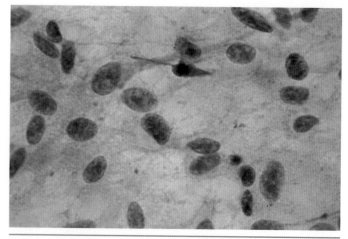

Figure 10-16 Malignant melanoma on a Pap test of a 66-year-old woman. The cells have a spindled appearance. The cytoplasmic boundaries are indistinct, and the nuclei have irregular nuclear membranes.

monly are noted. Immunohistochemical reactivity for HMB-45 and S-100 and negativity for keratin support the diagnosis of malignant melanoma.[100,101]

The differential diagnosis includes invasive squamous cell carcinoma, adenocarcinoma, and other sarcomas. Squamous cell carcinomas usually have more hyperchromatic nuclei, evidence of keratinization, an absence of a large prominent nucleolus, better-defined cytoplasmic borders, and an absence of melanin pigment. Adenocarcinomas generally show more cellular clusters (greater cohesion), more vacuolated cytoplasm, and an absence of melanin pigment. If malignant melanomas lack melanin pigment, separation from carcinomas may be impossible. Recall that benign melanocytic nevi also occur in the cervix and vagina and that benign melanocytes contain melanin pigment; these cells also could be mistaken on the Pap test for the cells of malignant melanoma.

GESTATIONAL TROPHOBLASTIC DISEASE

Gestational trophoblastic disease includes hydatidiform mole, invasive mole, choriocarcinoma, and placental site trophoblastic tumor. These lesions are characterized by abnormal proliferations of trophoblastic (e.g., cytotrophoblast, syncytiotrophoblast, and/or intermediate trophoblast) tissues.[102]

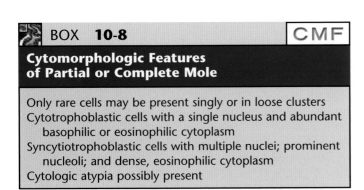

> **BOX 10-8**　　CMF
>
> ### Cytomorphologic Features of Partial or Complete Mole
>
> Only rare cells may be present singly or in loose clusters
> Cytotrophoblastic cells with a single nucleus and abundant basophilic or eosinophilic cytoplasm
> Syncytiotrophoblastic cells with multiple nuclei; prominent nucleoli; and dense, eosinophilic cytoplasm
> Cytologic atypia possibly present

Hydatidiform Moles

The incidence of hydatidiform mole in the United States and Europe ranges from 1:1000 to 1:2000.[103-105] In other areas of the world, such as Asia, the incidence is as high as 1:500.[104,106] Hydatidiform moles occur in women of reproductive age, particularly women younger than 20 years of age or older than 40 years of age.[105] Most often, hydatidiform moles originate in the uterus, but they also may arise in the fallopian tube or ovary. Clinically, women may have vaginal bleeding or excessive uterine enlargement.[107,108]

Hydatidiform moles may be subdivided into partial and complete moles. Complete moles comprise between 25% and 75% of all molar pregnancies.[109,110] Cytogenetic analysis has shown that most complete moles are 46XX and less often 46XY; in either instance, the chromosomes are androgenic (i.e., of paternal origin).[111,112] The karyotypes of partial moles most often are triploid (69XXY, 69XX, or 69XYY), but may be diploid or tetraploid.[112,113] Partial moles may be associated with an embryo or fetal tissue with congenital abnormalities.[113]

The greatest danger in women who have an hydatidiform mole is persistent or metastatic gestational trophoblastic disease. Postmolar trophoblastic disease includes persistent mole, invasive mole, and choriocarcinoma. In studies before the use of chemotherapy and sensitive assays for human chorionic gonadotropin (hCG), 16% of complete moles developed into invasive moles, and 2.5% into choriocarcinomas.[114,115] Some series have indicated that 5% of women with a partial mole have persistent or metastatic gestational trophoblastic disease.[110,116] The risk of progression to a choriocarcinoma is the same for an invasive mole as it is for a complete mole.[117]

The cytology of partial and complete moles is similar, although more atypia may be seen in complete moles. This atypia is insufficient to make a definitive separation. The neoplastic cells are of two kinds (Box 10-8). The first cell type is the cytotrophoblast, which is polygonal and has a large nucleus with a prominent nucleolus. Taki reported that the cytotrophoblast is similar in size to a decidual cell.[118] The nuclear chromatin is often open. The cytotrophoblastic cytoplasm is faint to clear and either basophilic or slightly eosinophilic (Figure 10-17). The second cell type

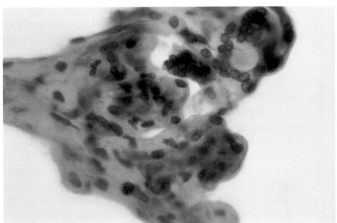
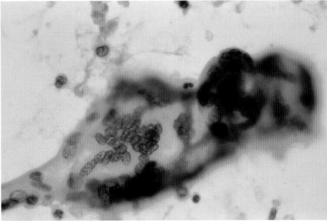

Figure 10-17　Complete mole on a Pap test of a 33-year-old woman. Cytotrophoblastic and syncytiotrophoblastic cells are present. The cytotrophoblastic cells are mononuclear and contain abundant basophilic cytoplasm. The syncytiotrophoblastic cells are multinuclear and contain dense cytoplasm.

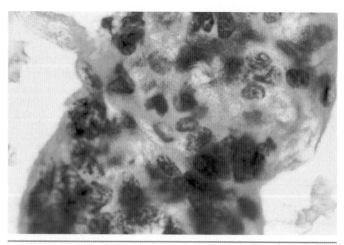

Figure 10-18 Choriocarcinoma on a Pap test of a 46-year-old woman. A cluster of malignant cytotrophoblastic and syncytiotrophoblastic cells is present. These cells have bizarre nuclei, and chorionic villi are not present.

is the syncytiotrophoblast, which is much larger than a cytotrophoblast and contains multiple nuclei with prominent nucleoli. The syncytiotrophoblastic cytoplasm is dense and eosinophilic.[118] On the Pap test, the cells may be seen in large clusters admixed with abundant blood.[118] Marked cytologic atypia may be seen, and on cytologic preparations, it may not be possible to separate a mole from a choriocarcinoma. In choriocarcinomas, villi are absent; although moles have villi, they usually are not present on the Pap test.

Invasive Moles

Invasive moles are hydatidiform moles in which molar tissue invades the myometrium or blood vessels and, in 20% to 40% of cases, metastasizes to extrauterine sites.[119] An invasive mole is the most common form of gestational trophoblastic disease after hydatiform mole. With chemotherapy, death from an invasive mole is very rare.[120] Histologically, molar villi and trophoblastic tissue are observed in the myometrium or at an extrauterine site. The cytologic preparations of invasive moles appear identical to the preparations of partial and complete moles.

Choriocarcinoma

Choriocarcinomas are malignant tumors that arise from trophoblastic tissue, most often from a preexisting mole. Hertig and Mansell reported that a choriocarcinoma may arise in one of 40 molar pregnancies but also may arise in ectopic pregnancies, abortions, and even in normal pregnancies.[121] Abnormal uterine bleeding is the most common presentation,[122] but patients also may present first with metastatic disease.[123] The survival rate for patients with choriocarcinoma who receive appropriate chemotherapy is approximately 80%.[124] Histologically, choriocarcinomas are characterized by sheets of trophoblastic cells (cytotrophoblasts, intermediate trophoblasts, and syncytiotrophoblasts) without chorionic villi (Figure 10-18). Choriocarcinomas demonstrate considerable cytologic atypia, and the nuclei in the trophoblastic cells may be markedly enlarged and mitoses may be easily identified. Multinucleated intermediate trophoblasts may be distinguished from syn-

cytiotrophoblasts by the lack of dense cytoplasm and eosinophilia (features seen in syncytiotrophoblasts). Extensive necrosis usually is present.

Placental Site Trophoblastic Tumor

Placental site trophoblastic tumors are composed mostly of intermediate trophoblast and are generally benign. They are the rarest forms of gestational trophoblastic disease. Clinically, women may present with signs and symptoms of a missed abortion and the serum hCG is low. Placental site trophoblastic tumors may be deeply invasive and may result in uterine perforation.[125] Ishi and colleagues reported that the cells of a placental site trophoblastic tumor are round or polygonal and have hyperchromatic, irregularly shaped nuclei.[126] However, the definitive diagnosis of placental site trophoblastic tumor is extremely difficult to make. The cells of a placental site trophoblastic tumor may be immunoreactive for human placental lactogen (hPL) and/or hCG.[126]

 ## HEMATOLYMPHOID MALIGNANCIES

Malignant lymphoma and leukemia may involve the gynecologic tract, most often as a manifestation of systemic disease. Leukemic involvement is a rather common occurrence in women dying of leukemia.[127] Approximately 6% of women dying of lymphoma have cervical involvement.[128] These women may exhibit vaginal bleeding or may have abdominal discomfort.[129] Most malignant lymphomas involving the gynecologic tract are of non-Hodgkin's type and of B-cell lineage.[130] Of malignant lymphomas of the cervix, 75% are large cell type, and 20% are low-grade follicular types.[131] Lathrop reported that 12% of all female genital tract malignant lymphomas were of the Hodgkin's type.[128] The sensitivity of detection of malignant lymphoma on the Pap test has been reported to range from 20% to 30%.[132,133] Ceelen and Sakurai reported the sensitivity of the Pap test for leukemic detection to be 28%.[134]

Pap tests of malignant large cell lymphoma shows a single cell population, high N:C ratios, small nucleoli, and coarse granular chromatin[135,136] (Figure 10-19). In small cell malignant lymphomas, a monomorphic population of small cells, roughly the size of red blood cells, is present (Figure 10-20). In Pap tests of Hodgkin's disease, Reed-Sternberg cells may be observed.[137] The differential diagnosis of malignant lymphoma on the Pap test includes follicular cervicitis, granulocytic sarcoma, small cell carcinoma, poorly differentiated carcinoma, and endometrial stromal sarcoma.[133,135,138-140] Myeloid leukemia is the most common type of leukemia to be seen on a gynecologic preparation; at a low power, the acute myeloid leukemic cells may resemble the cellular components seen in acute inflammation.

Lymphocytic cervicitis is the most common entity that may be confused with a malignant lymphoma or leukemia. In contrast with a hematolymphoid malignancy, lymphocytic cervicitis is characterized by a heterogeneous population of lymphoid cells and plasma cells; histiocytes may be prominent in lymphocytic cervicitis.

Cervical involvement by a granulocytic sarcoma, an extramedullary tumor of malignant granulocytes, needs to be separated from cervical involvement by leukemia. A Pap test of a granulocytic sarcoma (chloroma) is characterized

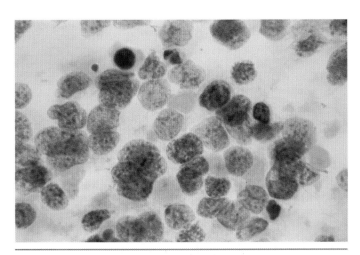

Figure 10-19 **Malignant large cell lymphoma on a Pap test of a 55-year-old woman.** The smear is cellular and shows numerous single cells. The cells have high N:C ratios, and the chromatin pattern is coarse. The nucleoli are small.

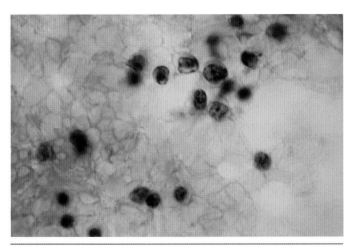

Figure 10-20 **Malignant well-differentiated lymphocytic lymphoma on a Pap test of a 66-year-old woman.** The smear is cellular and shows numerous monotonous small lymphoid cells. An absence of macrophages and larger lymphoid cells is evident.

by numerous large single cells and an absence of cell clusters.[141] The cells have a scant amount of eosinophilic cytoplasm and stain positively on a Leder stain.[141]

A more detailed discussion of the cytologic features of hematolymphoid malignancies is presented in Chapter 24.

 ## METASTATIC GERM CELL TUMORS

In addition to the ovary, malignant germ cell tumors may arise in the vagina, cervix, or endometrium and cells may be detected on the Pap test. Primary cervical germ cell tumors include teratomas and yolk sac tumors. Malignant germ cell tumors more often arise in the ovary, metastasize to other sites in the gynecologic tract, and subsequently shed cells. Hajdu and Nolan reported that the cytologic features of some germ cell malignancies such as dysgerminoma or embryonal carcinoma are sufficiently characteris-

tic for definitive diagnosis.[142] Chong and colleagues reported a case on a Pap test of a yolk sac tumor mimicking an adenocarcinoma that invaded the fallopian tube.[143] Chapter 25 contains a more in-depth description of the cytologic features of germ cell tumors.

References

1. Wright T, Ferenczy A, Kurman R. Carcinoma and other tumors of the cervix. In: Kurman RJ, editor. Blaustein's pathology of the female genital tract. New York: Springer-Verlag; 1994. pp.229-326.
2. Fetissof F, Serres G, Arbeille B. Argyrophilic cells and ectocervical epithelium. Int J Gynecol Pathol 1991; 10: 177-190.
3. Matsuyama M, Inoue T, Ariyoshi Y, et al. Argyrophil cell carcinoma of the uterine cervix with ectopic production of ACTH, beta-MSH, serotonin, histamine and amylase. Cancer 1979; 44:1813-1823.
4. Tateishi R, Wada A, Hayakawa K, et al. Argyrophil cell carcinomas (apudomas) of the uterine cervix: light and electron microscopic observations of 5 cases. Virchows Arch A 1975; 366:257-274.
5. Walker A, Mills S, Taylor P. Cervical neuroendocrine carcinoma: a clinical and light microscopic study of 14 cases. Int J Gynecol Pathol 1988; 7:64-74.
6. Silva E, Kott M, Ordonez N. Endocrine carcinoma intermediate cell type of the uterine cervix. Cancer 1984; 54:1705-1713.
7. Gersell D, Mazoujian G, Mutch D, et al. Small-cell undifferentiated carcinoma of the cervix: a clinicopathologic, ultrastructural, and immunocytochemical study of 25 cases. Am J Surg Pathol 1988; 12:684-698.
8. Lojek M, Fer M, Kasselberg A, et al. Cushing's syndrome with small cell carcinoma of the uterine cervix. Am J Med 1980; 69:140-144.
9. Scully R, Aguirre P, DeLellis R. Argyrophilia, serotonin and peptide hormones in the female genital tract and its tumors: review. Int J Gynecol Pathol 1984; 3:51-70.
10. Ambros R, Park J-S, Shah K. Evaluation of histologic, morphometric, and immunohistochemical criteria in the differential diagnosis of small cell carcinomas of the cervix with particular reference to human papillomavirus types 16 and 18. Mod Pathol 1991; 4:586-593.
11. Stoler M, Mills S, Gersell D, et al. Small cell neuroendocrine carcinoma of the cervix: A human papillomavirus type 18 associated cancer. Am J Surg Pathol 1991; 15: 28-32.
12. Barrett R, Davos I, Leuchter R, et al. Neuroendocrine features in poorly differentiated and undifferentiated carcinomas of the cervix. Cancer 1987; 60:2325-2330.
13. Groben P, Reddick R, Askin F. The pathologic spectrum of small cell carcinoma of the cervix. Int J Gynecol Pathol 1985; 4:42-57.
14. Joseph R, Enghardt M, Doiering D, et al. Small cell neuroendocrine carcinoma of the vagina. Cancer 1992; 70:784-789.
15. Fujii S, Konishi I, Ferenczy A, et al. Small cell undifferentiated carcinoma of the uterine cervix: histology, ultrastructure, and immunohistochemistry of two cases. Ultrastruct Pathol 1986; 10:337-346.
16. Kamiya M, Uei Y, Higo Y, et al. Immunocytochemical diagnosis of small cell undifferentiated carcinoma of the cervix. Acta Cytol 1993; 37:131-134.
17. Proca D, Keyhani-Rofagha S, Copeland L, et al. Exfoliative cytology of neuroendocrine small cell carcinoma of the endometrium: a report of two cases. Acta Cytol 1998; 42:978-982.

18. Ueda G, Shimizu C, Shimizu H, et al. An immunohisto-chemical study of small-cell and poorly differentiated car-cinomas of the cervix using neuroendocrine markers. Gynecol Oncol 1989; 34:164-169.

19. Habib A, Kaneko M, Cohen C. Carcinoid of the uterine cervix: a case report with light and electron microscopic studies. Cancer 1979; 43:535-538.

20. Stahl R, Demopoulos R, Bigelow B. Carcinoid tumor with a squamous cell carcinoma of the cervix. Gynecol Oncol 1981; 11:387-392.

21. Miles P, Herrara G, Mena H, et al. Cytologic findings in primary malignant carcinoid tumor of the cervix. Acta Cytol 1985; 29:1002-1008.

22. Lozowski W, Hajdu S, Melamed M. Cytomorphology of carcinoid tumors. Acta Cytol 1979; 23:360-365.

23. Albores-Saavedra J, Poucell S, Rodriquez-Martinez H. Primary carcinoid of the uterine cervix. Pathologica 1972; 10:185-193.

24. Albores-Saavedra J, Rodriquez-Martinez H, Larraza-Hernandez O. Carcinoid tumors of the cervix. Pathol Annu 1979; 14:273-291.

25. Kurman R, Norris H, Wilkinson E. Atlas of tumor pathol-ogy. 3rd series, Fascicle 4: tumors of the cervix, vagina and vulva. Washington, DC: Armed Forces Insititute of Pathology; 2000.

26. Zaloudek C, Norris H. Mesenchymal tumors of the uterus. In: Kurman RJ, editor. Blaustein's pathology of the female genital tract. New York: Springer-Verlag; 1994. pp.487-528.

27. Covens A, Nisker J, Chapman W, et al. Uterine sarcoma: an analysis of 74 cases. Am J Obstet Gynecol 1987; 156:370-374.

28. Wheelock J, Krebs H, Schneider V, et al. Uterine sarcoma: analysis of prognostic variables in 71 cases. Am J Obstet Gynecol 1985; 151:1016-1022.

29. Saksela E, Lampinen V, Precope B. Malignant mesenchy-mal tumors of the uterine corpus. Am J Obstet Gynecol 1974; 120:452-460.

30. Marchese M, Liskow A, Crum C, et al. Uterine sarcomas: a clinicopathologic study, 1965-1981. Gynecol Oncol 1984; 18:299-312.

31. Burns B, Curry R, Bell M. Morphologic features of prog-nostic significance in uterine smooth muscle tumors: a re-view of 84 cases. Am J Obstet Gynecol 1979; 135:109-114.

32. Curtin J, Saigo P, Slucher B, et al. Soft-tissue sarcoma of the vagina and vulva: a clinicopathologic study. Obstet Gynecol 1995; 86:269-272.

33. Hajdu S, Hajdu E. Cytopathology of sarcomas and other non-epithelial malignant tumors. Philadelphia: WB Saunders; 1976. pp.183-212.

34. Koss L. Uncommon malignant tumors of the female gen-ital tract. Philadelphia: JB Lippincott; 1992. pp.643-662.

35. Tavassoli F, Norris H. Mesenchymal tumors of the uterus. VII. A clinicopathological study of 60 endometrial stro-mal nodules. Histopathology 1981; 5:1-10.

36. Norris H, Roth E, Taylor H. Mesenchymal tumors of the uterus. II. A clinical and pathologic study of 31 mixed mesodermal tumors. Obstet Gynecol 1966; 28:57-63.

37. Berchuck A, Rubin S, Hoskins W, et al. Treatment of endometrial stromal tumors. Gynecol Oncol 1990; 36:60-65.

38. Chang K, Crabtree G, Lim-Tan S, et al. Primary uterine en-dometrial stromal neoplasms. A clinicopathologic study of 117 cases. Am J Surg Pathol 1990; 14:415-438.

39. Fekete P, Vellios F. The clinical and histologic spectrum of endometrial stromal neoplasms: a report of 41 cases. Int J Gynecol Pathol 1984; 3:198-212.

40. Larson B, Silfversward C, Nilsson B, et al. Endometrial stromal sarcoma of the uterus. A clinical and histopatho-logical study. The Radiumhemmet series 1936-1981. Eur J Obstet Gynecol Reprod Biol 1990; 35:239-249.

41. Clement P, Scully R. Uterine tumors resembling ovarian sex-cord tumors. A clinicopathologic analysis of 14 cases. Am J Clin Pathol 1976; 66:512-525.

42. Tang C, Toker C, Ances I. Stromomyoma of the uterus. Cancer 1979; 43:308-316.

43. Massoni E, Hajdu S. Cytology of primary and metastatic uterine sarcomas. Acta Cytol 1984; 28:93-100.

44. Morimoto N, Ozawa M, Kato Y, et al. Diagnostic value of mitotic activity in endometrial stromal sarcoma. Report of two cases. Acta Cytol 1982; 26:695-698.

45. Becker S, Wong J. Detection of endometrial stromal sar-coma in cervicovaginal smears: report of three cases. Acta Cytol 1980; 25:272-276.

46. Hsiu J-G, Stawicki M. The cytologic findings in two cases of stromal sarcoma of the uterus. Acta Cytol 1979; 23:487-489.

47. Becker S, Wong J. Detection of endometrial stromal sar-coma in cervicovaginal smears: reports of three cases. Acta Cytol 1981; 25:272-275.

48. Friedman M, Peretz B, Nissenbaum M, et al. Modern treat-ment of vaginal embryonal rhabdomyosarcoma. Obstet Gynecol Surv 1986; 41:614-618.

49. Hilgers D, Malkasian GJ, Soule E. Embryonal rhabdomyo-sarcoma (botryoid type) of the vagina: a clinicopatho-logic review. Am J Obstet Gynecol 1970; 107:484-502.

50. Bale P, Parsons R, Stevens M. Diagnosis and behavior of juvenile rhabdomyosarcoma. Hum Pathol 1983; 14:596-611.

51. Newton W, Soule E, Hamoudi A. Histopathology of child-hood sarcomas, intergroup rhabdomyosarcoma studies I and II: clinicopathologyc correlation. J Clin Oncol 1988; 6:67-75.

52. Zaleski S, Setum C, Benda J. Cytologic presentation of alveolar soft-part sarcoma of the vagina: a case report. Acta Cytol 1986; 30:665-670.

53. Macasaet M, Waxman M, Fruchter R, et al. Prognostic fac-tors in malignant mesodermal (müllerian) mixed tumors of the uterus. Gynecol Oncol 1985; 20:32-42.

54. Peters W, Kumar N, Fleming W, et al. Prognostic features of sarcomas and mixed tumors of the endometrium. Obstet Gynecol 1984; 63:550-556.

55. Shaw R, Lynch P, Wade-Evans T. Müllerian mixed tumour of the uterine corpus: a clinical and histopathological review of 28 patients. Br J Obstet Gynaecol 1983; 90:562-569.

56. Norris H, Taylor H. Post-irradiation sarcomas of the uterus. Obstet Gynecol 1965; 26:689-694.

57. Spanos W, Wharton J, Gomez L, et al. Malignant mixed müllerian tumors of the uterus. Cancer 1984; 53:311-316.

58. Schweizer W, Demopoulos R, Beller U, et al. Prognostic factors for malignant mixed müllerian tumors of the uterus. Int J Gynecol Pathol 1990; 9:129-136.

59. Vongtama V, Karlen J, Piver S, et al. Treatment, results and prognostic factors in stage I and II sarcomas of the corpus uteri. Am J Roentgenol 1976; 126:139-147.

60. Dinh T, Slavin R, Bhagavan B, et al. Mixed müllerian tu-mors of the uterus: a clinicopathologic study. Obstet Gynecol 1989; 74:388-392.

61. Silverberg S, Major F, Blessing J, et al. Carcinosarcoma (malignant mixed mesodermal tumor) of the uterus: a Gynecological Oncology Group pathologic study of 203 cases. Int J Gynecol Pathol 1990; 9:1-19.

62. Bitterman P, Chun B, Kurman R. The significance of ep-ithelial differentiation in mixed mesodermal tumors of the uterus: a clinicopathologic and immunohistochemi-cal study. Am J Surg Pathol 1990; 14:317-328.

63. An-Foraker S, Kawada C. Cytodiagnosis of endometrial malignant mixed mesodermal tumor. Acta Cytol 1985; 29:137-141.

64. Tenti P, Babilonti L, Fianza AL, et al. Cytology of malignant mixed mesodermal tumour of the uterus: experience of 10 cases. Eur J Gynaecol Oncol 1989; 10:125-128.

65. Costa M, Tidd C, Willis D. Cervicovaginal cytology in carcinosarcoma (malignant mixed müllerian [mesodermal] tumor) of the uterus. Diagn Cytopathol 1992; 8:33-40.

66. Kahanpaa K, Wahlstrom T, Grohn P, et al. Sarcomas of the uterus: a clinicopathologic study of 119 patients. Obstet Gynecol 1986; 67:417-424.

67. Barwick K, LiVolsi V. Malignant mixed müllerian tumors of the uterus: a clinicopathologic assessment of 34 cases. Am J Surg Pathol 1979; 3:125-135.

68. Holmquist N. The exfoliative cytology of mixed mesodermal tumors of athe uterus. Acta Cytol 1962; 6:373-375.

69. Barbazza R, Infantolino D, Blandamura S, et al. Malignant mixed müllerian tumor of the endometrium: report of a case with cytological diagnosis. Eur J Gynaecol Oncol 1988; 9:381-385.

70. Mitchard P, Swingler G, Cave D. Cytologic features of a mixed mesodermal tumor of the uterus demonstrated by cells obtained with the mi-mark endometrial sampler. Acta Cytol 1980; 24:363-365.

71. Izumi S, Hasegawa T, Tsutsui F, et al. Carcinosarcoma of the uterus: cytologic and ultrastructural features. Acta Cytol 1985; 29:602-606.

72. Clement P, Scully R. Extrauterine mesodermal (müllerian) adenosarcoma: a clinicopathologic analysis of five cases. Am J Clin Pathol 1978; 69:276-283.

73. Clement P, Scully R. Müllerian adenosarcoma of the uterus: a clinicopathologic analysis of ten cases of a distinct type of müllerian mixed tumor. Cancer 1974; 34:1138-1149.

74. Kaku T, Silverberg S, Major F, et al. Adenosarcoma of the uterus: a Gynecologic Oncology Group clinicopathologic study of 31 cases. Int J Gynecol Pathol 1992; 11:75-88.

75. Clement P, Scully R. Müllerian adenosarcoma of the uterus: a clinicopathologic analysis of 100 cases with a review of the literature. Hum Pathol 1990; 21:363-381.

76. Gast M, Radkins L, Jacobs A, et al. Müllerian adenosarcoma of the cervix with heterologous elements: diagnostic and therapeutic approach. Gynecol Oncol 1989; 32:381-384.

77. Imai H, Kitamura H, Nananura T, et al. Müllerian carcinofibroma of the uterus: a case report. Acta Cytol 1999; 43:667-674.

78. Das-Gupta F, D-Urso J. Melanoma of female genitalia. Surg Gynecol Obstet 1964; 119:1074-1078.

79. Levitan Z, Gordon A, Kaplan A, et al. Primary malignant melanoma of the vagina: report of four cases and review of the literature. Gynecol Oncol 1989; 33:85-90.

80. Fleming H, Mein P. Primary melanoma of the cervix: a case report. Acta Cytol 1994; 38:65-69.

81. Mordel N, Mor-Yosef S, Ben-Baruch N, et al. Case report: malignant melanoma of the uterine cervix (case report and review of the literature). Gynecol Oncol 1989; 32:375-380.

82. Yu H, Ketabchi M. Detection of malignant melanoma of the uterine cervix from Papanicolaou smears: a case report. Acta Cytol 1987; 31:73-76.

83. Chung A, Casey M, Flannery J, et al. Malignant melanoma of the vagina: report of 19 cases. Obstet Gynecol 1980; 55:720-727.

84. Hajdu S, Savino A. Cytologic diagnosis of malignant melamona. Acta Cytol 1973; 17:320-327.

85. Patel J, Kidolkar M, PIcren J, et al. Metastatic pattern of malignant melanoma: a study of 216 autopsy cases. Am J Surg 1978; 135:807-810.

86. Takeda M, Diamond S, DeMarco M, et al. Cytologic diagnosis of malignant melanoma metastatic to the endometrium. Acta Cytol 1978; 22:503-506.

87. Nagy P, Csaba I, Kadas I. Malignant melanoma mestastatic to the endometrium. Cytologic findings in a direct endometrial sample. Acta Cytol 1990; 34:382-384.

88. Holmquist N, Torres J. Malignant melanoma of the cervix: report of a case. Acta Cytol 1988; 32:252-256.

89. Santoso J, Kucera P, Ray J. Primary malignant melanoma of the uterine cervix: two case reports and a century's review. Obstet Gynecol Surv 1990; 45:733-740.

90. Jones H, Droegemuller W, Makowski E. A primary melanocarcinoma of the cervix. Am J Obstet Gynecol 1971; 111:959-963.

91. Hall D, Schneider V, Goplerud D. Primary malignant melanoma of the uterine cervix. Obstet Gynecol 1980; 56:525-529.

92. Krishnamoorthy A, Desai M, Simanowitz M. Primary malignant melanoma of the cervix: a case report. Br J Obstet Gynaecol 1986; 93:84-86.

93. Mudge T, Johnson J, MacFarlane A. Primary malignant melanoma of the cervix: a case report. Br J Obstet Gynaecol 1981; 93:1257-1259.

94. Podczaski E, Abt A, Kaminiski P, et al. A patient with multiple, malignant melanomas of the lower genital tract. Gynecol Oncol 1990; 37:422-426.

95. Schlosshauer P, Heller D, Koulos J. Malignant melanoma of the uterine cervix diagnosed on a cervical cytologic smear. Acta Cytol 1998; 42:1043-1045.

96. Bokun R, Perkovic M, Bakotin J, et al. Cytology and histopathology of metastatic melanoma involving a polyp on the uterine cervix: a case report. Acta Cytol 1985; 29:612-615.

97. Ehrmann R, Younge P, Lerch V. The exfoliative cytology and histogenesis of an early primary malignant melanoma of the vagina. Acta Cytol 1962; 6:245-254.

98. Garcia-Valdecasas R, Rodriguez-Rico L, linares J, et al. Malignant melanoma of the vagina: a case diagnosed cytologically. Acta Cytol 1974; 18:535-537.

99. Deshpande A, Munshi M. Primary malignant melanoma of the uterine cervix: report of a case diagnosed by cervical scrape cytology and review of the literature. Diagn Cytopathol. 2001; 25:108-111.

100. Takehara M, Ito E, Saito T, et al. HMB-45 staining for cytology of primary melanoma of the vagina: a case report. Acta Cytol 2000; 44:1077-1080.

101. Feichter G, Curschellas E, Gobat S, et al. Malignant melanoma of the uterine cervix; case report including cytology, histology and immunocytochemistry. Cytopathology 1995; 6:196-200.

102. Mazur M, Kurman R. Gestational trophoblastic disease and related lesions. In: Kurman RJ, editor. Blaustein's pathology of the female genital tract. New York: Springer-Verlag; 1994. pp.1049-1093.

103. Craighill M, Cramer D. Epidemiology of complete molar pregnancy. J Reprod Med 1984; 29:784-787.

104. Elston C. The histopathology of trophoblastic tumors. J Clin Pathol 1976; 29:111-131.

105. Yen S, MacMahon B. Epidemiologic features of trophoblastic disease. Am J Obstet Gynecol 1968; 101: 126-132.

106. Bracken M, Brinton L, Hayashi K. Epidemiology of hydatidiform mole and choriocarcinoma. Epidemiology 1984; 6:52-75.

107. Curry S, Hammond C, Tyrey L, et al. Hydatidiform mole: diagnosis, management, and long-term follow-up of 347 patients. Obstet Gynecol 1975; 45:1-8.

108. Morrow C, Kletzky O, Disaia P, et al. Clinical and laboratory correlates of molar pregnancy and trophoblastic disease. Am J Obstet Gynecol 1977; 128:424-430.

109. Szulman A, Surti U. The clinicopathologic profile of the partial hydatidiform mole. Obstet Gynecol 1982; 59: 597-602.

110. Czernobilsky B, Barash A, Lancet M. Partial moles: a clinicopathologic study of 25 cases. Obstet Gynecol 1982; 59:75-77.

111. Wake N, Takagi N, Sasaki M. Androgenesis as a cause of hydatidiform mole. J Natl Cancer Inst 1978; 60:51-57.

112. Szulman A, Surti U. The syndromes of hydatidiform mole. I. Cytogenetic and morphologic correlations. Am J Obstet Gynecol 1978; 131:665-671.

113. Lage J, Weinberg D, Yavner D, et al. The biology of tetraploid hydatidiform moles: histopathology, cytogenetics, and flow cytometry. Hum Pathol 1989; 20:419-425.

114. Brewer J, Torok E, Kahan B, et al. Gestational trophoblastic disease: origin of choriocarcinoma, invasive mole and choriocarcinoma associated with hydatidiform mole, and some immunologic aspects. Adv Cancer Res 1978; 27:89-147.

115. Hertig A, Sheldon W. Hydatidiform mole: a pathologicoclinical correlation of 200 cases. Am J Obstet Gynecol 1947; 53:1-36.

116. Goto S, Yamada A, Ishizuku T, et al. Development of postmolar trophoblastic disease after partial molar pregnancy. Gynecol Oncol 1993; 48:165-170.

117. Ober W, Edgcomb J, Jr. The pathology of choriocarcinoma. Ann NY Acad Sci 1971; 172:299-426.

118. Taki I. Cytology of hydatidiform mole, invasive mole, and choriocarcinoma. In: Wied GL, Keebler CM, Koss LG, et al., editors. Compendium of diagnostic cytology, 6th ed. Chicago: Tutorials of Cytology; 1988. pp.232-235.

119. Elston C. Trophoblastic tumors of the placenta. In: Fox H, editor. Pathology of the placenta. Philadelphia: WB Saunders; 1978. pp.368-425.

120. Brewer J, Eckman T, Dolkart R, et al. Gestational trophoblastic disease: a comparative study of the results of therapy in patients with invasive mole and with choriocarcinoma. Am J Obstet Gynecol 1971; 109:335.

121. Hertig A, Mansell H. Tumors of the female sex organs. I. Hydatidiform mole and choriocarcinoma. In: Hertig A, Mansell H, editors. Atlas of tumor pathology, Section 9, Fascicle 33. Washington, DC: Armed Forces Institute of Pathology; 1956.

122. Olive D, Lurain J, Brewer J. Choriocarcinoma associated with term gestation. Am J Obstet Gynecol 1984; 148:711-716.

123. Tsukamoto N, Kashimura Y, Sano M. Choriocarcinoma occurring within the normal placenta with breast metastasis. Gynecol Oncol 1981; 11:348-363.

124. Lurain J, Brewer J, Torok E, et al. Gestational trophoblastic disease: treatment results at the Brewer Trophoblastic Disease Center. Obstet Gynecol 1982; 60:354-360.

125. Kurman R, Scully R, Norris H. Trophoblastic pseudotumor of the uterus: an exaggerated form of "syncytial endometritis" simulating a malignant tumor. Cancer 1976; 38:1214-1226.

126. Ishi K, Suzuki F, Saito A, et al. Cytodiagnosis of placental site trophoblastic tumor: a report of two cases. Acta Cytol 1998; 42:745-750.

127. Lucia S, Mills H, Lowenhaupt E. Visceral involvement in primary neoplastic diseases of the reticuloendotelial system. Cancer 1952; 5:1193.

128. Lathrop J. Views and reviews: malignant pelvic lymphomas. Obstet Gynecol 1967; 30:137-145.

129. Hahn G. Gynecologic consideration in malignant lymphomas. Am J Obstet Gynecol 1958; 75:673-683.

130. al-Talib R, Sworn M, Ramsay A, Higchcock A, Herbert A. Primary cervical lymphoma: the role of cervical cytology. Cytopathology 1996; 7:173-177.

131. Muntz H, Ferry J, Flynn D. Stage IE primary malignant lymphomas of the uterine cervix. Cancer 1991; 68:2023-2032.

132. Whitaker D. The role of cytology in the detection of malignant lymphoma of the uterine cervix. Acta Cytol 1976; 20:510-513.

133. Harris N, Scully R. Malignant lymphoma and granulocytic sarcoma of the uterus and vagina: a clinicopathologic analysis of 27 cases. Cancer 1984; 53:2530-2545.

134. Ceelen G, Sakurai M. Vaginal cytology in leukemia. Acta Cytol 1962; 62:370-372.

135. Cahill L, Stastny J, Frable W. Primary lymphoma of the endometrium: a report of two cases diagnosed on cervicovaginal smears. Acta Cytol 1997; 41:533-538.

136. Katayama I, Hajian G, Evjy J. Cytologic diaagnosis of reticulum cell sarcoma of the uterine cervix. Acta Cytol 1973; 17:498-501.

137. Nasiell M. Hodgkin's disease limited to the uterine cervix: a case report including cytological findings in the cervical and vaginal smears. Acta Cytol 1964; 8:16-18.

138. Taki I, Aozasa K, Kurokawa K. Malignant lymphoma of the uterine cervix. Cytologic diagnosis of a case with immunocytochemical corroboration. Acta Cytol 1985; 29:607-611.

139. Matsuyama T, Tsukamoto N, Kaku T, et al. Primary malignant lymphoma of the uterine corpus and cervix: report of a case with immunocytochemical analysis. Acta Cytol 1989; 23:228-232.

140. Castaldo T, Ballon S, Lagasse L, et al. Reticuloendothelial neoplasia in the female genital tract. Obstet Gynecol 1979; 54:167-170.

141. Spahr J, Behm F, Schneider V. Preleukemic granulocytic sarcoma of cervix and vagina: initial manifestation by cytology. Acta Cytol 1982; 26:55-60.

142. Hajdu S, Nolan M. Exfoliative cytology of malignant germal tumors. Acta Cytol 1975; 19:255-260.

143. Chong S, Wee A, Yeoh S, et al. Retroperitoneal endodermal sinus tumor. Report of a case with abnormal cervicovaginal smear. Acta Cytol 1994; 38:562-567.

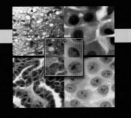

FLUIDS

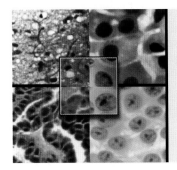

Urinary Tract Cytology

CHAPTER
11

Diagnostic urinary tract cytology may be divided into the study of cellular material and the study of the non-cellular, particulate matter (e.g., crystals and casts). This chapter focuses on the analysis of the cellular material. The investigation of the urinary particulate matter may be found in urinalysis texts.

The study of urinary tract cytology is mainly a study of cancer and its mimics. Urinary tract specimens generally are used for screening to determine if patients require more invasive diagnostic procedures. Advantages of urinary tract cytology are that it samples lesions that are difficult to see by cystoscopy (e.g., the renal pelvises, ureters, diverticuli) or lesions that are nearly cystoscopically invisible (e.g., flat lesions, such as carcinoma in situ), and it may sample the entire urothelial surface. A disadvantage of urinary tract cytology is that, for the most part, urinary cytology does not usually allow for lesion localization.[1] One exception is selective brushing of the upper tract. Urinary tract cytology and visualization through cystoscopy (with biopsy) are complementary.

THE URINARY TRACT

The urinary tract serves as a conduit to transmit and store urine and is lined by a specialized type of epithelium known as *urothelium,* or *transitional epithelium.* The term *transitional* implies an intermediary position between squamous and glandular, and urothelium exhibits properties of both types of epithelia. The structures lined by urothelium include the renal calyces and pelvises, ureters, bladder, and urethra; all or one of these structures may be sampled, depending on the specimen type. Given the transitional nature of urothelium, differentiation into true squamous or glandular epithelium may be seen along portions of the urinary tract. As with (or similar to) squamous epithelium, urothelium is impermeable to urine so that urine does not cross into the blood. In contrast to squamous and glandular epithelium, urothelium has a specialized cell membrane, which permits the urothelial cell to flex and contract. These tasks are particularly important in the bladder during expansion and contraction.

Similar to the cervicovaginal epithelium, the urothelial lining in these sites may be divided into three layers:

basal/parabasal, intermediate, and superficial. The thickness of the basal/parabasal layer is a single cell, and basal/parabasal cells are flattened to cuboidal. The cells in the intermediate layer are slightly larger than or similar in size to basal/parabasal cells, and the intermediate layer varies in thickness, depending on the site and functional state. The thickness of the superficial layer is a single cell. These superficial cells are large, often multinucleated, and referred to as *umbrella cells* by some. The total number of cell layers depends on the site, ranging from two to three in the renal pelvises to four to six in the ureters to five to six in the bladder.

The female urethra is lined primarily by stratified squamous epithelium separated by patches of pseudostratified urothelium. The male urethra is much longer and is divided into three parts. The prostatic portion of the urethra is lined by stratified urothelium. The membranous portion is lined by pseudostratified or stratified urothelium separated by patches of stratified squamous epithelium. At the orifice of the spongy (or penile) portion, the lining is entirely stratified squamous; the remainder of the spongy portion is lined by stratified or pseudostratified urothelium separated by patches of stratified squamous epithelium. Mucus-secreting glands are found in both the male (spongy portion) and female urethra.

Specimen Types

The three types of urinary tract specimens are (1) voided urine, (2) catheterized urine, and (3) washing or brushing samples. These specimens are used for different purposes.

Voided urine, sometimes called a *clean catch urine specimen,* is used mainly for screening in populations with specific signs and symptoms (e.g., hematuria); it is not used primarily to monitor patients with disease. Voided urine is superior to catheterized urine or bladder washings in detecting lesions of the urethra. Voided urine is usually sparsely cellular and may consist of desquamated cells from all three cell layers. Cellularity may increase with disease processes such as neoplasia or lithiasis. Voided urine specimens should be processed immediately, although refrigeration and 50% ethanol fixation helps with preservation[2] if this is not feasible. Alcoholic Carbowax prefixation also increases cellular yield.[3] Immediate processing limits degeneration, the main problem associated with voided urine specimens. Although urothelial cells are hardy and may remain intact even after several days at a warm temperature,[4,5] degenerative cellular features are extremely common in voided urine cytology.[6] Degeneration may be related to high acidity of the urine, normal cellular turnover, or disease processes, especially inflammation.[6,7] Degeneration is a cause of false-positive and false-negative diagnoses. First morning–voided urine specimens should be avoided, because these specimens are usually the most degenerated.[8] Specimens obtained from collection bags should be eschewed for a similar reason. A second problem with voided urine specimens is contamination, particularly in women. The main contaminant is squamous cells from the vagina or the skin, and infectious organisms such as bacteria and fungi also may be accompaniments. A rule of thumb in voided urine specimens is that if squamous cells and bacteria are present and an absence of inflammation is evident, the specimen is contaminated. Special fixatives such as Cyto Rich Red may be used to reduce the number of red blood cells (RBCs) and the amount of background material in urinary tract specimens.[9]

Catheterized urine specimens usually are more cellular and better preserved than voided urine specimens. The higher cellularity occurs as the catheter dislodges cells and may cause an inflammatory response that further results in cell sloughing. A catheterized urine specimen is used for surveillance in patients with known or suspected urothelial neoplasia. Contamination generally is not a problem in a catheterized urine specimen.

The wash specimen, either directed or undirected, is the most sensitive cytologic means to detect urothelial neoplasia. Most wash specimens are from the bladder, although wash specimens also may be obtained from the upper tract. Brushing specimens of a visualized bladder abnormality or of the upper tract may be obtained in conjunction with washes. A properly obtained wash specimen is cellular and uncontaminated, although lubricant (blobs of purple to green amorphous material; Figure 11-1) may hinder inter-

pretation. The disadvantages of washings are that they are uncomfortable to the patient and more expensive than voided or catheterized urine specimens. Washings are usually obtained during cystoscopy in patients with suspected urothelial neoplasia or as a means to monitor patients with disease.

Diagnostic Accuracy

The diagnostic accuracy of urinary tract cytology depends on the specimen type, prevalence of disease in the studied population, and tumor subtype. Accuracy also depends on the diagnostic schema, and one of the more commonly used schema is shown in Box 11-1.[10] Diagnoses of suspicious and malignant increase the probability of neoplasia[11] and generally result in aggressive follow-up. Interestingly, the diagnosis of atypia may decrease the risk of neoplasia, depending on the experience of the pathologist and specimen type. Unfortunately, this lack of uniformity of diagnostic criteria and especially terminology contributes to the lack of uniformity in patient management. A benign diagnosis may be followed aggressively, depending on the clinical signs and symptoms. The symptoms of bladder cancer include pain, urinary frequency and urgency, and hematuria. Other important clinical information that guides patient management is history of urothelial neoplasia and treatment, instrumentation, history of lithiasis, and cystoscopic findings.

The diagnostic sensitivity for the different tumor subtypes is discussed in the individual sections. For high-grade urothelial cell carcinomas the main cause of false-negative diagnosis is sampling (Box 11-2), and for low-grade urothelial cell carcinomas, the main causes are interpretation (low-grade cancers may cytologically look benign) and sam-

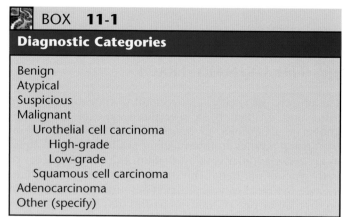

BOX 11-1

Diagnostic Categories

Benign
Atypical
Suspicious
Malignant
    Urothelial cell carcinoma
        High-grade
        Low-grade
      Squamous cell carcinoma
Adenocarcinoma
Other (specify)

BOX 11-2

Sources of False-Negative Diagnoses in Urinary Tract Cytology

Sampling of an insufficient number of cells
Degenerated specimens
Low-grade papillary urothelial cell carcinoma

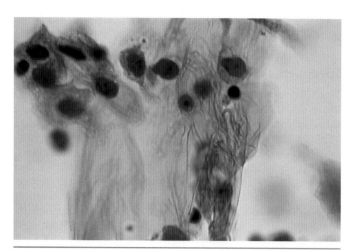

Figure 11-1 Lubricant in a catheterized urine specimen. Lubricant has a variable tint on Pap stain, ranging from blue to pink to purple. In this example, the lubricant has a pink cellophane appearance and is admixed with benign intermediate and parabasal urothelial cells. Mucin may have a similar appearance.

pling. Causes of false-positive diagnoses are listed in Box 11-3 and discussed throughout the rest of this chapter. The interobserver variability between cytologists examining urinary tract specimens is poor to good (Kappa [κ] values = 0.29 to 0.60).[12]

The main concern in urinary tract cytology is separating nonneoplastic from neoplastic disease. The rest of this chapter focuses on this separation.

Nonneoplastic Conditions

Benign Urine

A urine specimen is almost never completely *normal,* because most specimens are obtained in patients who have some disease process that leads to specimen collection in the first place. Fortunately, the majority of urinary tract specimens are benign, and the cytologic findings are nonspecific and often minimal. The diagnoses of *benign urine, no malignant cells,* or alternative terms may be used. The benign urine may contain a number of cell types, including urothelial, glandular, squamous, and inflammatory cells. Diagnostic difficulties arise when either these cells are degenerated or when some of these cells are present in groups architecturally suggestive of neoplasia.

Urothelial cells. The most commonly seen cell in urinary tract specimens is the urothelial cell. Basal/parabasal and intermediate urothelial cells appear similar and are easily distinguished from superficial urothelial cells (Figure 11-2). Voided urine specimens are composed predominantly of single superficial cells, whereas catheterized and wash urine specimens are composed of single cells from all cell layers and groups of intermediate and basal/parabasal cells (Figure 11-3).

Basal/parabasal and intermediate urothelial cells are approximately the size of lymphocytes and, compared with other benign cell types, have high nuclear to cytoplasmic (N:C) ratios (Box 11-4). Think of these cells as the counterparts to the basal cells in Papanicolaou (Pap) tests. The nuclei are round to oval with smooth membranes, although

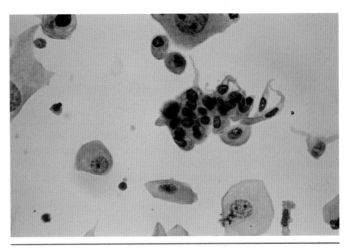

Figure 11-2 **Benign basal/parabasal, intermediate, and superficial urothelial cells in a bladder wash specimen.** Similar to parabasal cells seen in Pap tests, the parabasal cells in urinary tract specimens have high nuclear to cytoplasmic (N:C) ratios and hyperchromatic nuclei. However, the nuclei are generally small and not in the size range of high-grade urothelial cell carcinoma cells. The intermediate cell nuclei are slightly larger and the intermediate cell cytoplasm is slightly more abundant. The superficial cells are large and have abundant cytoplasm and large nuclei that may contain prominent nucleoli. Superficial cells also may be multinucleated. Parabasal cells generally are obtained by washing or other methods of instrumentation in which they are forcibly dislodged from the bladder wall. Superficial cells will exfoliate without instrumentation.

BOX 11-3

Sources of False-Positive Diagnoses in Urinary Tract Cytology

Lithiasis
Viral effects
Instrumentation artifact
Chemotherapy
Radiation therapy
Degenerated specimens
Inflammatory atypia
Inflammatory pseudotumor
Follicular cystitis
Ileal conduit specimen atypia

BOX 11-4   CMF

Cytomorphologic Features of Basal/Parabasal Cells and Intermediate Urothelial Cells

Round to oval nuclei with smooth nuclear membranes
Centrally placed nuclei
Finely granular anuclear chromatin
One to several inconspicuous nucleoli
Foamy or slightly bubbly cytoplasm

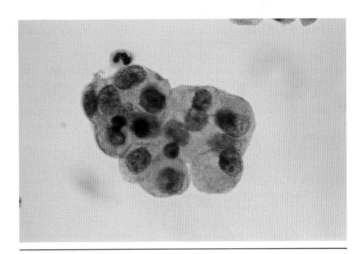

Figure 11-3 **Cell group of benign urothelial cells in a bladder wash specimen.** These benign urothelial cells contain a moderate to large amount of slightly granular basophilic cytoplasm and round to oval nuclei with slight nuclear membrane irregularities. The chromatin pattern of these cells is finely stippled to slightly hyperchromatic, and a lack of coarseness to the chromatin is evident. In wash specimens, urothelial cell groups may be variable in size. (Papanicolaou [Pap])

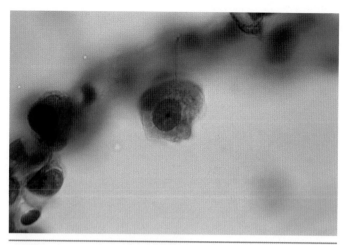

Figure 11-4 Benign urothelial cell in a bladder wash specimen. This cell shows a moderate amount of cytoplasm and an enlarged nucleus with a moderately sized nucleolus. The cytoplasm is granular and has a sharp cytoplasmic border. The N:C ratio is not significantly enlarged, and the nucleus is not significantly hyperchromatic. Note the bluish lubricant in the background. (Pap)

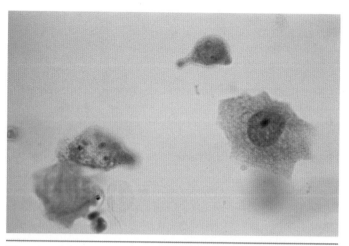

Figure 11-6 Benign superficial urothelial cell in a bladder wash specimen. Three benign urothelial cells are present in the field. The large cell on the right with a prominent nucleolus is a superficial cell and contains abundant cytoplasm and an enlarged nucleus. Prominent nucleoli with a lack of nuclear hyperchromasia is usually indicative of a reactive condition. (Pap)

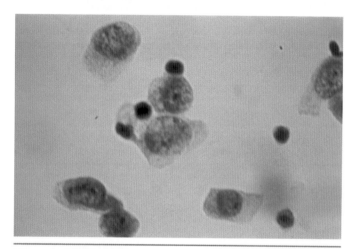

Figure 11-5 Benign urothelial cell with foamy cytoplasm in a catheterized urine specimen. These urothelial cells have high N:C ratios but lack the hyperchromasia sufficient for a diagnosis of high-grade urothelial cell carcinoma. The nuclei have granular chromatin and relatively regular nuclear membranes. Nucleoli may be observed. The cytoplasm of urothelial cells varies in texture and may be vacuolated or dense. Vacuolated cytoplasm is not typically characteristic of high-grade urothelial cell carcinoma. Several lymphocytes are in the background. (Pap)

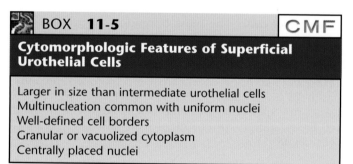

BOX 11-5 CMF

Cytomorphologic Features of Superficial Urothelial Cells

Larger in size than intermediate urothelial cells
Multinucleation common with uniform nuclei
Well-defined cell borders
Granular or vacuolized cytoplasm
Centrally placed nuclei

cells is important because these are the cells that must be distinguished from the neoplastic cells of urothelial cell carcinoma.

Superficial cells also are known as *umbrella cells* because they overlie and protect the intermediate cells from the toxic urine (Box 11-5). Superficial cells are larger than intermediate and basal/parabasal cells (Figure 11-6). Superficial cells may be greater than 100 microns in diameter, making superficial cells the biggest benign cells in the body! The N:C ratio is low, and on this feature alone, superficial cells, even very reactive ones, are easily separated from neoplastic cells. The cytoplasmic borders are well-defined, and the cells have a rounded appearance. The cytoplasm has a finely granular quality, and cytoplasmic vacuolization is often seen. Multinucleation is the norm, and superficial cells may contain up to 50 nuclei per cell (Figure 11-7). However, the majority of superficial cells contain from one to three nuclei and are about the size of an intermediate squamous cell. The nuclei of superficial cells may exhibit considerable reactive changes including hyperchromasia, membrane irregularity, and prominence of nucleoli. In some conditions, Murphy and colleagues describe the nuclei as resembling the nuclei of high-grade urothelial cell carcinoma (Figure 11-8), although the N:C ratio should not be increased sufficiently to warrant a neoplastic diagnosis.[6]

slight irregularities may be seen (Figure 11-4). The nuclei are centrally placed and if many cells contain eccentrically placed nuclei, a low-grade urothelial cell carcinoma may be suspected. The chromatin pattern is finely granular and often mildly hyperchromatic. Mitoses should not be seen. One to two small nucleoli are common. The cytoplasm is variable in tinctural quality and, with a Pap stain, ranges from gray to blue to green. Small cytoplasmic vacuoles give the cell a foamy cytoplasmic appearance, and the cytoplasmic membrane is well outlined (Figure 11-5). In reactive conditions the cytoplasm becomes denser in appearance, and the vacuoles may disappear. Knowledge of the spectrum of appearance of basal and intermediate urothelial

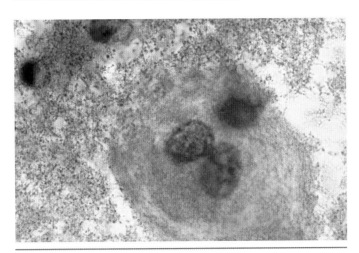

Figure 11-7 **Multinucleated urothelial cell in a bladder wash specimen.** Superficial urothelial cells are often multinucleated, and this binucleated cell contains abundant cytoplasm. The nuclei are slightly degenerated and show small gaps within the nuclear membrane. A large number of degenerated red cells and a few inflammatory cells are seen in the background. (Pap)

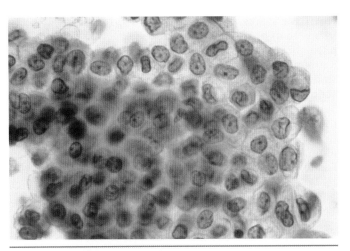

Figure 11-9 **Groups of benign urothelial cells in bladder wash specimen.** Large groups of benign urothelial cells may be seen in instrumented urines. A three-dimensional group of urothelial cells is present. It may be difficult to evaluate the nuclei in the areas of extreme cellular overlap. At the edges, the urothelial cells contain a moderate amount of cytoplasm, and the nuclei appear relatively monomorphic. Note the degree of nuclear membrane irregularities that may be seen in benign urothelial cells. These cells contain open chromatin and a prominent nucleolus. (Pap)

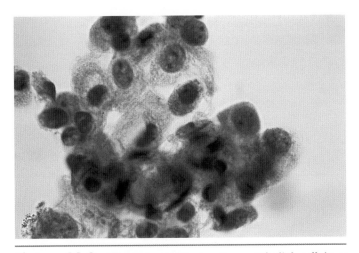

Figure 11-8 **Hyperchromatic benign urothelial cell in a bladder wash specimen.** Superficial, intermediate and parabasal urothelial cells are seen in this fragment. The parabasal cells may be markedly hyperchromatic, although their nuclei are small. This fragment most likely represents a full thickness portion of the mucosa with parabasal cells at the bottom, intermediate cells in the middle and superficial cells along the surface. The amount of cytoplasm and nuclear size increase from the parabasal level to the superficial level. (Pap)

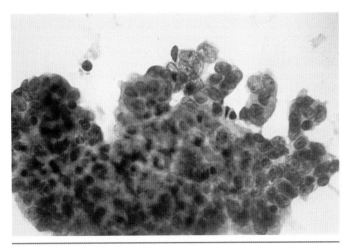

Figure 11-10 **Pseudopapillary group representing instrumentation artifact in a catheterized urine specimen.** Extremely large groups of urothelial cells may be obtained from instrumentation. In this group, considerable nuclear overlap occurs, although a true fibrovascular core is absent. The cells at the periphery of the fragment contain nuclei with hypochromatic chromatin. Scattered inflammatory cells are present within the pseudopapillary fragment and in the background. (Pap)

In catheterized urine and bladder wash specimens, large groups of urothelial cells may be observed (Figure 11-9). These groups often have a papillary appearance, although a true fibrovascular core is usually absent (Box 11-6).[273] Large groups should not cause concern in these types of specimens, although they should raise suspicion in voided urine specimens. In fact, some laboratories use the diagnosis of at least *atypical* if these groups are present in a voided urine; the reason for this is that in most benign processes, cell groups are not dislodged. The appearance of these groups, no matter how bland, raises the suspicion of a low-grade urothelial cell carcinoma. A contrasting viewpoint is provided by Goldstein and colleagues who argued that bland cell groups have little diagnostic use in voided urine specimens.[13]

In catheterized urine and bladder wash specimens, pseudopapillary groups often represent instrumentation artifact (Box 11-7 and Figure 11-10). A soft rule is that if the patient is known to have been instrumented, large groups of urothelial cells should not be cause for concern. Rather, the diagnostic money lies in the single cells or the slightly dissociated cells. In addition to forming pseudopapillary structures, the cells may slough in three-dimensional balls, in which considerable nuclear overlap may limit interpretation (Figure 11-11). Examination of the edges of the group, where the aggregates are less thick, helps in the evaluation. In a benign process, the cells at the edges have lower N:C ratios, bland nuclei, and distinct cytoplasmic membranes.[14] Kannan and colleagues described benign groups as having smooth borders (neoplastic groups do not) and a densely staining, well-defined cytoplasmic collar (Figure 11-12).[15] Superficial cells may be seen protruding from the large pseudopapillae.

In histologic specimens, superficial cells may cover papillomas and low-grade papillary urothelial cell carcinomas. Frable and colleagues reported the same findings in cyto-

logic specimens and suggested that one should not be too certain that a group is benign if it is lined by superficial cells.[274] However, when papillary groups are covered by superficial cells, a benign diagnosis is likely (at least in wash specimens) and therefore not much stock is placed in this potential pitfall.

When urothelial cells degenerate, the nuclei often appear more darkly stained with smudged chromatin. Pyknosis, karyorrhexis, and karyolysis may be observed (Figure 11-13). By contrast, well-preserved urothelial cells, including neoplastic cells, have distinctly granular chromatin pat-

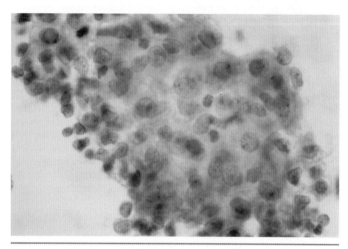

Figure 11-11   Pseudopapillary group of benign urothelial cells in a bladder wash specimen. This pseudopapillary fragment shows extensive nuclear overlap and is admixed with numerous small inflammatory cells. The cell nuclei vary in size although the chromatin pattern of the cells is relatively consistent and is not hyperchromatic. The nuclear membranes are round to moderately irregular in shape. (Pap)

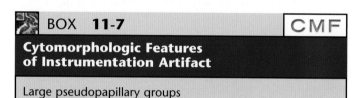

BOX 11-6

Sources of Papillary-Like Groups in Urine

Instrumentation artifact
Lithiasis
Infectious conditions
Low-grade urothelial cell carcinoma

BOX 11-7   CMF

Cytomorphologic Features of Instrumentation Artifact

Large pseudopapillary groups
Three-dimensional balls
Nuclear overlap
Individual cells with low nuclear-to-cytoplasmic (N:C) ratios
Evenly dispersed chromatin
Distinct cytoplasmic membranes
Cytoplasmic collars
Groups lined by superficial urothelial cells

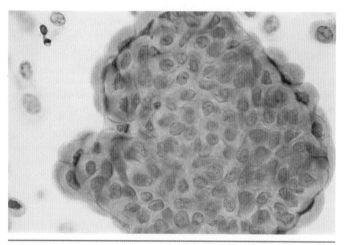

Figure 11-12   Cytoplasmic collars in a bladder wash specimen. This large group of benign urothelial cells contains an outer layer of superficial cells with basally placed nuclei and abundant cytoplasm. The cytoplasm at the edge of the fragment is referred to as a *cytoplasmic collar*. Cytoplasmic collars usually are indicative of a benign process although they have been described in low-grade urothelial cell carcinomas. Thus, in instrumented urine specimens, the cells outside of these large groups should be examined to make the diagnosis of a low-grade urothelial cell carcinoma. (Pap) (From Raab SS. Urinary cytology. In: Atkinson BF, Silverman JF, editors. Atlas of difficult diagnoses in cytopathology. Philadelphia: WB Saunders; 1998. p.243.)

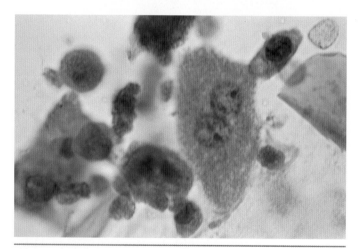

Figure 11-13   Degenerated cells in a catheterized urine specimen. These cells show variable degrees of degeneration. The large binucleated superficial cell shows cytoplasmic degeneration consisting of cytoplasmic fraying and slight nuclear degeneration consisting of loss of the crispness of the nuclear chromatin and gaps within the nuclear membrane. Other urothelial cells show greater degrees of nuclear degeneration including nuclear pyknosis and karyorrhexis. Nuclear hyperchromasia may be a worrisome feature of high-grade urothelial cell carcinoma, although in this case, the nuclear degeneration and the relatively low N:C ratios indicate that these cells most likely are degenerated benign cells rather than malignant cells. (Pap)

terns and a well-defined nuclear border. In degenerated urothelial cells, the nuclear membrane may have gaps or may appear frayed. The cytoplasm in degenerated cells tends to lyse, leaving only the nucleus with a thin rim of cytoplasm. These cells may make the N:C ratio appear increased, even though it is not. Cytoplasmic vacuolization also may become more prominent in degenerated urothelial cells (Figure 11-14). Overinterpreting degenerated urothelial cells as high-grade urothelial cell carcinoma is a cause of false-positive diagnoses in urinary tract cytology.

Glandular cells. Several types of glandular cells may be seen, most commonly in catheterized urine and bladder wash specimens (Box 11-8). Most of these arise from the urothelial lining itself (Figure 11-15). The urothelium is capable of differentiating along several pathways, and their presence may indicate cystitis glandularis (see p. 323). Glandular epithelium also may occur on the surface as a response to chronic irritation and in cases of bladder extrophy.[16] These glandular cells have basally placed oval nuclei with finely granular blue to green cytoplasm. Occasionally, the

cells have small cytoplasmic vacuoles that contain mucin droplets. They are usually seen singly or in small groups. These cells are rarely ciliated (Figure 11-16). Glandular cells are almost always benign, although their presence does not exclude a coexistent neoplasm. Glandular cells that shed from the periurethral glands may be seen in voided urine specimens. Cases of intestinal metaplasia of the entire urothelial surface associated with mucosuria have been described.[17]

Sources of extraneous benign glandular cells in urinary tract specimens include the kidney, prostate, epididymis, seminal vesicles, vas deferens, and female genital tract (contaminant from menses or the endocervix). Glandular cells from nephrogenic adenomas and endometriosis are

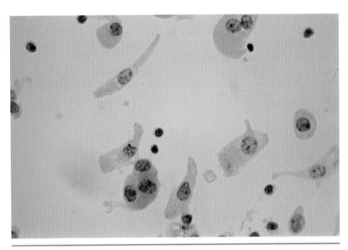

Figure 11-15 **Benign glandular cells in a bladder wash specimen.** Glandular cells are admixed with intermediate urothelial cells and superficial urothelial cells. The glandular cells show elongated cytoplasmic configurations with nuclei present either basally or centrally within the cytoplasm. The cytoplasm is granular and may be vacuolated. The chromatin pattern of these cells is finely stippled and nucleoli may be present. Glandular cells normally may be present within urinary tract specimens. (Pap)

BOX 11-8

Sources of Glandular Cells in Urinary Tract Specimens

Normal urothelial lining
Cystitis glandularis
Periurethral glands
Kidney
Prostate
Epididymis
Seminal vesicle
Vas deferens
Female genital tract
Nephrogenic adenoma
Adenocarcinoma
Urothelial cell carcinoma with glandular differentiation

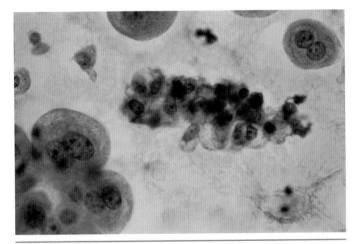

Figure 11-14 **Degenerated urothelial cells with cytoplasmic vacuolization in a bladder wash specimen.** Binucleated superficial cells are seen along the edge, and in the center is a group of degenerated intermediate urothelial cells with slight nuclear hyperchromasia and vacuolated cytoplasm. The hyperchromatic nuclei are small compared with the relatively intact superficial urothelial cells. The background contains abundant blood and rare inflammatory cells. (Pap)

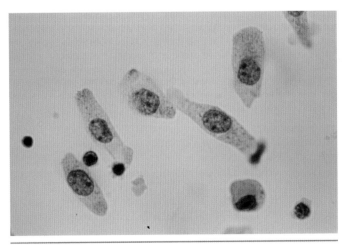

Figure 11-16 **Ciliated benign glandular cells in a bladder wash specimen.** The glandular cells seen in this photomicrograph contain abundant granular cytoplasm, and the nuclei are centrally placed. One of the cells shows cilia depicted by a dark blue-purple color at the edge of the cell. (Pap) (From Raab SS. Urinary cytology. In: Atkinson BF, Silverman JF, editors. Atlas of difficult diagnoses in cytopathology. Philadelphia: WB Saunders; 1998. p.243.)

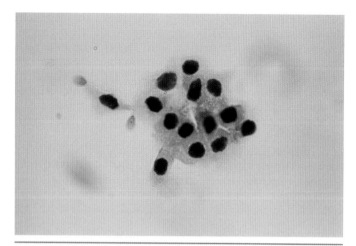

Figure 11-17 Collecting tubular cells in a clean catch urine specimen. Cells from the collecting tubule are polygonal and have round nuclei with granular chromatin. Often, as in this case, in clean catch urine specimens the nuclei show degeneration and are hyperchromatic. The N:C ratio is relatively low and the cytoplasm has an orangeophilic appearance. (Pap)

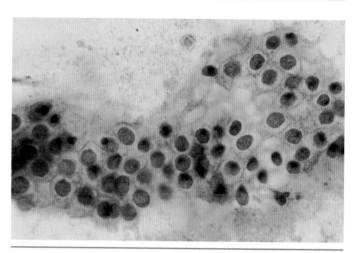

Figure 11-19 Prostatic cells in a catheterized urine specimen. Prostatic cells have a cuboidal appearance and generally are seen in small to moderately sized clusters. The nuclei are centrally placed and the cytoplasmic boundaries often are well-demarcated. The cytoplasm is granular and basophilic in tincture. The chromatin is often hyperchromatic to finely granular. Nucleoli in benign prostatic cells generally are not seen. (Pap)

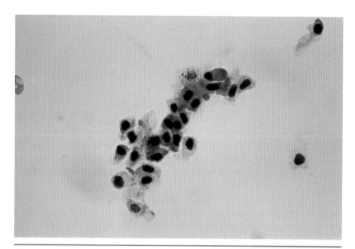

Figure 11-18 Convoluted tubular cells in a clean catch urine specimen. Similar to collecting tubular cells, convoluted tubular cells often are degenerated and show nuclear hyperchromasia and cytoplasmic fragmentation. Convoluted tubular cells are larger and contain more abundant cytoplasm than collecting tubular cells. The convoluted cell nuclei are round to oval and have a relatively low N:C ratio. Nucleoli generally are not seen. Cellular degeneration may make these cells difficult to separate from degenerated urothelial cells. (Pap)

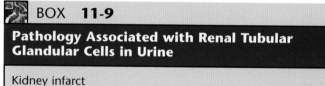

BOX 11-9

Pathology Associated with Renal Tubular Glandular Cells in Urine

Kidney infarct
Acute tubular necrosis
Allograft rejection
Trauma

BOX 11-10

Sources of Yellow Cellular Pigmentation in Urinary Tract Specimens

Lipofuscin pigment in seminal vesicular cells
Hematoidin pigment in macrophages
Malignant melanoma

discussed in the section on inflammatory conditions (see pp. 233-234).

Renal tubular glandular cells usually are observed in casts or small sheets (Box 11-9). Their presence is indicative of kidney disease, such as infarct, acute tubular necrosis, or allograft rejection.[18] Renal tubular cells differ in appearance, depending on their source and state of preservation.[19] Cells from the collecting tubule are round to polygonal and have round nuclei with granular chromatin (Figure 11-17). Cells from the convoluted tubule are bigger with abundant cytoplasm (Figure 11-18). Convoluted tubular cell nuclei also are round to oval; these cells have a lower N:C ratio. Nucleoli generally are not seen. The diagnosis of medical kidney disease is beyond the scope of this chapter.

Prostatic and seminal vesicular cells rarely are shed in the urine but may be seen following prostatic massage. Prostatic cells are cuboidal, contain round nuclei with dense chromatin, and present in small clusters (Figure 11-19). As in tissue sections, seminal vesicular cells may show considerable atypia, resulting in a false-positive diagnosis for the unwary. Cells from the seminal vesicle have enlarged nuclei, high N:C ratios, prominent nucleoli, and hyperchromasia (Figure 11-20). Seminal vesicular nuclei often have a degenerated appearance with smudging and nuclear breakdown. In contrast to high-grade urothelial cell carcinoma cells, seminal vesicular cells contain cytoplasm with yellow lipofuscin pigment. Thus, if the nuclei look atypical and the cytoplasm contains yellow granules, these cells are not malignant (Box 11-10).

Squamous cells. Squamous epithelium normally lines the urethra, but also may be seen in the bladder trigone in up to 10% of men and 50% of women.[20,21] Squamous cells

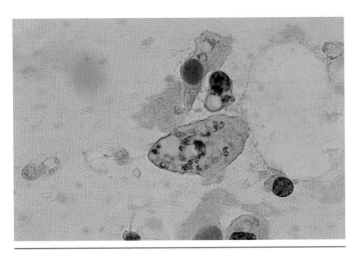

Figure 11-20 **Seminal vesicular cells in catheterized urine specimen.** Seminal vesicular cells may show considerable atypia with moderate to high N:C ratios. These seminal vesicular cells show nuclear degeneration and smudging. The cytoplasm is often vacuolated and lipofuscin pigment may be recognized. (Pap)

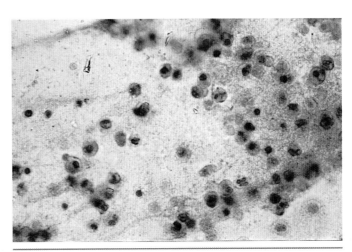

Figure 11-22 **Eosinophils in a clean catch urine specimen.** Eosinophils and chronic inflammatory cells are increased in number. When eosinophils lyse, a red granular tinge may be seen in the background. Eosinophils most often are the result of infection or acute interstitial nephritis. (Pap)

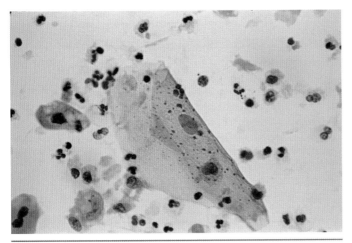

Figure 11-21 **Urine from a prepubescent girl showing increased squamous maturation.** A superficial squamous cell is seen in the center portion of the field. Degenerated urothelial cells, histiocytes, and acute inflammatory cells are seen in the background. Maturation indices may be performed on clean catch urine specimens and reflect the amount of endogenous or exogenous estrogens. (Pap)

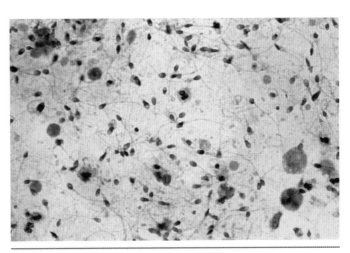

Figure 11-23 **Sperm in a bladder wash specimen.** Numerous sperm with degenerated urothelial cells and chronic inflammatory cells are seen in this specimen. Sperm may be seen after ejaculation or prostatic massage. (Pap)

undergo the same maturation process in the bladder and urethra as they do in the cervix and vagina. As stated previously, contamination from the female genital tract and perineum must be excluded, particularly in voided urine specimens, before reporting that true squamous epithelium is present. In addition to the normal state, squamous metaplasia may be seen in inflammatory diseases (e.g., lithiasis), infectious conditions (e.g., schistosomiasis), and with exogenous hormones (e.g., men being treated with estrogen or neonates secondary to maternal estrogen). A maturation index may be performed on urinary cytology specimens from prepubescent girls, similar to the maturation index performed on Pap tests (Figure 11-21).

Other cell types and structures. Other cells and structures in benign urinary tract specimens include RBCs, inflammatory cells, sperm, inclusion bodies, crystals, and casts. RBCs in the urine (e.g., micro- or macrohematuria) often are

taken as a sign and/or symptom of neoplasia[22]; however, less than 2% of patients with microhematuria turn out to have a carcinoma. More often, RBCs in the urine arise from a glomerular process.[23] RBCs also may be seen in patients with cystitis, trauma, menstrual shedding (e.g., contamination), and hypertension. Mentioning that RBCs are present may be clinically helpful, because microscopic examination is more sensitive than a urinary dipstick. Erythrocytes in washing specimens, however, may be related to the procedure and thus do not equate with clinical hematuria.

Inflammatory cells include lymphocytes, eosinophils, neutrophils, and histiocytes. The finding of these cell types is nonspecific, although most cases of eosinophilia are the result of infection or acute interstitial nephritis. Greater sensitivity of detecting eosinophils is provided using Hansel's stain (Figure 11-22).[24] Sperm may be seen after ejaculation or prostatic massage (Figure 11-23).

Large cytoplasmic inclusions may be seen in benign urinary tract cells and usually are a result of degeneration.[25,26] Thus, inclusions are most often seen in voided urine specimens. The inclusions are rounded with smooth borders and are variable in size (Figure 11-24). In some cells the nuclei are absent and single or multiple inclusions are observed. With the Pap test the inclusion usually stains red.

Corpora amylacea occasionally are seen in male urinary tract specimens (Figure 11-25). These structures generally arise from the prostate and may be seen after prostatic massage; these very rarely occur in the bladder. Corpora amylacea are concentrically laminated structures and usually are not calcified (a feature useful in the separation of corpora amylacea from psammoma bodies which are calcified). Corpora amylacea stain green to blue. These structures are not surrounded by prostatic or urothelial cells.

Inflammatory Conditions: Cystitis, Urethritis, Ureteritis, and Pyelonephritis

Lithiasis (Calculi)

Lithiasis, more than any other nonneoplastic lesion, is likely to be confused cytologically with either low- or high-grade urothelial cell carcinoma. Stones form when insoluble materials become supersaturated. Up to 85% of stones are composed of calcium oxalate or calcium phosphate. Other stones are formed from uric acid, cystine, or struvite. Clinically, stones may cause micro- or macroscopic hematuria. If x-rays are obtained, a radiographic filling defect or defects may be detected, thus mimicking carcinoma. If a stone is passed, the patient often has the classic symptom of almost unbearable pain. However, many patients with stones have no known symptoms. On the basis of the cytologic features alone, the separation of reactive urothelial cells, secondary to lithiasis, from either low- or high-grade urothelial cell carcinoma may be difficult. The clinical history (e.g., pain, previous history of stones, hematuria,

pyuria) and radiographic findings may prove invaluable in short circuiting an overinterpretation, although it should be remembered that urothelial cell carcinoma may arise in the setting of lithiasis.[27]

Fortunately, most urine specimens from patients with stones show changes that fall far short of neoplasia (Box 11-11). Some urinary tract specimens are hypercellular resulting from the abrasion of the mucosa by the stone (Figure 11-26). The urothelial cells are sloughed in large groups that form pseudopapillae or are observed singly.[14,28] The urothelial cells exhibit varying degrees of nuclear abnormalities, ranging from slight hyperchromasia to coarsely clumped, dark chromatin.[29] The nuclei invariably show somewhat irregular membranes and prominent nucleoli (Figure 11-27). The N:C ratios may be quite enlarged and mitotic figures may be seen with some frequency. The background usually consists of blood and inflammatory cells, mostly neutrophils that may obscure the specimen. Stone fragments, staining red to dark green, sometimes are observed (Figure 11-28). Stone fragments may be calcified and laminated. In

---

BOX 11-11   CMF

Cytomorphologic Features of Lithiasis

Hypercellularity
Pseudopapillary groups
Nuclear hyperchromasia
Increased N:C ratios
Regular nuclear membranes
Prominent nucleoli
Squamous metaplasia
Increased mitotic rate
Acute inflammation
Stone fragments
Calcifications

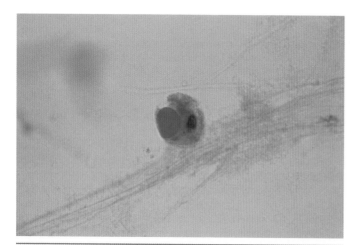

Figure 11-24 Cytoplasmic inclusion in a clean catch urine specimen. In this degenerated urothelial cell, a large cytoplasmic eosinophilic inclusion is seen. The inclusion has rounded borders and a relatively homogeneous appearance. The nucleus is small and hyperchromatic, and in some cells with cytoplasmic inclusions, nuclei are not seen. These inclusions must be differentiated from viral cytoplasmic or nuclear inclusions, which usually have a basophilic and less dense appearance. (Pap)

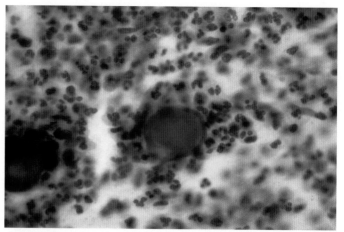

Figure 11-25 Corpora amylacea in a bladder wash specimen. Two corpora amylacea are admixed with a large amount of acute inflammation. These structures generally are not surrounded by epithelial cells and have a blue laminated appearance. Corpora amylacea should be differentiated from psammoma bodies, which have a calcified, purple appearance. These structures usually arise from the prostate, although occasionally they may arise from the bladder wall. (Pap)

rare instances, necrotic debris, mimicking a tumor diathesis is present. Squamous metaplasia of the bladder or renal pelvis may be a feature of long-standing lithiasis, particularly in men (Figure 11-29).[30]

· Lithiasis may mimic low-grade urothelial cell carcinoma in cases in which the obvious reactive changes are slight and the specimen is hypercellular with many cell groups (Box 11-12). Lithiasis is typified by a single population of slightly atypical urothelial cells (and acute inflammatory cells), whereas low-grade urothelial cell carcinoma shows a dual population of cells (both benign and atypical urothelial cells; Figure 11-30). Low-grade urothelial cell carcinoma should not be diagnosed in a background heavy with acute inflammation. For the most part, the urothelial cells in lithiasis lack homogeneous, nonvacuolated cytoplasm (seen in low-grade urothelial cell carcinoma) and exhibit N:C ratios that are too high for a low-grade urothelial cell carcinoma.

In contrast to high-grade urothelial cell carcinoma, the atypia resulting from lithiasis is usually not as severe, or a

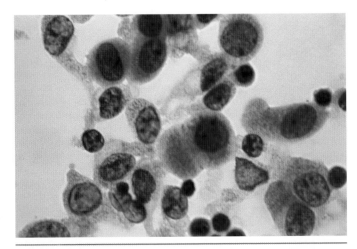

Figure 11-26 **Hypercellularity resulting from lithiasis in this catheterized urine specimen.** Stone fragments may cause hypercellularity by abrading the epithelial portion of the bladder wall. The urothelial cells may appear singly, in small groups, or in large fragments. Individual cells often show a degree of atypia with granular to slightly coarse chromatin and increased N:C ratios. The chromatin usually is not hyperchromatic enough to warrant a diagnosis of high-grade urothelial cell carcinoma and usually the cells are too atypical for a diagnosis of low-grade urothelial cell carcinoma. Scattered cells may show degenerative features, and the background usually contains inflammation and/or blood. (Pap)

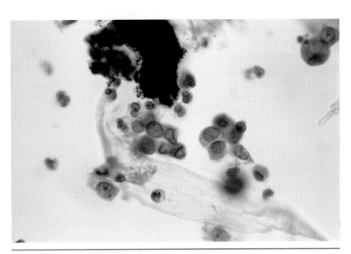

Figure 11-28 **Stone fragments in bladder wash specimen.** Stone fragments are seen in the upper central field of this photomicrograph and are usually accompanied by acute inflammation and reactive urothelial cells. The urothelial cells seen in this photomicrograph are parabasal cells most likely stripped from the bladder wall. These cells contain high N:C ratios but relatively bland-appearing chromatin. (Pap)

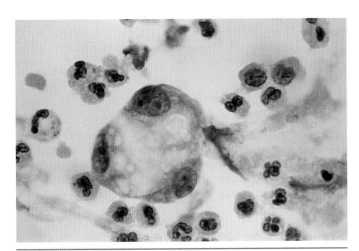

Figure 11-27 **Nuclear atypia resulting from lithiasis in a catheterized urine specimen.** Three urothelial cells with cytoplasmic vacuolization and nuclear atypia are admixed with abundant acute inflammation. Urothelial cells often show cytoplasmic and nuclear changes resulting from lithiasis. These nuclei are hyperchromatic, contain nucleoli, and show nuclear membrane irregularities. The N:C ratio here is relatively low and therefore reflects reactive changes rather than a high-grade urothelial cell carcinoma. (Pap)

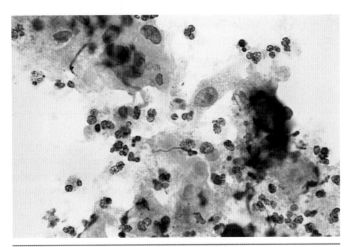

Figure 11-29 **Squamous metaplasia secondary to lithiasis in this bladder wash specimen.** Squamous metaplasia resulting from chronic irritation of the bladder wall may be seen in lithiasis. In this case, squamous metaplastic cells having orangeophilic, abundant cytoplasm are seen. In the center of the field is a large superficial urothelial cell showing reactive changes consisting of an enlarged nucleus and irregular cytoplasmic contours. Abundant acute inflammation also is seen in the background. (Pap)

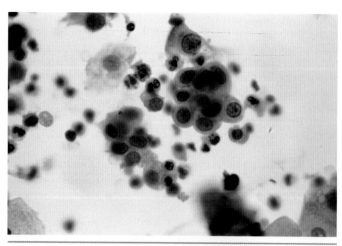

Figure 11-30 Acute inflammation resulting from lithiasis in a catheterized urine specimen. Parabasal cells, intermediate cells and neutrophils are seen. The parabasal cells often are seen in small clusters as a result of the abrasion. The acute inflammation is seen in the background, although acute inflammatory cells may infiltrate the small clusters. (Pap)

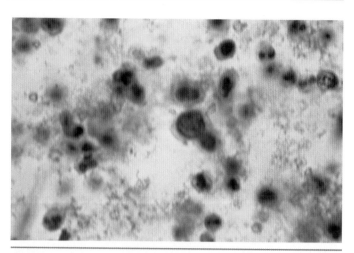

Figure 11-31 Tumor diathesis in high-grade urothelial cell carcinoma in a bladder wash specimen. In this photomicrograph, a high-grade urothelial carcinoma cell is seen in the center portion of the field. Necrotic debris and acute inflammatory cells surround this cell. The necrotic debris represents tumor diathesis, which generally is not seen in lithiasis. Thus, in lithiasis, acute inflammation predominates the background, whereas in high-grade urothelial cell carcinoma, diathesis predominates the background. (Pap)

BOX 11-12   CMF

Cytomorphologic Features Supportive of Lithiasis over Low-Grade Urothelial Cell Carcinoma

Acute inflammation
Spectrum of atypical changes rather than dual population
Nonhomogeneous cytoplasm

BOX 11-13   CMF

Cytomorphologic Features Supportive of Lithiasis over High-Grade Urothelial Cell Carcinoma

Absence of marked atypia
Absence of diathesis background
Acute inflammation
Smoothly bordered groups (rather than irregularly bordered groups)

BOX 11-14   CMF

Cytomorphologic Features of Bacterial Cystitis

Acute inflammation
Bacteria
Single cells and large groups of cells
Degenerative features
Cytoplasmic vacuolization
Stripped nuclei

---

concern, or the clinical and laboratory findings are not diagnostic of an infectious process. Cancer must then be excluded. This section primarily focuses on bladder infections. Infections elsewhere in the urinary tract have a similar appearance.

Bacterial Infections

Most cases of bacterial cystitis are caused by gram-negative bacteria, usually fecal flora, such as *Escherichia coli* (80% of cases), *Klebsiella, Proteus,* and *Pseudomonas aeruginosa.* Gram-positive organisms such as *Staphylococcus* and *Streptococcus,* rarely are the infectious agents. Bacterial urinary tract infections are largely a disease of adult females,[31] but also occur in men with benign prostatic hypertrophy, children, patients with stones (and other obstructions), and patients with nerve damage. Urinary tract infections are the most common bacterial infection in older adults and are a common source of bacteremia.[31] Signs and symptoms of cystitis include suprapubic tenderness, dysuria, frequency, nocturia, and malodorous urine.

The bacteria may be either absent or teeming on cytologic preparations, and the background contains copious numbers of neutrophils (Box 11-14 and Figure 11-32). In some cases, urothelial cells may not be seen. However, sin-

spectrum of atypical changes occur (Box 11-13). In high-grade urothelial cell carcinoma, the atypia is present in many cells. Although a tumor diathesis may be present in high-grade urothelial cell carcinoma, marked acute inflammation generally is absent (Figure 11-31). In lithiasis, the larger cell clusters have a smooth border, whereas in high-grade urothelial cell carcinoma, the groups have an irregular contour.

Infectious Conditions

More than 4 million patients in the United States annually are diagnosed with urinary tract infections. Specimens from the majority of these patients are not sent to the cytology laboratory for analysis. However, in some cases, cancer is a

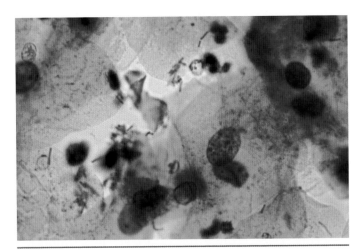

Figure 11-32 Bacteria and neutrophils in bacterial cystitis in a clean catch urine specimen. Intermediate squamous cells, urothelial cells, and bacterial rods are seen. A background of acute inflammation also is present. In bacterial cystitis, the bacteria usually are easily identifiable at high power. (Pap)

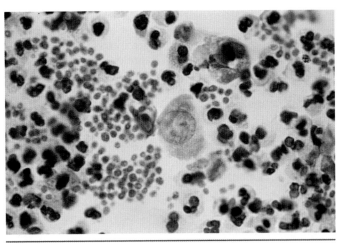

Figure 11-33 Urinary candidiasis in a catheterized urine specimen. A reactive degenerated urothelial cell is seen in the center of the field. The remainder of the photomicrograph shows numerous neutrophils and candidal yeast forms. Occasional pseudohyphae may be observed. In contrast with contaminated specimens, squamous cells are not seen in abundance in candidal cystitis. (Pap)

gle and large groups of urothelial cells may be sloughed, mimicking a high-grade urothelial cell carcinoma. In some cases the urothelial cells exhibit striking atypia resulting from inflammatory change and repair with increases in N:C ratios, nuclear hyperchromasia, and prominent nucleoli. More often, the urothelial cells are extensively degenerated and demonstrate nuclear smudging and breakdown. The cytoplasm may show extensive vacuolization, which is an unusual feature in most urothelial cell carcinomas. Stripped nuclei resulting from cytoplasmic destruction may be visible.

In contrast with high-grade urothelial cell carcinoma, the findings in bacterial cystitis include more abundant inflammation, bacteria, less cellular atypia, fewer atypical cells, and more degeneration. Although both bacterial cystitis and lithiasis may show similar epithelial changes and acute inflammatory backgrounds, bacteria generally are not present in lithiasis unless a superinfection is present. Acute pyelonephritis may show neutrophils, casts, and renal tubular cells that are observed in small clusters or individually.

Fungal Infections

Candida is the most common fungal organism seen in urinary tract specimens, and in most cases, *Candida* is a contaminant from the female genital tract. When it is a contaminant, *Candida* unfailingly is admixed with squamous cells, bacteria, and neutrophils. Yeast forms predominate, although occasional pseudohyphae are seen. True candidiasis of the urinary tract may be seen in individuals with diabetes and other immunosuppressed patients. Specimens from these patients are similar to those from patients with bacterial cystitis, although the bacteria are replaced by *Candida* (Figure 11-33). The urothelial cells may be shed in large clusters and exhibit marked reactive, atypical changes. Atypia may be overinterpreted in the context of fungal forms, so care must be taken to not do so.

Other fungal organisms that infect the urinary tract include *Histoplasma, Aspergillus, Cryptococcus,* and *Blastomyces* (Figure 11-34).[32] Infection may be localized or systemic and usually occurs in immunosuppressed patients. The fungal

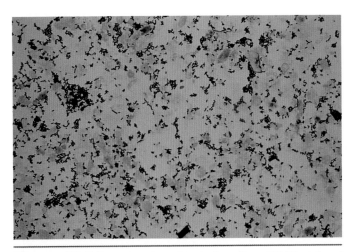

Figure 11-34 Gomori methenamine silver (GMS) stain of *Histoplasma capsulatum* in a bladder wash specimen. This low-powered image shows numerous *Histoplasma capsulatum* yeast forms in small clusters and individually.

organisms may be seen in cytologic preparations, although culture is a mainstay in reaching a definitive diagnosis. Urine specimens contain abundant acute inflammatory cells and reactive urothelial cells.

Mycobacterial Infections

The main mycobacterial agent which involves the urinary tract is *Mycobacterium tuberculosis*. The principal site of infection is the kidney although the bladder (adjacent to the ureteral orifices) may be involved secondarily. The bladder washing findings of primary tuberculosis are similar to findings associated with the *bacillus Calmette-Guérin (BCG)* vaccine used in the treatment of urothelial cell carcinoma. Bladder wash specimens are often cellular and show multinucleated giant cells and epithelioid histiocyte clusters that are consistent with granulomas.[33,34] The epithelioid histiocytes have elongated nuclei that are usually pale, although hyperchromasia is sometimes present and causes concern for carcinoma. The cytoplasm of these cells usually is finely vacuolated, and if clusters of cells are present, the cytoplasmic borders are indistinct. Tuberculosis infections of the urinary tract typically are associated with marked reactive epithelial atypia, a pitfall in the overdiagnosis of high-grade urothelial cell carcinoma. The urothelial cells may show considerable nuclear enlargement, membrane irregularities, and hyperchromasia. A clue that a carcinoma is not present lies in the observation of numerous histiocytes and granulomatous fragments, assuming the BCG vaccine is not being used as treatment.

Viral Infections

Human polyomavirus. Human polyomavirus is a DNA virus and a member of the papovirus family. Human polyomavirus is also known as *BK virus,* after the initials of the first patient diagnosed with the virus.[35] Infections with human polyomavirus may be detected in all urinary tract specimen types and are one of the classic pitfalls causing a false-positive diagnosis. Human polyomavirus is first acquired in

childhood. The virus may be reactivated and cause infection in patients who are immunocompromised (e.g., patients with cancer or undergoing chemotherapy, patients with acquired immune deficiency syndrome [AIDS]) or in those who have no underlying disorder.[36-40] In many patients, the disease is asymptomatic, and the infection resolves in several months.[37]

Human polyomavirus infects urothelial cells or renal tubular cells, particularly in renal transplant patients.[41] Urothelial cells infected with human polyomavirus are termed *decoy cells,* because they resemble high-grade urothelial carcinoma cells (Box 11-15).[37,42,43] Infected urothelial cells are variable in size, and the larger cells have nuclei rivaling the size of neoplastic cell nuclei (Figure 11-35). The cells may be difficult to separate from neoplastic cells, because the nuclei are hyperchromatic and the cells have a high N:C ratio. The nuclear hyperchromasia is a result of a nuclear inclusion that is homogeneous and blue to black.[39] The inclusion expands and occupies almost the entire nucleus and pushes the residual chromatin to the nuclear edge, resulting in the appearance of a thick nuclear rim (Figure 11-36). The nucleus retains a round to oval shape and lacks significant membrane irregularity. The cells may be few or plentiful but are always single.[44] The difficulty in the separation from high-grade urothelial cell carcinoma mainly lies in extensively degenerated specimens. Compared with nondegenerated cells infected with human polyomavirus, slightly degenerated cells may appear even more hyperchromatic and have a less homogeneous nuclear chromatin texture. Some of these cells show nuclear membrane irregularities and appear similar to the degenerated "coal-black" nuclei of high-grade urothelial cell carcinoma. The viral inclusion may degenerate to such an extent that the infected cells have a cleared or empty nuclear appearance. Cells infected with human polyomavirus are also known as *comet cells,* because only a thin, eccentric rim of blue to green cyto-

---

BOX 11-15 CMF

Cytomorphologic Features of Human Polyomavirus

Single urothelial cells with increased N:C ratios
Enlarged nuclei
Hyperchromasia with even dispersion of chromatin
Thick nuclear rim
Regular nuclear membranes
Eccentrically placed cytoplasm
Nuclear degeneration

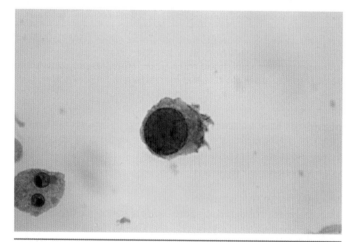

Figure 11-35 Human polyomavirus in a bladder wash specimen. Urothelial cells infected with human polyomavirus are known as *decoy cells* because the nuclei are hyperchromatic, thus mimicking a high-grade urothelial cell carcinoma. In contrast with a high-grade urothelial cell carcinoma, decoy cells show round nuclei with a lack of nuclear membrane irregularity. A nuclear inclusion that is blue-black in color occupies almost the entire nucleus, although the nuclear rim appears slightly hyperchromatic resulting from compressed chromatin. The nucleus is seen at the edge of the cell. (Pap)

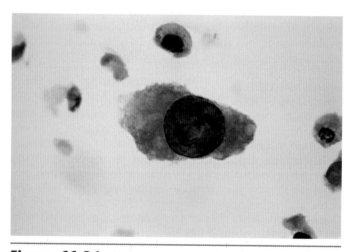

Figure 11-36 Human polyomavirus in a catheterized urine specimen. The nuclear inclusion has a homogeneous appearance, which contrasts from the irregular chromatin appearance seen in high-grade urothelial cell carcinoma. The cytoplasm seen in infected cells may have a degenerated appearance with indistinct cytoplasmic boundaries and slight cytoplasmic vacuolization. A lack of nuclear membrane irregularity is evident. (Pap)

plasm remains (Figure 11-37). The background often contains degenerated debris and scattered inflammatory cells; abundant acute inflammation generally is not present. Urothelial cells without inclusions may be admixed with infected cells.

High-grade urothelial cell carcinoma may be separated morphologically from human polyomavirus in nondegenerated specimens. In contrast with cells infected with human polyomavirus, high-grade urothelial carcinoma cells do not have a homogeneous chromatin pattern and display more nuclear membrane irregularities. Neoplastic cells also tend to be larger and may form large or small groups, which are not seen in urine specimens from patients with human polyomaviral infections. If only degenerated cells are present, caution should be taken with making a malignant diagnosis.

The differential diagnosis of human polyomavirus also includes other viruses, such as cytomegalovirus (CMV). In contrast with CMV infected cells, human polyomavirus infected cells are smaller and have an inclusion that extends almost to the nuclear rim. A larger halo typically surrounds the nuclear cytomegalic inclusion. Cytoplasmic inclusions, seen in CMV infected cells, are lacking in cells infected with human polyomavirus. Polymerase chain reaction may be used to confirm a CMV or human polyomavirus infection.[45,46]

Cytomegalovirus. As CMV tends to infect renal convoluted tubular cells, only rare infected cells may be found in most urinary tract specimens in patients with infections.[47] Cytomegalovirus infects immunocompromised patients such as the very young or immunosuppressed (patients with AIDS or cancer or transplant patients).[48] In many patients, the infection is life-threatening, although some individuals are carriers. The infected cells have a large nucleus with a prominent blue to black inclusion, surrounded by a region of perinuclear clearing (e.g., an "owl's eye"). The nuclear membrane appears thickened, although pronounced nuclear membrane irregularities are absent (Figure 11-38).

Cytoplasmic inclusions also may be observed. Similar to human polyomavirus–infected cells, CMV infected cells often show degenerative features.

Herpes simplex virus. Herpes simplex virus may infect urothelial cells but often is a contaminant from a genital herpes infection.[49,50] Herpes simplex infections may occur in transplant and cancer patients. The appearance of a herpetically infected cell in a urinary tract specimen is identical to the appearance of an infected cell in a Pap test (Figure 11-39). Multiple nuclei or multilobated nuclei with nuclear molding are seen. The chromatin may have a ground glass

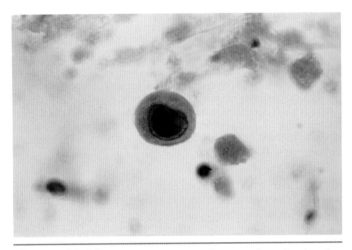

Figure 11-38 Cytomegalovirus in a catheterized urine specimen. Cytomegalovirus infects renal convoluted tubular cells and therefore only rare cells may be seen in urinary tract specimens. These cells have a large nucleus with a prominent blue-black inclusion surrounded by a region of perinuclear clearing. The nuclear membrane appears thickened although marked nuclear membrane irregularities are absent. Cytoplasmic inclusions also may be seen but are not present in this photomicrograph. Inflammatory cells and degenerated cells are seen in the background. (Pap)

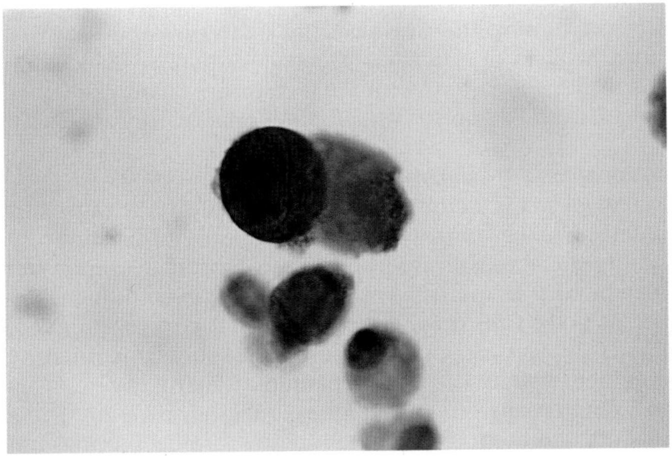

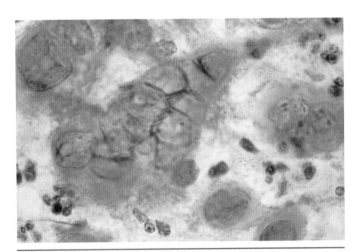

Figure 11-37 Human polyomavirus in a bladder wash specimen. Human polyomavirus–infected cells are sometimes referred to as *comet cells* because the nucleus is seen at one edge with cytoplasm trailing from the other edge of the cell. In this field, two infected cells are present along with a histiocyte. The infected cells may be few or plentiful but are always seen singly and not in large groups. (Pap)

Figure 11-39 Herpes simplex virus in a catheterized urine specimen. Herpes simplex virus may infect urothelial cells although contaminant from a genital herpes infection also must be considered. In this photomicrograph, numerous cells infected with herpes simplex virus are seen. These cells contain multilobated nuclei with nuclear molding; the nuclear chromatin has a ground glass, slightly eosinophilic appearance. Numerous acute inflammatory cells often are seen in the background. (Pap)

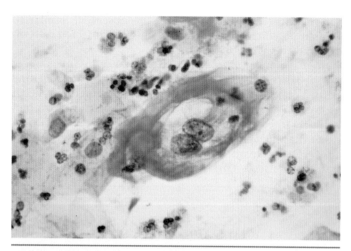

Figure 11-40 **Human papillomavirus in a bladder wash specimen.** A large koilocyte having a hyperchromatic, raisinoid nucleus, perinuclear clearing and peripheral cytoplasmic condensation is seen. Contamination from the genital tract must be excluded before a primary bladder or urethral condyloma diagnosis is made. In this case, several degenerated urothelial and squamous cells are seen. (Pap)

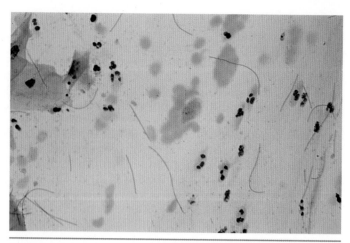

Figure 11-41 *Trichomonas vaginalis* **in a clean catch urine specimen from a male patient.** *Trichomonas* rarely may involve the bladder but in this case represents a nongonococcal urethritis in a male. The findings are similar to those seen in a Pap test. In this case, a *T. vaginalis* organism is seen in the center field and is surrounded by leptothrix organisms and acute inflammation. (Pap)

appearance,[51,52] or eosinophilic nuclear inclusions may be seen. In bladder infections, acute inflammatory cells may overwhelm the specimen and limit interpretation.

Human papillomavirus. Human papillomavirus (HPV) is a sexually transmitted DNA virus that infects both urothelial and squamous cells. In the bladder, types 6 and 11 are most commonly found. The incidence of HPV bladder infection increases in the immunosuppressed population.[53] Clinical cystitis or urethritis usually is not present, and more typically, HPV infection clinically manifests as a flat or exophytic condyloma. Genital condylomas are seen in conjunction with bladder condylomas in 20% of cases.[275] Condylomas appearing only in the bladder are rare. HPV infection is a risk factor for developing squamous cell carcinoma.[54]

Cytologically, the diagnostic cell is the koilocyte, and contamination must be excluded before a diagnosis of primary bladder or urethral condyloma is made (Figure 11-40). Typically, koilocytes have a hyperchromatic, raisinoid nucleus, perinuclear clearing and peripheral cytoplasmic condensation. Parakeratosis may be prominent. Immunohistochemical stains or hybridizing nucleic acid probes may be used to confirm the infection.

Other viruses. Other viruses that may infect the urinary tract include adenovirus and measles virus. Both viruses are associated with cytoplasmic inclusions.

Parasitic Infections
The principal parasites found in urinary tract specimens are *Trichomonas* and *Schistosoma*. In women, *Trichomonas* usually is a contaminant. Trichomonas rarely may involve the bladder but more likely is seen in the male urethra where it is a cause of nongonococcal urethritis.[55] The cytologic findings in urinary tract specimens are identical to those seen in Pap tests (Figure 11-41).

Schistosomiasis of the bladder is caused mainly by *Schistosoma hematobium* and occasionally by *Schistosoma mansoni*. The disease is much more common in the Middle East than in North America.[56] The ova initially are deposited in the veins of the muscularis propria leading to ul-

ceration of the overlying tissues. The eggs of *Schistosoma* may be observed in urinary tract specimens.[57] The eggs are oval and have a large nucleus with a pointed terminal spur. Miracidium also may be seen.[58] Schistosomal infections are characterized by pronounced acute inflammation, squamous metaplasia, blood, and reactive epithelial change. Granulomas and foreign body giant cells may be seen. Schistosomal infection is a risk factor for developing squamous cell carcinoma of the bladder.

Other parasites that may infect the urinary tract are *Entamoeba histolytica*, *Enterobius vermicularis* (pinworm), and *Echinococcus granulosis*. *E. histolytica* spreads to the bladder through the lymphatics. *E. histolytica* has two cytoplasmic zones, one at the periphery that is transparent and a central one that is dense. Ingested RBCs and one to four small nuclei are seen. *E. vermicularis* typically is seen in infected children; the ova have thick capsules and flattened sides. Scolices of *Echinococcus granulosis* may be detected in the urine of a patient with renal disease.[59] Filariasis may be diagnosed by demonstrating microfilariae, worms, or eggs.[60]

Malacoplakia (Malakoplakia)
Malacoplakia is a chronic granulomatous disease caused by a defect in the phagolysosomal processing of bacteria.[61] It occurs characteristically in middle-age or older women but may be seen in men and patients of any age and in a number of body sites (e.g., entire urogenital system, lungs, or brain).[62-64] Cystoscopically, the bladder surface is lined by confluent yellow nodules or plaques, ranging in size of up to 5 cm in diameter. The larger nodules may ulcerate. These plaques represent granulomas in the lamina propria and muscular wall.[65] On histologic examination, the granulomas consist of histiocytes, multinucleated giant cells known as von Hansemann histiocytes, lymphocytes, and plasma cells. The von Hansemann histiocytes contain abundant granular cytoplasm that stains positively with periodic acid Schiff (PAS). This staining results from the presence of numerous phagolysosomes containing partially digested bacteria. The definitive diagnosis of malacoplakia rests on the observation of the characteristic Michaelis-Gutmann body,

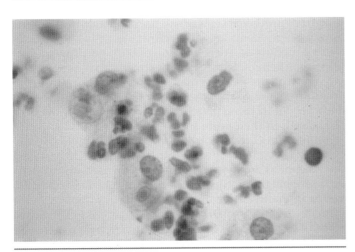

Figure 11-42 Malacoplakia in a bladder wash specimen. Specimens of malacoplakia generally contain histiocytes and acute inflammation. A Michaelis-Gutmann body is seen in the lower central portion of the field. The Michaelis-Gutmann body has a bird's-eye appearance and is a round, laminated cytoplasmic inclusion seen within the histiocyte. Michaelis-Gutmann bodies also are periodic acid Schiff (PAS) positive and may calcify or may be encrusted with iron. Similar structures may be seen in patients with hypercalciuria. Michaelis-Gutmann bodies even may be seen in voided urine specimens. (Pap)

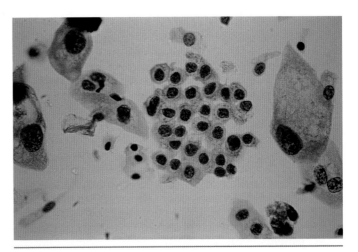

Figure 11-43 Cytologic atypia resulting from cyclophosphamide therapy in a catheterized urine specimen. Enlarged superficial urothelial cells are admixed with parabasal cells and inflammation. The cell on the right shows marked enlargement with abundant cytoplasm and a hyperchromatic nucleus. The nuclear membrane shows slight membrane irregularity, and the chromatin pattern is irregularly clumped. In this case the N:C ratio is not increased, indicating that the features most likely are reactive rather than neoplastic. (Pap)

which is a round, laminated cytoplasmic inclusion.[66] These inclusions range in diameter from 4 to 10 microns and usually are eosinophilic (Figure 11-42). Michaelis-Gutmann bodies are described as having a bird's-eye appearance, because the center of the structure has a dotlike appearance. Michaelis-Gutmann bodies are also PAS positive and may calcify and become encrusted with iron. Thus, they also may stain positively for calcium and iron. Ultrastructural features are diagnostic.[62,67] Michaelis-Gutmann bodies may be seen in voided urine.[68] Similar structures may be seen in patients with hypercalciuria.[68] Voided urine specimens from patients with malacoplakia may be highly cellular and contain neutrophils and histiocytes.

Chemotherapeutic Effect

Chemotherapeutic effect results from agents given either systemically or intravesically. Systemic agents include cyclophosphamide and busulfan (both alkylating agents) that are concentrated in the urine; their effect is primarily seen in the bladder where they are in contact with the urothelium for extended periods. These drugs are used for several purposes, including cancer treatment and immunosuppression for patients undergoing transplantation or with severe autoimmune disease. Intravesicular chemotherapeutic agents include cyclophosphamide, mitomycin C, thiotepa, adriamycin (doxyrubicin), epirubicin, ethoglucid, mitoxantrone, N-triflouroacetyladriamycin-14-valerate, and BCG vaccine.[69] The cytologic effects of some of these agents have been better described than others, and several of the main chemotherapeutic agents are discussed later in this chapter. Although all these agents may be used to treat patients with urothelial cell carcinoma, the current first-line treatment is BCG vaccine. However, BCG is not without significant side effects and some patients may not respond to BCG therapy.[69,70] Thus, patients still receive a variety of chemotherapeutic agents.

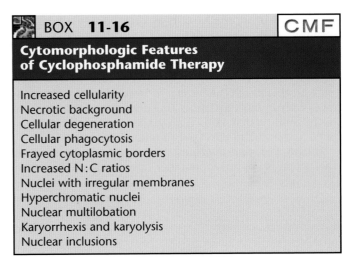

BOX 11-16   **CMF**

Cytomorphologic Features of Cyclophosphamide Therapy

Increased cellularity
Necrotic background
Cellular degeneration
Cellular phagocytosis
Frayed cytoplasmic borders
Increased N:C ratios
Nuclei with irregular membranes
Hyperchromatic nuclei
Nuclear multilobation
Karyorrhexis and karyolysis
Nuclear inclusions

Cyclophosphamide. Cyclophosphamide is used systemically for cancer or immunosuppressive therapy and intravesically for cancer therapy. Cyclophosphamide is a nitrogen mustard that prevents DNA replication in both tumor and nonneoplastic cells. When used systemically, cyclophosphamide is concentrated in the urine and causes necrosis, degeneration, and sloughing of normal urothelial epithelial cells. Cyclophosphamide usually results in hematuria.[71] Cyclophosphamide has been linked to hemorrhagic cystitis resulting in uncontrollable bleeding necessitating cystectomy.

Cytologically, the urothelial cells may exhibit severe atypia (Box 11-16), closely mimicking high-grade urothelial cell carcinoma.[72,73] These changes are seen in all specimen types. The urothelial cell nuclei may be greatly enlarged, and their nuclear membranes may be highly irregular (Figure 11-43). The N:C ratios usually are markedly increased. The nuclei may be multilobated, or the cells may be multinucleated. Degenerative nuclear features such as smudging, vacuolization, karyorrhexis, and karyolysis are common (Figure 11-44). One or several nucleoli may be visible and even atypical in shape. The cytoplasm also may be increased in size, frayed, and vacuolated or dense. Phagocytosis of debris is not unusual.[74] The background is often bloody or necrotic.

Separation from high-grade urothelial cell carcinoma may be difficult or impossible in some cases. Signs of cellular degeneration should suggest cyclophosphamide effect. The differential diagnosis includes human polyomavirus that also may be characterized by degenerative cellular features. True nuclear inclusions are absent in cyclophosphamide effect.[75] Superimposed viral infection may be seen in immunosuppressed patients treated with cyclophosphamide.

As patients with urothelial cell carcinoma may be treated with cyclophosphamide, both chemotherapeutic effect and urothelial cell carcinoma may be seen in the same specimen. If a patient has a known history of urothelial cell carcinoma, a diagnosis of at least atypia may be warranted in cases in which the source for the atypia is uncertain. In addition, cyclophosphamide treatment is a risk factor for developing urothelial malignancy. Consequently, just because a history of systemic cyclophosphamide treatment is provided, urothelial cell carcinoma is not necessarily excluded.[76-78]

Busulfan. Busulfan is given systemically and causes similar changes in urothelial cells as cyclophosphamide, and busulfan may also result in hemorrhagic cystitis.[276] Urothelial cells may be dramatically increased in size with corresponding nuclear hyperchromasia and membrane irregularity (Figure 11-45).[72,79] These cells may mimic high-grade urothelial cell carcinoma. As busulfan is not given intravesically in most instances, one does not have to exclude the possibility that both high-grade urothelial cell carcinoma and busulfan effect are simultaneously present.

Mitomycin C and thiotepa. Mitomycin C and thiotepa (triethylene thiophosphoramide) have been used to treat

superficial urothelial cell carcinoma, particularly carcinoma in situ. These agents are injected intravesically and initially cause sloughing and degeneration of both normal and neoplastic epithelium. Subsequent treatments may suppress tumor growth, and patients may be followed by obtaining repeat urine cytology specimens. Therapy generally is deemed unsuccessful in those patients who continue to show neoplastic cells in their urine specimens.[80]

Mitomycin C and thiotepa show similar changes in urine cytology specimens (Box 11-17). With initial treatments, the specimens are hypercellular and contain both neoplastic and benign urothelial cells. These chemotherapeutic agents primarily affect the superficial cells although intermediate and basal/parabasal cells also may exhibit changes. All urothelial cell types may increase in size, but an increased N:C ratio generally is not observed.[81-84] The cells may be multinucleated with round to oval nuclei with prominent nucleoli (Figure 11-46). Reparative features such as cytoplasmic polychromasia and streaming are seen. Difficulties in diagnosis arise when the cells show degenerative features. As with other chemotherapeutic agents, nuclear hyperchro-

---

BOX 11-17   **CMF**

Cytomorphologic Features of Mitomycin C and Thiotepa Therapy

Hypercellular specimen
Reparative features
Increased cell size
Normal N:C ratios
Multinucleation
Round nuclei with regular nuclear membranes
Prominent nucleoli
Degenerated nuclei
Cytoplasmic polychromasia
Vacuolated cytoplasm

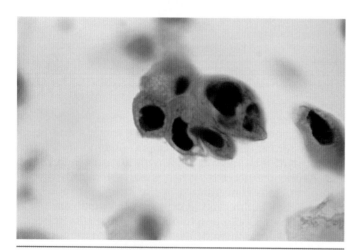

Figure 11-44 **Degenerated nuclei in cyclophosphamide therapy in a bladder wash specimen.** Nuclear degeneration and hyperchromasia may be pronounced in cyclophosphamide therapy. In the cluster of intermediate cells, the nuclei appear markedly irregular and coal black in color. These cells easily may be mistaken for high-grade urothelial cell carcinoma, indicating that a nondegenerated urothelial carcinoma cell should be observed before the diagnosis is made. (Pap)

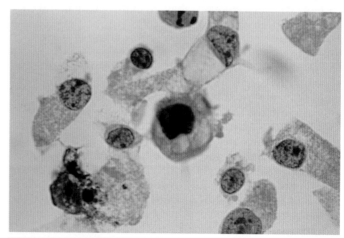

Figure 11-45 **Nuclear hyperchromasia resulting from busulfan therapy in a bladder wash specimen.** Marked nuclear hyperchromasia and degeneration is seen. The cytoplasm shows vacuolization, which is not typically characteristic of high-grade urothelial cell carcinoma. In some cases of busulfan therapy, the cells increase markedly in size, although this is not seen in the current photomicrograph. (Pap)

masia, smudging, membrane irregularity, and vacuolation may be present.[83,277] The cytoplasm occasionally shows fraying and large vacuoles. Atypical cells may be seen in patients undergoing mitomycin C or thiotepa treatment (similar to cyclophosphamide treatment), although it is the exception rather than the rule. If severely atypical cells are seen, recurrent or persistent high-grade urothelial cell carcinoma should be seriously considered.

Bacillus Calmette-Guérin vaccine. BCG vaccine is currently the linchpin chemotherapeutic agent for treating many bladder cancers, particularly urothelial cell carcinoma in situ. BCG vaccine is derived from *Mycobacterium bovis* and induces a granulomatous response with epithelial sloughing and degeneration. Patients undergoing BCG vaccine treatment are usually monitored for tumor recurrence with repeat urine specimens (usually bladder washes).[85]

The cytologic changes vary, depending on the time course of therapy (Box 11-18).[17] Initially, a neutrophilic response occurs with numerous sloughed epithelial cells (Figure 11-47). After the first week, neutrophils decrease in number and are replaced by lymphocytes, histiocytes, and histiocytic aggregates.[17,86,87] These aggregates vary in ap-

pearance from loose collections of histiocytes to true granulomas, identical to the findings in primary mycobacterial infection (Figure 11-48). In the granulomas, the histiocyte nuclei are elongated and boomerang in shape, and cytoplasmic borders are indistinct. Acid fast stains show the attenuated organisms (Figure 11-49). BCG vaccine may induce epithelial atypia, but generally not to the extent seen in cyclophosphamide therapy.[88] Benign urothelial cell nuclei may show enlargement and slight darkening of the chromatin. Degenerative features are customary. In contrast with urothelial cell carcinoma, the N:C ratios are maintained with BCG vaccine, and pronounced nuclear membrane irregularities are absent.

BOX 11-18 CMF

Cytomorphologic Features of Bacillus Calmette-Guérin Vaccine Therapy

Increased cellularity
Inflammatory cells including lymphocytes
Neutrophils and histiocytes
Granulomas
Mild epithelial atypia

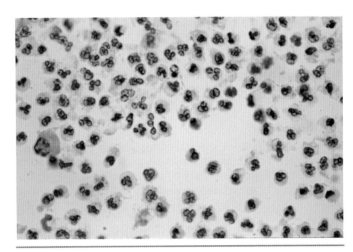

Figure 11-47 **Acute inflammation secondary to bacillus Calmette-Guérin (BCG) vaccine in a bladder wash specimen.** In the early stages of BCG therapy, numerous neutrophils are seen. Sloughed epithelial cells such as the one in the left central portion of the field may show degeneration. When abundant acute inflammation occurs, the epithelial cells may be few in number. (Pap)

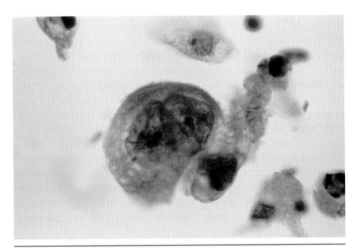

Figure 11-46 **Multinucleation resulting from chemotherapy in a bladder wash specimen.** Several multinucleated cells with enlarged, degenerated nuclei are seen. The nuclei exhibit slight nuclear membrane irregularities and in the central cell, prominent nucleoli are observed. The degenerated nuclear features include hyperchromasia, membrane irregularity, and slight vacuolization. The cytoplasm shows fraying and vacuolization. (Pap) (From Raab SS: Urinary cytology. In: Atkinson BF, Silverman JF, editors. Atlas of difficult diagnoses in cytopathology. Philadelphia: WB Saunders; 1998. p.245.)

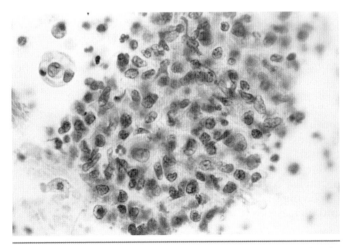

Figure 11-48 **Granulomas resulting from BCG vaccine in a bladder wash specimen.** After the first week of BCG therapy, the neutrophils decrease in number and chronic inflammation may be seen. Granulomas are variable in size and appearance, depending on their age. In this granuloma, numerous histiocytes admixed with other chronic inflammatory cells are seen. The histiocytes are elongated and irregular in shape and the chromatin pattern is hypochromatic. (Pap)

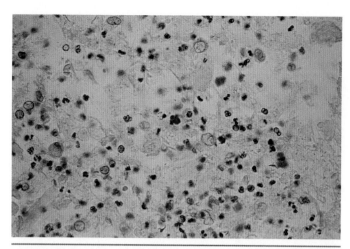

Figure 11-49 Acid fast stain showing attenuated organisms in BCG therapy in a cell block from a bladder wash specimen. Numerous organisms may be seen on acid fast stains on either cytospin or cell block preparations.

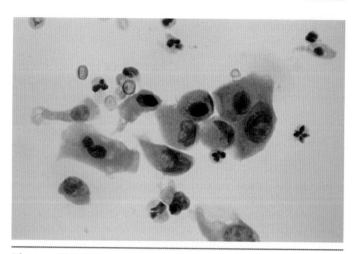

Figure 11-50 Radiation effect in a bladder wash specimen. In radiation effect the urothelial cells show nuclear and cytoplasmic enlargement with preservation of the N:C ratio. Nuclear hyperchromasia, vacuolization, polychromasia, and degeneration are seen. In addition, cytoplasmic vacuolization and fraying are observed. Although radiation effect may mimic high-grade urothelial cell carcinoma, in this case the lack of significant hyperchromasia and degenerated features are indicative of radiation change. Radiation change may be seen for many years following the therapy. (Pap)

Radiation Effect

Patients who are poor surgical candidates or those with recurrent pelvic or abdominal tumors may undergo radiation therapy. Bladder tumors may be the intended target, or the bladder may be irradiated secondarily for the treatment of other tumors. In either case, radiation cystitis with accompanying cytologic atypia may be seen.

The cytologic changes associated with radiation in the urinary tract mimic the changes seen in other sites (Box 11-19).[89] Immediately after radiotherapy, ulceration of the bladder mucosa and cellular degeneration are observed. These changes should disappear in the 3 to 4 months after radiotherapy.[90] Chronic changes, which may occur even after 10 years postradiotherapy, include nuclear and cytoplasmic enlargement with preservation of the N:C ratio; multinucleation; nuclear hyperchromasia, vacuolization, polychromasia, and degeneration; and cytoplasmic vacuolization and degeneration (Figure 11-50). Prominent and multiple nucleoli may be seen. One of the more common findings is the presence of massively enlarged epithelial cells.[91] Radiation changes may be seen for years after therapy.[92,93]

Radiation change must be distinguished from high-grade urothelial cell carcinoma, and in some cases the separation is impossible.[5] Features favoring radiation change include nuclear and cytoplasmic degeneration, multinucleation, and cytoplasmic and nuclear vacuolization. High-grade urothelial cell carcinoma is more likely in cases with cells displaying nuclear hyperchromasia, membrane irregularity, and increased N:C ratios.[94]

Other Inflammatory Conditions

Nonspecific cystitis (cystitis cystica and cystitis glandularis). The most common reactive change in the bladder is the formation of Brunn's nests, which are invaginations of the surface epithelium. Because of chronic irritation resulting from identifiable (e.g., stones) or unidentifiable causes, Brunn's nests may lose contact with the overlying surface and form cystic structures. This process is known as *cystitis cystica,* and because these structures are lined by normal urothelium, it is not diagnosable on cytology. It is believed that

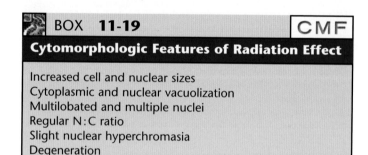

BOX 11-19 | CMF

Cytomorphologic Features of Radiation Effect

Increased cell and nuclear sizes
Cytoplasmic and nuclear vacuolization
Multilobated and multiple nuclei
Regular N:C ratio
Slight nuclear hyperchromasia
Degeneration

continued chronic inflammation may lead to replacement of the urothelium by glandular epithelium, and the end result of this process is known as *cystitis glandularis.* Benign glandular epithelium from cystitis glandularis may be observed in urine specimens, particular bladder washes. Thus, if glandular epithelium is seen, a chronic irritative process may be present. Cystitis glandularis also may be observed in the renal pelvis (pyelitis glandularis) and the ureter (ureteritis glandularis).[95] Because glandular epithelium may normally be present in urinary tract specimens and may not be the result of inflammation, most cytologists do not make an outright diagnosis of cystitis glandularis, although the condition may be suggested. Cystitis cystica and cystitis glandularis are not premalignant lesions.[96,97]

Inverted papilloma. Inverted papillomas are believed to be proliferative lesions that form as a result of noxious insults.[98] They are not premalignant. Inverted papillomas occur most commonly in the bladder but also are seen in other sites of the urinary tract.[99,100] Grossly, an inverted papilloma appears polypoid, and histologically, nests of urothelium fill the lamina propria. On cystoscopy, a urothelial cell carcinoma may be suspected, although on washing specimens, only normal epithelium, representing the benign surface, is seen.

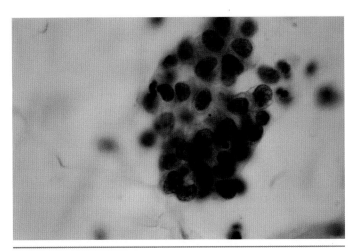

Figure 11-51 Endometrial cells in a clean catch urine specimen. The presence of endometrial cells in a clean catch urine specimen usually indicates contaminant, although endometriosis also must be considered. In this case a cluster of degenerated endometrial glandular cells is observed. These cells are tightly packed and contain small hyperchromatic nuclei. Considerable nuclear overlapping is seen. In some cases of endometriosis, only the glandular cells are observed (as in this case).

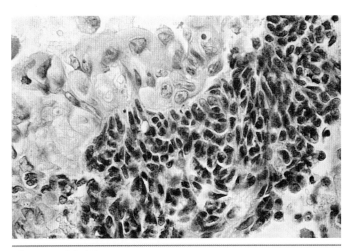

Figure 11-52 Endometriosis in a cell block of a bladder wash specimen. In this cell block, endometrial glandular cells and stromal cells are observed. The glandular cells have an atypical appearance with enlarged nuclei and prominent nucleoli. Abundant cytoplasm is seen. The stromal cells appear hyperchromatic and small and have a spindled appearance. Inflammation is seen in the lower right hand corner and is commonly seen in urinary tract specimens of endometriosis. (Hematoxylin and eosin [H&E])

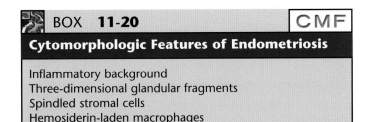

BOX 11-20   CMF

Cytomorphologic Features of Endometriosis

Inflammatory background
Three-dimensional glandular fragments
Spindled stromal cells
Hemosiderin-laden macrophages

Interstitial cystitis. Interstitial cystitis typically affects middle-age women who have classic cystitis symptoms (e.g., frequency, urgency, suprapubic pain, and so on). Urine cultures do not grow organisms. Cystoscopically, interstitial cystitis may resemble urothelial cell carcinoma in situ, raising the clinical concern.[275] Small petechial hemorrhages and ulcers (Hunner's ulcers) may be seen. The disease may be autoimmune and is diagnosed only after infectious processes have been excluded. Feltis and colleagues argue that mast cells observed histologically in the bladder wall may be a disease marker.[101] Mast cells also may be detected in bladder washes.[275] Others question the significance of mast cells as a marker for disease.[102] Neutrophils and eosinophils also may be seen in interstitial cystitis.[103] In cytologic specimens, although reactive changes may be seen in the urothelial cells, the atypia falls far short of neoplastic or pre-neoplastic change. A specific diagnosis of interstitial cystitis cannot be made cytologically.

Eosinophilic cystitis. Eosinophilic cystitis usually is seen in children and women and is associated with allergic disorders and eosinophilia,[104,105] but it also may be seen in older adult men and could be associated with trauma. Cystoscopically, ulcerated, nodular lesions may mimic carcinoma. The cytologic picture is variable, and the urothelium may appear reactive or squamous metaplasia may be present.[105] If ulcers are present, an inflammatory component, consisting of mixtures of neutrophils, eosinophils,

and lymphocytes may be seen in the background. These cytologic findings are nonspecific.

Follicular cystitis. The term *follicular cystitis* actually is a misnomer because it refers to the presence of lymphoid follicles in the wall and does not necessarily imply that inflammation is present.[106] However, chronic inflammatory conditions (e.g., lithiasis) may result in the true inflammatory form of follicular cystitis. Follicular cystitis cannot be diagnosed on cytology because the changes are seen beneath the mucosal surface. If an ulcer is present, the lymphocytes may be sampled on wash specimens, although the findings are completely nonspecific.

Urethral caruncle. Urethral caruncles usually are seen in older adult women and may be associated with hematuria and pain. On histologic examination, they resemble hemangiomas and may be ulcerated.[107] Cytologic findings are nonspecific and show variable numbers of inflammatory cells.

Inflammatory pseudotumor. Inflammatory pseudotumors often are polypoid and grossly mimic a malignant process. Histologically, they exhibit features reminiscent of a leiomyosarcoma or a high-grade spindle cell urothelial cell carcinoma. They may occur in a background of cystitis or after a recent operative procedure.[108,109] The cytologic findings are not constant and depend on whether the epithelial surface is ulcerated. Inflammatory cells and highly atypical spindle cells have been reported.[110] An outright diagnosis of inflammatory pseudotumor is best reserved for the histologic specimen.

Endometriosis. Foci of bladder or periurethral endometriosis may result in shedding of glandular cells. The bladder is the most common site of urinary tract involvement by endometriosis[111] and may even be seen in men receiving exogenous estrogen therapy.[112] The appearance of endometriotic shedding in urinary tract specimens is similar to the menstrual pattern in the Pap test (Box 11-20). The endometrial cells usually are degenerated, consist of glandular and stromal cells, and are heavily mixed with inflammation and blood (Figures 11-51 and 11-52).[113] In voided urine specimens, endometrial cells are first considered a contaminant rather than a sign of endometriosis. Endometriosis may involve the ureter, where it may cause obstruction and grossly mimic carcinoma.[114] Endometriosis of the urethra is rare.

Nephrogenic adenoma. Nephrogenic adenoma is a metaplastic lesion characterized by tubular and papillary aggregates of cuboidal cells with clear or eosinophilic cytoplasm (Box 11-21). The nuclei have prominent nucleoli.[115] Nephrogenic adenomas may be seen anywhere in the urinary tract and may result from inflammatory stimuli.[116,117] Cytologically, a definitive diagnosis of nephrogenic adenoma is difficult to make because the cells resemble those of a well-differentiated adenocarcinoma or even urothelial cell carcinoma. Cytologic specimens may be cellular with clusters of cells and scattered single cells.[118] The cytoplasm often is vacuolated and signet ring forms may be observed.[119] Pseudoglandular structures and papillary fragments also may be seen.[118,120] Although the cells may have a reactive appearance, on close inspection, they lack the necessary atypia for an outright diagnosis of adenocarcinoma. Usually, a diagnosis of atypical or suspicious is made.

Ileal Conduit

An ileal conduit may be constructed in patients with bladder cancer after resection of the primary tumor. Monitoring ileal conduit specimens is necessary to detect recurrence or, because of the multifocal nature of urothelial neoplasia, to detect a new tumor in the renal pelvis or calyces.[121] Some experts recommend that ileal conduit specimens be obtained at 3- to 6-month intervals.[122]

Ileal conduit specimens may be challenging to interpret as the cells undergo extensive degeneration that may mimic a high-grade urothelial cell carcinoma (Box 11-22). As urine causes sloughing of the normal ileal mucosa, ileal conduit specimens are highly cellular and contain many single cells and cell clusters.[123] The majority are glandular ileal lining cells, and urothelial cells from the upper tract are few in number (Figure 11-53). The glandular cells may form flat sheets similar to the findings in benign colonic brush specimens. When the glandular cells degenerate, they often dissociate and have vacuolated cytoplasm, sometimes containing debris. The nuclei often are pyknotic and eccentrically placed (Figure 11-54). The N:C ratio in these cells is not particularly alarming, but the nuclear hyperchromasia and smudging may cause concern. The background is cluttered with inflammatory cells, crystals, bacteria, and debris.

Ileal conduit specimens must be examined closely because the neoplastic cells, if present, are generally scarce.[123] Cells of high-grade urothelial cell carcinoma maintain their classic features of malignancy (e.g., hyperchromasia, irregular nuclear membranes, and so on) in ileal conduit speci-

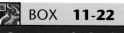

BOX 11-21 CMF

Cytomorphologic Features of Nephrogenic Adenoma

Hypercellular specimens with pseudopapillary fragments
Aggregates of glandular cells
Clear or eosinophilic cytoplasm
Round to oval nuclei with prominent nucleoli
Occasional signet-ring cell forms

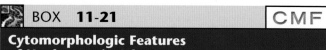

BOX 11-22 CMF

Cytomorphologic Features of Ileal Conduit Specimens

Hypercellular specimen
Extensive cellular degeneration
Single cells and groups of glandular cells
Macrophages, bacteria, crystalline debris

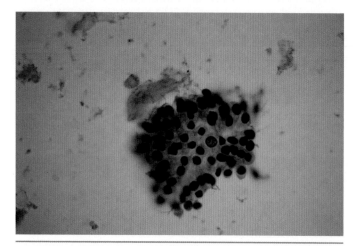

Figure 11-53 Ileal conduit specimen. A cluster of glandular ileal lining cells is seen admixed with degenerated debris. The cells appear hyperchromatic and small and are somewhat degenerated. The glandular cells generally are present in a flat sheet or honeycomb arrangement. (Pap)

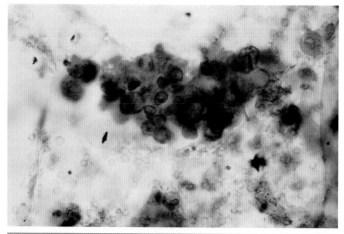

Figure 11-54 Ileal conduit specimen. A cluster of degenerated ileal cells and urothelial cells is seen. These cells exhibit slight nuclear overlap, although the nuclear features include hyperchromasia, vacuolization, and nuclear membrane irregularities. Degenerated debris is seen in the background. The nuclei are relatively small and therefore should not be confused with a high-grade urothelial cell carcinoma. (Pap)

mens.[122] Patients who have an ileal conduit also may undergo radiation therapy and or chemotherapy, which may make interpretation even more difficult.

Neoplastic Lesions

Bladder Cancer

An estimated 54,000 new bladder cancers occur yearly in the United States, and more than 12,000 patients die of their cancer.[124] Carcinoma of the bladder is the fourth most common type of cancer (after lung, colon, and prostate) in men and the eighth most common type in women.[125] The male to female ratio is approximately 3:1 for urothelial cell tumors.[98] Overall, 3% of all cancer deaths in the United States result from bladder cancer.[125] Bladder cancer is more common after the fifth decade of life with the median age of diagnosis in the late sixties. Although the incidence of bladder cancer has increased over the past several decades, the death rate has remained the same, probably as a result of increased detection and early treatment.[98]

Bladder cancer often presents insidiously. More than 75% of patients have hematuria, which is often painless.[125] Bladder irritability is seen in a minority of patients. Symptoms include dysuria, urinary frequency, and urgency, all of which occur in 25% of patients. A small number of patients have ureteral obstruction or pelvic pain. Occasionally, patients may present with signs of late disease, such as weight loss and bone or abdominal pain. Physical examination is usually unremarkable and the differential diagnosis includes lithiasis and urinary tract infection. Approximately 90% of bladder cancers are of urothelial cell origin, 5% squamous, and 5% mixed urothelial and squamous. Primary adenocarcinoma of the bladder is rare.

Risk factors for bladder carcinoma are several. Occupational exposure to toxins (or carcinogens) has been associated with one fourth to one third of all cases.[126-128] Exposure is primarily related to aromatic amines used in the production of rubber, plastic, and dyes in textiles, colored condom manufacturing, and printing. Thus, workers at higher risk include painters, truck drivers, machinists, textile workers, and automobile workers.[128] Bladder cancer occurs only after a long period of toxic exposure, estimated to be approximately 20 years. Urine cytology may be highly beneficial when targeted at these patients.[129]

Cigarette smoking is a risk factor for the development of bladder cancer, accounting for 25% to 65% of cases.[130] The risk of bladder cancer is up to four times greater among male cigarette smokers than among non-smokers.[98,123] Some argue that the risk of bladder cancer related to smoking is much higher than the risk related to industrial exposure.[131] An increased incidence of squamous cell bladder cancer is detected in patients who have a history of *S. hematobium* bladder infections. Up to 40% of all malignant tumors in Egypt, where *Schistosomal* infections are much more common, are squamous cell carcinomas.[98] The risk of bladder cancer correlates with the number of cigarettes smoked and the number of years smoked. Cancer risk is increased in men who smoke pipes and cigars and who use smokeless tobacco.[132] Increased cancer risk also is associated with long-term use of cyclophosphamide; analgesics, particularly in patients who use analgesics with phenacetin, and chronic irritation resulting from lithiasis.[125,133,134] Having a urothelial cell carcinoma is a risk factor for having synchronous or metachronous urothelial cell tumors. Approximately 2% to 7% of patients with bladder diverticuli develop an associated neoplasm.

Urothelial Cell Tumors

Urothelial cell tumors are the most common tumors of the urinary tract. The natural history of urothelial cell carcinoma may be correlated with several prognostic factors, including histologic grade, presence of carcinoma in situ, depth of invasion, and presence of lymphatic/vascular space invasion. Despite the knowledge of these indicators, the biologic basis for different subsets of carcinoma is not completely understood.[130] For example, some tumors with seemingly favorable histology are aggressive, whereas other neoplasms with unfavorable histology may be well controlled. Thus, histology, which is the gold standard for cytology, is not a sufficiently sensitive determinant to predict accurately biologic potential. The molecular biology and genetics of urothelial cell carcinoma are currently being assessed and suggest that tumor progression may occur along several pathways.

Simplistically, bladder neoplasms may progress along either a papillary pathway or a flat pathway. Genetic changes support these different pathways of carcinogenesis. In the papillary pathway, normal epithelium may progress through stages that are observed histologically as hyperplasia, low-grade papillary urothelial cell carcinoma, high-grade papillary urothelial cell carcinoma, and invasive carcinoma. Alternatively, in the papillary pathway, normal urothelial cell epithelium may progress directly to high-grade papillary urothelial cell carcinoma and then to invasive cancer. Defects in chromosome 9 and increased vascular endothelial growth factor expression support the hypothesis that normal urothelial cell epithelium may progress to either low- or high-grade papillary urothelial cell carcinoma.[130,135] Alterations in chromosome 17(p53) then may lead to an invasive carcinoma.[130]

In the flat pathway, normal urothelial cell epithelium may progress through the stages of dysplasia, carcinoma in situ, and invasive carcinoma. Alterations in chromosome 17(*p53*) support the hypothesis that normal urothelial cell epithelium may directly progress to carcinoma in situ, thereby bypassing the papillary stage.[130,135]

In pathology texts, the flat noninvasive lesions are often referred to as *dysplasia* or *carcinoma in situ,* and the papillary noninvasive lesions are referred to as *carcinoma.* This description encompasses those lesions that are pre-neoplastic. Any invasive lesion, regardless of the pathway that led to it, also is referred to as a *carcinoma.* In surgical pathology circles, this provides for some confusion because some flat lesions such as carcinoma in situ actually have a greater potential for progression to an invasive carcinoma, which may kill the patient, than many papillary lesions such as low-grade urothelial cell carcinoma. The surgical pathology literature is further complicated by the lack of agreement on grading the lesions, particularly in the papillary pathway. The 1998 World Health Organization/International Society of Urological Pathology (WHO/ISUP) grading system is outlined in Box 11-23.

For cytologists, these distinctions are simpler as all urothelial cell neoplasms are diagnostically categorized as either low-grade urothelial cell carcinoma or as high-grade urothelial cell carcinoma. This separation ignores the individual histogenetic pathways. This is a practical approach because it is based purely on cytomorphology rather than oncology. However, this discussion of urothelial cell neoplasia revolves around the two pathways and relates to how these tumors are placed in the two category cytologic system (low- vs. high-grade).

The Flat Pathway to Urothelial Cell Carcinoma

In the flat pathway, normal urothelial cells may progress to dysplasia (a premalignant process), which may progress to invasive urothelial cell carcinoma. Urothelial cell dysplasia is analogous to squamous cell dysplasia in the uterine cervix or in the head and neck region. In some conventional systems, urothelial cell dysplasia is divided into low- and high-grade dysplasia (alternatively called *severe dysplasia* or *carcinoma in situ*). The high-grade lesions have a greater likelihood of progression than the low-grade lesions. This theory is based on studies of chemically induced bladder cancer in animals and the observation of similar changes in humans.[136-139] These data indicate that the urothelium undergoes a progressive process from hyperplasia to low-grade dysplasia to high-grade dysplasia to invasive carcinoma.

Urothelial cell hyperplasia. Hyperplasia may be seen in inflammatory conditions and is not a preneoplastic lesion. On histologic examination, hyperplasia is characterized by an increased number of epithelial cell layers, beyond the five to six normally found in the bladder. The hyperplastic cells are described as *de-differentiated,* meaning that they resemble basal/parabasal cells. Hyperplastic change may be focal or multifocal. Significant epithelial cell atypia is absent, and therefore hyperplasia cannot be diagnosed by cytologic examination.

Low-grade urothelial cell dysplasia. Low-grade dysplasia is a better-recognized entity in the surgical pathology literature than in the cytology literature. It is a controversial diagnosis and not all pathologists use the term. In histologic

sections, low-grade dysplasia is characterized by a slightly increased N:C ratio, mildly irregular nuclear membranes, and slight nuclear hyperchromasia. Low-grade dysplasia bridges the gap between carcinoma in situ and hyperplasia, and it may be found in association with one or both of these lesions. The value of using the term *low-grade dysplasia* has not been ascertained, and no treatment is recommended for low-grade dysplasia. Murphy and colleagues report that patients with low-grade dysplasia should be followed conservatively.[140]

The ability of cytologists to make a diagnosis of low-grade dysplasia is questionable. Murphy and colleagues report that features of low-grade dysplasia include mildly enlarged nuclei, a slightly increased N:C ratio, and slightly irregular nuclear membranes.[140] These cytologic findings supposedly are the same as those seen in low-grade papillary carcinoma and urothelial cell papilloma. Studies showing the reproducibility of the term low-grade dysplasia and rigorous studies showing that the cytologic diagnosis of low-grade dysplasia correlates with histologic findings have yet to be performed.

High-grade urothelial cell dysplasia. High-grade urothelial cell dysplasia is a premalignant lesion and clinically may precede invasive carcinoma or may be found in conjunction with invasive carcinoma. Some investigators subclassify high-grade dysplasia into the categories of severe dysplasia and carcinoma in situ, based on the level of atypical basal cell hyperplasia (similar to lesions in the cervix). Cytologically, this separation is difficult or impossible to perform, and many authors use only the term *carcinoma in situ.* Carcinoma in situ appears cytologically identical to high-grade invasive or noninvasive papillary urothelial cell carcinoma.[141] Therefore, most cytologists use the term *high-grade urothelial cell carcinoma* to encompass carcinoma in situ and high-grade invasive and noninvasive tumors. Murphy and Irving report that invasive urothelial cell carcinoma of the bladder may develop without progression through a full thickness epithelial atypia stage.[82]

The majority of cases of carcinoma in situ are seen in men.[142] The severity of disease directly correlates with the symptoms. Hematuria may be the only presenting sign or symptom of a patient with carcinoma in situ.[143,144] Occasionally, patients have dysuria, frequency, and urgency. On cystoscopy, carcinoma in situ is notoriously difficult to recognize because carcinoma in situ is not exophytic. The gross findings are similar to those in the cervix where carcinoma in situ may appear normal. In the bladder, regions of carcinoma in situ grossly may appear erythematous, although this finding is nonspecific and mucosal erythema also may be seen in a number of inflammatory conditions.

Utz and colleagues report that more than 50% of patients with carcinoma in situ will develop an invasive carcinoma.[145,146] Presumably, some cases of carcinoma in situ persist and few regress. The time to progression from carcinoma in situ to invasive urothelial cell carcinoma has not been well studied and may be anywhere from months to years. Melamed and colleagues wrote that the time interval between in situ and invasive carcinoma is quite long[147] and that urine cytology may be used to detect lesions when they are potentially curable.[148] As with all bladder neoplasms, carcinoma in situ may be multifocal and when a patient is diagnosed as having carcinoma in situ, close follow-up is

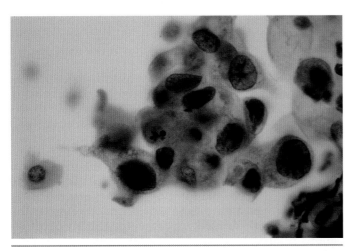

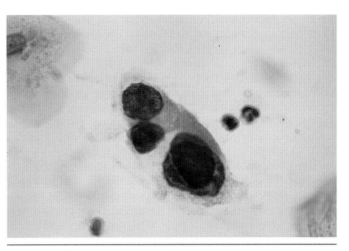

Figure 11-55 **High-grade urothelial cell carcinoma in a bladder wash specimen.** In bladder wash specimens, single cells of high-grade urothelial cell carcinoma usually are seen, although in this case a relatively large group of malignant cells is appreciated. These cells have large nuclei with increased N:C ratios and coarse chromatin. Variability in nuclear size is evident, and several of the malignant cells show nuclear degeneration. (Pap)

Figure 11-56 **High-grade urothelial cell carcinoma in a bladder wash specimen.** In this photomicrograph, three malignant cells are seen. The largest cell contains a huge nucleolus that is red in color. The nuclear membranes are irregular in shape and show thickening. (Pap)

recommended, even if the original lesion is successfully treated. Bladder biopsies may be negative even after a cytologic diagnosis of carcinoma in situ because the lesions are difficult to see or because the bladder epithelium is prone to sloughing and may not be seen on biopsy material.[149] Thus, the cytologic diagnosis of carcinoma in situ may precede the histologic diagnosis of carcinoma in situ by months, and the cytologic diagnosis is sometimes incorrectly viewed as a false-positive diagnosis.[150]

Because carcinoma in situ is difficult to see and hence biopsy, urinary tract cytology is the primary means to make the initial diagnosis. Cytology is also the most effective means to monitor patients with a known diagnosis of carcinoma in situ.[137] The sensitivity of detection on bladder wash specimens approaches 100%.[151-153] The majority of errors arise from sampling, although interpretive errors may occur when few cells are present. Wright and Halford reported that monolayer preparations were similar in sensitivity to cytospin preparations in neoplastic cell detection.[154]

Cytologically, the neoplastic cells vary in number depending on the specimen type, and bladder washings contain the most cells (Box 11-24). The neoplastic cells may be present individually or seen in small groups.[141,155] Large groups are only infrequently observed (Figure 11-55) although tissue fragments with attached cells may be seen.[156] The individual cells display "classic" features of malignancy, with high N:C ratios; nuclear enlargement, hyperchromasia, membrane irregularities and thickening; irregularly clumped chromatin; and nucleoli that are prominent, multiple, and enlarged (Figure 11-56).[8,157] The cells may exhibit extensive degeneration resulting in nuclei that are pitch-black and irregular in shape (coal-black nuclei). Mitoses may be either numerous or scarce. The cytoplasm tends to be scant and foamy, although in some cases, it may appear metaplastic. Some authors have described that the urine specimens from patients with carcinoma in situ appear *monomorphic,* meaning that a uniform population of malignant-appearing cells is present.[158]

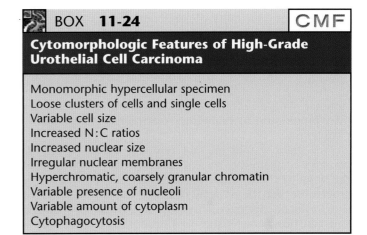

BOX 11-24 **CMF**

Cytomorphologic Features of High-Grade Urothelial Cell Carcinoma

Monomorphic hypercellular specimen
Loose clusters of cells and single cells
Variable cell size
Increased N:C ratios
Increased nuclear size
Irregular nuclear membranes
Hyperchromatic, coarsely granular chromatin
Variable presence of nucleoli
Variable amount of cytoplasm
Cytophagocytosis

Some investigators have provided criteria to cytologically separate carcinoma in situ from invasive carcinoma. The ability to prospectively make this separation is unclear and probably not warranted because patients with a diagnosis of high-grade urothelial cell carcinoma on cytology need further evaluation to locate the source of the neoplasia. Compared with invasive urothelial cell carcinoma, the cytologic features that are more indicative of carcinoma in situ include greater monotony of cells (i.e., less pleomorphism), smaller cells, cleaner background (i.e., no tumor diathesis), and fewer nucleoli.[141,157] Kojima and colleagues reported that cannibalism, or cytophagocytosis, was an important predictor of progression to invasion (Figure 11-57).[159]

Invasive carcinomas arising from the flat pathway appear cytologically identical to the invasive carcinomas arising from the papillary pathway and are discussed on p. 240.

The Papillary Pathway to Urothelial Cell Carcinoma

In the papillary carcinogenic pathway, normal urothelial cell epithelium may progress through noninvasive papillary carcinoma to invasive carcinoma. The histologic classification of papillary urothelial cell neoplasms is controversial, and different classification systems (essentially based on tumor grading) have been put forward (Table 11-1). The source of the controversy is the low-grade lesion, and this controversy spills over into the cytologic diagnostic arena. Papillary urothelial cell neoplasms may or may not be associated with pre-neoplastic (dysplastic), flat lesions, which also may give rise to invasive carcinomas. In the World Health Organization (WHO) diagnostic schema, papillary lesions are classified as papilloma, papillary urothelial neoplasm of low malignant potential, and grades I to III urothelial cell carcinoma. Other experts consider all papillary lesions as urothelial cell carcinomas (i.e., a papilloma category is excluded) and grade the tumors on a 0 to III scale or even other scales that reflect the degree of potential aggressiveness. The differences in these grading systems center on whether a truly benign category exists and on the number of grades necessary for accurate classification. In the WHO system, the histologic definition of a papilloma is restrictive, and few lesions (less than 2% of all bladder neoplasms) actually are classified as such. Also, some argue that no matter how benign a urothelial cell lesion may appear histologically, a risk of malignancy always exists, so all these lesions should be classified as urothelial cell carcinomas even though some will be low grade. Because the reproducibility of papilloma and grade I urothelial cell carcinoma is poor, some argue that separating these two lesions is not practical.[166] Regardless of the classification system used, all (or the vast majority, depending on individual pathologist's beliefs) of urothelial cell neoplasms are malignant or at least capable of metastasis or local recurrence. The recurrence of the low-grade carcinomas or their progression to high-grade carcinomas is particularly troublesome.

Two theories that are not mutually exclusive are espoused to explain the concept of recurrence. Proponents of the clonality theory argue that neoplastic cells give rise to a progenitor cell, the progeny of which implant at different sites in the urinary tract. These foci have the same cytologic and genetic characteristics as the mother tumor. Proponents of the field effect theory argue that disparate carcinogenic events occur independently at multiple foci. Tumors at these different foci may have different cytologic and genetic characteristics.

In cytology, lesions are classified as low-grade or high-grade urothelial cell carcinoma. If the histologic grading system of papilloma and three grades of urothelial cell carcinoma are used, low-grade lesions encompass grade I and II carcinomas and papillomas and high-grade lesions encompass grade III urothelial cell carcinomas, high-grade dysplasias, and most invasive carcinomas. However, not all cytologists place the category of papilloma in the low-grade urothelial cell carcinoma category. The majority of cytologists do not separately diagnose papilloma because (1) the criteria are poorly defined; (2) the reproducibility of the diagnosis is unestablished; and (3) philosophically, some do not believe that this separate category exists.

Low-grade papillary urothelial cell carcinoma. Jordan and colleagues estimated that only about 5% of patients with low-grade urothelial cell carcinomas die of their disease.[160] Thus, the majority of low-grade urothelial cell carcinomas do not behave aggressively.[161] However, from 50% to 75% of low-grade papillary urothelial cell carcinomas recur, and most recurrences are seen within 2 years of the initial diagnosis.[130] Low-grade urothelial cell carcinomas may progress to high-grade urothelial cell carcinomas in up to 20% of patients, so patients with low-grade urothelial cell carcinomas should be monitored closely.[8,160]

Low-grade papillary urothelial cell carcinomas often are identified on cystoscopy because they have a frondlike, exophytic appearance. These lesions may be biopsied and/or washed. The criteria for the cytologic diagnosis of low-grade papillary urothelial cell carcinoma primarily are derived from bladder wash, not voided urine studies. Making a diagnosis of low-grade urothelial cell carcinoma on voided urine specimens is difficult. On wash specimens the reported sensitivity of diagnosis varies from 0% to 73%, although a few studies indicate that with select criteria, the

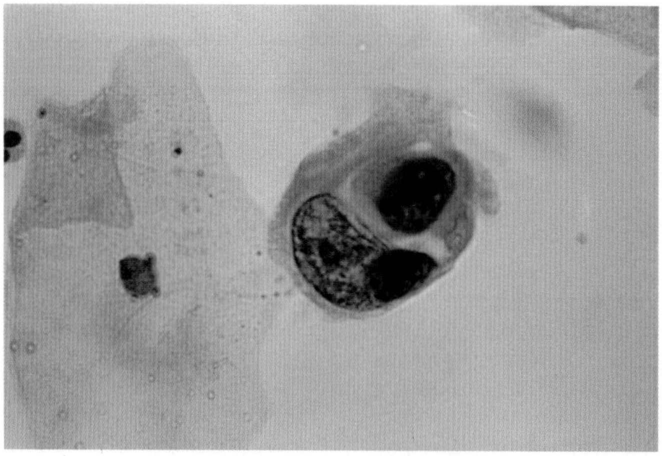

Figure 11-57 **Cannibalism in high-grade urothelial cell carcinoma in a bladder wash specimen.** In this photomicrograph, two malignant cells with a degenerated superficial squamous cell are seen. The larger malignant cell has engulfed the smaller malignant cell in a process known as *cytophagocytosis* or *cannibalism*. Some authors have suggested that this feature is a predictor of progression to an invasive carcinoma. (Pap)

TABLE 11-1	
Comparison of Histologic Classification Systems for Papillary Neoplasms	
WHO/ISUP (1999)	**WHO (1999)**
Papilloma	Papilloma
Papillary urothelial neoplasm of low malignant potential	Papillary urothelial neoplasm of low malignant potential
Low-grade urothelial carcinoma	Urothelial cell carcinoma I
High-grade urothelial carcinoma	Urothelial cell carcinoma II
High-grade urothelial carcinoma	Urothelial cell carcinoma III

From Epstein JI (and the World Health Organization). Histological typing of urinary bladder tumors. 2nd ed. Geneva: World Health Organization; 1999.
WHO, World Health Organization; *ISUP,* International Society of Urological Pathology.

sensitivity of diagnosis is over 50%.[6,162,163] The majority of these studies have focused on the diagnoses of grade II papillary urothelial cell carcinoma, indicating that grade I papillary carcinomas are more difficult or virtually impossible to diagnose. Renshaw and colleagues have argued that well-defined criteria for the correct identification of grade I papillary carcinomas are elusive.[164] The jury on whether the practicing cytologist may consistently diagnose low-grade papillary tumors is still out.

Low-grade papillary urothelial cell carcinoma is a well-differentiated neoplasm and the tumor cells, although exhibiting some degree of atypia, closely resemble normal urothelial epithelium. In histologic specimens, the connective tissue stalks are covered by an increased number of cell layers, increased N:C ratios, and mild nuclear changes. On cytologic specimens, papillary groups may or may not be present. The presence of papillary groups may be the only sign of a low-grade papillary carcinoma on voided urine specimens, although most cytologists would not make a definitive diagnosis on these groups alone. These groups may show crowding and slight cellular dissociation. The more

definitive cytologic features often are more clearly seen in individual cells, emphasizing that single cells in addition to cellular groups should be examined.[6,162,163,165]

In bladder wash specimens, criteria suggestive of a low-grade papillary carcinoma include irregular nuclear borders, nuclear enlargement, nuclear hypochromasia, atypical single cells, cell clusters with peripheral palisading, homogeneous cytoplasm, and irregular papillary fragments (Box 11-25).[6,162,163,166-168] The neoplastic cells should not be smaller than the normal basal/parabasal cells (Figure 11-58), and small, degenerated, hyperchromatic cells should not be mistaken for a low-grade urothelial cell carcinoma. Murphy and colleagues and Raab and colleagues have indicated that cytoplasmic homogeneity, or lack of vacuoles, is an important criterion for malignancy (Figure 11-59).[162,163] The nuclei may be eccentrically placed within the cytoplasm, and the cells show increases in N:C ratios and mild nuclear membrane irregularities (Figure 11-60).[162,163] In some cases,

---

BOX   11-25   C M F

Cytomorphologic Features of Low-Grade Papillary Urothelial Cell Carcinoma

Hypercellular specimen
Papillary clusters and single cells
Uniform cell size
Homogeneous cytoplasm
Increased N:C ratio
Enlarged nuclei
Irregular nuclear membranes
Finely granular to hypochromatic chromatin
Absent to small nucleoli
Eccentrically placed nuclei

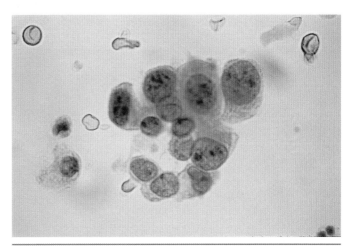

Figure 11-59 **Low-grade papillary urothelial cell carcinoma in a bladder wash specimen.** These low-grade malignant cells exhibit cytoplasmic homogeneity or an absence of cytoplasmic vacuoles. The nuclei contain irregular membranes, and the chromatin pattern is finely granular to hypochromatic. (Pap)

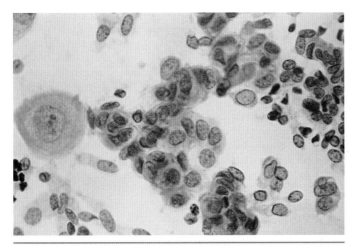

Figure 11-58 **Low-grade papillary urothelial cell carcinoma in a bladder wash specimen.** Numerous low-grade urothelial cell carcinoma cells are admixed with reactive urothelial cells. The low-grade malignant cells have more open-appearing chromatin with thickened irregular nuclear membranes. The low-grade urothelial cell carcinoma cells are less hyperchromatic than the parabasal cells. (Pap)

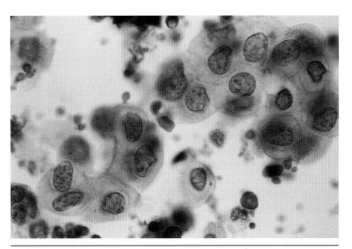

Figure 11-60 **Low-grade papillary urothelial cell carcinoma in a bladder wash specimen.** This cluster of low-grade urothelial carcinoma cells show cytoplasmic homogeneity with an absence of cytoplasmic vacuoles. The N:C ratios are slightly increased, and slight nuclear membrane irregularities are seen. (Pap)

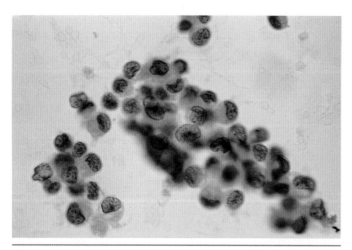

Figure 11-61 Low-grade papillary urothelial cell carcinoma. In this case of low-grade papillary urothelial cell carcinoma, the nuclei are eccentrically placed and contain homogeneous cytoplasm. The nuclear shape is elongated to oval, and notches within the nuclear membrane are seen. (Pap)

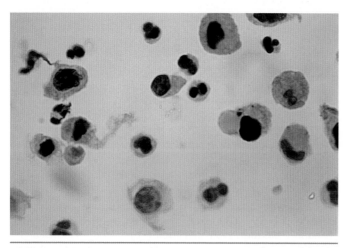

Figure 11-62 High-grade urothelial cell carcinoma in a bladder wash specimen. Numerous malignant single high-grade urothelial carcinoma cells are admixed with degenerated cells. The malignant cells have markedly hyperchromatic nuclei with irregular nuclear membranes and an increase in N:C ratio. Scattered inflammatory cells are seen in the background. (Pap)

the nuclei appear spindle shaped (Figure 11-61). The chromatin pattern tends to be finely granular and not hyperchromatic.[163] Raab and colleagues showed that using the criteria of increased N:C ratios, cytoplasmic homogeneity, and irregular nuclear membranes, experienced cytologists were able to diagnose a considerable percentage of low-grade papillary lesions.[165] Less experienced cytologists could not use these criteria with the same facility. In cytology specimens, low-grade papillary urothelial cell carcinomas do not display marked cytologic atypia. Thus, cases with marked anaplasia, mitoses, necrosis and other worrisome features are more likely to be high-grade urothelial cell carcinomas.

High-grade papillary and invasive urothelial cell carcinoma. High-grade papillary urothelial cell carcinomas are grade III lesions (or grades III and IV if grading is based on a I to IV scale).[137] High-grade urothelial cell carcinomas are aggressive neoplasms, and most cancer deaths resulting from pap-

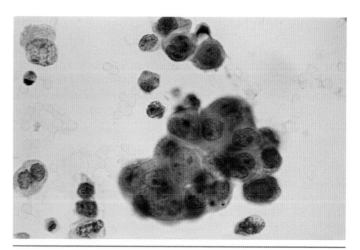

Figure 11-63 High-grade urothelial cell carcinoma in a catheterized urine specimen. A relatively large cluster of malignant cells is admixed with single malignant cells. These cells show variation in nuclear size, although most of the cells contain a prominent nucleolus. (Pap)

illary urothelial cell carcinoma are from the high-grade types.[160]

In cytologic specimens, the diagnosis is usually straightforward except in voided urine specimens where the tumor cells may be few in number. The diagnostic accuracy of voided urine increases as the number of specimens increases. Of neoplasms that may be diagnosed, Koss and colleagues reported that approximately 90% are detected on the first sample, with additional detection on second and third samples.[151] On bladder wash specimens, the sensitivity of diagnosis is more than 95%; difficulties may occur if extensive degeneration is present. The sensitivity of voided urine cytology for the detection of high-grade urothelial cell carcinoma is also high.[169]

Cytologic specimens of high-grade urothelial cell carcinoma are usually hypercellular (see Box 11-24), and the cells may be found in loose clusters or singly (Figure 11-62). Large papillary groups are generally absent. The malignant cells vary in size and shape (Figure 11-63), and in some cases, huge malignant cells are present. The N:C ratio is increased, and some cells have only a thin rim of cytoplasm.[170] High-grade urothelial cell carcinomas have either vacuolated or homogeneous cytoplasm (Figure 11-64).[6,163] Engulfed debris, blood products, and benign and malignant cells may be present (Figure 11-65). Tumor diathesis with background debris may be seen (Figure 11-66).

The malignant cell nuclei are enlarged and have irregular membranes. Multinucleated tumor cells may be present. The chromatin pattern is coarse and irregularly clumped with pronounced nuclear membrane thickening (Figure 11-67). Nuclear degeneration is common (Figure 11-68) and sometimes is manifested by a hyperchromatic coal-black nucleus. Nucleoli are enlarged and may be multiple. Mitoses with atypical forms may be seen.

High-grade urothelial cell carcinomas may exhibit differentiation along several lines, and foci of glandular or squamous differentiation are not uncommon (Figure 11-69).[6,8] In fact, in cytologic specimens, even if only malignant glandular or squamous differentiation is seen, the possibility of a high-grade urothelial cell carcinoma should be suggested. The highest-grade tumors may show sarcomatoid patterns,

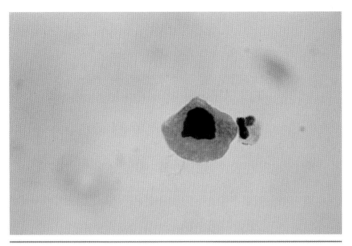

Figure 11-64 High-grade urothelial cell carcinoma in a clean catch urine specimen. In clean catch urine specimens, only a few malignant cells may be seen. These cells may exhibit more degeneration than the cells seen in bladder wash or catheterized urine specimens. Nonetheless, the more viable cells contain hyperchromatic, irregularly shaped nuclei. Here, the cytoplasm of the malignant cell has a homogeneous, nonvacuolated appearance. (Pap)

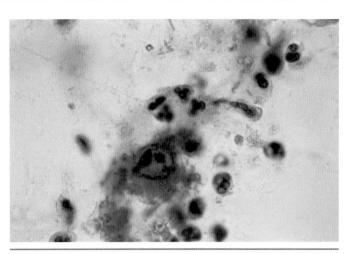

Figure 11-66 Tumor diathesis in a high-grade urothelial cell carcinoma in a bladder wash specimen. A single malignant cell with degenerated cytoplasm and an enlarged nucleus with a prominent nucleolus is seen. Surrounding the cell is necrotic debris, which is consistent with tumor diathesis. (Pap)

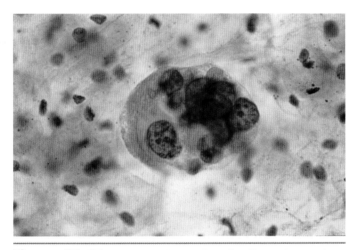

Figure 11-65 High-grade urothelial cell carcinoma in a bladder wash specimen. Scattered malignant cells are seen admixed with benign squamous cells in this bladder wash specimen. A large malignant cell has engulfed necrotic debris, hemosiderin, and other malignant cells in this case. (Pap)

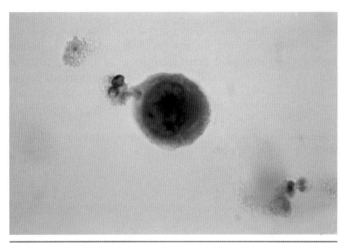

Figure 11-67 High-grade urothelial cell carcinoma in a clean catch urine specimen. This malignant cell shows a coarse chromatin pattern with nuclear membrane thickening and irregularity. The N:C ratio is high. (Pap)

and in cytology samples, spindle cells and bizarre-appearing tumor cells may be observed.

The differential diagnosis includes otherwise unremarkable degenerated benign specimens; reactive urothelial cells in cystitis resulting from lithiasis, chemotherapy, and radiation therapy, and so on; ileal conduit specimens; and human polyomavirus infection. Overcalling degenerated specimens as high-grade urothelial cell carcinoma is a principal cause of false-positive diagnoses. Thus, when such a diagnosis is being rendered, a few intact (nondegenerated) obviously malignant cells should be present. Reactive conditions typically do not show the marked anaplasia (e.g., high N:C ratios, nuclear hyperchromasia, mitoses, and so on) of high-grade urothelial cell carcinomas. As mentioned previously, human polyomavirus is a major pitfall, and to make matters more confusing, it may occur in conjunction with high-grade urothelial cell carcinoma. Although hyperchro-

matic, the nuclei of human polyomavirus infected cells show more evenly dispersed chromatin and regular nuclear membranes.

Other malignancies, such as metastases or prostatic adenocarcinoma, also may mimic a high-grade urothelial cell carcinoma. Prostate adenocarcinomas tend to be less anaplastic, show glandular differentiation throughout the entire specimen and contain more prominent nucleoli. Immunohistochemical stains for prostate-specific antigen (PSA) and prostate-specific acid phosphatase (PSAP) may be helpful. Poorly differentiated adenocarcinoma or squamous cell carcinoma metastases may be impossible to differentiate from a high-grade urothelial cell carcinoma, particularly if an accurate history is not provided.

High-grade papillary or invasive urothelial cell carcinoma is cytologically inseparable from high-grade urothelial cell dysplasia (carcinoma in situ). This distinction is a

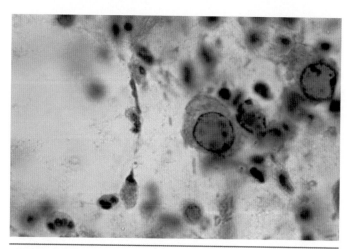

Figure 11-68 High-grade urothelial cell carcinoma in a bladder wash specimen. Nuclear and cytoplasmic degeneration commonly is seen in high-grade urothelial cell carcinoma. In this case, three degenerated malignant cells are seen. These cells actually exhibit nuclear hypochromasia with breakdown of the nuclear membranes. The N:C ratio is high and nuclear membrane irregularities still are appreciated. In this case, extensive tumor diathesis and inflammation is seen in the background. (Pap)

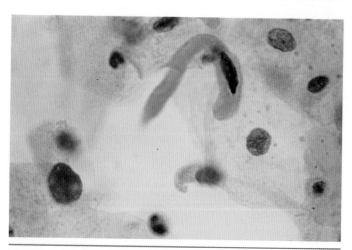

Figure 11-69 High-grade urothelial cell carcinoma in a bladder wash specimen. In this photomicrograph, a malignant cell exhibiting squamous differentiation is present. This cell has elongated cytoplasm, giving the cell a tadpolelike appearance. The nucleus is hyperchromatic and irregularly shaped, although the N:C ratio is not markedly increased. The differential diagnosis in this case includes a squamous cell carcinoma. (Pap)

clinical one and generally correlates with the presence of a mass, which is more consistent with a high-grade papillary or invasive urothelial cell carcinoma. If the diagnosis of high-grade urothelial cell carcinoma is made and no lesion is located in the bladder, the source of the malignant cells may be from the upper tract. Although invasive carcinomas are graded, the majority are of the higher grades. Cytologically, these invasive tumors are inseparable from their noninvasive counterparts.

Ancillary Studies

The greatest determinants of cytology sensitivity are sampling and cytopathologist/cytotechnologist expertise.[171] However, a number of ancillary studies have been proposed to increase the sensitivity of tumor detection. The development and application of ancillary studies is rapidly changing, and this survey summarizes the findings as of late 2001.

Bladder tumor antigen. Currently, three different assays for bladder tumor antigen (BTA) are on the market. These assays test for urothelial cell tumor secretory products that lyse the basement membrane into fragments of collagen, proteoglycans, and glycoproteins. The Bard BTA test (Bard Diagnostic Sciences, C.R. Bard; Redmond, Wash.), is positive when human immunoglobulin G (IgG)–coated latex particles combine with bladder tumor analytes.[171] The BTA stat test (Bard Diagnostic Sciences, C.R. Bard; Redmond, Wash.) is positive when monoclonal antibodies combine with human complement–related H-factor protein, which has been isolated from urine specimens of patients with cancer.[171] Both of these tests are qualitative. The BTA TRAK assay (Bard Diagnostic Sciences, C.R. Bard; Redmond, Wash.) is a quantitative test that detects the same antigen as the Bard BTA test.[171] Variable sensitivities and specificities have been reported. The sensitivity of the BTA stat test is higher than the Bard BTA test and ranges from 67% to 87%; the specificity, however, ranges from 40% to 70%.[171] The BTA TRAK assay also has a fairly high

sensitivity (72%) but also has a low specificity (43% to 48%), particularly in patients with infections or lithiasis.[171] As these tests lack sufficient specificity, they generally are not deemed appropriate to screen patients with potential urothelial cell carcinoma.[172,173] In addition, the sensitivity of urine for detection of urothelial cell carcinoma rivals that of the BTA tests. BTA tests may be more useful to predict tumor recurrence.[174]

Flow cytometry for ploidy. The majority of high-grade lesions are aneuploid, whereas the majority of low-grade lesions are diploid. Thus, flow cytometry is not helpful in detecting low-grade lesions. Although the reported sensitivity of flow cytometry for the detection of high-grade lesions is variable, recent data indicate that the combination of urine and bladder washing cytology is a more sensitive and specific test than flow cytometry alone.[175-178] Another limitation of flow cytometry is that a large number of aneuploid cells is necessary to establish a malignant diagnosis.[175] This limits the use of flow cytometry in voided urine specimens.

Image analysis for ploidy. DNA image analysis is better at detecting high-grade lesions than low-grade lesions. Some authors suggest that morphometric features such as nuclear size cannot be used to separate low-grade lesions from benign urothelial cells, and that cytology alone is more sensitive than image analysis.[164,171] Other authors report that morphometry may be useful to separate low-grade neoplastic cells from benign cells using large numbers of criteria.[171] DNA image analysis combined with conventional light microscopy has been shown to be helpful in detecting recurrences of high-grade lesions.[179-185] Currently, most image analyzers are used in conjunction with cytology and are not intended to replace conventional morphology.

Lewis X antigen. The Lewis X antigen, which is closely related to the ABO blood groups antigens, may be demonstrated immunohistochemically in up to 89% of urothelial cell carcinomas.[171] However, as has been demonstrated time again in other tissues, such immunohistochemical markers lack specificity and may be positive in up to 50% of cases with reactive changes.[171] Other glycoprotein antigens such as M344 and 19A211 also lack sufficient specificity to be helpful diagnostically.[186]

p53 Tumor suppressor gene. Overexpression of the *p53* tumor suppressor gene is an independent predictor of tumor aggressiveness and thus has prognostic significance.[187,188] The *p53* gene rarely is mutated in low-grade lesions and therefore cannot be used as a screening tool to detect low-grade lesions. The *p53* gene is altered more often in high-grade lesions, and the gene mutations may be detected in urine specimens.[171,189-191] However, *p53* immunohistochemical staining has a low sensitivity and specificity, and cannot be used as a method to detect high-grade urothelial cell cancer.[192] It is more useful as a prognostic indicator in histologic specimens.

Fibrin/fibrinogen degradation products. Urothelial cell carcinoma produces an angiogenic factor known as vascular endothelial growth factor (VEGF), which results in increased vascular permeability.[193] Plasma proteins such as fibrinogen and plasminogen are activated, and fibrinogen forms a fibrin clot. Urine contains a substance known as *urokinase,* which converts plasminogen to plasmin, which in turn breaks down fibrin and any fibrinogen into degradation products.[194] The AuraTek FDP assay (PerImmune; Rockville, Md.) qualitatively measures these degradation products and fibrinogen. The sensitivity of the AuraTek FDP assay ranges from 48% to 68%.[171,195,196] The assay has a high false-positive rate in patients with hematuria.[171,196]

Nuclear matrix proteins. Nuclear matrix proteins provide a structural framework for the nucleus and may be seen normally in the urine specimens of patients without cancer. The levels of nuclear matrix proteins may be increased in patients with urothelial cell carcinoma.[197-199] The NMP22 test (Matritech; Newton, Mass.) is a quantitative test that measures the level of nuclear matrix proteins.[171,196] The overall sensitivity is 66%, which is lower than that of conventional cytology.[171,200-202] The assay has a high false-positive rate[203] and may be indeterminate in patients with prostate cancer.[171]

Telomerase. Telomerase is a ribonucleoprotein that catalyzes the synthesis of telomeres, which are structures located at the ends of chromosomes that are normally shortened with each cell replication.[204] With progressive telomere shortening, somatic cells die. Neoplastic cells may become immortal through the disruption of telomerase activity.[171,196] Immortal cells have short but stable chromosomes and increased telomerase activity. Semiquantitative determination of telomerase activity may be performed using a fluorescence-based telomeric repeat amplification protocol (TRAP).[205] The sensitivity of telomerase ranges from 79% to 88%, although false-positive results may be seen in up to 34% of cases.[171,200,206-210] In addition to a high false-positive rate, as of late 2000, telomerase is not readily available in many laboratories and requires a high level of technical expertise.[171]

Hyaluronic acid and hyaluronidase. Hyaluronic acid is a glycosaminoglycan involved in tumor adhesion.[171] Hyaluronic acid may be detected in the urine of patients with bladder cancer, with the reported sensitivity of 92%.[171] Hyaluronidase activity is reported in patients with high-grade tumors but has not been shown to be useful in detecting low-grade tumors.[171,200]

Summary of ancillary studies. Many experts agree that ancillary studies have not replaced conventional urinary cytology as the primary means to detect urinary tract cancer.[171,211] Some ancillary studies are quite useful for the detection of high-grade carcinomas but are less effective in the detection of low-grade carcinomas. On the whole, most ancillary studies lack sufficient specificity to be used as a general screening tool and may be more effective in tracking patients with known disease. Ancillary studies are most useful when combined with conventional cytology. As new tests are developed and current tools improved, the use of ancillary studies may become more important in the detection of urothelial carcinoma.

Upper Tract Specimens

The upper tract consists of the ureters, renal pelvises, renal calyces, and renal collecting ducts. These regions may be sampled by voided urine specimens or by catheterization with brushing or washing.[212] In most cases, these regions cannot be visualized and clinical information is derived from the radiologic reports, symptoms, and signs. Up to 10% of urothelial tumors arise in the upper tract, and most tumors are papillary urothelial cell carcinomas. Patients with upper tract tumors have the same risk factors as patients with lower tract neoplasms. Patients who have lower tract tumors are at a higher risk than the general population to develop an upper tract tumor.[213,214] Hematuria is the major sign and symptom of upper tract neoplasms. Larger tumors may produce signs and symptoms similar to those seen in renal cell carcinoma.

The sensitivity of neoplastic detection depends on the specimen type and lesion grade.[11,215,216] Voided urine specimens may detect high-grade tumors but sometimes cannot detect low-grade tumors at all. Upper tract lesions, like their lower tract counterparts, shed neoplastic cells that are often degenerated.[217] Shedding may be sporadic, which results in false-negative specimens.[218-221] Hurle and colleagues recommended obtaining urine cytology to sample the upper tract every 4 months in patients who have a history of lower tract urothelial cell carcinoma.[213]

Direct sampling (washing or brushing) of the upper tract is a good means to detect high-grade urothelial cell tumors, but similar to voided urine, it is poor at detecting low-grade urothelial cell tumors.[11,212] The reason for this is that the benign cells of the upper tract have more atypical features than the benign cells of the lower tract (Figure 11-70), and overlap of the cytologic features of low-grade urothelial cell carcinoma and upper tract benign cells is high. The benign basal/parabasal, intermediate, and superficial cells of the upper tract, compared with their lower tract counterparts, show relatively high N:C ratios, enlarged nuclei, and more prominent nuclear membrane irregularities.[222] Benign superficial cells may show large nucleoli and have hyperchromatic nuclei. Inflammatory conditions such as lithiasis may result in greater cytologic atypia (Figure 11-71).[223] Instrumentation is associated with large groups of cells, mimicking the papillary clusters of urothelial cell carcinoma. For this reason, the diagnosis of low-grade urothelial cell carcinoma in the upper tract is virtually impossible.[11] In fact, the benign cells may exhibit more atypia than commonly is associated with low-grade urothelial cell carcinoma. Paradoxically, if an upper tract specimen shows only bland-looking cells, a low-grade lesion may be sus-

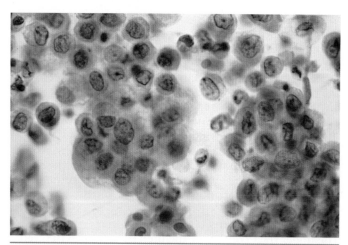

Figure 11-70 **Benign cells of renal pelvis in a renal pelvis barbotage specimen.** Wash specimens of the upper tract are often cellular, and the cells exhibit more cytologic atypia than the cells commonly seen in the urinary bladder. Similar to the cells in the bladder, the cells in the upper tract may be subclassified as parabasal, intermediate, and superficial. However, these cells exhibit increased N:C ratios and greater variability in nuclear size and shape. Benign cells of the upper tract lack the nuclear hyperchromasia seen in high-grade urothelial cell carcinoma cells. It may be difficult to separate a low-grade urothelial cell carcinoma from the benign cells of the upper tract. (Pap)

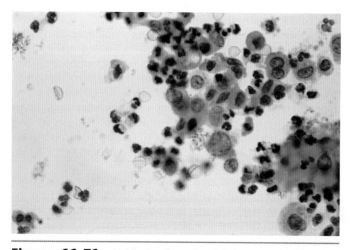

Figure 11-71 **Lithiasis of renal pelvis in a renal barbotage specimen.** Lithiasis of the upper tract is characterized by abundant acute inflammation and urothelial cell cytologic atypia. The atypia is characterized by variation in nuclear size and increased N:C ratios. The nuclear membranes are irregular in shape and may be thickened. Marked nuclear hyperchromasia generally is not seen in upper tract lithiasis. (Pap)

pected, although most cytologists will not make an outright diagnosis.

The cytologic diagnosis of upper tract high-grade urothelial cell carcinoma usually is easier. The reported cytologic features are the same as the features in the lower tract. The neoplastic nuclei show enlargement, hyperchromasia, pronounced membrane irregularities, and multilobation (Figure 11-72). Using statistical analysis in washings, Potts and colleagues showed that the criteria of anisonucleosis, high N:C ratios, and nuclear overlapping were key criteria

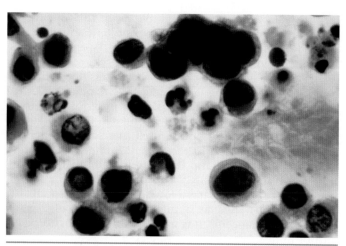

Figure 11-72 **High-grade urothelial cell carcinoma of the renal pelvis in a barbotage specimen.** Numerous malignant cells showing hyperchromatic nuclei with nuclear membrane irregularities are seen. These cells have increased N:C ratios and show nuclear enlargement. This degree of nuclear hyperchromasia generally is not seen in nonneoplastic conditions. (Pap)

for the identification of high-grade urothelial cell carcinoma.[11] Atypical mitoses are common, and tumor diathesis may be present in the background. If directly sampled, the specimen should be highly cellular and the characteristic coal-black nuclei often are present. The differential diagnosis is the same as for high-grade tumors of the lower tract.

Urethral Specimens

Urothelial cell carcinomas may develop in the urethra, particularly in patients with a history of urothelial malignancy. Sampling of the urethra occurs naturally in voided urine specimens, and the urethra may be specifically swabbed, washed, or brushed. Specimens are obtained to rule out malignancy and to determine if an infectious disease (e.g., gonorrhea, herpes, *Trichomonas, Chlamydia,* or HPV) is present.[224] With better understanding of cervical cancer risk factors, sampling of the urethra may increase to determine if HPV is present. The cytologic features of malignancies and infectious processes are the same in urethral specimens as they are in bladder specimens. Benign urethral specimens contain urothelial cell epithelium, glandular epithelium, and squamous epithelium. As with all urinary tract specimens, contamination must be excluded.

Squamous Cell Carcinoma

In North America, approximately 5% of primary bladder tumors are squamous cell carcinomas. More commonly, malignant squamous cells represent a component of a urothelial cell carcinoma. Thus, cytologists may suggest that a primary squamous cell carcinoma is present, but more sampling may be necessary to rule out a urothelial cell carcinoma. Squamous cell carcinomas arising in adjacent organs (e.g., gynecologic tract) and secondarily involving the urinary tract also must be excluded before a primary diagnosis is made.

Most squamous cell carcinomas arise in the anterior wall and are well differentiated. The cytologic appearance of a squamous cell carcinoma in a urinary tract specimen is similar to the appearance of this tumor in other sites

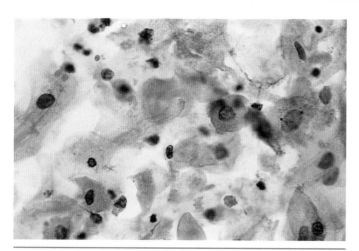

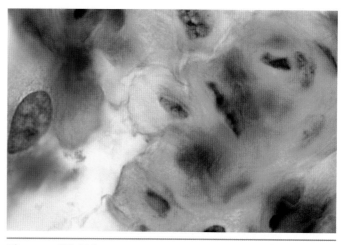

Figure 11-73 Squamous cell carcinoma in a bladder wash specimen. Most squamous cell carcinomas of the bladder are well differentiated and show parakeratosis, anucleated squamous cells, and rare intact definitively malignant cells. The nondegenerated malignant cells in this case show slightly hyperchromatic nuclei with irregular nuclear membranes. It may be difficult to separate well-differentiated squamous cell carcinomas of the bladder from reactive squamous cells. Generally, the nuclear atypia is seen in the absence of acute inflammation in squamous cell carcinoma. (Pap)

Figure 11-74 Squamous cell carcinoma in a bladder wash specimen. Malignant keratinized cells are seen. The malignant cell on the left resembles a dysplastic squamous cell with a hyperchromatic nucleus and nuclear membrane irregularities. The cluster of keratinized cells on the right shows extensive nuclear degeneration. (Pap)

BOX **11-26** | CMF

Cytomorphologic Features of Squamous Cell Carcinoma

Hypercellular specimen
Rare intact malignant cells with the following squamous
　features:
　Keratinized cytoplasm
　Bizarre shapes
　Pyknotic like chromatin
　"Pearls"
Parakeratosis
Anucleated squamous cells

BOX **11-27** | CMF

Cytomorphologic Features of Adenocarcinoma

Hypercellular specimen
Clusters of cuboidal to columnar cells with nuclear overlap
Hyperchromatic eccentric nuclei
Nuclei with regular membranes
Vacuolated cytoplasm
Occasional signet-ring cell forms

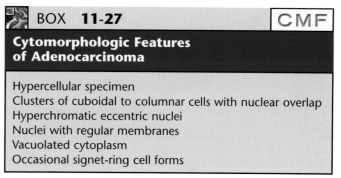

(Box 11-26). The cytologic features depend on the tumor grade. The well-differentiated tumors may be difficult to diagnose cytologically because they show little atypia. The majority of squamous cell carcinomas are keratinizing, and the well-differentiated ones for the most part show anucleated squamous cells, parakeratosis, and rare intact malignant cells (Figure 11-73). Well-differentiated squamous carcinoma cells usually are seen singly, although small clusters may be present. Specimens of well-differentiated squamous cell carcinoma may appear similar to specimens showing marked squamous metaplasia. Malignant squamous cells may mimic dysplastic cells seen in Pap tests. Thus, the differential diagnosis includes contaminating cervicovaginal lesions and reactive primary lesions of the bladder. The squamous cell carcinoma component of a urothelial cell carcinoma usually is not as well-differentiated.

The more poorly differentiated squamous cell carcinomas are either keratinizing or nonkeratinizing. Cytologically, the malignant cells are seen singly and in small and large groups (Figure 11-74). The single cells show unusual shapes (e.g., tadpole or spindle cells). High-grade keratiniz-

ing tumors have eosinophilic cytoplasm and bizarre, hyperchromatic nuclei that may exhibit degeneration. Keratin pearls and tumor diathesis may be present. Nonkeratinizing tumors show clusters of cells with high N:C ratios and enlarged nuclei. The cytoplasm may appear hard and metaplastic or have a more granular quality. Prominent nucleoli may be seen. The nonkeratinizing tumors are more likely to be confused with an adenocarcinoma or high-grade urothelial cell carcinoma.

Adenocarcinoma

Adenocarcinomas comprise less than 1% of all primary bladder carcinomas. Similar to squamous cell carcinomas, most bladder adenocarcinomas represent a component of a urothelial cell carcinoma rather than a primary. Adenocarcinomas may be subdivided into carcinomas that resemble colonic carcinomas, signet-ring cell carcinomas, and clear cell carcinomas (Box 11-27).

The carcinomas that resemble colonic adenocarcinomas are the most common subtype (more than 85% of primary adenocarcinomas). Cytologically, clusters of cuboidal or columnar cells with large, irregularly shaped, hyperchromatic nuclei, and vacuolated cytoplasm characterize these tumors (Figure 11-75). Nuclear crowding is seen, and the more poorly differentiated adenocarcinomas may be pleomorphic. The differential diagnosis includes prostatic adenocarcinoma and metastases, in addition to urothelial cell carcinoma with focal adenocarcinomatous differentiation. Criteria to separate this subtype of adenocarcinoma from metastatic adenocarcinomas have not been detailed.[225]

Approximately 25% of signet ring cell adenocarcinomas are of urachal origin. A signet ring cell component may be seen in conventional adenocarcinomas, metastases, and even urothelial cell carcinomas,[226] although the term *signet ring cell carcinoma* should be reserved for carcinomas showing exclusively signet ring cell differentiation. Cytologically, large pools of mucin may be present. The malignant cells may be small and usually are dissociated (Figure 11-76).

Clear cell carcinomas of the bladder may appear similar to signet ring cell carcinomas, although clear cell carcino-mas usually have more of an aggregate pattern (Figure 11-77). The background is inflamed (mucin is not present) and the cells have granular to vesicular chromatin with multiple nucleoli.[227] The cytologic detection of urethral clear cell carcinoma also has been described.[228]

Small Cell Carcinoma

Primary small cell carcinoma appears similar to small cell carcinoma found elsewhere.[229] Metastatic small cell carcinoma first must be excluded. Small cell carcinoma also may be combined with primary adenocarcinoma or squamous cell carcinoma.[230] The differential diagnosis includes malignant lymphoma and urothelial cell carcinoma with a predominance of small or degenerated malignant cells.

Cytologically, small cell carcinoma cells show high N:C ratios, naked nuclei, nuclear enlargement, nuclear molding, and frequent mitoses (Box 11-28).[231] The neoplastic cell nuclei have a neuroendocrine appearance with evenly dispersed granular chromatin (Figure 11-78). Neuroendocrine stains may assist in the diagnosis.

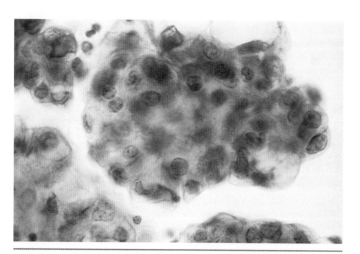

Figure 11-75 Adenocarcinoma in a bladder wash specimen. In this case of adenocarcinoma, three-dimensional groups of cells are seen in the cytospin preparation. Adenocarcinomas of the bladder may resemble adenocarcinomas in other fluid specimens. These groups show nuclear overlap and variability in nuclear size. The cytoplasm often has a vacuolated appearance and the vacuoles may indent the nuclei. (Pap)

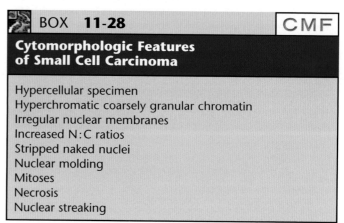

BOX   **11-28**   CMF

**Cytomorphologic Features
of Small Cell Carcinoma**

Hypercellular specimen
Hyperchromatic coarsely granular chromatin
Irregular nuclear membranes
Increased N:C ratios
Stripped naked nuclei
Nuclear molding
Mitoses
Necrosis
Nuclear streaking

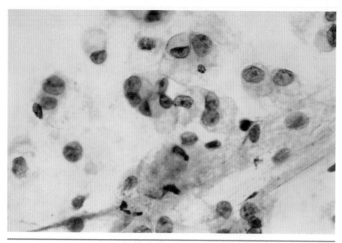

Figure 11-76 Signet ring cell carcinoma in a bladder wash specimen. Conventional adenocarcinomas may show signet ring cell differentiation, and the term *signet ring cell carcinoma* is reserved for carcinomas showing exclusively signet ring cell differentiation. The nuclei are relatively small, and a large cytoplasmic vacuole is seen at the edge of the cell. (Pap)

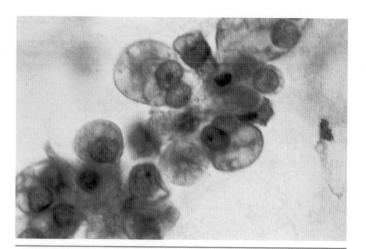

Figure 11-77 Clear cell adenocarcinoma in a bladder wash specimen. Clear cell carcinomas may resemble signet ring cell carcinomas, although they generally show cellular aggregates. Clear cell carcinoma cells have variably sized nuclei with occasional prominent nucleoli. The cytoplasm has a foamy, vacuolated appearance, and generally, the cells appear more anaplastic than the typical signet ring cell adenocarcinoma. Background mucin is not seen, and the chromatin pattern is granular to vesicular. (Pap)

Hematolymphoid Lesions

The main hematolymphoid lesions to be detected on urinary tract cytology are malignant lymphoma[232-235] and plasma cell dyscrasia.[236-238] Malignant lymphoma more commonly involves the urinary tract secondarily but rarely may present as a primary urinary tract neoplasm.[239,240] All subtypes of malignant lymphoma may involve the urinary tract, including Hodgkin's disease.[241] The differential diagnosis depends on the differentiation of the malignant lymphoma. Large cell malignant lymphoma may resemble small cell carcinoma and poorly differentiated urothelial cell carcinoma (Figure 11-79). The more well-differentiated malignant lymphomas may mimic reactive conditions such as follicular cystitis (Figure 11-80). Regardless of the malignant lymphoma subtype, the malignant cells are dissociated and have high N:C ratios. Cell clustering indicates that other processes are more likely. Large cell malignant lymphoma may be associated with abundant necrotic debris.

Plasma cell dyscrasias infrequently involve the urinary tract.[236] In cytologic specimens, cell clustering should not be found. Rare forms of urothelial cell carcinoma may mimic a plasma cell dyscrasia.[242] The appearance of the neoplastic plasma cells depends on the degree of differentiation (Figure 11-81). The more well-differentiated neoplastic cells have eccentrically placed nuclei and occasional binucleated forms. Perinuclear clearing and coarsely lumped chromatin ("clock-face" nucleus) may be observed. Invasion of the kidney by malignant plasma cells may result in renal tubular damage; the urine may contain granular myeloma casts and syncytial giant cells.[243] Leukemia also may be detected in urinary tract specimens.[244]

Tumors Secondarily Invading the Urinary Tract

Prostatic adenocarcinoma

Unfortunately, when a prostatic adenocarcinoma is diagnosed in a urinary tract specimen, the tumor usually is advanced.[245,246] Malignant cells have been detected after prostatic massage.[247]

Cytologically, the neoplastic cells usually are present in small clusters or pseudoacini with slight dissociation (Box 11-29). The nuclei may be eccentrically placed, and the cells show an increased N:C ratio and nuclear hyperchromasia (Figure 11-82).[248] The most discriminating features are the presence of prominent and sometimes multiple nucleoli, evenly dispersed chromatin, and an oval nucleus with smooth borders.[245,249] The more poorly differentiated tumors mimic urothelial cell carcinoma.[246] Prostatic duct adenocarcinoma also has been detected in urine specimens.[250]

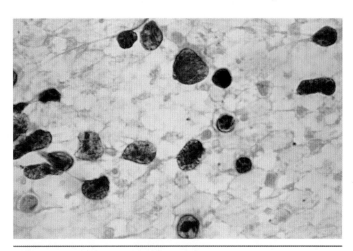

Figure 11-79 **Large cell malignant lymphoma in a bladder wash specimen.** Large cell malignant lymphomas may resemble high-grade urothelial cell carcinomas in urinary tract specimens. The malignant cells often are seen singly and show high N:C ratios, nuclear hyperchromasia and occasionally prominent nucleoli. Degenerated malignant lymphoma cells may exhibit a coal-black nucleus similar to high-grade urothelial cell carcinoma cells. Generally, most high-grade malignant lymphomas lack cellular cohesion, and all the malignant cells are seen singly. The cytoplasm of high-grade malignant lymphomas generally is more fragile than the cytoplasm of high-grade urothelial cell carcinoma cells. (Pap) (From Raab SS. Urinary cytology. In: Atkinson BF, Silverman JF, editors. Atlas of difficult diagnoses in cytopathology. Philadelphia: WB Saunders; 1998. p.251.)

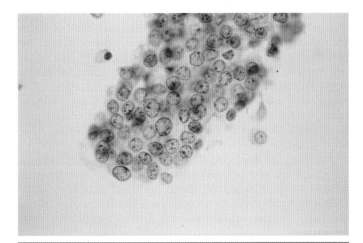

Figure 11-78 **Small cell carcinoma in a bladder wash specimen.** A three-dimensional group of small cell carcinoma is seen. These cells have a neuroendocrine appearance with finely granular, stippled chromatin. The cells have high N:C ratios, nuclear enlargement, and nuclear molding. The differential diagnosis includes a metastatic small cell carcinoma from another site. (Pap)

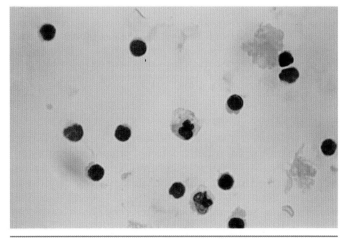

Figure 11-80 **Well-differentiated malignant lymphoma in a bladder wash specimen.** Well-differentiated malignant lymphomas may be difficult to diagnose in bladder wash specimens, because the malignant cells may resemble those cells seen in a lymphocytic cystitis. In this case, the cells have a monotonous appearance, are small, and show nuclear invaginations. (Pap)

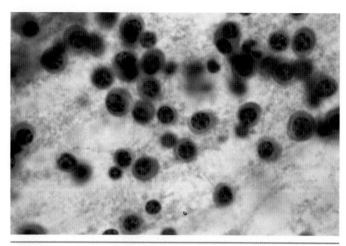

Figure 11-81 Plasma cell dyscrasia in a bladder wash specimen. In plasma cell dyscrasias, the cytospin preparations usually are cellular and show numerous plasma cells of varying degrees of differentiation. The nuclei are eccentrically placed, and occasional binucleated forms are seen. The chromatin pattern is irregular and coarse and scattered cells typically have a clock-face chromatin appearance. Clusters generally are not observed. (Pap)

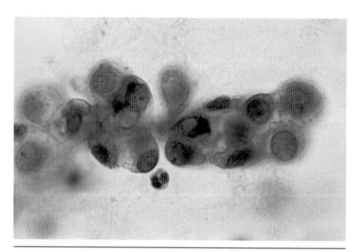

Figure 11-83 Renal cell adenocarcinoma in a bladder wash specimen. The presence of renal cell adenocarcinoma in bladder wash specimens depends on the shedding of the malignant cells from the renal pelvis. In this example the cells have a clear cell appearance with vacuolated cytoplasm and variably sized and shaped nuclei. The cells contain prominent nucleoli. (Pap)

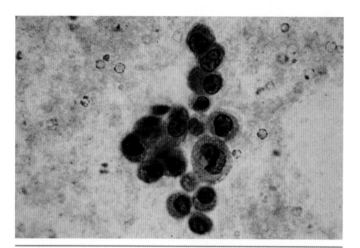

Figure 11-82 Prostatic adenocarcinoma in a bladder wash specimen. Prostatic adenocarcinomas resemble other adenocarcinomas when they invade the bladder wall. In this case the malignant cells have high N:C ratios, and occasional cells with prominent nucleoli are seen. The cytoplasm has a granular appearance. The background contains degenerated red blood cells, consistent with mucosal ulceration and bleeding. (Pap)

> **BOX 11-29** **CMF**
>
> **Cytomorphologic Features of Prostatic Adenocarcinoma**
>
> Small clusters and pseudoacinar groups
> Eccentrically placed, smooth round-oval, hyperchromatic nuclei
> Evenly dispersed chromatin patterns
> Prominent and multiple nucleoli
> Increased N:C ratios

higher nuclear grade, and the neoplastic cells of the well-differentiated cases may appear similar to benign renal tubular cells.[261] The more poorly differentiated clear cell variant tends to have abundant, vacuolated cytoplasm with hyperchromatic nuclei with prominent nucleoli.[262] Degeneration leads to greater nuclear hyperchromasia, nuclear breakdown, and cytoplasmic fragmentation.[253] The clear cell variant of renal cell adenocarcinoma must be distinguished from other clear cell carcinomas, mesonephric carcinoma,[263] and nephrogenic adenomas of the urinary tract.[119] The granular cell and sarcomatoid variants also have been described.[251] Collecting duct carcinomas have more granular cytoplasm.[255]

Staining for lipid (Oil-Red-O or Sudan IV) may help in the diagnosis of renal cell adenocarcinoma. Lipid staining should be performed on fresh, unfixed preparations.[264] However, lipid positivity may be seen in benign cells (tubular cells or macrophages) and other neoplastic cells (metastases).[265]

Colonic and gynecologic tumors

Cancers from the colon and the gynecologic tract may secondarily invade the urinary tract, resulting in shedding of neoplastic cells in the urine. These tumors may be inseparable from primary adenocarcinomas, squamous cell carci-

Renal tumors

Although renal tumors may be detected in urinary tract specimens, they are usually detected when the tumors are at a high stage.[4,251,252] If a renal tumor grows into the renal pelvis or collecting ducts, neoplastic cells may be shed in the urine. Renal cell adenocarcinoma, collecting duct adenocarcinoma, renal medullary carcinoma, renal carcinoid tumor, mucinous carcinoma, and Wilms' tumor have all been described in urinary tract specimens.[252-260]

The most commonly seen tumor is renal cell adenocarcinoma, which has several morphologic appearances (the clear cell variant being the most common). The neoplastic cells, which usually are degenerated, are seen in small groups or singly (Figure 11-83). Most reported cases are of

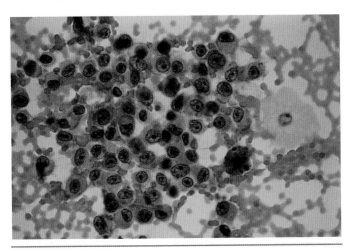

Figure 11-84 Metastatic malignant melanoma in a bladder wash specimen. A cluster of malignant cells with high N:C ratios, eccentrically placed nuclei and prominent nucleoli are seen. A fragment of melanin pigment is seen in the background. (Pap)

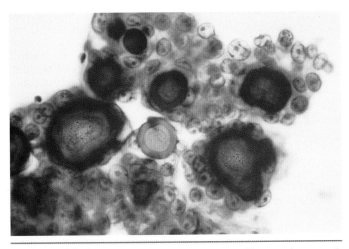

Figure 11-85 Metastatic serous papillary adenocarcinoma in a bladder wash specimen. Malignant cells and psammoma bodies are present. The cells contain prominent nucleoli and exhibit irregular nuclear shapes. This tumor is a metastasis from an ovarian primary. (Pap)

nomas, and urothelial cell carcinomas. Features suggestive of colonic origin include necrosis, columnar cell contours, and coarse nuclear chromatin.[225]

Metastases

Tumors may metastasize to the urinary tract. Some of the more common sites of origin of metastatic tumors are skin (melanoma), ovary, testes, and breast. Malignant melanoma may be primary of the urinary tract but more likely is metastatic. Malignant melanoma may present as melanuria without malignant cells[266] or may present with variable numbers of tumor cells.[267-269] The malignant cells are seen singly and contain enlarged nuclei with visible nucleoli (Figure 11-84). Cytoplasmic pigment granules may be present, which should be separated from hemosiderin and lipofuscin. The presence of malignant cells in the urine harbors a poor prognosis and is indicative of widespread dissemination.[267]

Testicular tumors and ovarian tumors may be poorly differentiated and difficult to separate from urothelial cell carcinoma (Figure 11-85).[270-272]

References

1. Sadek S, Soloway M, Hook S, et al. The value of upper tract cytology after transurethral resection of bladder tumor in patients with bladder transitional cell cancer. U Urol 1999; 161:77-79.
2. Ro J, Staerkel G, Ayala A. Cytologic and histologic features of superficial bladder cancer. Urol Clin North Am 1992; 19:435-453.
3. Tang C, Lau Y, Kung I. Alcoholic carbowax prefixation and formal alcohol fixation: a new technique for urine cytology. Acta Cytol 1997; 41:1183-1188.
4. Umiker W. Accuracy of cytologic diagnosis of cancer of the urinary tract. Acta Cytol 1964; 8:186-193.
5. Cowen P. The development of a urological cytodiagnosis service and an evaluation of its success. J Clin Pathol 1971; 24:107-112.
6. Murphy W. Current status of urinary cytology in the evaluation of bladder neoplasms. Hum Pathol 1990; 21:886-896.
7. Crabtree W, Murphy W. The value of ethanol as a fixative in urinary cytology. Acta Cytol 1980; 24:452-455.
8. Murphy W. Urinary cytology in diagnostic pathology. Diagn Cytopathol 1985; 1:173-175.
9. Weidmann J, Chaubal A, Bibbo M. Cellular fixation: a study of CytoRich Red and cytospin collection fluid. Acta Cytol. 1997; 41:182-187.
10. Ooms E, Veldhuizen R. Cytological criteria and diagnostic terminology in urinary cytology. Cytopathology 1993; 4:51-54.
11. Potts S, Thomas P, Cohen M, et al. Diagnostic accuracy and key cytologic features of high-grade transitional cell carcinoma in the upper urinary tract. Mod Pathol 1997; 10:657-662.
12. Paez A, Coba J, Murillo N, et al. Reliability of the routine cytological diagnosis in bladder cancer. Eur Urol 1999; 35:228-232.
13. Goldstein M, Whitman T, Renshaw A. Significance of cell groups in voided urine. Acta Cytol 1998; 42:290-294.
14. Kannan V, Gupta D. Calculus artifact. A challenge in urinary cytology. Acta Cytol 1999; 43:794-800.
15. Kannan V, Bose S. Low grade transitional cell carcinoma and instrument artifact: a challenge in urinary cytology. Acta Cytol 1993; 37:899-902.
16. Nielson K, Nielson K. Adenocarcinoma in extrophy of the bladder: the last case in Scandanavia? A case report and review of the literature. J Urol 1983; 130:1180-1182.
17. Betz S, See W, Cohen M. Granulomatous inflammation in bladder wash specimens after intravesical bacillus Calmette-Guérin therapy for transitional cell carcinoma of the bladder. Am J Clin Pathol 1993; 99:244-248.
18. Schumann G, Johnston J, Weiss M. Renal epithelial fragments in urine sediment. Acta Cytol 1981; 25:147-152.
19. Eggensperger D, King C, Gaudette L. Cytodiagnostic urinalysis: three years experience with a new laboratory test. Am J Clin Pathol 1989; 91:202-206.
20. Wiener D, Koss L, Sablay B, et al. The prevalence and significance of Brunn's nests, cystitis cystica and squamous metaplasia in normal bladders. J Urol 1979; 122:317-321.
21. Widran J, Sanchez R, Gruhn J. Squamous metaplasia of the bladder: a study of 450 patients. J Urol 1974; 112:479-482.
22. Whelan P, Britton J, Dowell A. Three-year follow-up of bladder tumours found on screening. Br J Urol 1993; 72:893-896.
23. Pellet H, Buernerd A, Minaire E. Clinical prevalence of glomerular hematuria: a nine-year retrospective study. Diagn Cytopathol 1991; 7:27-31.

24. Corwin H, Bray R, Haber M. The detection and interpretation of urinary eosinophils. Arch Pathol Lab Med 1989; 113:1256-1258.

25. Rouse B, Donaldson L, Goellner J. Intranuclear inclusions in urinary cytology. Acta Cytol 1986; 30:105-109.

26. Melamed M, Wolinska W. On the significance of intracytoplasmic inclusions in the urinary sediment. Am J Pathol 1961; 38:711-719.

27. Wynder E, Goldsmith R. The epidemiology of bladder cancer: a second look. Cancer 1977; 40:1246-1268.

28. Highman W, Wilson E. Urine cytology in patients with calculi. J Clin Pathol 1982; 35:350-356.

29. Beyer-Boon M, Cuypers L, et al. Cytological changes due to urinary calculi: a consideration of the relationship between calculi and the development of urothelial carcinoma. Br J Urol 1978; 50:81-89.

30. Salm R. Combined intestinal and squamous metaplasia of the renal pelvis. J Clin Pathol 1969; 22:187-191.

31. Swedlund S. Acute urinary tract infection in adults. Urinary Tract Disorders 1998; VIII:544-546.

32. Orr W, Mulholland S, Walzak M. Genitourinary tract involvement with systemic mycosis. J Urol 1972; 107: 1047-1050.

33. Piscioli F, Pusiol T, Polla E. Urinary cytology of tuberculosis of the bladder. Acta Cytol 1985; 29:125-131.

34. Kapila K, Verma K. Cytologic detection of tuberculosis of the urinary bladder. Acta Cytol 1984; 28:90-91.

35. Gardner S, Field A, Coleman D, et al. New human papovavirus (B.K.) isolated from urine after renal transplantation. Lancet 1971; i:1253-1257.

36. Koss L. Viruria and hemorrhagic cystitis. N Engl J Med 1987; 316:108-109.

37. Minassian H, Schinella R, Reilly J. Polyomavirus in the urine: follow-up study. Diagn Cytopathol 1994; 10: 209-211.

38. Kahan A, Coleman D, Koss L. Activation of human polyomavirus infection: detection by cytologic technics. Am J Clin Pathol 1980; 74:326-332.

39. Coleman D. The cytodiagnosis of human polyoma virus infection. Acta Cytol 1975; 19:93-96.

40. Arthur R, Shah K, Baust S, et al. Association of BK viruria with hemorrhagic cystitis in recipients of bone marrow transplants. N Engl J Med 1986; 315:230-234.

41. Drachenberg C, Beskow C, Cangro C, et al. Human polyoma virus in renal allograft biopsies: morphological findings and correlation with urine cytology. Hum Pathol 1999; 30:970-977.

42. Kupper T, Stoffels U, Pawlita M, et al. Morphological changes in urothelial cells replicating human polyomavirus BK. Cytopathology 1993; 4:361-368.

43. Crabbe J. "Comet" or "Decoy" cells found in urinary sediment smears. Acta Cytol 1971; 15:303-305.

44. Boon M, van Keep J, Kok L. Polyomavirus infection versus high-grade bladder carcinoma: the importance of cytologic and comparative morphometric studies of plastic-embedded voided urine sediments. Acta Cytol 1989; 33:887-893.

45. Itoh S, Irie K, Nakamura Y, et al: Cytologic and genetic study of polyomavirus-infected or polyomavirus-activated cells in human urine. Arch Pathol Lab Med 1998; 122: 333-337.

46. Boldorini R, Zorini E, Vigano P, et al. Cytologic and biomolecular diagnosis of polyomavirus infection in urine specimens of HIV-positive patients. Acta Cytol 2000; 44:205-210.

47. Bancroft J, Seybolt J, Windhager H. Cytologic diagnosis of cytomegalic inclusion disease: a case report. Acta Cytol 1961; 5:182-186.

48. Chang S. Urinary cytologic diagnosis of cytomegalic inclusion disease in childhood leukemia. Acta Cytol 1970; 14:338-343.

49. Person D, Kaufman R, Gardner H, et al. Herpes virus type 2 in genitourinary tract infections. Am J Obstet Gynecol 1973; 116:993-995.

50. Masukawa T, Garancis J, Rytel M, et al. Herpes genitalis virus isolation from human bladder urine. Acta Cytol 1972; 16:416-428.

51. Gomousa-Michael M, Rammou-Kinia R. Herpesvirus infection of the male urethra identified by cytology. Acta Cytol 1992; 36:270-271.

52. Murphy W. Herpes virus in bladder cancer. Acta Cytol 1976; 20:207-210.

53. DelMistro A, Koss L, Braunstein J, et al. Condylomata acuminata of the urinary bladder: natural history, viral typing, and DNA content. Am J Surg Pathol 1988; 12: 205-215.

54. Walther M, O'Brien D, Birch H. Condylomata acuminata and verrucous carcinoma of the bladder: case report and literature review. J Urol 1986; 135:362-365.

55. Krieger J. Urologic aspects of trichomoniasis. Invest Urol 1981; 18:411-417.

56. Clements M, Oko T. Cytologic diagnosis of schistosomiasis in routine urinary specimens: a case report. Acta Cytol 1983; 27:277.

57. Dimmette R, Sproat H, Klimt C. Examination of smears of urinary sediment for detection of neoplasms of bladder: survey of an Egyptian village infested with schistosoma hematobium. Am J Clin Pathol 1955; 25:1032-1042.

58. Procop G, Mendez J, Schneider S, et al. Diagnostic value of a miracidium in urinary sediment. Diagn Cytopathol 1999; 20:34-37.

59. Noi I, Cohen I, Loberant N. Renal hydatid cyst: urinary cytological diagnosis. Diagn Cytopathol 1995; 12: 152-154.

60. Jain S, Sodhani P, Gupta S, et al. Cytomorphology of filariasis revisited: expansion of the morphologic spectrum and coexistence with other lesions. Acta Cytol 2001; 45:186-191.

61. Stanton M, Maxted W. Malacoplakia: a study of the literature and current concepts of pathogenesis, diagnosis and treatment. J Urol 1981; 125:139-146.

62. Ho K. Morphogenesis of Michaelis-Gutmann bodies in cerebral malacoplakia: an ultrastructural study. Arch Pathol Lab Med 1989; 113:874-879.

63. Smith B. Malakoplakia of the urinary tract: a study of 24 cases. Am J Clin Pathol 1965; 43:409-417.

64. Chalvardjian A, Carydis B, Cohen S. Cytologic diagnosis of extravesical malacoplakia. Diagn Cytopathol 1985; 1:216-220.

65. Curran F. Malakoplakia of the bladder. Br J Urol 1987; 59:559-563.

66. Ashton P, Lambird P. Cytodiagnosis of malakoplakia: report of a case. Acta Cytol 1970; 14:92-94.

67. Lewis R, Jackson A, Murphy W, et al. Cytology in the diagnosis and follow-up of transitional cell carcinoma of the urothelium: a review with a case series. J Urol 1976; 116:443-446.

68. Melamed M. The urinary sediment cytology in a case of malakoplakia. Acta Cytol 1962; 6:471-474.

69. Duque J, Loughlin K. An overview of the treatment of superficial bladder cancer: intravesical chemotherapy. Urol Clin North Am 2000; 27:125-135.

70. Messing E, Catalona W. Urothelial tumors of the urinary tract. In: Walsh PC, AB Retik, Vaughan ED Jr, et al., editors. Campbell's urology. 1998; 3:2327-2410.

71. Stillwell T, Benson R. Cyclophosphamide-induced hemorrhagic cystitis: a review of 100 patients. Cancer. 1988; 61:451-457.

72. Stella R, Battistelli S, Marcheggiani F, et al. Urothelial cell changes due to busulfan and cyclophosphamide treatment in bone marrow transplantation. Acta Cytol 1990; 34:885-890.

73. Stella F, Battistelli S, Marcheggiani F, et al. Urothelial toxicity following conditioning therapy in bone marrow transplantation and bladder cancer: morphologic and morphometric comparison by exfoliative urinary cytology. Diagn Cytopathol 1992; 8:216-221.

74. Forni A, Koss L, Geller W. Cytological study of the effect of cyclophosphamide on the epithelium of the urinary bladder in man. Cancer 1964; 17:1348-1355.

75. Colandrea J, Elwood L, Solomon D. Identifications of polyoma virus antigens in urine from cyclophosphamide-treated patients. Acta Cytol 1990; 34:710.

76. Dale G, Smith R. Transitional cell carcinoma of the bladder associated with cyclophosphamide. J Urol 1974; 112:603-604.

77. McDougal W, Cramer S, Miller R. Invasive carcinoma of the renal pelvis following cyclophosphamide therapy for nonmalignant disease. Cancer 1981; 48:691-695.

78. Fuchs E, Kay R, Poole R, et al. Uroepithelial carcinoma in association with cyclophosphamide ingestion. J Urol 1981; 126:544-545.

79. Koss L, Melamed M. The effect of Busulfan on human epithelia. Am J Clin Pathol 1965; 44:385-397.

80. Cant J, Murphy W, Soloway M. Prognostic significance of urine cytology on initial follow-up after intravesical mitomycin C for superficial bladder cancer. Cancer 1986; 57:2119-2122.

81. Murphy W, Soloway M, Lin C. Morphologic effects of thiotepa on mammalian urothelium: changes in abnormal cells. Acta Cytol 1978; 22:550-554.

82. Murphy W, Irving C. The cellular features of developing carcinoma in murine urinary bladder. Cancer 1981; 47:514-522.

83. Rasmussen K, Peterson BL, Jacobo E, et al. Cytologic effects of thiotepa and adriamycin on normal canine urothelium. Acta Cytol 1980; 24:237-243.

84. Koshikawa T, Leyh H, Schenck U. Difficulties in evaluating urinary specimens after local mitomycin therapy of bladder cancer. Diagn Cytopathol 1989; 5:117-121.

85. Baltaci S, Suzer O, Ozer G, et al. The efficacy of urinary cytology in the detection of recurrent bladder tumours. Int Urol Nephrol 1996; 28:649-653.

86. Spagnolo D, Waring P. Bladder carcinoma after bladder surgery. Am J Clin Pathol 1986; 86:430-437.

87. Pagano F, Bassi P, Milani C, et al. Pathologic and structural changes in the bladder after BCG intravesical therapy in men. Prog Clin Biol Res 1989; 310:81-91.

88. Lage J, Bauer W, Kelley D, et al. Histological parameters and pitfalls in the interpretation of bladder biopsies in bacillus Calmette-Guérin treatment of superficial bladder cancer. J Urol 1986; 135:916-919.

89. Wiggishoff C, McDonald J. Urinary exfoliative cytology in the diagnosis of bladder tumors. Acta Cytol 1972; 16:139-141.

90. Koss L. Tumors of the urinary bladder. Washington, DC: AFIP; 1975:99-102.

91. Harris M, Schwinn C, Morrow J, et al. Exfoliative cytology of the urinary bladder irrigation specimen. Acta Cytol 1971; 15:385-388.

92. Weiss M, Mills S. Atlas of genitourinary tract disorders. Philadelphia: JB Lippincott; 1988.

93. O'Morchoe P, Riad W, Cowles L, et al. Urinary cytological changes after radiotherapy of renal transplants. Acta Cytol 1976; 20:132-136.

94. Loveless K. The effects of radiation upon the cytology of benign and malignant bladder epithelia. Acta Cytol 1973; 17:355-360.

95. Dabbs D. Cytology of pyelitis glandularis cystica: a case report. Acta Cytol 1992; 36:943-945.

96. Edwards P, Hurm R, Jaeschke W. Conversion of cystitis glandularis adenocarcinoma. J Urol 1972; 108:568-570.

97. Lin J, Tseng C, Choy C, et al. Diffuse cystitis glandularis associated with adenocarcinomatous change. Urology 1980; 15:411-415.

98. Cotran R, Kumar V, Robbins S. The lower urinary tract. 4th ed. Pathologic basis of disease. WB Saunders: Philadelphia; 1989. pp.1083-1097.

99. Caro D, Tesler A. Inverted papilloma of the bladder: a distinct urological lesion. Cancer 1978; 42:708-713.

100. Whitesel J. Inverted papilloma of the urinary tract: malignant potential. J Urol 1982; 127:539-540.

101. Feltis J, Perez-Marrero R, Emerson L, et al. Increased mast cells of the bladder in suspected cases of interstitial cystitis: a possible disease marker. J Urol 1987; 138:42-43.

102. Hanno P, Levin R, Monson F. Diagnosis of interstitial cystitis. J Urol 1990; 143:278-281.

103. Dodd L, Tello J. Cytologic examination of urine from patients with interstitial cystitis. Acta Cytol 1998; 42: 923-927.

104. Rubin L, Pincus M. Eosinophilic cystitis: the relationship of allergy in the urinary tract to eosinophilic cystitis and the pathophysiology of eosinophilia. J Urol 1974; 112:457-460.

105. Hellstrom H, Davis B, Shonnard J. Eosinophilic cystitis: a study of 16 cases. Am J Clin Pathol 1979; 72:777-784.

106. Sarma K. On the nature of cystitis follicularis. J Urol 1970; 104:709-714.

107. Elbadawi A, Malhoski W, Frank I. Mucinous urethral caruncle. Urology 1978; 12:587-590.

108. Nochomovitz L, Orenstein J. Inflammatory pseudotumor of the urinary bladder: possible relationship to nodular fasciitis. Am J Surg Pathol 1985; 9:366-373.

109. Proppe K, Scully R, Rosai J. Postoperative spindle-cell nodules of the genitourinary tract resembling sarcomas: a report of eight cases. Am J Surg Pathol 1984; 8:101-108.

110. Sonobe H, Okada Y, Sudo S, et al. Inflammatory pseudotumor of the urinary bladder with aberrant expression of cytokeratin: report of a case with cytologic, immunocytochemical and cytogenetic findings. Acta Cytol 1999; 43:257-262.

111. Lichtenfeld F, McCauley R, Staples P. Endometriosis involving the urinary tract: a collective review. Obstet Gynecol 1961; 17:762-768.

112. Randolph-Schrodt G, Alcorn M, et al. Endometriosis of the male urinary system: a case report. J Urol 1980; 124:722-723.

113. Schneider V, Smith M, Frable W. Urinary cytology in endometriosis of the bladder. Acta Cytol 1980; 24:30-33.

114. Rangmade C. Pelvic endometriosis and ureteral obstruction. Am J Obstet Gynecol 1975; 122:463-469.

115. Bhagavan B, Tiamson E, Wenk R, et al. Nephrogenic adenoma of the urinary bladder and urethra. Hum Pathol 1981; 12:907-916.

116. Stilmant M, Sivoky M. Nephrogenic adenoma associated with intravesical bacillus Calmette-Guérin treatment: a report of two cases. J Urol 1986; 135:359-361.

117. Navarre R, Loening S, Narayana A, et al. Nephrogenic adenoma: a report of nine cases and review of the literature. J Urol 1982; 127:775-779.

118. Rutgers J, Young R. Nephrogenic adenoma of the urinary bladder: a comparison of its cytologic and histopatholgic features in ten cases. Diagn Cytopathol 1988; 4:210-216.

119. Stilmant M, Murphy J, Merriam J. Cytology of nephrogenic adenoma of the urinary bladder: a report of four cases. Acta Cytol 1986; 30:35-40.

120. Troster M, Wyatt J, Alen-Halagah J. Nephrogenic adenoma of the urinary bladder: histologic and cytologic observations in a case. Acta Cytol 1986; 30:41-44.

121. Banigo O, Waisman J, Kaufman J. Papillary (transitional) carcinoma in an ileal conduit. J Urol 1975; 114:626-627.

122. Anagnostopoulou I, Rammou-Kinia R, Likourinas M. Urine cytology evaluation in cases of uretero-ileal cutaneous diversion. Cytopathology 1995; 6:268-272.

123. Wolinska W, Melamed M. Urinary conduit cytology. Cancer 1973; 32:1000-1006.

124. Landis S, Murray T, Bolden S, et al. Cancer statistics. CA Cancer J Clin 1999; 49:8-31.

125. Hall D. Bladder cancer: VIII urinary tract disorders. WB Saunders: Philadelphia; 1998. pp.563-565.

126. Matanoski G, Elliott E. Bladder cancer epidemiology. Epidemiology 1981; 3:203-229.

127. Schulte PA, Ringon K, Hemstreet GP, et al. Risk factors for bladder cancer in a cohort exposed to aromatic amines. Cancer 1986; 58:2156-2162.

128. Lower G. Concepts in causality: chemically induced human urinary bladder cancer. Cancer 1982; 49:1056-1066.

129. Crosby J, Allsbrook W, Koss L, et al. Cytologic detection of urothelial cancer and other abnormalities in a cohort of workers exposed to aromatic amines. Acta Cytol 1991; 35:263-268.

130. Lee R, Droller M. The natural history of bladder cancer: implications for therapy. Urol Clin North Am 2000; 27:1-13.

131. Cole P, Monson R, Haning H, et al. Smoking and cancer of the lower urinary tract. N Engl J Med 1971; 284:129-134.

132. Hartge P, Hoover R, Kantor A. Bladder cancer risk and pipes, cigars and smokeless tobacco. Cancer 1985; 55:901-906.

133. Piper J, Tonascia J, Matanoski G. Heavy phenacetin use and bladder cancer in women aged 20 to 49 years. N Engl J Med 1985; 313:292-295.

134. Veltman G, Bosch F, van der Plas Cats M, et al. Urine cytology as a screening method for transitional-cell carcinoma in dialysis patients with analgesic nephropathy. Nephrol Dial Transplant 1991; 6:346-348.

135. Droller M. Bladder cancer: state-of-the-art care. CA Cancer J Clin 1998; 48:269-284.

136. Koss L. Evaluation of patients with carcinoma in situ of the bladder. Pathol Annu 1982; 17:353-359.

137. Murphy W. Current topics in the pathology of bladder cancer. Pathol Annu 1983; 18:1-25.

138. Fukui I, Yokokawa M, Sekine H, et al. Carcinoma in situ of the urinary bladder. Cancer 1987; 59:164-173.

139. Hofstadter F, Delgado R, Jakse G, et al. Urothelial dysplasia and carcinoma in situ of the bladder. Cancer 1986; 57:356-361.

140. Murphy W, Soloway M. Developing carcinoma (dysplasia) of the urinary bladder. Pathol Annu 1982; 17:197-219.

141. Shenoy U, Colby T, Schumann G. Reliability of urinary cytodiagnosis in urothelial neoplasms. Cancer 1985; 56:2041-2045.

142. Farrow G, Utz D, Rife C, et al. Clinical observations of sixty-nine cases of in-situ carcinoma of the urinary bladder. Cancer Res 1977; 37:2794-2798.

143. Koss L. Precursor lesions of invasive bladder cancer. Eur Urol 1988; 14:4-6.

144. Utz D, Farrow G. Management of carcinoma in-situ of the bladder: the case for surgical management. Urol Clin North Am 1980; 7:533-541.

145. Utz D, Farrow G, Rife C, et al. Carcinoma in-situ of the bladder. Cancer 1980; 45:1842-1848.

146. Weinstein R, Miller A, Pauli B. Carcinoma in-situ: comments on the pathobiology of a paradox. Urol Clin North Am 1980; 7:523-531.

147. Melamed M, Koss L, Ricci A, et al. Cytohistiological observations on developing carcinoma of the urinary bladder in man. Cancer 1960; 13:67-74.

148. Melamed M, Whitmore W. Carcinoma in-situ of bladder: clinico-pathologic study of case with a suggested approach to detection. J Urol 1966; 96:466-471.

149. Boon M, Blomjous C, Zwartendijk J, et al. Carcinoma in-situ of the urinary bladder: cinical presentation, cytologic pattern and stromal changes. Acta Cytol 1986; 30:360-366.

150. Harving N, Petersen S, Melsen F, et al. Urinary cytology in the detection of bladder tumours: Influence of concomitant urothelial atypia. Scand J Urol Nephrol Suppl 1989; 125:127-131.

151. Koss L, Deitch D, Ramanathan R, et al. Diagnostic value of cytology of voided urine. Acta Cytol 1985; 29:810-816.

152. O'Donoghue J, Horgan P, Corcoran M, et al. Urinary cytology in the detection of bladder carcinoma. Irish J Med Sci 1991; 160:352-353.

153. Farrow G. Pathologist's role in bladder cancer. Sem Oncol 1979; 6:198-206.

154. Wright R, Halford J. Evaluation of thin-layer methods in urine cytology. Cytopathology 2001; 12:306-313.

155. Rosa B, Cazin M, Dalian G. Urinary cytology for carcinoma in-situ of the urinary bladder. Acta Cytol 1985; 29:117-124.

156. Nasuti J, Fleisher S, Gupta P. Significance of tissue fragments in voided urine specimens. Acta Cytol 2001; 45:147-152.

157. Highman W. Flat in-situ carcinoma of the bladder: cytological examination of urine in diagnosis, followup, and assesment of response to chemotherapy. J Clin Pathol 1988; 41:540-546.

158. Vousta N, Melamed M. Cytology of in-situ carcinoma of the human urinary bladder. Cancer 1963; 16:1307-1316.

159. Kojima S, Sekine H, Fukui I, et al. Clinical significance of "cannibalism" in urinary cytology of bladder cancer. Acta Cytol 1998; 42:1365-1369.

160. Jordan A, Weingarten J, Murphy W. Transitional cell neoplasms of the urinary bladder: can biologic potential be predicted from histologic grading? Cancer 1987; 60:2766-2774.

161. Brawn P. The origin of invasive carcinoma of the bladder. Cancer 1982; 50:515-519.

162. Raab S, Lenel J, Cohen M. Low grade transitional cell carcinoma of the bladder. Cytologic diagnosis by key features as identified by logistic regression analysis. Cancer 1994; 74:1621-1626.

163. Murphy W, Soloway M, Jukkola A, et al. Urinary cytology and bladder cancer: the cellular features of transitional cell neoplasms. Cancer 1984; 53:1555-1565.

164. Renshaw A, Nappi D, Weinberg D. Cytology of grade 1 papillary transitional cell carcinoma: a comparison of cytologic, architectural and morphometric criteria in cystoscopically obtained urine. Acta Cytol 1996; 40:676-682.

165. Raab S, Slagel D, Jensen C, et al. Low-grade transitional cell carcinoma of the urinary bladder: application of select cytologic criteria to improve diagnostic accuracy. Mod Pathol 1996; 9:225-232.

166. Kern W. The cytology of transitional cell carcinoma of the urinary bladder. Acta Cytol 1975; 19:420-428.
167. Boon M, Kurver P, Baak J, et al. Morphometric differences between urothelial cells in voided urine of patients with grade I and grade II bladder tumors. J Clin Pathol 1981; 34:612-615.
168. Sack M, Artymyshyn R, Tomaszewski J, et al. Diagnostic value of bladder wash cytology, with special reference to low grade urothelial neoplasms. Acta Cytol 1995; 39:187-194.
169. Bastacky S, Ibrahim S, Wilczynski S, et al. The accuracy of urinary cytology in daily practice. Cancer 1999; 87:118-128.
170. Ylagan L, Humphrey P. Micropapillary variant of transitional cell carcinoma of the urinary bladder: a report of three cases with cytologic diagnosis in urine specimens. Acta Cytol 2001; 45:599-604.
171. Brown F. Urine cytology: it is still the gold standard for screening? Urol Clin North Am 2000; 27:25-37.
172. Nasuti J, Gomella L, Ismial M, et al. Utility of the BTA stat test kit for bladder cancer screening. Diagn Cytopathol 1999; 21:27-29.
173. Leyh H, Marberger M, Conort P, et al. Comparison of the BTA stat test with voided urine cytology and bladder wash cytology in the diagnosis and monitoring of bladder cancer. Eur Urol 1999; 35:52-56.
174. van der Poel H, van Balken M, Schamhart D. Bladder wash cytology, quantitative cytology, and the qualitative BTA test in patients with superficial bladder cancer. Urology 1998; 51:44-50.
175. Bakhos R, Shankey T, Flanigan R, et al. Comparative analysis of DNA flow cytometry and cytology of bladder washing: review of discordant cases. Diagn Cytopathol 2000; 22:65-69.
176. Sole M, Alos L, Mallofre C, et al. Bladder wash flow cytometry in transitional cell carcinoma: useful or misleading? Urol Res 1995; 22:361-365.
177. Gourlay W, Chan V, Gilks C. Screening for urothelial malignancies by cytologic analysis and flow cytometry in a community urologic practice: a prospective study. Mod Pathol 1995; 8:394-397.
178. Eleuteri P, Grollino M, Pomponi D, et al. Bladder transitional cell carcinomas: a comparative study of washing and tumor bioptic samples by DNA flow cytometry and FISH analyses. Eur Urol 2000; 36:275-280.
179. de la Roza G, Hopkovitz A, Caraway N, et al. DNA image analysis of urinary cytology: prediction of recurrent transitional cell carcinoma. Mod Pathol 1996; 9:571-578.
180. van der Poel H, Boon M, van Stratum P, et al. Conventional bladder wash cytology performed by four experts versus quantitative image analysis. Mod Pathol 1997; 10:976-982.
181. Bonner R, Hemstreet G, Fradet Y, et al. Bladder cancer risk assessment with quantitative fluorescence image analysis of tumor markers in exfoliated bladder cells. Cancer 1993; 72:2461-2469.
182. Katz R, Sinkre P, Zhang H, et al. Clinical significance of negative and equivocal urinary bladder cytology alone and in combination with DNA image analysis and cystoscopy. Cancer 1997; 81:354-364.
183. Richman A, Mayne S, Jekel J, et al. Image analysis combined with visual cytology in the early detection of recurrent bladder carcinoma. Cancer 1998; 82:1738-1748.
184. Wiener H, Remkes G, Schatzl G, et al. Quick-staining urinary cytology and bladder wash image analysis with an integrated risk classification: a worthwhile improvement in the follow-up of bladder cancer? Cancer 1999; 87:263-269.
185. Desgrippes A, Izadifar V, Assailly J, et al. Diagnosis and prediction of recurrence and progression in superficial bladder cancers with DNA image cytometry and urinary cytology. BJU Int 2000; 85:434-436.
186. Sagerman P, Saigo P, Sheinfeld J, et al. Enhanced detection of bladder cancer in urine cytology with Lewis X, M344 and 19A211 antigens. Acta Cytol 1994; 38:517-523.
187. Zlotta A, Schulman C. Biological markers in superficial bladder tumors and their prognostic significance. Urol Clin North Am 2000; 27:179-189.
188. Kay E, Barry-Walsh C, Whelan D. Interobserver variation of p53 immunohistochemistry: an assessment of a practical problem and comparison with other studies. Br J Biomed Sci 1996; 53:101-107.
189. Sidransky D, Von-Eshenbach A, Tsai Y, et al. Identification of p53 gene mutations in bladder cancers and urine samples. Science 1991; 252:706-709.
190. Phillips H, Howard G, Miller W. p53 mutations as a marker of malignancy in bladder washing samples from patients with bladder cancer. Br J Cancer 2000; 82:136-141.
191. Prescott J, Montie J, Pugh T. Clinical sensitivity of p53 mutation detection in matched bladder tumor, bladder wash, and voided urine specimens. Cancer 2001; 91:2127-2135.
192. Righi E, Rossi G, Ferrari G, et al. Does p53 immunostaining improve diagnostic accuracy in urine cytology. Diagn Cytopathol 1997; 17:436-439.
193. Jones A, Crew J. Vascular endothelial growth factor and its correlation with superficial bladder cancer recurrence rates and stage progression. Urol Clin North Am 2000; 27:191-197.
194. Tsihlias J, Grossman H. The utility of fibrin/fibrinogen degradation products in superficial bladder cancer. Urol Clin North Am 2000; 27:39-46.
195. Schmetter B, Habicht K, Lamm D, et al. A multicenter trial evaluation of the fibrin/fibrinogen degradation products test for detection and monitoring of bladder cancer. J Urol 1997; 158:801-805.
196. Ramakumar S, Bhuiyan J, Besse J, et al. Comparison of screening, methods in the detection of bladder cancer. J Urol 1999; 161:388-394.
197. Grocela J, McDougal W. Utility of nuclear matrix protein (NMP22) in the detection of recurrent bladder cancer. Urol Clin North Am 2000; 27:47-51.
198. Mian C, Lodde M, Haitel A, et al. Comparison of the monoclonal UBC-ELISA test and the NMP22 ELISA test for the detection of urothelial cell carcinoma of the bladder. Urology 2000; 55:223-226.
199. Chahal R, Darshane A, Browning A, et al. Evaluation of the clinical value of urinary NMP22 as a marker in the screening and surveillance of transitional cell carcinoma of the urinary bladder. Eur Urol 2001; 40:415-420.
200. Grossman H. New methods for detection of bladder cancer. Semin Urol Oncol 1998; 16:17-22.
201. Hughes J, Katz R, Rodriguez-Villanueva J, et al. Urinary nuclear matrix protein 22 (NMP22): a diagnostic adjunct to urine cytologic examination for the detection of recurrent transitional-cell carcinoma of the bladder. Diagn Cytopathol 1999; 20:285-290.
202. Sozen S, Biri H, Sinik Z, et al. Comparison of the nuclear matrix protein 22 with voided urine cytology and BTA stat test in the diagnosis of transitional cell carcinoma of the bladder. Eur Urol 1999; 36:225-229.
203. Atsu N, Ekici S, Oge O, et al. False-positive results of the NMP22 test due to hematuria. J Urol 2001; 167:555-558.
204. Liu BC, Loughlin K. Telomerase in human bladder cancer. Urol Clin of North Am 2000; 27:115-123.

205. Ohyashiki K, Yahata N, Ohyashiki J, et al. A combination of semiquantitative telomerase assay and in-cell telomerase activity measurement using exfoliated urothelial cells for the detection of urothelial neoplasia. Cancer 1998; 83:2554-2560.

206. Kavaler E, Landman J, Chang Y, et al. Detecting human bladder carcinoma cells in voided urine samples by assaying for the presence of telomerase activity. Cancer 1998; 82:708-714.

207. Yoshida K, Sugino T, Tahara H. Telomerase activity in bladder carcinoma and its implication for noninvasive diagnosis by detection of exfoliated cancer cells in urine. Cancer 1997; 79:362-369.

208. Rahat M, Lahat N, Gazawi H, et al. Telomerase activity in patients with transitional cell carcinoma: a preliminary study. Cancer 1999; 85:919-924.

209. Lancelin F, Anidjar M, Villette J, et al. Telomerase activity as a potential marker in preneoplastic bladder lesions. BJU Int 2000; 85:526-531.

210. Saad A, Hanbury DC, McNicholas TA, et al. A study comparing various noninvasive methods of detecting bladder cancer in urine. BJU Int 2002; 84:369-373.

211. Boman H, Hedelin H, Holmang S. Four bladder tumor markers have a disappointingly low sensitivity for small size and low grade recurrence. J Urol 2002; 167:80-83.

212. Dodd L, Johnston W, Robertson C, et al. Endoscopic brush cytology of the upper urinary tract. Evaluation of its efficacy and potential limitations in diagnosis. Acta Cytol 1997; 41:377-384.

213. Hurle R, Losa A, Manzetti A, et al. Upper urinary tract tumors developing after treatment of superficial bladder cancer: 7-year follow-up of 591 consecutive patients. Urology 1999; 53:1144-1148.

214. Miller E, Eure G, Schellhammer P. Upper tract transitional cell carcinoma following treatment of superficial bladder cancer with BCG. Urology 1993; 42:26-30.

215. Bian Y, Ehya H, Bagley D. Cytologic diagnosis of upper urinary tract neoplasms by ureteroscopic sampling. Acta Cytol 1995; 39:733-740.

216. Kawakami H, Hoshida Y, Hanai J, et al. Voided urine cytology of papillary renal cell carcinoma and renal calculus: report of a case with emphasis on the importance of cytologic screening in high-risk individuals. Acta Cytol 2001; 45:771-774.

217. HIghman W. Transitional carcinoma of the upper urinary tract: a histological and cytopathological study. J Clin Pathol 1986; 39:297-305.

218. Zincke H, Aguilo J, Farrow G, et al. Significance of urinary cytology in the early detection of transitional cell cancer of the upper urinary tract. J Urol 1976; 116:781-783.

219. Sarnacki C, McCormack L, Kiser W, et al. Urinary cytology and the clinical diagnosis of urinary tract malignancy: a clinicopathologic study of 1,400 patients. J Urol 1971; 106:761-764.

220. Bibbo M, Gill W, Harris M, et al. Retrograde brushing as a diagnostic procedure of ureteral, renal pelvic and renal calyceal lesions: a preliminary report. Acta Cytol 1974; 18:137-141.

221. Hawtrey C. Fifty-two cases of primary ureteral carcinoma: a clinical-pathologic study. J Urol 1971; 105:188-193.

222. Prall R, Wernett C, Mims M. Diagnostic cytology in urinary tract malignancy. Cancer 1972; 29:1084-1089.

223. Kannan V. Papillary transitional-cell carcinoma of the upper urinary tract: a cytological review. Diagn Cytopathol 1990; 6:204-209.

224. Fralick R, Malek R, Goellner J, et al. Urethroscopy and urethral cytology in men with external genital condyloma. Urology 1994; 43:361-364.

225. Bardales R, Pitman M, Stanley M, et al. Urine cytology of primary and secondary urinary bladder adenocarcinoma. Cancer 1998; 84:335-343.

226. Shinagawa T, Tadokoro M, Abe M, et al. Papillary urothelial carcinoma of the urinary bladder demonstrating prominent signet-ring cells in a smear: a case report. Acta Cytol 1998; 42:407-412.

227. Doria M, Martin G, Wang H, et al. Cytologic features of clear cell carcinoma of the urethra and urinary bladder. Diagn Cytopathol 1996; 14:150-154.

228. Peven D, Hidvegi D. Clear-cell adenocarcinoma of the female urethra. Acta Cytol 1985; 29:142-146.

229. Young R, Eble J. Unusual forms of carcinoma of the urinary bladder. Hum Pathol 1991; 22:948-965.

230. Grignon D, Ro J, Ayala A, et al. Small cell carcinoma of the urinary bladder: a clinicopathologic analysis of 22 cases. Cancer 1992; 69:527-536.

231. Ali S, Reuter V, Zakowski M. Small cell neuroendocrine carcinoma of the urinary bladder: a clinicopathologic study with emphasis on cytologic features. Cancer 1997; 79:356-361.

232. Cheson B, Schumann G, Johnston J. Urinary cytodiagnosis of renal involvement in disseminated histiocytic lymphoma. Acta Cytol 1984; 28:148-152.

233. Cheson B, Schumann J, Schumann G. Urinary cytodiagnosis abnormalities in 50 patients with non-Hodgkin's lymphomas. Cancer 1984; 54:1914-1919.

234. Yam L, Janckila A. Immunocytochemical diagnosis of lymphoma from urine sediment. Acta Cytol 1985; 29:827-832.

235. Minicoine G. Primary malignant lymphoma of the urinary bladder with a positive cytologic report. Acta Cytol 1982; 26:69-72.

236. Geisinger K, Buss D, Kawamoto E, et al. Multiple myeloma: the diagnostic role and prognostic significance of exfoliative cytology. Acta Cytol 1986; 30:334-340.

237. Neal M, Swearingen M, Gawronski L, et al. Myeloma cells in the urine. Arch Pathol Lab Med 1985; 109:870-872.

238. Yang C, Motteram R, Sandeman T. Extramedullary plasmacytoma of the bladder: a case report and review of literature. Cancer 1982; 50:146-149.

239. Weimar G, Culp D, Loening S, et al. Urogenital involvement by malignant lymphomas. J Urol 1981; 125:230-231.

240. Andrion A, Gaglio A, Zai G. Bladder involvement in disseminated malignant lymphoma diagnosed by voided urine cytology. Cytopathology 1993; 4:115-117.

241. Bocian J, Flam M, Mendoza C. Hodgkin's disease involving the urinary bladder diagnosed by urinary cytology: a case report. Cancer 1982; 50:2482-2485.

242. Sahin A, Myhre M, Ro J, et al. Plasmacytoid transitional cell carcinoma: report of a case with initial presentation mimicking multiple myeloma. Acta Cytol 1991; 35:277-280.

243. Cheson B, DeBellis C, Schumann G, et al. The urinary myeloma cast: frequency of detection and clinical correlations in 30 patients with multiple myeloma. Am J Clin Pathol 1985; 83:421-425.

244. Kepner L, Cohen C. Monocytic leukemia cells in urine: a case report. Acta Cytol 1982; 26:335-337.

245. Rupp M, O'Hara B, McCullogh L, et al. Prostatic carcinoma cells in urine specimens: cytologic, histologic and immunocytochemical features. Acta Cytol 1990; 34:744-745.

246. Nguyen Ho P, Nguyen G, Villanueva R. Small cell anaplastic carcinoma of the prostate: report of a case with positive urine cytology. Diagn Cytopathol 1994; 10:159-161.

247. Sharifi R, Shaw M, Ray V, et al. Evaluation of cytologic techniques for diagnosis of prostate cancer. Urology 1983; 21:417-420.

248. Varma V, Kekete P, Franks M, et al. Cytologic features of prostate adenocarcinoma in urine: a clinicopathologic and immunocytochemical study. Diagn Cytolpathol 1988; 4:300-305.

249. Krishnan B, Truong L. Prostatic adenocarcinoma diagnosed by urinary cytology. Am J Clin Pathol 2000; 113:29-34.

250. Vandersteen D, Wiemerslage S, Cohen M. Prostatic duct adenocarcinoma: a cytologic and histologic case report with review of the literature. Diagn Cytopathol 1997; 17:480-483.

251. Piscioli F, Pusiol T, Scappini P, et al. Urine cytology in the detection of renal adenocarcinoma. Cancer 1985; 56:2251-2255.

252. Park C-H, Britsch C, Uson A, et al. Reliability of positive exfoliative cytologic study of the urine in urinary tract malignancy. J Urol 1969; 102:91-92.

253. Foot N, Papanicolaou G, Holmqist N, et al. Exfoliative cytology of urinary sediments: a review of 2,829 cases. Cancer 1958; 11:127-137.

254. Papanicolaou G. Cytology of the urine sediment in neoplasms of the urinary tract. J Urol 1947; 57:375-379.

255. Mauri M, Bonzanini M, Luciani L, et al. Renal collecting duct carcinoma: report of a case with urinary cytologic findings. Acta Cytol 1994; 38:755-758.

256. Rudrick B, Nguyen G, Lakey W. Carcinoid tumor of the renal pelvis: report of a case with positive urine cytology. Diagn Cytopathol 1995; 12:360-363.

257. Larson D, Gilstad C, Manson G, et al. Renal medullary carcinoma: report of a case with positive urinary cytology. Diagn Cytopathol 1998; 18:276-279.

258. Nguyen G, Schumann G. Cytopathology of renal collecting duct carcinoma in urine sediment. Diagn Cytopathol 1997; 16:446-449.

259. Fallick M, Hutchinson M, Alroy J, et al. Collecting-duct carcinoma presenting as upper tract lesion with abnormal urine cytology. Diagn Cytopathol 1997; 16:258-261.

260. Yonekawa M, Hoshida Y, Hanai J, et al. Catheterized urine cytology of mucinous carcinoma arising in the renal pelvis: a case report. Acta Cytol 2000; 44:442-444.

261. McDonald J. Exfoliative cytology in genitourinary and pulmonary diseases. Am J Clin Pathol 1954; 24:684-687.

262. Meisels A. Cytology of carcinoma of the kidney. Acta Cytol 1963; 7:239-244.

263. Hausdorfer G, Chandrasoma P, Pettross B, et al. Cytologic diagnosis of mesonephric adenocarcinoma of the urinary bladder. Acta Cytol 1985; 29:823-826.

264. Hajdu S, Savino A, Hajdu E, et al. Cytologic diagnosis of renal cell carcinoma with the aid of fat stain. Acta Cytol 1971; 15:31-33.

265. Milsten R, Frable W, Texter J, et al. Evaluation of lipid stain in renal neoplasms as adjunct to routine exfoliative cytology. J Urol 1973; 110:169-171.

266. Valente P, Atkinson B, Guerry D. Melanuria. Acta Cytol 1985; 29:1026-1027.

267. Woodard B, Ideker R, Johnston W. Cytologic detection of malignant melanoma in urine: a case report. Acta Cytol 1978; 22:350-352.

268. Zogno C, Schiaffino E, Boeri R, et al. Cytologic detection of metastatic malignant melanoma in urine: a report of three cases. Acta Cytol 1997; 41:1332-1336.

269. Piva A, Koss L. Cytologic diagnosis of metastatic malignant melanoma in urinary sediment. Acta Cytol 1964; 8:398-402.

270. Viddeleer A, Lycklama A, Nijeholt G, et al. A late manifestation of testicular seminoma in the bladder in a renal transplant recipient: a case report. J Urol 1992; 148: 401-402.

271. Rojewska J, Pykalo R, Czaplicki M. Urine and semen cytomorphology in patients with testicular tumors. Diagn Cytopathol. 1989; 5:9-13.

272. Edgerton M, Hoda R, Gupta P. Cytologic diagnosis of metastatic ovarian adenocarcinoma in the urinary bladder: a case report and review of the literature. Diagn Cytopathol 1999; 20:156-159.

273. Farrow GM. Urine cytology in the detection of bladder cancer: a critical approach. J Occup Med 1990; 32: 817-821.

274. Frable WJ, Paxson L, Barksdale JA, et al. Current practice of urinary bladder cytology. Cancer Res 1977; 37: 2800-2805.

275. Fall M, Johansson S, Aldengorg F. Chronic interstitial cystitis: a heterogeneous syndrome. J Urol 1987; 137:35-38.

276. Pode D, Perlberg S, Steiner D. Busulfan-induced hemorrhagic cystitis J Urol 1983; 130:347-348.

277. Droller M, Erozan Y. Thiotepa effects on urinary cytology in the interpretation of transitional cell cancer. J Urol 1985; 136:671-674.

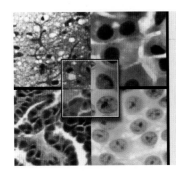

Effusions

CHAPTER
12

The body's cavities and visceral thoracic, abdominal, and pelvic organs are lined with a layer of mesothelial cells. Although mesothelial cells are derived from mesoderm, they are generally considered to have the appearance and many characteristics of epithelial cells. The mesothelial layer lining the organ surface is called *visceral mesothelium,* and the layer lining the thoracic, abdominal, and pelvic walls is called *parietal mesothelium.* This layer of mesothelial cells is only one cell thick, and rests on fibrovascular stromal tissue that is rich in vasculature and lymphatics (Figure 12-1). The lymphatic lacunae open onto the mesothelial surface through narrow gaps or stoma so that the body cavities are essentially an extension of the lymphatic system.[1]

The accumulation of fluid in a body cavity is referred to as an *effusion.* All effusions are pathologic regardless of their cellular constituents. The extravasation of fluid into the body cavities can occur under multiple clinical scenarios, including collagen vascular disorders, circulatory disorders, trauma, infections, and neoplasms.[1]

Normally, the pleural fluid is produced by the parietal pleura and absorbed by the visceral pleural capillaries and lymphatics. The parietal and visceral pleural surfaces are in apposition and slide easily along each other through the lubrication provided by this small amount of fluid. The pleural/pericardial cavities are not true cavities but only become so in the presence of a disease that leads to the accumulation of serous fluid. Effusions can be caused by increased intravascular hydrostatic pressure (e.g., congestive heart failure [CHF]), decreased osmotic pressure (e.g., cirrhosis and nephrotic syndrome), and altered lymphatic drainage (neoplasms). The extravasation of fluid into the pleural space may also be an inflammatory response of the serosal membrane (e.g., collagen vascular diseases or infections). Vasodilation and hyperpermeability of the microvasculature lead to the extravasation of inflammatory cells and serum. Neoplasms block and break down blood vessel walls. This leads to bloody effusions that may potentially contain tumor cells. It has been theorized that the increase in vascular permeability associated with malignant effusions may be the result of high levels of vascular endothelial growth factor (VEGF) which is elevated in malignant effusions.[201] Limited studies of antiangiogenesis factors such as VEGF antibodies and receptors have had some success in a subset of patients with advanced neoplastic disease.[2]

An effusion that is composed of an ultrafiltrate of plasma is designated a transudate. Transudates are caused by CHF, renal failure, and so on. An effusion rich in cells and protein is designated an exudate. Malignant and infectious effusions are exudates. General aspects of transudates and exudates and causes of transudative and exudative effusions of the pleura, pericardium, and peritoneum are listed in Tables 12-1 and 12-2. Transudates tend to be clear, whereas exudates can be cloudy, bloody, milky, chylous, or bilious, depending on the etiologic factors and duration. Generally, transudates do not require pathologic examination particularly when the underlying cause is known (e.g., CHF, cirrhosis). They tend to be the result of systemic disease and often are bilateral.[3] Malignant pleural effusions may be transudates in 1% to 10% of patients, thus, the inclusion of transudates for cytologic examination should be considered.[4] Exudates uniformly require cytologic examination.[3,5]

Clinically, when trying to distinguish a transudate from an exudate, if the serum albumin level is 1.2 gm/dl higher than in the pleural fluid, then the fluid is a transudate. Aside from a cytologic examination, an exudative effusion, particularly pleural, may be examined for Gram stain and cultures, cell counts with differential, glucose, amylase, lactic acid dehydrogenase, and a marker for tuberculous pleuritis (adenosine deaminase above 45 IU/L or gamma interferon level above 3.7 U/ml).[6]

Several recent texts have dealt comprehensively with the topics of effusion physiology and benign and infectious causes of effusions.[7,8] This chapter summarizes much of this information from these texts and focuses on what the authors view to be the major diagnostic dilemmas encountered most commonly in clinical practice.

Statistically, almost an equal distribution of the causes of pleural effusions are between malignant and nonmalignant etiologic factors (Tables 12-3 and 12-4).[9] The most common causes of benign pericardial effusions are infectious, usually of a viral (e.g., Coxsackie) or tuberculous origin. Adenocarcinomas of the breast and lung or hematopoietic malignancies are the most common causes of neoplastic pericardial effusions (Box 12-1).

More than 90% of cases of ascites are from portal hypertension, mostly as a result of cirrhosis. Resulting from malignancy are 10% of cases, with peritoneal carcinomatosis responsible for 50% of these[10] (Box 12-2).

OBTAINING A SPECIMEN FROM AN EFFUSION

When attempting to discover the etiologic factors of an effusion, cytologic examination of the fluid has been found to be the superior diagnostic mode as compared with biopsy, particularly with regard to pleural effusions. In cases of suspected malignancy, when the initial cytology of the effusion sample is negative, the performance of a pleural biopsy and a successive fluid evaluation can be performed. The diagnostic yield improves when both are done in conjunction after an initially negative effusion cytology.[11,12]

Fluid from the thorax, abdomen, and pericardium are fairly easily obtained. This is accomplished under local anesthesia, by the insertion of a wide bore needle or catheter through the body wall and into the effusion-laden cavity. These procedures are referred to as *thoracentesis, abdominal paracentesis,* and *pericardiocentesis,* respectively.

Alternatively, testing for the presence of abnormal cells along the mesothelial surfaces in the absence of an effusion (as in staging procedures, particularly for gynecologic malignancies) is accomplished through *washing.* This is performed through a similar catheter or directly (intraoperatively) by instilling physiologic saline solution into the area of interest, attempting to distribute it diffusely, withdrawing the fluid, and submitting it for cytologic examination.

SPECIMEN PREPARATION

Effusion samples can either be fixed in equal volumes of 50% ethanol or prepared fresh. Evaluation of smear/cytospin preparations along with a cell block is critical because a large proportion of diagnoses are missed or at least reported in a less specific manner by viewing the cytology in the absence of a cell block.[13,14] Multiple preparatory, particularly concentration, techniques may increase the

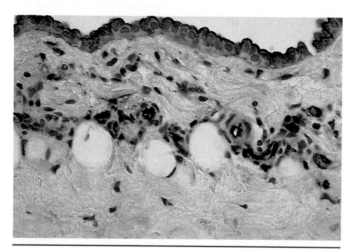

Figure 12-1 Mesothelial cells highlighted with cytokeratin. A single layer of mesothelial cells rests on fibrovascular stromal tissue that is rich in vasculature and lymphatics. (From Carter D, True L, Otis CN. Serous membranes. In: Sternberg SS. Histology for pathologists. 2nd ed. Philadelphia: Lippincott-Raven; 1997.)

TABLE 12-1		
Comparison of Transudates and Exudates		
Aspect	**Transudate**	**Exudate**
Specific gravity	≤1.015	>1.015
Total protein	≤3.0	>3.0
Appearance	Clear	Cloudy
Cellularity	Sparse	High
Organisms	(−)	(±)
Coagulation properties	Does not coagulate	Coagulates upon standing
LDH pleural ratio fluid:plasma	<0.6	>0.6

Modified from Bedrossian CWM. Malignant effusions: a multimodal approach to cytologic diagnosis. New York: Igaku-Shoin; 1994.

TABLE 12-2			
General Aspects of Pathologic Effusions			
Category	**Appearance**	**Cellular Components**	**Clinical Significance**
Serous	Clear, thin	Low cellularity	Transudate
Chylous	Milky	Lipid-laden cells	Lymphatic retention
Pseudochylous	Milky, green	Foamy cells	Cholesterol crystals
Cirrhotic	Thin, brown	Reactive mesothelial cells	Transudate
Eosinophilic	Thin, silky	Eosinophils	Allergic
Inflammatory	Yellowish, white, thick	Neutrophils, lymphocytes	Collagen-vascular disease
Infectious	Green, foul smelling	Lymphocytes	Tuberculosis or other infection
Hemorrhagic	Brown, thin	Malignant cells	Carcinoma
Hemorrhagic	Brown, viscous	Malignant cells	Mesothelioma
Pigmented	Dark brown, thick	Malignant cells	Melanoma

Modified from Bedrossian CWM. Malignant effusions: a multimodal approach to cytologic diagnosis. New York: Igaku-Shoin; 1994.

chance of detecting neoplasia in a single specimen.[15] With ethanol fixation it is only possible to do Pap stains and a hematoxylin and eosin (H&E) cell block. When an effusion is freshly prepared, a Diff-Quik (DQ), Pap, and an H&E cell block can be done. Generally, for the best cellular preservation, fresh specimens are kept in the refrigerator until they are prepared. When refrigerated, the cells are well preserved for at least several days (up to 1 week), unless the specimen is highly inflammatory.

The authors of this text believe in the processing of all effusion fluid fresh. A combination of all three stains and preparations is optimal for viewing effusion samples.[16] Cytologically, the air-dried, DQ–stained samples tend to be the most informative as the cytoplasmic features are expanded and better delineated than on Pap-stained preparations. The Pap stain, with ethanol fixation, highlights the nuclear features. The cell block produces tissue fragments that simulate histologic examination and affords the pathologist a myriad of special tests easily initiated at the time of evaluation. In addition, the cell block allows long-term storage of the specimen and the potential to perform tests at a later date (see the section in this chapter on Ancillary Techniques).

The ability to use the DQ stain is dependent on the fresh status of the sample. Samples can be made into cytospins (DQ or Pap), cell blocks (H&E), smears (DQ or Pap), or filter preparations, including monolayer preparations (Pap). Grossly bloody samples should be lysed and concentrated as needed.[16] These simple procedures enhance the numbers of cells of interest and facilitate ease of viewing by eliminating excess blood.[16] In highly inflammatory samples, subjecting the specimen to a Ficoll Hypaque gradient decreases the acute inflammatory cells while preserving the lymphoid population and possible malignant mesothelial/epithelial cells.[16]

BOX 12-1

Most Common Causes of Pericardial Effusions

Malignant	Benign
Breast carcinoma	Sarcoidosis
Lung carcinoma	Tuberculosis
Lymphoma	Viral
	Cystic hygroma
	Trauma
	Thrombosis of chest vessels

BOX 12-2

Most Common Causes of Ascites

Malignant	Benign
Mesothelioma	Portal hypertension
Gatrointestinal carcinoma	Cirrhosis
Ovarian carcinoma	Congestive heart failure
Breast carcinoma	Veno-occlusive disease
Lung carcinoma	Peritoneal tuberculosis
Lymphoma	Nephrotic syndrome
	Myxedema
	Meig's syndrome
	HIV-associated

From Bennett JC, Plum F, editors. Cecil's textbook of medicine. 20th ed., vol. I. Philadelphia: WB Saunders; 1996.
HIV, Human immunodeficiency virus.

TABLE 12-3

Etiologies of Effusions

	Pleural	Abdominal	Pericardial
Transudates	Obstruction of superior vena cava	Portal vein occlusion	
	Peritoneal dialysis	Diffuse hepatic metastasis	Uremia, myxedema
	Acute atelectasis		
	CHF	CHF	CHF
	Hypoproteinemia/cirrhosis	Hypoproteinemia/cirrhosis	
	Postoperative		
	Postpartum		
Exudates	Infectious diseases, viral, bacterial, parasitic, fungal	Infectious diseases, viral, bacterial, parasitic, fungal	Infectious diseases, viral, bacterial, parasitic, fungal
	Cancer	Cancer	Cancer
	Pulmonary emboli with or without infarct	Pulmonary emboli with or without infarct	Myocardial infarct
	Collagen vascular disease		Collagen vascular disease
	Gastrointestinal inflammation	Pancreatitis, peritonitis	
	Post–myocardial infarct		
	Chylous	Chylous	
	Trauma	Trauma	Trauma

From Kjeldsberg CR, Knight JA, editors. Body fluids: laboratory examination of amniotic, cerebrospinal, seminal, serous and synovial fluids. 3rd ed. Chicago: ASCP Press; 1993.; Tao L-C. Cytopathology of malignant effusions. Chicago: ASCP Press; 1996.
CHF, Congestive heart failure.

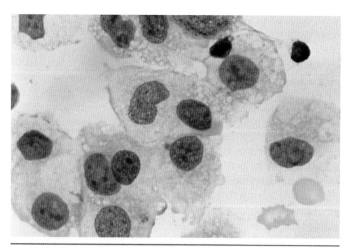

Figure 12-2 Macrophages. The cells have oval to bean-shaped nuclei, variable-appearing nucleoli, and abundant amphophilic, vacuolated cytoplasm with indistinct cell borders.

TABLE 12-4	
Relative Distribution of Causes of Pleural Effusions	
Cause	Percentage (%)
Malignancy	45
Infectious	22
Congestive heart failure	12
Indeterminate	10
Pulmonary embolism	3
Hepatic cirrhosis	2
Collagen vascular disease	1
Other	5

 NONNEOPLASTIC EFFUSIONS

Normal/Reactive Cells

Mesothelial Cells

The normal cells usually found in benign and malignant effusions are mesothelial cells, macrophages, and peripheral blood elements in traumatic taps (Figures 12-2 to 12-6). The cytopathology of these cells and a comparison with aberrant cells is summarized in Table 12-5. *For the purposes of this discussion, reactive and hyperplastic mesothelial cells are considered together.*

Mesothelial cells are best viewed by a combination of Pap and DQ stains. Nuclear morphology is better assessed on the Pap stain. Nuclei are generally central but may be peripherally located. The contours are round and smooth. Nucleoli are common and may be prominent; however, under nonneoplastic conditions macronucleoli (equal to one third the nuclear diameter in size) should usually not be seen. The chromatin pattern is usually finely stippled and nuclear chromasia is variable. Although nucleoli can also be noted on the DQ stain, it is harder to evaluate the degree of nuclear chromasia.

The DQ stain highlights the biphasic appearance of mesothelial cell cytoplasm that has commonly been referred to as the *endoplasmic-ectoplasmic* demarcation (Figure 12-7). This is visible in many mesothelial cells as an area of

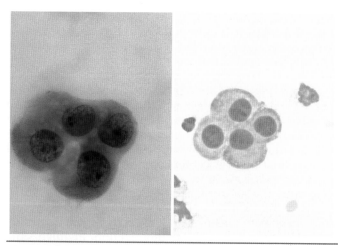

Figure 12-3 Mesothelial cells. The cells have round, central nuclei with visible nucleoli. The cytoplasm is abundant and shows a biphasic staining quality that is most visible on the DQ stain. A mesothelial window is evident in the Pap-stained portion of the figure. Because of the air drying of the DQ stained cells, the cytoplasm appears more voluminous than that of the Pap-stained material, which is actually at a higher magnification. (Diff-Quik [DQ], Papanicolaou [Pap])

perinuclear lightening/eosinophilia of the DQ stain, with a more peripheral cytoplasmic basophilia. This is the result of a greater density of intermediate filaments around the nucleus.[7] This biphasic appearance may be used to help distinguish mesothelial cells from other cells within an effusion; however, it is not specific to mesothelial cells and may be seen in nonmesothelial neoplasms, particularly malignant melanoma and adenocarcinoma of the breast.[17]

The cytoplasm of mesothelial cells does not always show biphasic staining with DQ. The cytoplasm often stains basophilic to varying degrees and is finely granular. At times, however, mesothelial cytoplasm may become pale and vacuolated, simulating the cytoplasm of accompanying macrophages. In this scenario, nuclear morphology should aid the pathologist in distinguishing these cell types from one another because mesothelial cells have round to oval nuclei with smooth contours and macrophages generally have reniform-shaped nuclei with irregular contours. When it is impossible to distinguish these cell types morphologically, immunohistochemical stains can be used if needed (see the section in this chapter on Ancillary Techniques).

The membranous surface of mesothelial cells exhibits a crowded array of long, slender microvilli. In Pap-stained material, this may be seen as a peripheral rim of pallor. On the ultrastructural level, this feature allows for the distinction of mesothelial cells from aberrant/malignant epithelial cells. Although these usually cannot be appreciated at the light microscopic level, when mesothelial cells appear in clusters, the tight intertwining of these microvilli gives rise to the phenomenon known as *mesothelial windows*. On the light microscopic level, windows correspond to the slitlike spaces present between mesothelial cells that are in apposition to each other, thus keeping the cell membranes from touching. Although characteristic of mesothelial cells, the appearance of these windows is in no way specific for mesothelial cells and can be seen in other pathologic processes at times as a result of cell-to-cell apposition with trapped secretions or because of fluid trapped between the

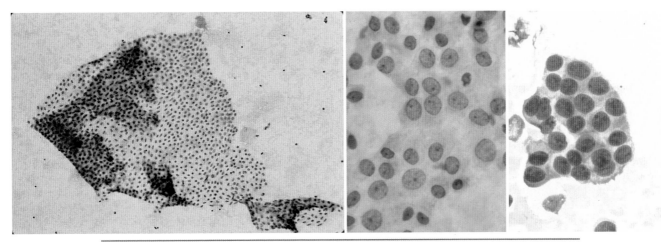

Figure 12-4 Sheets of mesothelial cells. The cells are arranged in a monolayer with a honeycombed appearance (i.e., the cells and nuclei are evenly spaced). The nuclei are round and centrally located and have visible nucleoli. Large sheets of mesothelial cells are often dislodged during washing procedures. (Pap, DQ)

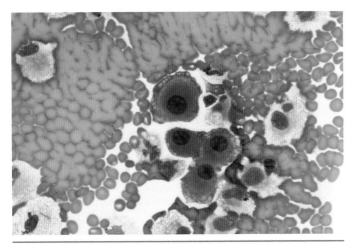

Figure 12-5 Mesothelial cells. The cells are present singly and in a small cluster. The nuclei are round, have visible nucleoli, and are central or eccentric in location. A window is present between two of the cells. The cytoplasm is abundant and finely granular and shows a "ruffled border" phenomenon peripherally, in which fluid is trapped between the microvilli. Several lighter-stained macrophages are present peripherally. (DQ)

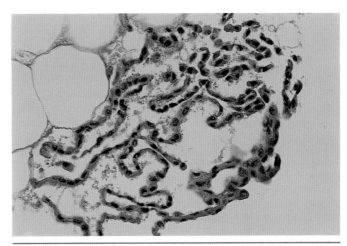

Figure 12-6 Mesothelial cells in a cell block. Mesothelial cells in a cell block can appear as chains of single cells that can mimic glandular formations. (Hematoxylin and eosin [H&E])

TABLE	**12-5**			CMF

Cytomorphologic Features of Normal/Benign and Abnormal Cells in an Effusion

Feature	Mesothelial Cells	Macrophages	Aberrant Cells
Cell shape	Round	Round	Aberrant
Nuclear shape	Round, oval	Reniform	Irregular
Nuclear location	Central	Peripheral	Variable
Chromatin	Variable	Finely granular	Irregular
Nucleolus	Distinct	Indistinct	Variable
Nuclear membrane	Regular	Regular	Irregular
Cytoplasm	Biphasic	Cyanophilic	Variable

cells (e.g., malignant melanoma, adenocarcinoma, or even plasma cell myeloma).

Mesothelial cells can show varying degrees of vacuolization (Figures 12-8 and 12-9). An interesting phenomena may take place whereby fluid gets trapped in between the microvilli, giving the cells a ruffled border appearance. This may simulate cytoplasmic vacuolization, although it is technically beyond the cell membrane. The longer the cells remain in the fluid medium, in general, the greater the degree of vacuolization. The cells actually imbibe the effusion fluid leading to the vacuolization. Although vacuoles in mesothelial cells are usually small and evenly distributed, they may occur at the periphery of the cell or centrally and appear to cover the nucleus. The more chronic the effusion, the larger the vacuoles may become, which may lead to difficulty in identifying the cells as being mesothelial in ori-

gin. Although conventional wisdom states that benign mesothelial cells with large vacuoles can be distinguished from adenocarcinoma cells with large vacuoles by the nuclear features, in actual practice this may not be possible because of obscuring of nuclear details by the vacuoles or compression of nuclei as in signet ring–type cells. Special studies may be necessary for this discrimination.

Mesothelial cells produce hyaluronic acid. This can be seen on the DQ stain as magenta-staining intracytoplasmic or extracytoplasmic material (Figure 12-10). At times, this magenta-staining material can appear within the center of small clusters of mesothelial cells, simulating an acinus with mucin secretion. This also results in positive staining with Alcian blue, without hyaluronidase digestion. Mesothelial cells may react histochemically with periodic acid Schiff (PAS) because of intracytoplasmic glycogen, and

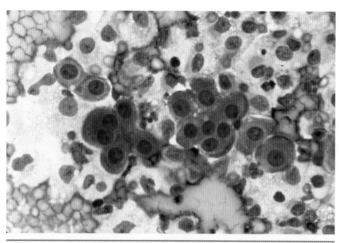

Figure 12-7 Mesothelial cells with biphasic cytoplasm. This is visible as an area of perinuclear lightening/eosinophilia of the DQ stain with a more peripheral cytoplasmic basophilia. This results from a greater density of intermediate filaments around the nucleus. The nuclei are central and the nucleoli are prominent. Small windows are present. Macrophages and scattered mesothelial cells are present in the background. (DQ)

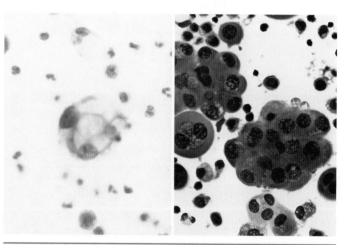

Figure 12-8 Mesothelial cells with vacuolization. These mesothelial cells show varying degrees of vacuolization from small, perinuclear vacuoles to large vacuoles that distort the nucleus and mimic adenocarcinoma cells. (DQ, Pap)

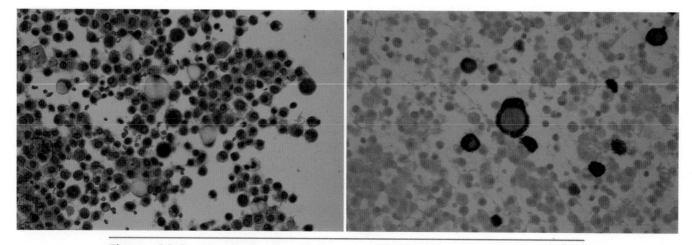

Figure 12-9 Mesothelial cells with vacuolization. This reactive effusion shows mesothelial cells with extensive vacuolization mimicking an adenocarcinoma. Calretinin staining clarifies that the cells with the balloonlike vacuolization are mesothelial in origin. (Pap, H&E, and diaminobenzidine [DAB])

weakly with mucin; however, the staining will be removed by diastase digestion.

The size spectrum of a normal mesothelial cell is from about 15 to 20 microns, which is about 1.5 to 2 times the size of a neutrophil. When reactive, they may enlarge to sizes of up to 40 to 50 microns with frequent multinucleation. Under normal circumstances, macrophages are slightly larger than mesothelial cells, measuring 20 to 25 microns.[7]

Alcohol fixation with Pap staining yields mesothelial cell viewing with less cytoplasmic volume and detail. Although intermesothelial cell windows and cytoplasmic vacuoles are still evident, cytoplasmic staining nuances noted on DQ stain are not easily visible. With the Pap stain, mesothelial cytoplasm stains light green with a variable degree of density and vacuolization as discussed above. Their nuclei are characteristically round to oval with smooth nuclear membrane contours. Even when malignant, mesothelial cells may maintain a perfectly rounded nucleus. The nuclear location is classically described as central; however, in any effusion, mesothelial cells may have both central and peripherally located nuclei. The peripheral nuclei cannot approximate the cytoplasmic membrane. The central location of the nucleus may help discriminate mesothelial cells from macrophages and malignant epithelial cells, which typically have peripherally located nuclei.

Mesothelial cells show frequent bi- and multinucleation (Figure 12-11). This phenomenon is more common in reactive effusions. The nuclei of mesothelial cells may have prominent nucleoli but only rarely approach the size of the macronucleoli that are seen in various malignancies (at least one third the diameter of the nucleus). The chromatin pattern is finely stippled, without significant chromatin clumping.

The issue of mitotic activity in benign effusions is an interesting one (see Figure 12-11). Mesothelial cells begin mitotic divisions while intact on the mesothelial surface. Although they may complete mitotic divisions after they are shed into an effusion fluid, they do not initiate new mitotic activity. Thus, brisk mitotic activity of mesothelial cells while on the serosal surface may be signaled by many mitotic figures within an effusion. The diagnostic significance

of this in terms of predicting possible mesothelial neoplasia is minimal. Abnormal-appearing mitotic figures should not be seen.

Washings, lavages, and scrapes, which are samples obtained for the investigation of microscopic disease on the peritoneal surfaces as part of staging procedures predominantly for neoplasms of gynecologic origin (e.g., ovarian carcinomas), usually also yield benign mesothelial cells. The mesothelial cells in these types of samples have a different appearance than those in effusions, however, because they are traumatically removed from their in situ location rather than having shed into a free-floating location in fluid. The cells are present in monolayered flat sheets that almost resemble squamous metaplastic cells. The cells have well-defined cytoplasmic outlines with obvious slits in between each cell. Rather than round outlines, the cells have a more triangular/rhomboidal/trapezoidal shape with central bland nuclei. At times the sheets of cells may roll over

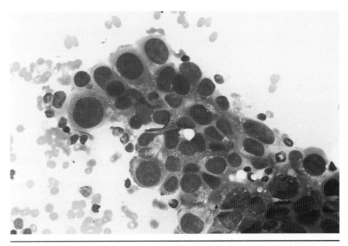

Figure 12-10 Mesothelioma, fine-needle aspiration (FNA). A thin layer of magenta-staining material consistent with hyaluronic acid surrounds these atypical mesothelial cells. At times, this can mimic the appearance of extra- or intracellular mucin, particularly when it is centrally placed in a group of mesothelial cells that simulate a gland. (DQ)

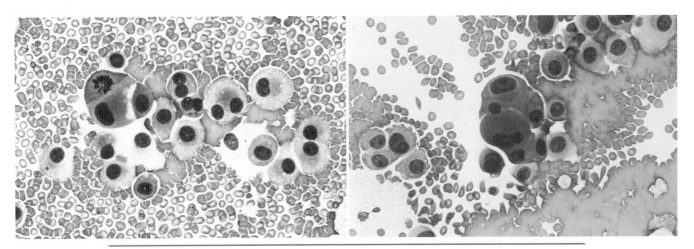

Figure 12-11 **Reactive mesothelial cells.** Although nuclear enlargement is evident, the N:C ratio remains low. Nucleoli are large and prominent. A rare mitotic figure may be seen, and multinucleation is present. (DQ)

TABLE 12-6

Cytolomorphologic Features of Mesothelial Cells in Effusions and Washings

Cytomorphologic Feature	Description
Uniform cell population	Single population of cells
Dense cytoplasm	Optically dense cytoplasm ± small perinuclear vacuoles
Cell-to-cell apposition	Mesothelial windows
Centrally placed nuclei	Nucleus in central or paracentral location
Multinucleation with atypia	Greater than two nuclei
Microvillus edge	Eosinophilic halo noted around the circumference (or part of the circumference) of mesothelial cytoplasm*
Cell-in-cell engulfment	Cells that appear to be engulfed or surrounded by the cytoplasm of adjacent cells
Macronucleoli	Nucleolus that is at least one third the diameter of the nucleus
Blebbing	Prominent cytoplasmic outpouchings
Nuclear pleomorphism	Significant variability in nuclear size and morphology
Irregular nuclear membrane	Nuclei with irregular, rounded borders
Proliferative cell balls	Cellular aggregates with overlapping nuclei or nuclei so close to one another that virtually no cytoplasm is visible in between the nuclei
True papillary aggregates	Papillary structures around a fibrovascular core or a core of central amorphous material
Monolayer cell aggregates	• Two-dimensional sheets with cells arranged in an orderly fashion and having distinct cell borders with the nuclei arranged regularly • Irregular syncytial fragments that are loosely arranged with no spaces obvious between the cells
Regular chromatin distribution	Evenly distributed chromatin pattern with minimal aggregates of chromatin
Fine chromatin granularity	Chromatin granules small and of uniform size
Acinus-like structures	Aggregates of cells arranged around a central lumen
Balloon-like vacuolization	Intracytoplasmic vacuoles twice the diameter of a neutrophil
Psammoma bodies	Lamellated concentric concretions

From Stevens MW, Leong AS-Y, Fazzalari NL, et al. Cytopathology of malignant mesothelioma: a stepwise logistic regression analysis. Diagn Cytopathol 1992; 8:333-341.
*For the purposes of the above referenced study, it was defined as being at least 1 μm in width on a Giemsa-stained cytospin.

onto themselves, importing a more three-dimensional quality to the cells. It is important to look at the edges of these aggregates to elucidate the origin of these folded sheets to determine the true nature of the cells and not mistake these cells for aggregates of neoplastic cells. The bland and regular nuclear features and the normal nuclear to cytoplasmic (N:C) ratios are clues to the benign mesothelial nature of the cells. Usually, small areas of the edges of these folded sheets show the monolayered appearance that one expects of benign mesothelium.

Cul-de-sac and peritoneal washing specimens may have tissue fragments of mesothelial cells with psammoma bodies. Cells are uniform and lack malignant features.

Peritoneal washings may yield an interesting cytologic finding called *collagen balls*. These consist of fragments of tissue made up of collagen covered with mesothelial cells. Although these are only found in a small percentage of specimens (2% to 6%), it is important to be able to recognize them and not misinterpret these nonspecific benign structures as being part of a papillary or mucinous gynecologic neoplasm. These structures are actually found on the surface of the ovaries and thus are not present in washings from males[18] (see the section in this chapter on Differential Diagnosis of Pelvic Washings).

Appearance of mesothelial cells in reactive effusions.
Normal/reactive mesothelial cells can assume a highly variable appearance in both their nuclear and cytoplasmic morphology. These cells and those of malignant mesothelial proliferations cannot be distinguished based on morphol-

ogy alone and can have considerable overlap with the cells of adenocarcinoma and other neoplasms in effusions. Cells of most neoplasms, regardless of their morphology on smears and cytospins, tend to round up in effusions and assume an epithelioid appearance, although this is certainly not true of all neoplasms (e.g., squamous cell carcinoma, lymphoma). The cytologic features of mesothelial cells often noted in benign and malignant effusions are described in Table 12-6. At times a malignant mesothelioma (MM) can have a bland cytologic appearance. Conversely a reactive effusion, particularly one that results from an inflammatory or reparative process (e.g., infection, myocardial infarction, pulmonary infarction, or culdocenteses), can have mesothelial cells that are highly atypical and assume what mimics a malignant morphology.

It is of the utmost importance to view the cytology of effusions that are composed predominantly of mesothelial cells in conjunction with the clinical history. Usually, an underlying cause for a reactive/benign or malignant effusion is evident (see Table 12-3). Reactive mesothelial cells can be present as a major or minor component of a malignant effusion of nonprimary mesothelial etiology. It can be a challenge to distinguish reactive mesothelial cells from malignant nonmesothelial cells. Likewise, in cases of MM a combination of factors, including cellularity of the sample, patient history, radiologic appearance, and ancillary studies, are all contributing factors toward generating the correct diagnosis (see the section in this chapter on Malignant Mesothelioma).

TABLE 12-7 CMF

Cytomorphologic Features of Mesothelial Cells in Reactive Effusions

Cytomorphologic Feature	Reactive Effusions that Exhibit this Feature (%)
Uniform cell population	100
Dense cytoplasm	100
Cell to cell apposition, or "windows"	97
Centrally placed nucleus	97
Microvillus edge	63
Regular chromatin distribution	100
Monolayer cell aggregates	93
Fine chromatin granularity	90
True papillary aggregates	23

From Stevens MW, Leong AS-Y, Fazzalari NL, et al. Cytopathology of malignant mesothelioma: a stepwise logistic regression analysis. Diagn Cytopathol 1992; 8:333-341.

TABLE 12-8

Cytomorphologic Comparison of Reactive and Malignant Mesothelial Cells

Cytomorphologic Feature	Mesothelioma	Reactive Mesothelial Cells
Nuclear pleomorphism	+	−
Macronucleoli	+	−
Cell-in-cell	+	±
Monolayers	−	+

From Stevens MW, Leong AS-Y, Fazzalari NL, et al. Cytopathology of malignant mesothelioma: a stepwise logistic regression analysis. Diagn Cytopathol 1992; 8:333-341.

Reactive changes in mesothelial cells can be seen in pulmonary infarction, cirrhosis, radiation, chemotherapy, systemic disease, traumatic irritation, underlying neoplasms, chronic inflammation, foreign substance, and infection. This is usually evidenced cytologically by an increase in the number of mesothelial cells in the effusion with mild nuclear variability, some prominence of the nucleoli, with maintenance of the usual N:C ratios (Box 12-3). The background cellular population is variable, depending on the etiologic factors of the effusion. Common cytologic features noted in reactive mesothelial cells are listed in Table 12-7. In the distinction of benign reactive mesothelial proliferations from malignant mesothelioma, the most important of these cytologic features (by logistic regression analysis) is the formation of monolayer cell aggregates in benign effusions[19] (Table 12-8). Conversely, the cytologic findings in mesothelial cells of multinucleation with atypia, cell-in-cell engulfment, macronucleoli, and cytoplasmic blebbing—although seen much more often in malignant mesothelioma—can also be seen in benign, reactive mesothelium in a small percentage of cases.[19] Effusions of MM are bloody, inflammatory, and highly cellular with huge clusters of mesothelial cells and large tissue fragments. Unfortunately, in some sam-

BOX 12-3

General Features of a Reactive Effusion

Moderate number of mesothelial cells singly or in small clusters
Mesothelial cells with mild nuclear variability
Prominent nucleoli
Maintenance of the usual N:C ratios and windows
Variable background inflammatory component

N:C, Nuclear to cytoplasmic.

BOX 12-4 CMF

Cytomorphologic Features of Atypical Mesothelial Cells

Mesothelial cells in large groups
Cell groups have scalloped borders
Cellular molding
Nuclear hyperchromasia
High N:C ratios
Coarse chromatin clumping
Prominent nucleoli
Extensive morphologic variability

From Bedrossian CW. Diagnostic problems in serous effusions. Diagn Cytopathol 1998; 19(2):131-137.
N:C, Nuclear to cytoplasmic.
NOTE: In the absence of a history predisposing to mesothelial neoplasia, most likely the cytologic features are purely reactive in nature.

ples, this is not the case; the malignant cells may present as mostly individual cellular elements.

Although irradiation and chemotherapy are associated with well-documented atypical/reactive changes in epithelial cells, the exact secondary changes in mesothelial cells are fairly nonspecific.[8,20] Four features, although not specific for postradiotherapy changes, tend to occur more often in this type of sample: (1) degenerative changes, (2) smudgy chromatin, (3) large cytoplasmic vacuoles deforming the nucleus, and (4) cytomegaly. The cytologic feature of "bizarre cells" was found to occur significantly more regularly in irradiated samples.[20] These changes, however, are not specific. The cellular changes associated with irradiation may also be seen with chemotherapy and immunotherapy treatment such as interleukin-2 (IL-2). The mesothelial cells are large, often multinucleated, with a proportional increase in the cytoplasmic and nuclear volumes. Vacuolization is common.[7] Mitotic figures may be seen. Depending on the amount of associated inflammation, the nuclei may appear homogenous and dark or open with a prominent nucleolus. These changes are not specific and can be seen in other nonneoplastic effusions.[20]

The spectrum of changes that can be seen in reactive mesothelial cells is great; however, mesothelial cells may be considered atypical when the following morphologic features are evident: cells in large groups, cell clusters with scalloped edges, molding of the cells, nuclear hyperchromasia, high N:C ratios, coarse chromatin clumping, prominent nucleoli, and extensive morphologic variability[21] (Box 12-4).

Clinical correlation is imperative, as in the absence of a history predisposing to mesothelial neoplasia, the cytologic features are likely purely reactive in nature (Figures 12-12 to 12-16).

Macrophages

Macrophages may comprise a majority of the cellular population in an effusion and can have an extremely variable appearance (see Figures 12-2, 12-5, and 12-7). As with mesothelial cells, macrophages are best viewed with a combination of DQ and Pap for reasons as outlined above. Typically, macrophages have a rounded cell shape with variable cell borders that can be well or ill defined. They may appear singly or in loose clusters. When in clusters the cytoplasmic borders may not be well maintained, and the peripheral contours of the group can appear irregular, as apposed to the smooth or "knobby" appearance of mesothelial cell clusters or clusters of most epithelial tumor cells.

Typically, the nuclei of macrophages are kidney shaped and peripheral in location. Nucleoli are indistinct. Multinucleation may occur. The cytoplasm is highly variable and may appear from pale homogeneously cyanophilic to extensively vacuolated. Depending on the associated pathologic process, macrophages may ingest many waste products or material that has been deposited extracellularly, such as melanin in cases of malignant melanoma or hemosiderin in cases with previous bleeding. In short the cytoplasmic appearance depends largely on what the cells have ingested. This may also include cellular debris such as nuclear particles, red blood cells (RBCs), whole inflammatory cells, and organisms.

Macrophages with extensive vacuolization and peripherally placed nuclei may resemble mesothelial cells or adenocarcinoma cells when present singly or in groups. A mucin stain on the cell block is negative in macrophages and potentially positive in adenocarcinoma cells. Alterna-

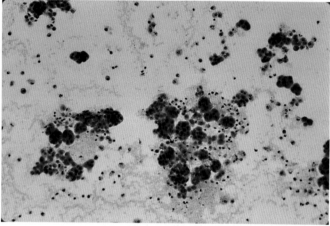

Figure 12-12   Reactive/atypical effusion. This reactive effusion is cellular with mesothelial cells primarily present as three-dimensional groups with scalloped edges. Although this case is benign, a similar appearance can be seen in mesothelioma. (Pap)

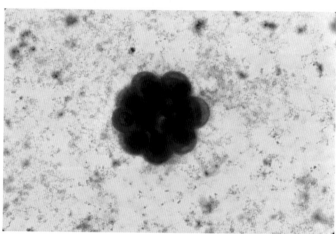

Figure 12-14   Reactive/atypical mesothelial cells. The cells are in a three-dimensional cluster with a scalloped edge. A peripheral rim of pallor is present. Nucleoli are prominent. (Pap)

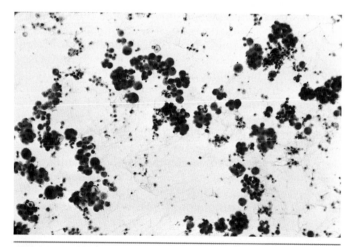

Figure 12-13   Mesothelioma. This cellular effusion appears similar to the effusion in Figure 12-12. The cells are present in three-dimensional groups with scalloped edges. Nuclear hyperchromasia is present, cell-in-cell engulfment is noted, and many cells maintain a normal nuclear-to-cytoplasmic (N:C) ratio. (Pap)

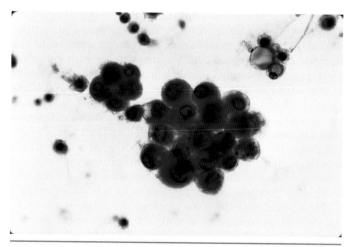

Figure 12-15   Mesothelioma. The cells are in three-dimensional clusters with a scalloped edge. A peripheral rim of pallor is present with focal vacuolization. Nucleoli are prominent and are large in some cells. Cytoplasmic windows can be seen. (Pap)

tively, immunohistochemistry for CD-68 is positive in the macrophages and negative in the mesothelial cells. Calretinin and HBME-1 are positive in mesothelial cells and negative in macrophages (see the section in this chapter on Ancillary Techniques).

Hematopoietic Cells

Depending on the nature of the effusion and whether peripheral blood contamination is present, various types of hematopoietic cells may be present within an effusion. The morphology resembles a peripheral blood smear, and cell staining is variable depending on whether they are viewed with Pap or DQ (Table 12-9). Benign lymphocytes may also be common cells noted in effusions. Lymphoid morphology is uniformly rounded in effusions. Megakaryocytes when present in an effusion are usually indicative of a myeloproliferative disorder or carcinomatous replacement of the bone marrow. Bleeding from the pulmonary microvasculature into the pleural cavity can also lead to the presence of megakaryocytes in an effusion.[8]

Detached Ciliary Tufts

The ciliated epithelial lining of the fallopian tubes may give rise to the presence of what are known as *detached ciliary tufts* (DCTs) in ascitic fluid or laparoscopic washing specimens of the peritoneum. These DCTs consist of ciliated, nonnucleated cellular fragments. Interestingly, these are fully motile on toluidine blue–stained wet preparations; however, they are extremely difficult to locate on conventionally prepared cytologic smears and are without pathologic significance.[8]

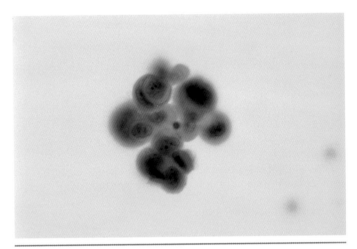

Figure 12-16 Mesothelioma. The cells are in a poorly formed three-dimensional cluster. Some of the cells have increased N:C ratios with focal irregularities of the nuclear membrane. Cell-in-cell engulfment is present. (Pap)

NONNEOPLASTIC EFFUSIONS ASSOCIATED WITH SPECIFIC ETIOLOGIC FACTORS

For a listing of the major cytomorphologic features of nonneoplastic effusions of a specific cause, see Table 12-10.

TABLE **12-9**

Possible Inflammatory Constituents of an Effusion

Cell	Source	Size	Pap	Diff-Quik
Red blood cells	Peripheral blood	6-8 μm	Rounded disc with central concavity Anucleated Eosinophilic	Eosinophilic
Neutrophils	Peripheral blood Inflammatory process	11 μm	Nucleus basophilic with two to five lobes Cytoplasm is granular and faintly cyanophilic	Nucleus basophilic with two to five lobes Cytoplasm granular and faintly eosinophilic
Eosinophils*	Peripheral blood Inflammatory process Collagen vascular disease Neoplasia Pulmonary infarct Trauma Pneumothorax Hemothorax Idiopathic	14 μm	Nucleus basophilic bi-lobed but can have up to 4 lobes Cytoplasm lightly eosinophilic to light green with granularity	Nucleus basophilic bi-lobed but can have up to four lobes Cytoplasm intensely eosinophilic and granular
Basophils†	Peripheral blood Inflammatory process Neoplasia	10 μm	Central rounded to irregularly shaped pale staining nucleus Cytoplasm granular and lightly eosinophilic to light green	Central rounded to irregularly shaped pale staining nucleus Cytoplasm has large, coarse basophilic granules Granules may overlie nucleus

From Bibbo M. Comprehensive cytopathology. 2nd ed. Philadelphia: WB Saunders; 1997. pp.551-621.
*See the section in this chapter on Eosinophilic Effusions.
†Basophils and mast cells, if present, are usually in very small numbers.

TABLE 12-10	CMF

Cytomorphologic Features of Nonneoplastic Effusions of Specific Cause

Clinical Diagnosis	Effusion Characteristics
Eosinophilic effusions	At least 10% eosinophils (see Boxes 12-5 and 12-6)
Rheumatoid disease	Multinucleated macrophages
	Multinucleated macrophages in large, spindled cell morphology
	Granular necrotic exudate
Systemic lupus erythematosus	Lupus erythematosus cells
	Hematoxylin bodies
	Tart cells
	Reactive mesothelial cells
	Background of nuclear fragments and necrotic cells
Bacterial pneumonia	Acute inflammation initially
	Chronic inflammation as pneumonia resolves
	Reactive mesothelial cells
Viral pneumonia	Chronic inflammation
	Reactive mesothelial cells
	Highly atypical mesothelial cells if virally infected
	Acute inflammation with secondary bacterial infection possible
Cirrhosis	Low cellularity composed of mesothelial cells with macrophages and some lymphocytes
	Reactive mesothelial cells
	Possible acute inflammation with secondary bacterial infection
Pneumothorax	Numerous eosinophils
	Reactive, large mesothelial cells
	Variable appearance
Infarction	Variable cellularity
	Acute or chronic inflammation
	Eosinophils may be numerous
	Reactive mesothelial cells
	Possible involvement of adjacent body cavity
Congestive heart failure	Variable cellularity
	Possible mixed inflammation
	Mesothelial cells and macrophages
	Possible progression to inflammatory or reactive effusion depending on duration and secondary infection

From Bibbo M. Comprehensive cytopathology. 2nd ed. Philadelphia: WB Saunders; 1997. pp.551-621.

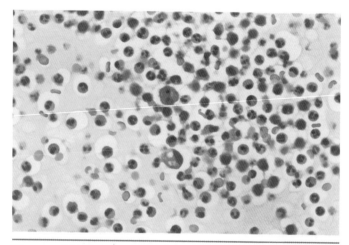

Figure 12-17 Eosinophilic effusion. Numerous eosinophils are seen scattered throughout the specimen, which also contains neutrophils, lymphocytes, reactive mesothelial cells, and red blood cells (RBCs). (DQ)

Eosinophilic Effusions

An effusion is considered to be an eosinophilic effusion (EE) if it is composed of at least 10% eosinophils[22] (Box 12-5 and Figure 12-17). Many EEs are associated with the etiologic factors shown in Box 12-6; a significant proportion are idiopathic.[23,24] These effusions usually occur in males, and most spontaneously resolve; however, it is possible to have a protracted clinical course depending on the cause.

EEs rarely have been reported to occur in the abdomen and peritoneum. In the abdomen they have been reported to occur with chronic dialysis. These effusions have also been associated with considerable atypical reactive mesothelial changes.[25]

It is theorized that the eosinophilia is the result of chemotaxis associated with particulate matter in air or RBCs. For infectious or hypersensitivity states, the chemotactic factors are most likely unique. In *Paragonimiasis westermani*, the eosinophilia associated with pleural effusions and the peripheral blood has been shown to be associated with IL-5.[26]

BOX 12-5

Summary of Eosinophilic Effusions

Composition of 10% or more eosinophils
Male preponderance
Most commonly pleural
Most spontaneously resolve
Possible protracted clinical course
Strong association with trauma (iatrogenic or spontaneous)
Presence of eosinophils resulting from chemotaxis from air and/or blood in pleural cavity
Pulmonary infarct, pneumonia, or neoplasm
Less common occurrence in hypersensitivity states, parasitic infections, or asbestos inhalation
Extremely rare, but may occur in abdomen or pericardium

From Bibbo M. Comprehensive cytopathology. 2nd ed. Philadelphia: WB Saunders; 1997.

BOX 12-6

Etiologies of Eosinophilic Effusions

Pleural
Pneumothorax
Parasites
Trauma
Autoimmune disease
Infectious pneumonitis
Eosinophilic pneumonia
Tuberculosis
Fungus
Hemothorax
Pulmonary infarction
Allergic
Neoplasia

Pericardial
Hypersensitivity reaction
Neoplasia
Pulmonary eosinophilia
Lymphoma

Peritoneal
Allergic
Parasites
Peritoneal dialysis
Eosinophilic gastroenteritis

From Bedrossian CVM. Malignant effusions: a multimodal approach to cytologic disease. New York: Igaku-Shoin; 1994.

General Inflammatory Effusions

Most benign and malignant effusions have an inflammatory component. Although it is generally the job of cytopathologists to render diagnoses that are as specific as possible, in most benign inflammatory effusions, the most specific diagnosis that can usually be rendered is *negative for malignant cells, inflammatory/reactive effusion*. Although this is clearly useful information for the clinician, in most benign effusions it is ultimately up to the clinician to piece the puzzle together of the clinical, imaging, and laboratory (microbiology and chemistry) findings, along with the cytology to establish the most likely cause for the effusion. Several primary inflammatory effusions do have characteristic features that are suggestive of specific diagnoses (e.g., rheumatic effusion, effusion associated with systemic lupus erythematosus).

The presence of inflammatory cells within an effusion does not necessarily reflect a primary inflammatory process of the mesothelial surfaces. In fact, the inflammation in most instances represents a serosal response to an underlying lesion. The presence and amount of mesothelial cells may vary greatly from virtually absent to numerous and atypical, simulating neoplasia.

Inflammatory changes of the mesothelial-lined surfaces are usually associated with the formation of a fibrinous exudate. This can be noted cytologically by the identification of fibrin strands or aggregates of fibrinous material. These fibrin strands are often stringy and trap cells. They may simulate fungal organisms to the untrained eye. On Pap stain, they are long cyanophilic strands or aggregates; in DQ–stained material, they are basophilic; on cell blocks, they are eosinophilic aggregates, which morphologically may simulate the frothy exudate seen with *Pneumocystis carinii* organisms.

The inflammatory population can either be at the extremes of acute, purulent inflammation or chronic lymphoid and is usually in between the two extremes with a mixed population of inflammatory cells. Effusions with a marked purulent population should be cultured to identify any potential infectious pathogens. Alternatively, predominantly lymphoid effusions should be evaluated for lymphoid markers when the etiologic factors are not obvious to rule out involvement with a hematologic neoplasm. Review of the peripheral blood smear may also be useful.

The presence and percentages of natural killer (NK) cells in effusions has been investigated as a potential aid to discriminate between benign and malignant effusions. Benign effusions have an average percentage of 5% NK cells. Alternatively, in adenocarcinomas the percentage of NK cells rises to 22%. Mesotheliomas tend to have an average of 3%.[27]

Although effusions with a nonspecific inflammatory component can occur in any of the serous cavities, the following general pattern emerges for several specific diagnoses: effusions associated with systemic lupus erythematosus may involve all three serous cavities (e.g., pleural, pericardial, and peritoneal), whereas effusions associated with rheumatoid arthritis usually involve only the pleural and pericardial cavities.[8]

Tuberculous Effusions

Tuberculous effusions (TE) usually contain more than 50% lymphocytes with an accompanying paucity of reactive mesothelial cells (Figure 12-18). However, in individuals with human immunodeficiency virus (HIV), it has been reported that mesothelial cells are numerous in tuberculous effusions.[28] The presence of reactive mesothelial cells in TE may, in fact, be a distinguishing feature between TE in patients with or without HIV.[29]

In addition to cytologic examination, a microbiologic workup is indicated for the diagnosis of TE. Unfortunately, if the acid-fast bacilli are not identified on the initial smear, it can take weeks for them to grow in culture. Recently, molecular techniques have been used in the hopes of making a more specific diagnosis in a smaller amount of time. A recent study evaluating the diagnostic efficacy of real-time and nested polymerase chain reaction (PCR) for the identification of acid-fast bacilli (AFB) has shown that PCR assay is more sensitive than AFB staining and mycobacteria culture for the diagnosis of TE; however, the specificity was lower than expected.[30]

A recent study evaluating subpopulations of lymphocytes in TE has shown the phenomenon known as *compartmentalization,* whereby specific subpopulations of lymphocytes are seen in the effusion reacting to the tuberculous infection. These subpopulations are different than those noted in the peripheral blood. A greater number of activated T lymphocytes are in the effusion fluid. The effusion fluid also shows a predominance of helper cells (CD4+), with a greater CD4+:CD8+ ratio in pleural fluid than in the peripheral blood.[31]

TE and malignant effusions are two main causes of exudative effusions, depending on the population studied. In a comparison of patients with TE and malignant effusions, the following determinations were made: the average age of patients with malignant effusions was greater than that of patients with TE (68 years of age vs. 34); both causes yielded effusions with right-sided dominance; large effusions were more common with malignant causes (44% vs. 12%); and lymphocyte-predominant effusions were more common with tuberculous causes.[32]

Effusions Associated with Rheumatoid Arthritis

Effusions associated with rheumatoid arthritis have pathognomonic cytologic features that allow the cytopathologist to make a specific diagnosis with such accuracy that the diagnosis of rheumatic disease in an effusion, at times, may even antedate the onset of the arthritis[33,34] (Figure 12-19). The granulomatous serositis associated with rheumatoid arthritis is reflected in the effusion cytology by several characteristic features: spindle-shaped multinucleated giant cells (macrophages); round multinucleated giant cells (macrophages); and necrotic granular background material. Not all three components are present in all effusions.[35]

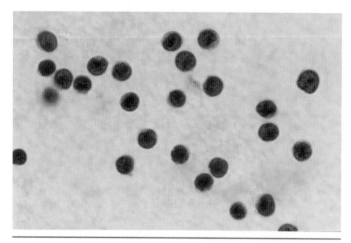

Figure 12-18   Tuberculous effusion. Numerous lymphocytes with a relative paucity of reactive mesothelial cells are characteristic of tuberculous effusions. (Pap)

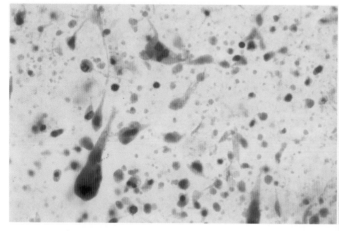
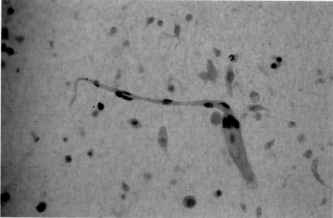
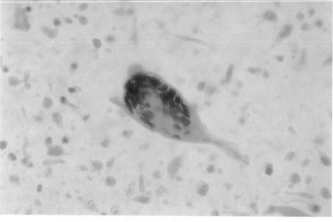

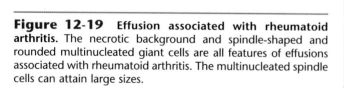

Figure 12-19   Effusion associated with rheumatoid arthritis. The necrotic background and spindle-shaped and rounded multinucleated giant cells are all features of effusions associated with rheumatoid arthritis. The multinucleated spindle cells can attain large sizes.

The multinucleated spindle-shaped cells can attain large sizes (up to 150 μm in length), which makes their appearance fairly distinctive, aside from the fact that spindled cells are rarely present in effusions. They are believed to be derived from the palisading histiocytes. Intermediate forms between the rounded and spindled multinucleated macrophages can often be seen. Nuclei can be numerous, attaining more than 20. On Pap stains, these cells appear to have densely staining eosinophilic or cyanophilic cytoplasm and basophilic oval nuclei, which may overlap and tend toward the center of the cells. In the spindled forms the nuclei are spindled as they conform to the shape of the cell.

The necrotic granular exudate is formed by necrotic cells derived from the necrobiotic core of the rheumatoid nodulelike granulomas and may contain numerous visible necrotic cells that can impart the appearance of a purulent effusion. Although it may appear amorphous and "fluffy" on Pap-stained smears, in cell blocks the necrotic material appears as large coalescing aggregates that appear densely eosinophilic.[33,35]

Cells referred to as *ragocytes* or RA cells may be seen in rheumatoid effusions. These cells, which are seen on wet preparations of rheumatoid joints and effusions are neutrophils or monocytes that contain small, spherical cytoplasmic inclusions that give the staining reaction of neutral fat. These are not specific for rheumatic disease.[8] Cholesterol crystals, another nonspecific finding, may also be seen. Mesothelial cells are conspicuously absent, present in only a small minority of reported cases.[8]

Effusions Associated with Systemic Lupus Erythematosus

The systemic lupus erythematosus (SLE) cell is a neutrophil or macrophage that has phagocytosed an injured, degenerated cell. Effusions associated with SLE can occur in the pleural, pericardial, and peritoneal cavities.[36] Large series of patients with SLE have reported that 29% of the patients, at some stage of the disease, develop a pleural effusion; 11% develop ascites; and 33% develop pericarditis, which may or may not be accompanied by an effusion.[37,38]

The cellular phenomenon most characteristic of the effusion cytology of SLE, the LE cell, was initially described more than 50 years ago in the bone marrow and subsequently the peripheral blood before it was noted in effusion samples.[39] *The LE cell is a neutrophil or less often a macrophage that has phagocytosed an injured cell, the cell supposedly damaged by the circulating antinuclear antibodies associated with SLE* (Figure 12-20). The nucleus does not appear homogeneously staining blue but maintains some of its original structure. A small rim of cytoplasm is present. These stain dark blue on Pap stain and pale red with the DQ stain. Originally thought to be an *in vitro* event, LE cells have been shown to form *in vivo*. Interestingly, the number of LE cells in an effusion from an SLE patient is said to increase as the effusion stands at room temperature.[23,40] LE cells have been reported in non-SLE patients who have developed a drug-induced SLE-like syndrome with effusions.[41] Although conventional wisdom considers LE cells to be diagnostic of SLE, rarely patients without SLE have LE cells in effusion or joint fluids.[42-44]

Although easy to miss, it is important to look for LE cells in effusions of unknown origin, particularly in young female patients, because LE cells can be a major clue to the correct cause and can precede the clinical diagnosis of SLE.[45] SLE can, however, occur in either gender and at any age.

The presence of LE cells in an effusion is usually accompanied by neutrophils and tart cells. A tart cell is a macrophage that has phagocytosed a stripped nucleus of a dead cell.

In a study of effusions on 33 patients with SLE, 27% of effusions actually showed LE cells, and in none of these patients did the effusion pre-date the diagnosis of SLE. This study was based on 34 years of cytology practice at the University of Michigan; thus, it appears as though the clinical diagnosis of SLE precedes the effusion.[36]

Unlike the typical picture of rheumatic effusions, mesothelial cells may be present in SLE effusions. The mesothelial cells can show reactive changes. Neutrophils in the effusion, although consistent with SLE, should raise the possibility of a secondary bacterial infection.[40]

Effusions Associated with Pneumonia

Pneumonia of various causes may be associated with a pleural effusion if the pulmonary inflammatory process ex-

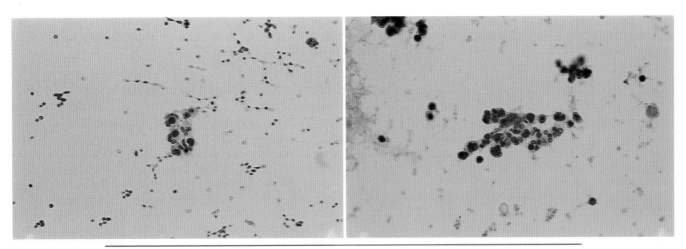

Figure 12-20 Systemic lupus erythematosus (SLE). Effusion showing a background of neutrophils and LE cells. (Pap)

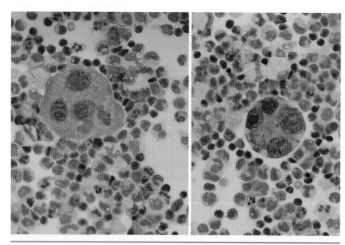

Figure 12-21 Reactive/atypical mesothelial cells in an effusion associated with a pneumonitis. These atypical, multinucleated cells show bizarre nuclear features including macronucleoli. (DQ)

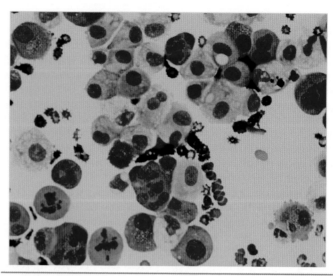

Figure 12-23 Atypical mesothelial cell in a background of chronic inflammation in a patient with Kaposi's sarcoma. (Pap)

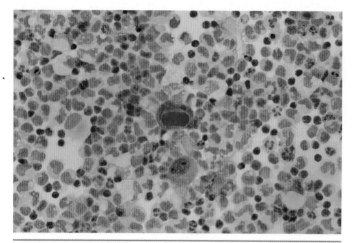

Figure 12-22 Cytomegalovirus (CMV) in effusion. Additional cytospins from the same cases as Figure 12-21, reveal cells with the characteristic features of CMV. (DQ)

tends to the pleura. As the nature and inflammatory population of the primary pneumonia are highly variable, so are the associated inflammatory effusions. Most inflammatory effusions include macrophages and mesothelial cells. The mesothelial cells can potentially become quite numerous and manifest striking reactive atypia (Figure 12-21).

Primary bacterial pneumonias may initially have associated purulent effusions composed predominantly of neutrophils; however, as the inflammatory infiltrate in the pneumonia progresses to lymphoid, so will the inflammatory population in the effusion. If, however, a secondary bacterial infection of the pleura is evident, an acute inflammatory reaction resumes.

Viral pneumonias are typically associated with a chronic inflammatory reaction in associated effusions. If, however, a secondary bacterial infection is in the pleural cavity, the effusion will become purulent.

The reactive changes in the mesothelial cells associated with viral effusions can produce cytologic features suggestive of neoplasia, particularly in cytomegalovirus (CMV)

pneumonia. Although the authors' experience with this phenomenon is limited to a handful of cases, they have been able to document through immunohistochemistry that some of the atypical mesothelial cells in CMV-associated viral pneumonias were actually infected with CMV (Figure 12-22). The nuclei, although large and atypical, did not show the characteristic nuclear features associated with CMV; however, a positive-staining reaction was elicited with antibodies to CMV. The authors have noted an interesting similar phenomena in patients with Kaposi's sarcoma and the associated human herpesvirus-8 (HHV-8) infection. Effusions have developed in these patients that are not the highly lethal HHV-8–associated primary body cavity lymphoma. Rather, these are effusions with mixed inflammation; a spectrum of lymphocytes, including plasma cells; and highly atypical mesothelial cells similar to those seen in viral infection. PCR conducted on these samples in the laboratory has shown the cases to be positive for HHV-8 DNA, despite the absence of Kaposi's and primary body cavity lymphoma in the samples. Flow cytometry has been polyclonal on all samples tested. PCR conducted on microdissected mesothelial cells has shown the cells to contain HHV-8 DNA. Thus, the mesothelial atypia may result from direct viral infection of the mesothelial cells with the HHV-8 (Figure 12-23).[202]

Effusions Associated with Infarct

The loss of blood supply to a segment of the pulmonary parenchyma resulting from a pulmonary embolism or other intravascular microembolic diseases (e.g., sickle cell anemia) has a characteristic pathologic sequela. This consists of a peripherally placed wedge-shaped area of infarction of the lung. The wedge-shaped lung tissue undergoes hemorrhagic necrosis with the base of the wedge formed by the pleural surface. The ensuing inflammatory reaction of the pleural tissue gives rise to an exudative pleural effusion, which actually may extend to the abdominal cavity and yield ascites with a similar cytologic picture. Likewise, infarction of abdominal organs yielding peritoneal inflammation may also result in ascites.

The cytologic picture of an effusion associated with a pulmonary infarct is variable; however, the effusions are usually cellular with a component of inflammation and a mixture of mesothelial cells and macrophages, some of which may be hemosiderin-laden. The inflammatory cells may be acute or chronic, but often a significant number of eosinophils is present.[8] Presumably, the inflammatory components vary with the age and degree of resolution of the infarct.

Mesothelial cells may be highly reactive appearing and numerous. It is important not to confuse these reactive mesothelial cells with neoplastic cells. This distinction is particularly important with an infarct at the lung base which may yield an abdominal effusion in which the reactive mesothelial cells could easily be mistaken for adenocarcinoma cells (see the section in this chapter on Nonneoplastic Effusions).

Effusions Associated with Surgery

The association of surgery and subsequent effusions is well known. A study performed 25 years ago evaluated postoperative pleural effusions through the performance of decubitus chest x-rays and measurements of visible pleural fluid between 48 and 72 hours after surgery. Of the patients, 97% had effusions; however, of these, only about 20% measured greater than 10 mm. The incidence of pleural effusions was higher in patients after upper abdominal surgery, patients with postoperative atelectasis (on the side where the surgery was performed), and patients with fluid in the abdominal cavity. In 16 of the 20 patients in whom thoracentesis was performed, the effusions were exudative. All of the effusions resolved spontaneously except one that was culture positive for *Staphylococcus aureus*. The conclusion of the study was that small pleural effusions were common after abdominal surgery and that most resolve spontaneously within a few days.[46]

A recent study evaluated the postsurgical effusions in patients who had undergone cardiac artery bypass graft (CABG) procedures. Effusions that occurred shortly after the surgery (<30 days) were characteristically bloody with a high eosinophil count. Later effusions (>30 days) were yellow exudates composed of primarily lymphocytes and monocytes. It is quite likely that these effusions result from different causes.[47] An unfortunate number of these patients have pleural effusions that do not resolve spontaneously.[48] The effusions and pleural tissue originally characterized by large numbers of lymphocytes eventually develop pleural fibrosis that leads to dyspnea and, in a certain percentage, trapped lungs that required surgical intervention.[48]

Ipsilateral pleural effusion occurs in all lung transplant recipients.[49] The effusions are exudates with abundant blood and marked acute inflammation. These effusions spontaneously resolve and may be related to the postoperative/posttransplant pulmonary edema.[49]

Effusions Associated with Cirrhosis

The abdominal and pleural effusions resulting from the hypoalbuminemia and decreased intravascular osmotic pressure of cirrhosis are usually sterile and low in cellularity with a predominance of mesothelial cells. At times, particularly in longstanding effusions, the mesothelial cells may be numerous and exhibit reactive changes. It is important not to misinterpret these cells as malignant epithelial cells

(see the section in this chapter on Nonneoplastic Effusions). Lymphocytes and macrophages may be present. In the absence of peripheral blood contamination, the numbers of neutrophils is usually small. *Because patients with longstanding cirrhosis are prone to spontaneous bacterial peritonitis, the presence of numerous neutrophils should alert the cytopathologist to the advent of this possible occurrence.*

Patients with cirrhosis and a pleural effusion are candidates for spontaneous bacterial empyema. Although the source of the microorganism may not be apparent, it may be through hematogenous seeding or possibly the transfer of infected ascites from the abdominal cavity. The patients may be asymptomatic or present with fever, chills, and dyspnea.[50]

Effusions Associated with Congestive Heart Failure

The fluid overload associated with CHF can lead to effusions of the thorax, pericardium, and/or abdomen, depending on the severity of the disease. Because the clinical etiologic factors of these effusions are usually obvious and the effusions are predominantly transudates rather than exudates, many of these samples may not be submitted for cytologic examination. When submitted, the main function of the cytopathologist is to rule out the presence of any previously undiscovered or known malignant disease.

The cytologic picture of these effusions is variable. Commencing with a sterile effusion of low cellularity (mixed inflammation, mesothelial cells, macrophages), after time they may evolve into inflammatory exudative effusions in the unlikely event of a secondary infection. In general, the cellularity of the effusion is proportional to the duration; longer standing effusions yield cellularity suggestive of a reactive effusion (see the section in this chapter on Nonneoplastic Effusions).

Effusions Associated with Fungal/Parasitic Infections

Disseminated fungal infections that yield effusions are, with rare exception, associated with an immunocompromised host.[7] Fungi that have been identified in effusions include *Aspergillus, Blastomyces dermatitidis, Candida, Coccidioides immitis, Cryptococcus neoformans, Histoplasmosis capsulatum, Paracoccidioides braziliensis, Mucormycosis,* and *P. carinii.* The authors have found attempts to cytologically identify fungal organisms in effusions through cytology essentially futile, despite clinical history suggestive of fungal causes for an effusion. This has been true even with the presence of a significant inflammatory background, the preparation of a cell block and stains for infectious organisms (e.g., Grocott methenamine silver). Although cytology has proven to be the superior modality for the identification of fungal organisms over microbiology in a distinct subset of patients, with respiratory disease[51,52] with regard to effusion cytology, the authors have generally relied heavily on microbiology for organism culture and identification.

Effusions associated with fungal infections show a mixed inflammatory population that may be predominantly acute or chronic, depending on the evolution and treatment of the infection, and are usually associated with a prominent number of eosinophils. Invariably, mixed numbers of reactive mesothelial cells are present. The mesothelial cells may show extensive reactive atypia such that the distinction from neoplasia may be difficult. This is true particularly in patients known to have epithelial malignancies and who are secondarily immunocompromised from chemotherapy. In these cases, the clinical history, microbiologic studies, and perhaps immunocytochemistry for calretinin (positive in mesothelial cells) elucidate the reactive nature of the cells.

Parasitic causation of an effusion is a rare event in the western world. Although the primary cause of the effusion may be initially parasitic, effusions most commonly result from secondary involvement of the pleural, abdominal, or pericardial cavities from direct extension, fistula formation, or lymphatic or hematogenous dissemination. Travel and immigration history plays a pivotal role in the cytologic and microbiologic investigation necessary for the proper organism identification (Table 12-11).

Effusions Associated with Viral Infections

The association between viral pneumonitis and secondary lymphocytic effusions is well known. Primary viral infections of the pleura or secondary extension of a pulmonary infection to the mesothelial surface leading to pleuritis is also a mechanism for the production of effusions, which are largely pleural in this case. Most of these patients are immunocompromised either primarily or secondarily from immunosuppressive agents.

Thus, direct viral infection of the mesothelial surface does occur and may present with an effusion. Interestingly, documentation of viral inclusions in mesothelial cells is inherently elusive, despite the fact that this phenomenon has been documented in the medical literature.[53] Infection with herpes virus, varicella zoster, and CMV have all been substantiated.[7] In these cases, immunohistochemistry on pre-pared cell block material for antibodies to possible etiologic viral agents may yield a definitive diagnosis or support a positive viral culture reported by the virology laboratory.

Effusions resulting from viral infections of the pleural surface (primary or from pulmonary extension) are challenging cytologic specimens (see Figures 12-21 to 12-23). The background inflammation may be variable in all respects (acute vs. chronic, marked vs. minimal, and so on) and is not where the diagnostic problem lies. The mesothelial cells may become large and show extensive nuclear enlargement, multinucleation, and pronounced atypia approaching that of a neoplasia. Nucleoli may also be large, simulating viral inclusions yet not diagnostic of viral inclusions. Some cells may actually show an increase in the N:C ratio, yet viral inclusions may not and usually are not found. This pattern has been seen in documented viral infections resulting from respiratory syncytial virus, CMV, herpes virus, and more currently, HHV-8 infection.[202] It is interesting that a similar pattern has been noted despite the different viral etiologic agents.

Effusions Associated with Pneumothorax

The presence of a pneumothorax, collapsed pulmonary tissue with accompanying air in the pleural cavity, often elicits an effusion. The effusion may be variable in appearance but is often associated with a large number of eosinophils and reactive, large mesothelial cells.[8]

Table 12-12 outlines briefly other pathologic entities or microscopic findings that may be associated with effusions.

TABLE 12-11

Effusions Associated with Parasitic Etiologic Factors

Organism	Geographic Distribution, Noteworthy Features
Echinococcus granulosus	East Africa, Mediterranean, Middle East
Paragonimus westermani	South Asia, Latin America, Africa
Strongyloides stercoralis	Tropical climates, southern United States
Trichomoniasis	Ubiquitous
Giardia lamblia	• Warm climates • Poor sanitation
Balantidium coli	Worldwide, tropical and subtropical regions
Schistosoma	Japan, Middle East, South America
Entamoeba histolytica	Worldwide
Wucheria bancrofti	India, Pacific islands, Asia
Leishmania donovani	South America, Africa, Mediterranean, Asia

From Bedrossian CWM. Malignant effusions: a multimodal approach to cytologic diagnosis. New York: Igaku-Shoin; 1994; Bibbo M. Comprehensive cytopathology. 2nd ed. Philadelphia: WB Saunders; 1997.

TABLE 12-12

Less Common Pathologic Entities Associated with Effusions

Entity	Associated Features
Fistula (lung, gastro-intestinal tract)	• Peculiar cytologic picture • Vegetable matter • Infectious organisms • Cells of origin of site of fistula

Endometriosis	• Rare in effusions; more commonly seen in abdominal washings; peritoneal fluid; culdocentesis
	• Cellular appearance variable:
	  • Small columnar cells with small, round cells
	  • Cells may be cohesive
	  • Hemosiderin-laden macrophages
	• Differential diagnosis: lymphoid, mesothelial cells
	• Diagnosis usually made retrospectively

Asbestos bodies	• Significant asbestos load • True effusion or aspiration of pulmonary tissue during tap
Curschmann's spirals Charcot-Leyden crystals	No pathologic significance

From Bibbo M. Comprehensive cytopathology. 2nd ed. Philadelphia: WB Saunders; 1997.

Pericardial Effusions

Although pericardial effusions are similar in most respects to effusions in general, a few issues need to be dealt with separately. Although mesothelioma may occur *de novo* in the pericardium, the vast majority of malignancies involving the pericardium are through direct extension (primaries of lung and thymus) or from retrograde lymphangitic spread.[54] Pericardial effusions are rare in comparison with pleural effusion and ascites samples. Usually the result of viral infections, tuberculosis, collagen vascular diseases, and various neoplasms, they can be a challenge for the cytopathologist because of reactive mesothelial cell changes that simulate malignancy. These effusions should rarely be called malignant without the prior history of neoplasia with complementary morphology to the atypical cells in the effusions, and should, if possible, be evaluated with confirmatory immunohistochemistry.[55]

A large scale study evaluating survival of patients with pericardial effusions and malignant disease concluded that subxiphoid pericardiotomy was a safe, effective treatment, relieving pericardial effusion in 99% of patients.[56] Survival was most closely related to extent of malignant disease and the chemo- or radiosensitivity of the neoplasm. Of the patients who survived longer than 1 year, 72% had breast cancer, leukemia, or lymphoma. In this group of patients, not all of whom had malignant effusions (etiologies also included radiation induced, infectious, hemorrhagic, no known etiology), pericardial fluid cytology had a sensitivity of 90%, whereas pericardial biopsy had a sensitivity of 56%.[56] This relative high degree of cytologic diagnostic sensitivity vs. biopsy sensitivity has been confirmed by other investigators.[57]

Pericardial effusions in individuals with acquired immune deficiency syndrome (AIDS), although the effusions may be associated with malignancies such as lymphoma and infections such as histoplasmosis, have also been found to exhibit a marked degree of mesothelial atypia with papillary formations simulating malignancy. The mesothelial atypia, however, is benign and should not be confused with adenocarcinoma.[58]

MALIGNANT EFFUSIONS

Cytologic evaluation of pleural fluid has a higher sensitivity ($P < 0.001$) than needle biopsy for the diagnosis of malignant effusions.[59,60] In patients who are ultimately diagnosed with a malignant effusion, the cytologic detection of cancer cells in an effusion can generally be made with the submission of a maximum of two samples. The examination of more than three samples is of little value.[15] Aside from malignant mesothelioma, which is a primary malignancy of the mesothelium commonly presenting with effusions, the presence of a malignancy in an effusion heralds an advanced stage of neoplasia. Although malignant effusions are often inflammatory and contain blood, this is not always the case, particularly with hematologic malignancies.

Generally speaking, the cytology of malignant effusions can be divided into the following three groups:

- *Group 1:* An obvious population of abnormal cells discreet from mesothelial cells, macrophages and inflammatory cells is seen. In this group it is easy to distinguish these cells as outsiders from the usual constituents of an effusion. The cells have abnormal cytology, whereas the background cells maintain the usual or reactive morphology. The cells may be present singly and/or in aggregates. This is a common pattern of epithelial, mesodermal, and melanomatous effusions (Figure 12-24).

- *Group 2:* A population of abnormal cells is present that is difficult to distinguish from mesothelial cells. A spectrum of atypia is present so that all of the cells appear to come from the same origin. The cells may be single or in aggregates. This pattern is commonly found in mesotheliomas, adenocarcinomas, and occasionally in nonepithelial neoplasms such as malignant melanoma (Figure 12-25).

- *Group 3:* The background population of inflammatory cells is abnormal with usual mesothelial cells and macrophages present in variable numbers. This heralds the presence of a hematopoietic malignancy, which can be missed if the cells are not evaluated carefully, particularly in mixed malignant/inflammatory samples (Figure 12-26).

Although this approach is a rather simplistic way to view initially any potentially malignant effusion, it may help categorize a sample. The main challenge is that a tremendous degree of cytologic overlap is present, not only between benign/reactive processes but also between malignancies of diverse origins. This is usually not a problem in patients with a previous history of a well-documented neoplasm in which the effusion heralds the progression of disease. However, the cytologic characterization of an effusion can be of the utmost importance in the unfortunate patient in which an effusion is the presenting symptom of a heretofore unknown underlying malignancy.

Categorizing the malignant cells in an effusion can be as simple as comparing the cells of interest to a previous specimen on the same patient and deeming the sample "morphologically compatible with a metastasis from the pa-

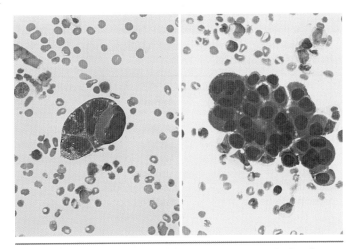

Figure 12-24 *Group 1:* **Adenocarcinoma of the breast with a background of reactive mesothelial cells.** This figure shows two distinct populations of cells that are easily distinguished from one another. The breast carcinoma cells show high N:C ratios with cellular and nuclear molding. The nuclear contours are irregular. The cluster of mesothelial cells shows reactive changes with multinucleation, but the nuclei are fairly uniform, and the low N:C ratios are maintained. (DQ)

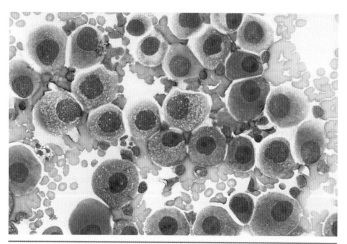

Figure 12-25 *Group 2:* **Metastatic carcinoma mimicking mesothelial cells.** A uniform population of cells can be seen with round, central nuclei, prominent nucleoli, and abundant cytoplasm. Some of the nuclei show slightly lobulated contours. Spaces resembling windows are present. Morphologically, these cells are difficult if not impossible to distinguish from mesothelial cells. (DQ)

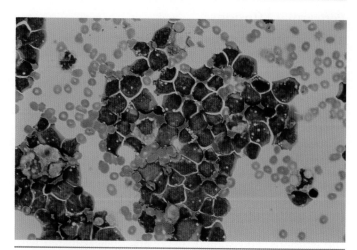

Figure 12-26 *Group 3:* **Burkitt's lymphoma in an effusion.** At low power, this may seem to be an inflammatory effusion, but on closer inspection the malignant nature of the lymphoid population is established. (DQ)

TABLE **12-13**		
Common Etiologies of Malignant Ascites and Pleural Effusions in Men and Women		
Primary Site of Neoplasia	**Pleural Effusions (%)**	**Ascites (%)**
Breast	51	7
Lung	16	
Ovary	10	26
Stomach		40
Undetermined	8.5	7

From Filho LA, Bisi H, Bortolan J, et al. Frequency of adenocarcinomas in serous effusions. Rev Assoc Med Bras 1999; 45(4): 327-336.

TABLE **12-14**			
Approximate Distribution of Malignancy in Pleural Effusions			
Male	**Distribution (%)**	**Female**	**Distribution (%)**
Lung	50	Breast	40
Hematologic	15	Lung	17
Miscellaneous	14	Gynecologic	15
Unknown	10	Unknown	7
Gastrointestinal	9	Miscellaneous	5
Mesothelioma	4	Gastrointestinal	4
		Mesothelioma	2

TABLE **12-15**			
Approximate Distribution of Malignancy in Peritoneal Effusions			
Male	**Distribution (%)**	**Female**	**Distribution (%)**
Lung	7	Gynecologic	55
Gastrointestinal	30	Breast	15
Miscellaneous	40	Lung	1
Unknown	15	Miscellaneous	14
		Unknown	6

description of various neoplastic entities in effusion cytology but also explores the use of ancillary techniques, at times the cytologist's best friend, for arriving at an accurate diagnosis.

Tables 12-13[61] to 12-15 deal with important clinical statistics that are associated with malignant effusions. Although the types of malignancies seen in effusions vary depending on the population base, these types of clinical statistics are vital for the cytopathologist to grasp particularly in instances when the effusion is the first sign of malignant disease. Breast and lung adenocarcinomas are the most common causes of pleural effusions, although gastric and ovarian carcinomas are the most common causes of ascites. Anatomically speaking, this is certainly a logical distribution. What the statistics also show is a significant number of cases with an unknown source for the malignant cells in the effusion. It is sobering knowledge that between 6% and 15% of malignant effusions are derived from neoplasms of unknown origin.

Malignant Mesothelioma

Histologically, the distinction of benign from malignant mesothelial proliferations is characterized by underlying stromal invasion.[62] The problem surgical pathologists face is

tient's known. . . ." However, the distinction between neoplasias and the identification of origin of the neoplasm on purely morphologic grounds may be difficult to impossible. The use of ancillary techniques such as immunocytochemistry is an invaluable tool to the cytopathologist. This portion of the chapter focuses not only on the morphologic

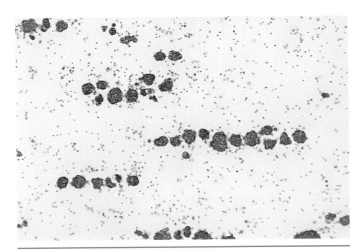

Figure 12-27   Mesothelioma. Tumor cell balls in streaks, most likely resulting from thick hyaluronic acid production. This phenomenon is rare but is characteristic of mesothelioma. (DQ)

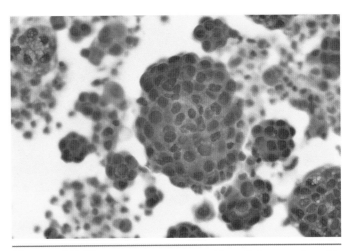

Figure 12-29   Mesothelioma. Highly cellular sample with cells in cell balls with fairly smooth edges and high N:C ratios. These cells appear similar to adenocarcinoma cells. (DQ)

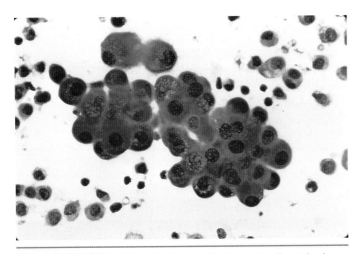

Figure 12-28   Mesothelioma. Clusters of cells with dense and vacuolated cytoplasm and scalloped edges. These cells do not have high N:C ratios and cytologically do not appear malignant. (Pap)

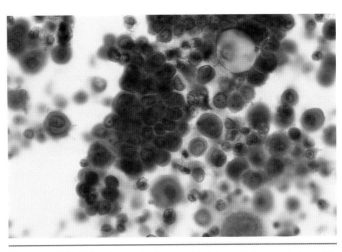

Figure 12-30   Mesothelioma. Highly cellular aspirate with malignant cells present both singly and in aggregates. (Pap)

the distinction of true stromal invasion from mesothelial cell entrapment as part of a reactive process or organizing effusion. This diagnostic distinction is perplexing in both the pleural and abdominal cavities. In these histologic dilemmas, distinguishing benign cytologic atypia from malignant mesothelial proliferations is decidedly deceptive because MM can be bland while reactive processes can be wildly atypical.[62] Histologically, the zonation of cells may be helpful in this discrimination. Densely packed mesothelial cells within the pleural space favor benignity, whereas densely packed mesothelial cells within the stroma favor a malignant cause. Also, in benign organizing fibrinous effusions, a zonation of the cells occurs with the area closest to the pleural space containing the most cells, with decreasing cellularity and increasing fibrosis toward the chest wall or lung. Mesotheliomas, in general, do not demonstrate this type of zonation.[62] Because the diagnostic sensitivity of cytologic examination from the initial diagnosis of MM has been documented at as low as 32%, it has been recommended that to avoid delay in diagnosis of patients with

potential MM and an initial negative cytologic examination, immediate pleural biopsy should be attempted.[63] One factor that should be entertained while attempting to make the diagnosis of MM cytologically is that effusions resulting from MM invariably recur. Although particularly in carcinomatoid MM, a slow progression of the disease may occur.[64]

Cytopathologists are faced with making this benign-vs.-malignant distinction without any histologic information. In the absence of a second alien population of cells that would render the diagnosis of metastatic neoplasia possible, when faced with solely atypical mesothelial cells, the cytologic distinction between benign and malignant mesothelial cells can be difficult (Figures 12-27 to 12-33). The florid hyperplasia occurring in cirrhosis or following a pulmonary infarct can be among the most challenging.[21] In general, a cytologic spectrum is evident from obviously benign to atypical in reactive effusions. Keeping in mind the cytologic features outlined in Tables 12-5 to 12-8 and Boxes 12-3 and 12-4, the cells of mesothelioma are generally more atypical

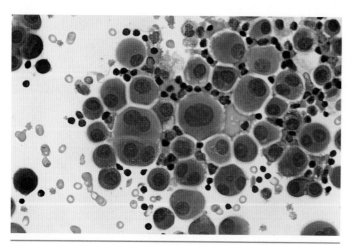

Figure 12-31   Mesothelioma. Malignant cells are present singly and are indistinguishable from reactive mesothelial cells. Multinucleation and prominent nucleoli are present. The background is bloody with inflammatory cells. (DQ)

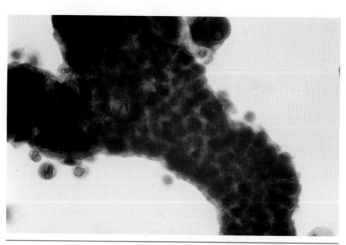

Figure 12-33   Mesothelioma. Well-formed papillary aggregate of cells with high N:C ratios similar to those seen usually in ovarian carcinoma. The cells have high N:C ratios. (Pap)

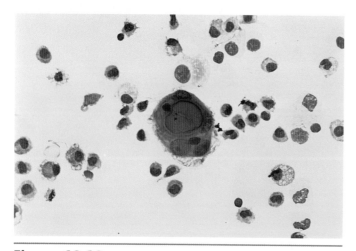

Figure 12-32   Mesothelioma. Malignant cells exhibiting cell-in-cell engulfment with central inspissated magenta-staining hyaluronic acid, which may simulate mucin. (DQ)

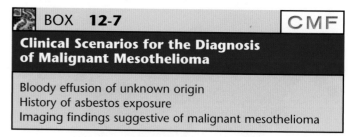

BOX   12-7   CMF

Clinical Scenarios for the Diagnosis of Malignant Mesothelioma

Bloody effusion of unknown origin
History of asbestos exposure
Imaging findings suggestive of malignant mesothelioma

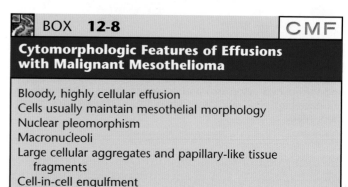

BOX   12-8   CMF

Cytomorphologic Features of Effusions with Malignant Mesothelioma

Bloody, highly cellular effusion
Cells usually maintain mesothelial morphology
Nuclear pleomorphism
Macronucleoli
Large cellular aggregates and papillary-like tissue fragments
Cell-in-cell engulfment

and numerous and come in larger cell groups and tissue clusters than those seen in reactive mesothelial proliferations. However, exceptions exist for each diagnostic category. For example, a single cell dominant picture may occur with MM.

The diagnosis of MM should be entertained in the following scenarios: history of asbestos exposure, imaging findings suggestive of MM (pleural/chest wall, or abdominal/omental diffuse or irregular plaque-like thickenings), or a bloody effusion without a cause[21] (Box 12-7). Most patients also have dyspnea and chest pain.[65] Interestingly, the clinical and radiographic findings among patients with MM are similar with and without a history of asbestos exposure.[65] Statistically, about 90% of mesotheliomas are pleural in origin, with the other 10% either abdominal alone or abdominal in combination with pleural. True pericardial mesotheliomas without involvement of the adjacent pleura and lung are extremely rare.[21]

The effusions of MM are characterized by abundant blood in a highly cellular effusion composed of a uniform population of cells (Box 12-8). Although the cellular morphology may vary from extremely bland to highly pleomorphic, no evidence is shown of a second population of cells or even much of a spectrum within a single population. Histologically, MM may be purely spindled or biphasic with spindled and epithelioid features, but in effusion fluid the cells round up and do not assume a spindled appearance. The aggregates of balled-up cells may contain thousands of cells and typically may demonstrate scalloped or "knobby" edges. The scalloping of edges, however, is not specific, and the cell balls may have smooth borders in MM. Likewise, in adenocarcinoma, characterized by cell groups with smooth borders, or "cannonballs," scalloping of edges may be seen.

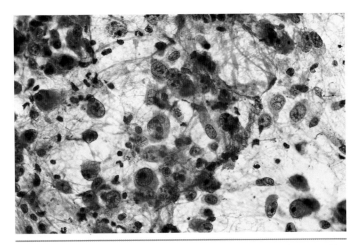

Figure 12-34 FNA of sarcomatoid mesothelioma. The cells are highly pleomorphic with variable epithelioid and spindled morphology. The nuclei are round to oval with macronucleoli, chromatin clumping, and fairly smooth nuclear contours. The cytoplasm is amphophilic and dense to variegated. (Pap)

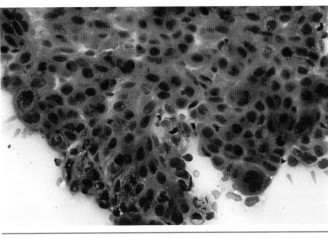

Figure 12-35 FNA of carcinomatous mesothelioma. The cells are arranged in a flat sheet. The nuclei are central and round to oval. Nucleoli are prominent in some of the cells. Windows may be seen. Multinucleation is focally present. (DQ)

The cells of MM retain the basic cytologic features seen in benign mesothelial cells (see the section in this chapter on Nonneoplastic Effusions). However, the cells of MM are generally larger, with significant variation in size, nuclear pleomorphism, macronucleoli, possibly irregular nuclear membrane contours, chromatin clumping, nuclear hyperchromasia, and cell-in-cell arrangements[19,21] (Table 12-16; see Box 12-8). A recent study has concluded that the use of antibodies to E-cadherin and calretinin can aid in the distinction of benign mesothelial cells from MM.[66] In this study, MM cells consistently expressed E-cadherin, whereas reactive mesothelial cells did not express E-cadherin in cytologic samples. Calretinin proves the mesothelial origin of the cells in question.[66]

In many instances, the distinction between MM and adenocarcinoma must be made on effusion cytology. There are many overlapping cytologic features that may make this distinction difficult. For an in depth discussion of this topic, see the sections in this chapter on Adenocarcinoma in Effusions, Distinguishing Adenocarcinoma from Mesothelia, and Ancillary Techniques.

Fine-Needle Aspiration of Malignant Mesothelioma

In conjunction with the clinical picture and imaging characteristics, FNA of pleural-based lesions can be used to diagnose benign and malignant mesothelial proliferations.

Mesotheliomas are plaquelike lesions that are superficially located on the mesothelial surfaces and invade the underlying soft tissues. A majority occur in the thoracic cavity. Although they usually present with effusions, this is not always the case, and at times, the effusion cytology may not be diagnostic. In such instances fine needle aspiration (FNA) of the lesion is an appropriate diagnostic tool[67,68] (Figures 12-34 and 12-35).

FNAs of mesothelioma have been subclassified into the following four categories based on their FNA appearance: benign, carcinomatous, sarcomatous, and undifferentiated.[69,70] Using this subclassification, it was noted that of patients with carcinomatous or undifferentiated types, 83% developed effusions, whereas only 42% of patients with be-

TABLE 12-16	CMF

Cytomorphologic Features of Mesothelial Cells in Malignant Mesothelioma Effusions

Cytomorphologic Feature	Malignant Mesothelioma Effusions that Exhibit this Feature (%)
Uniform cell population	100
Dense cytoplasm	95
Cell to cell apposition, or "windows"	95
Multinucleation with atypia	93
Centrally placed nucleus	93
Cell-in-cell engulfment	93
Microvillus edge	93
Macronucleoli	73
Cytoplasmic blebbing	73
Nuclear pleomorphism	70
Irregular nuclear membrane	68
Proliferative cell balls	68
Proliferative cell balls with scalloped edges	66
True papillary aggregates	23

From Stevens MW, Leong AS-Y, Fazzalari NL, et al. Cytopathology of malignant mesothelioma: a stepwise logistic regression analysis. Diagn Cytopathol 1992; 8:333-341.

nign mesothelial tumors or sarcomatous mesotheliomas developed effusions. Fibrous and sarcomatous mesotheliomas are not prone to effusions.[69] The cytologic characteristics of FNA of mesothelioma are highlighted in Table 12-17. In Tao's series of 39 cases, nine were benign, 14 were carcinomatous, 13 were sarcomatoid, and three were undifferentiated. Several interesting points were raised in this study. No benign epithelial mesotheliomas were located in the pleural cavity; of the nine benign cases, two were pleural and fibrous. The seven benign peritoneal lesions were epithelial.

This raises the common practical issue of distinguishing between reactive mesothelial hyperplasia and benign mesothelioma of the pleura, which is impossible morphologically. In practical terms, however, all benign mesotheliomas of the pleura in this study were of the fibrous type.[69] These fibrous tumors, known under many pseudonyms but most commonly as solitary fibrous tumor of pleura (SFTP), have been well described and have been shown to exhibit clinical aggression when signs of cytologic malignancy are encountered.[71] When the diagnosis is in question, it is useful to

---

TABLE 12-17   `CMF`

Cytomorphologic Features of Fine-Needle Aspiration of Mesothelioma

Type	Features
Benign	
Fibrous type: Solitary fibrous tumor of pleura	Bundles and loose groupings of spindle-shaped cells with uniform and regular elongated or ovoid nuclei
	Tissue fragments possibly present
	Naked small nuclei*
	Moderate amount of poorly defined cytoplasm in cells
	Finely granular chromatin pattern; nucleoli usually not seen
	Wirelike desmoplastic collagen pattern in cell blocks
	Metachromatic stroma on Diff-Quik
	Immunoreactive with CD34
	Nonimmunoreactive with cytokeratin
Epithelial	Abundant atypical mesothelial cells usually in sheets
	Prominent slits in between the cells
	Small nucleoli
	Small number of spindled cells
Malignant	
Carcinomatous	**Papillary epithelial cell type:**
	Papillary fragments and cohesive cell clusters mimicking papillary carcinoma
	Round to ovoid nuclei with prominent nucleoli and a moderate amount of cytoplasm
	Central fibrovascular core may be present
	Psammoma bodies infrequently seen associated with cores
	Cohesive epithelial cell type:
	Cohesive groupings or sheets with occasional slits between the cells
	Nuclei round or ovoid with some variation in size
	Nuclei often in eccentric positions
	Chromatin pattern slightly coarsely granular
	Multinucleation common
	± Prominent nucleoli
	± Mitotic figures
	Asbestos bodies occasionally seen
Sarcomatous	Spindle-shaped cells with elongated or ovoid nuclei
	Nuclei vary in size and shape
	Cells occur singly and in loose groupings
	Stripped nuclei
	Variable appearance and amounts of cytoplasm
	Chromatin coarsely granular
	± Conspicuous nuclei
	Cytokeratin positive
Undifferentiated/anaplastic	Fast growing and aggressive clinically
	Single tumor cells with bizarre morphology
	Pleomorphism
	Prominent nucleoli
	Some cells have abundant dense cytoplasm
	Chromatin pattern coarsely granular
	Multinucleated tumor cells common
	Mitotic figures common

From Tao LC. Aspiration biopsy cytology of mesothelioma. Diagn Cytopathol 1989; 5:14-21; Dusenbery D, Grimes MM, Frable WJ. Fine-needle aspiration cytology of localized fibrous tumor of pleura. Diagn Cytopathol 1992; 8:444-450.
*Similar to those of myoepithelial cells seen in fibroadenoma.

note that solitary fibrous tumors of the pleura stain immunohistochemically with CD34 and are nonimmunoreactive with cytokeratin. A general tendency for these tumors is not to shed cells into the pleural cavity, and thus, this diagnosis is not made with effusion cytology (Table 12-18).

To distinguish between reactive mesothelial hyperplasia and carcinomatous mesothelioma, the presence of many three-dimensional groupings of neoplastic cells with nuclear atypia and prominent nucleoli in irregular arrangements are most consistent with a malignant etiology.[69] On the other hand, the distinction between carcinomatous mesothelioma and a papillary adenocarcinoma can be difficult on morphologic grounds alone and may require ancillary studies including immunohistochemistry.

Carcinoma in Effusions

The discussion of carcinoma in effusions should not be read in isolation but rather needs to be read in conjunction with the previous sections on benign mesothelial cells, macrophages, reactive/atypical changes in mesothelial cells, and mesothelioma. This statement results from the significant amount of overlapping cytologic features of these entities. The misinterpretation of a sample as adenocarcinoma has far reaching implications for both the patient and cytopathologist. Prudence would also dictate that a familiarization with the ensuing discussion of immunocytochemistry in effusion cytology. Specimen preparation and the appropriate selection of a panel of antibodies can be key factors for diagnostic discrimination. For all effusions, particularly adenocarcinomas in effusions, the preparation of a cell block may be paramount in the rendering of a specific diagnosis. The architecture present on a cell block may clearly elucidate the nature of a malignant effusion obviating the need for additional studies. Although previously thought to herald the presence of malignant cells (particularly adenocarcinoma cells) in an effusion cell block, pericellular lacunae have been deemed to not be a reliable indicator of malignancy in body cavity fluids.[72,73]

Metastatic carcinoma, particularly adenocarcinoma is the leading cause of malignant effusions (see Tables 12-13 to 12-15). Because of gender and geographic disease demographics, the most common neoplasms noted in any given cytopathologist's practice vary; however, the most common adenocarcinomas that generate malignant effusions are lung and breast, causing mostly pleural effusions, and ovarian, producing largely abdominal effusions. Although each etiologic neoplasm has certain morphologic features that are suggestive of the specific diagnosis, considerable morphologic overlap occurs between adenocarcinomas, which may make the distinction impossible in cases with unknown primaries.

Malignant effusions with adenocarcinoma, in most cases, show two distinct populations of cells: reactive mesothelial cells and malignant adenocarcinoma cells. The proportions of the two populations differ from case to case. The background may also contain macrophages, inflammatory cells, and blood to variable extents. The reactive mesothelial cells and macrophages may be seen singly or in clusters (see the section in this chapter on Nonneoplastic Effusions). The malignant adenocarcinoma cells may also be present singly or in clusters that may deviate in size from a few cells to large three-dimensional cell balls, or cannonballs. Typically the edges of the cell balls are smooth, although they may appear knobby, similar to those seen in mesothelial cells. One of the main cytologic features of adenocarcinoma cells is increased N:C ratios. The nuclei in the cell balls show considerable overlapping and crowding and appear as though the cytoplasmic matrix they occupy is too small to support the number of atypical, variably sized nuclei. Cell-in-cell engulfment, which is indicative of a malignant population in general and not specific for adenocarcinoma, often may be seen. The cells may be present in monolayered aggregates. True papillary aggregates with or without connective tissue cores and in bizarre shapes with smooth outlines may be seen. Cell balls with fingerlike projections may also be present. The cell groups may be uniform or nonuniform in size. Some adenocarcinomas may appear to form true acini (i.e., contain a true central lumen) when focusing up and down on the three-dimensional clusters, although in the author's experience, this is rarely seen.[19] Box 12-9 lists the common cytologic features of adenocarcinoma cells in effusion cytology.

Distinguishing Adenocarcinoma from Reactive Mesothelial Cells

The distinction of adenocarcinoma from reactive mesothelial cells can be a challenging cytologic distinction, particularly in long-standing effusions with reactive mesothelial atypia. The individual cells of adenocarcinoma show the general features diagnostic of adenocarcinoma in other specimen types. The cells have somewhat high N:C ratios with irregularly shaped nuclear membranes with rounded contours. They may also demonstrate variable degrees of nuclear pleomorphism and multinucleation with atypia. The nuclei are usually eccentric with prominent nucleoli, including macronucleoli, which may stain brightly eosinophilic with Pap stain. The cytoplasm is usually delicate or vacuolated to at least a minor degree but may show balloonlike vacuolization with extreme peripheral displace-

TABLE 12-18	
Differential Diagnosis of Solitary Fibrous Tumor of Pleura	
Neoplastic Lesion	**Distinguishing Features**
Fibrosarcoma of chest wall	No evidence of mesothelial origin CD34 negative
Spindle-cell squamous carcinomas	Not peripheral in location Cytokeratin positive
Sarcomatoid renal cell carcinomas	Cytokeratin positive
Sarcomatous mesothelioma	SFTP has circumscribed radiologic appearance not associated with diffuse pleural thickening Cytokeratin positive
Peripheral nerve sheath tumors of the posterior mediastinum	Characteristic morphology on cell block S-100 positive

SFTP, Solitary fibrous tumor of pleura.

BOX 12-9   CMF

Cytomorphologic Features of Adenocarcinoma Cells in Malignant Effusions

Increased N:C ratios
Large nuclear size
Centrally placed nucleus
Irregular nuclear membrane
Nuclear pleomorphism
Variably sized nuclei
Atypical mitoses
Multinucleation with atypia
Macronucleoli
Sharply defined cytoplasmic outlines
Dense cytoplasm
Irregular, noncentral vacuoles
Acinus-like structures
Cell-in-cell engulfment
Balloonlike vacuolization
Uniform-size aggregates
Monolayer cell aggregates
True papillary aggregates
Proliferative cell balls
Proliferative cell balls with scalloped edge

From Stevens MW, Leong AS-Y, Fazzalari NL, et al. Cytopathology of malignant mesothelioma: a stepwise logistic regression analysis. Diagn Cytopathol 1992; 8:333-341.
N:C, Nuclear to cytoplasmic.

BOX 12-10

'Best' Criteria to Differentiate Adenocarcinoma in a Pleural Effusion from a Benign Pleural Effusion as per Logistic Regression Analysis

Increased N:C ratios
Large nucleoli
Irregular nuclear borders
Sharply defined cytoplasmic boundaries
Three-dimensional aggregates

From Bottles K, Reznicek MJ, Holly EA, et al. Cytologic criteria to diagnose adenocarcinoma in pleural effusions. Mod Pathol 1991; 4(6):677-681.
N:C, Nuclear to cytoplasmic.

TABLE 12-19

Morphologic Distinction of Adenocarcinoma and Mesothelioma

Cytomorphologic Feature	Mesothelioma and Adenocarcinoma	Adenocarcinoma
True papillary aggregates	+	
Multinucleation with atypia	+	
Acinus-like structures	+	+
Balloonlike vacuolization	+	+
Cell-to-cell apposition (cell in cell)	+	

though nucleoli may be prominent in reactive mesothelial cells, they are not usually cherry red and are rarely what one would describe as macronucleoli. In fact they are rather small but stand out because of the pale chromatin. The nuclear outlines of reactive mesothelial cells are smooth and oval or round. Although rare mesothelial cells may show nuclear grooves, they do not show the irregular nuclear lobulations noted in adenocarcinoma. Conversely, reactive mesothelial cells have central nuclei, mesothelial windows, and the biphasic cytoplasm noted prominently on DQ stain, all of which are not features of ACA cells. ACA cells may also exhibit intercellular spaces in approximately 13% of cases, which appear as "windows." These spaces contain extracellular mucin.[75]

The true three-dimensional aggregates characteristic of adenocarcinoma (cell balls, or cannonballs) appear as many overlapping nuclei in an ill-defined sea of cytoplasm. Because the cells of adenocarcinoma typically have high N:C ratios, it virtually appears as though there are too many nuclei for the given amount of cytoplasm. To the contrary, in the cellular aggregates associated with reactive mesothelial cells, the cytoplasm is more abundant, and the nuclei are not as numerous nor as overlapping. Small aggregates of mesothelial cells may show magenta-staining hyaluronic acid material present in the middle of groups of cells. Mucin generally is not present.

Distinguishing Adenocarcinoma from Mesothelioma

The morphologic distinction of adenocarcinoma from mesothelioma is one of the most difficult diagnostic dilemmas in cytopathology (Table 12-19). Because the cells can be morphologically identical, in this situation the cytopathologist must rely heavily on clinical history and the presence of previously known malignancy, as well as possibilities for asbestos exposure. In cases where the distinction cannot be made on morphology alone, the use of a panel of antibody markers that may distinguish adenocarcinoma from mesothelioma (as is outlined in the section in this chapter on Ancillary Techniques) is of paramount importance. It is prudent to employ immunocytochemistry for diagnostic support in any case where the origin of the malignant cells is in question. The panel should consist of ep-

ment and deforming of the nucleus. The cytoplasmic boundaries may be sharply defined. Depending on the primary neoplasm, the cytoplasm could actually be dense rather than vacuolated. Atypical mitoses can be seen[19] (Box 12-10; see Tables 12-5 through 12-8 and Boxes 12-3, 12-4, and 12-9).

As reactive mesothelial cells may cytologically mimic adenocarcinoma cells, the best criteria to distinguish malignant adenocarcinoma cells are the following: increased N:C ratios, large nucleoli, irregular nuclear outlines, sharply defined cytoplasmic boundaries and the presence of true three-dimensional aggregates with rather smooth outlines.[74] Reactive mesothelial cells usually have abundant cytoplasm and thus do not have an increased N:C ratio. Al-

TABLE 12-20

Cellular Patterns in Effusions Associated with Specific Diagnoses

Cellular Pattern	Commonly Associated Etiologies
Cell balls, or "cannonballs"	Breast adenocarcinoma
	Ovarian adenocarcinoma
Acini	Gastric adenocarcinoma
	Colorectal adenocarcinoma
	Lung adenocarcinoma
	Breast adenocarcinoma
	Ovarian adenocarcinoma
	Uterine adenocarcinoma
	Mesothelioma
	Reactive mesothelial proliferations
Signet ring cells	Gastric adenocarcinoma
	Colorectal adenocarcinoma
Intracytoplasmic lumina	Breast adenocarcinoma
Extreme vacuolization	Ovarian adenocarcinoma
	Lung adenocarcinoma
	Pancreatic adenocarcinoma
	Benign mesothelial cells
	Conventional renal cell adenocarcinoma
Principally single malignant cells	Lobular breast adenocarcinoma
	Gastric adenocarcinoma
	Melanoma
	Sarcoma
	Lymphoma
Tumor cell chains, or Indian filing	Lobular and ductal breast adenocarcinoma
	Gastric adenocarcinoma
	Small cell adenocarcinoma
Bizarre giant cells	Pancreatic adenocarcinoma
	Melanoma
	Lung adenocarcinoma
	Thyroid anaplastic carcinoma
	Squamous cell carcinoma
	Pleomorphic sarcoma

From DeMay RM. Pleura. In: Demay RM, editor. The art and science of cytopathology: exfoliative cytology. Chicago: ASCP Press; 1996; Bernard N. Pleural, peritoneal and pericardial fluids. In: Bibbo M, editor. Comprehensive cytopathology. 2nd ed. Philadelphia: WB Saunders; 1997.

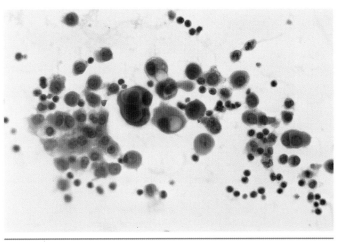

Figure 12-36 **Lobular breast adenocarcinoma.** Macrophages and chronic inflammatory cells are present in the background. The tumor cells are present singly and in small clusters exhibiting cell-in-cell engulfment. Some of the single cells exhibit characteristic large vacuoles. The N:C ratios are high, and the nuclei are fairly hyperchromatic. (Pap)

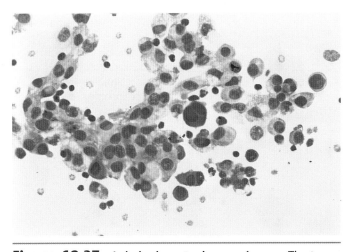

Figure 12-37 **Lobular breast adenocarcinoma.** The tumor cells are scattered singly throughout the aggregates of histiocytes and mesothelial cells. The tumor cells have deeply basophilic cytoplasm and high N:C ratios. One tumor cell is multinucleated. (DQ)

ithelial and mesothelial markers to get appropriate positive and negative reactions.

In general, the cells of adenocarcinoma have increased N:C ratios, large nucleoli, irregular nuclear borders, and sharply defined cytoplasmic boundaries. Usually the cells are present in three-dimensional aggregates or cell balls that appear as though too many nuclei are present for the amount of cytoplasm. The nuclei show variation in size and shape, depending on the level of differentiation and anaplasia of the neoplasm, and usually show noticeable overlapping. The cell balls may have smooth or less often scalloped edges (see Box 12-9).

Although MM and adenocarcinoma will show true papillary aggregates, multinucleation with atypia, acinus-like structures, balloonlike vacuolization, and cell-to-cell apposition, acinus-like structures and balloonlike vacuolization are more common in adenocarcinoma.[74]

Characteristic Features of Specific Types of Adenocarcinoma and Carcinoma

The previously discussed cytologic descriptions are generalizations that are useful in terms of categorizing a malignant effusion as adenocarcinoma. Within the spectrum of adenocarcinoma, there are cytologic features that are common (although in most cases are not unique) for specific subcategories of adenocarcinoma and may also be seen in other malignancies as indicated (Table 12-20).[203,76]

The diagnosis of adenocarcinoma of breast origin in an effusion is suggested by the presence of cell balls, acini, intracytoplasmic lumina, many single malignant cells, and tumor cell chains (Figures 12-36 to 12-41). Although the presence of tumor cell chains, intracytoplasmic lumina,

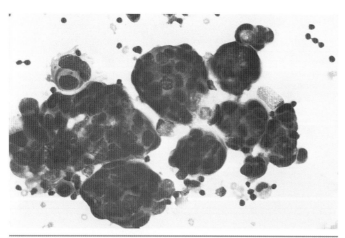

and principally single malignant cells may suggest a lobular etiology, these are not completely reliable indicators. In general, lobular carcinomas present with cells in effusions that are quite monotonous, with high N:C ratios and fairly uniform bland nuclei. It may be a real challenge to differentiate these cells from benign mesothelial cells. Ductal carcinomas tend to produce effusions with large cell balls with smooth borders and acini. Nuclei are typically eccentric and N:C ratios are fairly high. The cytoplasm is basophilic and variably vacuolated (Box 12-11).

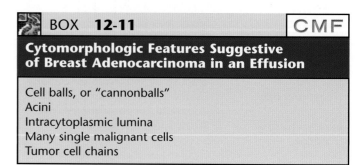

BOX 12-11   CMF

Cytomorphologic Features Suggestive of Breast Adenocarcinoma in an Effusion

Cell balls, or "cannonballs"
Acini
Intracytoplasmic lumina
Many single malignant cells
Tumor cell chains

Figure 12-38   Breast adenocarcinoma. The cells are present in cell balls. These cell balls have fairly smooth contours and appear to be aggregates of three-dimensional nuclei admixed with a minimal amount of cytoplasm. The N:C ratios of the individual cells are high and the intercellular borders are not distinct. Nuclear contours are rounded to irregular. Nucleoli can be seen in some of the cells. (DQ)

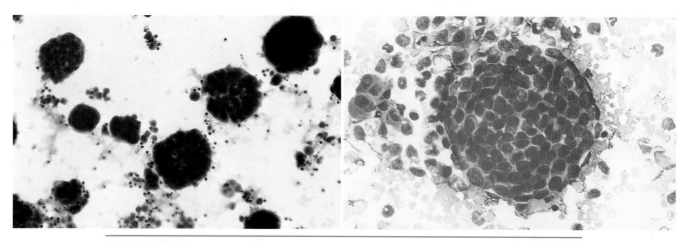

Figure 12-39   Breast adenocarcinoma. Cell balls characteristic of cells of breast and ovarian adenocarcinoma. Individual tumor cells are present singly in the background admixed with macrophages and mesothelial cells. (Pap, DQ)

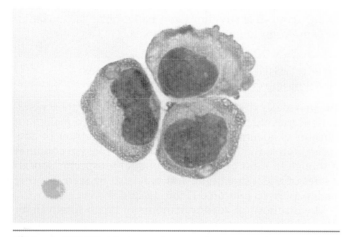

Figure 12-40   Breast adenocarcinoma. In this cerebrospinal fluid, the individual breast carcinoma cells show eccentric nuclei are variable shapes, and biphasic cytoplasm, mimicking that of mesothelial cells. (DQ)

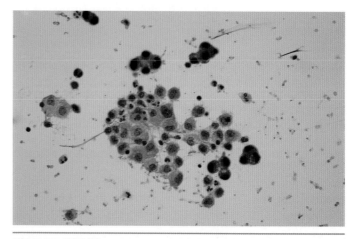

Figure 12-41   Breast adenocarcinoma. Centrally placed aggregate of macrophages and neutrophils surrounded by small aggregates of breast adenocarcinoma cells. Note the high N:C ratios and the peripherally placed hyperchromatic oval nuclei. (Pap)

Ovarian adenocarcinoma yields effusions that are among the most characteristic (Figures 12-42 and 12-43). The cells are present singly, in small groups, and in large cell balls with smooth edges, similar to those seen in breast adenocarcinoma. Ovarian ACA, however, yields cells with abundant large vacuoles that push the nuclei to a perimembranous locale. Papillary formations, often large and irregularly shaped with smooth edges, may be prominent. Mucin may or may not be present, depending on the histologic subclassification of the tumor. With clear cell carcinomas, the huge cells may have optically clear cytoplasm, huge nuclei, and a hobnail pattern.

Lung carcinomas are the most common source of malignant pleural effusions (Figures 12-44 to 12-46). The appear-

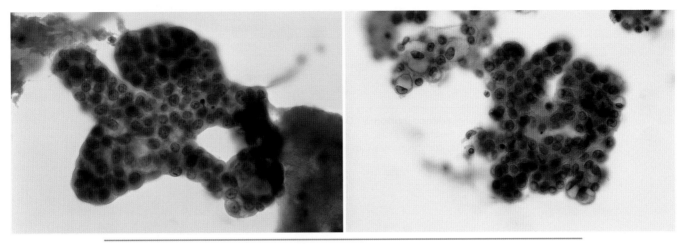

Figure 12-42   Ovarian adenocarcinoma. Complex, smooth-bordered papillary aggregates show monolayers of cells with high N:C ratios, round nuclei of different sizes, and visible nucleoli. Glandlike spaces are noted. Many of the nuclei exhibit grooves and small irregularities of the nuclear envelope. (Pap)

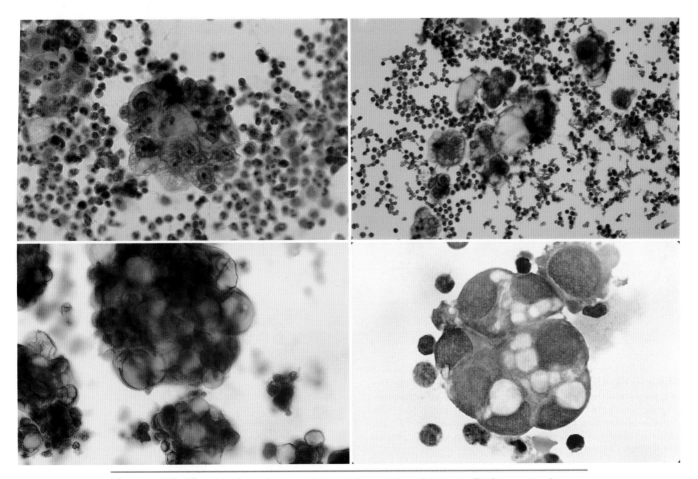

Figure 12-43   Ovarian adenocarcinoma. Aggregates of tumor cells show extensive vacuolization, which can obscure cellular detail. The nuclei are rounded and eccentric with prominent nucleoli. (Pap, DQ)

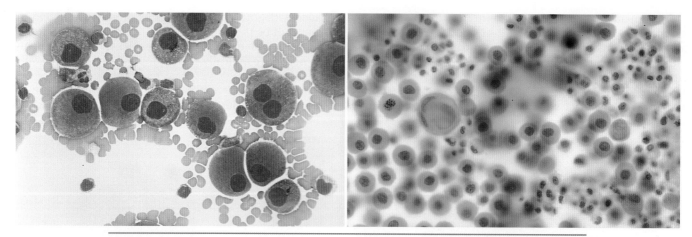

Figure 12-44   Lung adenocarcinoma. The cells of this adenocarcinoma are similar morphologically to reactive mesothelial cells. A mucicarmine stain reveals the cells to be strongly positive with mucicarmine, consistent with an adenocarcinoma. (DQ, mucicarmine)

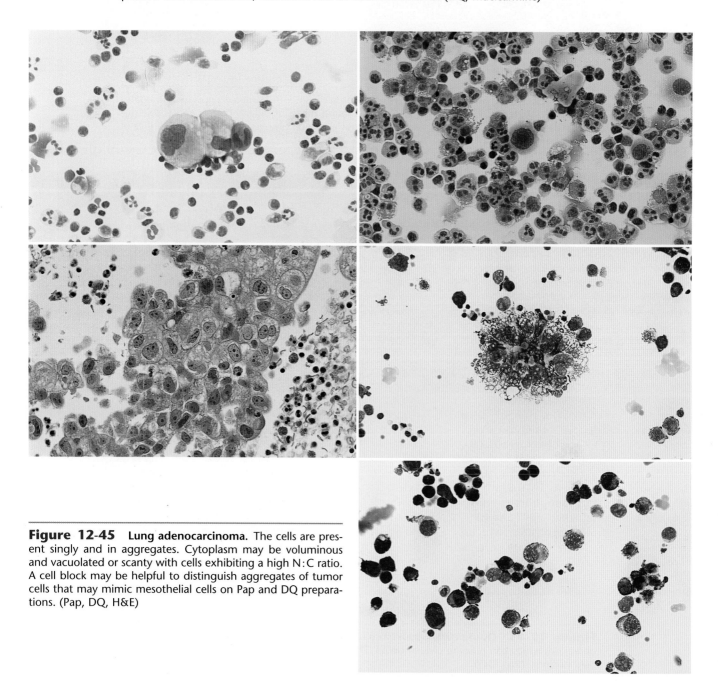

Figure 12-45   Lung adenocarcinoma. The cells are present singly and in aggregates. Cytoplasm may be voluminous and vacuolated or scanty with cells exhibiting a high N:C ratio. A cell block may be helpful to distinguish aggregates of tumor cells that may mimic mesothelial cells on Pap and DQ preparations. (Pap, DQ, H&E)

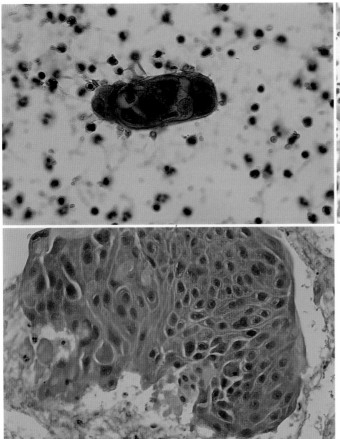

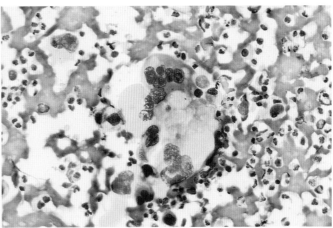

Figure 12-46 **Squamous carcinoma.** Although typically eosinophilic or cyanophilic on Pap-stained material, the cytoplasm of squamous carcinoma on DQ is robin's-egg blue, a bright blue color. The nuclei are typically irregular and darkly hyperchromatic. Depending on the duration of the effusion, the cells may be vacuolated and show significant variability in nuclear size and contours. Some cells have prominent nucleoli. Cells may be present singly or in clusters of different size. Cell block may show characteristic morphology. (DQ, Pap, H&E)

ance of lung carcinomas in effusion cytology depends on the cell type of the neoplasm. Squamous cell carcinomas, which may originate not only in the lung but also can come from the skin, head and neck area, esophagus, and genital tract, rarely cause effusions. However, when well differentiated, the squamous etiology is made obvious by the easily visualized cytoplasmic denseness, opaqueness, and keratinization, which are classically squamous, as well as the densely hyperchromatic, jaggedly irregular basophilic nuclei. The cells usually have abundant cytoplasm. Keratinization is seen as robin's-egg blue on DQ stain and as eosinophilic/orangeophilic on Pap stain. Squamous carcinomas may show cell-in-cell engulfment and may also appear vacuolated, depending on the duration of the effusion. Nonkeratinized neoplasms and long-standing effusions tend to show more cellular vacuolization. This vacuolization can lead to misinterpretation of the cells as adenocarcinoma or reactive mesothelial cells. Mucin stains are negative.

Malignant pleural effusions occurring after resection of pulmonary adenocarcinoma are associated with lymph node disease or pleural involvement by tumor.[77] Interestingly, malignant effusions developing in patients more than 2 years after the primary tumor resection are likely to be the result of involvement with a second primary.[77] Recent studies touting the use of preoperative pleural lavage in pulmonary adenocarcinoma patients noted that a positive pleural lavage at the time of operation may predict a poorer survival and is especially useful in determining high-risk patients with an early stage of disease.[78,79] Effusions associated with lung adenocarcinoma have diverse mor-

phologies, depending on the appearance of the primary neoplasm and the degree of differentiation. For instance, non–small cell carcinomas that show histologic features of adenocarcinoma and squamous carcinoma may show cytology compatible with one or both tumor types in the malignant effusion. Well-differentiated adenocarcinomas such as bronchiolar-alveolar carcinoma may show a uniform population of bland-appearing cells with or without vacuoles. These cells may mimic reactive mesothelial cells because of their striking homogeneity. Papillary clusters, acini, three-dimensional aggregates, and single cells may be seen. Less well-differentiated lung adenocarcinoma generates cells that exhibit variable degrees of atypia, inconsistent N:C ratios, and other cytologic features previously described for adenocarcinoma. Extreme pleomorphism may be seen in poorly differentiated tumors, particularly those with tumor giant cell morphology. Perinucleolar chromatin clearing may be prominent. Mucin may be seen as magenta with the DQ stain and amphophilic with Pap stain.

Small cell carcinomas in effusions appear as small, hyperchromatic cells with high N:C ratios and scant basophilic cytoplasm (Figure 12-47). The cells often show extensive cellular and nuclear molding. The distinguishing features that allow discrimination from lymphoma is the usual presence of at least some degree of cytoplasmic or nuclear elongation, angulation, or spindling, attributes that are not present in lymphoma. Cytoplasm is usually sparse but appears more abundant on air-dried smears and cytospins resulting from preparation artifacts. Cells appear singly but are also present in aggregates of different size. Tumor cell chains or "Indian filing" may be prominent.

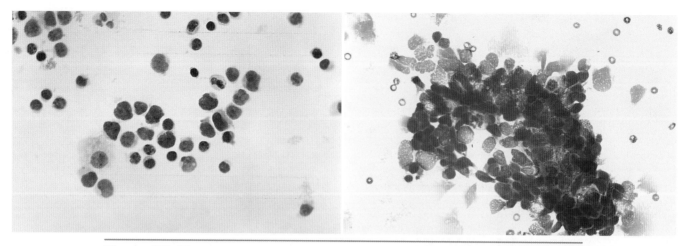

Figure 12-47   Small cell lung carcinoma. The cells appear singly and in aggregates and are slightly larger than the adjacent lymphocytes. Chains of tumor cells are evident. They exhibit high N:C ratios with hyperchromatic, smudged chromatin. In the aggregate, nuclear molding is present. (Pap, DQ)

Lymphoma cells as a rule are present singly and do not aggregate to the same extent, although clustering may seen as a part of cytospin artifact.

Pancreatic/pancreaticobiliary tract adenocarcinoma is characterized by highly atypical large cells with variably vacuolated cytoplasm (Figure 12-48). A columnar or cuboidal morphology may be present. Squamous features may be present, depending on the metaplastic leanings of the primary. The degree of differentiation within an effusion can be highly variable. Mucin production may be seen.

Malignant effusions resulting from renal cell carcinoma occur most often in patients with clear cell/conventional or papillary primaries[80] (Figure 12-49). In a recent study of the subject, it was noted that patients with high-grade tumors with sarcomatoid features presented early in their disease with benign effusions, whereas patients with papillary primaries presented later in the course of the disease with malignant effusions.[80] Depending on the histologic subtype of the primary neoplasm, renal carcinoma may show characteristic findings in an effusion; however the distinction between clear cell/conventional and papillary renal cell carcinoma may be difficult unless papillae, especially with central histiocytes, are present.[80] Clear cell or conventional renal cell carcinoma may show large cells with abundant clear or eosinophilic granular cytoplasm, round nuclei, and prominent nucleoli. Papillary carcinoma shows papillary aggregates, although this type of carcinoma is rarely seen in effusion cytology.

Cellular effusions with large numbers of single signet ring cells are highly suggestive of a gastric primary (Figure 12-50). Although a similar picture may be seen in lobular breast carcinoma, the cells in gastric adenocarcinoma are generally larger and more pleomorphic than those seen in breast adenocarcinoma. Ductal breast adenocarcinoma may also contain signet ring cells, as may pancreatic and other gastrointestinal adenocarcinomas.

Malignant effusions resulting from prostatic adenocarcinoma occur most commonly in patients with high-grade, high-stage tumors. The cells have a fairly characteristic appearance of prominent nucleoli, high N:C ratios, and small, loosely cohesive group arrangements.[81] Interestingly less than 50% of these effusions when studied with immunocytochemistry are immunoreactive with prostate-specific antigen (PSA) or prostatic alkaline phosphatase. The prostatic small cell anaplastic carcinoma has also been reported to occur in effusion cytology, resembling small cell carcinoma of the lung with a mixture of cells typical of prostatic adenocarcinoma.[81]

The presence of a cell block is of the utmost importance for the diagnosis of colorectal carcinoma in an effusion (Figure 12-51). The characteristic columnar morphology is readily identified on cell block material. The cells may appear columnar or rounded within the effusion milieu. This may make the discrimination more difficult on smears or cytospin preparations as opposed to the cell block. Mucus within the cells is usually obvious. Necrosis in the background may or may not be seen.

The ease with which one may diagnose pseudomyxoma peritonei (PMP) in effusion cytology may depend entirely on whether clinical history is available (Figure 12-52). With an appropriate clinical history the presence of an effusion composed of largely mucoid material with isolated bland-appearing columnar cells has been considered diagnostic for this peculiar neoplasm. The characteristic paucity of these bland columnar tumor cells is what makes the neoplasm difficult to diagnose in the absence of an appropriate history. Despite the abundant mucoid background the cells may or may not contain obvious mucus vacuoles. In the last several years, neoplasms previously termed *PMP* have been reclassified based on histologic data into diagnostically and prognostically distinct categories: disseminated peritoneal adenomucinosis (DPAM) and peritoneal mucinous carcinomatosis (PMCA).[82] DPAM is characterized by superficial implants; rare parenchymal or nodal involvement; and a fairly benign, indolent clinical course. In pelvic wash cytology DPAM is seen as variably sized, cohesive clusters or monolayered sheets of cells with discreet cell borders and fairly uniform nuclei with smooth nuclear outlines.[83] PMCA is characterized by more extensive lymph node involvement, visceral invasion, and metastasis remote from the abdominal cavity.[82] In pelvic wash cytology, PMCA is seen as small, three-dimensional clusters or irregular sheets

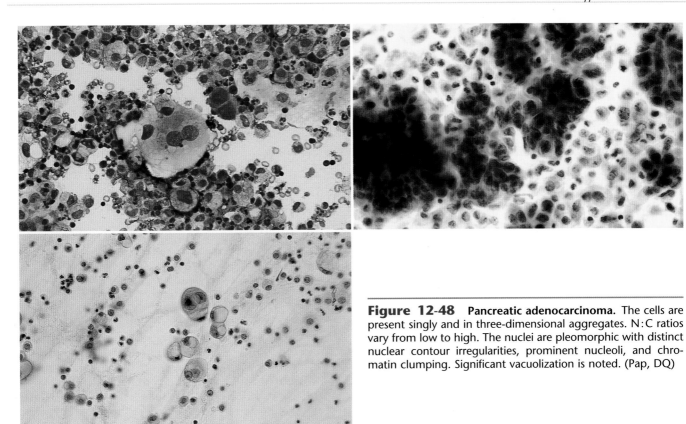

Figure 12-48 **Pancreatic adenocarcinoma.** The cells are present singly and in three-dimensional aggregates. N:C ratios vary from low to high. The nuclei are pleomorphic with distinct nuclear contour irregularities, prominent nucleoli, and chromatin clumping. Significant vacuolization is noted. (Pap, DQ)

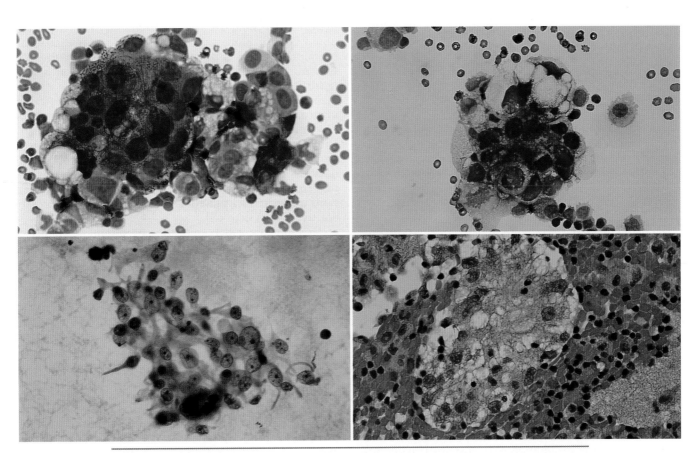

Figure 12-49 **Renal carcinoma, conventional type.** These cells are in aggregates with abundant vacuolated cytoplasm. The nuclei are large and round with prominent nucleoli. The degree of vacuolization is variable. The preparation of a cell block may enhance the neoplastic etiology of the cells when they are well differentiated and mimic mesothelial cells with vacuoles. (DQ, Pap, H&E)

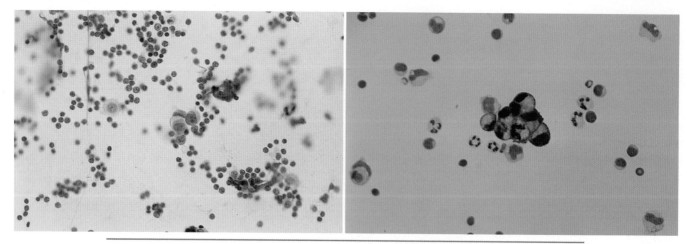

Figure 12-50 Gastric adenocarcinoma. These cells are highly pleomorphic and show prominent vacuolization. They occur singly and in groups. The nuclei are eccentric and are distorted by the vacuole, and the nucleoli are prominent. (Pap, DQ)

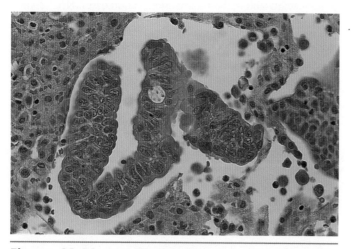

Figure 12-51 Colonic adenocarcinoma. The cell block exhibits the histologic features that are characteristic of this primary tumor. The cells are present in strips with pseudostratified, elongated, oval nuclei with prominent nucleoli. Mucin is focally present. (H&E)

of cells with enlarged, overlapping nuclei, irregular nuclear outlines, irregular chromatin distribution, nucleoli of various sizes, irregular chromatin distribution, and malignant signet ring cells.[83] Although this classification is not uniformly used in general pathology practice, it is interesting to note that the distinction between these two variants of PMP with reported prognostic differences can be attempted and made on pelvic washings.[83] It remains to be seen whether this distinction can be made on ascitic fluid.

Hematologic Neoplasms in Effusions

The authors believe, as do others, that the cytologic review of effusions with the potential for involvement with hematologic neoplasms is facilitated by the preparation of DQ smears or cytospins in addition to Pap-stained material[84] (Figures 12-53 to 12-56; see Figure 12-26). As a high percentage of hematologic malignancies may involve the peripheral blood during the course of the disease, it is important for the cytopathologist to establish that a potentially malignant effusion is not merely a bloody tap representing hematogenous involvement. When necessary, a differential count of the malignant cells can be done on the effusion and compared with that of the peripheral blood.

The detection of non-Hodgkin's lymphoma in effusion cytology is not a rare event in any cytopathology laboratory. In cellular samples the abnormal lymphoid population is easily identifiable and at least partially classifiable as to size and morphology based on parameters discussed in Chapter 24. It may be difficult to identify malignant lymphoid cells in bloody or malignant effusions that have a prominent reactive lymphoid component. In these instances, the malignant etiology of the effusion at least needs to be suspected to avoid misinterpreting the scattered malignant lymphoma cells as reactive cells. The performance of immunocytochemistry, flow cytometry, and/or PCR studies for heavy chain gene rearrangement, clonality, and/or framework 3 abnormalities may be vital diagnostic tools in cases with nebulous cytologic findings.[85-87] Immunocytochemical studies of paraffin blocks of effusions have proven to be a highly effective method of evaluating effusions associated with malignant lymphoma, with no false-positive results detected.[88]

This same approach and rationale should be applied for the evaluation of effusions with possible involvement with the various subtypes of leukemia.[89] With leukemia, however, it is of the utmost importance to rule out that the malignant cells in the effusion merely represent peripheral blood involvement. It is also consequential to recognize malignant leukemic cells in effusions that may contain malignant cells from another primary. Several cases have been noted, in which malignant effusions have contained cells from both chronic lymphocytic leukemia and metastatic epithelial neoplasms, as unlikely and rare as that occurrence may be.

The unfortunate advent of AIDS has been accompanied by an array of previously undescribed phenomena, among them primary body cavity–based AIDS-related lymphomas.[90-93] This malignant effusion is unique as it is unassociated with identifiable tumor masses.[92] HHV-8 sequences have been identified in three AIDS-related diseases: Kaposi's sarcoma, multicentric Castleman's disease, and primary body cavity lymphoma (PBCL). PBCL may occur in patients

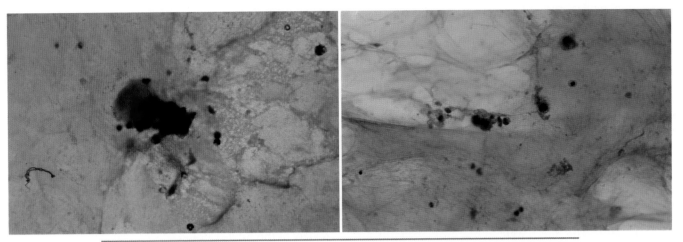

Figure 12-52 **Pseudomyxoma peritonei.** This effusion is composed of largely mucoid material with isolated bland-appearing columnar cells that are largely obscured by the mucin. A paucity of these bland columnar/cuboidal tumor cells is charateristic. (Pap, DQ)

with either Kaposi's or multicentric Castleman's disease.[93] The malignant lymphoma cells are said to ". . . bridge features of large cell immunoblastic and anaplastic large cell lymphomas. . . ."[92] These cells are large- to medium-sized and highly pleomorphic. The nuclei are peripherally located with prominent nucleoli. Their abundant, deeply basophilic cytoplasm is best visualized on DQ stain. Mitoses, apoptotic bodies, and bi- and multinucleation of the malignant lymphoid cells are also seen. These cells lack pan-B and pan-T cell markers but are immunoreactive for CD45, CD20, CD138 and may show lambda or kappa light chain restriction. The cells are immunoreactive with activation antigens CD30, CD38, CD71, and HLA-DR.[90,92] PCR studies for HHV-8 and Epstein-Barr virus (EBV) are positive.[92]

Hodgkin's disease may lead to pleural effusions in more than 20% of cases, usually resulting from obstruction of lymphatic drainage of the mediastinum or lung, systemic disease, or direct pleural involvement.[94] As with all neoplastic disease causing malignant effusions, this bodes poorly for the patient's prognosis. Most such effusions are negative for malignant cells. The effusions associated with Hodgkin's disease usually contain a nonspecific background of inflammatory cells with a mixture of lymphocytes, plasma cells, and eosinophils. Characteristic, diagnostic Reed-Sternberg cells may be sparse but must be present to definitively classify the effusion as involved with Hodgkin's disease. Confirmatory immunohistochemistry for CD15 and CD30 in the Reed-Sternberg cells should probably be done in most cases to avoid diagnostic pitfalls.[94] The differential diagnosis would be malignant non-Hodgkin's lymphoma, metastatic melanoma, carcinoma, and reactive inflammatory nonneoplastic effusions if the Reed-Sternberg cells are overlooked.[94]

Malignant effusions associated with multiple myeloma are a rare late complication of the disease associated with grave prognostic implications.[84,204] Identification of the malignant plasma cells is facilitated by the preparation of DQ stains.[84] Low cellularity, obscuring blood, or a paucity of the malignant plasma cells may lead to false-negative diagnoses. Because of the potential difficulties associated with correctly classifying plasma cells in these effusions, when this diagnosis is suspected, cytopathology should be performed in conjunction with flow cytometry for the best diagnostic outcome.[84]

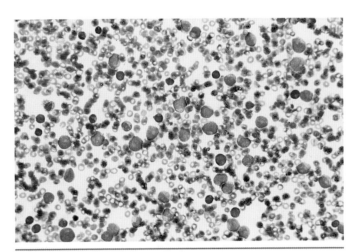

Figure 12-53 **Acute myeloid leukemia.** Scattered blasts of acute myelogenous leukemia (AML) are present in a bloody background. The cells have high N:C ratios. Cytoplasmic magenta-colored granules are present focally. (DQ)

A case of posttransplantation lymphoproliferative disorder (PTLD) mimicking a nonspecific lymphocytic pleural effusion in a bone marrow transplant recipient has been reported.[95] As with all potentially involved PTLD infiltrates, masses, or body fluids in this immunosuppressed patient population, lymphocyte markers and PCR for EBV-latent membrane protein are useful ancillary tests for aiding in the diagnosis.[94-96]

Melanoma in Effusions

Effusions resulting from metastatic malignant melanoma are not an uncommon event (Figure 12-57). A review of this topic evaluating 32 cases described the effusions due to melanoma as bloody and inflammatory. The melanoma cells were largely discohesive, round to oval in shape, and exhibited an extreme degree of variability in size, ranging from one to five times the size of background mesothelial cells.[17] The cytoplasm was abundant and usually vacuolated with a vast majority showing fine, even distribution of the vacuoles and rare cases showing both large and small vacuoles. One case actually had signet ring–type cytoplasmic vacuolization. With the DQ stain in 12% of Beaty's[17] cases, the melanoma cells showed a biphasic staining pattern simulating mesothelial cells.[17]

Cytoplasmic melanin was only present in a minority of the cases. When present, it was also noted in the associated background histiocytes. In the tumor cells the melanin pigment was present as fine, black-to-navy blue, tiny, equivalent-size cytoplasmic granules in the DQ–stained material.[17]

The nuclei of the malignant cells were large, round to oval, and eccentrically placed within the cell and exhibited frequent multinucleation with rare nuclear irregularities. As the cytoplasm was abundant, the cells did not exhibit high N:C ratios. The nuclei were hyperchromatic with single to multiple prominent macronucleoli. Cytoplasmic intranuclear pseudoinclusions were present in 25% of cases.[17]

The diagnostic challenge involved in establishing the diagnosis of melanoma in an effusion is that the melanoma cells strongly resemble both reactive mesothelial and adenocarcinoma cells. Cytoplasmic vacuolization, multinucleation, prominent nucleoli, and cell-in-cell engulfment are cytologic features common to all three. Utilization of immunocytochemistry for melanoma markers such as MART-1, HMB45, and Melan A may be imperative for arriving at the correct diagnosis.[17]

Sarcomas in Effusions

Sarcomas, which account for less than 6% of malignant effusions, usually present with effusions after the initial diagnosis of the tumor type has been generated.[97, 205] A recent review of the subject noted the general cytologic features of a diverse group of sarcomas (e.g., osteogenic sarcoma, rhabdomyosarcoma, leiomyosarcoma, malignant fibrous histio-

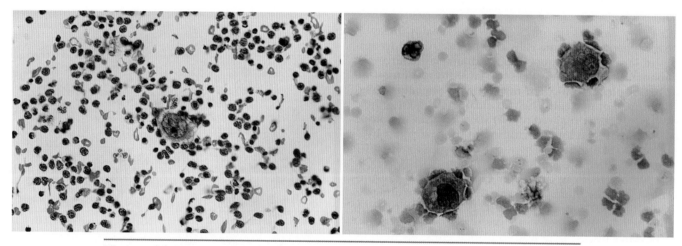

Figure 12-54 Hodgkin's lymphoma. A Reed-Sternberg variant is present in the foreground of an inflammatory background. The cytoplasm is abundant, and the nucleolus is large. An immunocytochemical study reveals the large cells to be immunoreactive with LeuM1, which is characteristic of Reed-Sternberg cells. (Pap, H&E, DAB)

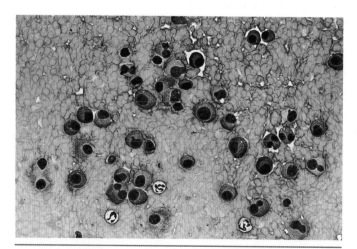

Figure 12-55 FNA of plasmacytoma of chest wall. The cells of this plasmacytoma mimic mesothelial cells. The cells have abundant basophilic cytoplasm and round nuclei that are often central. The "clock-face" chromatin pattern is characteristic of plasma cells. (DQ)

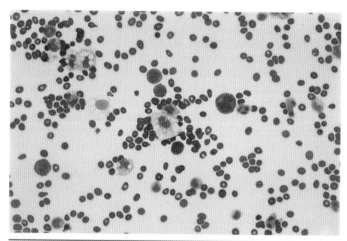

Figure 12-56 Primary body cavity lymphoma. Scattered among the RBCs and histiocytes are large- to intermediate-size, atypical lymphocytes with deeply basophilic cytoplasm and irregular nuclear contours. (DQ)

cytoma, liposarcoma, high-grade sarcoma not otherwise specified, synovial sarcoma, and chondrosarcoma) to be scant cellularity, single cell arrangement, indistinct cell borders, nuclear pleomorphism, multinucleation, and a proteinaceous background.[97] Nuclear features varied with each diagnosis; however, multinucleation, prominent nucleoli, nuclear pleomorphism, and coarse or clumped chromatin were seen for several different types of sarcomas. Interestingly, although cells of most other neoplasms round up in effusions, many of the different sarcomas exhibited spindled, fusiform or oval-shaped cells.[97] The authors state that it is usually not feasible to determine the exact histologic subtype of the sarcoma in an effusion; however, the importance of subclassification of sarcomas in effusions is superseded by the correct distinction of the cells as malignant[97] (Figures 12-58 and 12-59).

Neoplasms that May Give Rise to Effusions

Essentially any malignant neoplasm may lead to a malignant effusion. Although the cytology of the cellular origin of the malignant cells is preserved, it is important to remember that all cells have the capacity to "round up" in the fluid milieu, thus, characteristic cytoplasmic features such as spindling may be clouded. As cells in effusions often imbibe effusion fluid, the cells in any malignant effusion may appear vacuolated regardless of whether vacuolization is part of the usual visual spectrum of the tumor. Tumors that usually fall into this category are germ cell tumors, transitional cell carcinomas, and sarcomas. Ancillary studies for immunoperoxidase as performed in surgical pathology material may be necessary to reach a definitive diagnosis. Clinical information is imperative, particularly in effusions associated with small round blue cell tumors in children.

Effusions associated with esophageal carcinoma, although rare, are more likely to occur in patients with adenocarcinoma rather than squamous carcinoma.[98]

DIFFERENTIAL DIAGNOSIS OF PELVIC WASHINGS

A short discussion on peritoneal washing/lavages has been included in the section in this chapter on Mesothelial Cells. A recent study evaluating the use of pelvic washing cytology concluded the following three major appropriate indications for collecting and examining washing fluids: a prior diagnosis of a gynecologic or intraperitoneal cancer, an in-

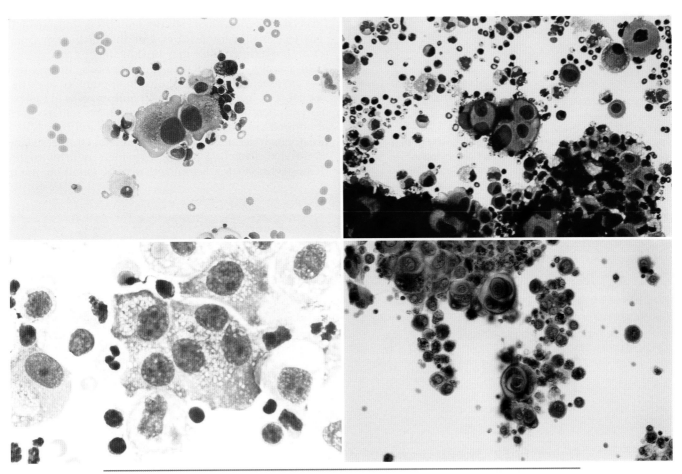

Figure 12-57 **Malignant melanoma.** The cells are large with abundant cytoplasm and round eccentric nuclei with prominent nucleoli. Mulitnucleation and variable degrees of vacuolization are present. Cells are present singly and in clusters. Cell-in-cell engulfment may be a prominent feature. (DQ, Pap)

traoperative suspicion of cancer, and reassessment of a patient's tumor status.[99] With the exception of a single patient, cancer was detected in concurrently obtained histologic material; thus, cytologic evaluation in isolation did not elevate the stage of any patient.[99] Other studies have concluded that although the increase in diagnostic yield for cytology when compared with histology alone was low, a positive cytology was strongly predictive of an adverse outcome.[100]

Based on the indications for pelvic washings and the diseases associated with the indications, the differential diagnosis encountered with these specimens includes atypical/reactive mesothelial cells, ovarian tumors of low malignant potential, serous carcinomas, endosalpingiosis, and endometriosis. Benign mesothelial cells in these samples are typically characterized by large flat sheets with smooth borders and a honeycomb-like appearance. The nuclei are

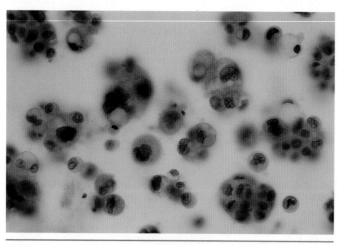

Figure 12-58 **Embryonal carcinoma.** The cells appear singly and in aggregates with an appearance similar to that of adenocarcinoma. Vacuoles are present, and the cytoplasm is abundant. Nuclei are irregular with prominent nucleoli. (Pap)

evenly spaced, and the cell borders are distinct. Individually, they may be multinucleated. Normal appearing mitotic figures may be evident. These cells may have small vacuoles that do not indent *the nuclear outline. Abnormal mitotic figures can be seen in washes performed during second-look procedures in patients that have had chemotherapy.[206]

Mesothelial cells may become quite atypical, however, because of reactive processes. This atypia may be characterized by elevated N:C ratios with normal chromatin pattern; large, irregular or multiple nucleoli; irregular nuclear outlines; prominent multinucleation with uniform nuclei; and prominent cytoplasmic vacuolization. A single population of cells with a morphologic continuum, along with preservation of the basic mesothelial architecture, helps distinguish benign reactive cells from adenocarcinoma. The presence of small, uniform nuclei in cells with high N:C ratios favors a diagnosis of borderline tumor.[101] The combination of windows, irregular outline of cell groups, and only slight nuclear atypia favor the diagnosis of benign mesothelial cells.[102] Additional discriminating factors and features characteristic of serous carcinoma are present in Table 12-21.

Endosalpingiosis presents in pelvic washings as cellular clusters and papillary fragments, often with centrally located psammoma bodies. The cells are tightly cohesive and present in only a few layers. The nuclei are uniform with finely granular and evenly distributed chromatin. The nucleoli are inconspicuous. The cells have high N:C ratios. Dispersion of individual cells does not occur. In general, the cells lack malignant features, but the distinction from a serous borderline tumor may be difficult.[103]

In samples involved with endometriosis, the epithelial cells are usually sparse and similar in appearance to those of vaginal pool specimens (i.e., small uniform cells in tight, cohesive spheres). The individual cells have solitary nuclei, nonprominent nucleoli, dark chromatin, and high N:C ratios. Cellular degeneration may be present. Distinct diagnostic stromal elements may be extremely difficult to find. Hemosiderin laden macrophages may be found but are not

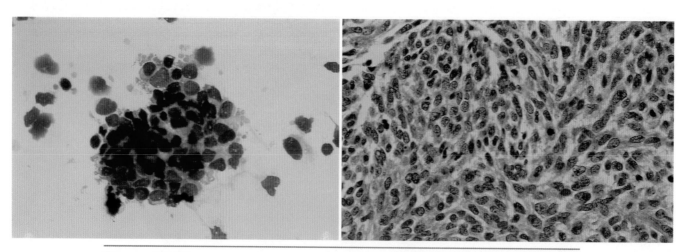

Figure 12-59 **Synovial sarcoma.** The cells of synovial sarcoma, when in a fluid milieu, may aggregate and appear similar to those of small cell carcinoma. This loosely formed aggregate shows cells with high N:C ratios, extreme nuclear hyperchromasia, and significant pleomorphism. Scant basophilic cytoplasm is evident. The characteristic spindle-cell morphology can be appreciated in the cell block rather than in smear or cytospin preparations in which the cells round up. (DQ, H&E)

TABLE 12-21

Distinction of Benign Mesothelial Cells from Serous Borderline Tumor and Serous Carcinoma in Pelvic Washings

Cytomorphologic Feature	Benign Mesothelium	Serous Borderline Tumor	Serous Carcinoma
Large smooth papillae	−	++	±
Many single cells	±	−	+
Large cell size	−	−	++
Pleomorphism	+	−	+++
High N:C ratios	−	+	−
Macronucleoli	−	−	+
Mitotic figures	+	−	−
Windows	+	−	−

diagnostic because they may be seen in other conditions. The differential diagnosis includes borderline neoplasm of the ovary; however, endometriosis does not have papillary fragments, which are prominent in serous borderline tumors. A discussion of the use of pelvic washings in pseudomyxoma peritonei is included in the section in this chapter on Characteristic Features of Specific Types of Adenocarcinoma and Carcinoma.

ANCILLARY TECHNIQUES

Electron Microscopy

In general, immunocytochemistry is used to discriminate among adenocarcinoma, MM, and reactive mesothelial cells. However, electron microscopy remains the "gold standard" for this distinction, with potential misinterpretations, for the most part, a result of sampling errors. A recent ultrastructural study performed for the discrimination of these three diagnostic entities concluded the following: reactive and neoplastic mesothelial cells contained more abundant cytoplasmic intermediate filaments and fewer free ribosomes than cells of adenocarcinoma; reactive mesothelial cells had fewer mitochondria than MM cells; MM cells had longer, thinner microvilli on the cell surfaces than adenocarcinoma (length-to-diameter ratios of microvilli for MM were 19, whereas for adenocarcinoma, they were nine); giant intercellular junctions were associated with some cases of MM; and core filaments or rootlets were found in a few cases of adenocarcinoma. Based on these findings, the authors believe that ultrastructural cytology is useful for this diagnostic discrimination.[104]

Immunocytochemistry

Immunocytochemistry is indispensable for the diagnostic workup of all but the most obvious benign and malignant effusions.[105,106] Significant morphologic overlap exists between diverse pathologic processes in the effusion milieu. Reactive mesothelial cells can mimic malignant cells. Malignant mesothelial cells can be indistinguishable from met-

astatic carcinoma cells.[8,107-109] In many cases a definitive diagnosis cannot be reached based on morphology alone. Immunocytochemistry can play a pivotal role in clarifying the origin of benign and malignant cells in effusions; however, effusions are samples that present unique challenges for this type of ancillary technique. Additionally, in practice, no standardization of methods for immunocytochemistry for effusions or cytology, in general, exist.

Reference studies for the antibodies used for the diagnostic discrimination of adenocarcinoma from MM from reactive mesothelial cells were performed on formalin-fixed, paraffin-embedded histologic surgical pathology specimens. However, evaluation of the same antibodies in effusions has been performed on several cytologic preparations (e.g., ethanol-fixed smears and cytospins, ThinPrep, air-dried cytospins, and formalin-fixed cell blocks). This may account for less than reliable and reproducible results. A wide variety of opinions exists among pathologists regarding the relative effectiveness of certain markers used for the differential diagnoses presented by most effusions.

Standardization of immunohistochemical methods is essential for reliable and reproducible results. Based on this premise, the authors' extensive experience with benign and malignant effusions, and the notion that immunocytochemistry on cytopathology samples should approximate the findings on surgical pathology material, the authors present what they have found to be the optimal approach for the use of ICC in effusion cytology. This view most closely approximates the current procedures used in surgical pathology samples.[110-113] It should be noted, however, that other investigators have claimed excellent or superior results performing immunocytochemistry on direct smear cytologic samples in lieu of paraffin embedding.[110,114-118]

Specimen Processing

For optimal specimen handling for potential immunocytochemistry, effusion samples should be received fresh in the cytology laboratory (Box 12-12). With refrigeration (2° to 8° C), cellular integrity is well preserved for at least 72 hours. The previous standard of fixation with equal volumes of 50% ethanol should be retained for only those samples requiring initial long-term storage before processing. Ethanol fixation impedes the use of DQ stains and immunocytochemistry markers for lymphoid processes.[105]

Immunocytochemistry can be done on other cytologic preparations (e.g., cytospins, smears, ThinPrep) as is necessary; however, it is optimally performed on formalin-fixed, paraffin-embedded cell blocks for effusion samples.[110,115,116]

BOX 12-12

Optimal Approach to Effusion Cytopathology for Neoplastic Disease

Prepare samples in fresh state
Lyse grossly bloody effusions
Stain slides with both Diff-Quik and Papanicolaou
Always make a cell block
Perform immunocytochemistry on cell blocks
Positively identify mesothelial cells

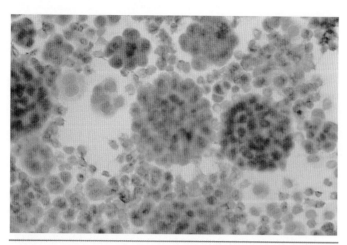

Figure 12-60 **Mesothelioma (cytospin).** This cytospin was stained with B72.3. The brown staining in the clusters can easily be interpreted as a positive result. However, this is an example of false-positive staining associated with cytospins. (Hematoxylin [H], DAB)

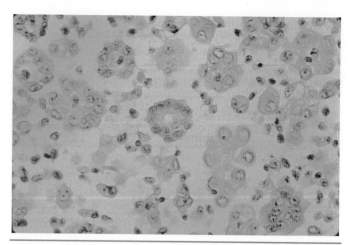

Figure 12-61 **Mesothelioma (cell block).** This cell block section from the same case as Figure 12-60 was also stained with B72.3 and shows a negative immunostaining result. This case illustrates how cell block preparations are optimal for immunocytochemistry in effusions because of the false background staining associated with cytospins, smears, and ThinPreps that is not encountered with cell block sections. (H, DAB)

 BOX   12-13

Effusion Immunocytochemistry on Cytospins/Smears

Cytospins are air-dried when the sample volume is low.
Red blood cells are lysed for sample optimization.
Cytospins are prepared using charged or silanated microscope slides.
Slides are air-dried for 30 minutes at room temperature.
Slides are refrigerated with desiccant.
Slides are equilibrated to room temperature for 30 minutes before opening.
Fixation is antibody-specific.
Carcinoma markers generally require alcohol fixation for 5 minutes.
Lymphoid markers generally require acetone fixation for 10 minutes.
Fixation performed immediately before immunostaining
Manufacturer's antibody specification sheet provides information on appropriate fixation methods.
Fixation time is critical.

From Fetsch PA, Abati A. Immunocytochemistry of effusion cytology: a contemporary review. Cancer Cytopathol 2001; 93:293-308.

Cytospins, Smears, and ThinPreps Versus Cell Blocks

Although cytospin preparations are often used successfully for immunocytochemistry in many types of specimens, they are less than ideal for effusions (Box 12-13). Cytospins are best used when the sample volume is small. Nonspecific and unexpected immunoreactivity can be a major problem in effusion samples resulting from the nature of the protein-rich fluid within which the cells are floating. Large, three-dimensional cell groups commonly encountered in cytospins may entrap immunologic reagents in the center leading to false-positive results. In addition, crushed, degenerated or necrotic cells may also contribute to background staining[115] (Figures 12-60 and 12-61).

The immunoreactivity of nine mesothelioma cell lines in air-dried cytospins and their corresponding cell block sections was investigated to determine the optimal type of sample preparation for mesothelial cells.[119] Using a panel of markers often used in effusion samples, it was determined that the expected results were seen in the cell block sections, whereas significant nonspecific immunoreactivity was observed in the cytospin samples.[119]

Although excellent results using smears and ThinPreps for immunocytochemistry have been claimed by some laboratories, these preparations may yield high background staining similar to cytospins because of the three-dimensional clusters of cells.[120-123] Cellular shrinkage resulting from fixation can also lend difficulty to the interpretation of staining patterns.[123] The methanol fixation of ThinPrep samples does not preserve antigens necessary for lymphoid marker studies, thus limiting antibody panels when using this type of preparation.[121]

A recent publication reports excellent results obtained on air-dried smears that are rehydrated and then postfixed in formal saline for 2 to 14 hours, followed by a 10-minute alcohol fixation. For all antibodies used, a short, heat-induced antigen retrieval pretreatment step was incorporated.[114,116] The authors have no experience with this technique.

Formalin-fixed cell block sections are the optimal form of sample preparation when performing immunostains on effusions due to ease of morphologic interpretations, standardized comparison with histologic material, minimal background staining, and expected immunostaining patterns (Box 12-14; see Figures 12-60 and 12-61). In addition, numerous sections may be obtained from a single sample, thus allowing for the evaluation of a large number of antigens. Archival material is also then available for future studies.[105]

Antibody Panels

Variations in immunoreactivity may be the result of technical issues such as sample size and type, fixation, pretreatment method (e.g., heat-induced epitope retrieval, enzyme

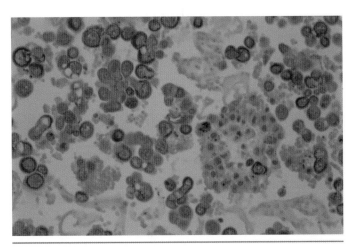

Figure 12-62 Adenocarcinoma, cytokeratin stain (cell block). This illustrates the strong staining of both adenocarcinoma and mesothelial cells for cytokeratins. The aggregates of macrophages are nonimmunoreactive. (H, DAB)

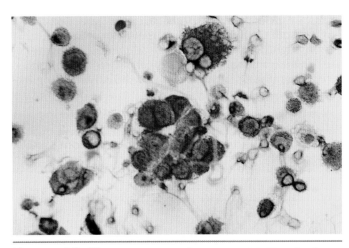

Figure 12-63 Malignant melanoma, HMB45 stain (cytospin). The HMB45 stain is immunoreactive with the melanoma cells, which may mimic mesothelial cells. (H, DAB)

BOX 12-14

Effusion Immunocytochemistry on Cell Blocks

Results are comparable to that of surgical pathology material.
Fixation should be avoided with formalin substitutes.
Charged slides are used.
Manufacturer's recommendations should be followed for pretreatment steps.
Overuse of microwave pretreatment can cause erroneous results.

From Fetsch PA, Abati A. Immunocytochemistry of effusion cytology: a contemporary review. Cancer Cytopathol 2001; 93: 293-308.

TABLE 12-22

General Immunocytochemistry Panel in Malignant Effusions with Unknown Primary

	Keratin	LCA	Calretinin*	HMB45/ MART-1
Carcinoma	+	−	−	−
Lymphoma	−	+	−	−
Melanoma	−	−	−	+
Mesothelioma	+	−	+	−

LCA, Leukocyte common antigen.
*Nuclear and cytoplasmic staining required for true immunoreactivity.

---

digestion, and so on), procedural technique, interlaboratory sensitivity, study size, and antibody clone. Differences in antigen expression may also be due to the effusion itself, where cells are floating in highly proteinaceous cavitary fluid which may contribute to nonspecific and unexpected immunoreactivity.[105,124,125]

Interpretation of immunoreactivity among pathologists also varies; in some studies, immunoreactivity in a single cell may be considered positive, whereas in others, immunoreactivity in a certain percentage of the cells is required for positivity.

An initial antibody screen may be performed when dealing with a neoplasm of unknown etiology to determine whether the malignancy is epithelial, lymphoid, melanoma, etc., with antibodies to cytokeratin (Figure 12-62). Leukocyte common antigen (LCA), S-100, and HMB45/ MART-1[17,115,126,127] (Table 12-22 and Figure 12-63). Additional antibodies can be tailored to the results of this initial test group.[115] A minimum of two markers should be used because of potentially heterogeneous antigen expression. Overlapping immunoreactivity in tumors may occur, so it is best to use several substantiating antibodies. In this scenario, monoclonal antibodies provide the greatest specificity with the least amount of background staining.[105]

Through the use of cell block preparations and a panel of antibodies appropriate for the differential diagnosis in question, immunocytochemistry conditions used in surgical pathology can be most closely replicated.

Reactive Mesothelial Cells Versus Adenocarcinoma Versus Malignant Mesothelioma

The identification of mesothelial cells in cytologic samples is often a diagnostic challenge (Tables 12-23 and 12-24; Boxes 12-15 and 12-16; see Table 12-22). This is particularly true in potentially malignant effusions in which reactive mesothelial cells may simulate adenocarcinoma cells and in the differentiation of adenocarcinoma from MM. However, the diagnosis of mesothelial proliferations, whether reactive or malignant, has traditionally been based on a negative pattern of immunostaining.[8,107,108] Reliable confirmatory markers of mesothelial cells were scarce until recently. Two mesothelium-related antibodies, calretinin and HBME-1, have shown promise for the positive identification of mesothelial cells[128] (see Table 12-24 and Boxes 12-15 and 12-16).

Calretinin typically stains with a stronger level of intensity and in a greater proportion of mesothelial cells than does HBME-1 in effusion samples. Calretinin shows a unique cytoplasmic and nuclear staining pattern which is characteristic of cells of mesothelial origin[128] (see Box 12-10) but does not distinguish benign from malignant cells.

Although neither HBME-1 nor calretinin can differentiate benign from malignant mesothelial cells in effusion cytology, the distinct advantage of consistently marking mesothelial cells is of great significance. This is particularly apparent when distinguishing between single adenocarcinoma cells and benign reactive mesothelial cells. For this clarification, anticalretinin is invaluable in a panel of markers in diagnostic effusion cytology.[128] Other positive

---

TABLE 12-23

Typical Immunoreactivity of Adenocarcinoma and Malignant Mesothelioma in Effusion Samples

NOTE: Unexpected reactivity has been reported for virtually all antibodies.

	CK	EMA	CEA	LeuM1	B72.3	BerEP4	CA19-9	Calretinin	E-cadherin	HBME-1
ACA	+	+	±	±	+	+	+	−	+	+
MM	+	+	−	−	−	−	−	+	±	+

From Fetsch PA, Abati A. Immunocytochemistry of effusion cytology-a contemporary review. Cancer Cytopathol 2001; 93:293-308.
CK, Cytokeratin; *EMA*, epithelial membrane antigen; *CEA*, carcinoembryonic antigen.

TABLE 12-24

Immunoreactivities of Commonly Used Antibodies for the Differentiation of Adenocarcinoma, Mesothelioma, and Reactive Mesothelial Cells

Antibody	Staining Pattern	Normal Tissue	Adenocarcinoma (%)	MM (%)	RM (%)
CEA	C/S	Mature PMN leukocytes	21-79	0-3	0-3
LeuM1	C/S	Myeloid cells, monocytes, macrophages, epithelial cells	32-51	0-14	0-4
B72.3	S	Secretory endometrium	44-80	0-8	0
BerEP4	C/S	Epithelial cells	32-96	0-17	0-8
CA19-9	C/S	Columnar epithelium of pancreas, stomach, gall bladder	27-86	0-3	13
BG-8		Bronchial glands of lung			
E-cadherin	S	Epithelial cells	87-100	0-100	0-14
Calretinin	C/N	Neural, mesothelial, Leydig/Sertoli endometrium/ovarian stromal, adrenal cortical cells; eccrine glands, kidney tubules	0-9 (focal)	88-100	80-100
HBME-1	S	Mesothelial cells	38-65	89	83

From Fetsch PA, Abati A. Immunocytochemistry of effusion cytology: a contemporary review. Cancer Cytopathol 2001; 93:293-308.
MM, Malignant mesothelioma; *RM*, reactive mesothelial cells; *CEA*, carcinoembryonic antigen; *C*, cytoplasmic; *S*, surface; *N*, nuclear; *PMN*, polymorphonuclear.

BOX 12-15

Comparison of Calretinin and HBME-1 for the Identification of Mesothelial Cells

All samples of mesothelial cells are immunoreactive with both antibodies.
Calretinin immunoreactivity is shown as both nuclear and peripheral cytoplasmic staining (biphasic staining).
Calretinin biphasic staining is specific for mesothelial cells.
Calretinin stains a larger percentage of mesothelial cells with a stronger degree of intensity than does HBME-1.
HBME-1 immunoreactivity is evidenced as membrane staining.
HBME-1 membrane staining is not specific for mesothelial cells.
Benign and malignant mesothelial cells stain with both antibodies.

HBME-1, Human mesothelial cell antibody.

BOX 12-16

Distinction of Mesothelial Cells from Adenocarcinoma Cells

It is difficult to distinguish reactive mesothelial cells from adenocarcinoma cells.
It is difficult to distinguish malignant mesothelioma cells from adenocarcinoma cells.
Adenocarcinoma markers are B72.3, BerEP4, CEA, LeuM1, and CA19-9.
Mesothelial markers are HBME-1 and calretinin.
Electron microscopy shows long, bushy microvilli in mesothelial cells.

HBME-1, Human mesothelial cell antibody.

mesothelial markers have been introduced, including OV632, thrombomodulin, cytokeratin 5/6, N-cadherin, CD44S, and WT1, with variable results.* There has also been speculation that markers such as p53, E-cadherin, and MOC-31 may be useful for the identification of reactive mesothelial cells.[138,140,141,156]

Some of the more commonly used antibodies in the differentiation of adenocarcinoma from MM are listed in Table 12-24.† Before the advent of calretinin and HBME-1, the diagnosis of MM had been that of a negative staining pattern with antibodies to BerEP4, LeuM1, B72.3, and carcinoembryonic antigen (CEA).‡ However, unexpected staining of mesothelial cells (benign or malignant) in a small proportion of samples caused difficulties with this panel.[119,135,163,164] Over the last several years, other epithelial/carcinoma markers, including MOC-31, blood group-related antigens, HMFG-2, and E-cadherin have been studied but often with conflicting results.§

The authors recommend an antibody panel consisting of B72.3, BerEP4, CA 19-9, and calretinin for the differentiation of adenocarcinoma from MM in effusions[105] (see Table 12-23). Of course, more extensive panels have been recommended by other authors for sound reasons that vary based on clinical scenarios and practice styles.[167] Although they are highly specific for adenocarcinoma, CEA, and LeuM1 are not recommended for the panel because the sensitivity of these antibodies is quite low and the staining of inflammatory cells can interfere with interpretation. In most cases, this panel can differentiate adenocarcinoma from MM.[105] This panel cannot determine the primary tumor site in cases of metastatic adenocarcinoma. A brief description and immunoreactivity rates of the most commonly used antibodies is in Table 12-24.

Cytokeratins and epithelial membrane antigen (EMA) are immunoreactive with reactive mesothelial cells, MM, and adenocarcinoma and thus are not usually considered to be diagnostic discriminators. These antibodies may be used to test general sample immunoreactivity (Figure 12-64; see Figure 12-62). A distinctive EMA pattern in MM has been described, which shows thick cell membrane staining at the edge of cell clusters highlighting the long microvillus projections,[133,168] whereas the staining of ACA cells is diffusely cytoplasmic.[133,168] This contrast in staining patterns is notoriously unreliable. Effusion studies have shown EMA positivity rates of 75% to 100% for MM, 91% for adenocarcinoma, and 6% for reactive cases.[149,157]

TAG-72 (B72.3). B72.3 recognizes a tumor-associated oncofetal antigen that is present in many adenocarcinomas, including lung, gastrointestinal tract, pancreas, breast, endometrium, and ovary.[169] It is not immunoreactive with leukemias, lymphomas, sarcomas, melanomas, or benign neoplasms. B72.3 can be seen on normal secretory endometrium but not on other normal tissues.[109,125,149,157,163] Immunoreactivity is indicated through a membrane staining pattern[169] (Figure 12-65).

On surgical samples adenocarcinoma immunoreactivity rates of 44% to 83% have been reported, whereas positivity rates of MM have been less than 5%.[124,129,134,158] Similar results have been noted in effusions; adenocarcinoma positivity rates fluctuate from 44% to 80%,[157,163] whereas MM and reactive effusions are usually negative or rarely positive (less than 10%).[149,157,163]

Human epithelial antigen (BerEP4). BerEP4 is produced by the immunization of mice with cells from the MCF7 breast cancer cell line. It reacts with two glycoproteins on the surface and in the cytoplasm of epithelial cells.[125,157,163,170] In contrast to other antiepithelial antibodies, it does not label benign mesothelial cells and only infrequent cases of MM are positive. BerEP4 does not react with nerve, glial, muscle, mesenchymal, or lymphoid tissues.[170] Immunoreactivity is typically demonstrated by membrane staining and may be accompanied by cytoplasmic staining (Figure 12-66).

BerEP4 immunoreactivity is variable, with ranges from 0% to 88% in MM and 32% to 100% in adenocarcinoma.[129,134,157-159,163,164] BerEP4 immunoreactivity in effu-

---

*References 120, 122, 124, 125, and 128-155.
†References 109, 124, 130, 132-135, and 157-162.
‡References 109, 124, 129, 133, 134, 136, 137, and 159.
§References 120, 124, 130, 134, 136-144, 163, 165, and 166.

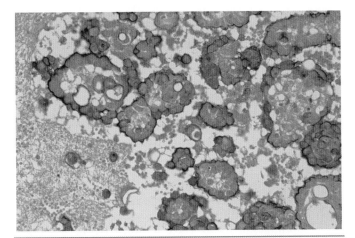

Figure 12-64 **Mesothelioma, epithelial membrane antigen stain (cell block).** The thick membrane staining of this mesothelioma is characteristic of mesothelial cells but can also be seen in other epithelial malignancies. (H, DAB)

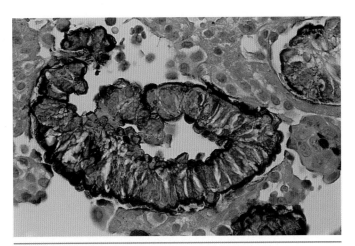

Figure 12-65 **Colonic adenocarcinoma, B72.3 stain (cell block).** The tumor cells are centrally located in a ribbon of characteristic morphology. The B72.3 exhibits a membranous pattern of staining, whereas the background macrophages and mesothelial cells are nonimmunoreactive. (H, DAB)

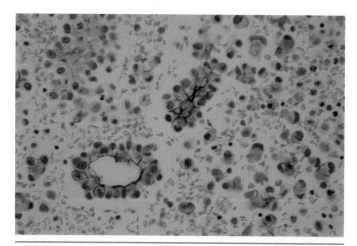

Figure 12-66 Micropapillary adenocarcinoma of the breast, Ber-EP4 stain (cell block). The malignant cells are present singly, in small papillary groups and in glandlike structures. Membranous and focally cytoplasmic staining is present with the Ber-EP4 stain. (H, DAB)

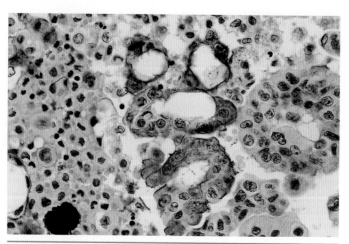

Figure 12-67 Pancreatic adenocarcinoma, CA19.9 (cell block). The adenocarcinoma cells in the central portion of the figure exhibit strong membranous staining and some cytoplasmic staining with CA19.9. Not all of the tumor cells are immunoreactive. (H, DAB)

sions have shown essentially negative immunostaining with MM and reactive mesothelial cells and immunoreactivity in adenocarcinoma from 32% to 96%.[157,159,163,164] A large scale effusion study revealed an 83% positivity in adenocarcinomas tested, which included immunoreactivity rates of 93% ovary, 88% gastrointestinal, 81% lung, and 73% breast.[164] A recent surgical pathology study reported immunoreactivity rates of 26% in MM with focal patterns of staining and 92% in adenocarcinoma with strong and diffuse patterns of staining in some samples and focal staining in others.[134] Ber-EP4 has a benefit over CEA, B72.3, and Leu-M1 with its high sensitivity, ease of interpretation (because of the high percentage of tumor cells stained), characteristic membranous staining pattern, and lack of cross-reactivity with background inflammatory cells.[171]

Blood group–related antigens (CA19-9/BG8). CA19-9 is biochemically related to the Lewis A blood group substance.[172] BG8 is a monoclonal antibody raised against the SK-LU-3 lung cancer that recognizes the blood group antigen Lewis Y.[129,173] These antibodies have shown positive staining in most adenocarcinoma of the pancreas and stomach and in a large proportion of colon and gallbladder tumors.* They are also present in approximately half of primary and metastatic ovarian tumors and salivary gland mucoepidermoid carcinomas.[133,174]

This antibody can be used as part of a panel for the differentiation of adenocarcinoma and MM because of their high specificity, with the knowledge that the sensitivity of these antibodies is variable.[134,142,148] As CA19-9 is a relatively specific marker for gastrointestinal tumors, it may potentially be used to determine the primary site of metastatic tumors of unknown origin; however, this organ-specificity for digestive cancers could not be confirmed.[165,174] Lung carcinomas and MM are most often nonimmunoreactive with anti-CA19-9[130,172] (Figure 12-67).

Immunoreactivity rates in surgical samples of adenocarcinoma are from 39% to 84%, with only rare positivity in MM.[144,148] Effusion studies have shown a similar pattern of immunoreactivity, with immunoreactivity rates in adeno-

carcinoma from 49% to 86% and only rare immunoreactivity in MM.[130,163] A positive staining reaction with CA19-9 would make the diagnosis of MM doubtful.

Carcinoembryonic antigen. CEA was initially used as a specific marker for colon cancer.* Although highly specific for adenocarcinoma cells, it is typically negative in benign, reactive, and malignant mesothelial cells.[157,175] Little or no reactivity occurs with nonmalignant tissues, except for granulocytes and mature neutrophils.[175] Colorectal carcinomas, lung, breast, and gastric cancers all show immunoreactivity with this antibody, which is evidenced by cytoplasmic staining.

CEA immunoreactivity varies considerably depending on the antibody clone used and the range of tumor types tested in various studies.[157] Polyclonal antibodies are the most sensitive; however, they have a disadvantage of strong staining of neutrophils and macrophages. They have also shown cross-reactivity with nonspecific cross-reacting antigens.[134,157] This cross-reactivity of polyclonal anti-CEA may lead to reported reactivity of mesothelial cells, as immunoreactivity for CEA in MM is not usually encountered with monoclonal CEA.[133,135] In surgical pathology, CEA is considered the most widely accepted marker for the differential diagnosis of adenocarcinoma and MM.[124] Surgical pathology studies have reported positivity rates in adenocarcinoma from 85% to 94%, whereas MM remains essentially nonimmunoreactive.[124,129,158]

Reactive and MM effusions are also usually negative for CEA.[149,156,157,163] However, immunoreactivity rates of adenocarcinoma in effusions range from 21% to 79%, which is considerably lower than that of tissue studies. This is most likely because of the type of antibody used, as monoclonal antibodies to CEA are typically less sensitive than polyclonal antibodies.[156,157,163,165] The use of polyclonal CEA in effusion cytology leads to strong background staining yielding a great deal of difficulty in interpretation, thus, CEA is not an optimal marker for the discrimination between MM and adenocarcinoma in effusion cytology.

Cluster designation group 15 (LeuM1). Cluster designation group 15 (CD15), a granulocyte-associated antigen, is

---

*References 124, 130, 133, 148, 163, 165, and 174.

*References 109, 125, 149, 156, 157, 163, and 165.

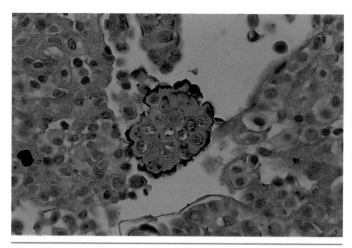

Figure 12-68 Colonic adenocarcinoma, LeuM1 stain (cell block). The centrally placed tumor cells exhibit a membrane pattern of staining. (H, DAB)

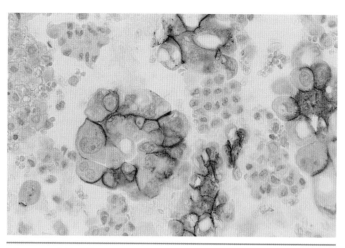

Figure 12-69 Breast adenocarcinoma, E-cadherin stain (cell block). The malignant cells show a strong membrane-staining pattern with some cytoplasmic staining. Background macrophages and mesothelial cells are nonimmunoreactive. (H, DAB)

associated with a variety of monoclonal antibodies including LeuM1.[176] These immunoglobulin M (IgM) isotype antibodies share immunoreactivity patterns and are reactive with mature neutrophils. Leu M1 reacts with human myelomonocytic antigen and lacto-N-fucopentose III, which is present on Reed Sternberg cells of Hodgkin's disease, many adenocarcinomas, and selective peripheral blood elements, exhibiting immunoreactivity with both a membrane and cytoplasmic immunostaining pattern.[109,125,157,176,177] LeuM1 is used as part of a panel for acute leukemias, diagnosis, and classification of Hodgkin's disease and in the differential diagnosis of adenocarcinoma vs. MM[176] (Figure 12-68; see Figure 12-54, *B*).

In surgical pathology studies the immunoreactivity rates for adenocarcinoma are from 50% to 78% and for MM, from 0% to 34%.[124,136,141,158] Reactive pleural tissue (i.e., reactive mesothelial cells) is typically nonreactive.[141]

The sensitivity of LeuM1 staining for adenocarcinoma in effusions does not achieve the same results as it does in histologic studies.[133] One effusion study found only 32% immunoreactivity in adenocarcinomas (showing only focal staining). However, all reactive mesothelial and MM cells were nonimmunoreactive.[157,176] This focal staining pattern may contribute to negative results seen in small-sized samples.[133] For effusion samples, the main drawback of LeuM1 is staining heterogeneity that causes limited use in samples of moderate to low cellularity. Although LeuM1 is an excellent marker for separating adenocarcinomas from MMs in surgical material, it is not recommended for the panel to distinguish between adenocarcinomas and MM in effusions.[129,134]

E-cadherin. E-cadherin (epithelial cadherin or uvomorulin; HECD-1) is expressed on the cell surfaces of nonneoplastic epithelial cells and their malignant counterparts; thus, it is potentially useful for the distinction of reactive mesothelial cells from well-differentiated carcinoma cells. It may also be helpful in the differentiation of adenocarcinoma from MM* (Figure 12-69).

Histologic studies have shown negative or rare immunoreactivity in MM, with positivity in 81% to 93% of adenocarcinomas.[139,148] Effusion studies have not been as conclusive, in large part because of antibody clones used.[129,148] E-cadherin has been found in 97% of adenocarcinomas, 46% of MMs, and 14% of reactive mesothelial cells.[138] A distinct membranous pattern has been observed in ductal breast adenocarcinoma, whereas in other adenocarcinomas and MMs, both cytoplasmic and membranous staining was observed.[138,178]

Additional studies evaluating cell block sections of effusions noted that all MM tested were nonimmunoreactive, whereas all adenocarcinomas were immunoreactive.[139]

Other cytologic sample preparations have also yielded conflicting results. In previously Pap-stained smears, 100% of MM were positive, 87% of adenocarcinomas were positive, and all reactive effusions were negative.[120]

Calretinin. Calretinin, a neuron-specific calcium-binding protein, is strongly expressed in neural tissues and a few non-neural cell types, including mesothelium.* Antibodies to this antigen are strongly reactive with malignant and benign mesothelial cells, showing both nuclear and cytoplasmic staining.[155] In adenocarcinomas, calretinin is usually nonimmunoreactive or may show weak cytoplasmic staining.[132,147,179,180] The diagnostic reliability of calretinin immunostaining for a positive identification of MM in histologic and cytologic preparations is becoming increasingly evident with the advent of purified antibodies[134,152] (Figures 12-70 and 12-71).

Histologic studies have yielded immunoreactivity rates for MM ranging from 92% to 100%, with rare adenocarcinomas showing nuclear staining.[132,147] Effusion studies utilizing various cytologic preparations (cell blocks, cytospins, and Pap-stained smears) have also shown calretinin to be a sensitive and specific marker of reactive and malignant mesothelial cells, with immunoreactivity rates of 88% to 100% for MM and 80% to 100% for reactive effusions.[120,153-155,180] Calretinin is an important marker in diagnostic effusion cytology, particularly when there is a need to distinguish between single adenocarcinoma cells and reactive mesothelial cells. This view has been corroborated by other investigators.[181]

---

*References 120, 134, 138, 139, 148, and 178.

*References 120, 132, 136, 141, 147, 152, 179, and 180.

Human mesothelial cell antibody (HBME-1). The human mesothelial cell antibody, HBME-1, originated from a suspension of human mesothelioma cells from patients with malignant epithelioid mesothelioma. This antibody reacts with an antigen present on the membrane of mesothelial cells.[130,141,150,182] No immunoreactivity has been observed in normal cells other than mesothelial cells; however, immunoreactivity has been found in some sarcomas, chordomas, lymphomas, and papillary and follicular carcinomas of the thyroid.[129,150] Epithelioid mesotheliomas stain in a thick membrane pattern, whereas in adenocarcinoma, this pattern is cytoplasmic, or thin surface staining.[130,182] Desmoplastic/sarcomatous MM cells are usually nonimmunoreactive, which has been attributed to the loss of cell surface microvilli in these variants[150] (Figure 12-72).

Many tissue studies have shown overlapping staining patterns with anti-HBME-1 in MM and adenocarcinoma.[129,134,142,183] One study found a sensitivity of 89% and a specificity of 70% of HBME-1 for MM and concluded that it was less efficient than other markers for the positive identification of MM.[141] Similarly, another investigation reported immunoreactivity in 76% of MM tested, 73% of adenocarcinomas, and 83% of reactive pleural tissue.[141]

Likewise, an effusion study showed immunoreactivity of 89% with MM and 65% with adenocarcinoma. The staining pattern elicited was both thick and thin membrane staining present in selected cases of both entities.[130] Thus, in general, the use of HBME-1 is limited because of its relative lack of specificity for cells of mesothelial origin and overlapping staining patterns.

Less commonly used mesothelial and adenocarcinoma-associated markers are listed in Tables 12-25 and 12-26. A short list of recent immunocytochemical applications to the diagnosis of effusions follows (Table 12-27).

 # ADDITIONAL ANCILLARY STUDIES

Fluorescence in Situ Hybridization

Because of the known numerical abnormalities present in the chromosomes of malignant cells, fluorescence in situ hybridization (FISH) has been used for the detection of cellular populations exhibiting aneusomy. Theoretically, this should be a highly sensitive and specific way to evaluate equivocal effusions as has been shown with mesothelioma cell lines.[188] Common numerical and structural aberrations in malignant mesothelial cells involve chromosomes 1, 3, 6, 7, and 9.[119,189]

FISH studies performed on ThinPrep slides of effusions, evaluating hyperdiploidy for chromosomes 3, 8, 10 and 12, showed that FISH can detect hyperdiploid malignant cells and is especially helpful when the majority of the cells cannot be distinguished from a benign atypical or a malignant population of cells. It has been found to be less helpful for detecting a small population of malignant cells obscured by an inflammatory or reactive background.[190]

The chromosome 17 alpha satellite probe may also prove useful for distinguishing benign from malignant effusions. Done on alcohol fixed specimens with pretreatment with

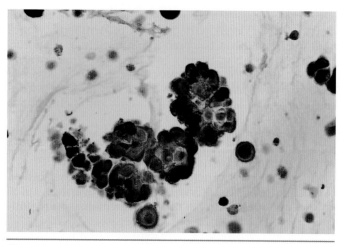

Figure 12-70 Malignant mesothelioma (MM), calretinin stain (cell block). The malignant cells exhibit strong nuclear and cytoplasmic staining. (H, DAB)

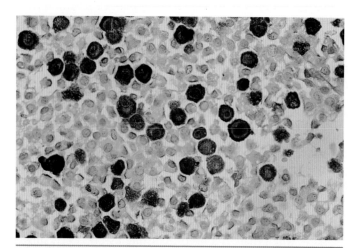

Figure 12-71 Reactive mesothelial cells, calretinin stain (cell block). This low-power view of a cell block highlights the reactive mesothelial cells, which show strong immunostaining in a nuclear and cytoplasmic pattern for calretinin. (H, DAB)

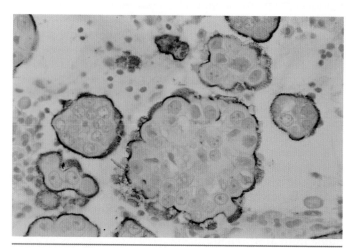

Figure 12-72 Mesothelioma, HBME stain (cell block). This highlights the thick membrane pattern of staining, which may be seen in mesotheliomas. (H, DAB)

protease K before hybridization, the chromosome index of malignant specimens was 2.23, and that of benign samples was 1.98. Benign samples showed a diploid population of cells in more than 85% of samples; however, bizarre signals were seen in a small percentage of benign samples.[191] Using centromeric probes for chromosomes 7 and 9 in cytologic samples of MM and benign effusions with reactive mesothelial cells, investigators noted that polysomy for chromosomes 7 or 9 is a common finding in MM and uncommon in reactive effusions. Thus, in cases of indeterminate morphology, FISH may potentially be a diagnostic adjunct.[189]

Histochemistry

The detection of significant mucicarmine in malignant samples generally signifies the diagnosis of adenocarcinoma. A recently performed evaluation of histochemical methods for the detection of intracytoplasmic mucin was done looking at different types of mucin stains performed on cytospins and cell blocks of known malignancies.[192] The study made several important conclusions: PAS with diastase is a more sensitive test for the detection of intracytoplasmic mucin in both cell blocks and cytospins; mucicarmine shows preferential staining for cell

---

TABLE 12-25

Less Commonly Used Mesothelium-Associated Markers

Marker	Description
CD44[146,147,148,151]	Transmembrane protein that acts as the principal receptor for hyaluronic acid
	Recently developed probe found to be predictive for MM in tissue samples but unreliable for use in effusions
CK5/6[129,134,147]	Relatively select expression of cytokeratin 5 in mesothelial cells compared to adenocarcinoma
	No published studies regarding effusions using this antibody
Thrombo-modulin*	Glycoproteins normally present in mesothelial cells
	Variable staining rates in both tissue and effusion studies
WT-1[129,134,141,148]	Tumor suppressor gene involved in the development of MM
	Potentially useful in the differentiation of MM from pulmonary adenocarcinoma
	No published studies regarding effusions using this antibody
N-Cadherin†	Expressed in mesothelial cells
	Variable sensitivity and specificity for MM

MM, Malignant mesothelioma.
*References 129, 130, 133, 134, 142, and 147.
†References 125, 129, 134, 138, 139, and 159.

TABLE 12-26

Less Commonly Used Adenocarcinoma Markers

Marker	Description
HMFG-2[124,125,133]	Cell surface glycoprotein used to distinguish adenocarcinoma and MM
	Strong cytoplasmic stain characteristic of adenocarcinoma
	Conflicting results from antibody source and disagreement in interpretation
MOC-31[129,134,140-142,184]	Present on most normal and malignant epithelia
	Reacts with the majority of adenocarcinomas and rarely with MM and reactive mesothelial cells
TTF-1[148]	Tissue-specific transcription factor expressed in thyroid and lung
	MM-negative with 75% of lung adenocarcinoma-positive

MM, Malignant mesothelioma.

TABLE 12-27

Recent Immunocytochemical Findings

Marker	Description
HLA class I antigens	Mesothelial cells and macrophages are strongly positive for HLA antigens A, B, and C
	Metastatic breast carcinoma cells show paucity of HLA class I staining
	Can be used as potential diagnostic discriminator in effusions[185]
Combining ICC for Ber-EP4 only and DNA-cytometry in equivocal effusions	Sensitivity for positive identification of malignant cells is 89%, with 95% specificity
	Positive predictive value of 98%
	Negative predictive value 79%[186]
CA15-3	High sensitivity and specificity for adenocarcinomas, particularly of breast etiologic factors in cell block material from effusions[187]

blocks; and by prolonging incubation time of staining protocols, an increase in the mucicarmine detection rate was seen.[192]

Flow Cytometry

Flow cytometry has been shown to be a rapid and effective method for the evaluation of effusions and peritoneal washings. The detection of Ber-EP4 positive cells using flow cytometry is highly indicative of carcinoma cells in effusions, whereas false positives in benign effusions are relatively infrequent.[193] Other studies have shown the ability of flow cytometry to detect malignant populations of cells in cytologically benign effusions.[194]

Imaging

Controversy in the recent literature exists over the use of DNA image cytometry for the distinction of benign versus malignant cell populations in effusions. Although some authors claim that the combination of morphology and DNA cytometry results in a highly specific and sensitive prediction of malignancy, others believe that the additional diagnostic value of DNA image cytometry is limited.[194-196]

Confocal laser scanning microscopy has been used for three-dimensional reconstruction of cell clusters in serous fluids.[197] Using this technology, distinct architectural differences were noted between cell clusters of MM and adenocarcinoma. In MM, the clusters were in one of the following four configurations: obvious central collagen cores by light microscopy, randomly coiled cords of cells, tissue fragments with pseudoacinar formations, and small papillae with central cores.[197] Conversely, adenocarcinomas showed tightly cohesive cells with true acinar formation and exhibited a more orderly pattern in general.[197]

Telomerase

Telomerase is inactive in most somatic cells but has been found to be reactivated in a majority of cancers. It is a ribonucleoprotein that synthesizes telomeric DNA on chromosome ends and appears to be related to the aging and immortality of cells. The telomerase repeat amplification protocol (TRAP) has been used along with cytologic examination in effusion samples.[198,199] The results of initial studies are intriguing, with excellent correlation with malignant cytology samples aside from those with poor cellular preservation (poor preservation of RNA). Cytologically benign samples in patients with advanced metastatic malignancies were positive for TRAP, raising questions regarding TRAP being beyond the detection of morphologic malignancies.[198] This may represent a useful addition to immunohistochemistry in the future but awaits further study.[198-200]

References

1. Carter D, True L, Otis CN. Serous membranes. In: Sternberg SS, editor. Histology for pathologists. 2nd ed. Philadelphia: Lippincott-Raven; 1997. pp.223-239.
2. Sherer DM, Eliakim R, Abulafia O. The rule of angiogenesis in the accumulation of peritoneal fluid in benign conditions and the development of malignant ascites in the female. Gynecol Obstet Invest 2000; 50(4):217-224.
3. Kjeldsberg CR, Knight JA, editors. Body fluids: laboratory examination of amniotic, cerebrospinal, seminal, serous and synovial fluids. 3rd ed. Chicago: ASCP Press; 1993. pp.159-222.
4. Porcel JM, Alvarez M, Salud A, et al. Should a cytologic study be ordered in transudative pleural effusions? Chest 1999; 116:1836-1837.
5. Light RW. Management of pleural effusions. J Formos Med Assoc 2000; 99(7):523-531.
6. Light RW. Useful tests on the pleural fluid in the management of patients with pleural effusions. Curr Opin Pulm Med 1999; 5(4):245-249.
7. Bedrossian CWM. Malignant effusions: a multimodal approach to cytologic diagnosis. New York: Igaku-Shoin; 1994.
8. Bibbo M. Comprehensive cytopathology. 2nd ed. Philadelphia: WB Saunders; 1997. pp.551-621.
9. Tao L-C. Cytopathology of malignant effusions. Chicago: ASCP Press, 1996.
10. Bennett JC, Plum F, editors. Cecil's textbook of medicine. 20th ed., vol. 1. Philadelphia: WB Saunders; 1996.
11. Nance KV, Shermer RW, Askin FB. Diagnostic efficacy of pleural biopsy as compared with that of pleural fluid examination. Modern Pathol 1991; 4:320-324.
12. Ong KC, Indumathi V, Poh WT, et al:. The diagnostic yield of pleural fluid cytology in malignant pleural effusions. Singapore Med J 2000; 41(1):19-23.
13. Dekker A, Bupp PA. Cytology of serous effusions: an investigation into the usefulness of cell blocks versus smears. Am J Clin Pathol 1978; 70(6):855-860.
14. Dhundee J, Cotter M, Gibbs AR. Examination of cytological smears and clot sections prepared from pleural fluids: a comparative study. Cytopathology 1996; 7(6):406-413.
15. Garcia LW, Ducatman BS, Wang HH. The value of multiple fluid specimens in the cytological diagnosis of malignancy. Mod Pathol 1994; 7(6):665-668.
16. Filie A, Copeland C, Wilder AM, et al. Individual specimen triage of effusion samples: an improvement in the standard of practice, or a waste of resources? Diagn Cytopathol 2000; 22(1):7-10.
17. Beaty M, Fetsch PA, Wilder AM, et al. Effusion cytology of malignant melanoma. Cancer Cytopathol 1997; 81(1):57-63.
18. Wojcik EM, Naylor B. Collagen balls in peritoneal washings: prevalence, morphology, origin and significance. Acta Cytol 1992; 36(4):446-470.
19. Stevens MW, Leong AS-Y, Fazzalari NL, et al. Cytopathology of malignant mesothelioma: a stepwise logistic regression analysis. Diagn Cytopathol 1992; 8:333-341.
20. Wojono KJ, Olson JL, Sherman ME. Cytopathology of pleural effusions after radiotherapy. Acta Cytol 1994; 38:1-8.
21. Bedrossian CW. Diagnostic problems in serous effusions. Diagn Cytopathol 1998; 19(2):131-137.
22. Koss LG. Diagnostic cytology and its histopathologic bases. 4th ed. Philadelphia: JB Lippincott; 1992.
23. Spriggs AI, Boddington MM. Atlas of serous fluid cytopathology: a guide to the cells of pleura, pericardial, peritoneal and hydrocele fluids. In: Gresham GA, editor. Current histopathology series, vol. 14. Kluwer Academic Publishers: Dordrecht, Netherlands; 1989.
24. Veress JF, Koss LG, Schreiber K. Eosinophilic pleural effusions. Acta Cytol 1979; 23:40-44.
25. Selvaggi SM, Midgal S. Cytologic features of atypical mesothelial cells in peritoneal dialysis fluid. Diagn Cytopathol 1990; 6:22-25.
26. Taniguchi H, Mukae H, Matsumoto N, et al. Elevated IL-5 levels in pleural fluid of patients with paragonimiasis westermani. Clin Exp Immunol 2001; 123(1):94-98.

27. Laurini JA, Garcia A, Elsner B. Relation between natural killer cells and neoplastic cells in serous fluids. Diagn Cytopathol 2000; 22(6):347-350.

28. Jones D, Lieb T, Narita M, et al. Mesothelial cells in tuberculous pleural effusion of HIV-infected patients. Chest 2000; 117(1):289-291.

29. Ellison E, Lapuerta P, Martin SE. Cytologic features of mycobacterial pleuritis: logistic regression and statistical analysis of a blinded, case-controlled study. Diagn Cytopathol 1998; 19(3):173-176.

30. Reechaipichitkul W, Lulitanond V, Sungkeeree S, et al. Rapid diagnosis of tuberculous pleural effusion using polymerase chain reaction.Southeast Asian J Trop Med Public Health 2000; 31(3):509-514.

31. San Jose ME, Valdes L, Saavedra MJ, et al. Lymphocyte populations in tuberculous pleural effusions. Ann Clin Biochem 1999; 36(4):492-500.

32. Liam CK, Lim KH, Wong CM. Differences in pleural fluid characteristics, white cell count and biochemistry of tuberculous and malignant pleural effusions. Med J Malaysia 2000; 55(2):21-28.

33. Naylor B. The pathognomonic cytologic picture of rheumatoid pleuritis: the 1989 Maurice Goldblatt Cytology Award Lecture. Acta Cytologica 1990; 34(4):465-473.

34. Fernandez-Muixi J, Vidal F, Razquin S, et al. Pleural effusion as initial presentation of rheumatoid arthritis: cytological diagnosis. Arch Bronconeumol 1996; 32(8):427-429.

35. Nosanchuk JS, Naylor B. A unique cytologic picture in pleural fluid from patients with rheumatoid arthritis. Am J Clin Pathol 1968; 50:330-335.

36. Naylor B. Cytological aspects of pleural, peritoneal and pericardial fluids from patients with systemic lupus erythematosus. Cytopathology 1992; 3(1):1-8.

37. Dubois EL. Lupus erythematosus. 2nd ed. Los Angeles: University of Southern California Press; 1974.

38. Jones PE, Rawcliffe P, White N, et al. Painless ascites in systemic lupus erythematosus. Br Med J 1977; 1(6075):1513.

39. Hargraves MM, Richmond H, Morton R. Presentation of two bone marrow elements: the "tart cell" and the "LE" cell. Proc Staff Meet Mayo Clin 1948; 23:25-28.

40. Reda MG, Baigelman W. Pleural effusion in systemic lupus erythematosus. Acta Cytol 1980; 24(6):553-557.

41. Kaplan AI, Zakher F, Sabin S. Drug-induced lupus erythematosus with *in vivo* lupus erythematosus cells in pleural fluid. Chest 1978; 73:875-876.

42. Chao T-Y. Lupus erythematosus cells in pleural effusions: diagnostic of systemic lupus erythematosus? Acta Cytologica 1997; 41(4):1231-1233.

43. Greis M, Atay Z. Zytomorphologische begleitreaction bei malignen pleuraergüssen. Pneumatologie 1990; 44(Suppl):262-264.

44. Hunder GG, Pierre RV. In vivo LE cell formation in synovial fluid. Arthritis Rheum 1970; 13:448-451.

45. Fazio J, Friedman HD, Swerdlow J, et al. Diagnosis of systemic lupus erythematosus in an elderly male of pericardial fluid cytology: a case report. Diagn Cytopathol 1998; 18(5):346-348.

46. Light RW, George RB. Incidence and Significance of pleural effusions after abdominal surgery. Chest 1976; 69(5):621-625.

47. Sadikot RT, Rogers JT, Cheng DS, et al. Pleural fluid characteristics of patients with symptomatic pleural effusion after coronary artery bypass graft surgery. Arch Intern Med 2000; 160(17):2665-2668.

48. Lee YC, Vaz MA, Ely KA, et al. Symptomatic persistent post-coronary artery bypass graft pleural effusions requiring operative treatment: clinical and histologic features. Chest 2001; 119(3):795-800.

49. Judson MA, Handy JR, Sahn SA. Pleural effusions following lung transplantation. Time course, characteristics, and clinical implications. Chest 1996; 109(5):1190-1194.

50. Xiol X, Castellote J, Baliellas C, et al. Spontaneous bacterial empyema in cirrhotic patients: analysis of eleven cases. Hepatology 1990; 11(3):365-370.

51. Vezza PR, Wilder AM, Holland SM, et al. Detection of fungal organisms in pulmonary cytology samples of chronic granulomatous disease: a comparison of alternate techniques. Diagn Cytopathol 2001; 24(3):226-227.

52. Abati A, Cajigas A, Holland SM, et al. Chronic granulomatous disease of childhood: respiratory cytology. Diagn Cytopathol 1996; 15(2):98-102.

53. Goodman ZD, Gupta PK, Frost JK, et al. Cytodiagnosis of viral infections in body cavity fluids. Acta Cytol 1979; 23:204-208.

54. Warren WH. Malignancies involving the pericardium. Semin Thorac Cardiovasc Surg 2000; 12(2):119-129.

55. Chen LM, Chao TY, Chiang JH, et al. Examination of pericardial effusions by cytology and immunocytochemistry. Zhonghua Yi Xue Za Zhi (Taipei) 1996; 58(4):248-253.

56. Wilkes JD, Fidias P, Vaickus L, et al. Malignancy-related pericardial effusion: 127 cases from the Roswell Park Cancer Institute. Cancer 1995; 76(8):1377-1387.

57. Bardales RH, Stanley MW, Schaefer RF, et al. Secondary pericardial malignancies: a critical appraisal of the role of cytology, pericardial biopsy, and DNA ploidy analysis. Am J Clin Pathol 1996; 106(1):29-34.

58. Zakowski MF, Ianuale-Shanerman A. Cytology of pericardial effusions in AIDS patients. Diagn Cytopathol 1993; 9(3):266-269.

59. Prakash UB, Reiman HM. Comparison of needle biopsy with cytologic analysis for the evaluation of pleural effusion: analysis of 414 cases. Mayo Clin Proc 1985; 60(3):158-164.

60. Kumar ND, Bhatia A, Misra K, et al. Comparison of pleural fluid cytology and pleural biopsy in the evaluation of pleural effusion. J Indian Med Assoc 1995; 93(8):307-309.

61. Filho LA, Bisi H, Bortolan J, et al. Frequency of adenmocarcinomas in serous effusions. Rev Assoc Med Bras 1999; 45(4):327-336.

62. Churg A, Colby TV, Cagle P, et al. The separation of benign and malignant mesothelial proliferations. Am J Surg Pathol 2000; 24(9):1183-1200.

63. Renshaw AA, Dean BR, Antman KH, et al. The role of cytologic evaluation of pleural fluid in the diagnosis of malignant mesothelioma. Chest 1997; 111(1);106-109.

64. Koss L. Benign and malignant mesothelial proliferations. Am J Surg Pathol 2001; 25(4):548-549.

65. Garcia-Lopez MP, Barrera-Rodriguez R. Malignant mesothelioma: clinical and radiological description of 45 cases with and without asbestos exposure. Salud Publica Mex 2000; 42(6):511-519.

66. Kitazume H, Kitamura K, Mukai K, et al. Cytologic differential diagnosis among reactive mesothelial cells, malignant mesothelioma, and adenocarcinoma: utlility of combined E-cadherin and calretinin immunostaining. Cancer Cytopathol 2000; 90(1):55-60.

67. Reuter K, Raptopolous V, Reale F, et al. Diagnosis of peritoneal mesothelioma: computed tomography, sonography and fine needle aspiration biopsy. Am J Radiol 1984; 140:1189-1194.

68. Sterrett G, Whitaker D, Shilkin KB, et al. Fine-needle aspiration cytology of malignant mesothelioma. Acta Cytol 1987; 31:185-193

69. Tao LC. Aspiration biopsy cytology of mesothelioma. Diagn Cytopathol 1989; 5(X):14-21.

70. Tao LC. The cytopathology of mesothelioma. Acta Cytol 1979; 23:209-213.

71. Dusenbery D, Grimes MM, Frable WJ. Fine-needle aspiration cytology of localized fibrous tumor of pleura. Diagn Cytopathol 1992; 8:444-450.

72. Thomas T, Hayes MM. Pericellular lacunae in the diagnosis of metastatic carcinoma in effusions: is this a useful sign? Diagn Cytopathol 1996; 15(3):193-196.

73. Price BA, Ehya H, Lee JH. Significance of pericellular lacunae in cell blocks of effusions. Acta Cytologica 1992; 36(3):334-337.

74. Bottles K, Reznicek MJ, Holly EA, et al. Cytologic criteria to diagnose adenocarcinoma in pleural effusions. Mod Pathol 1991; 4(6):677-681.

75. Yu GH, Sack MJ, Baloch ZW, et al. Occurrence of intercellular spaces (windows) in metastatic adenocarcinoma in serous fluids: a cytomorphologic, histochemical, and ultrastructural study. Diagn Cytopathol 1999; 20(3): 115-119.

76. Bernard N. Pleural, peritoneal and pericardial fluids. In Bibbo M, editors. Comprehensive cytology. 2nd ed. Philadelphia: WB Saunders; 1997.

77. Renshaw AA, Madge R, Sugarbaker DJ, et al. Malignant pleural effusions after resection of pulmonary adenocarcinoma. Acta Cytol 1998; 42(5):1111-1115.

78. Dresler CM, Fratelli C, Babb J. Prognostic value of positive pleural lavage in patients with lung cancer resection. Ann Thorac Surg 1999; 67(5):1435-1439.

79. Kjellberg SI, Dresler CM, Goldberg M. Pleural cytologies in lung cancer without pleural effusions. Ann Thorac Surg 1997; 64(4):941-944.

80. Renshaw AA, Comiter CV, Nappi D, et al. Effusion cytology of renal cell carcinoma. Cancer Cytopathol 1998; 84:148-152.

81. Renshaw AA, Nappi D, Cibas ES. Cytology of metastatic adenocarcinoma of the prostate in pleural effusions. Diagn Cytopathol 1996; 15(2):103-107.

82. Ronnett BM, Zahn CM, Kurman RJ, et al. Disseminated peritoneal adneomucinosis and peritoneal mucinous carcinomatosis: a clinicopathologic analysis of 109 cases with emphasis on distinguishing pathologic features, site of origin, prognosis and relationship to pseudomyxoma peritonei. Am J Surg Pathol 1995; 19:1390-1408.

83. Jackson SL, Fleming RA, Loggie BW, et al. Gelatinous ascites: a cytohistologic study of pseudomyxoma peritonei in 67 patients. Mod Pathol 2001; 14(7):664-671.

84. Palmer HE, Wilson CS, Bardales RH. Cytology and flow cytometry of malignant effusions of multiple myeloma. Diagn Cytopathol 2000; 22(3):147-151.

85. Simsir A, Fetsch P, Stetler-Stevenson M, et al. Immunophenotypic analysis of non-Hodgkin's lymphomas in cytologic specimens: a correlative study of immunocytochemical and flow cytometric technique. Diagn Cytopathol 1999; 20(5):278-284.

86. Murphy M, Signoretti S, Nasser I, et al. Detection of concurrent/recurrent non-Hodgkin's lymphoma in effusions by PCR. Hum Pathol 1999; 30(11):1361-1366.

87. Dunphy CH. Combined cytomorphologic and immunophenotypic approach to evaluation of effusions for lymphomatous involvement. Diagn Cytopathol 1996; 15(5): 427-430.

88. Santos GC, Longatto-Filho A, de Carvalho LV, et al. Immunocytochemical study of malignant lymphoma in serous effusions. Acta Cytol 2000; 44(4):539-542.

89. Bourantas KL, Tsiara S, Panteli A, et al. Pleural effusion in chronic myelomonocytic leukemia. Acta Haematol 1998; 99(1):34-37.

90. Perez MT, Cabello-Inchausti B, Viamonte M Jr, et al. Pleural body cavity-based lymphoma. Ann Diagn Pathol 1998; 2(2):127-134.

91. Matolcsy A. Primary effusional lymphoma: a new non-Hodgkin's lymphoma entity. Pathol Oncol Res 1999; 5(2):87-89.

92. Ansari MQ, Dawson DB, Nador R, et al. Primary body cavity-based AIDS-related lymphomas. Am J Clin Pathol 1996; 105(2):221-229.

93. Ascoli V, Signoretti S, Onetti-Muda A, et al. Primary effusion lymphoma in HIV-infected patients with multicentric Castleman's disease. J Pathol 2001; 193:200-209.

94. Olson PR, Silverman JF, Powers CN. Pleural fluid cytology of Hodgkin's disease: cytomorphologic features and the value of immunohistochemical studies. Diagn Cytopathol 2000; 22(1):21-24.

95. Lechapt-Zalcman E, Rieux C, Cordonnier C, et al. Post-transplantation lymphoproliferative disorder mimicking a nonspecific lymphocytic pleural effusion in a bone marrow transplant recipient: a case report. Acta Cytol 1999; 43(2):239-242.

96. Hoffmann H, Schlette E, Actor J, et al. Pleural post-transplantation lymphoproliferative disorder following liver transplantation. Arch Pathol Lab Med 2001; 125(3): 419-423.

97. Abadi MA, Zakowski MF. Cytologic features of sarcomas in fluids. Cancer Cytopathol 1998; 84:71-76.

98. Renshaw AA, Nappi D, Sugarbaker DJ, et al. Effusion cytology of esophageal carcinoma. Cancer 1997; 81(6): 365-372.

99. Walts AW. Optimization of the peritoneal lavage. Diagn Cytopathol 1998; 18:265-269.

100. Zuna RE, Behrens A. Peritoneal washing cytology in gynecologic cancers: long-term follow-up of 355 patients. J Natl Cancer Inst 1996; 88:980-987.

101. Johnson TL, Kumar NB, Hopkins M, et al. Cytologic features of ovarian tumors of low malignant potential in peritoneal fluids. Acta Cytol 1988; 32:513-518.

102. Weir BB, Bell DA. Cytologic identification of serous neoplasm in peritoneal fluids, Acta Cytol 1998; 42:1220.

103. Sidawy MK, Silverberg SG. Endosalpingiosis in female peritoneal washings: a diagnostic pitfall. Intern J Gynecol Pathol 1987; 6:340-346.

104. Sakuma N, Kamei T, Ishihara T. Ultrastructure of pleural mesothelioma and pulmonary adenocarcinoma in malignant effusions as compared with reactive mesothelial cells. Acta Cytol 1999; 43(5):777-785.

105. Fetsch PA, Abati A. Immunocytochemistry of effusion cytology: a contemporary review. Cancer Cytopathol 2001; 93:293-308.

106. Bedrossian CWM. Special stains, the old and the new: the impact of immunocytochemistry in effusion cytology. Diagn Cytopathol 1998; 18(2):141-149.

107. Koss LG. Diagnostic cytology and its histopathologic bases. Philadelphia: JB Lippincott; 1961. pp.272-302.

108. Tao L-C. Cytopathology of malignant effusions. Chicago: ASCP Press; 1996.

109. Kho-Duffin J, Tao L-C, Cramer H, et al. Cytologic diagnosis of malignant mesothelioma, with particular emphasis on the epithelial noncohesive cell type. Diagn Cytopathol 1999; 20(2):57-62.

110. Abati A, Fetsch PA, Filie A. If cells could talk: the application of new techniques to cytopathology. Clin Lab Med 1998; 18(3):561-583.

111. Fetsch PA, Abati A. Overview of the clinical immunohistochemistry laboratory: regulations and troubleshooting guidelines. In: Javois LC. Methods in molecular biology (vol. 115): immunocytochemical methods and protocols. Humana Press: Totowa, NJ; 1998. pp.405-414.

112. Department of Health and Human Services, Health Care Financing Administration. Clinical Laboratory Improvement Amendments of 1988: Final Rule. *Fed Reg* 1992; 57:7001-7288.

113. College of American Pathologists Laboratory Accreditation Program. Standards for Laboratory Accreditation, Commission of Laboratory Accreditation Inspection Checklist. Sec. 1, 8; 2000.

114. Leong A S-Y. Immunostaining of cytologic specimens. Am J Clin Pathol 1996; 105(2):139-140.

115. Nadji M, Ganjei P, Morales A. Immunocytochemistry in contemporary cytology: the technique and its application. Lab Med 1994; 25(8):502-508.

116. Leong A S-Y, Suthipintawong C, Vinyuvat S. Immunostaining of cytologic preparations: a review of technical problems. Appl Immunohistochem 1999; 7(3):214-220.

117. Lozano MD, Panizo A, Toledo GR, et al. Immunocytochemistry in the differential diagnosis of serous effusions: a comparative evaluation of eight monoclonal antibodies in Papanicolaou-stained smears. Cancer 2001; 93(1):68-72.

118. Jensen ML, Johansen P. Immunocytochemical staining of smears and corresponding cell blocks from serous effusions: a follow-up and comparative investigation. Diagn Cytopathol 1996; 15(1):33-36.

119. Pass H, Stevens E, Oie H, et al. Characteristics of nine newly derived mesothelioma cell lines. Ann Thorac Surg 1995; 59:835-844.

120. Kitazume H, Kitamura K, Mukai K, et al. Cytologic differential diagnosis among reactive mesothelial cells, malignant mesothelioma, and adenocarcinoma: utility of combined E-cadherin and calretinin immunostaining. Cancer Cytopathol 2000; 90(1):55-60.

121. Leung SW, Bedard YC. Immunocytochemical staining on ThinPrep-processed smears. Mod Pathol 1996; 9(3):304-306.

122. Han AC, Filstein MR, Hunt JV, et al. N-cadherin distinguishes pleural mesotheliomas from lung adenocarcinomas: a ThinPrep immunocytochemical study. Cancer 1999; 87(2):83-86.

123. Fetsch PA, Brosky K, Simsir S, et al. Preparation of effusion cytology samples for optimal immunocytochemistry: a comparison of cytospins, vs. Thin Preps, vs. cell blocks. Mod Pathol 2001; 14(1):52A.

124. Ordonez NG. The immunohistochemical diagnosis of mesothelioma: differentiation of mesothelioma and lung adenocarcinoma. Am J Surg Pathol 1989; 13(4):276-291.

125. Betta P-G, Andrion A, Donna A, et al. Malignant mesothelioma of the pleura: the reproducibility of the immunohistological diagnosis. Pathol Res Pract 1997; 193:759-765.

126. Fetsch PA, Marincola FM, Filie A, et al. Melanoma-associated antigen recognized by T-cells (MART-1): the advent of a preferred immunocytochemical antibody for the diagnosis of metastatic malignant melanoma in fine needle aspirations. Cancer Cytopathol 1999; 87(1):37-42.

127. DAKO Corporation. Monoclonal mouse anti-human leukocyte common antigen package insert. Carpinteria, Calif: DAKO; 1998.

128. Fetsch PA, Simsir A, Abati A. Comparison of antibodies to HBME-1 and calretinin for the detection of mesothelial cells in effusion cytology. Diagn Cytopathol 2001; 25(3):158-161.

129. Ordonez NG. The immunohistochemical diagnosis of epithelial mesothelioma. Hum Pathol 1999; 30(3):313-323.

130. Fetsch PA, Abati A, Hijazi Y. Utility of the antibodies CA 19-9, HBME-1, and thrombomodulin in the diagnosis of malignant mesothelioma and adenocarcinoma in cytology. Cancer Cytopathol 1998; 84(2):101-108.

131. Roberts F, Harper CM, Downie I, et al. Immunohistochemical analysis still has a limited role in the diagnosis of malignant mesothelioma. A study of thirteen antibodies. Am J Clin Pathol 2001; 116(2):253-262

132. Ordonez N. Value of calretinin immunostaining in differentiating epithelial mesothelioma from lung adenocarcinoma. Mod Pathol 1998; 11(10):929-933.

133. Leong A, Vernon-Roberts E. The immunohistochemistry of malignant mesothelioma. Pathol Annu 1994; 29(2):157-179.

134. Ordonez NG. Role of immunohistochemistry in differentiating epithelial mesothelioma from adenocarcinoma. Am J Clin Pathol 1999; 112:75-89.

135. Brockstedt U, Gulyas M, Dobra K, et al. An optimized battery of eight antibodies that can distinguish most cases of epithelial mesothelioma from adenocarcinoma. Am J Clin Pathol 2000; 114:203-209.

136. Ordonez NG, Mackay B. Glycogen-rich mesothelioma. Ultrastruct Pathol 1999; 23:401-406.

137. Dejmek A, Brockstedt U, Hjerpe A. Optimization of a battery using nine immunocytochemical variables for distinguishing between epithelial mesothelioma and adenocarcinoma. APMIS 1997; 105(11):889-894.

138. Simsir A, Fetsch PA, Mehta D, et al. E-cadherin, N-cadherin, and calretinin in pleural effusions: the good, the bad, the worthless. Diagn Cytopathol 1999; 20(3):125-130.

139. Han A, Peralta-Soler A, Knudsen K, et al. Differential expression of N-cadherin in pleural mesotheliomas and E-cadherin in lung adenocarcinomas in formalin-fixed, paraffin-embedded tissues. Hum Pathol 1997; 28(6):641-645.

140. Morgan RL, DeYoung BR, McGaughy VR, et al. MOC-31 aids in the differentiation between adenocarcinoma and reactive mesothelial cells. Cancer Cytopathol 1999; 87(6):390-394.

141. Oates J, Edwards C. HBME-1, MOC-31, WT1, and calretinin: an assessment of recently described markers for mesothelioma and adenocarcinoma. Histopathology 2000; 36(4):341-347.

142. Chenard-Neu MP, Kabou A, Mechine A, et al. Immunohistochemistry in the differential diagnosis of mesothelioma and adenocarcinoma. Evaluation of 5 new antibodies and 6 traditional antibodies. Ann Pathol 1998; 18(6):460-465.

143. Leers MP, Aarts MM, Theunissen PH. E-cadherin and calretinin: a useful combination of immunochemical markers for differentiation between mesothelioma and metastatic adenocarcinoma. Histopathology 1998; 32(3):209-216.

144. Carella R, Deleonardi G, D'Errico A, et al. Immunohistochemical panels for differentiating epithelial malignant mesothelioma from lung adenocarcinoma: a study with logistic regression analysis. Am J Surg Pathol 2001; 25(1):43-50.

145. Abati A, Fetsch PA. OV632 as a possible marker for malignant mesothelioma: high expectations, low specificity. Diagn Cytopathol 1995; 12:81-82.

146. Filie A, Abati A, Fetsch PA, et al. Hyaluronate binding probe and CD44 in the differential diagnosis of malignant effusions-disappointing results in cytology material. Diagn Cytopathol 1998; 18(6):473-474.

147. Cury PM, Butcher DN, Fisher C, et al. Value of the mesothelium-associated antibodies thrombomodulin, cytokeratin 5/6, calretinin, and CD44H in distinguishing epithelioid pleural mesothelioma from adenocarcinoma metastatic to the pleura. Mod Pathol 2000; 13(2): 107-112.

148. Ordonez N. Value of thyroid transcription factor-1, E-cadherin, BG8, WT1, and CD44S immunostaining in distinguishing epithelial pleural mesothelioma from pulmonary and nonpulmonary adenocarcinoma. Am J Surg Pathol 2000; 24(4):598-606.

149. Donna A, Betta P-G, Bellingeri D, et al. Cytologic diagnosis of malignant mesothelioma in serous effusions using an antimesothelial-cell antibody. Diagn Cytopathol 1992; 8(4):361-365.

150. Miettinen M, Kovatich A. HBME-1: a monoclonal antibody useful in the differential diagnosis of mesothelioma, adenocarcinoma, and soft-tissue and bone tumors. Appl Immunohistochem 1995; 3(2):115-122.

151. Azumi N, Underhill CB, Kagan E, et al. A novel biotinylated probe specific for hyaluronate: its diagnostic value in diffuse malignant mesothelioma. Am J Surg Pathol 1992; 16(2):116-121.

152. Doglioni C, Dei Tos AP, Laurino L, et al. Calretinin: a novel immunocytochemical marker for mesothelioma. Am J Surg Pathol 1996; 20(9):1037-1046.

153. Wieczorek TJ, Krane JF. Diagnostic utility of calretinin immunohistochemistry in cytologic cell block preparations. Cancer 2000; 90(5):312-319.

154. Nagel H, Hemmerlein B, Ruschenburg I, et al. The value of anti-calretinin antibody in the differential diagnosis of normal and reactive mesothelia versus metastatic tumors in effusion cytology. Pathol Res Pract 1998; 194(11):759-764.

155. Chhieng DC, Yee H, Schaefer D, et al. Calretinin staining pattern aids in the differentiation of mesothelioma from adenocarcinoma in serous effusions. Cancer 2000; 90(3):194-200.

156. Stoetzer OJ, Munker R, Darsow M, et al. P53-immunoreactive cells in benign and malignant effusions: diagnostic value using a panel of monoclonal antibodies and comparison with CEAstaining. Oncology Rep 1999; 6:433-436.

157. Shield PW, Callan JJ, Devine PL. Markers for metastatic adenocarcinoma in serous effusion specimens. Diagn Cytopathol 1994; 11(3):237-245.

158. Koss MN, Fleming M, Przgodzki RM, et al. Adenocarcinoma simulating mesothelioma: a clinicopathologic and immunohistochemical study of 29 cases. Ann Diagn Pathol 1998; 2(2):93-102.

159. Dejmek A, Hjerpe A. Reactivity of six antibodies in effusions of mesothelioma, adenocarcinoma and mesotheliosis: stepwise logistic regression analysis. Cytopathology 2000; 11(1):8-17.

160. Dejmek A, Hjerpe A. Immunohistochemical reactivity in mesothelioma and adenocarcinoma: a stepwise logistic regression analysis. APMIS 1994; 102(4):255-264.

161. Moran CA, Wick MR, Suster S. The role of immunohistochemistry in the diagnosis of malignant mesothelioma. Semin Diagn Pathol 2000; 17(3):178-183.

162. Lucchi I, Morigi F, Naldi S, et al: Cell-block immunocytochemical characterization of effusions. Use of antibody panel: calretinin, Ber-EP4, keratin and CD68. Pathologica 1999; 91(6):447-452.

163. Davidson B, Risberg B, Kristensen G, et al. Detection of cancer cells in effusions from patients diagnosed with gynaecological malignancies: evaluation of five epithelial markers. Virchows Arch 1999; 435:43-49.

164. Diaz-Arias AA, Loy TS, Bickel JT, et al. Utility of BER-EP4 in the diagnosis of adenocarcinoma in effusions: an immunocytochemical study of 232 cases. Diagn Cytopathol 1993; 9(5):516-521.

165. Miedouge M, Rouzaud P, Salama G, et al. Evaluation of seven tumour markers in pleural fluid for the diagnosis of malignant effusions. Br J Cancer 1999; 81(5):1059-1065.

166. Schofield K, D'Aquila T, Rimm DL. The cell adhesion molecule, E-cadherin, distinguishes mesothelial cells from carcinoma cells in fluids. Cancer 1997; 81(5):293-298.

167. Gupta RK, Kenwright DN, Fauck R, et al. The usefulness of a panel of immunostains in the diagnosis and differentiation of metastatic malignancies in pericardial effusions. Cytopathology 2000; 11(5):312-321.

168. DAKO Corporation. Monoclonal mouse anti-human epithelial membrane antigen, package insert. Carpinteria, Calif: Author; 1998.

169. BioGenex. Monoclonal antibody to tumor-associated glycoprotein (TAG-72) package insert. San Ramon, Calif: BioGenex; 1998.

170. DAKO Corporation. Monoclonal mouse anti-human epithelial antigen, clone Ber-EP4, package insert. Carpinteria, Calif: DAKO; 1998.

171. Bailey ME, Brown RW, Mody DR, et al. Ber-EP4 for differentiating adenocarcinoma from reactive and neoplastic mesothelial cells in serous effusions: comparison with carcinoembryonic antigen, B72.3 and Leu-M1. Acta Cytol 1996; 40(6):1212-1216.

172. Signet Pathology Systems. Monoclonal mouse CA 19-9 package insert. Dedham, Calif: Signet; 1994.

173. Signet Laboratories. Monoclonal mouse anti-BG-8 (murine) package insert. Dedham, Mass: Author; 1994.

174. Gatalica Z, Miettinen M. Distribution of carcinoma antigens CA19-9 and CA15-3: an immunohistochemical study of 400 tumors. Appl Immunohistochem 1994; 2(3):205-211.

175. Anti-carcinoembryonic antigen package insert. Indianapolis, Ind: Boehringer-Mannheim, 1995.

176. Arber DA, Weiss LM. CD15: a review. Appl Immunohistochem 1993; 1(1):17-30.

177. Becton-Dickinson Immunocytometry Systems. CD15 (Leu-M1) package insert. San Jose: Becton-Dickinson; 1993.

178. Zymed Laboratories. Monoclonal mouse anti-E-cadherin antibody package insert. San Francisco: Zymed; 1999.

179. Zymed Laboratories. Polyclonal rabbit anti-calretinin package insert. San Francisco: Zymed; 1999.

180. Simsir A, Fetsch PA, Abati A. Calretinin immunostaining in benign and malignant pleural effusions. Diagn Cytopathol 2001; 24(2):149-152.

181. Nagel H, Hemmerlein B, Ruschenburg I, et al. The value of anti-calretinin antibody in the differential diagnosis of normal and reactive mesothelia versus metastatic tumors in effusion cytology. Pathol Res Pract 1998; 194(11):759-764.

182. DAKO Corporation. Monoclonal mouse anti-human mesothelial cell (HBME-1), package insert. Carpinteria, Calif: DAKO; 1998.

183. Ascoli V, Carnovale-Scalzo C, Taccogna S, et al. Utility of HBME-1 immunostaining in serous effusions. Cytopathology 1997; 8(5):328-335.

184. Morgan RL, De Young BR, McGaughy VR, et al. MOC-31 aids in the differentiation between adenocarcinoma and reactive mesothelial cells. Cancer 1999; 87(6):390-394.

185. Magyarosy E, Martin WJ, Chu EW, et al. Differential diagnostic significance of the paucity of HLA-I antigens on metastatic breast carcinoma cells in effusions. Pathol Oncol Res 1999; 5(1):32-35.

186. Motherby H, Friedrichs N, Kube M, et al: Immunocytochemical and DNA-image cytometry in diagnostic effusion cytology. II. Diagnostic accuracy in equivocal smears. Anal Cell Pathol 1999; 19(2):59-66.

187. Zimmerman RL, Fogt F, Goonewardene S. Diagnostic value of a second generation CA 15-3 antibody to detect adenocarcinoma in body cavity effusions. Cancer 2000; 90(4):230-234.

188. Abati A, Sanford J, Fetsch P, et al. Detection of aneuploidy in mesothelioma cell lines by fluorescence in situ hybridization (FISH). Diagn Cytopathol 1997; 16(4): 375-377.

189. Shin HJC, Shin DM, Tarco E, et al. Detection of numerical aberrations of chromosomes 7 and 9 in the effusion fluids of pleural malignant mesothelioma (MM). Mod Pathol 2001; 14(1):61A. (Abstract).

190. Florentine BD, Sanchez B, Raza A. Detection of hyperdiploid malignant cells in body cavity effusions by fluorescence in situ hybridization on thinprep slides. Cancer 1997; 81(5):299-308.

191. Zimmerman RL, Bibbo M. Clinical utility of chromosome 17 alpha satellite probe in distinguishing benign mesothelium from malignant cells: a pilot study using routinely fixed specimens. Oncol Rep 1999; 6(3): 695-698.

192. Yu GH, De Frias DV, Horcher AM. Evaluation of histochemical methods for the detection of intracytoplasmic mucin in serous effusions. Cytopathology 1999; 10(5): 298-302.

193. Risberg B, Davidson B, Dong HP, et al. Flow cytometric immunophenotyping of serous effusions and peritoneal washings: comparison with immunocytochemistry and morphological findings. J Clin Pathol 2000; 53(7):513-517.

194. Saha I, Dey P, Vhora H. Role of DNA flow cytometry and image cytometry on effusion fluid. Diagn Cytopathol 2000; 22(2):81-85.

195. Thunnissen FB, Buchholtz RT, Woutersen DP. Clinical value of DNA image cytometry in effusions with atypia. Diagn Cytopathol 1999; 21(2):112-116.

196. Decker D, Stratmann H, Springer W. Benign and malignant cells in effusions: diagnostic value of image DNA cytometry in comparison to cytological analysis. Pathol Res Pract 1998; 194(11):791-795.

197. Michael CW, King JA, Hester RB. Confocal laser scanning microscopy and three-dimensional reconstruction of cell clusters in serous fluids. Diagn Cytopathol 1997; 17(4): 272-279.

198. Braunschweig R, Yan P, Guilleret I, et al. Detection of malignant effusions: comparison of a telomerase assay and cytologic examination. Diagn Cytopathol 2001; 24(3):174-180.

199. Dejmek A, Yahata N, Ohyashiki K, et al. In situ telomerase activity in pleural effusions: a promising marker for malignancy. Diagn Cytopathol 2001; 24(1):11-15.

200. Toshima S, Arai T, Yasuda Y, et al. Cytological diagnosis and telomerase activity of cells in effusions of body cavities. Oncol Rep 1999; 6(1):199-203.

201. Zebrowski BK, Yano S, Liu W. Vascular endothelial growth factor levels and induction of permeability in malignant pleural effusions. Clin Cancer Res 1999; 5(11):3364-3368.

202. Bryant-Greenwood P, Sorbara L, Filie AC, et al. Infection of mesothelial cells with human herpes virus 8 in human immunodeficiency virus–infected patients with Kaposi's sarcoma, Castleman's disease, and recurrent pleural effusions. Mod Pathol 2003; 16(2):145-153.

203. DeMay RM. Pleura. In: Demay RM, editor. The art and science of cytopathology: exfoliative cytology. Chicago: ASCP Press; 1996.

204. Geisinger KR, Buss DH, Kawamoto EH, et al. Multiple myeloma: the diagnostic role and prognostic significance of exfoliative cytology. Acta Cytol 1986; 30(4): 334-340.

205. Geisinger KR, Hajdu SI, Helson L. Exfoliative cytology of nonlymphoreticular neoplasms in children. Acta Cytol 1984; 28(1):16-28.

206. Geisinger KR, Ng LW, Hopkins MB, III, et al. Tenckhoff catheter cytology in patients with ovarian cancer. Cancer 1988; 62(8):1582-1585.

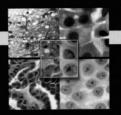

NEUROLOGY

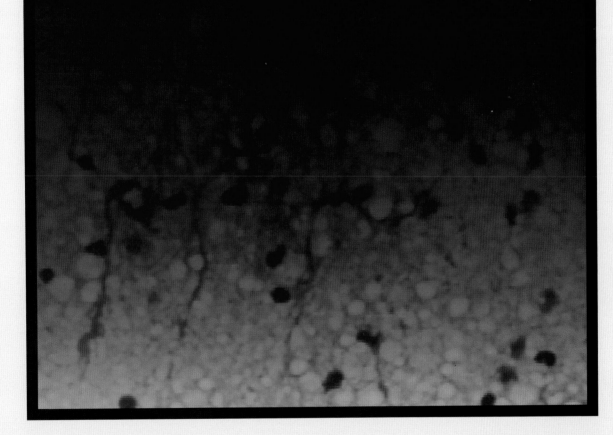

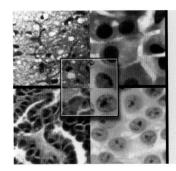

CHAPTER
13

Cerebrospinal Fluid

The cerebrospinal fluid (CSF) originates in the choroid plexus, which is present in the floor of the lateral ventricles and the roof of the third and fourth ventricles. It flows out of the ventricular system at the base of the brain and into the subarachnoid space through the foramina of Luschka and Magendie.[1]

The clinical settings in which lumbar punctures are indicated for the evaluation of CSF are seemingly ambiguous, yet all are signs and symptoms (such as headache) of potential cerebral pathology (Box 13-1). The cytologic and biochemical evaluations of the CSF may be the critical tests obtained for the diagnosis of a treatable yet potentially fatal disease such as meningitis. CSF cytology may herald the initial manifestation of widely metastatic neoplastic disease such as breast cancer. The evaluation of CSF may also be part of a protocol of ongoing monitoring of the cellular components contained therein, such as tumor cell burden variations during treatment. The latter case is particularly true in patients receiving intrathecal chemotherapy for central nervous system (CNS) primary or secondary neoplasia delivered through an Ommaya reservoir. In these patients CSF samples are routinely and easily obtained periodically through the Ommaya.

A recent article reviewing quality improvement issues pertaining to CSF samples yielded several conclusions that the authors found thought-provoking[2]:

1. *Encouraging clinicians to submit CSF to cytopathology only when indicated rather than ordering multiple tests on the same sample.* In other words, cytology is best ordered when a tumor rather than neurosyphilis is suspected. Ordering every test on each sample is not cost effective.
2. *Recommending that fewer samples be submitted to both hematology and cytology because studies have found them to be essentially diagnostic equivalents.* Malignant samples are reviewed by pathologists, and minimal patient benefit is obtained for having the sample submitted to both laboratories.
3. *Encouraging clinicians to provide accurate clinical histories and working diagnoses on clinical forms, with feedback provided to noncompliant clinicians.*
4. *Discouraging clinicians from ordering CSF samples on patients unless therapy will be altered by the result.*
5. *Establishing a system whereby samples thought to be malignant and evaluated by the hematology laboratory will be reviewed and reported by the hematopathologist and having additional studies performed on the remainder of the sample.*[2] Alternatively, this sample could be brought directly to the cytology laboratory for evaluation and special studies.

This chapter discusses the cytologic aspects of CSF evaluation rather than those aspects that are performed predominantly by the clinical pathology laboratory, such as cell counts, microbiology, and clinical chemistries.

 ## PREPARATION AND STAINING OF CEREBROSPINAL FLUID FOR CYTOLOGIC EXAMINATION

Technical considerations that need to be addressed when processing CSF samples for cytology are aimed at the maximum conservation of cellular preservation and sample viewing through various concentration and staining techniques, as well as reducing the potential for intersample contamination. Although Pap stain is widely used for cytologic samples, CSF samples are routinely processed in some laboratories using a Diff-Quik (DQ) stain solely. This rationale was developed based on the procedural protocols of the clinical hematology laboratory where CSF samples are routinely stained with a Giemsa stain, presumably because of the greatest potential for the highest quality cellular visualization. As a majority of the differential diagnoses within the spectrum of CSF cytology are inflammatory, hematologic malignancies and metastatic malignancies, the authors believe that this staining philosophy enhances the ability to evaluate accurately the cells in question.

Optimal cellular preservation is maintained via a system that rapidly transports the sample to the laboratory and the prompt preparation of cytologic slides. The best results have been reported when this occurs within the first 30 minutes postprocurement.[3] This may be particularly important with neoplastic samples such as high-grade lymphomas in which cells may rapidly degenerate. Degenerated cells appear as simply stained smudges devoid of cellular detail. If samples cannot be processed within this time frame then rapid refrigeration is recommended. With rapid refrigeration, scanning electron microscopic studies on CSF samples have demonstrated maintenance of cellular preservation for up to 72 hours.[4] Because of the potential for cross contamination from other specimens, some laboratories adhere to a policy of the separate processing of CSF samples.[3,5] Regular filtration of stains or the maintenance of a designated stain line may also be advocated.

Air-dried CSF samples may be stained with DQ, whereas those that have been fixed in 95% ethanol may be Pap stained. Although the DQ stain enhances the viewing of cytoplasmic features, the Pap stain enhances nuclear detail.[6] Alcohol prefixation of CSF is not recommended. This may lead to limitations of staining options (i.e., it may preclude DQ and immunohistochemistry for lymphoid markers), decreased cellular adherence to slides, and potentially poor staining quality.[5] In the authors' laboratory, all of the slides are stained with DQ unless special studies such as those for infectious organisms, immunocytochemistry, flow cytometry, or molecular studies are indicated. Although some cytopathologists believe that there is a place for use of both stains in the laboratory, the authors feel DQ is the preferred stain for CSF material because of the augmented viewing of hematologic cells with this stain. Pathologists are trained to view hematologic neoplasms with Romanowsky/Wright/Giemsa stains. The DQ is the cytology equivalent of these stains, thus, most pathologists are more comfortable viewing hematologic cells with DQ rather than with Pap. In addition, metastatic neoplasms of nonhematologic derivation are also easily recognized with the DQ stain.

Due to the low cellularity inherent in many CSF samples, concentration techniques assume an important role in specimen preparation. A triage approach may be used in the laboratory to maximize potential use of ancillary techniques when necessary. In general, the first 2 ml yield two cytospins. Any volume greater than 2 ml is concentrated and made into two additional cytospins. A drop of 22% bovine albumin (approximately 0.05 ml) is added to each cytospin chamber to improve cellular adherence and to cushion the cells from the force of the cytocentrifuge. The material is used in its entirety. Cytocentrifugation yields a flattened appearance to the cells, and when combined with the air-drying necessary for DQ staining, it yields cells that appear larger and have enhanced cytoplasmic volume. The morphology is slightly different yet comparable with cells in smears.[7] The optimal cytocentrifugation for all samples is 500 RPM for 5 minutes.

Membrane filtration may be performed on prefixed material. Both filtration and cytocentrifugation methods are associated with small false negative rates, most likely due to low numbers of pathologic cells.[7,8] The small number of false-negative results may be lowered by utilization of both techniques run in tandem; however, this is not deemed

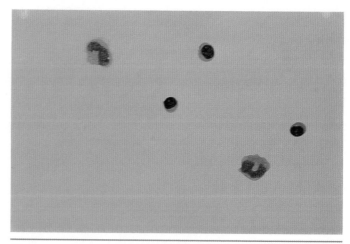

Figure 13-1 Normal cerebrospinal fluid (CSF). This sparsely cellular sample reveals benign lymphocytes that have round, deeply basophilic nuclei with clumped chromatin and a rim of peripheral, lightly basophilic cytoplasm. Two monocytes are present that show characteristic bean- to horseshoe-shaped nuclei and lightly basophilic-vacuolated cytoplasm. (Diff-Quik [DQ])

necessary by all authors.[7] Although millipore filters have been shown to yield the greatest number of cells per sample, some cytopathologists prefer the cytomorphology of cytocentrifuge preparations.[8] Samples prepared with membrane filtration must be evaluated with Pap stain, which some feel limits the detailed visualization of hematopoietic cells. Membrane filtration also causes the lysis of red blood cells (RBCs). Although this may be an aid in the interpretation of some bloody specimens, it can potentially be an impediment to the accurate interpretation of traumatic taps that may be composed partly of circulating tumor cells. Circulating tumor cells may be prominent in lymphoma and leukemia. In these instances, it is important to be aware of the peripheral blood contamination and note it in the report rather than diagnose CSF involvement with neoplastic disease. A formula supplied by Kjeldsberg and Knight has been used by some laboratories for the determination of a corrected total white cell count for the CSF sample[97]:

$$W = WBC_f - \left(WBC_b - \frac{RBC_f}{RBC_b}\right)$$

In this formula:

W = CSF white blood cell count before the addition of blood
WBC_f = Total CSF white cell count
WBC_b = White blood cell count in blood
RBC_f = Red blood cell count in CSF
RBC_b = Red blood cell count in blood

CSF samples are inherently of low cellularity under normal circumstances. Any stray cells, which appear out of context to the usual milieu may rouse the suspicion for malignancy, thus, importance is placed on separate processing, as discussed previously.

Normal Cells

Normal CSF is inherently paucicellular (Figure 13-1). Cells usually present are small, benign-appearing lymphocytes, monocytes, pia-arachnoid cells, and perhaps rare neutrophils and RBCs (owing to the trauma of the tap itself). Small capillaries, isolated choroid plexus, or ependymal

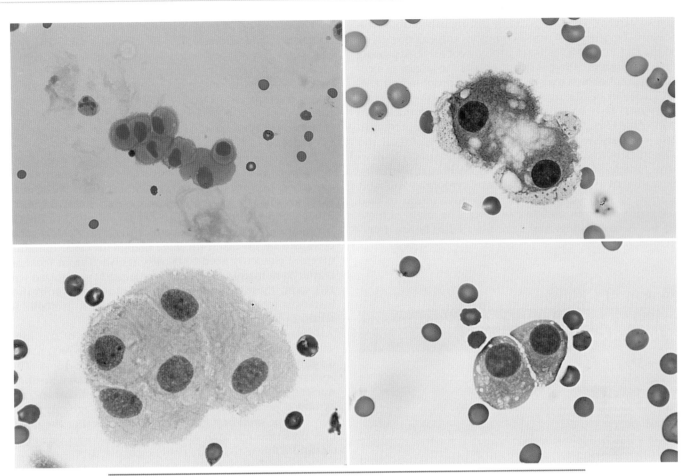

Figure 13-2   Choroidal/ependymal cells. Because of similar cytologic morphology, it may be virtually impossible to distinguish choroidal cells from ependymal cells in CSF samples. The cells may be single or in clusters with abundant cytoplasm and round to oval eccentric nuclei. Cytoplasmic borders are prominent. The cytoplasm may be vacuolated in areas and may assume a biphasic staining pattern with DQ-simulating mesothelial cells. Nucleoli may be inconspicuous or prominent. (DQ)

cells may also be seen (Figure 13-2). Samples drawn from Ommaya reservoirs may have small aggregates of actual brain tissue and choroid plexus or ependymal cells in small aggregates (Figure 13-3). The brain tissue may include glial cells, neurons, and capillaries. Rare reports of blastlike cells from CSF samples of young infants with hydrocephalus who have had ventriculoperitoneal (VP) shunts implanted have been described, representing germinal matrix cells (GMCs).[9,10] Cells that may be introduced by the tap itself include cartilage, muscle, adipose tissue, and cutaneous squamous cells (Figure 13-4). Occasionally bone marrow elements can be seen. Talc, corpora amylacea, and acellular fragments of bone or cartilage may also be present (Box 13-2). It is important to recognize these elements as they may be erroneously interpreted as malignant cells (choroid plexus, ependyma, bone marrow elements, squamous cells, chondrocytes, brain tissue, GMCs) or infectious organisms (corpora amylacea).[11]

Pia-arachnoid cells, although rarely seen in CSF, appear as clusters of small, bland spindle cells. Choroid plexus and ependymal cells may be impossible to distinguish from each other in routine preparations (see Figure 13-2). They appear as small cellular clusters of bland, plump, round to columnar cells with abundant cytoplasm and small, round

nuclei that may or may not have small round nucleoli. The cells may form a syncytium without obvious cell borders.[12,13] The cells may be present as flat sheets or in three-dimensional papillary aggregates. These cells usually appear more numerous in Ommaya taps. In cases of choroid plexus papilloma, a neoplasm of the ventricles in the pediatric population, numerous papillary clusters of these cells will be seen, but on a cell-for-cell basis may be indistinguishable from normal.[14]

Albeit rarely seen, GMCs, when present, may pose a diagnostic dilemma. A recent study compared these cells from 12 patients with VP shunts to the GMCs from a 22-week fetus, noting that the origin of the cells were the same. It is speculated that the placement of the VP shunt leads to the displacement of these cells into the CSF.[9] These blastlike cells usually present in clusters. They have high N:C ratios with prominent nuclear molding. The chromatin pattern is homogeneous and finely reticular. Small nucleoli may be present. On immunohistochemistry these cells are positive for neuron-specific enolase and negative for leukocyte common antigen. The differential diagnosis includes medulloblastoma and lymphoblasts. Although the clinical scenario and cytologic appearance of medulloblastoma may be similar, the claim has been made that cells of medulloblastoma are larger.[10] The GMCs can be distinguished from lymphoblasts by their leukocyte common antigen negativity and the fact that GMC cells are strongly cohesive, appearing largely in clusters, whereas lymphoblasts are largely noncohesive. Lymphoblasts may also have more prominent nucleoli.[9] They can be distinguished from choroidal/ependymal cells, which have abundant cytoplasm and low nuclear to cytoplasmic (N:C) ratios, by the high N:C ratios present in GMC. Of course when dealing with these cells, clinical and radiologic information plays a key role. Additionally in newborns, lumbar punctures may yield notochordal remnants, which present as large cells with foamy cytoplasm and faint indistinct cellular borders. These cells have round to oval nuclei with coarse chromatin clumping. The origin of these cells has been histologically demonstrated to be the intervertebral disc.[15]

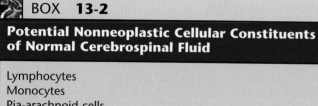

BOX 13-2

Potential Nonneoplastic Cellular Constituents of Normal Cerebrospinal Fluid

Lymphocytes
Monocytes
Pia-arachnoid cells
Choroid plexus cells
Capillaries
Red blood cells (traumatic)
Neutrophils (traumatic)
Brain tissue, including germinal matrix
Ependymal cells
Cartilage
Bone
Soft tissue (muscle, adipose tissue)
Bone marrow elements
Squamous cells

The presence of peripheral blood elements needs to be recognized and addressed in all traumatic taps. This is of particular importance when many inflammatory cells or circulating tumor cells are present. In these instances, CNS involvement with infection or neoplasia cannot be reliably assessed. Preparations that lyse RBCs such as membrane filtration make this evaluation difficult to impossible. Freshly prepared cytospins stained with DQ remain the preparation of choice.

During the process of obtaining a CSF, the needle may come in contact with bone, cartilage, or bone marrow that can then become part of the CSF sample.[16,17] Although extramedullary hematopoiesis may rarely involve the meninges, bone marrow elements can be admitted to the CSF in a manner similar to bone and cartilage.[18,19,20] Megakaryocytes can be mistaken for large malignant cells. Immature myeloid elements need to be distinguished from leukemic blasts. As hematologic elements are readily recognized with DQ stain, these distinctions remain more of a problem in instances where only Pap-stained material is available for review.[7]

Chondrocytes from the nucleus pulposus of the intervertebral disc appear as large polygonal cells, which may be misinterpreted as malignant[11,16,17] (see Figure 13-4). They appear as single cells or in small groups and have shrunken nuclei devoid of detail. The cytoplasm is abundant and may exhibit a perinuclear halo. Bone and cartilaginous matrix may also be present. Other tissue elements that the needle may pass through such as superficial squamous cells, muscle, and adipose tissue are easily recognized.

Corpora amylacea may appear as laminated blue concretions and talc as crystal-like structures with areas of central clearing. It is important not to mistake these for organisms, particularly yeast. Starch granules, which are commonly seen, exhibit a characteristic Maltese-cross configuration with polarized light.

Squamous cells, although most commonly resulting from the procedure itself, in isolated events have been as-

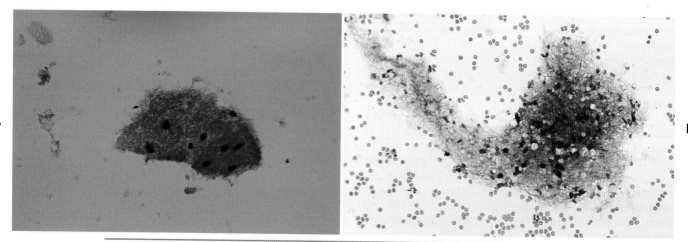

A **B**

Figure 13-3 **Brain tissue obtained from an Ommaya reservoir tap.** These figures show neuropil, which stains green with Pap and purple with DQ. The neuropil has a fibrillar appearance and contains scattered astrocytic and oligodendroglial cell nuclei. The oligodendroglial nuclei are best distinguished from the astrocytes in **A.** The oligodendroglial nuclei are small and dark while the astrocytic nuclei are larger and more lightly basophilic. (**A,** Papanicolaou [Pap]; **B,** DQ)

sociated with ruptured craniopharyngioma, CNS dermoid, and squamous carcinoma of the sphenoid sinus.[15]

Cellular Components

Under normal circumstances in an adult CSF sample, up to 5 cells per ml^3 are present, with lymphocytes predominating over monocytes. Infants may show up to 10 cells per ml^3, with monocytes predominating over lymphocytes.

A significant increase of any single cell type within the CSF brings to mind a specific differential diagnosis. A marked increase in the number of neutrophils may signify a bacterial meningitis or the early stages of an infectious meningitis from other causes (e.g., viral, tuberculous, fungal). It is always best when reporting these types of cytologic findings to comment on the need for clinical and microbiologic correlation. The presence of many neutrophils may also signify damage to cerebral tissue from ischemia, neoplasia, or recent surgery[11] (Figures 13-5 and 13-6).

The presence of many benign lymphocytes may herald nonbacterial infections but may also signify chronic or subacute primary CNS pathology such as multiple sclerosis (MS) or syringomyelia (Figure 13-7). These conditions are accompanied by mixed inflammation with many lymphoid cells with atypical/reactive and plasmacytoid forms present.

A similar picture also may be seen in individuals with acquired immune deficiency syndrome (AIDS) (Figure 13-8). A large proportion of plasma cells and plasmacytoid cells may be associated with MS or neurosyphilis.

The presence of many eosinophils, although nonspecific, may portend a myriad of diagnostic possibilities from drug reactions, foreign material, foreign bodies within the subarachnoid space (e.g., shunt placement), or neoplasia[21-24] (Figure 13-9).

The discrimination between benign inflammatory cells and malignant hematopoietic elements is probably the most important consideration for what appears to be an inflammatory tap sample. In the setting of a fairly uniform population of lymphoid cells, or a polymorphous setting with large blastlike forms and without an appropriate clinical history (e.g., syringomyelia or multiple sclerosis), a primary hematologic process should be excluded. As a general cytologic rule, reactive hematopoietic or lymphoid processes reveal a polymorphous population of cells, whereas malignant processes yield a monotonous population of cells (Figures 13-10 and 13-11). Flow cytometry or molecular diagnostics may be used to enhance this diagnostic discrimination (see Chapter 24).

Macrophages recruited largely from bone marrow reservoirs are called on to respond to foreign materials within

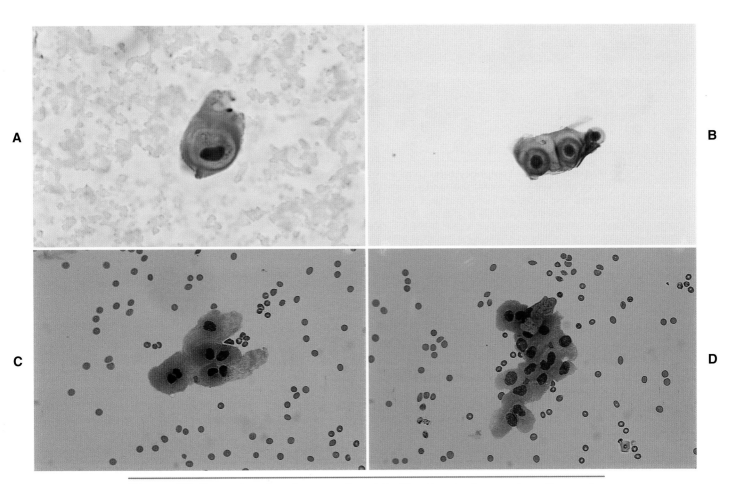

Figure 13-4   Benign chondrocytes. **A** and **B,** Chondrocytes have mature, dense cytoplasm with a visible lacuna and a central oval, irregular pyknotic nucleus. **C** and **D,** Cytoplasm appears less mature and forms more of a magenta fibrillar matrix. Some of these cells are binucleated. **C** and **D** appear to show focal chondroid formation. (Pap and DQ)

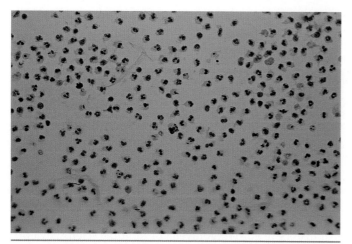

Figure 13-5   Marked acute inflammation. This picture of many neutrophils may signify an acute meningitis. (Pap)

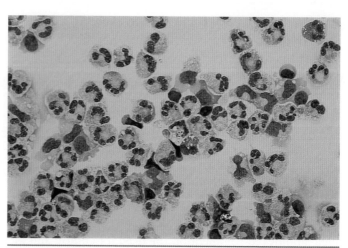

Figure 13-6   Marked acute and focal chronic inflammation with intracellular bacteria. Diplococci are present within the neutrophil in the central portion of the figure, signaling that the cause of this acute meningitis is most likely bacterial. (DQ)

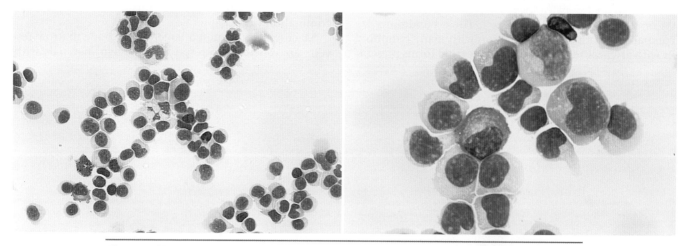

Figure 13-7   Lymphocytosis. Large numbers of reactive, benign lymphocytes of varying sizes admixed with monocytes and plasmacytoid forms may be seen in chronic inflammatory states. The nuclei are bland and largely central. The cells have abundant cytoplasm. The degree of cytoplasmic basophilia is variable. (DQ)

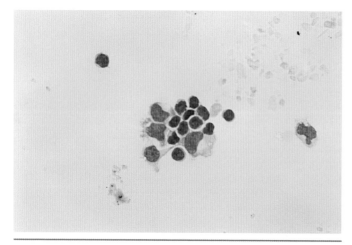

Figure 13-8   Reactive lymphocytosis in a patient with acquired immune deficiency syndrome (AIDS). These lymphocytes show high nuclear to cytoplasmic (N:C) ratios and nuclear irregularities. Adjacent monocytes are present. (DQ)

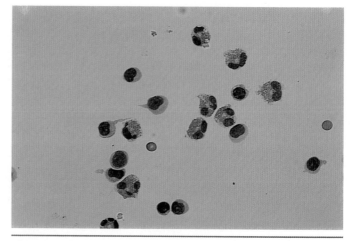

Figure 13-9   Chronic inflammation with eosinophilia. Reactive lymphocytes are admixed with eosinophils. (DQ)

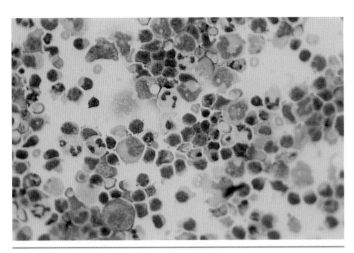

Figure 13-10 **Reactive pleocytosis.** This highly cellular sample contains a polymorphous spectrum of lymphoid cells, some of which are quite large and atypical. The polymorphous population suggests a benign origin. (DQ)

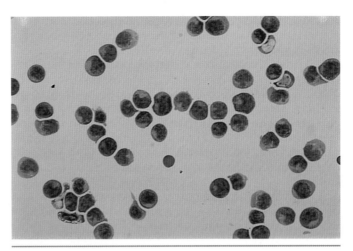

Figure 13-11 **Lymphoma involving the central nervous system (CNS).** This cellular sample shows a monotonous population of mid-size lymphoid cells, all of which show similar morphologic features. The cells have high N:C ratios with deeply basophilic cytoplasm and paranuclear hofs. The nuclei have irregular contours, irregularly clumped chromatin, and prominent nucleoli. (DQ)

the CSF. Macrophages may be numerous after cerebral damage resulting from trauma, hemorrhage, or infarction. They may show well-developed cytoplasmic vacuolization or hemosiderin deposition resulting from the phagocytosis of the offending agent and thus may appear extremely foamy. Vacuolated macrophages may mimic vacuolated carcinoma cells. Multinucleated giant cells may be seen postmyelography, during surgical manipulations, in association with foreign material or in patients with sarcoidosis.[23,25,26] Nuclear morphology and potential use of immunocytochemistry should aid in the diagnostic discrimination when the clinical history is ambiguous.

After an intracerebral hemorrhage secondary to primary ischemic or traumatic incidents, macrophages play a key role in antigen processing and presentation and may be accompanied by neutrophils. The RBCs within the CSF will first appear free floating and intact and then later, within the macrophage cytoplasm; they will eventually leave large round uniform intracytoplasmic vacuoles (Figure 13-12). The macrophages subsequently contain green-brown hemosiderin or yellow hematoidin pigmentation, which can persist for many months after the event.[1,27] In lumbar punctures performed on neonates, the discrimination between fresh (e.g., traumatic tap) and old blood can aid in the discrimination of a previous hemorrhage resulting from birth trauma or germinal matrix hemorrhage.

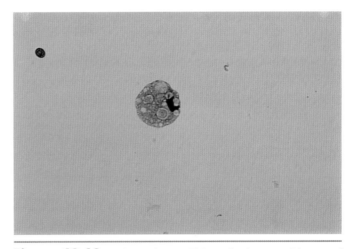

Figure 13-12 **Macrophage.** This cell shows evidence of previous phagocytosis of red blood cells (RBCs). (DQ)

 NONNEOPLASTIC CONDITIONS

Infections

Although the diagnosis of an infectious process can be suspected by the population of inflammatory cells within the CSF, a specific diagnosis cannot be given without direct visualization of the causative organism, thus, microbiologic cultures should always be obtained.

The presence of many neutrophils may suggest a bacterial meningitis (see Figures 13-5 and 13-6). Actual bacterial organisms can occasionally be identified in cytologic samples. Although better visualized with the DQ stain, they can also be seen with Pap stain. The bacterial elements stain dark blue with both stains; however, this dark coloration bears no relationship to the Gram-staining characteristics of the organism. One can, however, discern the morphology of the organism (i.e., coccoid, bacillary, etc.), report the location (intracellular or extracellular), and determine whether many or few organisms are present. Although extracellular organisms may represent contaminant, intracellular organisms should be considered pathologic. The exact characterization of the infectious agent requires a workup by the clinical microbiology laboratory.

As in effusion fluid, meningitis resulting from mycobacterial infection yields a marked chronic inflammation, dominated by a lymphocytic response (see Figure 13-7). The actual visualization of the acid-fast organisms may remain elusive; thus, identification usually rests with the microbiology laboratory where polymerase chain reaction (PCR) for the rapid detection, as well as culture, remains highly useful. Although classically yielding a persistent lymphocytic response, early cases of mycobacterial infection may actually cause a marked neutrophilic response and may be a cause of *persistent neutrophilic meningitis.*[28]

In clinical practice the fungal organism most often encountered in CSF samples is *Cryptococcus;* however, in the immunosuppressed population, particularly with AIDS, *Aspergillus, Mucormycosis, Coccidiomycosis,* and *Candida* may also be encountered[29,30] (Figure 13-13). Aside from cytologic identification of *Cryptococcus* in the CSF, the identification of these other organisms resulting from primarily parenchymal disease usually necessitates tissue biopsy or culture.[30]

The inflammatory response generated by the *Cryptococcus* organism within the CSF is highly variable. In some individuals an acute inflammatory response may be seen. Other patients may yield a highly reactive lymphocytic response, simulating lymphoma (see Figures 13-7 and 13-8). This inflammatory reaction is an important diagnostic pitfall for the erroneous interpretation of lymphoma. At times, however, the absence of an inflammatory response is striking. The definitive diagnosis of *Cryptococcus* within the CSF relies heavily on the appropriate fungal stain reactivity coupled with morphology. The morphology on standard stains alone is insufficient to make the diagnosis as the organisms may resemble degenerated nuclei of inflammatory cells, talc granules, and the vacuoles created by depigmented RBCs that have been phagocytosed by macrophages.[27] Because of the distinctive appearance and staining characteristics of *Cryptococcus,* the diagnosis can be made with confidence on

cytologic preparations.[31,32] Although the yeast itself is round with a diameter of 7 to 10 microns (RBC to neutrophil range), the surrounding mucoid capsule can reach 20 microns in diameter. In Pap-stained samples, the capsule is pale and lucid, whereas on DQ preps the capsule is pale to dark blue. The budding progeny, which remain attached to the parent organism, have a pinched-off teardrop appearance. The yeast may appear in both intracellular and extracellular locations. When intracellular, it may resemble an intracytoplasmic vacuole. Cryptococcus has the unusual feature of mucicarmine positivity in its capsule, which, when coupled with Grocott methenamine silver (GMS) positivity, is pathognomonic. The capsule also stains with Fontana Masson and Alcian blue. The diagnostic appearance of the teardrop-shaped bud is best highlighted with the GMS stain. A true challenge is presented with the capsule-deficient form of *Cryptococcus,* which may be present in AIDS patients.[33,34] In this format, the yeasts are small (2.4 microns) and resemble those of *Candida* and *Histoplasma* (particularly when present intracellularly). The organisms as such do remain positive with India ink and Fontana Masson.

Toxoplasmosis, a not infrequent CNS infection in AIDS, is usually treated presumptively. When patients with CNS toxoplasmosis are submitted to lumbar puncture, the crescent-shaped, basophilic, free-floating bradyzoites and tachyzoites are only rarely seen in CSF cytology. A recent report on this issue evaluated 6090 CSF samples over a 12-year period and found two cases with diagnostic tachyzoites.[35] The authors noted that in patients with obstructive

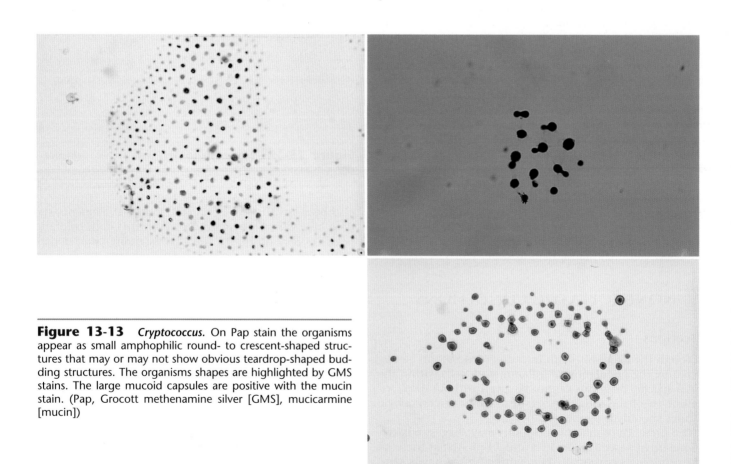

Figure 13-13 *Cryptococcus.* On Pap stain the organisms appear as small amphophilic round- to crescent-shaped structures that may or may not show obvious teardrop-shaped budding structures. The organisms shapes are highlighted by GMS stains. The large mucoid capsules are positive with the mucin stain. (Pap, Grocott methenamine silver [GMS], mucicarmine [mucin])

hydrocephalus the tachyzoites were more likely to be found in ventricular rather than lumbar taps.[35] The organisms may be seen on tissue sections and in brain aspirates. Inflammatory cells that have engulfed several organisms may yield a pseudocyst-like appearance.[36,37] The accompanying inflammatory response may be mixed and, like *Cryptococcus*, may need to be distinguished from a lymphomatous process, which is also in the clinical and radiographic differential diagnosis.

Aside from the distinctive morphology of cytomegalovirus, which may rarely be diagnosed in CSF specimens, the presence of a primary viral meningitis usually cannot be made without the assistance of the virology laboratory. Immunoperoxidase may be helpful in suspected cases. The usual cytologic pattern seen in CSF samples is one of a brisk lymphocytosis.

The cytologic picture of recurrent aseptic meningitis (Mollaret meningitis) is characterized by an initial neutrophilic response that progresses to a lymphocytic infiltrate and gradually fades. The lymphocytic response may be accompanied by Mollaret cells, which are large monocytes with abundant vacuolated cytoplasm (Figure 13-14). As with the clinical symptoms, the cytologic picture is cyclical and varies with the clinical picture.[38] Epstein-Barr virus (EBV) and herpes simplex I have both been associated with this condition.[38,39]

Other infections of the CNS that may yield inflammatory responses within the CSF but that may not usually be directly diagnosed by CSF visualization are: Lyme disease, infectious mononucleosis, cryptosporidiosis, cysticercosis, and *Pneumocystis carinii*.[29,40,41] In the clinical setting of AIDS, multiple primary cerebral inflammatory processes may be represented by reactive inflammatory responses within the CSF.[42,43] In AIDS encephalopathy, many mono- or multinucleated macrophages may be seen.[42]

The diagnosis of aseptic meningitis may present a perplexing picture on CSF cytology. Conflicting reports have indicated a prevalence of both neutrophils and mononuclear cells in CSF samples. A recent study of this disease in children concluded that a predominance of neutrophils in the CSF is not limited to the first 24 hours, thus, the preponderance of neutrophils cannot discriminate between bacterial and aseptic etiologies.[44]

Autoimmune, Reactive, and Miscellaneous Processes

Autoimmune processes involving the CNS such as MS and Guillain-Barré syndrome are associated with a brisk polymorphous inflammatory response. These may include highly atypical lymphocytes that are nonetheless reactive.[45]

The etiology of MS, a chronic inflammatory and demyelinating disease of the CNS, remains speculative. Several recent studies have evaluated CSF findings with patient subgroups and disease progression.[46,47] One study investigated CSF cytology from 60 patients with MS by use of flow cytometry and determined that the CSF B cell to monocyte ratios, which remained stable during different phases of the disease, correlated with progression but not with the level of disability or disease duration. A high ratio (predominance of B cells) was associated with more rapid disease progression, whereas a low ratio (predominance of monocytes) was noted in patients with slower rates of disease progres-

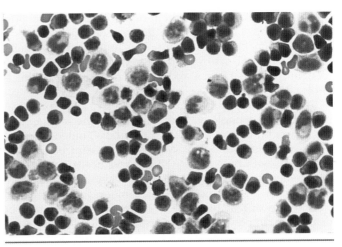

Figure 13-14 **Chronic aseptic meningitis.** The reactive background of lymphocytes also contains many scattered, large monocytes with abundant cytoplasm. Some of the monocytes show vacuolization. (DQ)

sion.[46] Another study evaluated the CSF of 77 patients with MS and found differences that allowed for the division of the patients into several subgroups, as follows:

- Patients in the primary progressive MS subgroup demonstrated a higher prevalence of mitotic activity.
- The more severely disabled patients demonstrated a higher presence of foam cells and mononuclear cells (referred to in the publication as *lymphophages*), with a lower prevalence of lymphoid pleocytosis.
- Treated patients showed a lower cell count, lower prevalence of CSF pleocytosis, lower lymphocyte to monocyte ratio, and a lower prevalence of plasmacytoid lymphocytes.

In addition, patients with disease of longer duration had a higher prevalence of mature plasma cells and lipophages.[47]

An interesting side note is the recently reported finding of an increased number of macrophages/phagocytes in the CSF of schizophrenic patients during acute psychotic episodes. The high number of macrophages was not associated with a significantly higher total cell count and reverted to normal in some patients during therapy.[48]

NEOPLASMS

At least 5% of patients with disseminated cancer develop leptomeningeal metastases[49] (Figures 13-15 to 13-19). Malignant cells may reach the subarachnoid space through direct extension or by hematogenous or lymphatic routes.[49] When evaluating a CSF, an accurate clinical history is imperative. History not only provides information regarding symptomatology, but also data concerning past medical history and previous or ongoing neoplastic disease. This information also provides guidance with regard to the necessity of possible ancillary studies. Because of the high percentage of malignant CSF samples in cytology practice, it is prudent to do an initial evaluation of CSF with volumes over 8 to 10 ml, using a cytospin prepared from 2 to 3 ml. Whether ancillary studies are required and the sample can be divided accordingly is then decided. The application of immunocytochemistry, flow cytometry, and molecular diagnostics are invaluable tools to achieve the most specific diagnoses possible. Table 13-1 is a general outline of sample preparation for various ancillary techniques. It is important to remember that with CSF cytospins to be evaluated for immunocytochemistry, the fixation and treatment of the cytospins is antibody specific.[50]

The advantage of immunocytochemistry is the preservation of cytomorphology, which results in the requirement for a lower number of neoplastic cells and a limited, targeted panel of antibodies.[51] This is especially useful in necrotic neoplasms with only a few well-preserved cells. In hematologic neoplasms, the advantages of flow cytometry are in the detection of a small population of monoclonal cells in a background of reactive cells.[51] The low number of cells in many CSF samples may limit the utility of flow cytometry.[52] A study by Cibas showed a 69% positive correlation of positive flow cytometry with positive cytology; however, it identified nine of 10 cytologically negative cases that were later found to have radiologic or laboratory evidence of meningeal involvement.[53] Additional studies have confirmed a markedly improved sensitivity with flow cytometry when used in combination with conventional cytology for CSF evaluation.[54] Reaner found the combination of nucleic acid and cell surface marker flow cytometry to be at least as sensitive as conventional cytology for the identification of CNS involvement by lymphomas or leukemia.[55,56] Evaluations have suggested that a sample not be used for flow cytometry if the WBC count was less than 1000 cells/mm³ on complete blood count (CBC) and if any of the following situations exist: less than 20% is comprised of lymphocytes; less than five lymphocytes are noted on cytocentrifuge preparation; or the sample is older than 3 days.[54]

The use of immunocytochemistry for positive and negative diagnoses has been found to be useful in CSF cytology. This view has been collaborated by others, although not all are in agreement.[57,58] Immunocytochemistry is most useful when dealing with small specimen volumes and sparse cellularity that preclude flow cytometry and also when visualization of the cells labeled with the specific markers is necessary.

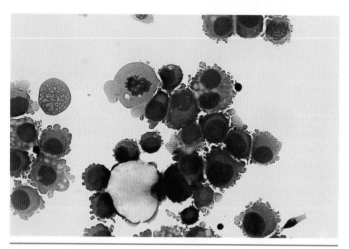

Figure 13-15 **Metastatic malignant melanoma.** The cells have abundant basophilic cytoplasm and eccentric round, regular nuclei. Cytoplasmic pseudopodia are evident and are not specific for melanoma; they can be seen with any cells in a fluid milieu. A single cell reveals a large cytoplasmic vacuole, whereas other cells have several smaller vacuoles. These are the result of pinocytosis of CSF. (DQ)

TABLE 13-1	
Preparation of Cerebrospinal Fluid for Ancillary Tests	
Ancillary Test	**Optimal Cerebrospinal Fluid Preparation**
Immunoperoxidase	Cytospins fixed as required by antibodies to be used
Flow cytometry	Fresh material given to flow laboratory
Molecular markers	Fresh material given to molecular laboratory
	Microdissected cells from previously stained cytospins

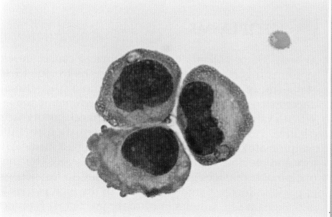
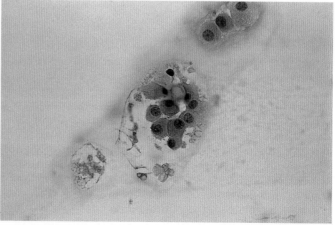

Figure 13-16 **Metastatic breast adenocarcinoma.** These three large cells have formed a semiaggregate. Their nuclei are large and irregular. Nucleoli are prominent and are best seen on the Pap-stained material. Curiously, their cytoplasm reveals a biphasic pattern similar to choroidal/ependymal and mesothelial cells on the DQ. (DQ and Pap)

Cytologic examination of CSF is the primary tool used for the diagnosis of meningeal carcinomatosis. Metastatic cerebral lesions often achieve entrance into the subarachnoid space and shed malignant cells into the CSF. The presence of neoplastic disease involving the leptomeninges may be heralded by a myriad of clinical presentations, including signs of increased intracerebral pressure (headache, nausea, vomiting, papilledema), cranial nerve signs, mental status changes, and gait disturbances.[59-61] Symptoms may or may not be localized; however, it is more often the combination of nonlocalizing symptoms that suggests a neoplastic meningitis.[59,61]

Examination of CSF is associated with a known false-negative rate.[59,61-63] A recent study revealed that false-negative CSF cytology correlated with small CSF volume, delayed sample processing, lack of obtaining CSF from a site of demonstrated disease, and submission of less than two taps. Thus, this false-negative rate can potentially be minimized through submission of at least 10.5 ml of CSF for cytologic analysis, processing the CSF specimen expeditiously, sampling CSF from a site of known leptomeningeal disease, and submission of multiple samples if the initial sample is negative.[64] With sampling of ventricles vs. lumbar taps, the tap closer to the site of the suspected disease is more likely to yield the diagnostic cells.[49] Interestingly, during the course of treatment of CNS neoplastic disease, the presence of tumor cells may wax and wane on repeated taps. However, a series of successive negative taps may be considered indicative of successful treatment.[63] Multifocal microscopic CNS disease is considered more likely to result in malignant CSF cytology than is less extensive involvement.[63]

The most common neoplasms encountered in CSF cytology are those of metastatic epithelial, melanomatous, and hematopoietic origins. However, any neoplastic process, primary or metastatic, may gain access into the subarachnoid space and thus be shed into the CSF. Primary CNS neoplasms are less commonly seen in CSF than are metastases.

The majority of malignant CSF samples are from patients with a previous history of known neoplasia and thus represent documentation of metastatic disease. Many of these patients are symptomatic, and the identification of the ma-lignant cells is not difficult. When CSF disease represents the initial manifestation of metastatic disease from an unknown primary cause, the exact source of the malignant cells may be more problematic and require immunocyto-chemical stains, flow cytometry, or molecular studies, which may be helpful.

Meningeal involvement by malignant cells may or may not be associated with parenchymal involvement of the CNS. A large autopsy study evaluated the incidence of negative CSF cytology in patients with CNS malignancy, incidence of false-positive cytology, and whether any relationship existed between a true-positive cytology and neoplastic distribution at autopsy.[63] Their data indicate that multifocal involvement is more likely to yield a malignant CSF sample than is less extensive disease. Of 117 patients with CNS tumor and premortem CSF cytology, 26% were positive, and 74% were negative. Of 66 patients with neoplastic disease that did not involve the CNS, only one had

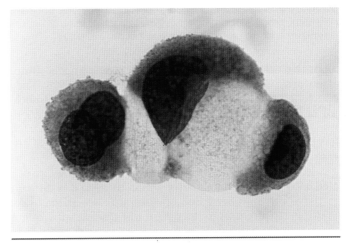

Figure 13-17 Metastatic bronchioloalveolar carcinoma. These three large cells have prominent mucin vacuoles with small magenta-colored granules. The vacuoles of mucin displace the nuclei to peripheral locations. The nuclei are round and may show grooves. (DQ)

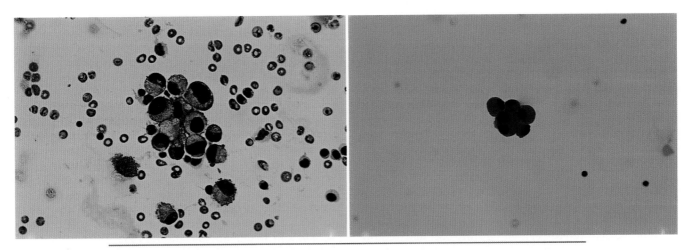

Figure 13-18 Metastatic colonic adenocarcinoma. These atypical cells are showing typical clustering of malignant epithelial cells. The cytoplasm is more rounded in CSF than in fine-needle aspiration (FNA) of metastatic colonic adenocarcinoma where the cells are characteristically columnar and elongated. The cytoplasm contains mucinous vacuoles that are highlighted on the mucin stain. (DQ, mucin)

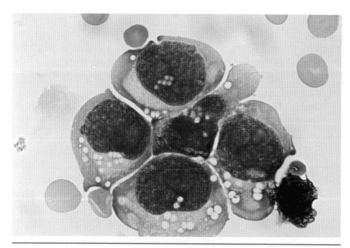

Figure 13-19 **Metastatic rhabdomyosarcoma.** These large bizarre cells have formed an aggregate, as is usually seen in small, round blue cell tumors present within cytospins of the CSF. Prominent intercellular borders and irregular outlines of the cytoplasm are present. The nuclei are rounded to irregular but have consistent prominent multiple nucleoli. Vacuoles are noted in the cytoplasm and are probably pinocytotic in nature. (DQ)

a positive cytology. In patients with leptomeningeal tumor at autopsy, malignant cytology was found in 59%. They concluded that a positive CSF cytology is a reliable indicator of CNS malignancy and usually reflects neoplastic leptomeningeal involvement.[63] Another study showed that less than 6% of autopsied patients with leptomeningeal disease do not have parenchymal involvement.[60]

Although reported rates of positive CSF cytology associated with systemic malignancy are up to 30%, it is difficult to prove this number based on several issues. It may take multiple tap attempts to document CSF disease; subsequent tissue follow-up is hardly ever obtained and treatment may eradicate disease.[59,61-63,65] It has been proven by multiple investigators that malignant diagnostic yields increase (from 45% to 80%) with multiple CSF examinations.[59,61,62] Diagnostic yield is also increased by doing the tap closer to the region of the suspected disease (i.e., cisternal vs. lumbar puncture). When the yield of ventricular taps is compared to that of lumbar taps, the diagnostic yield of the former is more likely to be higher.[61]

The search for abnormal cells begins with the knowledge of the presence and appearance of the expected cellular constituents. Beyond reactive lymphoid cells and monocytes, peripheral blood elements from trauma, and occasional choroidal/ependymal or cartilage, few other cells are part of the usual CSF population (Box 13-3). Thus, the identification of abnormal cells should, in theory, in most cases be fairly easy. When looking at the cells in question, the cytopathologist can inquire as to whether these cells even belong there; if not, chances are it is a malignancy. Regarding differential diagnoses, only choroidal/ependymal cells or vacuolated macrophages could potentially be in the differential diagnosis of a nonhematopoietic malignancy. Atypical lymphoid cells require careful scrutiny that may require additional studies.

Although conventional wisdom states that neoplasms involving the CSF appear largely as single cells (even those of epithelial origin), this is not necessarily true. In many instances of nonhematopoietic tumors, if only two malignant

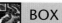

Benign Mimics of Carcinoma Cells in Cerebrospinal Fluid

Choroidal/ependymal cells
Vacuolated macrophages

BOX 13-4

Approach to a Positive Cerebrospinal Fluid in a Patient with No History of Malignancy

Commonly results from melanoma, lung, or stomach primary
Less commonly from breast or hematopoietic etiology
Avoid false-positive diagnoses due to reactive lymphoid processes
Determine if cells are hematopoietic
Morphologic evaluation
Immunocytochemical panel based on differential diagnoses
Flow cytometry if hematopoietic origin is suspected

cells are evident, they seem to manage to "find each other" on the slide. This may be because of cytospin artifact but is a helpful phenomenon regardless. This appears true of most neoplasms, including carcinomas; melanomas; small, round blue cell tumors; and primary CNS neoplasms (see Figures 13-15 to 13-19).

Metastatic Neoplasms

Nonhematologic Neoplasms

The diagnostic examination of CSF in patients with suspected CNS disease and as part of monitoring during treatment is a routine practice in cytology. The most common neoplasms encountered are adenocarcinomas of the breast and lung, malignant melanoma, and small cell lung carcinoma (Box 13-4). Primary CNS neoplasms may also be encountered.[65] In the authors' experience, the presence of CNS symptomatology is more commonly associated with a positive cytology than in patients without global or focal findings. The spread of a carcinoma to the meninges, as is documented through CSF cytology, is usually a grave prognostic indicator.[57,61] When a positive CSF is obtained as part of disease monitoring and is indicative of recurrent disease, it may also indicate that the patient has tumor in regions in addition to the CNS.[61] A large-scale study evaluating malignant CSF samples in patients with nonhematologic neoplasms was performed at Memorial Sloan-Kettering Cancer Center.[62] The most common neoplasms to involve the CSF in this study were breast carcinoma (37%), lung carcinoma (27%), and malignant melanoma (18%). Interestingly, the interval between initial diagnosis and CSF involvement was distinctive to the tumor type, with breast carcinoma and malignant melanoma having a significantly longer delay period (52 months), compared with lung and bladder carcinoma (11 and 9 months, respectively). In this group, 75%

of patients with follow-up died within 100 days of the first malignant CSF sample.[62]

For most cytopathologists, the majority of CSF samples evaluated in daily practice are benign and contain a mixture of lymphocytes and monocytes with occasional peripheral blood elements, depending on the level of trauma incurred by the tap. The presence of most malignancies within the CSF is usually quite easily detected by the presence of large, single or clumped cells that appear out of context (see Figures 13-15 to 13-19). As in other cytologic samples, hematologic neoplasms exhibit a more significant degree of cellular dispersion. The malignant cells should maintain diagnostic cytologic malignant features, and most patients will have a prior history of malignancy that sheds light on the interpretation. If ancillary studies are necessary as part of a diagnostic workup, additional material may be submitted, or immunoperoxidase studies may be attempted directly on to Pap-stained slides. (This cannot be done for lymphoma markers, which are inactivated through ethanol fixation.) Alternatively laboratories may wish to initially process only a part of the sample so that some remains in the event of necessity of additional studies. For flow cytometry or immunoperoxidase, submission of at least 10 ml is recommended. In most institutions, it is important to recognize that for cytologic review of additional material from any given sample, the hematology laboratory will, in a majority of instances, have additional slides prepared from the same sample stained with Giemsa for microscopic review.

Generally speaking, the appearance of metastatic neoplastic cells within the CSF will have appearances similar to those in other fluid mediums, such as in effusions. The main difference is that a tendency exists toward single malignant cells within the CSF, the groups may be smaller, and the actual number of malignant cells may be meager. Because of the relatively scanty number of diagnostic cells, careful scrutiny is of the utmost importance. Normal cells should be used as a guideline for comparison with the large size of most tumor cells.

In a fluid milieu, any cell may become vacuolated, and thus, vacuoles do not necessarily denote adenocarcinoma. Likewise, the benign nature of large, vacuolated monocytes/macrophages can be inferred by the low N:C ratio and the bean-shaped nucleus devoid of malignant characteristics.

The appearance of breast adenocarcinoma varies with the grade of tumor (see Figure 13-16). Generally, the malignant cells are present as single cells and loose clusters with variable amounts of eosinophilic or lightly basophilic cytoplasm. The cells should have high N:C ratios and prominent nucleoli. The cells may be identifiable as breast based on past medical history or previous sample review. With a history of no known primary, the cells may need to be distinguished from other metastatic sources, particularly lung adenocarcinoma. Lobular carcinoma presents as small cells with hyperchromatic nuclei, micronucleoli, and scanty cytoplasm, either singly or in loosely cohesive clusters. At times, they may line up in a single-file pattern.

Although typically a history of breast carcinoma precedes the detection of malignant cells in the CSF, rare cases occur where CNS symptoms and a positive CSF are the initial steps in a diagnostic hunt to identify a primary neoplasm that turns out to be breast. The authors have seen several such cases in the last 5 years, and most of the patients were young women who presented with headaches and were thought to have infectious meningitis.

A significant proportion of patients with primary lung carcinoma have CNS metastases during the course of their disease (see Figure 13-17). Often, CNS metastases are present at the time of the initial diagnosis or are even the presenting problem. Of primary neoplasms of the lung, squamous cell carcinoma is the least likely type to be found in the CSF. Lung adenocarcinoma appears as large cells present singly or in groups with variable amounts of eosinophilic or lightly basophilic cytoplasm that may have well-defined vacuoles and discreet cell borders. Their nuclei have rounded to lobulated contours with prominent eosinophilic nucleoli with chromatin clearing.

Squamous cell carcinoma, which is not often seen in CSF, is characterized by cells with dense cytoplasm with variable amounts of keratinization; central nuclei with irregular, angulated contours; and dense hyperchromasia. The presence of nucleoli is variable.

The appearance of small cell/neuroendocrine carcinoma depends on the subtype. The cells, which are usually small, are present singly or in small groups. They have angulated, basophilic, hyperchromatic nuclei with variable nucleoli and small amounts of basophilic cytoplasm. Molding may or may not be present.

As in cytology samples from other locations, when malignant melanoma is present in CSF, the cells rarely exhibit cytoplasmic pigment (see Figure 13-15). When present, the pigment appears as fine, evenly distributed black cytoplasmic granules. Pigmented tumor cells must be distinguished from pigment-laden macrophages that may contain hemosiderin or melanin. In macrophages, melanin often appears as coarse black granules of variable size. Hemosiderin is likewise chunky but has a refractile, golden brown, greenish hue. The cells usually appear singly, but also occur in small, loose groups. As in other cytologic preparations, they have abundant cytoplasm with a large, round eccentric nucleus and a prominent nucleolus. Cytoplasmic intranuclear pseudoinclusions may be seen.

The declining incidence of gastric adenocarcinoma in the United States and much of the world has led to its decreased appearance in CSF samples. However, in meningeal carcinomatosis of unknown origin, along with lung carcinoma, gastric adenocarcinoma is a prime contender in males[65] (see Box 13-4). These cells appear in the CSF singly, may be highly pleomorphic with prominent nucleoli, and show variable amounts of cytoplasmic vacuolization.

Small round blue cell tumors, including rhabdomyosarcoma and Ewing's/PNET (primitive neuroectodermal tumor) may involve the CSF. The cells of these neoplasms have a distinct similarity within the CSF. The tumor cells are small with high N:C ratios and scant amounts of deeply basophilic cytoplasm that may or may not be vacuolated. The nuclei are eccentric. These cells are often found in clusters of at least two cells. The nuclei may be angulated and are large and hyperchromatic[98] (see Figure 13-19).

Hematologic Neoplasms Involving the Cerebrospinal Fluid

Of tumor types that involve the CNS, lymphoma and leukemia are among the most frequent. The infiltration of the meninges by these processes lends itself to CSF sampling as

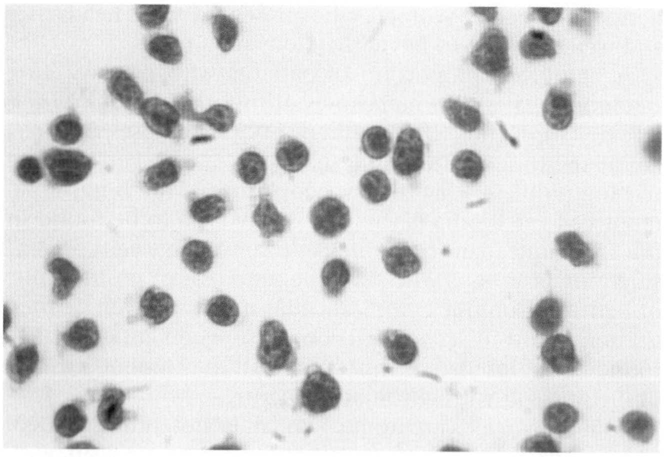

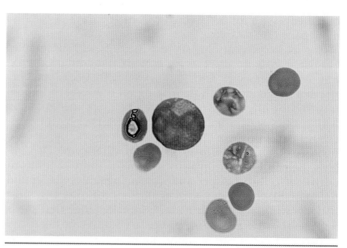

Figure 13-20 **Acute lymphoblastic leukemia/lymphoma.** This cellular sample reveals primitive blastlike cells with high N:C ratios, irregular nuclear contours, and prominent nucleoli. The population is monomorphous, and the cell size is relatively small. (Pap)

Figure 13-21 **Leukemic blast of acute myeloid leukemia (AML).** This large, primitive cell has deeply basophilic cytoplasm; a large bean-shaped nucleus; a prominent nucleolus; and focal cytoplasmic azurophilic granules. (DQ)

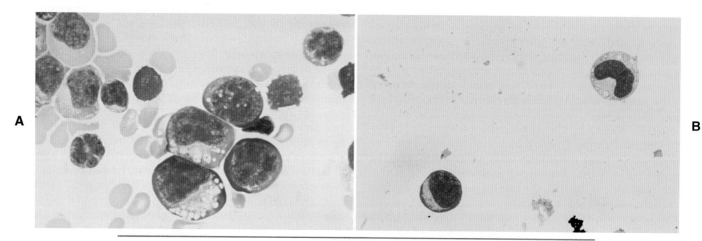

Figure 13-22 **Malignant cells of adult T-cell leukemia/lymphoma. A,** These bizarre lymphoid cells of varying size have abundant deeply basophilic cytoplasm, focal vacuolization, irregular nuclear contours, and prominent nucleoli. The typical nuclear floral outline of T cells is present in a few of the cells. **B,** Contrasting of a leukemic cell with a normal monocyte. (DQ)

a practical and easily implemented diagnostic procedure.[66] Diagnostic leukemia cells most commonly seen in the CSF are those from acute lymphocytic leukemia (ALL), and acute myeloid leukemia (AML). Thus, blast forms, which have high N:C ratios, fine chromatin, and prominent nucleoli, are the most commonly visualized cells (Figures 13-20 to 13-23).

The cytologic appearance of malignant hematopoietic cells within the CSF does not differ significantly from their appearance elsewhere (see Chapter 24). The differences that are noted, however, are mainly because of two phenomena: in CSF the cells are floating in a fluid, and in cytospins, they have been cytocentrifuged. When cells are floating in fluid, they have more pronounced, rounded contours. Cytospin preparations with associated air-drying required for DQ staining cause the cells to flatten out considerably, yielding the appearance of increased size due to increased cytoplasmic volume. The authors have found that the optimal cytocentrifuge speed for CSF samples and all other samples is 500 RPM for 5 minutes.

CSF samples containing hematologic malignancies can exhibit both high and low cellularity. Within any neoplasm, particularly hematologic neoplasms, a spectrum of cells is evident, with some obviously malignant and others having ambiguous morphology. When evaluating primary sites of origin such as lymph node fine-needle aspirations (FNAs) the advantage is being able to look at numerous cells spread over one or more slides on which the pattern and degrees of polymorphism can be assessed. This is not the case with CSF samples; only a few malignant cells may be on each slide, so the usual parameters by which we make the diagnosis of lymphoma are gone. The possibility exists, for example, that in a sample with 10 cells that are malignant on the genetic level, only two cells may be morphologically malignant. This represents the dilemma of the diagnosis of hematologic neoplasms in the CSF, particularly lymphomas. In many instances, neoplastic cells may be beyond the detection rate of conventional cytology. Ancillary studies such as flow cytometry and molecular diagnostics have assumed an expanding role in this regard. Specific tests as-

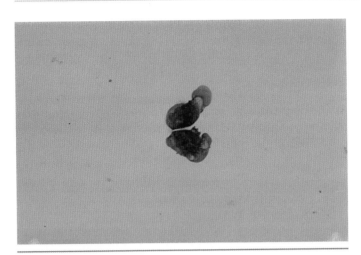

Figure 13-23 **Large cell lymphoma.** These two cells are typical of large cell lymphomas appearance in the CSF. They have abundant deeply basophilic cytoplasm in irregular shapes and large irregularly shaped nuclei with prominent nucleoli. The N:C ratio of these two cells is not particularly high. (DQ)

sociated with each diagnosis have been reviewed in detail in Chapter 24. When a hematologic neoplasm is suspected clinically in a CSF, 8 to 10 ml should be submitted with an initial evaluation done on a cytospin of 1 to 2 ml. Based on these findings, preparations may be made for immunocytochemistry, or material can be submitted for flow cytometry or molecular diagnostics. If the material is used in its entirety for cytology, molecular diagnostics, particularly for lymphomas, can be done on previously stained cytology samples through microdissection and polymerase chain reaction (PCR).[67] This approach can also be used in paucicellular samples with only a few cells that are beyond the detection rate of flow cytometry or immunocytochemistry.[53,67]

A significant percentage of hematologic neoplasms, particularly leukemias, have peripherally circulating tumor cells. The presence of these cells within the peripheral blood can wreak diagnostic havoc on the interpretation of CSF samples that are traumatic taps and contaminated with peripheral blood. As a rule of thumb, traumatic taps in patients with circulating tumor cells can be evaluated in a satisfactory manner, thus, the search on the cytospin for RBCs should be as careful as the search for abnormal cells. Because traumatic taps are usually not grossly bloody, it is of the utmost importance to not lyse these samples but to use fresh material and Giemsa-based stains that make the recognition of RBCs much easier. Rohlfing and associates illustrated this phenomenon in a 1981 publication.[68] Based on serial dilutions of CSF with blood from leukemic patients down to a 1:1.6 million dilution, with membrane filter techniques using 0.000000125 ml of leukemic blood spiking, leukemic cells were seen. They concluded that CSF could be contaminated with minute amounts of blood, leading to erroneous diagnoses.[68] A repeat tap may be useful, but days or weeks may be necessary to resolve changes induced by the traumatic tap.[69]

Other issues to keep in mind in the evaluation of CSF for a hematologic neoplasm are the potentials for false-positive and false-negative diagnoses. The risk of a false-positive diagnosis in leukemia or lymphoma is much greater than the risk of false-positive for carcinoma.[63] Intuitively this makes

sense as carcinoma cells appear much more alien in the CSF milieu. False-positive results in this scenario occur most often with reactive lymphocytoses that appear monomorphous or have atypical reactive forms. Major culprits include cryptococcal meningitis and MS; the latter is associated with reactive plasmacytoid cells. The presence of low numbers of reactive lymphoid cells within the CSF can also lead to false-positive diagnoses of ALL and chronic lymphocytic leukemia (CLL) in patients without any hematologic neoplasms.[70] False-negative diagnoses may be considered in polymorphous populations with rare atypical cells, which may be a source of false-negative diagnoses in lymphoma, and in AML when the cells have monocytic differentiation and resemble benign monocytes. In diagnostic dilemmas, the problem is compounded by the fact that repeat taps and intrathecal chemotherapy may give rise to atypical lymphocytes.[69,71] It is of the utmost importance to compare cells in CSF with previous diagnostic cells in patients with hematologic neoplasms.

Common clinical signs of leptomeningeal involvement with leukemia or lymphoma include cranial nerve palsies, visual changes, papilledema, and amyotrophy from nerve root lesions.[72] CNS involvement is usually suggested by any or all of this complex of symptoms and may or may not be accompanied by supporting imaging studies. For information regarding the diagnostic use of ancillary studies such as immunocytochemistry and PCR for hematologic neoplasms, the reader is referred to Chapter 24.

 ## LEUKEMIA

Issues surrounding CSF testing for leukemia involve not only initial diagnosis but relapse, as the CNS and testicles represent sanctuary sites where cells can avoid the effects of treatment. Improved prognosis associated with intrathecal therapy must be weighed against unnecessary treatment that has notable clinical side effects. Up to 10% of children with ALL relapse in the CNS despite appropriate therapy, and a significant percentage of these cases go on to bone marrow relapse and death.[73-75] ALL cells may enter the CNS through veins or direct extension from adjacent cranial bone marrow.[74] Interestingly, a low platelet count has been associated with CNS disease possibly through the precipitation of small hemorrhages. It is unclear whether CNS disease reseeds the bone marrow or vice versa (see Figures 13-20 and 13-21).

The cells of ALL exhibit a spectrum as related to the type of ALL (e.g., L1, L2, or L3). The cells of L1 are the smallest with finely stippled chromatin and scant, basophilic cytoplasm. The nuclei may be round or cleaved or assume a floret configuration, particularly in T-cell ALL. The cells of L3 are at the other end of the spectrum. They are large with abundant, deeply basophilic, sometimes vacuolated cytoplasm and large, round, or convoluted nuclei, often with several small nucleoli. These cells resemble those of Burkitt's lymphoma. The cells of L2 are intermediate in morphology.[76] Interestingly, an increased CSF protein concentration or an increased cell count in the absence of blasts is associated with a decreased probability of event-free 2-year survival, perhaps suggesting that these patients have undetectable CNS disease.[77] The use of ancillary techniques in seemingly negative samples (immunocytochemistry for CD10 [CALLA] and terminal desynucleotidyl transferase [TdT]) increases the diagnostic yield; however, the clinical relevance of occult disease identified in this manner is not always clear.[78-82]

TdT is a nuclear enzyme usually found in thymocytes and is present in 90% of ALL and 10% of AML cases.[83] Immunofluorescence and flow cytometry have been the mainstays for TdT identification, although immunocytochemistry stains are available. Results with immunocytochemistry for TdT have been unsatisfactory because of nonspecific nuclear staining in benign cells.[78,79,81,83,84] Rare instances of TdT and CALLA immunoreactive cells have been found in normal children without ALL.[82,84,85] The applications of flow cytometry require a large number of cells for analysis and have shown DNA aneuploidy of around 40%, which correlates with cytologic malignancy.[86]

Cells of AML are not detected as often in the CSF as are cells of ALL. Clinical findings in AML patients associated with CNS disease are high peripheral WBC count, splenomegaly, and skin or gingival involvement.[87] It has been observed that cases with a monocytic component are more likely to be associated with a positive CSF cytology.[88] From the cytopathologist's perspective, characteristic features may be recognized with a Giemsa/DQ stain to diagnose AML. The cells are large with basophilic cytoplasm that may contain Auer rods or eosinophilic granules. The nuclei are rounded, peripherally located, have a blastlike chromatin pattern, and may contain one or more prominent nucleoli. With the Pap stain, unfortunately, these features are not easily recognized and the cells may be indistinguishable from those of lymphoma, prompting the diagnostic categorization of *positive for malignant cells, consistent with lymphoma or leukemia*. Diagnostic stains for AML may be done on air-dried cytospins (e.g., myeloperoxidase, Sudan Black B).

Chronic myelogenous leukemia (CML) infrequently affects the CNS; however cases in blast transformation may yield positive CSF samples.[11,66] In this scenario, blast forms accompanied by eosinophils may be seen.[66]

CLL rarely involves the CNS.[70] In a patient with CLL and a small monomorphic lymphoid population in the CSF, an infection should be ruled out because these patients are immunocompromised and the likelihood of an infection involving the CNS is greater than that of CLL involvement.[70]

The cells of ATL often involve the CNS and may be detected through CSF cytology. They have characteristic deeply basophilic cytoplasm with atypical eccentric nuclei, prominent nucleoli, and irregular nuclear contours that may be prominent. The size of cells exhibiting these features ranges from small to large, a feature that is characteristic for this neoplasm[89] (see Figure 13-21).

 ## LYMPHOMA

Among nonprimary CNS lymphomas, those most likely to involve the CNS include high-grade variants (large B cell, peripheral T-cell, Burkitt, lymphoblastic) and lower-grade lymphomas, which have undergone high-grade transformation. Although the morphology in individual cases may make specific diagnostic discrimination possible especially in cases where previous material is available for comparison, ancillary tests such as immunocytochemistry (performed on air-dried cytospins), flow cytometry, and PCR are invaluable for the subcategorization and immunophenotyping of these samples. Immunocytochemistry on cytospins is preferable to flow cytometry when the sample volume is low. PCR can be done on fresh samples or on archival samples microdissected from DQ-stained cytospins.[51,67]

Patients with non-Hodgkin's lymphoma may develop CNS involvement in a small percentage of cases. The morphology of the cells within the CSF parallels the morphology of the diagnostic material and should always be compared for diagnostic accuracy. One should also keep in mind that involvement of the CNS may occur with a high-grade transformation of a previously low- to intermediate-grade lymphoma. In this instance the cells within the CSF will appear larger and more pleomorphic than those of the patient's original diagnostic material.

Primary CNS or metastatic lymphoma cells that may be seen in the CSF are mostly B cell neoplasms. These cells have abundant deeply basophilic cytoplasm, which may or may not have scattered vacuoles, large peripherally placed nuclei, rounded or irregular contours, chromatin clumping, and single or multiple nucleoli (see Figure 13-23). Although nuclear contours may be irregular, they do not approach the extreme degree of irregularity noted with T-cell lymphomas/leukemias. An exception is acute lymphoblastic leukemia/lymphoma, which is morphologically similar to ALL.

The presence of cells diagnostic for Hodgkin's disease has been described in CSF[72] (Figure 13-24). As in other peripheral lymphomas, CNS involvement with Hodgkin's disease is rare and is associated with widespread systemic disease. The diagnosis of Hodgkin's disease within the CSF requires the presence of the large atypical mononuclear Hodgkin's cells or binucleate Reed-Sternberg cells with an appropriate background of small benign lymphoid cells, eosinophils, and plasma cells.[72] For the initial diagnosis of Hodgkin's disease within the CNS, the presence of binucleated Reed-Sternberg cells is required.[72] Immunocytochemistry and PCR can be done on CSF samples to confirm the diagnosis, or if the diagnosis is suspected but characteristic Reed-Sternberg cells have not been seen.[72]

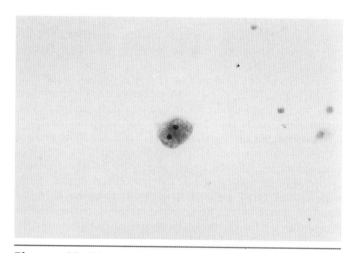

Figure 13-24 **Reed-Sternberg cell.** This characteristic Reed-Sternberg cell displays two nuclei each with a single prominent eosinophilic nucleolus. The cytoplasm in this preparation is wispy and lightly amphophilic. (Pap)

Primary CNS lymphomas are rare in the general population but are seen more often in patients with immunosuppression, such as transplant organ recipients or patients with AIDS. Although rarely involving the CSF, patients with AIDS generally may have a reactive lymphocytosis in which cells may be quite atypical. This may serve as a potential source of false-positive samples (i.e., mistaken for lymphoma) that one should keep in mind. In this population, cryptococcoses may yield a highly atypical brisk lymphocytosis that may also be a source for a false-positive lymphoma interpretation. The morphology of primary CNS lymphoma is that of a large B-cell lymphoma. The cells have abundant deeply basophilic cytoplasm, a large, rounded or irregular peripherally located nucleus and one or more prominent nucleoli.

Other peripheral hematologic processes have been found to involve the CSF and include multiple myeloma and lymphomatoid granulomatosis. In multiple myeloma the diagnostic cell is an atypical plasmacytoid cell, whereas in lymphomatoid granulomatosis the diagnostic cells are B-cell lymphoma cells that should show evidence of EBV infection through in situ hybridization or PCR.

PRIMARY CENTRAL NERVOUS SYSTEM NEOPLASMS

Considering the fact that initial interpretation of primary CNS neoplasms based on CSF cytology can be virtually impossible, it is fortuitous that in most instances, this is preceded by a histologic examination (Figures 13-25 and 13-26). In general, these samples fall into one of three categories: highly anaplastic tumor that is difficult to classify exactly, low-grade neoplasm that may be hard to classify as malignant, or a rare tumor that is hard to classify. Clinician submission of appropriate clinical information remains paramount. Usually, cytopathologists are only called upon in their practices to document extension of previously characterized CNS neoplasms in the CSF. As documented by a Mayo Clinic autopsy study more than 60 years ago, the most common CNS neoplasms to involve the meninges are medulloblastoma (47.6%), glioblastoma multiforme (14.3%), ependymoma (11.9%), oligodendroglioma (11.9%), astrocytoma (7.1%), retinoblastoma (4.8%), and primary pineal tumor (2.4%).[90] In clinical practice the most common primary CNS neoplasms encountered in CSF cytology are medulloblastomas (in the pediatric population) and high-grade astrocytomas (in the adult population) (Boxes 13-5 and 13-6). Cytologic examination of lumbar CSF has been shown to be superior to cytologic examination of the VP shunt CSF in the detection of leptomeningeal metastases in pediatric patients with primary CNS tumors.[91]

The diagnoses of low-grade gliomas are based on cellular tissue patterns rather than individual cellular cytology. Because these processes are notoriously difficult to distinguish from reactive gliosis histologically, the distinction on CSF cytology is impossible.[92,93] These cells have round to slightly ovoid, regular nuclei with a fine chromatin pattern and small nucleoli. The cytoplasm is wispy. Alternatively, the cells may be elongated and have a bipolar appearance.

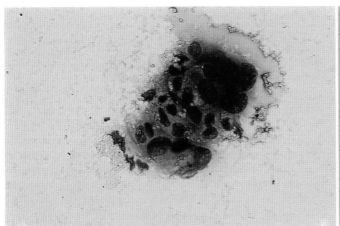

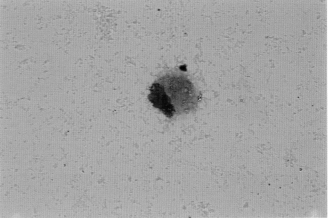

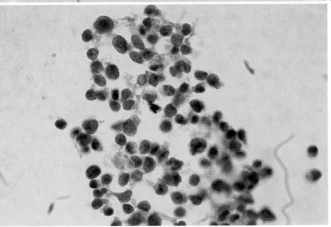

Figure 13-25 **High-grade astrocytoma.** These show a partial spectrum of what can be expected with astrocytoma in the CSF. The cells may be large and pleomorphic and may appear in aggregates or singly. The cells are extremely variable appearing and have inconstant nuclear features. (DQ and Pap)

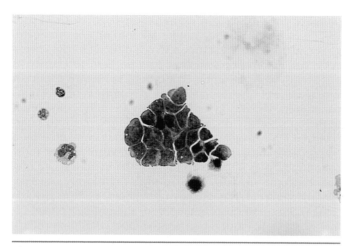

Figure 13-26 Medulloblastoma. Cells of medulloblastoma characteristically cluster in cytospins of CSF samples. Cellular molding is evident. The cells have high N:C ratios with small dark nucleoli. The cytoplasm is deeply basophilic. (DQ)

BOX 13-5

Most Common Primary Central Nervous System Neoplasms Encountered in Cerebrospinal Fluid Cytology

Medulloblastoma
High grade astrocytoma
Low grade astrocytoma
Anaplastic ependymoma
Anaplastic oligodendroglioma

From Chamberlain MC, Kormanik PA, Glantz MJ. A comparison between ventricular and lumbar cerebrospinal fluid cytology in adult patients with leptomeningeal metastases. Neuro-oncol 2001; 3(1):42-45; Bigner SH. Cerebrospinal fluid cytology: current status and diagnostic applications. J Neuropathol Exp Neurol 1992; 51(3):235-245.

BOX 13-6

Less Common Central Nervous System Neoplasms Previously Documented in Cerebrospinal Fluid Cytology

Pineal germ cell tumor
Choroid plexus carcinoma
Malignant teratoma
Olfactory neuroblastoma
Sarcoma
Meningioma
Craniopharyngioma
Hemangioblastoma
Pituitary adenoma

Modified from Chamberlain MC, Kormanik PA, Glantz MJ. A comparison between ventricular and lumbar cerebrospinal fluid cytology in adult patients with leptomeningeal metastases. Neuro-oncol 2001; 3(1):42-45.

The virtual identical appearance of these low-grade tumor cells to normal or reactive astrocytes or potentially macrophages renders a specific diagnosis infeasible[11,49,94] (see Figure 13-25).

The diagnosis of high-grade astrocytomas is based on histologic features such as vascular hyperplasia and necrosis that are not present in a CSF cytology. The cellular appearance is highly variable such that gemistocytic variants contain large, potentially multinucleated atypical cells with abundant cytoplasm and hyperchromatic pleomorphic nuclei, to small cells that can mimic those of small cell carcinoma. Thus, the morphology of these cells in the CSF varies from large, multinucleated, highly pleomorphic cells with hyperchromatic irregular nuclear contours to small cells with scant cytoplasm and hyperchromatic, irregular nuclear outlines, with a wide spectrum in between. The cells tend to cluster on cytospin preparations. Immunocytochemical stains for glial fibrillary acidic protein (GFAP) helps in the diagnosis (see the section on Direct Sampling Cytology of Central Nervous System Neoplasms).

The anaplastic variants of oligodendroglioma and ependymoma are characterized by individual cells or tissue fragments with anaplastic features. Although the presence of GFAP suggests a glial origin, it is not helpful in arriving at a specific diagnosis in the absence of a prior or concurrent histologic study.

The initial clinical presentation of medulloblastoma in the subarachnoid space may mimic meningitis. Medulloblastomas show a tendency for cellular adherence in cytospin preparations (see Figure 13-26). These cells closely mimic those of small cell carcinoma, with molding, scant cytoplasm, hyperchromatic nuclei and irregular nuclear contours. The cells may appear in tissue fragments. Although indistinguishable from the cytology of retinoblastoma, pineoblastoma, and neuroblastoma, the age of the patient and location of the tumor aid in the differential diagnosis.[66]

The presence of a midline mass in a patient with a CSF containing a dual population of cells that contain large polygonal cells with round nuclei, prominent nucleoli, coarse chromatin, and a lymphocytic background, is suggestive of germinoma.[66]

Choroid plexus papillomas, as mentioned previously, present mainly in children with cells that are similar to their normal counterparts. The diagnosis may be based on the finding of a ventricular mass. Choroid plexus carcinomas, however, appear as high-grade papillary carcinomas that are indistinguishable cytologically from papillary carcinomas from other locations. Because of the paucity of carcinomas in the pediatric age group, the diagnosis of choroid plexus carcinoma may be suspected based on this cytologic appearance.[66]

The low incidence of CSF spread and nonspecific cytologic appearance make the CSF examination of pituitary adenoma and craniopharyngioma, respectively, of limited value, although isolated reports have been made of such occurrences.[15,95]

It has recently been reported that specific matrix metalloproteinase (MMP) profiles in the CSF correlated with the presence of malignant astrocytomas, brain metastases, and carcinomatous meningitis.[96] These MMPs, especially gelatinases A and B, have been found in tumor tissue, and correlate with the grade and level of aggression of primary and metastatic brain tumors. The authors evaluated the presence and level of activation of MMPs in the CSF samples of healthy controls, patients with primary brain tumors, and individuals with metastatic tumors (some in the CNS, some not in the CNS). The study analyzed the premise that perhaps detection of MMPs in the CSF could correlate with the presence of brain tumors. They concluded that the precursor and activated forms of gelatinases A and B could be detected in the CSF of patients with primary and metastatic brain tumors. They also determined that the distribution of gelatinases distinguishes patients with malignant gliomas and brain metastases from patients without brain tumors, as well as distinguishing patients with meningeal carcinomatosis from patients without CSF spread of tumor, regardless of their brain tumor status. They claimed this may be a sensitive technique for the diagnosis of CNS tumors and may also provide information regarding tumor recurrence during treatment.[96]

References

1. Truex RC, Carpenter MB. Human neuroanatomy. 6th ed. Baltimore: Williams and Wilkins; 1969. pp.12-25.
2. Walts AE, Strigle S. Toward optimal use of the cytology laboratory: quality improvement and cerebrospinal fluid specimens. Diagn Cytopathol 1995; 13:357-361.
3. Rosenthal DL, Mandell DB. Central nervous system. In: Keebler CM, Somrak TM, editors. The manual of cytotechnology. 7th ed. Chicago: American Society of Clinical Pathologists Press; 1993. pp.208.
4. Beals TF. Scanning electron microscopy of body fluids. Diagn Cytopathol 1992; 8(3):266-271.
5. Keebler CM. Cytopreparatory techniques. In: Bibbo M, ed. Comprehensive cytopathology. Philadelphia: WB Saunders; 1991. pp.883-884.
6. Stanley MW, Löwhagen T. Fine needle aspiration of palpable masses. Boston: Butterworth-Heinemann; 1993. p.46-56.
7. Davey DD, Foucar K, Giller R. Millipore filter vs cytocentrifuge for detection of childhood central nervous system leukemia. Arch Pathol Lab Med 1986; 110:705-708.
8. Barrett DL, King EB. Comparison of cellular recovery rates and morphologic detail obtained using membrane filter and cytocentrifuge techniques. Acta Cytol 1976; 20: 174-180.
9. Jaffey PB, Varma SK, DeMay RM, et al. Blast-like cells in the cerebrospinal fluid of young infants: further characterization of clinical setting, morphology and origin. Am J Clin Pathol 1996; 105:544-547.
10. Fischer JR, Davey DD, Gulley ML, et al. Blast-like cells in cerebrospinal fluid of neonates: possible germinal matrix origin. Am J Clin Pathol 1989; 91:255-258.
11. Stanley MW. Cerebrospinal fluid: cytology and biochemical alterations. In: Garcia J, editor. Neuropathology: a diagnostic approach. St. Louis: Mosby; 1997.
12. Wilkins RH, Odom GL. Ependyma-choroid cells in cerebrospinal fluid: increased incidence in hydrocephalic infants. J Neurosurg 1974; 41:555-560.
13. Simon G. Der wert der liquorzelluntersuchung für die diagnostische klärung des hydrozephalus. Zentralbl Neurochir 1968; 29:197-202.
14. Yettou H, Marchal JC, Vinikoff L, et al. Papilloma of the choroid plexus: apropos of 11 cases. Neurochirurgie 1994; 40(4):227-232.
15. Takeda M, King DE, Choi HY, et al. Diagnostic pitfalls in cerebrospinal fluid cytology. Acta Cytol 1981; 25(3): 245-250.
16. Chen KTK, Moseley D. Cartilage cells in cerebrospinal fluid. Arch Pathol Lab Med 1990; 114:212.
17. Leiman G, Klein C, Berry AV. Cells of the nucleus pulposus in cerebrospinal fluid: a case report. Acta Cytol 1980; 24:347-349.
18. Kruskall MS, Carter SR, Ritz LP. Contamination of cerebrospinal fluid by vertebral bone-marrow cells during lumbar puncture. N Engl J Med 1983; 308:697-700.
19. Craver RD, Carson TH. Hematopoietic elements in cerebrospinal fluid in children. Am J Clin Pathol 1991; 95: 532-535.
20. Anderson C, Duggan C, Kealy WF. Extramedullary hematopoiesis in the central nervous system: an unusual cause of epilepsy. J Neurol Neurosurg Psychiatry 1987; 50: 640-641.
21. Tzvetanova EM, Tzekov CT. Eosinophilia in the cerebrospinal fluid of children with shunts implanted for the treatment of internal hydrocephalus. Acta Cytol 1986; 30:277-280.
22. Kuberski T. Eosinophils in the cerebrospinal fluid. Ann Intern Med 1979; 91:70-75.
23. Conrad KA, Gross JL, Trojanowski JQ. Leptomeningeal carcinomatosis presenting as eosinophilic meningitis. Acta Cytol 1986; 30:29-31.
24. Coleman A, Schumann GB. Cytodiagnosis of acute lymphocytic leukemia and eosinophilia in cerebrospinal fluid. Diagn Cytopathol 1987; 3:330-334.
25. Bigner SH, Elmore PD, Dee AL, et al. Unusual presentations of inflammatory conditions in cerebrospinal fluid. Acta Cytol 1985; 29:291-296.
26. Bigner SH, Elmore PD, Dee AL, et al. The cytopathology of reactions to ventricular shunts. Acta Cytol 1985; 29: 391-396.
27. Stanley MW, Henry-Stanley MJ, Ibe C. Bronchoalveolar lavage: cytology and clinical applications. New York: Igaku-Shoin; 1991. pp.65-119.
28. Peacock JR, McGinnis MR, Cohen MS. Persistent neutrophilic meningitis: report of four cases and review of the literature. Medicine 1984; 63:379-395.
29. Strigle SM, Gal AA. Review of the central nervous system cytopathology in human immunodeficiency virus infection. Diagn Cytopathol 1991; 7:387-401.
30. Ehni WF, Ellison RT. Spontaneous *Candida albicans* meningitis in a patient with the acquired immune deficiency syndrome. Am J Med 1987; 83;806-807.
31. Saigo P, Rosen PP, Kaplan MH, et al. Identification of *Cryptococcus neoformans* in cytologic preparations of cerebrospinal fluid. Am J Clin Pathol 1977; 67:141-145.
32. Bernad PG, Szyffelbein WM, Weiss HD, et al. Diagnosis of cryptococcal meningitis by cytologic methods: an old technique revisited. Neurology 1980; 30:102-105.
33. Gal AA, Evan S, Meyer PR. The clinical evaluation of cryptococcal infections in the acquired immunodeficiency syndrome. Diagn Microbiol Infect Dis 1987; 7:249-254.
34. Ro JY, Lee SS, Ayala AG. Advantages of Fontana-Masson stain in capsule-deficient cryptococcal infection. Arch Pathol Lab Med 1987; 111:53-57.
35. Brogi E, Cibas ES. Cytologic detection of *Toxoplasma gondii* tachyzoites in cerebrospinal fluid. Am J Clin Pathol 2000; 114(6):951-955.
36. Wheeler RR, Bardales RH, Tricot G, et al. Toxoplasma pneumonia: cytologic diagnosis by bronchoalveolar lavage. Diagn Cytopathol 1994; 11:52-55.
37. DeMent SH, Cox MC, Gupta PK. Diagnosis of central nervous system *Toxoplasma gondii* from the cerebrospinal fluid in a patient with acquired immunodeficiency syndrome. Diagn Cytopathol 1987; 3:148-157.
38. Evans H. Cytology of Mollaret meningitis. Diagn Cytopathol 1993; 9:373-376.

39. Steel JG, Dix RD, Baringer JR. Isolation of herpes simplex virus type I in recurrent (Mollaret) meningitis. Ann Neurol 1982; 11:17-21.

40. Wilbur RR, King EB, Howes EL. Cerebrospinal fluid cytology in five patients with cerebral cysticercosis. Acta Cytol 1980; 24:421-426.

41. Razavi-Encha R, Fleury-Feith J, Gherandi R, et al. Cytologic features of cerebrospinal fluid in Lyme disease. Acta Cytol 1987; 31:439-440.

42. Katz RL, Alappattu C, Glass PJ, et al. Cerebrospinal fluid manifestations of the neurologic complications of human immunodefidiency virus infection. Acta Cytol 1989; 33:233-244.

43. Lobenthal SW, Hajdu SI, Urmacher C. Cytologic findings in homosexual males with acquired immunodeficiency. Acta Cytol 1983; 27:597-604.

44. Negrini B, Kelleher KJ, Wald ER. Cerebrospinal findings in aspetic versus bacterial meningitis. Pediatrics 2001;105(2):316-319.

45. Polman CH, de Groot CJA, Koestsier JC, et al. Cerebrospinal fluid cells in multiple sclerosis and other neurological diseases: an immunohistochemical study. J Neurol 1987; 234:19-22.

46. Cepok S, Jaconsen M, Schock S, et al. Patterns of cerebrospinal fluid pathology correlate with disease progression in multiple sclerosis. Brain 2001; 124(11):2169-2176.

47. Zeman D, Adam P, Kalistova H, et al. Cerebrospinal fluid cytologic findings in multiple sclerosis: a comparison between patient subgroups. Acta Cytol 2001; 45:51-59.

48. Nikkila HV, Muller K, Ahokas A, et al. Accumulation of macrophages in the CSF of schizophrenic patients during acute psychotic episodes. Am J Psychiatry 1999; 156(11):1725-1729.

49. Chamberlain MC, Kormanik PA, Glantz MJ. A comparison between ventricular and lumbar cerebrospinal fluid cytology in adult patients with leptomeningeal metastases. Neuro-oncol 2001; 3(1):42-45.

50. Abati A, Fetsch P, Filie A. If cells could talk: the application of new techniques to cytopathology. Clin Lab Med 1998; 18(3):561-583.

51. Simsir A, Fetsch P, Stetler-Stevenson MA, et al. Immunophenotypic analysis of non-Hodgkin's lymphomas in cytologic specimens: a correlative study of immunocytochemical and flow cytometric techniques. Diagn Cytopathol 1999; 20(5):278-284.

52. Moriarty AT, Wiersma L, Snyder W, et al. Immunotyping of cytologic specimens by flow cytometry. Diagn Cytopathol 1993; 9:252-258.

53. Cibas ES, Malkin MG, Posner JB, et al. Detection of DNA abnormalities by flow cytometry in cells from cerebrospinal fluid. Am J Clin Path 1987; 88:570-577.

54. French CA, Dorfman DM, Shaheen G, et al. Diagnosing lymphoproliferative disorders involving the cerebrospinal fluid: increased sensitivity using flow cytometric analysis. Diagn Cytopathol 2000; 23:369-374.

55. Redner A, Melamed MR, Andreef M. Detection of central nervous system relapse in acute leukemia by multiparameter flow cytometry of DNA, RNA and CALLA. Ann NY Acad Sci 1986; 468:241-255.

56. O'Leary TJ. Flow cytometry in diagnostic cytology. Diagn Cytopathol 1998; 18:41-46.

57. Boogerd W, Vroom TM, van Heerde P, et al. CSF cytology versus immunocytochemistry in meningeal carcinomatosis. J Neurol Neurosurg Psychiatry 1988; 51:142-145.

58. Bigner S. Central nervous system. In: Bibbo M, editor. Comprehensive cytopathology. 2nd ed. Philadelphia: WB Saunders; 1997. pp.477-492.

59. Olson ME, Chernik NL, Posner JB. Infiltration of the leptomeninges by systemic cancer. Arch Neurol 1974; 30I:122-137.

60. Gonzalez-Vitale JC, Garcia-Bunuel R. Meningeal carcinomatosis. Cancer 1976; 37:2906-2911.

61. Wasserstrom WR, Glass JP, Posner JB. Diagnosis and treatment of leptomeningeal metastases from solid tumors: experience with 90 patients. Cancer 1982; 49:759-772.

62. Ehya H, Hajdu SI, Melamed MR. Cytopathology of non-lymphoreticular neoplasms metastatic to the central nervous system. Acta Cytol 1981; 25:599-610.

63. Glass JP, Melamed M, Chernik NL, et al. Malignant cells in cerebrospinal fluid (CSF): the meaning of a positive CSF cytology. Neurology 1979; 29:1369-1375.

64. Glantz MJ, Cole BF, Glantz LK, et al. Cerebrospinal fluid cytology in patients with cancer: minimizing false-negative results. Cancer 1998; 82(4):733-739.

65. Bigner SH, Johnston WW. The cytopathology of cerebrospinal fluid II: meningeal carcinomatosis and primary central nervous system neoplasms. Acta Cytol 1981; 25:461-479.

66. Bigner SH. Cerebrospinal fluid cytology: current status and diagnostic applications. J Neuropathol Exp Neurol 1992; 51(3):235-245.

67. Moses D, Sorbara L, Raffeld M, et al. Epstein-Barr virus in air-dried archival cerebrospinal fluid cytology: detection via conventional polymerase chain reaction. Mod Pathol 1999; 12(1):49A.

68. Rohlfing MB, Barton TK, Bigner SH, et al. Contamination of cerebrospinal fluid specimens with hematogenous blasts in patients with leukemia. Acta Cytol 1981; 25(6):611-615.

69. Bigner SH, Johnston WW. The cytopathology of cerebrospinal fluid (I): nonneoplastic conditons, lymphoma and leukemia. Acta Cytol 1981; 25:335-353.

70. Borowitz M, Bigner SH, Johnston WW. Diagnostic problems in evaluation of cerebrospinal fluid for lymphoma and leukemia. Acta Cytol 1981; 25:665-674.

71. McIntosh S, Ritchey K. Diagnostic problems in cerebrospinal fluid of children with lymphoid malignancies. Am J Pediatric Hematol Oncol 1986; 8:28-31.

72. Perez-Jaffe LA, Salhany KE, Green RJ, et al. Cerebral spinal fluid involvement by Hodgkin's disease diagnosed by CSF cytology and immunocytochemistry. Diagn Cytopathol 1999; 20:219-223.

73. Pochedly C. Meningeal leukemia: current concepts in biology and treatment (introduction to seminar). Am J Pediatric Hematol Oncol 1989; 11:55-56.

74. Bleyer WA. Biology and pathogenesis of CNS leukemia. Am J Pediatric Hematol Oncol 1989; 11:57-63.

75. Odom LF, Wilson H, Cullen J, et al. Significance of blasts in low-cell-count cerebrospinal fluid specimens from children with acute lymphoblastic leukemia. Cancer 1990; 66:1748-1754.

76. Cotran SR, Kumar V, Robbins SL. Pathologic basis of disease. 4th ed. Philadelphia: WB Saunders; 1989. p.724.

77. Rautonen J. Elevated cerebrospinal fluid leukocyte count and protein concentration at diagnosis: independent risk factors in children with acute lymphoblastic leukemia. Blut 1988; 56:265-268.

78. Tani E, Costa I, Svedmyr E, et al. Diagnosis of lymphoma, leukemia, and metastatic tumor involvement of the cerebrospinal fluid by cytology and immunocytochemistry. Diagn Cytopathol 1995; 12:14-22.

79. Yam LT, English MC, Janckila AJ, et al. Immunocytochemistry of cerebrospinal fluid. Acta Cytol 1987; 31:825-833.

80. Casper JT, Lauer SJ, Kirchner PA, et al. Evaluation of cerebrospinal fluid mononuclear cells obtained from children with acute lymphoblastic leukemia: advantages of combining cytomorphology and terminal deoxynucleotidyl transferase. Am J Clin Pathol 1983; 80:666-670.

81. Hooijkaas H, Hählen K, Adriaansen HJ, et al. Terminal deoxynucleotidyl transferase (TdT)-positive cells in cerebrospinal fluid and development of overt CNS leukemia: a 5-year follow-up study of 113 children with a TdT-postive leukemia or non-Hodgkin's lymphoma. Blood 1989; 74:416-422.

82. Homans AC, Barker BE, Forman EN, et al. Immunophenotypic characteristics of cerebrospinal fluid cells in children with acute lymphoblastic leukemia at diagnosis. Blood 1990; 76:1807-1811.

83. Lauer SJ, Kirchner PA, Camitta BM. Identification of leukemic cells in the cerebrospinal fluid from children with acute lymphoblastic leukemia: advances and dilemmas. Am J Pediatric Hematol Oncol 1989; 11:64-73.

84. Kranz BR, Thiel E, Thierfelder S. Immunocytochemical identification of meningeal leukemia and lymphoma: poly-L-Lysine-coated slides permit multimarker analysis even with minute cerebrospinal fluid cell specimens. Blood 1989; 73:1942-1950.

85. Homans AC, Forman EN, Barker BE. Use of monoclonal antibodies to identify cerebrospinal fluid lymphoblasts in children with acute lymphoblastic leukemia. Blood 1985; 66:1321-1325.

86. Redner A, Melamed M, Andreeff M. Detection of central nervous system relapse in acute leukemia by multiparameter flow cytometry of DNA, RNA, and CALLA. Ann NY Acad Sci 1986; 468:241-255.

87. Meyer RJ, Ferreira PPC, Cuttner J, et al. Central nervous system involvement at presentation in acute granulocytic leukemia. Am J Med 1980; 68:691-694.

88. Stanley MW, McKenna, RW, Ellinger G, et al. Classification of 358 cases of acute myeloid leukemia by FAB criteria: analysis of clinical and morphologic features. In: Bloomfield C, editor. Chronic and acute leukemias in adults. Dordrecht, The Netherlands: Martinus-Nijhott; 1985. pp.147-174.

89. Dahmoush Y, Hijazi E, Barnes MA. Adult T-cell leukemia/lymphoma: a cytopathological, immunocytochemical and flow cytometric study. Cancer Cytopathol 2002; 96(2):110-116.

90. Polmetyeer FE, Kernohan JW. Meningeal gliomatosis: a study of 42 cases. Arch Neurol Psychiatry 1947; 57: 593-616.

91. Gajjar A, Fouladi M, Walter AW, et al. Comparison of lumbar and shunt cerebrospinal fluid specimens for cytologic detection of leptomeningeal disease in pediatric patients with brain tumors. J Clin Oncol 1999; 17(6):1825-1828.

92. Burger PC, Vogel FS. Surgical pathology of the nervous system and its coverings. New York: John Wiley and Sons; 1976.

93. Watson CW. Hajdu SI. Cytology of primary neoplasms of the central nervous system. Acta Cytol 1977; 21:40-47.

94. EL-Batata M. Cytology of cerebrospinal fluid in the diagnosis of malignancy. J Neurosurg 1968; 28:317-326.

95. Zaharopoulos P, Wong JY. Cytology of common midline primary brain tumors. Acta Cytol 1980; 24:384-390.

96. Friedberg MH, Glantz MJ, Klempner MS, et al. Specific matrix metalloproteinase profiles in the CSF correlated with the presence of malignant astrocytomas, brain metastases and carcinomatous meningitis. Cancer 1998; 82(5):923-930.

97. Kjeldsberg CR, Knight JA. Body fluids: laboratory examination of cerebrospinal, synovial and serous fluids: a textbook atlas. Chicago: American Society of Clinical Society Press; 1982. pp.65-143.

98. Geisinger KR, Hajdu SI, Helson L. Exfoliative cytology of nonlymphoreticular neoplasms in children. Acta Cytol 1984; 28(1):16-28.

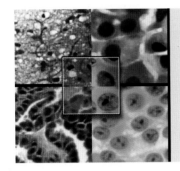

CHAPTER
14

Direct Sampling of the Central Nervous System

irect sampling techniques of central nervous system (CNS) mass lesions that lend themselves to cytologic examination include squash preparations, touch preparations (touch preps), and fine-needle aspirations (FNA). Squash and touch preparations may be performed on surgically removed tissue and used in lieu of or in addition to a frozen section. These preps have the benefit of not suffering from freezing artifact, which distorts the histology, particularly in brain tumors with edema. Burger has stated that cytologic preparations of lesions of the CNS "capture the fine cellular detail that frozen sections often obscure."[1] The use of these cytologic preparations is highly variable and depends largely on the expertise and experience of the surgeons, neuropathologists, and pathologists involved. The precision of cytologic preparations used in this regard compares well with that of intraoperative frozen sections. However, for the acquisition of the maximum amount of information, both techniques may be used together.[2]

The utility of FNA of cerebral mass lesions was originally hampered by unacceptably high morbidity and mortality rates resulting from elevated intracranial pressure and subsequent hemorrhage. Since the mid-1980s, the morbidity was reduced to 2% to 4% and mortality to 1% to 2%, primarily because of the use of steroids to decrease intracranial pressure, the use of image (stereotactic) guidance, and the employment of small-gauge needles.[3] The technical problems encountered are generally the result of sample inadequacy or tumor necrosis. A 1986 review of the subject on 221 published FNAs of the CNS, stated the false-negative and false-positive rates to be 24% and 2%, respectively. The sensitivity and specificity were at 92% and 100%, respectively.[3]

Familiarity with the clinical history, tumor location, differential diagnosis of lesions in a particular location, and cytohistologic appearance of the potential etiologies of CNS mass lesions is imperative for an accurate differential diagnosis. Based on primary familiarity with hematoxylin and eosin (H&E) tissue sections of brain tumors, these authors prefer to process CNS direct sampling cytology preparations with H&E or Papanicolaou (Pap) stains. Silverman recommends, however, that an initial Diff-Quik (DQ) stain be performed for an immediate assessment and, potentially, a rapid preliminary diagnosis, particularly with metastatic lesions.[4] He also claims that the utilization of FNA leads to a better triage of the sample for special studies, particularly in

cases with small amounts of tissue.[4] The potential disadvantages of FNA of the CNS include lack of architectural pattern within the sample, sampling errors, and erroneous grading due to heterogeneity.[4] Potential diagnostic problems and pitfalls are addressed in Box 14-1.[4-7]

The indications for brain FNA include patients with potentially radiosensitive lesions or deeply located lesions that are not resectable[3,4] (Box 14-2). FNAs are performed with a 22-gauge needle attached to a 20-ml syringe.[4]

Touch preps may be useful in diagnosing rare lesions and hematologic neoplasms. For the preparation of touch preps, the biopsy should be gently held with a forceps or laid on a table and touched with a glass slide. In the case of a needle biopsy, it should gently be rolled over the glass slide. These procedures need to be done in a very delicate manner due to the fragile nature of the cells.[2] In the case of crush preps, a scalpel is used to scrape a small portion of the biopsy material. The material is then placed on a slide, and another slide is placed on top of it and compressed. The sample is then squashed between the two slides, which are pulled apart until a thin film of cells is created.[2] Tissue in cases of reactive gliosis, nerve sheath tumors, and meningiomas resist smearing.[2] Other tumors are fragile and yield cells easily. Crush smears are extremely reliable with an accuracy rate of up to 95%.[4]

EPIDEMIOLOGY

A survey performed in the United States based on hospital stays and intracranial neoplasms concluded the annual incidence for primary and secondary intracranial neoplasms to be 8.2 and 8.3 per 100,000 population, respectively, with the rates of primary neoplasms increasing steadily with age.[8] A similar study was recently published evaluating the incidence and etiologic factors of primary intracranial tumors in Japan.[9] In this population group 5.1% were younger than 15 years of age, and 22.5% were older than 70. The distribution is outlined in Table 14-1. During the 1990s, the proportion of asymptomatic tumors increased from 24.5% to 33% with a majority of these being meningiomas (62.8%), followed by pituitary neoplasms.[9]

A recent analysis surveying the location, gender distribution, and pathologic types of pediatric brain tumors found

Potential Diagnostic Problems and Pitfalls in Direct Sampling of Central Nervous System Cytology

Distinction of reactive gliosis from low-grade astrocytoma
Correct interpretation of granular cell layer of cerebellum as normal rather than medulloblastoma; lymphoma; or other small, round, blue cell tumor
Distinction of meningioma and astrocytoma
Distinction of grade 4 astrocytoma (glioblastoma multiforme [GBM]) from metastatic carcinoma
Accuracy of tumor grading

From Silverman JF. Cytopathology of fine needle aspiration biopsy of the brain and spinal cord. Diagn Cytopathol 1986; 2:312-3193; Liwnicz BH, Rodriguez, CA. The central nervous system. In: Koss LG, Woyke S, Olszewski W, editors. Aspiration biopsy: cytologic interpretation and histologic basis. New York: Igaku-Shoin; 1984. pp.457-490; Liwnicz BH, Henderson KS, Masakawa T, et al. Needle aspiration cytology of intracranial lesions: a review of 84 cases. Acta Cytol 1985; 29:279-285; Rosenthal DL. Cytology of the central nervous system. In: Wied GL, editor. Monographs in clinical cytology. Karger: Basel; 1984. pp.160-171.

BOX 14-2

Indications for Fine-Needle Aspiration of the Central Nervous System

Lesion in deep cerebrum, including basal ganglia and thalamus
Lesion in area surrounding third ventricle
Malignant gliomas in parietal lobe of dominant hemisphere
Pineal germinoma
Metastatic carcinoma
Patient inoperable because of poor general condition

From Silverman JF. Cytopathology of fine needle aspiration biopsy of the brain and spinal cord. Diagn Cytopathol 1986; 2:312-319.

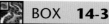

BOX 14-3   CMF

Cytomorphologic Features of Normal Neurons

Largest are Purkinje cells in cerebellum
Smallest are granular cells in cerebellum
Angulated shape of cell body
Highly variable in size
Branching cytoplasmic processes with multiple dendrites and a single axon
Abundant granular cytoplasm
Large, round central nucleus with a prominent nucleolus

From Frias-Hidvegi D, Hessel G, Cajulis R, et al. Neurocytology. In: Demay RM, editor. The art and science of cytopathology: exfoliative cytology. Chicago: ASCP Press; 1996.

TABLE 14-1

Distribution of Primary Brain Tumors in Kumamoto, Japan

Tumor Type	AGE GROUP		
	All Patients	Children	Elderly
Meningioma	33.3%		51.7%
Astrocytomas		37.6%	2.7%
Pituitary adenoma	18.3%		11.4%
Germ cell tumors		16.5%	
Malignant gliomas	14.8%		13.7%
Craniopharyngiomas		11.9%	
Schwannomas	9.8%		7.7%
Medulloblastoma		11.0%	
Ependymoma		4.6%	
Lymphoma			4.6%

Modified from Kuratsu J, Takeshima H, Ushio Y. Trends in the incidence of primary intracranial tumors in Kumamoto, Japan. Int J Clin Oncol 2001; 6(4):183-191.

the prevalence to be higher in boys (60.9%), with supratentorial locations being more common (53.3%). In this group, a fairly even distribution of low- and high-grade lesions was found. High-grade tumors seemed to be more common in patients 5 years of age or younger (53.2%).[10] In the pediatric age group, the most commonly encountered diagnoses were astrocytomas (37.6%), medulloblastomas (17.7%), ependymomas (9.9%), craniopharyngiomas (7.3%), and germ cell tumors (4.4%).[10]

CYTOLOGIC APPEARANCE

Normal Appearance

In direct cytologic preparations of the brain, the neuropil is a prominent feature of the background. It represents the supporting framework/intercellular matrix of processes on which the neurons and glia rest. Neuropil has a fibrillar appearance and stains cyanophilic with Pap, eosinophilic with H&E, and blue-purple in DQ. The cytologic appearance of normal brain cells is outlined in Boxes 14-3 to 14-8[2] (Figures 14-1 to 14-6).

Several of the primary cellular components of normal brain tissue resemble each other cytologically. Astrocytes may superficially appear similar to neurons; however, on closer inspection, astrocytes have oval nuclei, whereas neurons have round nuclei. Granular cells of the cerebellum, the smallest of neurons, mimic lymphocytes in cytologic preparations. Oligodendrocytes, which appear as small, round nuclei devoid of cytoplasm, may also be mistaken for lymphocytes. Oligodendrocytes, however, have a finer chromatin pattern than lymphocytes. Because of the apparent lack of cytoplasm, they may also be confused with astrocytes; however, astrocytes have oval nuclei, whereas those of oligodendrocytes are round.[2]

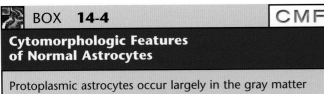

BOX 14-4 — CMF

Cytomorphologic Features of Normal Astrocytes

Protoplasmic astrocytes occur largely in the gray matter
Fibrillary astrocytes occur largely in the white matter
Stellate shaped cell bodies
Small, oval nuclei with open chromatin pattern and minute nucleoli
Delicate, thin cytoplasmic processes
Appear as naked nuclei in normal brain

From Frias-Hidvegi D, Hessel G, Cajulis R, et al. Neurocytology. In: Demay RM, editor. The art and science of cytopathology: exfoliative cytology. Chicago: ASCP Press; 1996; Okazaki H, Scheithauer BW. An atlas of neuropathology. New York: JB Lippincott; 1988.

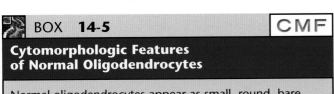

BOX 14-5 — CMF

Cytomorphologic Features of Normal Oligodendrocytes

Normal oligodendrocytes appear as small, round, bare nuclei with fine chromatin in the fibrillary background of the neuropil

From Frias-Hidvegi D, Hessel G, Cajulis R, et al. Neurocytology. In: Demay RM, editor. The art and science of cytopathology: exfoliative cytology. Chicago: ASCP Press; 1996; Silverman JF. Cytopathology of fine needle aspiration biopsy of the brain and spinal cord. Diagn Cytopathol 1986; 2:312-3193; Okazaki H, Scheithauer BW. An atlas of neuropathology. New York: JB Lippincott; 1988.

BOX 14-6 — CMF

Cytomorphologic Features of Microglia

Microglia appear as small hyperchromatic, elongated nuclei seemingly devoid of cytoplasm

From Frias-Hidvegi D, Hessel G, Cajulis R, et al. Neurocytology. In: Demay RM, editor. The art and science of cytopathology: exfoliative cytology. Chicago: ASCP Press; 1996.

Neoplastic Appearance

For the evaluation of any CNS mass lesion, knowledge of a past history of neoplasia, endocarditis, demyelinating disease, or any medical condition known to potentially produce a mass lesion in the CNS is imperative.[12] The distinctions between the lesions outlined in Box 14-9 depend not only on cytologic appearance but also on clinical information. The cytologic appearance of recent and remote hemorrhage, acute and granulomatous inflammation, lymphoma and metastatic neoplasms parallels that of other cytologic samples and is not the focus of this discussion.

Bigner takes a clever, practical approach to the cytologic evaluation of FNAs of supratentorial masses, concentrating on the level of cellularity (see Box 14-9).[12] Normal brain may be aspirated if the lesion is not sampled appropriately

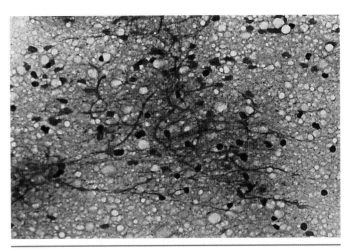

Figure 14-1 **Normal brain: white matter.** This touch preparation (prep) of normal brain white matter shows the background neuropil and oligodendrocytes. The neuropil stains a light purple and appears fibrillar with round holes. The oligodendrocytes appear as nuclei largely devoid of cytoplasm. Dark purple neuronal cellular processes are seen coursing through the neuropil. (Diff-Quik [DQ])

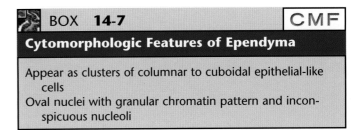

BOX 14-7 — CMF

Cytomorphologic Features of Ependyma

Appear as clusters of columnar to cuboidal epithelial-like cells
Oval nuclei with granular chromatin pattern and inconspicuous nucleoli

From Frias-Hidvegi D, Hessel G, Cajulis R, et al. Neurocytology. In: Demay RM, editor. The art and science of cytopathology: exfoliative cytology. Chicago: ASCP Press; 1996; Okazaki H, Scheithauer BW. An atlas of neuropathology. New York: JB Lippincott; 1988.

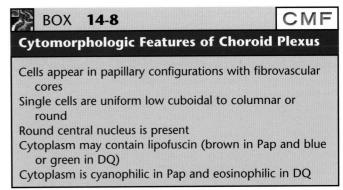

BOX 14-8 — CMF

Cytomorphologic Features of Choroid Plexus

Cells appear in papillary configurations with fibrovascular cores
Single cells are uniform low cuboidal to columnar or round
Round central nucleus is present
Cytoplasm may contain lipofuscin (brown in Pap and blue or green in DQ)
Cytoplasm is cyanophilic in Pap and eosinophilic in DQ

From Frias-Hidvegi D, Hessel G, Cajulis R, et al. Neurocytology. In: Demay RM, editor. The art and science of cytopathology: exfoliative cytology. Chicago: ASCP Press; 1996.
DQ, Diff-Quik.

and if areas surrounding the mass lesion are sampled. Although the relative cellularity of the sample will vary based on smear thickness, in normal brain this may appear as largely glial nuclei. In most H&E or Pap preps, normal glial cytoplasm may not be visible. In reactive or neoplastic tissue, glial processes are usually evident.

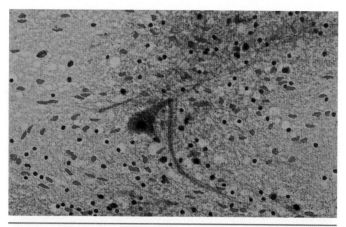

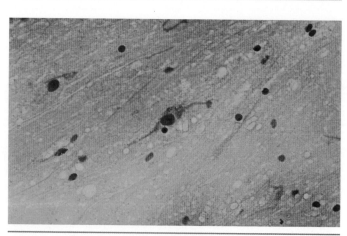

Figure 14-2   Normal brain: cerebellum. This touch prep of normal cerebellum reveals the neuropil staining in the background as moderately amphophilic. Small, round holes are present in the background. A large Purkinje cell is present in the center. It has abundant, deeply basophilic granular cytoplasm and a prominent axon. The central nucleus is round, hyperchromatic and contains a prominent eosinophilic nucleolus. Many granular cell nuclei are present in the background. (Papanicolaou [Pap])

Figure 14-3   Normal brain: gray matter. This touch prep of normal gray matter reveals background neuropil with scattered, small oligodendroglia and several neurons. The largest neuron is located centrally and has an elongated shape with a rounded, bulging central cell body. The cytoplasm is granular and deeply basophilic. The oval nucleus is central and hyperchromatic and has a prominent nucleolus. (DQ)

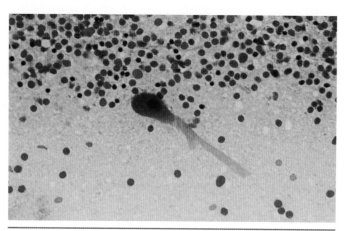

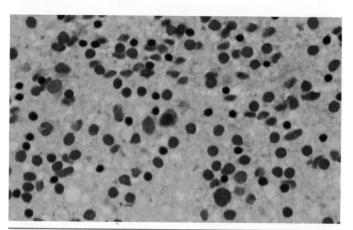

Figure 14-4   Normal brain: cerebellum. This touch prep of normal cerebellum reveals the neuropil staining in the background as light purple. A large Purkinje cell is present in the center. It has abundant deeply basophilic granular cytoplasm and a prominent axon. The central nucleus is round and hyperchromatic and contains a prominent eosinophilic nucleolus. Many granular cell nuclei are present in the background. (DQ)

Figure 14-5   Normal brain: cerebellum. This touch prep of normal cerebellum reveals an admixture of granular cells and astrocytes. The astrocytes have larger, more pale nuclei than the granular cells. Some of the astrocytes have a small rim of basophilic cytoplasm. (DQ)

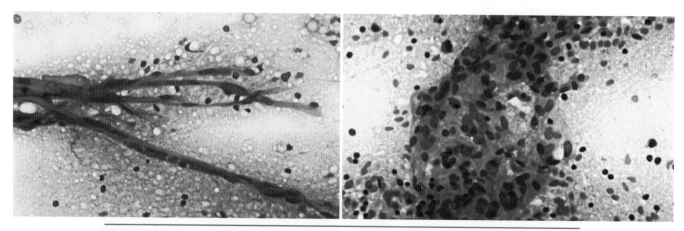

Figure 14-6   Normal brain: white matter. This touch prep of normal white matter reveals neuropil; oligodendrocytes; and prominent, central capillaries. (DQ)

The immunocytochemical approach to primary CNS neoplasms is outlined in Table 14-2. On the molecular level, the most consistent genetic abnormalities in gliomas have been documented in oligodendrogliomas and most often involve losses of 1p and 19q.[13-16] Interestingly, these genetic abnormalities have been associated with treatment responses, as well as prognosis, particularly loss of 1p, which has been associated with an improved response to chemotherapy and overall survival in patients with anaplastic oligodendroglioma.[13,15] Combined loss of 1p and 19q is a statistically significant predictor of increased survival in patients with oligodendroglioma, regardless of tumor grade.[17] Tumors without loss of 1p and without TP 53 mutations (at exons 5-8 of the TP 53 gene), which may be present in some oligodendrogliomas, tend to act like high-grade astrocytomas.[14] These abnormalities can be detected using floresence in situ hybridization (FISH), polymerase chain reaction (PCR) for loss of heterozygosity, and comparative genomic hybridization, all of which may be accomplished on cytologic material.[16]

CENTRAL NERVOUS SYSTEM NEOPLASMS

Astrocytoma

Astrocytomas can be divided into four histologic grades. In grades 1 and 2 astrocytomas the neoplastic cells are well differentiated and are distinguished largely by the degree of cellularity (Figure 14-7). Grade 3 astrocytomas (anaplastic astrocytomas) reveal high cellularity, mitoses,

---

BOX 14-9

Cytologic Approach to Direct Sampling of Supratentorial Masses Based on Cellularity

Low cellularity	High cellularity/malignant cytology
Normal brain	Lymphoma
Reactive gliosis	Metastatic carcinoma
Low-grade astrocytoma	Melanoma
	Sarcoma
High cellularity/benign cytology	High-grade astrocytoma
Abscess	
Granuloma	
Infarct	
Hemorrhage	
Oligodendroglioma	
Ependymoma	

From Bigner SH. Central nervous system. In: Bibbo M, editor. Comprehensive cytopathology. 2nd ed. Philadelphia: WB Saunders; 1997. pp.551-621.

TABLE 14-2

Immunocytochemical Reactivity of Common Primary Central Nervous System Neoplasms

Tumor	Antibodies
Astrocytoma (all grades)	GFAP +; Cytokeratins +/− (AE1/AE3)
Ependymoma	GFAP+/−; Cytokeratins +/− (AE1/AE3) S-100 and EMA inconsistent
Oligodendroglioma	GFAP+/−; S-100 +
Meningioma	EMA+, Vimentin +, E-Cadherin +/−
Medulloblastoma	GFAP− (without obvious differentiation) GFAP+ (astrocytic differentiation) Synaptophysin + (neuronal differentiation)

GFAP, Glial fibrillary acidic protein; *EMA*, epithelial membrane antigen.

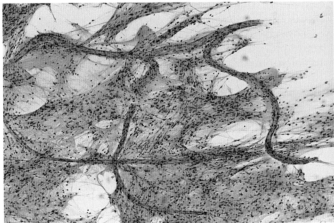 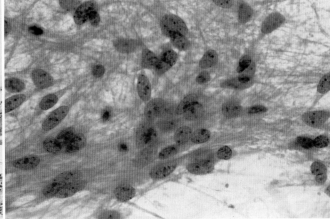

Figure 14-7 **Low-grade astrocytoma.** Prominent capillaries course through this sample of moderate cellularity. The background neuropil appears fibrillary. The nuclei are oval and elongated with a prominent central eosinophilic nucleoli. The chromatin is clumped. (Hematoxylin and eosin [H&E])

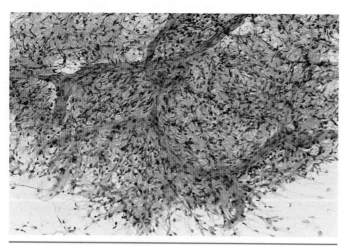

Figure 14-8 **Grade 4 astrocytoma.** This smear appears similar to Figure 14-7; however, the degree of tumor cellularity is much greater in this example. (H&E)

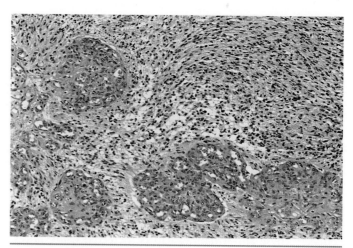

Figure 14-10 **Vascular hyperplasia/endothelial proliferation in grade 4 astrocytoma.** This histologic section reveals a grade 4 astrocytoma with glomeruloid aggregates of endothelial proliferation. (H&E)

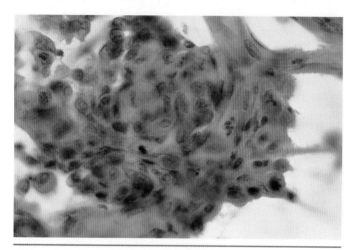

Figure 14-9 **Vascular hyperplasia/endothelial proliferation.** Prominent capillaries are seen to the periphery of this glomeruloid knot of hyperplastic endothelial cells. The endothelial nuclei are variable in shape and appear significantly clefted. Nucleoli are noted. (H&E)

vascular/endothelial hyperplasia, and increased atypia compared with the two lower grades (Figures 14-8 to 14-11). Grade 4 astrocytoma (glioblastoma multiforme [GBM]) is marked by a high degree of anaplasia and necrosis in addition to the attributes of grade 3 tumors (see Figure 14-11). Fibrillary, protoplasmic, gemistocytic (Figure 14-12), and pilocytic (Figure 14-13) are histologic subtypes that may be diagnosed cytologically.

The nuclei of reactive astrocytes tend to be similar to those of normal astrocytes, but their cytoplasm is more voluminous, and the nucleus appears obviously eccentric. The difference between low-grade astrocytoma and reactive gliosis is a difference in the cellularity (higher in astrocytoma) with the nuclei in astrocytoma showing a greater degree of hyperchromasia and irregularity of nuclear contours.[12] However, in practice, this cytologic distinction may be subtle, difficult, or even impossible in some instances.

In addition, mixed inflammatory cells may be present in a reactive process.[2] In general, the cells of astrocytoma are more pleomorphic than their reactive counterparts. In well-differentiated variants the differential features are the neoplastic cells' larger size and increased sample cellularity in comparison with normal cells.[18] In addition, the presence of atypical mitotic figures is deemed to be diagnostic of a glial neoplasm.[2,19] As stated previously, this distinction may be beyond the domain of cytopathology because it may be impossible in some cases for experienced neuropathologists to make this distinction accurately on histologic samples. Intratumoral heterogeneity with areas of divergent glial differentiation is common in glial neoplasms and can also lead to misclassification or diagnosis of lesions of a falsely lower grade than when the entire tumor is sampled.

The periphery of any CNS neoplasm may show an admixture of reactive astrocytes (Figure 14-14). It is important to know the origin of the sample from within or around the tumor to avoid erroneously diagnosing a mixed glioma with an astrocytic component.[2] Immunoperoxidase may be helpful for the distinction between primary gliomas and metastatic lesions (see Table 14-2).

Low-grade astrocytomas tend to be more cellular than reactive processes and show slight nuclear pleomorphism and hyperchromasia (see Figure 14-7). In pilocytic astrocytomas the cellular processes are prominent, and the nuclei are elongated[18] (see Figure 14-13). Higher grades of astrocytoma are associated with increasing anaplasia of the cells evidenced by angulation of the nuclei, pleomorphism, and hyperchromasia.[18] The prominence of nucleoli is variable (see Figures 14-7 to 14-13).

Cytologically the distinction between grades 2 and 3 astrocytomas (anaplastic astrocytomas) may be resolved by increased cellularity, increased pleomorphism, mitoses, numerous blood vessels and endothelial hyperplasia. Anaplastic astrocytomas show scattered bizarre large cells that may be multinucleated.[4] It is always wise, however, to remember that smear thickness affects the sample's overall appearance of cellularity. The prominent vasculature may

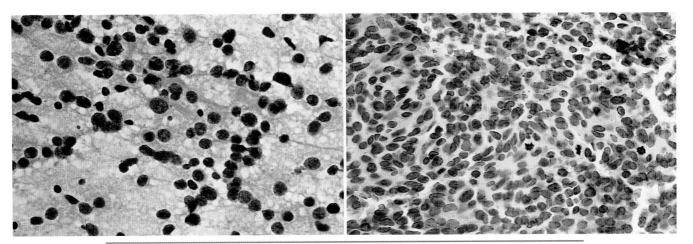

Figure 14-11 **High-grade astrocytoma.** The tumor nuclei dispersed against a background of neuropil are deeply hyperchromatic. The chromatin is clumped with multiple chromocenters. The shape and size of the nuclei are variable. Cytoplasm is inconspicuous. Mitotic figures are evident in the histologic section. (H&E)

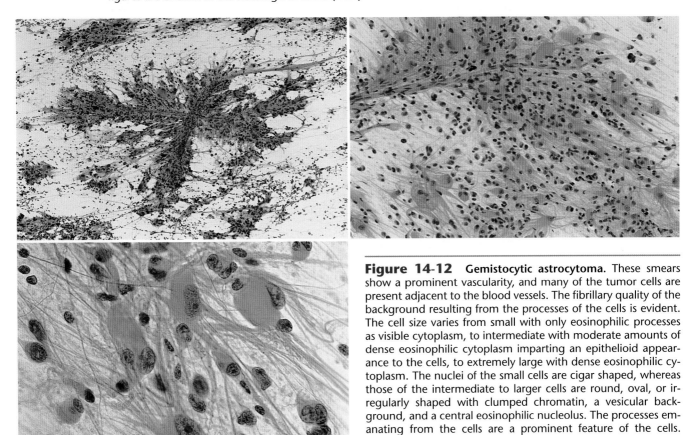

Figure 14-12 **Gemistocytic astrocytoma.** These smears show a prominent vascularity, and many of the tumor cells are present adjacent to the blood vessels. The fibrillary quality of the background resulting from the processes of the cells is evident. The cell size varies from small with only eosinophilic processes as visible cytoplasm, to intermediate with moderate amounts of dense eosinophilic cytoplasm imparting an epithelioid appearance to the cells, to extremely large with dense eosinophilic cytoplasm. The nuclei of the small cells are cigar shaped, whereas those of the intermediate to larger cells are round, oval, or irregularly shaped with clumped chromatin, a vesicular background, and a central eosinophilic nucleolus. The processes emanating from the cells are a prominent feature of the cells. (H&E)

appear as delicate branching capillaries.[4] Vessels with endothelial proliferation display a tangled and irregular appearance with prominent endothelial nuclei that are larger than usual.[4] The discrimination between grade 3 and grade 4 astrocytomas may be challenging on cytology because of the difficulty of distinguishing tumor necrosis from fibrin and other debris within the sample.[12]

Cells of GBM (grade 4 astrocytoma) are usually large and exceptionally pleomorphic with sizeable, indented, or cleffed nuclei displaying irregular, dense chromatin and prominent nucleoli. The cytoplasm may be dense and glassy with blatant processes. These high-grade tumors tend to yield very cellular smears.[18] Although the astrocytic nature of the cells may be evident, the presence of extreme pleomorphism with cells ranging from large to small, necrosis, and endothelial hyperplasia may potentially make it hard to classify. In addition, these tumors may greatly resemble metastatic carcinomas. GBMs composed of smaller anaplastic

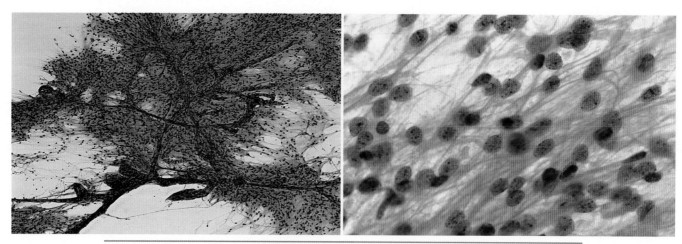

Figure 14-13 Pilocytic astrocytoma. The low-power view simulates that of the last case; however, all of the cells in this sample have fibrillary cytoplasm, and no globoid or epithelioid forms with abundant cytoplasm are noted. The lesion has an obvious rich vascularity and is fairly cellular with a fibrillary background. The higher power view highlights the bland nuclear features. The nuclei are largely oval and hypochromatic with finely stippled chromatin and several chromocenters. Some of the cells have small eosinophilic nucleoli. The cytoplasm is in the form of fibrillary processes. (H&E)

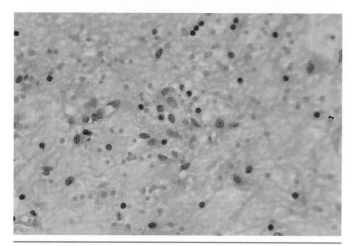

Figure 14-14 Reactive astrocytes adjacent to a brain tumor. These reactive astrocytes have vesicular elongated nuclei and small amounts of irregular eosinophilic cytoplasm. Oligodendroglial nuclei are present in the background. (H&E)

cells with less cytoplasm, irregular hyperchromatic nuclei, and significant pleomorphism may also be seen alone or as a component of a more typical GBM.

Gemistocytic astrocytomas (grade 4) are made up of cells with voluminous eosinophilic cytoplasm with many cytoplasmic processes. Their nuclei are large, eccentric, and hyperchromatic. They have prominent nucleoli with a coarse chromatin pattern (see Figure 14-12).

Pilocytic astrocytomas are low-grade tumors that occur most commonly in the cerebellum of the pediatric population. In cytologic preps, the cells exhibit a certain degree of variability and pleomorphism, with nuclei ranging from round to oval to elongated. Some of the cells have rounded ends, which makes them difficult to distinguish from oligodendroglial cells and endothelial cells.[2] A distinguishing feature from endothelial nuclei is the chromatin granularity in

the neoplastic astrocytes. Single or multiple nucleoli may be noted. The background is fibrillary[2] (see Figure 14-13).

A rare tumor, glial sarcoma, has both malignant glial and sarcomatous elements. The glial component, generally high-grade astrocytoma, can be highlighted by a glial fibrillary acidic protein (GFAP) stain, and the sarcomatous component usually assumes the pattern of angiosarcoma or fibrosarcoma.[1]

Oligodendroglioma

Oligodendrogliomas are typically hemispheric and show calcification on imaging studies. The calcification may lead to a gritty sensation when smeared.[2] Smears are usually highly cellular and are composed of low-grade–appearing small cells with uniform, round nuclei devoid of obvious cytoplasm, thus appearing as naked nuclei[2] (Figure 14-15). The chromatin pattern is finely granular, and nucleoli may be distinct.[2,11,12,20] Calcification may be seen in the smears as may numerous capillaries, with the latter giving rise to the histologic appearance of "chicken wire" vasculature.[2] The differential diagnosis includes lymphoma, although the cells of lymphoma have visible cytoplasm and clumped chromatin and may be distinguished through immunocytochemical lymphoid marker studies. Oligodendrogliomas stain variably with GFAP, but immunoreactivity for GFAP is not specific for these neoplasms because it is also detected in astrocytomas and ependymomas (see Table 14-2).

Ependymoma

Ependymomas are neoplasms derived from the ependymal lining of the ventricles and central canal. They may occur within the brain and spinal cord, most commonly in a periventricular or a lumbosacral location. In most instances the tumor cells are fairly monotonous and resemble their benign counterparts (Figures 14-16 and 14-17). They have abundant cytoplasm with uniform, round nuclei and finely

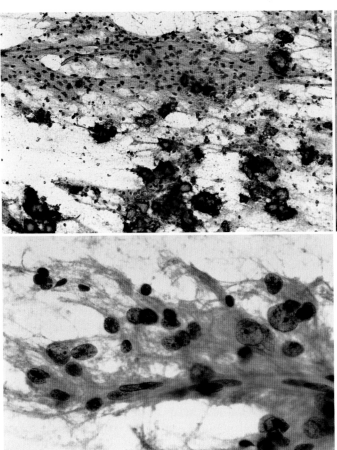

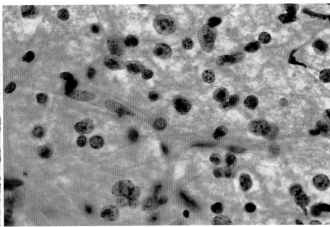

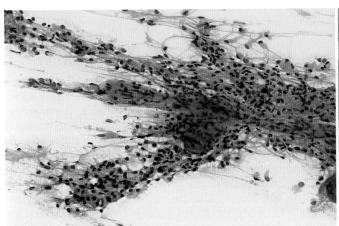

Figure 14-15 **Oligodendroglioma.** Calcification may be an obvious feature of the low-power view of an oligodendroglioma. The background may appear smudged or fibrillary. On closer inspection the tumor nuclei can be differentiated easily from endothelial nuclei of the capillaries coursing through the tumor. The endothelial nuclei are elongated and teardrop or cigar shaped, whereas the tumor nuclei are perfectly round with central, dark, basophilic nucleoli and finely stippled and focally clumped chromatin. (H&E)

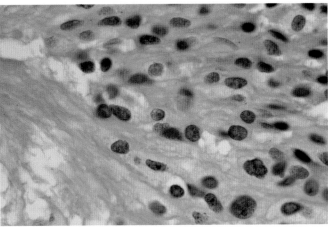

Figure 14-16 **Ependymoma.** The low-power view of this ependymoma with atypia reveals a cellular vascular neoplasm composed of cells with both fibrillary and epithelioid cytoplasm. A high-power view of a different area reveals a fibrillary background and cells with round to oval nuclei with coarse chromatin stippling. Some variability in nuclear size is evident. (H&E)

stippled chromatin. The cytoplasm is light purple with DQ, cyanophilic in Pap, and eosinophilic on H&E.[2] Cytologic preparations are usually cellular and are remarkable for the uniform appearance of the cells and their frequent perivascular location, imparting an almost papillary appearance to the tumor. In addition, the cells may form true rosettes in which cellular processes surround an actual lumen. Other rosettes appear around vascular cores (pseudorosettes).[2] Peculiar structures known as *blepharoplasts* can aid in the identification of a neoplasm as ependymal in etiology. Blepharoplasts are intracytoplasmic round- to rod-shaped structures that correspond to the basal bodies of cilia. These

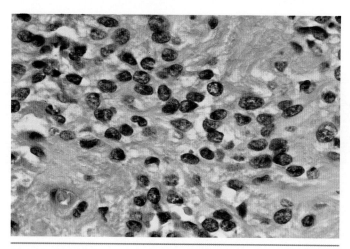

Figure 14-17 **Ependymoma with anaplasia.** This ependymoma with anaplasia exhibits a background similar to the previous example. However, the cellularity is greater, the nuclei are smaller and more hyperchromatic, and most of the nuclei have prominent eosinophilic nucleoli. (H&E)

structures are highlighted by the phosphotungstic acid hematoxylin (PTAH) stain and are best visualized under oil immersion. They are usually seen in the apical portion of neoplastic ependymal cells forming a rosette. Although helpful in the diagnosis, they are rarely seen.[19]

In ependymomas with malignant degeneration, the cells are anaplastic and may have irregular nuclear contours (see Figure 14-17). Vascular or endothelial hyperplasia may be seen, and necrosis and mitotic figures may be evident.[2]

Myxopapillary ependymoma (MPE) occurs in the region of the filum terminale and has a distinctive histology and cytology (Figure 14-18). The tumor cells lie in an abundant extracellular matrix that is mucin positive. Many of the bland-appearing tumor cells are in ball-like formations, whereas others are attached to blood vessels. Rare ependymal rosettes may be seen. The tumor has a characteristic biphasic pattern with the tumor cells arranged around cords and balls of this myxohyaline material.[45]

Based on both the location and the prominent matrix, the differential diagnosis includes metastatic mucin secreting adenocarcinoma and chordoma. The distinction is made on the GFAP positivity of the ependymoma, whereas the other two neoplasms are negative. Also, adenocarcinomas are usually immunoreactive with cytokeratins and exhibit a greater degree of nuclear pleomorphism than the cells of MPE. The cells of chordoma are immunoreactive with cytokeratins and S-100, whereas the background is negative for mucin. The characteristic physaliphorous cells of chordoma are not seen in MPE.[2]

Central Neurocytoma

Central neurocytoma, a neoplasm with neuronal differentiation that histologically resembles oligodendroglioma, has only been characterized fairly recently[21] (Figure 14-19). Cytologically the neoplastic cells appear in sheets. The cells are round with finely stippled nuclear chromatin and perinuclear halos. The smear background is finely fibrillar, although cell processes are not obvious. Calcospherites and

rosettelike formations may be seen.[22] These tumors are immunoreactive with synaptophysin.

Primitive Neuroectodermal Tumors

Primitive neuroectodermal tumors (PNET) of the brain are small, round, blue cell tumors of pluripotential primitive cells that have the ability to differentiate along glial or neuronal cell pathways (Figures 14-20 to 14-22). Within the CNS, based on location and particular histologic features, they may be subclassified as medulloblastomas, medulloepitheliomas, neuroblastoma (central or esthesio-), retinoblastoma, pineoblastoma, or ependymoblastoma. They share several features in common, including cellular samples composed of uniform, small, discohesive cells with high nuclear to cytoplasmic (N:C) ratios, angular nuclear contours, inconspicuous cytoplasm, high mitotic index, and individual cellular necrosis. The nuclei possess hyperchromatic, granular chromatin.[2] Astrocytic differentiation may be indicated by an increase in the cell size with a more vesicular pattern to the nuclei and a fibrillar background. Rosettes and cells resembling ganglion cells may suggest neuronal differentiation. In these instances, GFAP and synaptophysin should confirm astrocytic or neuronal differentiation, respectively.[2] In PNETs devoid of obvious differentiation, these markers would generally be negative. Medulloblastoma, the most common PNET of the CNS, is usually cerebellar and needs to be distinguished from cells of the internal granular cell layer (see Figures 14-21 and 14-22). The differential diagnosis includes lymphoma, which can be ruled out by an immunohistochemical stain for leukocyte common antigen, and metastatic small cell carcinoma, which is uncommon in the pediatric population and is usually positive with immunohistochemical stains for cytokeratin and possibly Leu7.[2,23]

Meningioma

Meningiomas are relatively common intracranial neoplasms that usually become evident after the third decade. They are more common in women than in men, particularly in spinal locations. Etiologically arising from the meninges, they usually occur in several locations: parasagittally, over the cerebral convexities, along the wings of the sphenoid ridge, and near the olfactory groove.[19] Meningiomas are usually single and can be cured by surgical excision in the majority of cases.[19] Histologically, there are a variety of subtypes. Cytologically, meningiomas are composed of cells arranged in syncytial clusters, whorls, and sheets with lightly eosinophilic, wispy cytoplasm that does not have clearly defined boundaries[4,24] (Figure 14-23). Nuclei are oval, sharply outlined, and slightly eccentric with homogeneous, evenly distributed chromatin. Small nucleoli that are centrally located are present. Other nuclear features include the presence of grooves and cytoplasmic pseudoinclusions. A characteristic attribute is the presence of cells in whorls with psammoma bodies. Scattered cells may have larger and more hyperchromatic nuclei.[4,24] The differential diagnosis of this epithelial-appearing tumor includes, metastatic neoplasms of squamous and papillary thyroid origins.[24] Generally, the diagnosis of a malignant meningioma rests on histologic criteria, including mitotic rate. Interestingly, E-cadherin, typically thought to be an

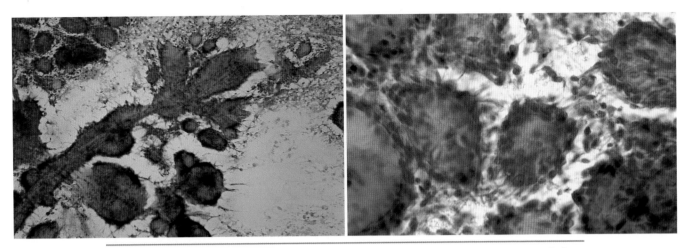

Figure 14-18 **Myxopapillary ependymoma.** This tumor exhibits a biphasic morphology with nests and aggregates of epithelioid malignant cells and branching cords of myxohyaline material. Tumor cells surround distinct myxohyaline globules. The nuclei are round to oval and have single, central, small nucleoli. (H&E)

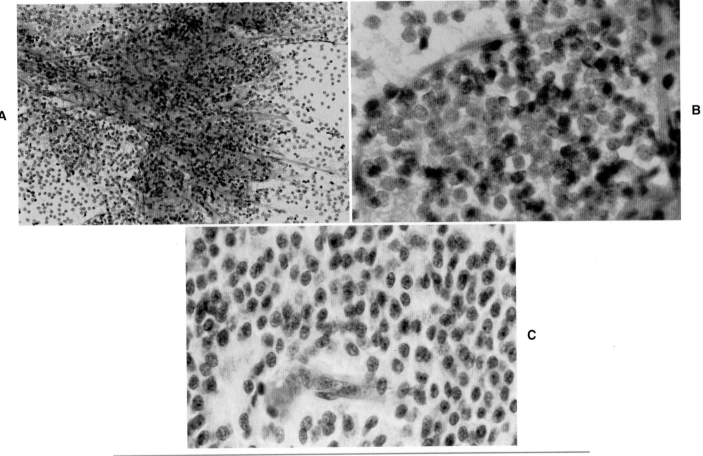

Figure 14-19 **Central neurocytoma. A,** Aside from the prominent vascularity of thin-walled vessels, the obvious low-power feature of this tumor is the large number of uniform, round nuclei, apparently devoid of cytoplasm. **B,** The high-power view confirms the low-power impression of the nuclear homogeneity. The nuclei have finely stippled chromatin and focal chromocenters but are devoid of obvious nucleoli. The background is finely fibrillar. **C,** The nuclei in this high-power view of a histologic section are oval and slightly irregular. The chromatin is clumped. Many of the cells have basophilic nucleoli. The background is finely fibrillar. Several poorly formed rosettelike formations are present. (H&E)

immunohistochemical marker for epithelial neoplasms, is positive in benign meningiomas. Recurrent and malignant meningiomas seem to lose this reactivity with E-cadherin.[25]

Pituitary Adenoma

Surprisingly, incidental pituitary adenomas have been found in about a quarter of all autopsy cases. Those that acquire sufficient size or exhibit clinically noticeable hormonal activity comprise 10% to 20% of all intracranial neoplasms.[19] The exact cell of origin of adenomas of the anterior pituitary is determined by clinically aberrant hormonal activity detected in blood tests and/or immunohistochemistry for the presence of thyroid-stimulating hormone (TSH), prolactin, or growth hormone in tumor samples.

Cytologic preps show polygonal cells with well-defined cytoplasmic outlines and round to oval nuclei of varying sizes (Figure 14-24). Cells are present singly and in loosely cohesive clusters. Isolated tumor cells may assume a plasmacytoid appearance with DQ stain.[4] A diagnostic pitfall is the distinction of a pituitary adenoma from a meningioma in a suprasellar mass with epithelial-appearing cells in nests with round nuclei and the presence of psammoma bodies.[4]

Choroid Plexus Papilloma

Choroid plexus papilloma (CPP), a rare neoplasm of predominantly the first decade of life, usually presents with hydrocephalus. The lateral ventricles are the most common location, although they may occur in the fourth ventricles in the adult population.[19]

The cytologic appearance of CPP is one of a papillary neoplasm with fibrovascular cores lined by layers of cuboidal epithelial cells. Psammoma bodies may be seen. The nuclei are round, bland, and strikingly uniform. In fact, significant degrees of pleomorphism may herald the presence of a choroid plexus carcinoma, although the cytology within these lesions can be variable from one portion of the tumor to another (Figure 14-25). The main differential diagnosis is with ependymoma. Both neoplasms may show papillary and acinar-like arrangements, a mosaic pattern of cells, and calcifications. Ependymomas are more likely to have bipolar cells with fibrillary cytoplasm, perivascular pseudorosettes, rare blepharoblasts (with PTAH stain), nuclear grooves, and intranuclear cytoplasmic pseudoinclusions.[26] CPP is positive immunohistochemically with cytokeratin, carbonic anhydrase C, prealbumin, and laminin, whereas ependymoma is positive with GFAP. Focal staining with GFAP may be seen in CPP, and focal staining with cytokeratins may be seen in ependymoma.[26] Other papillary tumors within the CNS that enter into the differential diagnosis include papillary meningioma and metastatic carcinoma. Metastatic carcinoma usually has a more anaplastic appearance. Papillary meningioma is an invasive neoplasm

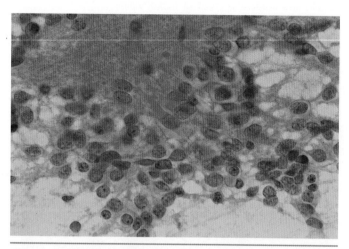

Figure 14-20 **Neuroblastoma.** The eosinophilic fibrillary matrix is abundant and a prominent feature of this neuroblastoma. The nuclei are oval and fairly regular in shape and size, with fine chromatin stippling and one or more chromocenters. Fibrillary cytoplasm is obvious in some of the cells. (H&E)

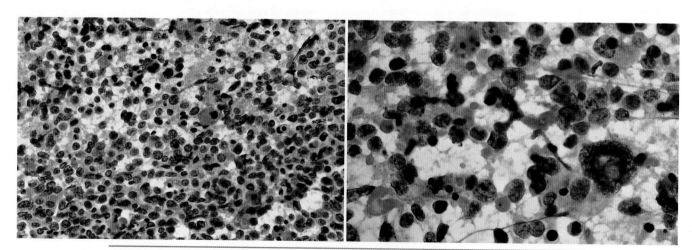

Figure 14-21 **Medulloblastoma.** The obvious cytologic features here are of high cellularity and individual cellular necrosis. The background is fibrinous and broken apart. The cells appear either devoid of cytoplasm or have small amounts of peripherally placed eosinophilic cytoplasm. The nuclei are mostly small and variably sized and are hyperchromatic with coarsely clumped cytoplasm. Some of the cells have prominent central eosinophilic nucleoli. (H&E)

with meningothelial features.[26] Interestingly, choroid plexus epithelium, both normal and neoplastic, expresses reactivity with synaptophysin, another distinguishing feature.[27] In addition, along with meningioma, CPP is immunoreactive with E-cadherin.[25] Choroid plexus carcinomas tend to express carcinoembryonic antigen (CEA), which is not evident in CPP, whereas they do not express prealbumin.[28]

Hemangioblastoma

Hemangioblastoma, a predominantly cerebellar neoplasm associated with von Hippel Lindau syndrome and renal cell carcinoma, has a characteristic cytologic appearance consisting of a thin capillary network with dispersed stromal cells that appear in sheets and clusters (Figure 14-26). The stromal cells have abundant, clear, vacuolated cytoplasm and central, round nuclei with variable-appearing nucleoli. The differential diagnosis includes conventional renal cell carcinoma; however the large cells in renal cell carcinoma should be immunoreactive with epithelial

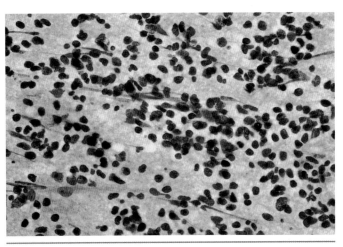

Figure 14-22 **Medulloblastoma.** This high-power view shows a prominent fibrillary matrix with some of the cells arranged in poorly formed pseudo-rosettelike structures is reminiscent of a neuroblastoma and may signify neuronal differentiation. (H&E)

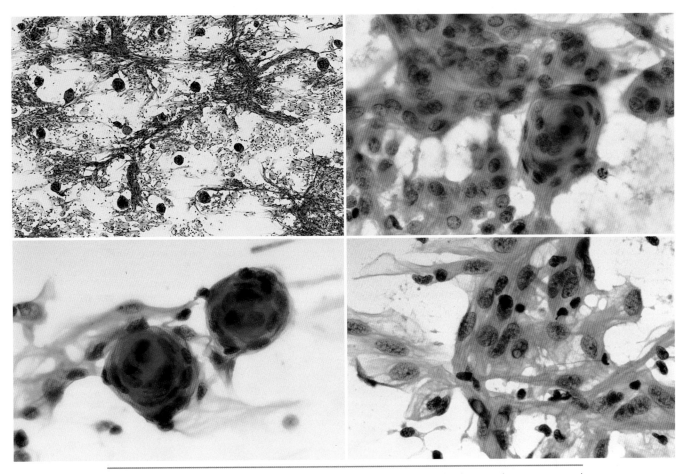

Figure 14-23 **Meningioma.** Prominent vascularity and whorls are the pronounced features of this neoplasm. The cells have variable amounts of dense fibrillar to epithelial-appearing cytoplasm. The nuclei are distinctly uniform and round to oval. They are normochromatic with small or no nucleoli. Whorls are formed by the concentric lamellations of tumor cells. Cytoplasmic intranuclear inclusions may be seen. Atypia may be noted in some meningiomas manifested by nuclear enlargement, irregularities, and nucleolar prominence. (H&E)

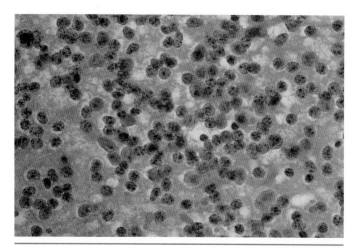

Figure 14-24 **Pituitary adenoma.** The eosinophilic fibrillar matrix and round nuclei are suggestive of an endocrine origin. The nuclei are round, with clumped chromatin and prominent eosinophilic nucleoli. Size variability of the nuclei is expected. (H&E)

membrane antigen (EMA), whereas those of hemangioblastoma should not.

Craniopharyngioma

Craniopharyngiomas occur almost exclusively in the first two decades of life and are easily visualized on imaging studies because of their sellar location and usual calcification.[19] Their suprasellar location yields symptoms of obstructive hydrocephalus, visual disturbances, and potential endocrine abnormalities.[19]

The cytology of craniopharyngioma may be confounded by a cystic component, the fluid of which is highly thick and viscous. Cytologically, this cystic fluid may contain necrotic debris, red blood cells (RBCs), histiocytes, keratinaceous debris, cholesterol crystals, and necrotic brain tissue[2] (Figure 14-27). The smears show squamous cells, anucleated squamous cells, keratin, and possibly calcium. As with keratinizing processes elsewhere, foreign body giant cells and histiocytes may be seen. When elements are present, such

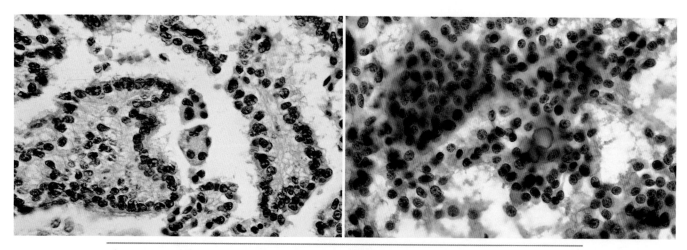

Figure 14-25 **Choroid plexus papilloma.** The architecture of this neoplasm is obviously papillary with vascular cores evident in this cell block section. The cells lining the papillae are cuboidal with round nuclei. A psammoma body is focally seen in the smear. The nuclei are round and uniform, with visible, central nucleoli and clumped chromatin. (H&E)

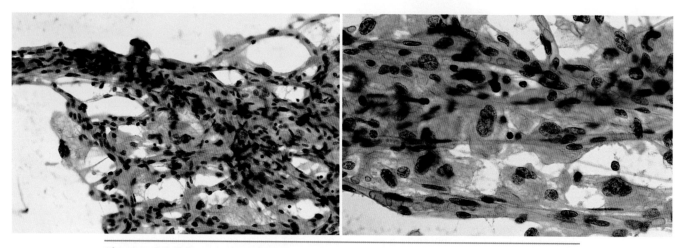

Figure 14-26 **Hemangioblastoma.** These smears show prominent vascularity, a biphasic population composed of endothelial cells comprising the capillaries, and larger interspersed cells with voluminous vacuolated cytoplasm and round nuclei. Red blood cells (RBCs) are visible in the capillaries. (H&E)

as anucleated squames, histiocytes, squamous epithelial fragments, and cholesterol crystals, it may be impossible to distinguish craniopharyngioma from dermoid and epidermoid cysts. The presence of hair, however, points to a dermoid.[2]

Lymphoma

Lymphoma involving the CNS can be primary or secondary. Primary CNS lymphoma (PCNSL) and peripheral body cavity lymphoma are much more prevalent in the immunocompromised population than in the population at large. The incidence is increased by approximately 100-fold in patients with advanced human immunodeficiency virus (HIV) infection.[29] In patients with acquired immunodeficiency syndrome (AIDS) the most common type is an intermediate or high-grade B-cell lymphoma that is usually extranodal in origin, with about 20% being primary CNS in location.[29] Patients with PCNSL are usually extremely immunosuppressed, with two thirds previously showing symptoms of AIDS-defining conditions.[30,31] PCNSL usually presents with one to three lesions of 2 to 4 cm in diameter, which are usually contrast enhancing on imaging and cerebral hemispheric in location, although they can also be seen infratentorially.[32-34]

Histologically, the lymphoma cells are disseminated in a perivascular distribution. The cells are of a germinal center B cell origin, and uniformly express Epstein-Barr virus (EBV)–associated DNA.[35] A cytologic study of 23 cases of PCNSL, including both HIV patients and those without the disease (20 HIV positive, two HIV negative, and one of unknown status) revealed 12 cases with immunoblastic morphology, 10 large cell, and one mixed small and large cell lymphoma. Of the cases, 19 were of B-cell origin, with two T-cell and one biphenotypic case identified. In situ hybridization for Epstein-Barr RNA virus early region (EBER-1) was performed on Pap-stained smears from each case and detected nuclear positivity for EBV RNA in 19 of 23 cases (83%).[36] A positive EBV DNA PCR test in the CSF has been recommended as a screening tool for PCNSL.[37] This test has a sensitivity of nearly 100% and a specificity of 98%.[36,37] Although the prognosis is poor in patients with AIDS who have PCNSL, recent evidence suggests that the addition of highly active antiretroviral therapy (HAART) has led to a decrease in the incidence of lymphoma in these patients and has improved the prognosis. The differential diagnosis in the CNS presentation of primary or secondary lymphoma, particularly in patients with AIDS, is infection.[29]

Other Neoplasms

Germ cell neoplasms may occur in the region of the pineal gland. These neoplasms are identical to their analogues in the gonads (Figure 14-28).

Because of the distinct eighth nerve location, characteristic dumbbell shape, and clinical symptomatology (tinnitus and dizziness), the diagnosis of acoustic neuroma or

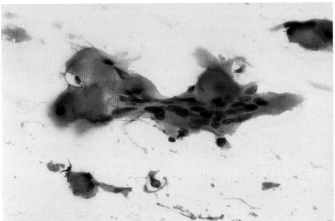

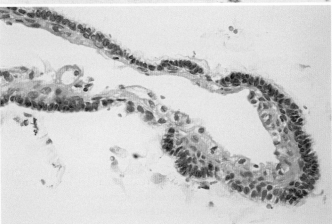

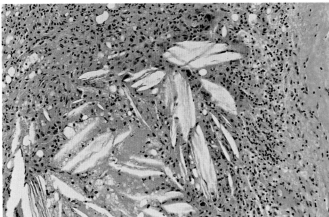

Figure 14-27 Craniopharyngioma. This smear and cell blocks reveal several features of this neoplasm. The keratin formed by the squamous cells leads to dense eosinophilic material, which, when ruptured, can yield hemorrhage, a foreign body giant cell reaction, and cholesterol clefts. The cells may be mature squamous cells or may appear to be more primitive basaloid epithelium. (H&E)

schwannoma is rarely a surprise. Thus, it only infrequently warrants an intraoperative consultation. The cytopathology of this benign peripheral nerve sheath tumor is described in Chapter 28 (Figure 14-29).

Metastatic Central Nervous System Neoplasms

The most common neoplasms to metastasize to the CNS are from the lung, breast, skin (malignant melanoma), kidney, and gastrointestinal (GI) tract. Although choriocarcinoma is a rare neoplasm, it metastasizes to the brain with a high frequency.[19,38]

Occasional reports of metastatic CNS neoplasms diagnosed by FNA have been documented.[20,23,24,39,40] Most instances of spread of primary gliomas outside of the CNS have occurred after surgical intervention, biopsy, or diversionary shunt.[40]

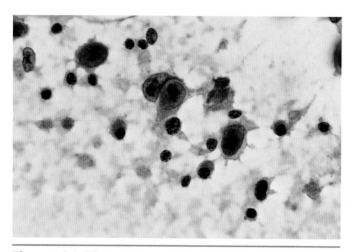

Figure 14-28   **Germinoma.** This tumor has a biphasic population composed of small plasmacytoid lymphocytes and larger tumor cells that have large, round nuclei with prominent nucleoli and perinucleolar clearing. The cytoplasm has clearly delineated boundaries. The background would appear characteristically tigroid on DQ but appears necrotic in this sample. (H&E)

 INFECTIONS

Since the 1980s and the emergence of AIDS, pathologists have been faced with making diagnoses on neoplastic and infectious processes within the CNS on these patients. The malignancies most commonly seen within the CNS of patients with AIDS are primary CNS lymphoma and secondary involvement of the CNS with peripheral lymphomas. The infections most commonly diagnosed in the CNS in AIDS that may require tissue sampling are progressive multifocal leukoencephalopathy (PML), toxoplasmosis, *Cryptococcus,* and *Mycobacterium avium intracellulare.*[2]

Most samples of CNS infections that can potentially be diagnosed on cytology include toxoplasmosis (trophozoites), bacteria, yeast, fungi, and viruses. Evaluation of cells on the DQ stain is optimal for the visualization of many of these organisms. In addition, in patients with AIDS where the differential diagnosis may be between infection and lymphoma, the DQ stain is the optimal stain for viewing hematologic neoplasms.

Progressive Multifocal Leukoencephalopathy

John Cunningham virus (JCV), the infectious agent implicated in PML is transactivated by HIV-1 and is associated with profound immunosuppression.[41] Although the disease has characteristic clinical and imaging findings (without mass effect) including focal neurologic defects with subcortical white matter abnormalities with scalloped edges and peripheral contrast enhancement, a definitive diagnosis usually requires brain biopsy. With the appropriate clinical and imaging findings, the use of PCR for the JCV in the CSF can now be used for diagnostic confirmation. PCR tests for JCV have a sensitivity and specificity of 92% or higher.[41-43] In lieu of PCR on CSF, if a direct brain sampling technique is used, the diagnosis of PML has several cytologic features that make the diagnosis possible. JCV infects oligodendrocytes, increasing their sizes and yielding a large, smudged, hyperchromatic, glassy, intranuclear inclusion that occupies the entire nucleus. The astrocytes in the surrounding parenchyma become large and reactive and may appear

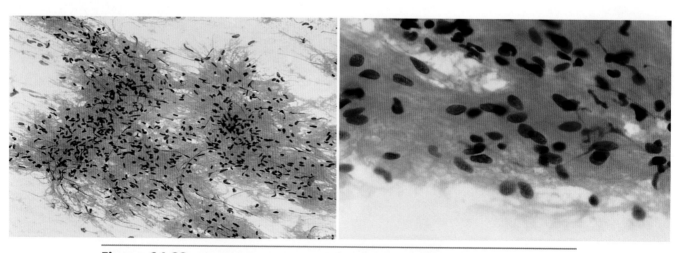

Figure 14-29   **Neurilemmoma.** The cells in this tumor assume a granuloma-like appearance, where the elongated and boomerang-shaped nuclei are arranged in aggregates of a fibrillary matrix. (H&E)

quite atypical. The viral-induced myelin destruction leads to the presence of lipid-laden macrophages. A lack of accompanying necrosis and inflammatory cells is evident.[2] Immunocytochemical stains for polyoma virus and electron microscopy can aid in the diagnosis in questionable cases.

Toxoplasmosis

Toxoplasmosis, a disease caused by the intracellular protozoan parasite *Toxoplasma gondii,* leads to a necrotizing encephalitis that is most commonly seen in immunocompromised hosts such as individuals with HIV. Clinically, the infection presents as space occupying lesions, usually bilaterally, in the basal ganglia region. The lesions are ring-enhancing on computed tomography (CT) scan, simulating the imaging appearance of lymphoma. The treatment paradigm for these types of lesions dictates initial treatment for toxoplasmosis in an attempt to avoid brain biopsy. Failure to respond to therapy leads to tissue sampling. Cytologically, the preferred stain is the DQ stain because it highlights the tiny crescent-shaped tachyzoites blue. Cytologic samples show a mixture of intact and disintegrating glial cells with abundant necrotic debris. Astrocytes may be present and show mild reactive atypia (not as pronounced as it is in PML) or may appear to be disintegrating. Histiocytes are also present. The organisms may be present in groups within histiocytic cytoplasm and/or may be present extracellularly. The organism is crescent or comma shaped, measuring 4 to 8 nm in length and 2 to 3 nm in width. On DQ the cytoplasm is dark blue with the nucleus staining dark purple to red. On Pap stain, the trophozoites may appear rounded.[44]

Cryptococcus Infection

Cryptococcus infection, although mostly seen in immunocompromised patients, may also be present in seemingly immunocompetent patients. It is thought that infection reaches the brain from an established pulmonary infection. These organisms are described in the section of the chapter on Cerebrospinal Fluid.

 # DIRECT SAMPLING OF THE ORBIT, OCULAR ADNEXA, AND GLOBE

Compared with most other organs, the cytopathology literature dealing with direct sampling techniques of the orbit, ocular adnexa, and globe is fairly sparse. This undoubtedly reflects the lack of experience that ophthalmologists and cytopathologists have with samples from the eye, as a majority of publications come from less than a handful of referral centers. An excellent review of this topic has been published by Rosenthal, Mandell, and Glasgow, reflective of their experience at University of California at Los Angeles.[46] When initially requested to render cytologic interpretations on vitreous samples, they obtained eyes from autopsy samples for simulated washings to collect nondiseased cells as a learning tool to become familiar with the morphology of the normal cellular constituents[47] (Table 14-3). For illustrations of these normal elements, the reader is referred to Rosenthal and Mandell[46,47] (Figure 14-30).

Sampling of the Eyelid and Cornea

The eye and surrounding structures can be sampled by scrape, FNA, or vitrectomy-washing cytology.[46] Lesions of the globe, eyelid, and orbit or adnexa may be sampled through FNA, whereas lesions of the conjunctiva and cornea are scraped.[46] Scraping requires a local anesthetic and must be done carefully to avoid damage to the delicate ocular tissues.[46] Ideally, this material should be fixed promptly in ethanol for Pap staining. The lack of moisture in the area may lead to general problems with air-drying of these samples.[46] Because the etiology of many scrape samples of the conjunctiva and cornea may be viral in origin and the viral inclusions are best visualized on Pap stain, air-drying should be kept to a minimum (Tables 14-4 and 14-5).

Fine-Needle Aspiration of the Orbit and Ocular Adnexa

FNA of the orbit and ocular adnexa has been deemed a safe and effective method for the sampling of orbital processes in lieu of an open biopsy[48,49] (Table 14-6). It is particularly useful when a

---

TABLE 14-3

Cytomorphologic Features of Normal Cells of the Eye

Area of Eye	Features
Cornea	Intermediate squamous cells
Conjunctiva	Basal columnar cells, goblet cells
Uvea	Retinal pigment and epithelial cells
Retina	Rods and cones (clusters of small dark nuclei, at the periphery of neuropil matrix)
	Large neurons
Ocular chambers	Histiocytes and lymphocytes (scarce)

Modified from Rosenthal DL, Mandell DB, Glasgow BJ. Eye. In: Bibbo M, editor. Comprehensive cytopathology. 2nd ed. Philadelphia: WB Saunders; 1997. pp.551-621.

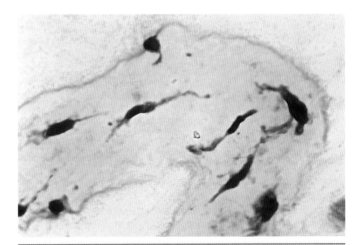

Figure 14-30 Cells in vitrectomy specimen. Cells are present here singly. They are slender and elongated but may be present in parallel groups. (DQ)

TABLE 14-4
Lesions of the Eyelid

Lesion	Cytomorphologic Findings

Viral:
  Molluscum contagiosum
  Herpes zoster
  Herpes simplex I and II
	Characteristic viral inclusions

Xanthalasmas	Lipid-laden macrophages
Melanocytic tumors	Features of malignant melanoma Features of benign melanocytic lesions have not been well defined cytologically
Chalazion	Granulomas with lipid-laden macrophages and neutrophils

From Rosenthal DL, Mandell DB, Glasgow BJ. Eye. In: Bibbo M, editor. Comprehensive cytopathology. 2nd ed. Philadelphia: WB Saunders; 1997. pp.551-621.

TABLE 14-5
Lesions of the Conjunctiva

Lesion	Cytomorphologic Findings

Viral:
  Molluscum contagiosum
  Herpes zoster
  Herpes simplex I and II
	Characteristic viral inclusions

Bacterial infection	Variable; acute inflammation Culture recommended
Allergic (vernal) reaction	Eosinophils, mast cells, and lymphocytes; goblet cells if chronic
Chlamydia	Inconsistent inflammatory pattern; polymerase chain reaction recommended

From Rosenthal DL, Mandell DB, Glasgow BJ. Eye. In: Bibbo M, editor. Comprehensive cytopathology. 2nd ed. Philadelphia: WB Saunders; 1997. pp.551-621.

TABLE 14-6
Lesions of the Orbit

Kennerdall* (156 Orbital Lesions)	Glasgow† (83 Orbital Aspirates)	Cangiarella‡ (22 Cases)	Zeppa§ (51 Cases)
Carcinomas (28%)	Lymphoid lesions (43%): benign and malignant	Metastatic neoplasms (36%): lung, breast, salivary gland, skin, renal, lymphoma, esophageal	Lymphoid lesions (50%) • Hyperplasia (8%) • Inflammatory pseudotumor (16%) • Non-Hodgkin's lymphoma (20%)
Inflammations (19%)	Miscellaneous tumors (27%): melanoma, meningioma, soft tissue neoplasms	Primary malignant lesions (23%): lymphoma, sarcoma, adenoid cystic carcinoma	Metastatic adenocarcinoma (12%)
Lymphoid lesions (17%)	Epithelial tumors (20%): adenocarcinoma, squamous carcinoma, adenoid cystic, miscellaneous	Benign neoplasms (9%): meningioma	Squamous cell carcinoma (14%)
Neural tumors (6%)	Granulomatous lesions (8%): granulomas, chalazion, Wegener's granulomatosis, eosinophilic granulomatosis	Inflammatory (27%): infectious	Miscellaneous benign and malignant lesions (30%)
Other neoplasms (6%)	Small cell tumors (4%): oat cell carcinoma, neuroblastoma, rhabdomyosarcoma)	Nasal chondrosarcoma (5%): malignant, locally invasive	
Miscellaneous (3%)			

*Kennerdall J, Inge E, Wang S: Orbital fine-needle aspiration biopsy. Ophthalmol Clin North Am 1996; 9:573-580.
†Glasgow, BJ, Goldberg RA, Gordon LK, et al. Fine needle aspiration of orbital masses. Ophthalmol Clin North Am 1995; 8:73-82.
‡Cangiarella JF, Cajigas A, Savala E, et al. Fine needle aspiration cytology of orbital masses. Acta Cytol 1996; 6:1205-1211.
§Zeppa Z, Tranfa F, Errico ME, et al. Fine needle aspiration biopsy of orbital masses: a critical review of 51 cases. Cytopathology 1997; 8:366-372.

definitive diagnosis cannot be made based on clinical and imaging studies. Technically, FNA in this area is performed in the same manner as superficial FNA elsewhere on the body; however, aspirates in this location must be performed by a physician who is familiar with the anatomy of the area to avoid perforation of the globe and other serious sequelae.[50,52] Complications of FNA of the orbit include ptosis, intraocular hemorrhage, movement disturbances and scarring.[52] The diagnosis can usually be achieved with two FNA passes.[53]

Primary tumors of the orbital region can arise from the lacrimal glands, lymphoid tissue, central nervous system, connective tissue, or bone.[50] Orbital masses can also be caused by cysts, infectious processes, and inflammatory conditions.[50] Metastatic neoplasms may also lead to mass lesions in this area. Because of the extreme cosmetic relevance of the area, FNA has assumed significant importance as a diagnostic procedure to avoid unnecessary surgery and to aid in potential surgical planning.[46,50]

Indications for Intraocular Fine-Needle Aspiration

Nonpigmented fundus or iris mass in which the differential diagnosis includes amelanotic melanoma, metastatic carcinoma, lymphoma, leukemia, or an inflammatory process

Nonpigmented fundus or iris mass suspected to be a metastatic carcinoma devoid of an obvious systemic neoplasm

Melanocytic iris mass with secondary glaucoma with the differential diagnosis of diffuse nevus or a diffuse melanoma

Nonpigmented fundus lesion in an immunocompromised patient without an obvious differential diagnosis

Leukocoria in a child with diagnostic uncertainty, but where retinoblastoma is not considered a diagnostic consideration*

Intraocular mass in which patient requests that a diagnosis be established prior to enucleation

From Shields JA, Shields CL, Ehya H, et al. Fine needle aspiration of suspected intraocular tumors. Ophthalmology 1993; 100:1677-1684.

*Fine-needle aspiration (FNA) should generally be avoided in retinoblastoma because of the potential of FNA tract seeding by tumor.

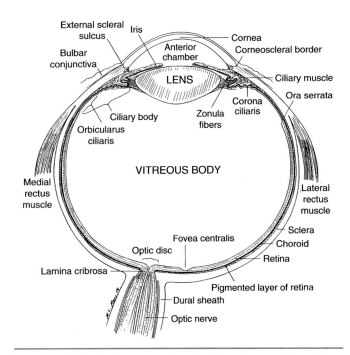

Figure 14-31 Anatomic landmarks of the globe. (From Bibbo M, editor. Comprehensive cytopathology. 2nd ed. Philadelphia: WB Saunders; 1997. p.495.)

The most commonly diagnosed lesions in this area are hematolymphoid diseases. The most common solid neoplasms of the lacrimal and ocular adnexal glands are benign mixed tumors and adenoid cystic carcinomas. The diagnostic accuracy of FNA of orbital or adnexal masses is between 70% and 75%.[48-51]

Direct Sampling of the Globe

". . . The contents of the eye are the lens, supported and controlled by the uvea, and two liquid-filled compartments that are separated by the lens. The anterior chamber contains a thin fluid, the aqueous humor, and the major portion of the globe contains a viscous gel, the vitreous body. Both fluids must be free of cells and color to optimally transmit light to the retina. . . ."[46] (see Figure 14-31).

The two main procedures for the sampling of the globe are FNA and vitrectomy. FNA of the globe must be done under direct visualization and performed by a trained ophthalmologic surgeon.[46] The indications for intraocular FNA are outlined in Box 14-10.

The most common lesions diagnosed from aspirates of this location in the adult population are lymphoma and malignant melanoma, whereas in the pediatric population, it is retinoblastoma. A recent study outlining the anatomic and diagnostic distribution of 20 intraocular aspirates is highlighted in Table 14-7.[55] Another study reporting 140 adequate intraocular FNAs revealed a distribution of pathology as follows: uveal melanoma (38%), uveal metastases (20%), nonspecific inflammation (9%), neutrophils consistent with infection (6%), eosinophils consistent with toxocariasis (4%), macrophages consistent with Coats disease (4%), erythrocytes consistent with hemorrhage (4%), uveal nevus (melanocytoma) (3%), lymphoma (3%), leukemia (2%), retinoblastoma (2%), histiocytes (possible xanthogranuloma) (2%), and benign cells unclassifiable (2%).[56]

In short, a vitrectomy is an intraocular washing. Initially, vitreous fluid can be removed through an FNA-like procedure that yields an undiluted vitreous humor sample. When the vitreous is actually washed or irrigated, the sample will be of a diluted vitreous or vitrectomy sample. These samples are handled in the cytopreparation laboratory using standard concentration and cytospin techniques. They are initially spun down through cytocentrifugation, and the sediment may be requested by the ophthalmologist for additional studies. Pap and DQ stains are used. As with other cytologic samples, DQ is deemed to be superior for the diagnosis of inflammatory and lymphoid processes of the vitreous (Figure 14-32).

The goals of a vitrectomy may be diagnostic (e.g., uveitis vs. lymphoma) or therapeutic (removal of vitreal opacities or fibrous strands).[46] This technique has been used therapeutically in patients with diabetic retinopathy and sickle cell anemia. It has also been used for the evacuation of hemorrhage in postidiopathic hemorrhagic and traumatic events.[46] A recent study of 20 intraocular aspirates revealed a disease distribution of adequate samples in which 37% were malignant lymphoma, 21% were malignant melanoma, and 42% were benign.[55] The benign lesions included a cyst of the iris and mixtures of macrophages and epithelial cells in the other cases.[55] The usual entities evaluated by vitrectomy are outlined in Table 14-8 (Figure 14-33).

Cytology of Unique Neoplasms

The cytologic appearance of two neoplasms unique to this area of the body warrant description: retinoblastoma and melanocytoma. Retinoblastoma may be encountered in an orbital FNA, although head and neck soft tissue and lymph nodes may also harbor metastatic tumor[57] (Figure 14-34). Two types of cells are noted in the aspiration smears. Type I cells do not show obvious differentiation, and type II cells re-

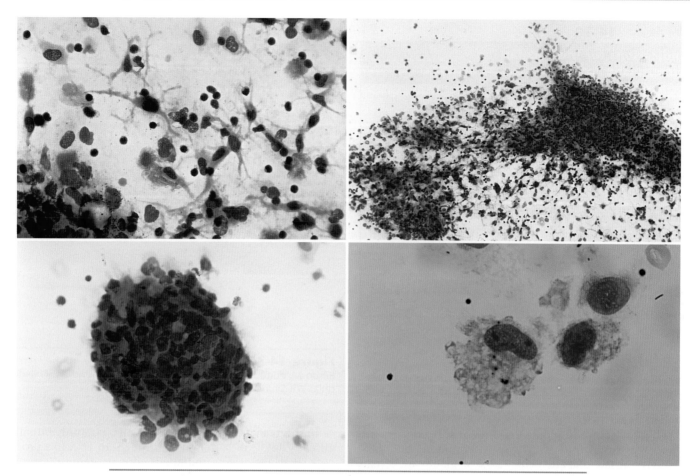

Figure 14-32   **Inflammatory samples from vitrectomies.** The cells are a mixture of reactive lymphocytes, monocytes, and macrophages that may be pigmented. The monocytes and histiocytes may form clusters and aggregates that simulate free-floating granulomas. (DQ)

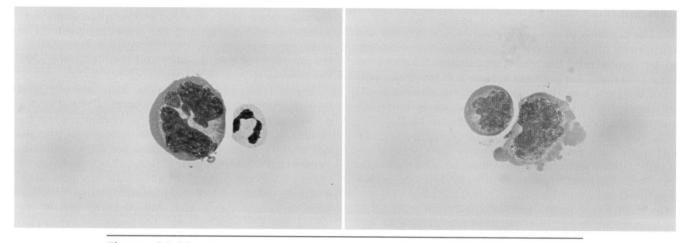

Figure 14-33   **Malignant lymphomas from vitrectomies.** These show markedly enlarged, atypical lymphocytes with a neutrophil present for size comparison. The cells have abundant, deeply basophilic cytoplasm and markedly pleomorphic, irregular, hyperchromatic nuclei. (DQ)

veal prominent cytoplasmic processes that probably indicate early photoreceptor differentiation. Flexner-Wintersteiner rosettes may be found in approximately 63% of cases.[57]

Melanocytoma of the ciliary body, a rare lesion, usually occurs in heavily pigmented adults. FNA of the tumor reveals polygonal tumor cells that are heavily pigmented with small vesicular nuclei and abundant cytoplasm packed with melanin granules.[58] The cells are round to plump. Other cells are present in the sample, including branching dendritic cells with short cytoplasmic processes. The differential diagnosis is malignant melanoma. The cytologic difference is in the cellular morphology and in the size of the granules: melanocytomas have benign nuclei and pigment granules that are larger than those of melanoma.[58]

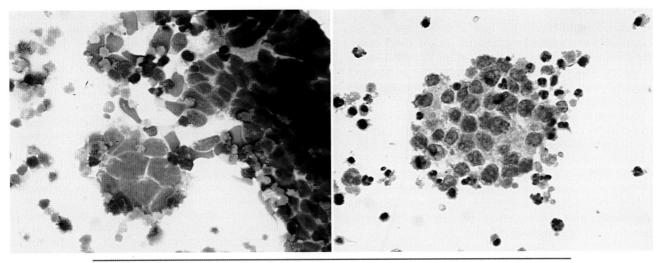

Figure 14-34 **Retinoblastoma obtained from a vitrectomy sample.** These cells show features of a small, round, blue cell tumor without any obvious photoreceptor or neuronal differentiation. The cells are small and round with hyperchromatic, irregular nuclei; abundant nuclear molding; and sparse cytoplasm. (DQ, Pap)

TABLE 14-7

Distribution of 20 Intraocular Aspirates

Cytologic Diagnosis	Vitreous	Anterior Chamber	Iris	Ciliary Body	Choroid
Malignant lymphoma	6	1			
Malignant melanoma				1	3
Benign	2	3	2		1
Unsatisfactory	1				
Total	9	4	2	1	4

From Spitz DJ, Reddy V, Kluskens L, et al. Fine needle aspiration of intra- and extraocular masses. Diagn Cytopathol 2000; 22:199-200.

TABLE 14-8

Entities Noted in Vitrectomy Samples

Entity	Cytomorphologic Description and Comments
Infections: viral, bacterial	Inclusion bodies or inflammatory cells:
Noninfectious inflammatory: proliferative diabetic retinopathy, blood induced glaucoma	• Fibrovascular membranes • Ghost erythrocytes, hemolytic cells, macrophages with engulfed red blood cells
Mechanical blockade of the anterior chamber	Proteinaceous debris, large macrophages with ingested lens material
Uveitis associated with collagen vascular disease	Lymphocytes and clusters of macrophages
Malignant melanoma	Epithelioid and spindled morphologies
Metastatic carcinoma	Most common: breast, lung, colon, prostate
Lymphoma	Large B cell; 75% develop involvement elsewhere in the CNS
Retinoblastoma	Most common pediatric neoplasm of the eye: small blue cell tumor with or without rosettes
Neuroblastoma	Metastatic in the pediatric population; small blue cell tumor with or without pseudorosettes

From Rosenthal DL, Mandell DB, Glasgow BJ. Eye. In: Bibbo M, editor. Comprehensive cytopathology. 2nd ed. Philadelphia: WB Saunders; 1997. pp.551-621.
CNS, Central nervous system.

Ancillary Studies

Immunohistochemistry (IHC), flow cytometry, PCR, and FNA have all been applied successfully to the diagnosis of orbital disease.[59] IHC has been most commonly used for the diagnosis of lymphoma; leukemia; metastatic adenocarcinoma, particularly breast or prostate; melanoma; and mesenchymal neoplasms.[59] Flow cytometry and IHC can be used together or separately, depending on sample cellularity, to diagnose lymphoma. The majority of orbital and ocular adnexal lymphomas have a B-cell phenotype and a large cell morphology.[60]

The use of the PCR is also particularly useful in this area of cytology, as it can be used to diagnose infectious agents (e.g., HIV, cytomegalovirus, Herpes simplex, chlamydia, and *Bartonella*) and can be extremely useful in the correct characterization of lymphoid lesions.[61-65]

References

1. Burger PC. Use of cytological preparations in the frozen section diagnosis of central nervous system neoplasms. Am J Surg Pathol 1985; 9:344-354.
2. Frias-Hidvegi D, Hessel G, Cajulis R, et al. Neurocytology. In: Demay RM, editor. The art and science of cytopathology: exfoliative cytology. Chicago: ASCP Press; 1996.
3. Sliverman JF, Timmons RL, Leonard JR III, et al. Cytologic results of fine-needle aspiration of the central nervous system. Cancer 1986; 58:1117-1121.
4. Silverman JF. Cytopathology of fine needle aspiration biopsy of the brain and spinal cord. Diagn Cytopathol 1986; 2:312-319.
5. Liwnicz BH, Rodriguez, CA. The central nervous system. In: Koss LG, Woyke S, Olszewski W, editors. Aspiration biopsy: cytologic interpretation and histologic basis. New York: Igaku-Shoin; 1984. p.457-490.
6. Liwnicz BH, Henderson KS, Masakawa T, et al. Needle aspiration cytology of intracranial lesions: a review of 84 cases. Acta Cytol 1985; 29:279-285.
7. Rosenthal DL. Cytology of the central nervous system. In: Wied GL, editor. Monographs in clinical cytology. Karger: Basel; 1984. pp.160-171.
8. Walker AE, Robins M, Weinfeld FD. Epidemiology of brain tumors: the national survey of intracranial neoplasms. Neurology 1985; 35(2):219-226.
9. Kuratsu J, Takeshima H, Ushio Y. Trends in the incidence of primary intracranial tumors in Kumamoto, Japan. Int J Clin Oncol 2001; 6(4):183-191.
10. Rickert CH, Paulus W. Epidemiology of central nervous system tumors in childhood and adolescence based on the new WHO classification. Childs Nerv Syst 2001; 17(9):503-511.
11. Okazaki H, Scheithauer BW. An atlas of neuropathology. New York: JB Lippincott; 1988.
12. Bigner SH. Central nervous system. In: Bibbo M, editor. Comprehensive cytopathology. 2nd ed. Philadelphia: WB Saunders; 1997. p.551-621.
13. Cairncross JG, Ueki K, Zlatescu MC, et al. Specific genetic predictors of chemotherapeutic response and survival in patients with anaplastic oligodendrogliomas. J Natl Cancer Inst 1998; 90(19):1473-1479.
14. Ino Y, Betensky RA, Zlatescu MC, et al. Molecular subtypes of anaplastic oligodendroglioma: implications for patient management at diagnosis. Clin Cancer Res 2001; 7(4):839-845.
15. Bauman GS, Ino Y, Ueki K, et al. Allelic loss of chromosome 1p and radiotherapy plus chemotherapy in patients with oligodendrogliomas. Int J Radiat Oncol Biol Phys 2000; 48(3):825-830.
16. Smith JS, Alderete B, Minn Y, et al. Localization of common deletion regions on 1p and 19q in human gliomas and their association with histological subtype. Oncogene 1999; 18(28):4144-4152.
17. Smith JS, Perry A, Borell TJ, et al. Alterations of chromosome arms 1p and 19q as predictors of survival in oligodendrogliomas, astrocytomas, and mixed oligoastrocytomas. J Clin Oncol 2000; 18(3):636-645.
18. Crain BJ, Bigner SH, Johnston WW. Fine needle aspiration biopsy of deep cerebrum—a comparison of normal and neoplastic morphology. Acta Cytol 1982; 26:772-778.
19. Burger PC, Scheitauer BW, Vogel FS. Brain: tumors. In: Burger PC, Scheitauer BW, Vogel FS, editors. Surgical pathology of the nervous system and its coverings. New York: Churchill Livingstone; 1991.
20. Lopez-Rios F, Alberti N, Ballestin C, et al. Extracranial metastasis of a glioma: diagnosis by fine needle aspiration and immunocytochemistry. Diagn Cytopathol 2000; 23:43-45.
21. Townsend JJ, Seaman JP. Central neurocytoma: a rare benign intraventricular tumor. Acta Neuropathol (Berl) 1986; 71(1-2):167-170.
22. Ng HK. Cytologic features of central neurocytomas of the brain: a report of three cases. Acta Cytol 1999; 43(2):252-256.
23. New KC, Bulsara KR, Dodd LG, et al. Fine needle aspiration diagnosis of medulloblastoma metastatic to the pelvis. Diagn Cytopathol 2001; 24:361-363.
24. Solares J, Lacruz C. Fine needle aspiration cytology diagnosis of an extracranial meningioma presenting as as a cervical mass. Acta Cytol 1987; 31(4):502-504.
25. Schwechheimer K, Zhou L, Birchmeier W. E-cadherin in human brain tumours: loss of immunoreactivity in malignant meningiomas. Virchows Arch 1998; 432(2):163-167.
26. Pai RR, Kini H, Rao VS, et al. Choroid plexus papilloma diagnosed by crush cytology. Diagn Cytopathol 2001; 25(3):165-167.
27. Kepes JJ, Collins JJ. Choroid plexus epithelium (normal and neoplastic) expresses synaptophysin. A potentially useful aid in differentiating carcinoma of the choroid plexus from metastatic papillary carcinomas. Neuropathol Exp Neurol 1999; 58(4):398-401.
28. Kato T, Fujita M, Sawamura Y, et al. Clinicopathological study of choroid plexus tumors: immunohistochemical features and evaluation of proliferative potential by PCNA and Ki-67 immunostaining. Noshuyo Byori 1996; 13(2):99-105.
29. Sparano JA. Clinical aspects and management of AIDS-related lymphoma. Eur J Cancer 2001; 37(10):1296-1305.
30. Gill PS, Levine AM, Meyer PR, et al. Primary central nervous system lymphoma in homosexual men: clinical, immunologic, and pathologic features. Am J Med 1985; 78:742-748.
31. Goldstein JD, Dickson DW, Moser FG, et al. Primary central nervous system lymphoma in acquired immunodeficiency syndrome: a clinical and pathologic study with results of treatment with radiation. Cancer 1991; 67:2756-2765.
32. Fine HA, Mayer RJ. Primary central nervous system lymphoma. Ann Intern Med 1993; 119:1093-1104.
33. Loureiro C, Gill PS, Meyer PR, et al. Autopsy findings in AIDS-related lymphoma. Cancer 1988; 62:735-739.
34. MacMahon EME, Glass JD, Hayward SD, et al. Epstein Barr virus in AIDS-related primary central nervous system lymphoma. Lancet 1991; 338:969-973.
35. Schlegel U, Schmidt-Wolf IG, Deckert M. Primary CNS lymphoma: clinical presentation, pathological classification, molecular pathogenesis and treatment. J Neurol Sci 2000; 181(1-2):1-12.

36. Yu GH, Montone KT, Frias-Hidvegi D, et al. Cytomorphology of primary CNS lymphoma: review of 23 cases and evidence for the role of EBV. Diagn Cytopathol 1996; 14(2):114-120.

37. Cinque P, Vago L, Dahl H, et al. Polymerase chain reaction on cerebrospinal fluid for diagnosis of virus-associated opportunistic diseases of the central nervous system in HIV-1–infected patients. AIDS 1996; 10:951-958.

38. Olasode BJ. A pathological review of intracranial tumours seen at the University College Hospital, Ibadan between 1980 and 1990. Niger Postgrad Med J 2002; 9(1):23-28.

39. Sunita, Kapila K, Singhal RM, et al. Extracranial metastasis of an astrocytoma detected by fine-needle aspiration: a case report. Diagn Cytopathol 1991; 7(3):290-292.

40. Vural G, Hagmar B, Walaas L. Extracranial metastasis of glioblastoma multiforme diagnosed by fine-needle aspiration: a report of two cases and a review of the literature. Diagn Cytopathol 1996; 15(1):60-65.

41. Goodkin K, Wilkie FL, Concha M, et al. Aging and neuro-AIDS conditions and the changing spectrum of HIV-1–associated morbidity and mortality. J Clin Epidemiol 2001; 54(Suppl 1):S35-43.

42. Whiteman M, Post MJD, Berger JR, et al. PML in 47 HIV-1–positive patients. Radiology 1993; 187:233-240.

43. McGuire D, Barhite S, Hollander H, et al. JC virus DNA in cerebrospinal fluid of human immunodeficiency virus-infected patients: predictive value for progressive multifocal leukoencephalopathy. Ann Neurol 1995; 37:395-399.

44. Hidvegi DF, Yungbluth P, Cajulis R, et al. Stereotactic needle biopsy diagnosis of brain lesions in patients infected with human immunodeficiency virus: ASCP check sample. Cytopathology No. C92-520(5); 1992.

45. Kulesza P, Tihan T, Ali SZ. Myxopapillary ependymoma: cytomorphologic characteristics and differential diagnosis. Diagn Cytopathol 2002; 26(4):247-250.

46. Rosenthal DL, Mandell DB, Glasgow BJ. Eye. In: Bibbo M, editor. Comprehensive cytopathology. 2nd ed. Philadelphia: WB Saunders; 1997. pp.551-621.

47. Mandell DB, Levy JJ, Rosenthal DL: Preparation and cytologic evaluation of intraocular fluids. Acta Cytol 1987; 31:150-158.

48. Kennerdall J, Inge E, Wang S: Orbital fine-needle aspiration biopsy. Ophthalmol Clin North Am 1996; 9:573-580.

49. Glasgow, BJ, Goldberg RA, Gordon LK, et al. Fine needle aspiration of orbital masses. Ophthalmol Clin North Am 1995; 8:73-82.

50. Cangiarella JF, Cajigas A, Savala E, et al. Fine needle aspiration cytology of orbital masses. Acta Cytol 1996; 6:1205-1211.

51. Zeppa Z, Tranfa F, Errico ME, et al. Fine needle aspiration biopsy of orbital masses: a critical review of 51 cases. Cytopathology 1997; 8:366-372.

52. Liu D: Complications of fine needle aspiration biopsy of the orbit. Ophthalmology 1985; 92:1768-1771.

53. Sturgis CD, Silverman JF, Kennerdel JS, et al. Fine-needle aspiration for the diagnosis of primary epithelial tumors of the lacrimal gland and ocular adnexa. Diagn Cytopathol 2001; 24:86-89.

54. Shields JA, Shields CL, Ehya H, et al. Fine needle aspiration of suspected intraocular tumors. Ophthalmology 1993; 100:1677-1684.

55. Spitz DJ, Reddy V, Kluskens L, et al. Fine needle aspiration of intra- and extraocular masses. Diagn Cytopathol 2000; 22:199-200.

56. Shields JA, Shields CL, Ehya H, et al. Fine needle aspiration of suspected intraocular tumors. Int Ophthalmol Clin 1993; 33(3):77-82.

57. Akhtar M, Ashraf Ali M, Sabbah R, et al. Aspration cytology of retinoblastoma: light and electron microscopic correlations. Diagn Cytopathol 1988; 4:306-311.

58. El-Harazi SM, Kellaway J, Font RL. Melanocytoma of the ciliary body diagnosed by fine needle aspiration biopsy. Diagn Cytopathol 2000; 22:394-397.

59. Diaz CE, Grossniklaus HE: Pathology techniques: current opinion in ophthalmology. 1997; 8(4):52-57.

60. Laucirica R, Font RL.: Cytologic evaluation of lymphoproliferative lesions of the orbit/ocular adnexa: an analysis of 46 cases. Diagn Cytopathol 1996; 15:241-245.

61. Garcia-Ferrer FJ, Blatt A, Laycock KA, et al. Molecular biologic techniques in ophthalmic pathology. Ophthalmla Clin North Am 1995; 8:25-36.

62. Hogan RN, Jakobiec FA. Molecular pathological diagnosis of ocular infections. Int Ophthalmol Clin 1996; 36(3):223-246.

63. Della NG. Molecular biology in ophthalmology: a review of principles and recent advances. Arch Ophthalmol 1996; 114(4):457-463.

64. Hammerschlag MR, Roblin PM, Gelling M, et al. Use of polymerase chain reaction for the detection of *Chlamydia trachomatis* in ocular and nasopharyngeal specimens from infants with conjunctivitis. Pediatr Infect Dis J 1997; 16(3):293-297.

65. Dondey JC, Sullivan TJ, Robson JM, et al. Application of polymerase chain reaction assay in the diagnosis of orbital granuloma complicating atypical oculoglandular cat scratch disease. Ophthalmology 1997; 104(7):1174-1178.

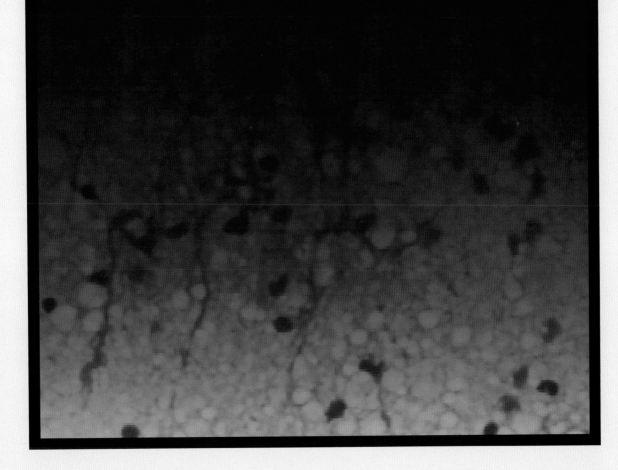

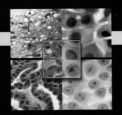

THORAX

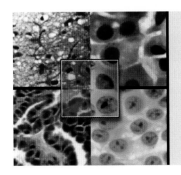

Normal Pulmonary Cytology and Diffuse Lung Diseases

Together with gynecologic cytopathology, pulmonary cytology has been investigated for a sufficient period and presents sufficient morphologic diversity to form much of the intellectual underpinnings of diagnostic cytopathology. From these areas arise the concepts about traditional cytomorphologic characteristics useful in distinguishing reactive processes from malignant neoplasms. Not until relatively uncommon problems in fine-needle aspiration (FNA) are encountered does the need arise to recognize malignancies that lack these traditional cytomorphologic characteristics of malignancy. Furthermore, it is in pulmonary samples that the cytopathologist most often searches for infectious agents.

 ## SAMPLING METHODS IN PULMONARY CYTOLOGY AND THE IMPORTANCE OF PREPARATORY METHODS

One reason for the broad use of cytologic methods in pulmonary disease is the variety of applicable sampling methods and the degree to which these can be tailored to both the disease process under investigation and the limitations that arise as a consequence of the patients' compromised state (Box 15-1). These range from completely noninvasive methods (examination of spontaneously expectorated sputum) to those that are minimally invasive but still applicable to even severely ill patients (bronchial brushings and washings). Except for bronchoalveolar lavage, these techniques are largely directed toward centrally located mass lesions and may leave unaddressed more diffuse infiltrates or peripherally situated tumefactions. In many clinical circumstances, direct cytopathologist involvement in specimen preparation and triage can be highly valuable (Box 15-2).

Induced sputum production requires minimal patient intervention, and involves nebulization by breathing a mist of hypertonic saline solution for 30 minutes. The primary use of this method is study of potential lung infections in patients who do not spontaneously produce adequate sputum. This technique is most commonly employed in patients at risk for pneumonia resulting from *Pneumocystis carinii*, for whom it is viewed as a rapid, inexpensive, and safe alternative to bronchoscopic exploration.

A sputum sample has traditionally been regarded as satisfactory if it contains macrophages. However, this does not guarantee sampling of the pulmonary parenchyma because such cells are also present in the larynx, trachea, and large bronchi. The most common type of nondiagnostic sputum sample shows mostly acute inflammatory cells, often to the exclusion of other elements, with the possible exception of squamous cells from the upper aerodigestive tract.

Bronchial brushing and washing are directed toward mucosal or submucosal lesions that are directly visualized at the time of bronchoscopy. In most instances the goal is diagnosis of suspected malignancy. Brushing attempts to dislodge cells from an ulcerated lesion or an abnormal mucosa and often provides large amounts of tissue in an excellent state of preservation. In most cases the material is smeared immediately onto glass slides and fixed at once by either spraying or immersion in 95% ethanol. Technical staff in the bronchoscopy suite must be instructed in the necessity of rapid fixation. In some institutions, the brush is also submitted in saline. Cells removed from this in the cytology laboratory can be used for preparation of additional smears, paraffin-embedded cell blocks, cytocentrifuge slides, or monolayer slides.

Bronchoalveolar lavage (BAL) can address many lesions that are diffuse or peripherally situated. It is usually added to a bronchoscopic examination and incurs little additional procedure time or risk to the patient. The goal of BAL is investigation of pathologic conditions situated beyond the range of bronchoscopic visualization. Most modern fiberoptic instruments have a diameter of approximately 0.5 cm so that only the proximal portion of subsegmental bronchi can be visualized directly.

During BAL, the bronchoscope is physically wedged into the bronchus. Warmed saline is then used to flood the bronchial and alveolar tissue distal to this point. Up to one million alveoli may thus be sampled. Fluid is introduced in aliquots that may range from 20 to 100 or more milliliters. After each fluid instillation, the bronchus is aspirated, and in most instances, up to 50% of the initial fluid volume is recovered. A series of four or five separate instillations follows in rapid succession. The returned fluid can be used for cytologic examination and enumeration, with differential counting of inflammatory cells, and in microbiologic studies.

BOX 15-1

Methods for Cytologic Sampling of the Lung

Sputum
- Spontaneously expectorated
- Induced

Bronchoscopic procedures
- Bronchial brushing
- Bronchial washing
- Bronchoalveolar lavage

Pulmonary artery catheter sampling

Fine-needle aspiration, including transbronchial aspirations

Core biopsy with imprint preparation

BOX 15-2

Cytopathologist and Cytotechnologist Intervention during Sampling of the Lung

Sample preparation

Fine-needle aspiration: prepare smears and formalin-fixed cell blocks

Core biopsy: prepare imprints and place cores in formalin or other media

Specimen triage by rapid staining of smears or imprints

Is the material adequate for diagnosis?

Is the initial diagnosis reasonable in the light of the clinical and radiographic findings, or is additional material required?

Does specimen triage indicate that additional studies may be needed to reach a final diagnosis?

Should material be submitted for cultures?

Should material be submitted for lymphocyte immunophenotyping?

Is there a diagnostic dilemma that might be addressed by immunocytochemistry?

BOX 15-3

Bronchoalveolar Lavage Specimen Adequacy

Adequacy assessment based primarily on cell counts

At least 2×10^6 total cells obtained

More than ten macrophages per high power microscopic field

More than 25 macrophages per high-power field in the presence of upper tract contamination or acute inflammatory exudate

Unsatisfactory, based primarily on other criteria

Excessive squamous or bronchial cells (epithelial cells > macrophages)

Excessive degeneration

Excessive red blood cells, especially if other adequacy problems exist

Laboratory artifacts

TABLE 15-1

Bronchoalveolar Lavage Contrasted with Bronchial Washing

Bronchoalveolar Lavage	Bronchial Washing
Large total fluid volume ($\geq$ 100 ml)	Small fluid volume (approximately 20 ml)
Pathologic process of interest not directly visualized	Directed toward a visible lesion
Mostly used to study distal or diffuse disease	Mostly used to study central lesions
Used in the absence of a mass or mucosal abnormality	Usually employed to evaluate a mass or mucosal abnormality
Most often used to investigate infectious processes or interstitial disease	Most often used to evaluate neoplastic masses

Preparation of BAL samples varies among institutions. The first aliquot is often heavily contaminated with upper aerodigestive tract material, the presence of which makes it difficult to evaluate pulmonary parenchymal disorders. Thus, many investigators suggest excluding this first sample and then pooling the remaining three or four aliquots for the studies listed previously.

In general, a good BAL sample is one that shows numerous macrophages with little mucus and few cells of other types, including epithelial and inflammatory cells. The normal ranges of BAL fluid inflammatory cell content are discussed later in this chapter when this method is applied to evaluation of the chronic interstitial lung diseases and other more specific inflammatory states.

Various approaches to BAL adequacy assessment have been advocated. In one scheme the absolute cell count is used as the sole criterion, with more than 2×10^6, indicating a good sample.[1] Others base their assessment on the fluid's contents (Box 15-3).[2] Low cellularity, excessive upper tract contamination, and marked acute inflammation indicate an unsatisfactory examination. The most common problem is extensive acute inflammation. Such lavage samples usually show neutrophils and mucus with few macrophages or epithelial cells.

It is conceptually important to contrast BAL with bronchial washings (Table 15-1). Both are obtained at the time of bronchoscopy, and both return a volume of saline containing various tracheobronchial and pulmonary components. Bronchial washing uses a small fluid volume to investigate a centrally located lesion under direct bronchoscopic visualization. BAL uses a larger volume to study more peripheral conditions that are not visualized by the bronchoscopist.

Pulmonary artery catheterization is not commonly used, but can effectively address lymphangitic tumor cell dissemination. Because this type of lung sampling is most often performed in patients already bearing a pulmonary artery catheter for the purpose of hemodynamic monitoring, it entails virtually no additional risk. A 20- to 25-ml sample of blood is removed from the catheter and either discarded or used for other laboratory evaluations. The next sample is collected in a standard ethylenediaminetetraacetic acid (EDTA) tube and prepared in the hematology laboratory as a standard buffy coat smear. This is enriched for leukocytes, megakaryocytes, and any malignant cells collected from the pulmonary interstitium.

Transthoracic FNA is used to sample all pulmonary lesions except those that are too small to be targeted accurately or those in which proximity to major mediastinal structures suggest that the procedure places the patient at risk for a significant complication. As discussed more fully below, the greatest risk of this procedure is pneumothorax. The magnitude of risk is directly proportional to the number of times the pleura is crossed by the needle and the time spent in breeching this surface. Thus, the risk to the patient can be minimized, if cytopathology staff are on site in the radiology suite during the procedure and use a rapid stain for specimen adequacy determinations. By these means, the number of needle passes can be minimized, and many lesions can be adequately addressed by a single aspiration. Furthermore, as with FNA of other sites, immediate evaluation reduces the number of patients who need to undergo an additional procedure because the first FNA was diagnostically unsatisfactory. An additional advantage of this approach is that the material can be triaged into broad diagnostic categories on an immediate basis. Additional studies such as microbiologic cultures or flow cytometry can be instituted at once, and the need for further procedures can be eliminated (see Box 15-2).

Transbronchial FNA is used to address mediastinal lymphadenopathy. In most instances the target is an enlarged subcarinal lymph node associated with a pulmonary mass. The needle is advanced through the carinal wall, as directed by the bronchoscope. On-site interpretation of the sample optimizes diagnostic yield.

Another application of cytologic methods to rapid specimen triage and adequacy determinations has recently emerged. Some radiologists and pathologists prefer core biopsy samples to smear material for evaluation of various mass lesions. In this setting, imprints of the tissue cores can be prepared on site by the cytopathology team and examined as indicated above. In all cases, except the most necrotic or most sclerotic neoplasms, these imprints have been found to be highly diagnostic and have been used to meet the need for rapid specimen evaluation.

In this light, it is important to note that when FNA is skillfully performed and the material is optimally prepared, even a single needle pass often provides material sufficient for both smears and a paraffin-embedded cell block for histologic sections. The latter is useful for hematoxylin and eosin (H&E)–stained sections, special stains, and immunohistochemistry. Furthermore, the nature of FNA can make this a more diagnostic sample than many core biopsies while still providing a histologic preparation. Many core biopsy samples yield a tumor sample that is extensively sclerotic and contains only a minor component of neoplastic cells. FNA, however, leaves much of the tumor's connective tissue scaffolding behind and returns tumor cells and tissue fragments in a highly enriched form.

For this reason, the apparently smaller gross yield of FNA is often diagnostically superior to many core biopsy samples. When provided with high-quality FNA laboratory services, many radiologists prefer this method to core biopsies. However, all of the potential advantages of FNA are lost if the radiology staff is not provided with help from laboratory personnel who are highly skilled in specimen preparation. Leaving these niceties to the busy radiologist and her assistants will minimize the use of FNA, unless someone among them is specifically trained in and dedicated to proper cytopreparatory techniques.

Although addressed in more detail when specific diagnoses are considered, the method of sampling can alter prominently the cytologic presentation of a given disease process. For example, the cytologic presentations of both bronchioloalveolar carcinoma and small cell anaplastic carcinoma differ enormously between sputum and FNA samples.

 ## NORMAL CELLS, NONCELLULAR ELEMENTS, AND CONTAMINANTS FOUND IN PULMONARY CYTOLOGY SAMPLES

A variety of normal cells, noncellular elements, and contaminants can be seen in various pulmonary cytology preparations (Box 15-4). The components of a sample depend largely on the type of specimens submitted and on the skill and vigor with which it has been obtained.

Spontaneously expectorated sputum and all bronchoscopically obtained samples can show each of the components listed in Box 15-4, except those specifically designated as being picked up by a needle at the time of FNA. In these types of samples, either the specimen (sputum) or the sampling device (bronchoscope) passes through various portions of the bronchi, trachea, larynx, pharynx, and the mouth or nose. Materials from any of these areas can be admitted to the cytologic specimen and may cause diagnostic difficulties.

During transthoracic FNA, the needle passes through the skin, various soft tissues (including skeletal muscle) pleural surfaces, any collection of fluid between the parietal and visceral pleural surfaces, and frequently normal lung parenchyma before entering the target lesion. Almost always, the target of FNA is a mass lesion usually suspected to represent a neoplasm or a localized infectious process. The surrounding uninvolved lung tissue often shows alterations, including lipoid pneumonia with collections of macrophages, bronchiolitis obliterans with reactive mesenchymal elements, and various degrees of type II pneumocyte hyperplasia. The latter can be troubling in cytologic samples and is discussed more fully in the following section on reactive alterations in pulmonary cells.

Diagnostic difficulties related to contamination of FNA samples by normal or reactive cells and tissues are summarized in Table 15-2. The most common error is mistaking normal or reactive mesothelial cells for evidence of a non–small cell carcinoma. This issue arises in other body sites where an aspirating needle crosses a mesothelial surface. For example mesothelial cells are often mistaken for carcinoma in aspirates of the liver. Such cells should be compared with their more common presentation in intraoperative washings from body cavity surfaces. Flat sheets with a squamoid or cobblestone arrangement emphasized by sharp cells borders and intercellular clearings, or "windows," are typical. Few neoplasms present such a high degree of architectural organization.

Bone marrow elements may also be inadvertently aspirated. In the absence of hematopoietic disease, these show the expected trilineage hematopoiesis. Small immature cells of the erythroid or myelocytic series can be mistaken for leukemia or malignant lymphoma, whereas large megakaryocytes can suggest various other types of malignancy. The key to correct diagnosis is recognition of the cells' polymorphism. Romanowsky-stained slides have an appearance that is familiar to most pathologists and highlights the myelocytic series by showing cytoplasmic granules of various tinctorial types.

In some right lower lobe lung aspirations, hepatic tissue is inadvertently collected. Hepatocytes are large, with prominent nucleoli and occasional nuclear clearing that resembles intranuclear cytoplasmic invaginations. The unwary sometimes mistake these cells for evidence of a non–small cell carcinoma, either primary or metastatic. Clues to the correct interpretation can include finely granular perinuclear lipofuscin pigment or an admixture of these large cells with small cuboidal bile duct elements. Furthermore, cell block sections may show normal hepatic architectural arrangements that are not expected in carcinomas.

BOX 15-4

Normal Cells, Noncellular Elements, and Contaminants in Various Pulmonary Cytology Preparations

Tracheobronchial level cells
Ciliated columnar cells with associated goblet cells and basal cells
Lymphocytes
Neutrophils
Mast cells
Macrophages
Bronchial smooth muscle cells

Alveolar level cells
Alveolar lining cells (type I and type II pneumocytes)
Macrophages, including multinucleated forms

Additional cells from the pulmonary interstitium
Megakaryocytes

Noncellular materials
Mucus, including Curschmann's spirals
Ferruginous bodies
Carbon particles
Hemosiderin
Stainable lipid
Charcot-Leyden crystals

Contaminants
Talc
Pollen
Nonpathogenic fungi (Alternaria)
Oral squamous cells, bacteria, yeast, and food particles
Corpora amylacea
Calcospherites

Materials picked up during fine-needle aspiration
Skin cells
Muscular or fatty soft tissue
Mesothelial cells
Small fragments of bone or cartilage
Bone marrow cells
Hepatocytes

TABLE 15-2

Diagnostic Difficulties Related to Normal Tissues Incidentally Present in Pulmonary Fine-Needle Aspiration Samples

Cellular Finding	Erroneous Diagnosis	Diagnostic Clues for Nonneoplastic Cells or Tissue
Cutaneous squamous cells	Squamous cell carcinoma	No malignant nuclei All cells are mature Bacteria on some cells No inflammatory cells No necrosis
Adipose tissue	Pulmonary hamartoma	Many hamartomas have adipose tissue, but other elements are required for confident diagnosis*
Skeletal muscle	Squamous cell carcinoma	Cross striations Small peripheral nuclei No malignant nuclei No necrosis
Mesothelial cells	Non–small cell carcinoma	Flat sheets† Uniform cell size and shape Squamoid appearance Sharp cell borders Uniform nuclei No malignant nuclei
Reactive type II pneumocytes	Non–small cell carcinoma‡	Uniform appearance Soap-bubble vacuoles Low N:C ratio
Normal bone marrow	Malignant lymphoma or leukemia	Polymorphous cytology with all three cell lines¶

N:C, Nuclear to cytoplasmic.
*The cytology of pulmonary hamartoma is discussed more fully in Chapter 16.
†As discussed more fully during consideration of body cavity fluids in Chapter 12, mesothelial cells that are directly sampled by fine-needle aspiration or intraoperative washing of body cavity surfaces have different cytologic features than cells spontaneously shed into an existing fluid collection.
‡This complex problem is discussed more fully in the section on reactive alterations.
¶This is best appreciated with Romanowsky-stained material.

Tracheobronchial Level Cells

Ciliated pseudostratified columnar epithelium with goblet cells and basal cells is typical of respiratory epithelium from the laryngeal glottis to the terminal bronchioles. It may be spontaneously shed or directly sampled. The morphologic features of the component cells are summarized in Box 15-5. Single cells may be numerous, but tissue fragments, or microbiopsies, are often encountered, in which ciliated cells, goblet cells, and basal cells can be appreciated in their normal architectural relationships (Figure 15-1). In general, the ratio of ciliated to goblet cells is approximately 5:1 or 6:1 but can be altered in favor of goblet cells. Increased proliferation of reserve cells is another reactive alteration. Both types of hyperplasia are discussed more fully in the subsequent section.

Bronchial brushing samples may show fragments of smooth muscle from the bronchial wall. These are basophilic in Romanowsky-stained samples and eosinophilic in fixed material. Single spindle cells are not seen. Instead, cohesive tissue particles consist of numerous uniform spindle cells with pale nuclei and low nuclear to cytoplasmic (N:C) ratios. The tissue fragments are highly organized, with uniformly distributed nuclei that are all oriented parallel to the long axis of the fragment (Figure 15-2). These features contrast with those of spindle cell malignancies discussed in Chapter 16.

Alveolar Level Cells

In the normal lung, alveolar lining cells are thin and highly attenuated, as they spread out to cover the alveolar surfaces. These normal cells are not readily appreciated in samples lacking evidence of lung injury and resemble macrophages, especially in sputum studies. When these cells are damaged, reparative proliferation of type II pneumocytes can lead to

striking cytologic atypia that can be mistaken for malignancy (see Table 15-2). This is especially true when they are recovered in large numbers and in a good state of preservation by BAL. This problem is discussed more fully in the next section.

Inflammatory Cells and Macrophages

Neutrophils, lymphocytes, eosinophils, mast cells, and rarely plasma cells can be seen in various lung samples. Specific alterations in their numbers may be associated with certain disease states, as noted subsequently in reference to BAL. Their morphology does not differ from that seen in other sites and is not addressed in detail here. However, one

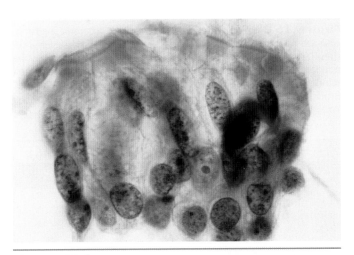

Figure 15-1 Normal respiratory epithelium. This tissue fragment shows a microbiopsy of ciliated respiratory epithelium. At the upper (luminal) surface, these tall columnar cells show a dense horizontal terminal bar and a covering of cilia. The base of the tissue fragment shows small, round basal cell nuclei. In the central portion, oval collections of lightly basophilic mucin can be seen within the cytoplasm of goblet cells. All nuclei in this tissue fragment are essentially identical with finely divided chromatin and occasional small nucleoli. (Papanicolaou [Pap])

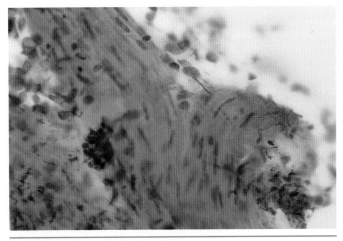

Figure 15-2 Normal bronchial smooth muscle. This cohesive tissue particle is composed of uniform spindle cells organized in a long fascicle. They feature bland oval nuclei and abundant eosinophilic cytoplasm. This represents smooth muscle removed from the bronchial wall by vigorous brushing. (Pap)

BOX 15-5   C M F

Cytomorphologic Features of Normal Tracheobronchial Epithelial Cells

Ciliated cells
May shed singly or in clusters
Pseudostratified (overlapping) in cell clusters
Columnar shape
Surface terminal bar and cilia
Basally located nucleus
Uniformly dispersed chromatin
May show small nucleoli

Goblet cells
Usually seen in cell clusters with ciliated cells
Normally one per five or six ciliated cells
Nuclear features similar to ciliated cells
Apical mucin goblet

Basal cells
Most easily seen in cell clusters as nuclei beneath taller ciliated cells
Basally located nuclei
Nuclear features similar to ciliated cells

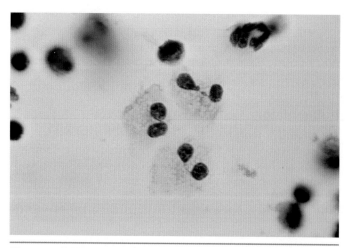

Figure 15-3 Eosinophils. In Pap-stained material, eosinophils do not show their characteristic red granules. However, after these are removed during processing, fine vacuolization may be apparent. Furthermore, eosinophils can be recognized by their bilobed nuclei. (Pap) (From Stanley MW, Henry-Stanley MJ, Iber C. Bronchoalveolar lavage: cytology and clinical applications. New York: Igaku-Shoin; 1991.)

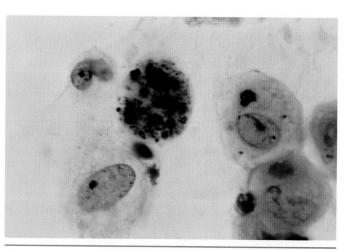

Figure 15-4 **Pulmonary macrophages.** This image shows several typical pulmonary macrophages with the cytologic features noted in Box 15-6. One of these cells contains abundant, dark anthracotic pigment. This material consists of nonrefractile granules that vary widely in size. (Pap) (From Stanley MW, Henry-Stanley MJ, Iber C. Bronchoalveolar lavage: cytology and clinical applications. New York: Igaku-Shoin; 1991.)

BOX 15-6   CMF

Cytomorphologic Features of Macrophages

Low nuclear to cytoplasmic (N:C) ratio
Frothy cytoplasm
Pale cytoplasmic staining
Ill-defined cytoplasmic borders
Various cytoplasmic inclusions (e.g., hemosiderin, anthracotic pigment, lipid)
Round, oval, or reniform nucleus with delicate membrane
Fine, pale, or vesicular nuclear chromatin
Multinucleation
Small nucleolus
Nucleoli may enlarge in reactive states
Always occur singly*

---

*Macrophages do not have the subcellular equipment necessary to form cohesive cell clusters or tissue fragments. However, they may appear cohesive when converging together on a target or when thrown together artifactually by cytopreparatory processes such as centrifugation.

---

observation should be made in the context of lung cytology, where the Pap stain is used most commonly. Eosinophils often have diagnostic significance or at least certain clinical associations. Without air-dried, Romanowsky-stained material, their distinctive red granules are not seen. In fixed material, these may be echoed by fine, round uniform cytoplasmic vacuoles. However, the nuclei are bilobed, which helps distinguish these cells from neutrophils (Figure 15-3).

As noted previously, macrophages are found in many levels of the aerodigestive tract and often play a role in specimen adequacy assessment. Their morphology tells us nothing about their residence before sampling, but may reflect their activity (Box 15-6 and Figure 15-4). Their frothy, ill-defined cytoplasm and eccentric, reniform nuclei are most useful in distinguishing these cells from epithelial elements of any type. Macrophages always occur singly because they do not possess the subcellular equipment needed to bind one another in true tissue fragments. However, they may artifactually appear to cluster after centrifugation. Multinucleation is common and nonspecific; it should not be interpreted as evidence of tuberculosis, foreign body reaction, or other pathologic states.

The cytoplasm of macrophages may contain carbon particles (anthracotic pigment), hemosiderin, or lipid. Hemosiderin is probably most common in patients with congestive heart failure. Its significance and evaluation in cases of suspected pulmonary hemorrhage is discussed later in this chapter. Lipid-containing macrophages may be an expression of tissue damage associated with pulmonary infarction, tuberculosis, or aspiration. Their use is for evaluation of aspiration pneumonias and is also discussed later in this chapter.

Mast cells are rare in lavage fluids from healthy controls. In fixed preparations, they resemble macrophages because their granules wash out completely during processing. In air-dried material, mast cells show a central, oval nucleus and a moderate amount of cytoplasm. Small basophilic granules fill the cytoplasm and partially obscure the nucleus.

Megakaryocytes and Other Bone Marrow Elements

Megakaryocytes are normal residents of the lungs' interstitium and should be anticipated in any type of cytologic preparation. These large complex cells are often mistaken for evidence of malignancy by the unwary. Most pathologists are comfortable with their appearance in air-dried preparations, but when these cells are encountered in fixed material, they appear large, hyperchromatic, and complex to an extent that suggests carcinoma or a sarcoma (Box 15-7 and Figure 15-5). They are rare to absent in most lung cytology specimens but may be numerous in pulmonary artery samples. Because one usually examines these aspirates in the setting of clinically suspected lymphangitic carcinoma, the danger of a false-positive diagnosis can be significant.

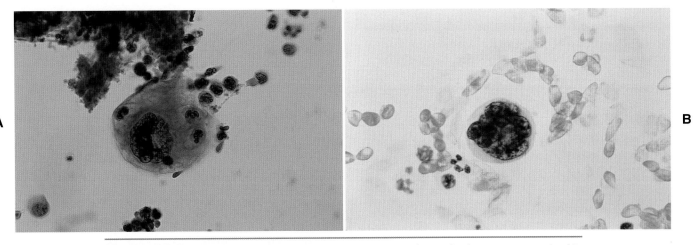

Figure 15-5 **Megakaryocytes.** **A,** This megakaryocyte shows the features summarized in Box 15-7. This example has a low nuclear to cytoplasmic (N:C) ratio resulting from abundant cytoplasm. At the periphery, this cytoplasm shows a ruffled border corresponding to platelet demarcation membranes. (Pap) **B,** This megakaryocyte shows a much higher N:C ratio because of a thin rim of cytoplasm. Its nucleus is large, hyperchromatic, and complex with prominent clearing and clumping of chromatin. (Pap)

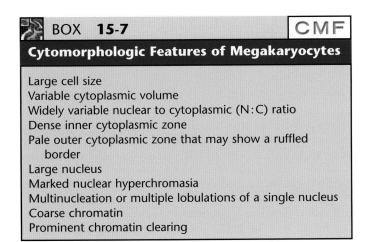

BOX 15-7 — CMF

Cytomorphologic Features of Megakaryocytes

Large cell size
Variable cytoplasmic volume
Widely variable nuclear to cytoplasmic (N:C) ratio
Dense inner cytoplasmic zone
Pale outer cytoplasmic zone that may show a ruffled border
Large nucleus
Marked nuclear hyperchromasia
Multinucleation or multiple lobulations of a single nucleus
Coarse chromatin
Prominent chromatin clearing

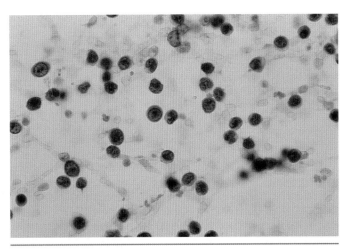

Figure 15-6 **Bone marrow.** This Pap-stained bone marrow shows uniform cells with scanty cytoplasm and hyperchromatic nuclei. Individual cells show varying degrees of chromatin clumping and nucleolar prominence. Such cells can easily be mistaken for evidence of malignant lymphoma or leukemia.

The most helpful diagnostic clues are multiple or single lobulated nuclei, nuclear hyperchromasia, chromatin clearing, and zonated cytoplasm. The inner cytoplasmic zone is denser than the outer rim, and the latter may show a vacuolated-appearing or distinctly ruffled border. This presumably corresponds to platelet demarcation membranes. Because this problem occurs in other areas of cytology, it is useful to study the cytology of megakaryocytes by applying alcohol fixation and the Pap stain to bone marrow aspirate smears. In studying the smaller hematopoietic elements, the nuclear lobulation of maturing myelocytes can be helpful in avoiding an inappropriate diagnosis of malignant lymphoma or leukemia (Figure 15-6).

Noncellular Materials

As noted in Box 15-4, various noncellular materials can be found in pulmonary cytology samples. Each of these can be seen incidentally but can assume greater significance in certain clinical situations that are discussed more fully as specific disease entities are considered (Table 15-3).

Mucus can be spread diffusely over the smear or occur as more localized, denser stringy or wispy material in the background. It is pale in fixed material and more darkly basophilic and thus easier to visualize and semiquantitate on air-dried samples. It can be quantitatively prominent in some inflammatory states and in the mucinous type of bronchioloalveolar carcinoma.

Curschmann's spirals are dense, impacted mucus extruded from bronchiolar-level obstructions, most commonly in smokers and asthmatics. These long, thin curved or spiraled structures show basophilic staining. They have a dense central, almost linear, core that is surrounded by a pale corona of more lightly staining material that thins progressively as the distance from the core increases (Figure 15-7).

TABLE 15-3
Clinical Conditions that May Be Associated with Various Otherwise Nonspecific, Noncellular Materials

Noncellular Material in Pulmonary Cytology*	Potential Clinical Condition†
Mucus (abundant)	Bronchioloalveolar carcinoma
Curschmann's spirals	Bronchiolar-level obstruction, including asthma and smoking-related disease
Ferruginous bodies	Asbestosis
Hemosiderin	Pulmonary hemorrhage, heart failure
Stainable (neutral) lipid	Aspiration pneumonia
Granular material with sparse cellularity	Pulmonary alveolar proteinosis
Charcot-Leyden crystals	Asthma, eosinophilic pneumonia, allergic bronchopulmonary *Aspergillosis*
Psammoma bodies	Suggestive of carcinoma (bronchioloalveolar or metastatic papillary carcinoma)‡

*Each of these is most commonly nonspecific but may suggest the indicated clinical associations.
†Each of these is considered in more detail in the chapter text.
‡Not all cases harbor a carcinoma, but the presence of Psammoma bodies should prompt an evaluation of these diagnostic possibilities.

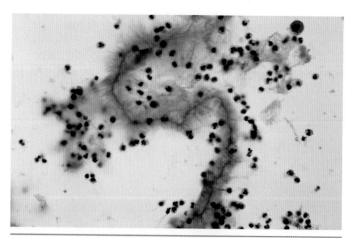

Figure 15-7 **Curschmann's spiral.** This represents dense mucus extruded from a bronchiole. It has a densely staining central core and a thinner basophilic corona of mucus. Inflammatory cells are present in the background. (Pap) (From Stanley MW, Henry-Stanley MJ, Iber C. Bronchoalveolar lavage: cytology and clinical applications. New York: Igaku-Shoin; 1991.)

Ferruginous bodies represent mineral fibers encrusted with proteins and iron salts. Not all represent asbestos so that adherence to strict morphologic criteria for the identification of asbestos bodies is essential (Figure 15-8).[3] Typical examples have a linear core that may be straight or curved. The encrusted material shows a variety of beaded or knoblike expansions, sometimes in a vertebrae-like pattern. More detailed analyses, including x-ray studies, may be needed for definitive identification of asbestos. The significance of asbestos bodies in pulmonary cytology samples is dependent in part on the type of specimen under investigation. In BAL, they are sufficiently common as to be nonspecific, whereas in sputum, their identification almost always indicates heavy occupational asbestos exposure that places the patient at risk for the complications of asbestosis.[4]

Hemosiderin is usually nonspecific, and some is seen in many pulmonary samples, especially if the patient has an element of cardiac failure. It is most often seen within macrophage cytoplasm, where it has a green-tinted golden color (ochre) and occurs as granules of variable size. When abundant, hemosiderin often consists in part of large, dense cytoplasmic droplets. Presumptive identification is improved when the material is shown to glow or glisten when the microscope's substage condenser is lowered. The large particle size and reaction to altered illumination are not characteristics of hemosiderin's major morphologic competitor, which is melanin. When necessary, iron stains highlight this iron-containing substance. Attempts to evaluate hemosiderin semiquantitatively as a

tool in diagnosing pulmonary hemorrhage are discussed in the next section. These are based on iron stains and have limited specificity. When identified, pulmonary hemorrhage has a broad clinical differential diagnosis so that this type of analysis is most effectively applied to highly selected patients.

Neutral lipids are usually identified on cytologic preparations using the Oil-Red-O (ORO) stain applied to air-dried material. Any fixation or other processing in organic solvents removes this material and invalidate attempts at special staining. Semiquantitation of ORO staining has been suggested as a means of identifying patients with aspiration pneumonias (see the next section). This test has limited specificity and is best applied to highly selected patients.

Charcot-Leyden crystals and psammoma bodies are occasionally seen in pulmonary cytology samples, with the clinical associations noted in Table 15-3.

Contaminants

These are summarized in Box 15-3. Radio and associates were able to identify either macroconidia or hyphae of *Alternaria* in BAL fluid from both immunosuppressed patients and healthy volunteers, but in no instance was lung disease attributable to this organism. These investigators concluded that it is either a contaminant or a saprophyte in virtually all instances. The hyphae are rarely seen in clinical material. They closely resemble those of *Aspergillus* spp. but differ by 90 degrees branching (as opposed to 45 degrees for *Aspergillus*) and by showing a bulbous swelling at each hyphal septum.[5]

As noted previously, sputum and samples obtained bronchoscopically can be contaminated with oral material of various types. The most common is mature squamous cells. These often occur in variably sized cohesive plaques and are frequently decorated by bacterial clusters. The latter are basophilic in routine cytologic preparations, a feature that bears no relationship to their status with the Gram stain.

When oral yeast are present, they are usually morphologically consistent with *Candida* spp. BAL samples from

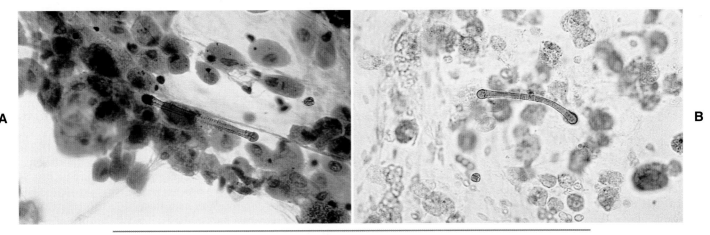

Figure 15-8 Ferruginous bodies. These illustrations show two examples of ferruginous bodies. Both feature a central linear region and terminal knob-like expansions. The central region has a beaded appearance. (**A,** Pap; **B,** Gomori methenamine silver [GMS]) (From Stanley MW, Henry-Stanley MJ, Iber C. Bronchoalveolar lavage: cytology and clinical applications. New York: Igaku-Shoin; 1991.)

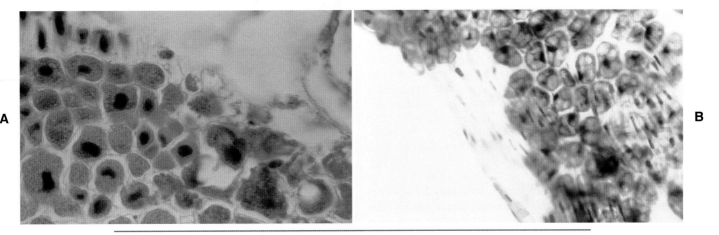

Figure 15-9 Vegetable matter. A, This example shows square eosinophilic cells arranged in linear palisades. Their nuclei are dense and hyperchromatic. Such cells can be mistaken for squamous cell carcinoma. (Pap) **B,** In these vegetable cells, cytoplasmic starch granules can give the impression of vacuoles. (Pap)

more than 30% of normal controls contain such yeast.[6] *Candida* should almost always be considered an oral contaminant, even in the face of immunosuppression. Invasive candidiasis cannot be diagnosed without histologic examination of surgically excised tissue that shows invasion by the organism.

Dietary meat fibers present as degenerated skeletal muscle. These are basophilic in air-dried preparations and eosinophilic to orangeophilic in Pap-stained material. Most show a rectangular shape. Degeneration is manifest by loss of cross striations and nuclei. This morphology contrasts with the well-preserved muscle fragments that can be encountered in FNA samples (see Table 15-2). These orangeophilic bodies should not be mistaken for evidence of squamous cell carcinoma. Even when they are numerous, the diagnosis of carcinoma should be reserved for those cases showing at least occasional well-preserved cells with squamous cytoplasmic differentiation and distinct nuclear features of malignancy.

Vegetable matter may also contaminate pulmonary samples, where it is commonly regarded as at least suspicious for carcinoma. The cells can be large, with distinct edges and smudgy hyperchromatic nuclei. The latter is

TABLE 15-4	CMF
Cytomorphologic Features of Vegetable Matter	

Morphologic Feature	Cytologic Representation
Thick cellulose cell wall	Thick, clear or pale layer around each cell
Square or rectangular cell shapes and palisading cells in linear files	Square and rectangular regimented arrangements within tissue particles
Good cellular cohesion	Tissue particles with few single cells
Degenerated nuclei that lack detail and are more uniform than carcinoma	Darkly staining uniform nuclei
Cytoplasmic starch granules	Vacuole-like appearance

probably degenerative in nature. Such findings are most commonly mistaken for squamous cell carcinoma. The square to rectangular cells with palisading arrangement and thick cell walls are helpful diagnostic clues (Figure 15-9 and Table 15-4).

BENIGN AND REACTIVE ALTERATIONS IN RESPIRATORY CELLS

A wide variety of reactive and reparative changes can affect the epithelial cells seen in respiratory samples. These range from alterations that leave the parent cell readily identifiable to striking transfigurations that may result in false-positive diagnoses of malignancy. This section considers changes that are not associated with specific infectious processes.

The authors' conceptualization of these cellular alterations reflects the anatomic distinction between tracheobronchial level cells and alveolar lining cells (see Box 15-3). The former can show a wide range of changes that include reactive alterations, metaplasias, and hyperplasias, whereas the latter consists of type II pneumocyte hyperplasia (Table 15-5). The type I pneumocytes are difficult to identify in their unaltered state and are apparently too labile to survive significant alveolar level lung injury. Thus, in this compartment only type II cells need be considered.

Tracheobronchial Level Cells

As noted previously, these include ciliated pseudostratified columnar cells, basal cells, and goblet cells. Table 15-5 summarizes the type of benign cellular changes that may overtake each cell type. Separation of reserve cell hyperplasia from other ciliated cell changes is somewhat artificial because it probably represents the earliest recognizable stage in the process of squamous metaplasia. However, this rarely encountered finding is distinctive and may raise a particularly important differential diagnostic consideration (see following section).

The most trivial reactive change in ciliated columnar cells is that which has been designated simple reactive columnar cell atypia. This includes both nuclear and cytoplasmic alterations (Box 15-8 and Figure 15-10). Variable

degrees of nuclear enlargement lead to a range of nuclear sizes. Other reactive nuclear alterations include multinucleation, increased chromatin clumping with minor abnormalities of distribution (clearing), and increased nucleolar prominence. When multiple, the nuclei are generally uniform within a given cell, even having a "mirror-image" quality. As nuclei enlarge, the cells become less columnar and take on a more rectangular or even square shape that departs from the usual tall columnar configuration. Such cells have been described as *boxcars*. Retention of the terminal bar is an important key to identifying these cells as benign. Cilia also indicate benign cells but may be lost as a part of the degenerative process that affects exfoliated cells. When large cell groups are studied, only the cluster's edge may show terminal bars and cilia. Finally, groups of reactive cells often show a spectrum of morphologic findings that ranges from nearly normal cells to others that may require careful study to exclude the suspicion of malignancy. These

---

BOX 15-8	CMF

Cytomorphologic Features of Simple Reactive Columnar Cell Atypia

Nuclear enlargement
Increased nucleocytoplasmic ratio
Multinucleation
Minor variability in nuclear size
Increased chromatin clumping
Minor irregularities in chromatin distribution
Small nucleoli
Cell shape shorter than normal
Terminal bars retained
Cilia may be lost because of degeneration

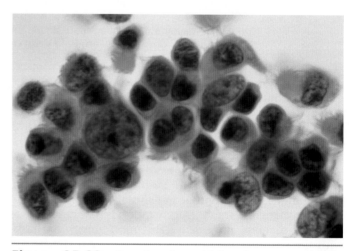

Figure 15-10 Reactive bronchial cells. These reactive bronchial cells show many of the features outlined in Box 15-8. Variability in nuclear size is evident, and overall decrease in cytoplasm contributes to an elevation of N : C ratio. Some of the larger nuclei feature mild degrees of chromatin clearing, and nucleoli are more prominent than those noted in Figure 15-1. At the edge of this cluster, occasional cells with intact cilia can be identified. This fact allows confident identification of even the most atypical nuclei as benign. (Pap) (From Stanley MW, Henry-Stanley MJ, Iber C. Bronchoalveolar lavage: cytology and clinical applications. New York: Igaku-Shoin; 1991.)

TABLE 15-5

Benign and Reactive Alterations in Respiratory Cells

Type of Cell	Alterations
Tracheobronchial level cells	
Ciliated columnar cells	Simple reactive columnar cell atypia
	Papillary mucosal hyperplasia (Creola bodies)
	Repair-like atypia
	Ciliocytophthoria and detached single cilia
	Therapy-related alterations
	Squamous metaplasia
	Goblet cell hyperplasia
Basal cells	Reserve cell hyperplasia (an initial stage of squamous metaplasia)
Alveolar level cells	
Type I pneumocytes	Not identified
Type II pneumocytes	Type II pneumocyte hyperplasia

are often bridged by intermediate forms so that a spectrum of increasing cytologic derangement unites the clearly normal to the frighteningly abnormal.

Mucosal hyperplasia that may include papillary outgrows of mucosal cells is a feature of clinical conditions, including smoking-related chronic bronchitis, asthma, and bronchiectasis of many causes (Box 15-9 and Figure 15-11). The cell clusters are formed completely by mucosal cells and, lacking fibrovascular cores, do not represent true papillae. Terminal plates, cilia, and banal nuclear features are important clues to the benign nature of these cells. However, each of these features may be difficult to recognize in thick, three-dimensional cell groups. Careful study of the clusters' edges remains the most efficient means to avoid an inappropriate diagnosis of papillary adenocarcinoma. The term *Creola body* honors the family name of the first patient in whom these structures were reported as a cause of false-positive carcinoma diagnosis.

The cytologic features of repair were described in detail in Chapter 4 where benign cellular changes in gynecologic cytology were considered (Box 15-10 and Figure 15-12).

This process is ubiquitous, affecting most mucosal surfaces in a wide variety of conditions. One of its most striking features is large nucleoli. As in many other cytologic situations, giving too much emphasis to this single feature can lead to inappropriate diagnoses of malignancy. The most common error is interpreting this finding as a feature of adenocarcinoma. Recognition of the other cytologic findings is essential and includes cohesive cell groups, pale nuclear chromatin, mosaic cytoplasmic configurations between adjacent cells, and frequent association with acute inflammatory cells. Furthermore, evaluation of the clinical findings often reveals a reason for inflammation and repair rather than the mass that usually heralds adenocarcinoma.

Ciliocytophthoria is encountered rarely and occurs when a bronchial cell sheds its entire ciliary tuft as an intact unit. This can occur as a response to several types of lung injury. A related but probably degenerative phenomenon is the release of single detached cilia. This is discussed below, when these structures are contrasted with bacterial organisms.

Therapy-related cytologic alterations include changes resulting from radiation treatment and chemotherapy. The

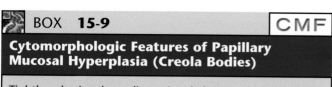

BOX 15-9 CMF

Cytomorphologic Features of Papillary Mucosal Hyperplasia (Creola Bodies)

Tightly cohesive three-dimensional clusters of mucosal cells
Smooth group border
No fibrovascular cores (not true papillae)
Nuclear details are the same as those seen in normal or reactive bronchial cells
Nuclei may be difficult to visualize in larger cell clusters
Terminal bars may be seen at the groups' edges
Cilia usually carpet the surface of cell groups
Differential diagnosis: Papillary adenocarcinoma

BOX 15-10 CMF

Cytomorphologic Features of Reparative Atypia

Cohesive cell clusters
Most groups arranged as flat sheets
Few if any single cells with similar morphology
Nuclei may be multiple
Pale nuclear chromatin
No significant abnormalities of chromatin distribution (no clumping or clearing)
Prominent nucleoli
Nucleoli may be multiple
Associated with neutrophils
Mitotic figures may be present

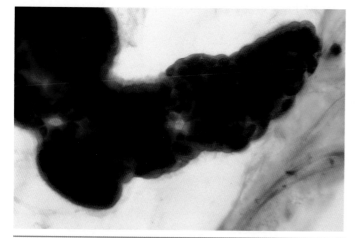

Figure 15-11 **Creola bodies.** This low-magnification image shows a large tissue particle representing papillary mucosal hyperplasia. The cell cluster is three-dimensional but lacks a fibrovascular core and is thus not a true papilla. The thickness of this cell cluster makes it difficult to appreciate the details of individual cells. However, some portions are covered with a carpet of cilia indicating the benign nature of this architecturally complex tissue fragment. (Pap) (From Stanley MW, Henry-Stanley MJ, Iber C. Bronchoalveolar lavage: cytology and clinical applications. New York: Igaku-Shoin; 1991.)

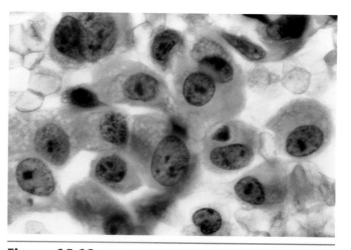

Figure 15-12 **Repair.** This example shows the features outlined in Box 15-10. Nuclear pallor, prominent nucleoli, increased N:C ratio, and the occurrence of these cells in a cohesive cluster are typical features. (Pap) (From Stanley MW, Henry-Stanley MJ, Iber C. Bronchoalveolar lavage: cytology and clinical applications. New York: Igaku-Shoin; 1991.)

latter are often radiomimetic so that both are discussed together. Understanding of these alterations is grounded in gynecologic cytology. However, an additional feature in pulmonary cytology is the large, often multinucleated columnar cells with cilia. The cytologic findings are summarized in Box 15-11 and Figure 15-13. Cytologic samples may not be taken in the acute postradiation period, but if available, such preparations can show evidence of tissue damage, including necrotic material, neutrophils and damaged red blood cells (RBCs). Distinction between therapy-related alterations and recurrent or persistent malignancy can be difficult because of the wide range of the alterations

that occur after therapy. In general, a diagnosis of malignancy must rest on the presence of well-preserved neoplastic cells that lack the more degenerative features listed in Box 15-11 (smudging, hyperchromasia, polychromasia, and vacuolization).

Squamous metaplasia was introduced in Chapter 3, where its central importance in gynecologic cytology was considered. Most glandular epithelia can participate in this process, when inflammation or other stress factors require surface protection stronger than afforded by a single layer or pseudostratified glandular cells. Conceptually, the process proceeds through three stages as summarized in Table 15-6.

Reserve cell hyperplasia (RCH) is rarely seen in pulmonary cytologic preparations. Most examples that are sufficiently well preserved for definitive identification are encountered in BAL samples. Clusters of small darkly staining cells feature high N:C ratios. The nuclei are usually hyperchromatic. The apparent degree of chromatin structure depends on the state of preservation because degeneration results in loss of detail and a smudgy appearance in many examples. Sources differ as to whether nucleoli can be seen. They are inconspicuous or inapparent even in well-preserved material. Another feature of degeneration is cytoplasmic loss. With the attendant cell shrinkage comes collapse of groups with nuclear molding. Such cells may be reminiscent of small cell anaplastic carcinoma.

Table 15-7 compares the cytology of small cell carcinoma with RCH (Figure 15-14). It is important to note that the morphology of both entities is preparation dependent. Degeneration in sputum samples alters the expected appearance considerably from that expected in the better-preserved cells collected by bronchial brushing, BAL, and FNA. The key differential diagnostic features are the small number of abnormal cell groups in RCH and the absence of the background necrosis and apoptotic bodies that typify small cell carcinoma. Furthermore, correlation with the clinical findings will almost always show a central pulmonary mass in cases of carcinoma.

BOX 15-11   CMF

Cytomorphologic Features of Therapy-Related Atypia

Overall cellular alterations
Cell enlargement
Nuclear enlargement
Maintenance of nuclear to cytoplasmic (N:C) ratio
Squamous metaplasia
Enlarged ciliated cells

Cytoplasmic alterations
Abnormal cell shape, including bizarre forms
Cytoplasmic vacuolization
Cytoplasmic polychromasia

Nuclear alterations
Multinucleation
Nuclear hyperchromasia
Irregular nuclear shape
Smudging of nuclear detail
Nuclear vacuolization
Nucleolar prominence

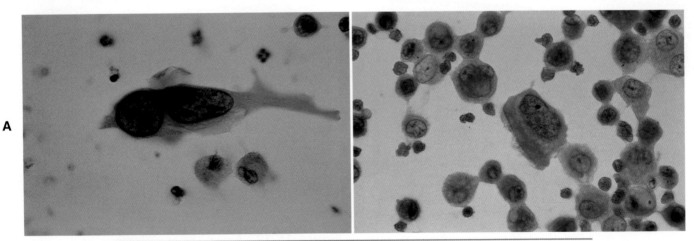

Figure 15-13   **Therapy-associated atypia. A,** The background macrophages in this image indicate how extremely enlarged the central atypical cell has become. This enlargement, the cells' bizarre shape, cytoplasmic vacuoles, and nuclear hyperchromasia with chromatin abnormalities are typical of therapy-related alterations. (Pap) **B,** This image shows a markedly enlarged bronchial cell with intact terminal plate and cilia. It is much larger than the surrounding macrophages. (Pap)

The remaining stages of squamous metaplasia closely resemble their counterparts in the uterine cervix. In some clinical situations, severe nuclear atypia and abnormal cell shapes that suggest squamous cell carcinoma can be superimposed on benign metaplastic squamous epithelium, leading to challenging diagnostic difficulties (Figure 15-15). In such instances, clinical correlation is essential and may be the only means by which a false-positive diagnosis can be avoided (Box 15-12). In these cases the atypical cells are clearly squamous and should not be confused with the equally troubling reactive type II pneumocytes that are discussed subsequently.

Problems related to identification of atypical but not clearly malignant squamous cells are considered in Chapter 16 when squamous cell carcinoma and its precursors are discussed in detail. Such cells are generally interpreted as atypical squamous metaplasia.

A related problem is identification of benign-appearing mature squamous cells in any pulmonary cytologic sample obtained by means other than FNA. In most instances, these represent contaminants from the upper aerodigestive tract, as discussed previously. However, the possibility of a well-differentiated squamous cell carcinoma may be considered in some cases. In the absence of clearly malignant nuclei, this diagnosis is not possible. Radiographic findings that include mass, particularly with cavitation, may compel the clinical team to further investigation because some squamous cell carcinomas shed mostly benign-appearing keratinized cells.

Well-differentiated squamous cells in an FNA sample may represent cutaneous contamination, as discussed previously, especially if they are associated with bacteria in the

TABLE 15-6
Stages of Squamous Metaplasia

Stage	Histologic Features	Cytomorphology
Reserve cell hyperplasia (RCH)	Immature cells No apparent cell borders Proliferate below preexisting glandular cells	Small, uniform cells Tightly cohesive clusters High N:C ratio Delicate chromatin* Small nucleoli* Variable nuclear molding†
Immature squamous metaplasia	Immature cells Larger than RCH cells More cytoplasm than RCH Glandular cells may persist Distinct cell borders	Resembles immature squamous Metaplasia in gynecologic cytology Polygonal cells Higher N:C ratio than mature squamous cells Small nucleoli may persist
Mature squamous metaplasia	Resembles normal squamous epithelium	Shows all features of normal mature squamous epithelium

N:C, Nuclear to cytoplasmic.
*These features require good cell preservation. Most examples show hyperchromatic, even smudgy nuclei lacking apparent internal substructure.
†As degeneration becomes prominent, the cells shrink, and group collapse causes nuclear molding.

TABLE 15-7
Cytomorphologic Comparison of Reserve Cell Hyperplasia and Small Cell Anaplastic Carcinoma

Well-Preserved*	Degenerated†
Reserve cell hyperplasia	
Very few abnormal cells present	Very few abnormal cells present
No background necrosis or apoptosis	No background necrosis or apoptosis
Very small round cells	
Finely stippled chromatin	Densely hyperchromatic chromatin
Small nucleoli possibly visible	Inapparent nucleoli
Minimal nuclear molding	More advanced nuclear molding
Small cell anaplastic carcinoma	
Abnormal cells usually numerous	Abnormal cells may be numerous
Background necrosis and apoptosis	Background necrosis or apoptosis
Very small round cells	
Finely stippled chromatin	Densely hyperchromatic chromatin
Small nucleoli possibly visible	Inapparent nucleoli
Some nuclear molding	Prominent nuclear molding

*This cytologic picture is typically associated with sampling methods that give well-preserved specimens, including bronchial brushing, bronchoalveolar lavage, and fine needle aspiration.
†This cytologic picture is typically associated with sputum cytology.

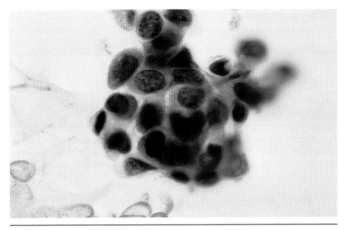

Figure 15-14 **Reserve cell hyperplasia.** This high-magnification image shows uniform small cells with scanty cytoplasm. In areas of degeneration, smudging of nuclear chromatin is evident, as is slight nuclear molding as group collapse. The red blood cells (RBCs) in this image indicate the small size of these cells. (Pap) (From Stanley MW, Henry-Stanley MJ, Iber C. Bronchoalveolar lavage: cytology and clinical applications. New York: Igaku-Shoin; 1991.)

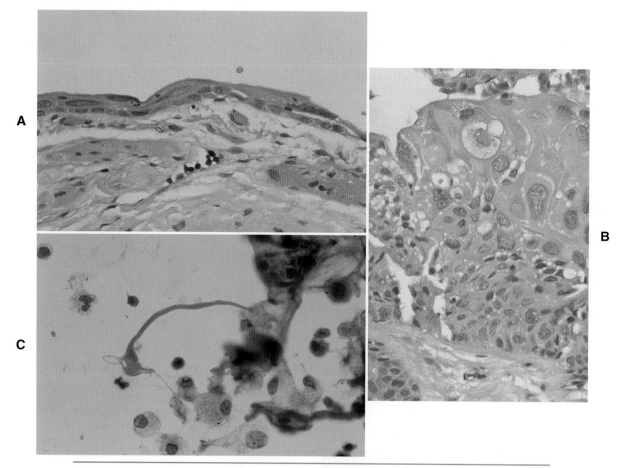

Figure 15-15   Atypical squamous metaplasia. These illustrations summarize the degree of abnormality that occurs in the clinical settings noted in Box 15-14. **A** and **B,** These histologic sections show therapy-related atypical squamous metaplastic alterations in bone marrow transplant patients. In neither instance was carcinoma a consideration during the patient's follow-up. (Hematoxylin and eosin [H&E]) **C,** These abnormally shaped and spindled squamous cells were obtained by bronchoalveolar lavage. The patient's biopsy is illustrated in Figure 15-15, *A.* These abnormal shapes and uneven tinctorial qualities are superimposed on cells that are much larger than the surrounding macrophages. (Pap)

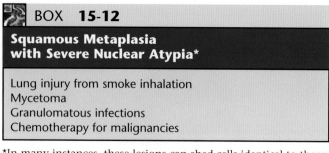

BOX   15-12

**Squamous Metaplasia
with Severe Nuclear Atypia***

Lung injury from smoke inhalation
Mycetoma
Granulomatous infections
Chemotherapy for malignancies

*In many instances, these lesions can shed cells identical to those of squamous cell carcinoma. Correlation with clinical and radiographic findings is the best way to avoid false-positive diagnoses.

absence of acute inflammation. Because such studies are virtually always directed at a mass lesion, finding only well-differentiated cells should prompt further sampling. Many such aspirates in which well-differentiated squamous cells are numerous are associated with only rare clusters of clearly malignant cells. These issues are discussed more fully in Chapter 16, when carcinomas are considered in more detail.

Goblet cell hyperplasia often accompanies chronic bronchitis and is defined histologically by an increased ratio of goblet cells to ciliated cells (Figure 15-16). The nuclear features within cell clusters are either normal or show the previously described benign reactive alterations. Furthermore, close association of these cells with ciliated cells helps underscore their benign nature.

Alveolar Level Cells

As noted previously, type I pneumocytes are difficult or impossible to appreciate in cytologic samples but may resemble macrophages. Histologically, these cells are highly attenuated and spread thinly to line alveolar surfaces specialized for efficient gas exchange. Type I cells are highly labile and are damaged in a wide range of clinical conditions (Box 15-13 and Figure 15-17). The lung's response to this type of injury includes covering the damaged alveolar lining with reactive type II pneumocytes. These cells show the morphologic features of rapid proliferation and intense, albeit reparative, metabolic activity.[7] (Box 15-14 and Figure 15-18.)

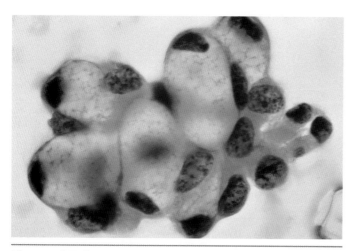

Figure 15-16 **Goblet cell hyperplasia.** This tissue particle contains occasional small columnar ciliated cells at its edge. However, most of the cells in this group represent goblet cells. In this preparation, the mucin was removed during specimen processing but has left behind a fine reticulum of cytoplasmic septations. Benign qualities of these nuclei and the intimate association of these cells with ciliated columnar elements, should prevent an inappropriate diagnosis of mucinous carcinoma. (Pap)

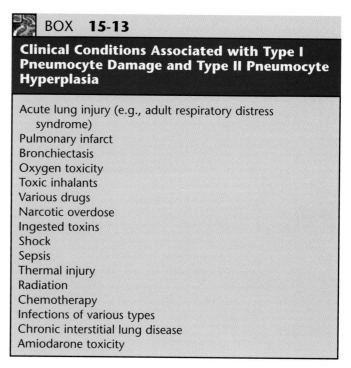

BOX 15-13

Clinical Conditions Associated with Type I Pneumocyte Damage and Type II Pneumocyte Hyperplasia

Acute lung injury (e.g., adult respiratory distress syndrome)
Pulmonary infarct
Bronchiectasis
Oxygen toxicity
Toxic inhalants
Various drugs
Narcotic overdose
Ingested toxins
Shock
Sepsis
Thermal injury
Radiation
Chemotherapy
Infections of various types
Chronic interstitial lung disease
Amiodarone toxicity

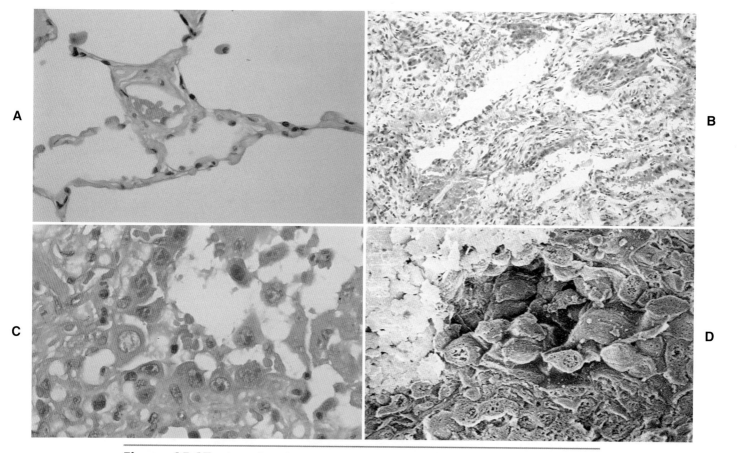

A

B

C

D

Figure 15-17 **Acute lung injury in contrast with normal alveolar level lung histology.** **A,** This image shows the thin, delicate alveolar septa of the uninjured lung. (H&E) **B,** This low-magnification image shows the marked loss of air space and interstitial widening in the proliferative phase of acute lung injury. The alveolar septa are expanded by edema, hemorrhage, and inflammatory cells. (H&E) **C,** Marked proliferation, cellular enlargement, and nuclear atypia of reactive type II pneumocytes in acute lung injury are shown here. (H&E) **D,** This scanning electron micrograph shows an expanded pulmonary interstitium. In the center of the image, a narrowed air space is lined by large hyperplastic type II pneumocytes, which bulge as rounded masses into the air space.

Cytomorphologic Features of Reactive Type II Pneumocytes

Sampling by sputum
Few abnormal cells
Lack of single cells
Flat sheets lacking depth of focus
Nuclear degeneration
Chromatin smudging

Sampling by bronchoalveolar lavage or fine-needle aspiration
Abnormal cells may be very numerous
Large cells
Single cells and small clusters
Three-dimensional (glandlike) cell groups
Moderate to abundant cytoplasm
Prominent ("soap bubble") cytoplasmic vacuoles
Nuclear enlargement
Nuclear hyperchromasia
Irregularities of nuclear contour
Prominent nucleoli
Nucleoli may be multiple
Mitotic figures
Irregular chromatin distribution with areas of clearing

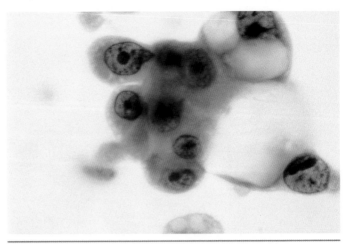

Figure 15-18 Hyperplastic type II pneumocytes. This cell cluster was obtained by bronchoalveolar lavage from a patient with acute lung injury and no evidence of malignancy. The cytomorphologic features summarized in Box 15-14 are shown here. This cluster of cells shows variability in size, irregularities of nuclear contour, prominent nucleoli, chromatin clearing, and prominent vacuolization. (Pap) (From Stanley MW, Henry-Stanley MJ, Gajl-Peczalska K, et al. Hyperplasia of type II pneumocytes in the adult respiratory distress syndrome: study of cell-shedding by sequential bronchoalveolar lavage. Am J Clin Pathol 1992; 97:669-677.)

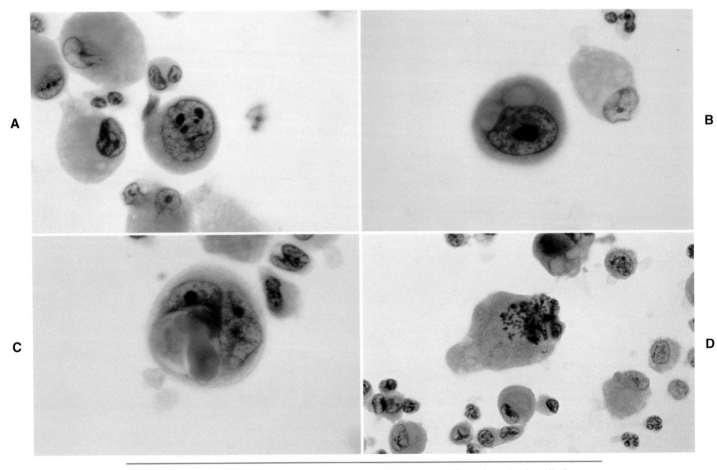

Figure 15-19 Hyperplastic type II pneumocytes. **A** to **D,** These four single cells from an acute lung injury patient represent free-lying hyperplastic type II pneumocytes. Their large size is apparent by comparison with adjacent macrophages. (Pap) **D,** A mitotic figure. (From Stanley MW, Henry-Stanley MJ, Gajl-Peczalska K, et al. Hyperplasia of type II pneumocytes in the adult respiratory distress syndrome: study of cell-shedding by sequential bronchoalveolar lavage. Am J Clin Pathol 1992; 97:669-677.)

Such cells are most often encountered in the clinical setting of an intense, rapidly evolving decrease in pulmonary function, when investigations directed at identification of possible infectious agents are undertaken. However, they may be seen in a wide variety of conditions, as emphasized in Box 15-13. The older cytology literature describes these cells as raising the possibility of malignancy and cautions that smudgy nuclei lacking in chromatin detail and a low number of abnormal cells are keys to avoiding a false-positive diagnosis of adenocarcinoma.

It seems paradoxical that newer sampling methods may actually exacerbate the diagnostic difficulties with type II cells. BAL and rarely FNA can yield large numbers of these bothersome elements and can render the nuclear features of well-preserved cells in frightening detail. In such samples, all the morphologic features noted in Box 15-14 can be seen. Furthermore, the presence of numerous abnormal cells can strengthen the impression of malignancy. Small cell clusters can mimic adenocarcinoma of either the acinar or bronchioloalveolar type. Single cells may be numerous. This feature alone is provocative and in marked contrast with the findings described in older literature based largely on sputum cytology. Individual cells may mimic signet-ring carcinoma or large cell malignant lymphoma (Figure 15-19).

Repeat samples in doubtful cases have long been recommended as an important means of avoiding an inappropriate diagnosis of malignancy; benign cells disappear over time, whereas malignant cells persist through further sampling. This was emphasized in a study of sequential BAL specimens in 38 individuals who survived well-documented episodes of acute lung injury. This clinical setting is useful in evaluating the type II cell shedding over time because most such patients are severely ill and under careful hemodynamic and respiratory monitoring. Thus, the onset of lung injury can be defined within a few hours and the follow-up shedding of abnormal cells carefully timed. The results of this evaluation are summarized in Table 15-8. A total of 62 lavages were performed from 1 to 435 days after the onset of acute lung injury. Hyperplastic type II cells were identified in 12 individuals but were never encountered in lavages performed after day 32.

Careful clinical correlation is also essential in patients with this type of atypia in one or more pulmonary cytologic samples. Great caution should be exercised in evaluating such material from patients experiencing clinical conditions known to be associated with type II cell hyperplasia (see Box 15-13). Other clues to the benign nature of the process include diffusely abnormal or rapidly evolving chest radiographic findings and the absence of a mass lesion by chest x-ray or tomographic scan. In such instances, most respiratory samples are submitted for evaluation of possible infections, and careful discussions with the clinical team often suffice to alleviate the cytologist's concern about atypical cells. As noted above, even when doubt persists, repeat cytologic samples should be considered before rushing to more invasive maneuvers.

 ## NONSPECIFIC INFLAMMATORY PATTERNS

As noted in Box 15-4, inflammatory cells of various types are common in pulmonary cytologic samples. In the appropriate clinical setting, a predominance of neutrophils is often felt to herald a bacterial infection. However, as noted in the following text, when BAL findings in various noninfectious chronic interstitial lung diseases are considered, this picture can be associated with pulmonary fibrosis in the absence of infection. Prominent eosinophilia with or without Charcot-Leyden crystals can be associated with asthma, eosinophilic pneumonia, allergic bronchopulmonary aspergillosis, or parasitic infestations. In BAL samples, eosinophilia is most often associated with either *Pneumocystis carinii* or a drug reaction.

Lymphocytes are also common. In the setting of BAL-based evaluations of various noninfectious chronic interstitial lung diseases, their presence is a sign of an active "alveolitis" stage of the disorder. This is considered more fully in the section on sarcoidosis and the interstitial pulmonary fibrosis group of conditions.

Follicular bronchitis is most often identified in bronchial brushing samples, where sufficiently vigorous sampling gives access to bronchial wall cells situated deep to the surface epithelium. Its cytologic features are identical to those of follicular cervicitis or the reactive lymphocytes seen in FNA of benign lymph nodes. The hallmark of this process is a polymorphous pattern with a spectrum of lymphocyte size and maturation. Tingible body macrophages are usually present.

Granulomatous inflammation is most commonly identified in FNA samples, where it has the same cytomorphology noted in lymph node aspirates. Granulomata have rarely been encountered in bronchial brushings, and this is largely confined to patients with sarcoidosis. In these individuals, the lesions are well formed and often lie immediately below the bronchial mucosa.

 ## SPECIFIC INFECTIOUS PROCESSES

Some infections can be identified in immunocompetent patients or in those with common types of immunosuppression resulting from conditions such as advanced age or diabetes. Chief among these are bacterial pneumonias. Other agents are responsible for infections in patients with various types of more severe immunosuppression. Within this large, diverse group, different clinical conditions are commonly associated with a specific profile of infections. For example, *P.*

TABLE	**15-8**

Identification of Hyperplastic Type II Pneumocytes in 62 Sequential Bronchoalveolar Lavage Samples from 36 Patients with Acute Lung Injury

Days After Onset of Acute Lung Injury	Patients Studied by BAL	Number of BAL Studies Performed	Number of BAL Studies with Hyperplastic Type II Pneumocytes (%)
1 to 3	22	24	6 (25)
4 to 10	8	9	4 (44)
11 to 32	10	11	2 (18)
33 to 435	8	13	0 (0)
Not recorded	5	5	0 (0)

BAL, Bronchoalveolar lavage.

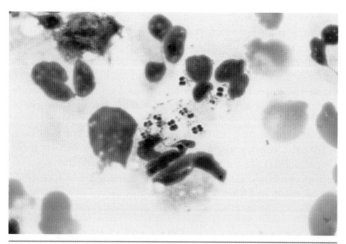

Figure 15-20 Bacterial pneumonia. This high-magnification image represents bronchoalveolar lavage fluid from a patient with proven pneumococcal pneumonia. The cells recovered in this preparation are mostly neutrophils, many of which show some degree of damage. In the center of the image are numerous clusters of basophilic cocci. (Diff-Quik [DQ]) (From Stanley MW, Henry-Stanley MJ, Iber C. Bronchoalveolar lavage: cytology and clinical applications. New York: Igaku-Shoin; 1991.)

carinii and cytomegalovirus (CMV) infections are common in patients with acquired immune deficiency syndrome (AIDS), whereas both of these are relatively rare in those experiencing acute leukemia. Invasive candidiasis occurs in exactly the opposite distribution. Some agents affect various hosts in different ways in an immune status–dependent fashion, as noted in the sections on *Aspergillus* and histoplasmosis.

Widespread application of BAL was contemporaneous with the rising incidence of AIDS. The initial experience with diagnosis of infections in BAL material centered around recognition of *P. carinii* and CMV in these patients. Because both disorders show cytologically characteristic features and most AIDS-related cases are characterized by the shedding of numerous organisms or inclusion-bearing cells, optimism regarding BAL for evaluation of pulmonary infections in general was initially significant. Subsequent information has shown that such optimism should not be extended uncritically to other types of infections or to other patient groups. Furthermore, as the care of AIDS patients has improved, even these agents are encountered much less frequently than in the 1980s.

Bacterial Pneumonias

Several problems make it difficult to recognize bacterial pneumonias based on cytologic samples, even with microbiologic culture. Various bacteria of upper aerodigestive tract origin contaminate most pulmonary cytology samples. Culture of these specimens for bacterial pathogens is simple but of limited value. Even with BALs, cultures may show suspect organisms isolated by study of healthy controls. Organisms identified in BAL fluids from immunosuppressed patients on antibiotics often prove to be of little clinical consequence. The situation is even more complex when one considers patients with endotracheal tubes in place. This permits colonization by a variety of organisms, and standard microbiologic techniques cannot distinguish between colonization and disease. When patients with AIDS are considered, bacterial pneumonias may be clinically mistaken

for *P. carinii*. Careful consideration of alternative diagnoses is necessary, if correct therapy is to be instituted.

Various types of quantitative culture, similar to those used to diagnose urinary tract infections can be applied to BAL samples. Certain counts of directly visualized organisms may correlate with a higher incidence of actual infection. Most such methods do not affect the cytology laboratory on a daily basis. However, the entire specimen is often sent to the cytology laboratory with no provision having been made for cultures or other microbiologic assessment. If any doubt exists about the adequacy of test requests, communication with the clinical team and other areas of the laboratory can prevent problems that occur when all necessary testing has not been ordered.

When numerous, bacteria can be visualized with either fixed or air-dried material and tend to be basophilic with both (Figure 15-20). It is important to note that this blue staining has nothing to do with the actual reaction the organisms will show on a Gram stain. This type of evaluation cannot be based on routine cytologic stains.

Release of single cilia probably represents a degenerative alteration of columnar bronchial cells. These tiny structures are almost exclusively seen in the clear background of some BAL specimens and are not usually visualized in other pulmonary cytology specimens. Their small size and linear configuration may suggest organisms, particularly bacteria, but they are eosinophilic and commonly entrapped in mucus.[8]

Most cytologic suspicions of bacterial pneumonia are based on increased numbers of neutrophils coupled with a failure to identify evidence of other types of infection caused by morphologically identifiable viral or fungal agents. In severely neutropenic patients, however, samples may show only macrophages so that clinical findings form the basis for suggesting this type of process.

Pneumocystis Carinii

Previously diagnosed in severely malnourished infants (plasma cell pneumonia) or rarely in other types of immunosuppression, *P. carinii* became prominent with the advancing AIDS epidemic. In this group of patients, it has always been one of the criteria by which the disease is defined. Recent genetic information suggests that this organism is more closely related to fungi than to the protozoa with which it was initially classified. Study remains difficult because it cannot be cultured outside a living host.

The cytology of *P. carinii* is complicated by the fact that it reflects a wide range of tissue responses that can be identified in histologic samples (Box 15-15). Still, the most common pattern is filling of alveolar spaces with a frothy eosinophilic exudate that is actually produced by the organisms. These foamy alveolar casts (FACs) of material approximate the size of distended alveoli and appear large when viewed against a background of macrophages in a typical cytologic sample (Box 15-16). The frothy appearance is imparted to the FAC matrix by a large number of uniform, RBC-size cysts that do not stain with routine methods. Each cyst typically contains from two to 10 minute trophozoites. In many examples, one or two can be seen in each cyst within an FAC. Trophozoites are eosinophilic dotlike structures in the Pap stain and are darkly basophilic in Romanowsky preparations. Some feel that they are more easily visualized with the latter methods (Figure 15-21). Their identi-

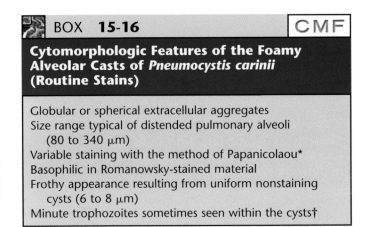

BOX 15-15

Histologic Tissue Responses to Infection by *Pneumocystis carinii*

Alveolar filling by frothy eosinophilic material (foamy alveolar casts)*†
Granulomatous inflammation
Fibrosis
Calcification
Giant cells
Cavitary mass lesions
No tissue response

*Associated with various degrees of interstitial inflammation, hemorrhage, or hyaline membrane formation.
†May be rare.

BOX 15-16 CMF

Cytomorphologic Features of the Foamy Alveolar Casts of *Pneumocystis carinii* (Routine Stains)

Globular or spherical extracellular aggregates
Size range typical of distended pulmonary alveoli (80 to 340 μm)
Variable staining with the method of Papanicolaou*
Basophilic in Romanowsky-stained material
Frothy appearance resulting from uniform nonstaining cysts (6 to 8 μm)
Minute trophozoites sometimes seen within the cysts†

*Large foam alveolar casts are typically cyanophilic at their periphery, with a central eosinophilic area.
†Eosinophilic in fixed material and basophilic with Romanowsky stains.

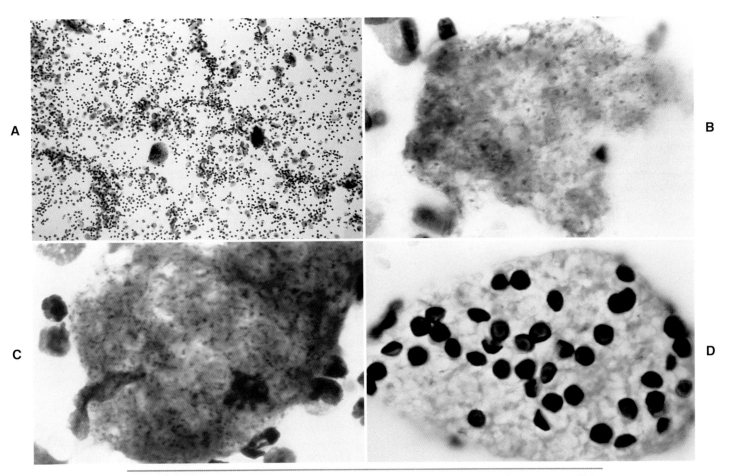

Figure 15-21 *Pneumocystis carinii.* **A,** This low-magnification image shows a very cellular bronchoalveolar lavage fluid. Most of the small, darkly staining objects represent macrophages. Interrupting this pattern are larger collections of material that represent foamy alveolar casts of pneumocystis, as seen at low-magnification. (Pap) **B,** This foamy alveolar cast is shown at high magnification. The cyanophilic background material represents a pneumocystis exudate. This has a lacy appearance and is filled with round, nonstaining cysts. Numerous tiny eosinophilic dotlike structures represent trophozoites that are themselves housed within the cysts. (Pap) **C,** This air-dried preparation shows a foamy alveolar cast. The FAC matrix is basophilic and has numerous round uniform clear openings due to the presence of non-staining cysts. Added uniformly through the entire fragment are very darkly staining tiny trophozoites. (DQ) **D,** This silver stain of BAL lavage fluid shows round and helmet-shaped pneumocystis cysts within the light-green counter stained FAC matrix. (GMS) (From Stanley MW, Henry-Stanley MJ, Iber C. Bronchoalveolar lavage: cytology and clinical applications. New York: Igaku-Shoin; 1991.)

fication is not essential but strengthens the diagnosis by completing the expected picture.

Identification of FACs by careful application of these criteria is diagnostic of *P. carinii*, and special stains are not necessary. Thus, when this picture is present, a cytologic preparation can give a rapid and inexpensive diagnosis of this condition. However, some workers still prefer to base the diagnosis on silver stains. These methods do not stain the FAC matrix, which is rendered pale with a counterstain (usually light green) and does not show trophozoites. Instead, they provide the precise mirror image of routine stains by highlighting the cyst walls. These are cup-, or helmet-shaped and about the size of an RBC. Many contain a central dotlike area of dense silver positivity. This is much larger than a trophozoite and corresponds to an area of cyst membrane collapse. It is important to note that an FAC is a relatively large structure that contains a number of cysts. For this reason, silver stains that are positive for *P. carinii* virtually always show clusters of RBC-size silver positive cups, helmets, and circles. Small isolated silver-positive structures should be regarded as nondiagnostic, or as possible fungi.

Monoclonal antibody stains vary in the extent to which the FAC matrix and the cysts are highlighted.[9] One interesting property of the Pap-stained FAC matrix is that it is autofluorescent. This method is of limited usefulness because other structures show this property as a result of their reactions with the cytoplasmic counterstains in this formulation (Box 15-17).

All methods for identification of *P. carinii* by recognition of FACs can be confounded by other materials in a given cytologic preparation (see Box 15-17). Most such difficulties relate to mucus, to small, rounded droplets of lubricant, to clusters of depigmented RBCs, or to aggregates of bacteria. Any of these may appear as oval or spherical structures in the size range of FACs (Figures 15-22 and 15-23). However, when examined in detail, they lack the internal details summarized in Box 15-16. When difficulties arise with spe-

---

BOX   15-17

Structures, Materials, and Cells that Can Be Mistaken for the Foamy Alveolar Casts of *Pneumocystis carinii*

Routine stains
Mucus
Lubricant
Clumps of bacteria
Clusters of red blood cells

Silver stains
Mucus
Talc
Clumps of bacteria
Clusters of red blood cells
Neutrophils
Hemosiderin-filled macrophages

Autofluorescence*
Mucus
Epithelial cells
Fungi
Clusters of red blood cells

*Pap-stained material viewed with ultraviolet light.

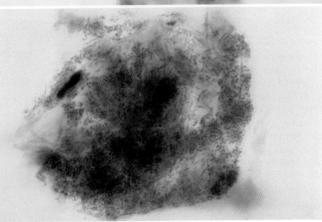
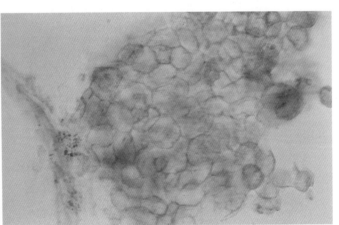
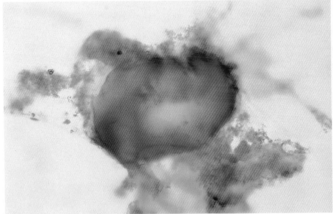

Figure 15-22 Artifacts that can be mistaken for *Pneumocystis carinii.* These images summarize the appearance of material sometimes mistaken for the foamy alveolar casts (FACs) of pneumocystis on Pap-stained preparations. All have been photographed at the same magnification. **A,** A droplet of lubricant is rounded and three dimensional but lacks the internal structure of an FAC. **B,** This aggregate of depigmented RBCs lacks the matrix material and trophozoites of a typical FAC. **C,** Careful examination reveals that this darkly staining ovoid structure is actually a mass of tiny basophilic bacteria. This cluster lacks the internal substructure typical of FACs, as illustrated in Figure 15-21. (From Stanley MW, Henry-Stanley MJ, Iber C. Bronchoalveolar lavage: cytology and clinical applications. New York: Igaku-Shoin; 1991.)

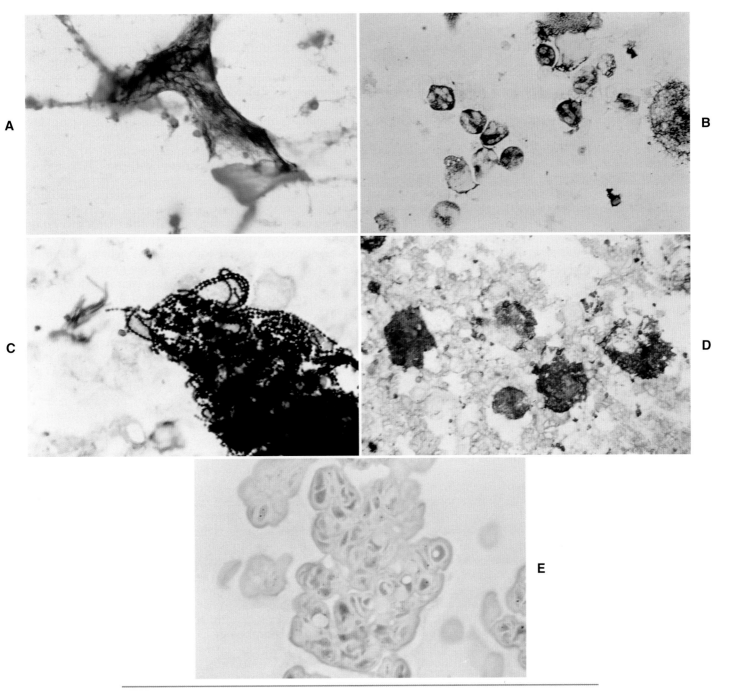

Figure 15-23 **Silver-staining artifacts.** This series of images summarizes artifacts sometimes mistaken for pneumocystis or other organisms on silver-stain preparations. All are stained with the GMS method and photographed at the same magnification. **A,** Wisps of mucous are often silver positive. These may have some laciness that superficially mimics the internal substructure of an FAC. However, they lack the globular shape and distinctive spheres and helmets of pneumocystis. **B,** The cytoplasmic granules of these neutrophils are positive with this silver stain. A nonstaining negative image of the lobulated nucleus can be seen in each cell. Furthermore, pneumocystis spheres occur in clusters where they are bound together within the matrix of the foamy alveolar cast while these cells lie singly. **C,** This cluster of large bacteria presumably from the mouth are strongly silver positive. However, the constituent spheres are much more crowded and smaller than the cysts of pneumocystis. **D,** These macrophages are dark because they are filled with hemosiderin. They do not show silver positivity and have no spherical or helmet-shaped objects. **E,** This clump of RBCs has retained sufficient pigment to appear dark against a light green background of this silver stain. No true silver positivity is demonstrated here, but the repetitive round shapes within this aggregate might be confusing. In such instances, it is most useful to refer to routinely stained material that will probably also show clumps of RBCs. (From Stanley MW, Henry-Stanley MJ, Iber C. Bronchoalveolar lavage: cytology and clinical applications. New York: Igaku-Shoin; 1991.)

cial stains, a look back to the routinely stained slides often clarifies the nature of any questionable materials.

Silver-stained neutrophils have been mistaken for *P. carinii*. These are positive on such stains because of staining of the cytoplasmic granules. Closer examination reveals the negative (nonstaining) image of the typical lobated nucleus that quickly betrays the cells' true nature. This type of error also violates the rule that cysts virtually always occur in clusters rather than as small isolated circles.

Problems in the cytologic diagnosis of *P. carinii* include cases with few FACs, those in which the other patterns summarized in Box 15-15 prevail, and those in which previous treatment has been given. In the first two settings, it is doubtful that most cases can be recognized without the more specific methods of monoclonal antibody staining or polymerase chain reaction (PCR).[10,11] This is because the presence of FACs is the basis for cytologic diagnosis. In some instances of low organism burden, rare FACs may be highlighted by a silver stain.

After treatment, the expected findings can be altered in a number of significant ways.[12] FACs may be rare and can be missed altogether because of sampling error. When identified with routine stains, they may lack trophozoites. Silver stains can show the limited number of such structures that may be present and can reveal degeneration of any remaining cysts that they contain.

Many *P. carinii* patients are unable to produce sputum spontaneously and a desire to obtain diagnostic samples without resorting to bronchoscopy has led to the use of induced sputum, as described previously. In most instances, laboratory diagnosis of *P. carinii* in this material has been based on direct immunofluorescence staining with monoclonal antibodies, but immunoperoxidase methods can also be used. The yield has been similar to that observed when these stains are applied to expectorated samples.[13]

It is important to note that the commonly used pick-and-smear method of sputum processing is not applicable to this technique. The mucinous background makes routinely stained slides difficult to examine for FACs. Furthermore, it is often densely black on silver stains and can give unacceptable background staining with immunologic methods. Alternatives involve treating the specimen with a chemical mucolytic agent (e.g., dithiothreitol [Sputolysin; Behring Diagnostics; La Jolla, Calif.]). The material of interest is then collected by centrifugation and used for smear preparation.[14]

In many institutions, most diagnoses of *P. carinii* have passed from the cytology laboratory with its routine and silver stains to the laboratory of microbiology where immunologic methods or PCR is usually employed. The fact remains, however, that this organism is often readily diagnosed in cytologic samples, and that when this is accomplished, it is the most rapid and least expensive route to identification of *P. carinii*.

Fungal Infections

Identification of fungal elements in a respiratory cytology sample is usually possible with routinely stained preparations. This is especially true when one encounters the larger hyphal forms (*Aspergillus*, *Candida*, and the *Zygomycetes*), whereas some small yeasts may be difficult to identify unless they are numerous (e.g., histoplasmosis,

blastomycosis, and *Cryptococcus*). In the latter instance, silver stains may help locate rare organisms. The previously noted difficulties in silver stain evaluation apply here and to *P. carinii*. Such preparations help identify yeast forms, especially when they are not numerous but show no internal structure, so that evaluation of routinely stained slides is still helpful in many cases. Table 15-9 summarizes the cytologic appearances of common fungi on routinely stained slides. In contrast to *P. carinii* and CMV, most literature describing application of BAL to fungal diseases involves patients with non-AIDS types of immunosuppression.

Several types of material can be mistaken for fungal forms, particularly yeast, as summarized in Box 15-18. One added complication is that talc is positive with silver stains. However, the central hole or defect and the characteristic appearance when viewed with polarized light are diagnostic. The recent widespread use of talc-free gloves has lessened the degree to which this material is seen in cytologic samples. Hemosiderin has been described in detail earlier. Its staining qualities, lack of the internal structure of yeasts, and variability in particle size help distinguish it from fungi. Neutrophils spend themselves by participating in inflammatory exudates. The residua of damaged cells include bits of basophilic nuclear material. Because these normally consist of small, rounded lobes joined by thin strands of chromatinic material, a resemblance to yeast may be noted. The small size of these particles, the presence of other neutrophils, and the presence of a blocklike nuclear chromatin structure (when preserved) all aid proper identification of these structures.

During processing for Pap or silver stains, RBCs often undergo varying degrees of depigmentation. Such cells have been misinterpreted as fungal organisms. They can be seen in clusters or singly and may be situated within the cytoplasm of macrophages. Often, a spectrum of increasing loss of pigment is seen so that the nature of the cleared, ringlike forms can be extrapolated from the more typical RBCs elsewhere on the slide.

Table 15-9 lists the most common types of fungi identified in respiratory cytology samples. However, many more possibilities exist but difficulties in classification cannot be resolved by morphology alone. Instead various characteristics noted in culture or from biochemical testing form the basis for speciation. Thus, definitive identification may not be possible so that a report should be issued that describes fungal elements without more detailed information. In some instances, one organism may be morphologically identical to another. For example, *Pseudoalleceria boydii* looks the same as *Aspergillus*, but does not respond to therapy with amphotericin. Fusarium is also cytologically identical to *Aspergillus*. This type of problem has prompted diagnoses with terms such as *fungal elements morphologically consistent with Aspergillus*.

Candida is commonly present as a contaminant from the upper aerodigestive tract and can be seen in virtually any respiratory cytology preparation. Its presence in BALs can be diminished by separate collection and preparation of the first aliquot, as previously described. It can be seen in samples from normal individuals and those with pulmonary disease. Even when it is encountered, it is usually not the cause of any lung pathology. Attempts have been made to increase the probability that this yeast is the cause of a pa-

TABLE 15-9

Cytomorphologic Features of Fungi Most Commonly Seen in Pulmonary Cytology Samples

Fungi	Forms	Hyphal Branches	Average Diameter (μm)	Budding Pattern	Special Features
Candida spp.	Budding yeast (BY) Pseudohyphae (PH)	Not applicable (NA)	BY: 4 PH: 4	Constricted neck	Often red or orange with Pap stain
Blastomycosis	Yeast	NA	8 to 15	Broad-based	Thick wall; internal dotlike nuclear material
Aspergillus spp.	SH* with 45-degree branches Spores†	45 degrees	SH: 5 to 10 Spores: 3 to 6	NA	Can be associated with oxylate crystals
Histoplasma capsulatum	BY	NA	2 to 4	Constricted neck	Most easily identified within macrophage cytoplasm
Coccidioides imitis	Endospores (ES) Spherules	NA	ES: 2 to 5 Spherules: up to 100	NA	Collapsed empty spherules diagnostic
Cryptococcus neoformans	Yeast	NA	5 to 8‡	Constricted neck	Positive capsule staining with mucicarmine

*The individual spores and fruiting heads are rarely encountered.
†Aspergillus spores are rarely seen in cytologic samples.
‡The total organism size can be up to 20 mm due to the presence of a variable-sized capsule.

BOX 15-18

Structures, Materials, and Cells that Can Be Mistaken for Fungi

Talc*
Pollen
Hemosiderin
Anthracotic pigment
Nuclear lobes from damaged neutrophils
Red blood cells in various states of depigmentation†
True fungal elements that are present only as contaminants (*Alternaria*)‡

*Silver stain positive.
†Less fully depigmented cells, often showing a range of clearing, are usually present.
‡Usually only one or two per case are seen sitting in a microscopic plane of focus above the other material on the slide.

tient's lung disease by setting thresholds for the number of organisms seen in a BAL sample.[15,16]

The cytology of *Candida* is as described in gynecologic material. As noted in Table 15-9, its yeast and pseudohyphae are often red or orange on Pap-stained preparations. This helpful feature excludes such contaminants as talc, hemosiderin, and neutrophil lobes from consideration.

Invasive pulmonary candidiasis features invasion of bronchial or vascular walls and lung parenchyma by yeast and pseudohyphae with variable degrees of hemorrhage. This type of destructive growth is much less common than noninvasive mucosal colonization and is encountered most often in patients with acute leukemia. This type of diagnosis is better reserved for histologic material. Reasons for this include (1) the high frequency of contamination in cytology material; (2) the dangers inherent in systemic antifungal therapy; and (3) the high fatality of untreated cases.

Colonization and infection with *Aspergillus* take several clinical forms (Box 15-19).[17] In general, the degree of invasiveness is inversely proportional to the patient's immunocompetence. In otherwise healthy individuals, the identification of the typical hyphae may have no significance, and the diagnosis of aspergillosis must rest on combined clinical, radiographic, and culture data. Hyphae have been identified in BAL specimens from patients ultimately shown to have other lung diseases, not all of which were infectious in origin.

The hyphal morphology summarized in Table 15-9 is readily appreciated in routine, silver, and Gram stains and in rapid preparations based on toluidine blue (Figure 15-24). The diagnostic yield of bronchoscopy with brushings, washing, and transbronchial biopsy in patients with confirmed aspergillosis has ranged from 15% to 50% in various series. In some series, this yield has been improved by culture and cytology of BAL samples.[18,19]

When *Aspergillus* grows on a surface that is exposed to air it develops fruiting heads that will produce and release the

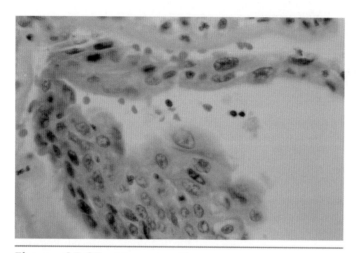

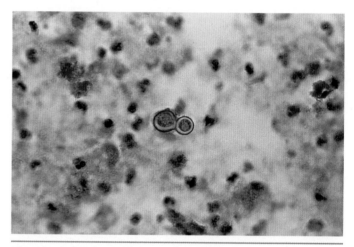

Figure 15-24 *Aspergillus.* **A,** This cluster of hyphae is typical of *Aspergillus* with septations and branching at 45-degree angles. The large fragment of material represents a three-dimensional mass formed by tangled hyphae. The individual hyphae are better seen in the center of the image where they spread out from this large mass. This material represents one of many such fragments aspirated from a pulmonary mycetoma. (Pap) **B,** *Aspergillus* spores that have rarely been encounter but which, in this case, may be seen germinating. (DQ)

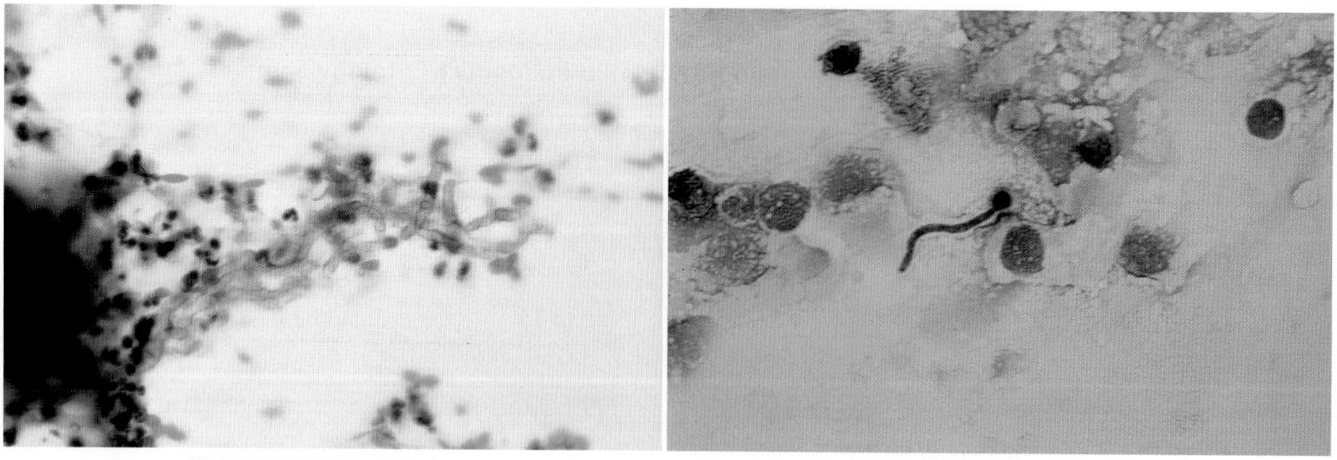

Figure 15-25 Mycetoma. The markedly atypical squamous metaplastic epithelium lining mycetomas is shown in this surgical resection specimen. (H&E)

Figure 15-26 Blastomycosis. This sputum smear shows a background of acute inflammatory cells and debris. In the center is an eosinophilic-staining yeast of blastomycosis. This features a thick outer cell wall and a broad-based bud. (Pap)

BOX 15-19

Clinical Forms of *Aspergillus* Colonization and Infection

Incidental
- Asymptomatic colonization

Immunologic reactions
- Extrinsic allergic alveolitis
- Allergic bronchopulmonary aspergillosis

Noninvasive mycetoma

Invasive disease
- Chronic necrotizing pulmonary aspergillosis*
- Angioinvasive aspergillosis

*This is distinguished from mycetoma by invasion of the pulmonary parenchyma and from angioinvasive aspergillosis by the absence of vascular involvement.

conidia on which speciation is based. This happens when a mycetoma-containing cavity retains its communication with the bronchial tree and continues to be at least partially aerated.[17] Another cytologic manifestation of mycetoma is recovery of enormous amounts of hyphal material, with or without fruiting heads by FNA. The radiographic features of these fungus balls are usually characteristic, and in this setting, FNA is diagnostic.[20] It is important to remember that mycetomas can be associated with atypical squamous metaplasia, which can be mistaken for carcinoma, if the underlying nature of the patient's condition is not appreciated (Figure 15-25). Diagnosis of *Aspergillus* by antigen detection in BAL fluids has been disappointing, whereas a recently described PCR test appears much more promising.[21,22]

Pulmonary blastomycosis is often tumefactive, and patients may undergo cytologic sampling ranging from expectorated sputum to FNA under a clinical suspicion of carcinoma. In geographic areas where this infection is common, it may be seen often in BAL material.[23] The conidia of blastomycosis resemble pollen, in that they have a thick, double-contoured outer wall, but they are smaller than most pollen grains (Figure 15-26). Furthermore, they have tiny central dotlike bits of basophilic nuclear material. Buds have a broadly based attachment to the parent yeast. The substructure of these conidia is much clearer in fixed than in air-dried material. The latter preparations tend to render the yeast as deeply basophilic spheres that lack internal detail to the extent that they are difficult to recognize. Furthermore, in Pap-stained material, the yeast are often somewhat eosinophilic, making them relatively easy to see during low-magnification slide screening. Another feature of blastomycosis that is nearly unique among the non-*Candida* fungi is its association with acute inflammatory cells. In smear material, the yeast can often be readily detected when the small organisms are surrounded by a much larger aggregate of neutrophils.

Infection with *Histoplasma capsulatum* is common in endemic areas, and many individuals harbor the organism without signs or symptoms. Its most common manifestation is as well-circumscribed, centrally necrotic granulomas, often with a thick hyaline capsule. These can be located in many areas but are most common in the lung, lymph nodes, liver, and spleen. This form of the disease is not commonly addressed by cytologic techniques but can be studied by FNA. Such specimens show mostly necrotic debris and may include small amounts calcific material or a few histiocytes. Organisms are usually not numerous in these samples and, if cytologically identified at all, usually require a silver stain. In many instances, it is necessary to wait for culture results. This is not a common specimen because the diagnosis is often apparent from clinical and radiographic findings. When aspirated, the clinical situation is often unclear, and it is necessary to exclude the possibility of carcinoma or another type of infection.

Disseminated histoplasmosis is usually encountered in immunosuppressed patients, including those with AIDS, but may occasionally be seen in normal hosts after massive acute inhalational exposure. Numerous small yeast fill the cytoplasm of macrophages in all affected tissues (Figure 15-27). In the lung, BAL readily recovers these. The organism's small size, intracellular location, and lack of hyphal forms help distinguish it from other fungi. Numerous organisms fill the cytoplasm of a macrophage and appear to be surrounded by a clear (nonstaining) narrow capsule. Each organism has a biphasic appearance with lighter and darker poles.

Problems in the diagnosis of histoplasmosis relate to the fact that the organism is small, and although numerous yeast may fill a macrophage, the cell is not obviously enlarged. Furthermore, the affected macrophages may be few in number. These features may cause the organisms to be missed when slides are reviewed at a screening magnification; the yeast are mistaken for nonspecific macrophage vacuoles or are missed altogether. Silver stains may be helpful in identifying rare affected cells. Distinction of histoplasmosis from *Penicillium marneffei* is discussed later in this chapter.

Coccidioidomycosis is seen primarily in residents of or travelers to arid regions of the southwestern United States. It represents a common infection in patients with AIDS in those areas, and may disseminate widely to involve the liver, spleen, kidneys, brain, adrenal glands, and other sites. Characteristic organisms can be detected in a variety of cytologic specimens, including BALs, but transbronchial biopsy has shown a greater sensitivity in some hands.[24] Although resulting in a delay of final diagnosis by days to weeks, culture is probably the most sensitive diagnostic test.

Coccidioidomycosis features spherules that are among the largest structures encountered in cytology, measuring up to 100 μm in diameter. These have a distinctive double contoured wall and contain up to several hundred small (2 to 5 μm) endospores (Figure 15-28). After rupture and release of endospores, empty spherules appear as large wrinkled structures that resemble collapsed ping-pong balls (Figure 15-29). These structures are considered to be diagnostic, even in the absence of their well-preserved, endospore-filled

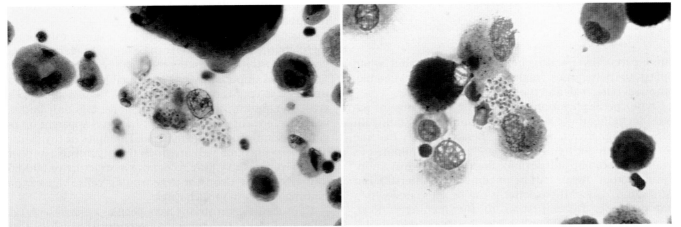

Figure 15-27 Histoplasmosis. **A** and **B,** These images show macrophages obtained by bronchoalveolar lavage. In the center of each image, one cell is filled with numerous yeast of histoplasmosis. In the DQ-stained slide **(B),** these have a biphasic appearance with one clear and one dark-staining end each. Many of the adjacent macrophages are filled with anthracotic pigment. **(A,** Pap; **B,** DQ)

A

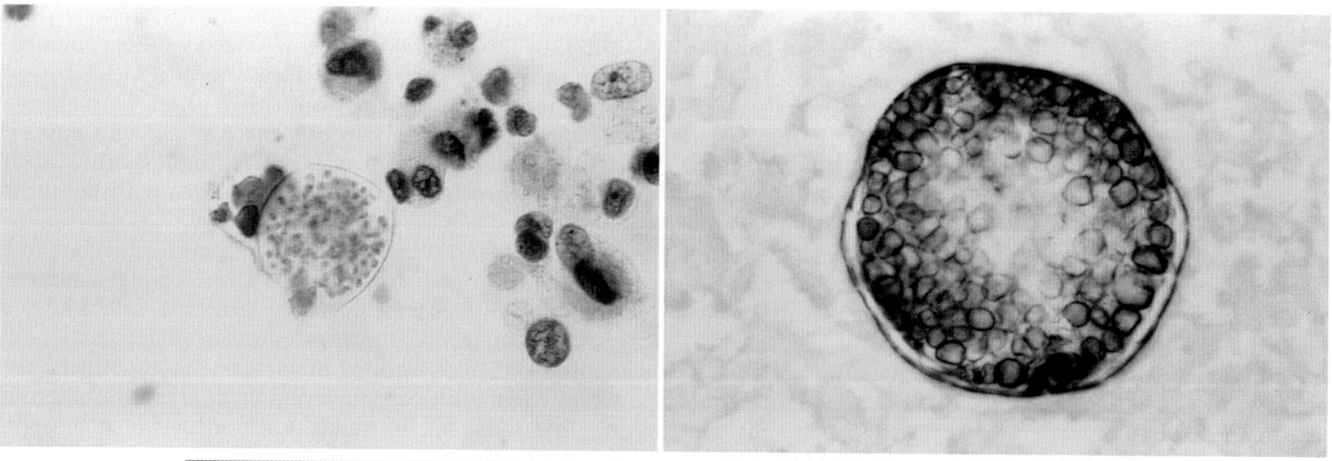

B

Figure 15-28   Coccidioidomycosis. **A,** The large structure in the center of this image is a spherule of coccidioidomycosis. Its size is greater than that of the surrounding macrophages. This spherule is filled with numerous small endospores. (Pap) **B,** The silver stain highlights the double wall of the spherule in the numerous internal endospores. (GMS)

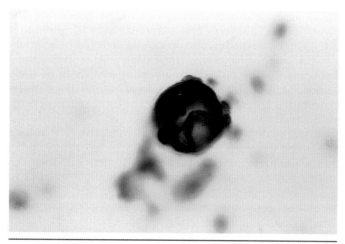

Figure 15-29   **Empty spherule of coccidioidomycosis.** This is sufficiently large so that it sits above the surrounding cells' plane of focus. This image was also selected to emphasize its wrinkled upper surface. These structures are diagnostic of coccidioidomycosis, even in the absence of better preserved, endospore-filled spherules. (Pap)

counterparts. Silver stains are rarely necessary but when applied to these cases, highlight the spherules' double-contoured outer wall and the numerous endospores.

Cryptococcal pneumonia occurs in a wide range of patients, including those with various chronic debilitating illnesses, malignancies, or steroid therapy. It has become more common during the AIDS pandemic. Granulomatous involvement can be diffuse or localized, and extensive non-granulomatous disease can be pneumonic or interstitial in distribution. Any of these patterns can be associated with a fatal outcome. Dissemination to the meninges, liver, spleen, kidneys, and lymph nodes has been described.[25] Antemortem recognition of this infection can be difficult in patients who lack meningeal involvement and is usually based on culture of lung samples including sputum. Cryptococcal antigen detection has been successfully applied to cerebrospinal fluid and serum but may not be

needed for evaluation of pulmonary cytology material, particularly BALs.[26]

Cytologic and histologic diagnoses of *Cryptococcus* can be accomplished with bronchial brushings, bronchial washings, BAL, and transbronchial biopsies. In patients with AIDS the organisms tend to be widely distributed in an interstitial pattern and are usually accompanied by macrophages without any other inflammatory cell types. As noted in Table 15-9, buds with constricted, teardrop-shaped attachments to the parent yeast are typical (Figure 15-30). The most striking and characteristic cytologic feature of *Cryptococcus* is its capsule. In Romanowsky-stained material, this is densely basophilic to the extent that the internal yeast is usually not visible. The details are much clearer in fixed preparations. The yeast often lie together in small clusters that seem to be held together by a common mass of fused capsular material. In Pap-stained samples, this is clear, or minimally basophilic. When the yeast are located within the cytoplasm of a macrophage, the clear capsule appears as a nonstaining halo. If fungi are situated immediately adjacent to a macrophage, the capsule often causes a concave indentation of the cells' cytoplasm.

Mucicarmine staining is a rapid and inexpensive way to highlight the capsule, which can be useful in identifying rare yeast forms or for confirming the identification of organisms. The latter is important when the variable size of this organism leads to confusion with *Candida, H. capsulatum,* or other yeast. In contrast, silver staining demonstrates only budding yeast, the presence of which often has been apparent on previously examined routine material. Examples of *Cryptococcus* have been encountered, in which the organisms are poorly preserved and show little recognizable structure or budding, thus resembling debris or degenerating cells. Mucicarmine staining is helpful in such cases.

Capsule-deficient strains have been associated with both AIDS and non-AIDS types of immunosuppression. Cytologic diagnosis can be difficult in these cases, but Watts and Chandler emphasized that at least some yeast have carminophilic capsules and can be easily identified among the more numerous nonencapsulated organisms with this stain[27] (Figure 15-31).

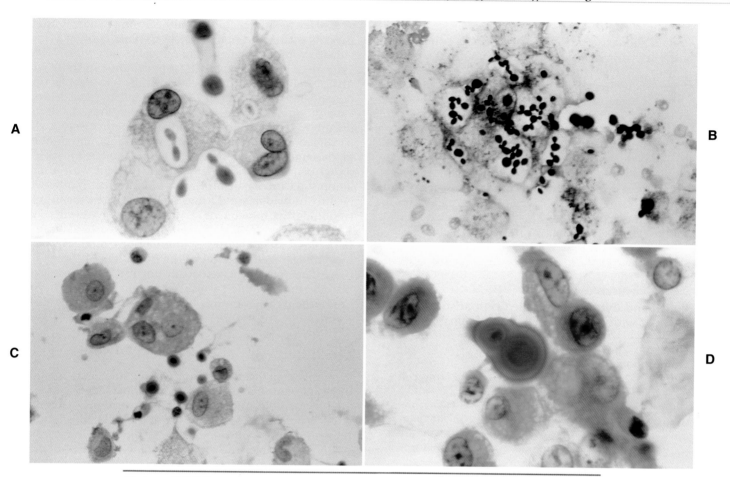

Figure 15-30 *Cryptococcus.* **A,** At the top of the image, two yeast are joined together by a thin, connecting mantle of mucinous capsular material. In the center, two yeast that are joined by a thin teardrop-like bud occupy the cytoplasm of a macrophage. The capsule appears as a clear surrounding vacuole. In the lower part of the image, cryptococcal organisms lie outside but adjacent to macrophages and their clear capsular material indents the cytoplasm of the larger cells. (Pap) **B,** In this silver-stained preparation, numerous budding yeast typical of *Cryptococcus* are present. (GMS) **C,** A mucin stain highlights the red-staining cryptococcal yeast in the center if the image (Mucicarmine stain [Mucin]). **D,** At high magnification a mucicarmine stain shows a budding cryptococcal organism. (Mucin) (From Stanley MW, Henry-Stanley MJ, Iber C. Bronchoalveolar lavage: cytology and clinical applications. New York: Igaku-Shoin; 1991.)

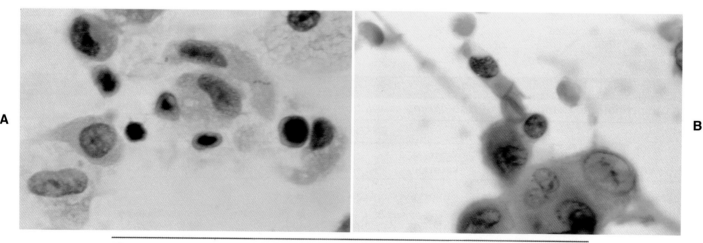

Figure 15-31 *Cryptococcus* **with degeneration. A,** The small darkly staining objects in this image most resemble degenerated nuclei of lymphocytes or bronchial cells. (Pap) **B,** The mucin stain shows that a few of these are carminophilic, representing a capsule-deficient strain of *Cryptococcus* recovered by bronchoalveolar lavage from an AIDS patient. (Mucin)

The family of fungi designated the *Zygomycetes* includes the genera *Rhizopus*, *Absidia*, and *Mucor*. The latter is most often identified in clinical samples, where it can be associated with several patterns of infection[28] (Table 15-10). Although these fungi are widely distributed in nature and can exist as saprophytes, identification in clinical material almost always indicates a significant infection, rather than colonization. Angioinvasive pulmonary involvement can be rapidly fatal and is associated with radiographic and pulmonary function studies that mimic thromboembolism. In this way, it can clinically resemble infection with *Aspergillus*.

Diagnosis of mucormycosis remains difficult, as attempts to culture it are often unsuccessful. BAL, bronchial brushings, and bronchial washings may show the characteristic hyphae as described in Table 15-10.[28]

P. marneffei is endemic in Southeast Asia, where it infects patients with AIDS approximately 10 times as often as individuals without human immunodeficiency virus (HIV). Untreated, it causes rapidly fatal pneumonia in those with AIDS.[29,30] It has recently been identified in people from nonendemic areas who have an appropriate travel history. Patients present with various combinations of diffuse pneumonia, generalized lymphadenopathy, sepsis, hepatosplenomegaly, anemia, fever, weight loss, and multiple molluscum-like skin lesions. The latter are often a marker of disseminated infection. Rare patients present with a mass lesion.[31] A carrier state for this organism exists in otherwise healthy individuals and forms the basis for reactivation infection during subsequent immunosuppressive events.

Diagnosis of *P. marneffei* can be achieved by culture of skin, blood, bone marrow, sputum, or BAL fluid, as well as by cytologic identification of the organisms in these samples. Care must be taken to distinguish this yeast from histoplasmosis (Table 15-11). Distinction from other types of *Penicillium* relies on microbiologic rather than cytologic features.

Viral Infections

Clinically significant infection with these agents is much more common than reflected in occasional identification of viral cytopathic effects in cytologic material. However, when cellular changes diagnostic of a specific infection are present, cytology provides the most rapid and inexpensive diagnosis possible. The primary cytologic manifestation of viral cytopathic effect is the presence of inclusions in the infected cells. These may be present in the nucleus or both the nucleus and the cytoplasm (Box 15-20). These alterations are associated with various degrees of cellular enlargement and multinucleation.

Numerous agents can be identified by culture or PCR and are not associated with specific cytologic alterations. As methods for viral detection become more sensitive, an uncoupling of positive test results may be perceived from clinically significant infection. This is especially true when a patient has multiple infections that require different therapeutic approaches. It may be clinically difficult to assess the significance of any viral infection that is identified. Furthermore, the significance of virus identification in respiratory material may not be clear for other reasons. Frequent

TABLE **15-10**		
Clinical and Cytomorphologic Comparison of Mucor with *Aspergillus* (Routine Stains)		
Clinical or Cytomorphologic Feature	*Aspergillus*	**Mucormycosis**
Clinical presentation	Refractory pneumonia Mimics thrombo-embolism	Refractory pneumonia Mimics thrombo-embolism
Tissue involvement	Mostly pulmonary	Rhinocerebral Pulmonary Cutaneous Gastrointestinal Disseminated
Relative frequency of disease	Common	Uncommon
Hyphal diameter	5 to 10 μm	10 to 30 μm
Hyphal septa	Yes	No*
Hyphal branching	45 degrees	90 degrees

*The broad septa of mucormycosis are often described a ribbon-like. They may fold and thereby appear to acquire septa, but these are not uniformly distributed.

TABLE **15-11**					
Cytomorphologic Comparison of *Histoplasma capsulatum* with *Penicillium marneffei* (Routine Stains)					
	CYTOMORPHOLOGIC FEATURE				
Type of Yeast	**Inflammatory Response**	**Yeast Location**	**Yeast Diameter (μm)**	**Hyphae**	**Reproduction**
Histoplasma capsulatum	Histiocytes	Histiocyte cytoplasm	2 to 4	None	Budding
Penicillium marneffei	Initial: histiocytes Subsequent: abscess formation	Histiocyte cytoplasm	Ovoid: 2 to 3 × 2 to 7	Rare: curved; length = 20 μm	Fission (schizogony)*

*This results in demarcation of a cell by one (or rarely, two) transverse septa.

contamination of these samples with cells and material from other sites has been discussed. This can be important, when considering, for example, that herpetic bronchitis and esophagitis are more common than pneumonitis due to this agent.

CMV is the most commonly identified pulmonary virus, regardless of the means of detection. Its significance varies considerably among various types of immunosuppression. It is less common, as a fraction of all serious pulmonary events, in bone marrow or solid organ transplant recipients than in patients with AIDS. However, in the former groups, it is often fatal, whereas patients with AIDS often harbor the infection for long periods and go on to die from other causes. The importance of rapid diagnosis by cytology, immunocytochemistry, or PCR is underscored by the fact that many seriously ill CMV patients do not survive for the days to weeks required for traditional techniques of viral culture.[32,33]

Cells showing CMV cytopathic effect are usually enlarged, with abundant cytoplasm. Cytoplasmic inclusions are difficult to visualize and usually appear as granularity rather than as distinct structures. The nuclear inclusion is distinctive and has been described as resembling an owl's eye (Figure 15-32). The nuclear membrane is thickened and may show a beaded pattern of small chromatin clumps along its inner surface. Much of the nucleus is filled by a large, round to oval, homogeneously eosinophilic inclusion, separated from the nuclear membrane by a narrow concentric clear zone. In some cells, a few small ragged bits of chromatinic material may remain within the otherwise clear halo. Reactive macrophages or type II pneumocytes with cellular enlargement and prominent nucleoli may be suggestive of CMV cytopathic effect. However, their nucleoli do not rival the size of the viral inclusions, and the features of nuclear membrane thickening and a clear halo are not present.

CMV can involve the lung in a nonuniform, multifocal fashion. Viral DNA can be identified in many cells from several organs, but most of these do not show cytopathic alterations. In fact, the morphologically identifiable CMV cell represents a small minority of the cells that are actually infected. Furthermore, in non-AIDS types of immunosuppression, inclusions can be rare, even when CMV is responsible for the patient's lung disease.

These observations probably account for relatively frequent false-negative interpretations, when cytologic samples or tissues biopsies are compared with viral identification by more sensitive means. The corollary for cytology is that inclusions must be carefully sought. Several cases have been noted in which a single diagnostic cell was identified after careful examination of six or more cytocentrifuge pellets. Diagnostic sensitivity can probably be improved by immunohistochemistry.[32] It has been suggested that, in bone marrow transplant recipients, positive CMV PCR in either blood or BAL fluid may predict a subsequent clinically significant CMV infection.[33]

Infection with the herpes simplex virus (HSV) can result in esophagitis, tracheitis, bronchitis, pneumonitis, or various combinations of these disease distributions. As noted previously, issues of sampling and contamination in pulmonary material can make it necessary to rely on clinical findings to determine the nature of the patient's condition.

The affected cells lack cytoplasmic inclusions. They are often multinucleated, but uninucleate bronchial cells with nuclear HSV cytopathic effect can be seen. In some cells, intranuclear inclusions may appear similar to those in CMV. However, it is more common to see complete transformation of the karyoplasm into a homogeneous "ground-glass" appearance that is less eosinophilic than the inclusions of CMV. The nuclear membrane can be thickened, beaded, or angulated[34] (Figure 15-33).

The inclusions of some adenovirus-infected cells can be mistaken for those of herpes. However, these are accompanied by large cells with distinctive, dark, smudgy inclusions that fill the nucleus or are attached to the nuclear membrane by chromatin threads.[35]

Mycobacterial Infections

Under most clinical circumstances, cytology plays a minor role in diagnosis of mycobacterial infections. Identification of granulomas by FNA occasionally occurs when a mass lesion is investigated under a suspicion of malignancy. Such aspirates show the cytologic features described in the chapter on lymph node cytology. With the exception of patients with AIDS harboring atypical mycobacterial infections,

---

BOX 15-20

Inclusions Associated with Viral Infections

Nuclear inclusions
Herpesvirus*
Adenovirus
Varicella-zoster virus
Respiratory syncytial virus*

Cytoplasmic and nuclear inclusions
Cytomegalovirus
Measles virus*

*These inclusions may be associated with the formation of multinucleated giant cells.

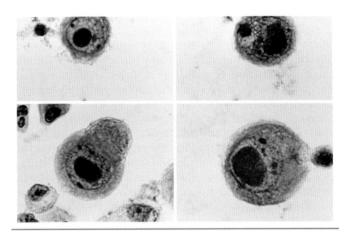

Figure 15-32   Cytomegalovirus (CMV). This composite image shows four cells with CMV viral cytopathic effect. The nuclei feature large, densely eosinophilic occlusions surrounded by a clear halo and rimmed with a thickened, focally beaded nuclear membrane. One cell shows a bulging granular cytoplasmic expansion that corresponds to cytoplasmic viral inclusions. (Pap)

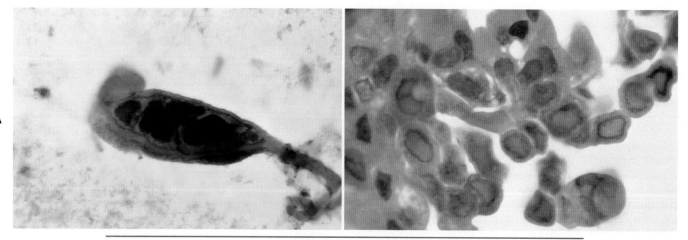

Figure 15-33 **Herpesvirus. A,** Each nucleus shows a dense inclusion and thickened nuclear membrane. These changes are typical of herpesvirus cytopathic effect; however, the gray slatelike appearance of the karyoplasm may be present without the inclusions noted in this example. (Pap) **B,** This bronchoscopic biopsy shows mucosal cells with the same viral cytopathic effect in a histologic preparation. (H&E) (From Stanley MW, Henry-Stanley MJ, Iber C. Bronchoalveolar lavage: cytology and clinical applications. New York: Igaku-Shoin; 1991.)

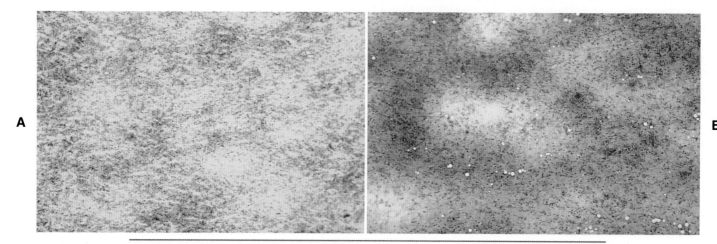

Figure 15-34 **Necrotizing granulomatous inflammation.** This granular necrotic material is typical of aspirates from tuberculous masses. However, positive stains or culture results are required for definitive diagnosis. (**A,** Pap; **B,** DQ)

most cytologic samples, including sputum and aspirates from tuberculous individuals, show the appropriate inflammatory pattern but contain few, if any identifiable organisms, even when special stains are applied. With FNA, much of the aspirated material consists of a characteristic, but not diagnostic granular precipitate that usually contains a few poorly preserved chronic inflammatory cells (Figure 15-34). In this setting, unless organisms are identified, the cytologic interpretation should be descriptive and note the presence or absence of granulomata, necrosis, and acute inflammation. The ultimate diagnosis rests on further evaluation in the microbiology laboratory. As noted in Box 15-2, cytologist involvement at the time of computed tomography (CT)–guided FNA can insure that appropriate cultures or other studies are instituted on a timely basis without the need for additional procedures.

When stains for acid-fast bacilli are considered, it is important to note that several types exist. The traditional Ziehl-Neelsen method is appropriate for *Mycobacterium tu-berculosis* but does not stain atypical mycobacteria that are much more weakly acid-fast. When such organisms are suspected, alternative techniques should be considered. The most common is the Fite stain. This method improves recognition of the atypical organisms by binding the dye to their lipid-rich capsules with peanut oil as a mordant. Furthermore, fluorescence stains for mycobacteria are now widely used in microbiology laboratories. These are rapid, simple to prepare, and easier to screen for rare organisms than traditional stains for acid-fast bacilli.

Patients thought to have *M. tuberculosis* but who have negative sputum cultures often undergo bronchoscopy. The ultimate diagnoses includes *M. tuberculosis*, other infectious processes, and malignancies. The yield of culture is higher for BAL than for bronchial washings or for postbronchoscopy sputum.

In many published studies, it is not possible to determine the extent to which reported yields for diagnosis of mycobacterial infections are based on cytology, including

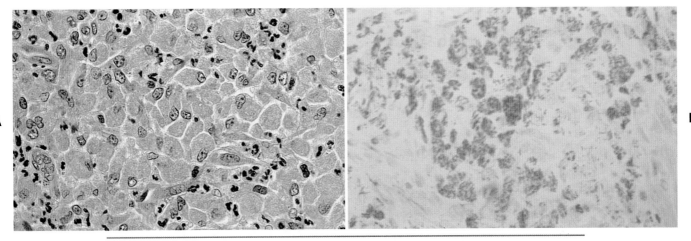

Figure 15-35 **Atypical mycobacterial infection of acquired immune deficiency syndrome (AIDS): histology. A,** This atypical mycobacterial infection in a patient with AIDS shows a sheetlike proliferation of large granular histiocytes interspersed with a few smaller chronic inflammatory cells. Well-formed granulomas are not present. (H&E) **B,** A special stain for acid fast bacilli demonstrates large numbers of these red-staining organisms within the cytoplasm of the enlarged histiocytes. (Fite)

cell block sections, with special stains or on culture. Mycobacteria can be associated with BAL lymphocytosis, but this finding is too nonspecific to be of diagnostic use.

Infection with atypical mycobacteria are common in AIDS and may disseminate widely in these patients. The associated impaired T-cell response leads to greatly reduced ability to form granulomata and to kill the organisms, despite a sometimes brisk histiocytic response. This results in a tissue pattern of a sheetlike histiocytic proliferation with few other inflammatory cells. The organisms may be numerous, filling the cytoplasm of histiocytes. Histologically, these cells show abundant granular eosinophilic cytoplasm, and stains for the organisms show enormous numbers of bacilli (Figure 15-35). This condition histologically resembles the granular cell infiltrations of Whipple's disease or Gaucher's disease.

Cytologic representation of this condition has been described in FNA of various sites, bone marrow aspirations, and BAL. Fixed slides show the histiocytes, but the presence of bacilli is difficult to discern. In air-dried material the large cells are filled with clear, nonstaining bacilli of the appropriate size. This imparts a Gaucher's cell-like appearance that is quite characteristic. During preparation of cytologic samples, some of the large, fragile cells are inevitably damaged. This releases naked nuclei, cytoplasmic debris, and large numbers of bacilli. The latter litter the smear and can be seen in the basophilic background staining typical of Romanowsky methods as clear negative images of bacilli (Figure 15-36). AIDS patients may harbor both *M. tuberculosis* and one or more atypical mycobacteria.

Other Infections

Strongyloides stercoralis, an intestinal nematode, is endemic in the southeastern United States and other parts of the world. Immunosuppressed patients are certainly at increased risk. Pulmonary involvement may result in hemoptysis, cough, and chest x-ray infiltrates and has been cytologically recognized in sputum and BAL (Figure 15-37).

Identification of the characteristic rhabditiform larvae is diagnostic.[36]

Serologic studies indicate that many healthy individuals harbor asymptomatic *Toxoplasmosis gondii* infections that may become activated during various types of immunosuppression, including AIDS. Acute infection through organ transplantation has also been described.[37] Numerous tissues can be involved, but the brain is the most common. Tissue involvement includes three forms: (1) bradyzoite-filled cysts measuring up to 200 μm in diameter, (2) free tachyzoites, and (3) parasitized host cells designated pseudocysts. Cytologic diagnosis of pulmonary involvement has been achieved with BAL, in which tachyzoites and pseudocysts but not true cysts have been described. The pseudocysts represent intracellular involvement of macrophages or neutrophils.[38]

Cytologic diagnosis of toxoplasmosis is difficult, unless one specifically seeks the organism, usually with high-magnification study. The small, crescent-shaped organisms are easily overlooked as cellular debris, especially at screening magnification. Furthermore, they are very pale in fixed material, whereas air-dried preparations highlight their shape, darkly staining nuclear material and overall basophilia (Figure 15-38). Diagnosis can also be accomplished by PCR, but careful study of cytologic material can sometimes achieve the same result quickly and at little cost.[39]

Cryptosporidium was originally described as a bovine diarrheal agent but has subsequently been identified in patients with AIDS and in occasional large community outbreaks associated with contamination of water supplies. Pulmonary involvement has been infrequently described in patients with AIDS. It is usually associated with intestinal disease but can be isolated. Cytologic diagnosis is rarely described and may be based on sputum and imprints of lung biopsy tissue. The organisms measure 4 to 6 μm and most closely resemble yeast or *P. carinii*. However, they are acid-fast and occasionally situated within the cytoplasm of macrophages. Romanowsky-stained preparations show tiny internal red granules.[40-42]

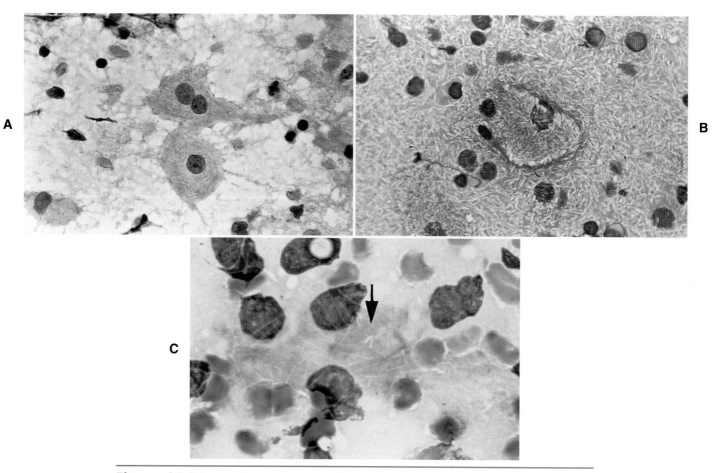

Figure 15-36   Atypical mycobacterial infection of AIDS: cytology. A, This Pap-stained preparation shows mostly macrophages with granular-appearing cytoplasm. Some nonspecific granular debris is in the background. The smudgy, damaged nuclei may represent macrophages damaged in the smearing processes. (Pap) **B,** The same material when stained by a rapid Romanowsky method shows that the granularity is actually large numbers of non-staining bacillary organisms. These fill the cytoplasm of a central macrophage, giving it a Gaucher cell–like appearance. They also litter the smear background. (DQ) **C,** This smear shows a cluster of macrophages. At the *arrow* a pair of nonstaining bacillary images is apparent. (DQ)

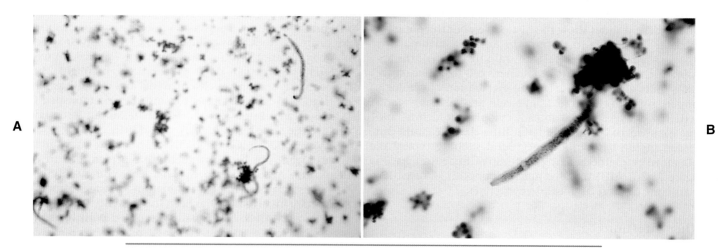

Figure 15-37   *Strongyloides.* A, This low-magnification image from a sputum sample shows a background of inflammatory cells. Scattered through this are several large larvae of *Strongyloides.* (Pap) **B,** This high-magnification image shows a typical rhabditiform larva in a background of inflammatory cells. (Pap) (From Stanley MW, Henry-Stanley MJ, Iber C. Bronchoalveolar lavage: cytology and clinical applications. New York: Igaku-Shoin; 1991.)

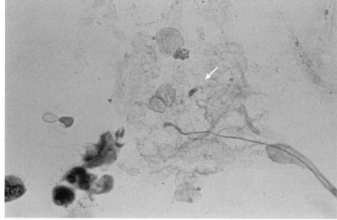

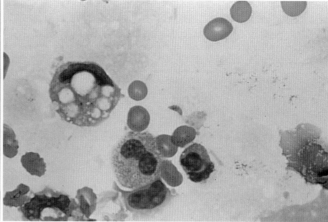

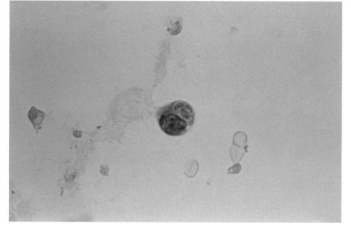

Figure 15-38 Toxoplasmosis. **A,** In fixed material the organisms are small and lightly cyanophilic and tend to blend in with background material so that high-magnification study is required for identification of this infection. (Pap) **B,** In air-dried material the organisms stain more darkly. Their basophilia, crescent shape, and densely staining nuclear material are characteristic. (DQ) **C,** This macrophage contains three spindle-shaped *Toxoplasma* organisms within its cytoplasm, thus representing a pseudocyst. (Pap)

 ## SPECIAL ISSUES RELATED TO BRONCHOALVEOLAR LAVAGE

BAL has the ability to sample deep pulmonary tissue by nonsurgical means and reflects conditions at levels otherwise far beyond the bronchoscopist's reach. Examination of changing immune effector cell content in samples representing various diseases has suggested that the method can help in the evaluation of inflammatory pulmonary disease. Thus, relative increases and decreases in a sample's content of neutrophils, eosinophils, lymphocytes, or macrophages are considered reflective of conditions in the air spaces and interstitium of deep lung tissue.

However, it is difficult to determine normal values. In the typical study, 40% to 60% of the instilled fluid is returned; it contains millions of cells, and macrophages predominate. Box 15-21 summarizes factors that alter the cellular yield, even in healthy volunteer controls. A previously published review of control series noted wide variation in all technical aspects and cellular yields of volunteer BALs (Table 15-12).[43] Interpretation of these highly variable data is further complicated by the fact that repeated lavage of the same lung segment in a given volunteer can show isolated increases in lymphocytes or neutrophils in the absence of lung disease.

When BAL is used to evaluate interstitial lung disease, it is reasonable to question the extent to which cells washed from the alveoli and small airways reflect immunologic events in the interstitium. Studies comparing BAL differential cell counts with cells obtained by disaggregation of lung biopsy tissue have shown contradictory results.[44] However,

 BOX 15-21

Factors Affecting the Cellular Yield of Bronchoalveolar Lavage in Healthy Controls

Patient factors
Smoking without chronic bronchitis yields more macrophages
Smoking with chronic bronchitis yields more neutrophils*

Procedural factors
Lung area studied†
Volume instilled (aliquot size and number of aliquots)

Preparatory factors
Separate processing of the first (bronchial) aliquot
Gauze filtration to remove mucus and bronchial cells
Cytocentrifugation causes selective loss of lymphocytes
Membrane filtration causes selective loss of neutrophils‡

*Mild to moderate BAL neutrophilia in these patients need not imply infection or interstitial fibrosis.
†Lavage of the lingula or the right middle lobe tends to give the most cellular samples.
‡This method of specimen concentration is no longer widely used.

a correlation is suggested by the fact that, at least in sarcoidosis patients, the most significantly abnormal cell counts occur when areas of greatest radiographic abnormality are lavaged. A recirculation of these cells between the interstitium and the air space has been postulated.

TABLE 15-12
Cellular Yields of Bronchoalveolar Lavage in Healthy Controls

	Total Instilled Lavage Volume	Total Cells Recovered × 10⁶	Macrophages	Lymphocytes	Neutrophils	Eosinophils
Low value	100 ml	1.9	78.3%	3.2%	0.4%	0.1%
High value	540 ml	64.3	95.6%	18.0%	11.2%	0.2%

From Stanley MW, Henry-Stanley MJ, Iber C. Bronchoalveolar lavage: cytology and clinical applications. New York: Igaku-Shoin; 1991. pp. 50-57.

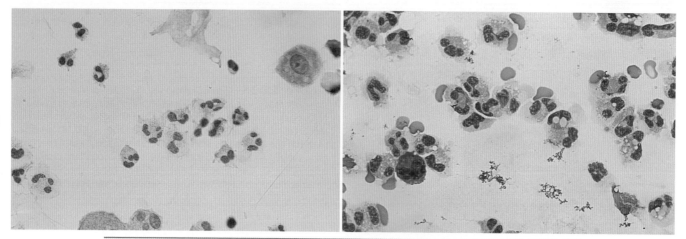

Figure 15-39 Eosinophilic pneumonia. Both images feature occasional macrophages and large numbers of eosinophils with their characteristic bilobed nuclei. (**A,** Pap; **B,** DQ)

Many of the interstitial lung diseases share a progression from an early alveolitis stage to a later fibrotic stage. In BAL samples this is associated with a shift from lymphocyte predominance to increased numbers of neutrophils. Examples include idiopathic pulmonary fibrosis and sarcoidosis. Other conditions typically show lymphocytosis (i.e., hypersensitivity pneumonitis, berylliosis, disseminated tuberculosis), whereas neutrophilia predominates in some settings such as Langerhans cell histiocytosis and bronchiolitis obliterans-organizing pneumonia.

The foregoing data on cell counts suggest that BAL cytology may form part of the total diagnostic pattern in some of these conditions. However, great overlap and variability exist and a given cellular pattern does not justify sweeping diagnostic conclusions. It is also inadvisable to emphasize changes in a patient's cytologic finding in the assessment of disease progression from alveolitis to fibrosis.

Despite its limited use in the chronic interstitial lung diseases, BAL continues to enjoy a role in the evaluation of acute and chronic eosinophilic pneumonias. Many cases show lavage fluid eosinophilia as high as 40% that decreases rapidly with steroid therapy[45] (Figure 15-39).

Active sarcoidosis may show a BAL lymphocytosis with predominantly helper T-cells.[43] This is in contrast with hypersensitivity pneumonitis in which a majority of the lymphocytes are T-suppressor cells. The major role of BAL in patients thought to have sarcoidosis is in excluding infectious disorders from the differential diagnosis.

BOX 15-22
Conditions Associated with the Histologic Pattern of Pulmonary Alveolar Proteinosis

Cytomegalovirus infections
Mycobacterial infections
Other infections
Hematologic malignancies
Massive acute silica exposure (acute silicoproteinosis)
Acquired immunodeficiency syndrome
Other immunodeficiency states
Idiopathic pulmonary alveolar proteinosis

Pulmonary Alveolar Proteinosis

The histologic pattern of pulmonary alveolar proteinosis (PAP) represents a particular response to lung injury in the conditions summarized in Box 15-22. In the setting of immunosuppression, these patients are often thought to have an infection. This picture is complicated by the fact that once a diagnosis of PAP of any etiologic factor is established, the patient is at risk for a variety of secondary infections.

BAL yields a characteristic milky-appearing sample. Cytologically, it shows granular proteinaceous precipitate that is usually sparsely cellular, with scattered macrophages[46] (Fig-

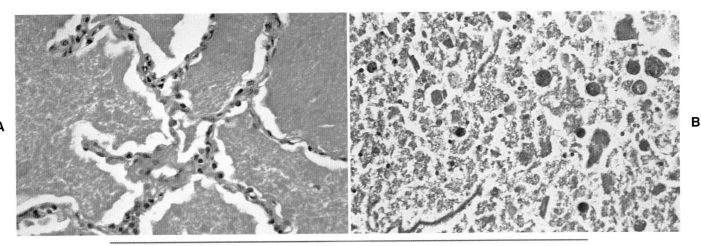

Figure 15-40 **Pulmonary alveolar proteinosis. A,** Histologically, the alveolar septal architecture remains intact. The air spaces are filled with a granular eosinophilic material. (H&E) **B,** In bronchoalveolar lavage samples, pulmonary alveolar proteinosis shows the cyanophilic to eosinophilic granular material depicted in this image. Most such samples are sparsely cellular with occasional macrophages. (Pap)

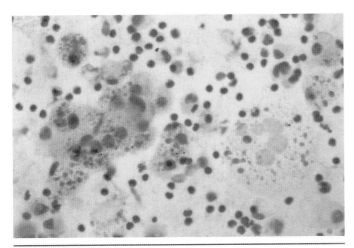

Figure 15-41 **Aspiration pneumonia.** This bronchoalveolar lavage sample from a patient with clinically suspected aspiration shows a background of acute inflammatory cells. Most of the macrophages contain abundant red-staining neutral lipid consistent with this clinical picture. (Oil-Red-O [ORO])

BOX 15-23

Conditions Associated with Pulmonary Hemosiderosis

Congestive heart failure*†
Mitral valve disease*
Smoking
Goodpasture's syndrome
Other types of glomerulonephritis
Chemotherapy
Radiation therapy
Vasculitis
Diffuse alveolar damage
Trauma
Pulmonary venous hypertension
Idiopathic pulmonary hemosiderosis

---

*Usually lower macrophage hemosiderin content than other conditions in this box.
†Clinically distinguished from occult pulmonary hemorrhage by a rapid response to diuretics.

---

ure 15-40). In some instances, it may be necessary to distinguish this material from the exudate of *P. carinii*. Careful attention to the details of pneumocystis and judicious use of silver stains usually suffice. Electron microscopy may also be helpful.[47]

Whole lung lavage remains the treatment of choice for PAP, and often achieves dramatic improvements in lung function.[48]

Exogenous Lipid Pneumonia

Many patients thought to have aspiration pneumonia have histories of previous aspirations, upper gastrointestinal difficulties, or neurologic impairments. In the absence of these findings, the radiographic features of aspiration pneumonia can mimic those of an infection or malignancy.

The cytologic finding of foamy macrophages is nonspecific. It has been suggested that ORO-positive material within the cytoplasm of macrophage supports a clinical impression of aspiration (Figure 15-41). Those who advocate use of this method count 100 macrophages and grade the ORO staining intensity from 0 to 4+, to generate a score between 0 and 400. Aspirators tend to have scores from 100 to 300. However, similar levels are noted in numerous other types of pulmonary disease, so this test is limited in diagnostic use.[49] This test may be most useful in neonates.[50] Those wishing to use this method must apply the stain to air-dried slides. Fixation removes stainable neutral lipids so that ORO staining is always negative.

Pulmonary Hemorrhage

Many BAL samples show some hemosiderin within the cytoplasm of macrophages, and this can be prominent in numerous clinical conditions (Box 15-23). Hemosiderin can be highlighted and quantitated using both an iron stain and the same semiquantitative approach described previously for evaluation of stainable lipids.

This approach is most commonly used in an effort to distinguish occult pulmonary hemorrhage (OPH) from infectious processes in immunocompromised patients. Results have been variable, but overall correlation of semiquantitative iron studies with coagulation profiles, and the patients' ultimate diagnosis has been poor.[51] In the proper clinical setting, including rapidly evolving chest x-ray abnormalities, large macrophage hemosiderin burdens are suggestive but not diagnostic of OPH. If BAL findings can be used to lower the likelihood of an infection, the probability of OPH may be higher.

Lung Transplantation

The most common use of BAL in lung or heart-lung transplant recipients is infection diagnosis or surveillance. The primary differential diagnosis is rejection. Once infections have been excluded, the cellular content of the lavagate

suggests certain findings (Table 15-13). However, the correlation of BAL findings with rejection as assessed by multiple transbronchial biopsies is poor, and universal agreement now exists that the latter method is essential for diagnosis of rejection.[52,53]

Ohori noted atypical cells in posttransplant BALs in association with harvest injury (i.e., diffuse alveolar damage or acute lung injury, as was previously discussed in this chapter), acute cellular rejection, and infections.[54] Many of the abnormal cells closely resembled the hyperplastic type II pneumocytes discussed earlier in this chapter. Clinical correlation is essential in distinguishing atypical cells in these conditions from those of a non–small cell carcinoma.

Amiodarone Pulmonary Toxicity

Hepatic and pulmonary toxicity sometimes limits use of the antiarrhythmic drug amiodarone and may be associated with a variety of other side effects. Pulmonary toxicity can manifest with local or diffuse x-ray infiltrates and fever in a manner that mimics an infectious condition. The histologic manifestations of pulmonary toxicity include interstitial fibrosis, interstitial lymphocytes, increased airspace and interstitial macrophages, type II pneumocyte hyperplasia, and bronchiolitis obliterans.

BAL yields large numbers of macrophages. At the light microscopic level, these are floridly vacuolated because of the presence of numerous clear inclusions that are not ORO positive (Figure 15-42). However, such inclusions are typical of patients on the drug but do not represent a manifestation of toxicity and do not correlate with clinical or radiographic evidence of toxicity. Biopsy demonstration of interstitial fibrosis and inflammation is required for assessment of actual lung damage. Given the clinical presentation cited above, exclusion of an infectious condition is usually BAL's most important role.[55,56]

When studied ultrastructurally, many types of cells, including type II pneumocytes, macrophages, lymphocytes, and numerous nonpulmonary tissues are found to contain large numbers of membrane bound inclusions. These are filled with osmiophilic laminated membrane whorls that mimic myelin figures and are typical of all patients on the drug, presumably as a result of widespread phospholipase inhibition (Figure 15-43).

TABLE	15-13
Conditions Associated with Bronchoalveolar Lavage Findings in Lung or Heart-Lung Transplant Recipients	

BAL Finding	Possible Clinical Association(s)
Neutrophilia	Early posttransplant period (3 months)
	Bacterial pneumonia or other infection
Lymphocytosis	Long-term posttransplant
Combined lymphocytosis and neutrophilia	Obliterative bronchiolitis (chronic rejection)
Lymphocytosis with decreased CD4/CD8 ratio	Acute rejection
	Viral pneumonia
	Chronic rejection with obliterative bronchiolitis

BAL, Bronchoalveolar lavage.

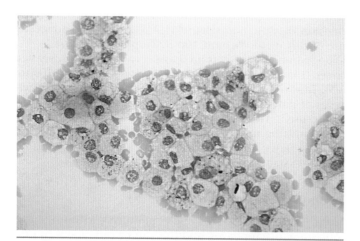

Figure 15-42 Amiodarone effect. Bronchoalveolar lavage findings in patients taking the antiarrhythmic drug amiodarone include large numbers of highly vacuolated macrophages. (DQ)

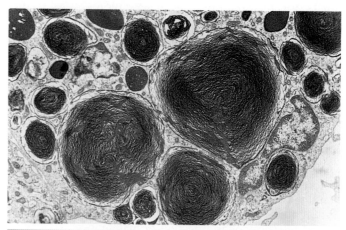

Figure 15-43 Amiodarone effect: ultrastructure. Macrophages show large numbers of membrane-bound inclusions. These are filled with membranous whorls and resemble myelin figures.

References

1. Rankin JA, Naegel GP, Reynolds HY. Use of a central laboratory for analysis of bronchoalveolar lavage fluid. Am Rev Respir Dis 1986; 133:186-190.
2. Chamberlain DW, Braude AC, Rebuck AS. A critical evaluation of bronchoalveolar lavage: criteria for identifying unsatisfactory specimens. Acta Cytol 1987; 31:599-605.
3. Churg AM, Warnock ML. Asbestos and other ferruginous bodies: their formation and clinical significance. Am J Pathol 1981; 102:447-456.
4. Roggli VL, Greenberg SD, McLarty JW, et al. Comparison of sputum and lung asbestos body counts in former asbestos workers. Am Rev Respir Dis 1980; 122:941-945.
5. Radio SJ, Rennard S, Ghafouri MA, et al. Cytomorphology of *Alternaria* in bronchoalveolar lavage specimens. Acta Cytol 1987; 31:243-248.
6. Ness MJ, Rennard SL, Vaughn WP, et al. Detection of *Candida* antigen in bronchoalveolar lavage fluid. Acta Cytol 1988; 32:347-352.
7. Stanley MW, Henry-Stanley MJ, Gajl-Peczalska KJ, et al. Hyperplasia of type II pneumocytes in acute lung injury: cytologic findings of sequential bronchoalveolar lavage. Am J Clin Pathol 1992; 97:669-677.
8. Stanley MW, Mrak RE, Bardales RH. Detached single cilia: another potential pseudomicrobe seen in bronchoalveolar lavage specimens. Diagn Cytopathol 1995; 8:225-228.
9. Wazir JF, Macrorie SG, Coleman DV. Evaluation of the sensitivity, specificity, and predictive value of monoclonal antibody 3F6 for the detection of *Pneumocystis carinii* pneumonia in bronchoalveolar lavage specimens and induced sputum. Cytopathology 1994; 5:82-89.
10. Leibovitz E, Pollack H, Moore T, et al. Comparison of PCR and standard cytological staining for detection of *Pneumocystitis carinii* from respiratory specimens from patients with or at high risk for infection by human immunodeficiency virus. J Clin Microbiol 1995; 33:3004-3007.
11. Tuncer S, Erguven S, Kocagoz S, et al. Comparison of cytochemical staining, immunofluorescence and PCR for diagnosis of *Pneumocystitis carinii* on sputum samples. Scand J Infect Dis 1998; 30:125-128.
12. Naryshkin S, Daniels J, Freno E, et al. Cytology of treated and minimal *Pneumocystis carinii* pneumonia and a pitfall of the Grocott methenamine silver stain. Diagn Cytopathol 1991; 7:41-47.
13. Metersky ML, Aslenzadeh J, Stelmach P. A comparison of induced and expectorated sputum for the diagnosis of *Pneumocystitis carinii* pneumonia. Chest 1998; 113:1443-1445.
14. Rocha P, Awe RJ, Guy ES, et al. A rapid and inexpensive method for processing induced sputum for detection of *Pneumocystis carinii*. Am J Clin Pathol 1996; 105:52-57.
15. Saito H, Anaissie EJ, Morice RC, et al. Bronchoalveolar lavage in the diagnosis of pulmonary infiltrates in patients with acute leukemia. Chest 1998; 94:745-749.
16. Linder J, Vaughn WO, Armitage JO, et al. Cytopathology of opportunistic infections in bronchoalveolar lavage. Am J Clin Pathol 1987; 88:421-428.
17. Stanley MW, Davies S, Deike M. Pulmonary aspergillosis: an unusual cytologic presentation. Diagn Cytopathol 1992; 8:585-589.
18. Kahn FW, Jones JM, England DM. The role of bronchoalveolar lavage in the diagnosis of invasive pulmonary aspergillosis. Am J Clin Pathol 1986; 86:518-523.
19. Fischler DF, Hall GS, Gordon S, et al. *Aspergillus* in cytology specimens: a review of 45 specimens from 36 patients. Diagn Cytopathol 1997; 16:26-30.
20. Stanley MW, Deike M, Knoedler J, et al. Diagnosis of pulmonary aspergillomas by fine needle aspiration. Diagn Cytopathol 1992; 8:577-579.
21. Rath PM, Oeffelke R, Muller KD, et al. Non-value of *Aspergillus* antigen detection in bronchoalveolar lavage fluids of patients undergoing bone marrow transplantation. Mycoses 1996; 39:367-370.
22. Skladney H, Buchheidt D, Baust C, et al. Specific detection of *Aspergillus* species in blood and bronchoalveolar lavage samples of immunocompromised patients by two-step PCR. J Clin Microbiol 1999; 37:3865-3871.
23. Lemos LB, Baliga M, Taylor BD, et al. Bronchoalveolar lavage for diagnosis of fungal disease. Five years' experience in a southern United States rural area with many blastomycosis cases. Acta Cytol 1995; 30:1101-1111.
24. DiTomasso JP, Ampel NM, Sobonya RE, et al. Bronchoscopic diagnosis of pulmonary coccidioidomycosis: comparison of cytology, culture, and transbronchial biopsy. Diagn Microbiol Infect Dis 1994; 18:83-87.
25. Maesaki S, Kohno S, Mashimoto H, et al. Detection of *Cryptococcus neoformans* in bronchial lavage cytology: report of four cases. Intern Med 1995; 34:54-57.
26. Kralovic SM, Rhodes JC. Utility of routine testing of bronchoalveolar lavage fluid for cryptococcal antigen. J Clin Microbiol 1998; 36:3088-3089.
27. Watts JC. Infection by capsule-deficiency cryptococci. Arch Pathol Lab Med 1987; 111:688.
28. Mousa AA, Russo K, Wilkinson EJ. Pulmonary mucormycosis diagnosed by bronchoalveolar lavage: a case report and review of the literature. Pediatr Pulmonol 1997; 23:222-225.
29. Cooper CR, McGinnis MR. Pathology of *Penicillium marneffai*: an emerging acquired immunodeficiency syndrome-related pathogen. Arch Pathol Lab Med 1997; 121:798-804.
30. Sirisanthana T. Infection due to *Penicillium marneffei*. Ann Acad Med 1997; 26:701-704.
31. McShane H, Tang CM, Conlon CP. Disseminated *Penicillium marneffei* infection presenting as a right upper lobe mass in an HIV positive patient. Thorax 1998; 53:905-906.
32. Solans EP, Yong S, Husain AN, et al. Bronchioloalveolar lavage in the diagnosis of CMV pneumonitis in lung transplant recipients: an immunocytochemical study. Diagn Cytopathol 1997; 16:350-352.
33. Fajac A, Stephan F, Ibrahim A. Value of cytomegalovirus detection by PCR in bronchoalveolar lavage routinely performed in asymptomatic bone marrow recipients. Bone Marrow Transplant 1997; 20:581-585.
34. Bedrossian CW, De Arce EA, Bedrossian UK, et al. Herpetic tracheobronchitis detected at bronchoscopy: cytologic diagnosis by the immunoperoxidase method. Diagn Cytopathol 1985; 1:292-299.
35. Bayon MN, Drut R. Cytologic diagnosis of adenovirus bronchopneumonia. Acta Cytol 1991; 35:181-182.
36. Sidoni A, Polidori GA, Alberti PF, et al. Fatal *Strongyloides stercoralis* hyperinfection diagnosed by Papanicolaou-stained sputum smears. Pathologica 1994; 86:87-90.
37. Jacobs R, Depierreux M, Goldman M, et al. Role of bronchoalveolar lavage in diagnosis of disseminated toxoplasmosis. Rev Infect Dis 1991; 13:637-641.
38. Bretagne S, Costa JM, Fleury-Feith J, et al. Quantitative competitive PCR with bronchoalveolar lavage fluid for diagnosis of toxoplasmosis in AIDS patients. J Clin Microbiol 1995; 33:1662-1664.
39. Wheeler RR, Bardales RH, North PE, et al. Toxoplasma pneumonia: cytologic diagnosis by bronchoalveolar lavage. Diagn Cytopathol 1994; 11:52-55.
40. Meynard JL, Meyohas MC, Binet D, et al. Pulmonary cryptosporidiosis in the acquired immunodeficiency syndrome. Infection 1996; 24:328-331.
41. Pellicelli AM, Palmieri F, Spinazzola F, et al. Pulmonary cryptosporidiosis in patients with acquired immunodeficiency syndrome. Minerva Medica 1998; 89:173-175.

42. Ma P, Villanueva TG, Kaufman D, et al. Respiratory cryptosporidiosis in the acquired immunodeficiency syndrome. JAMA 1984; 252:1298-1301.

43. Stanley MW, Henry-Stanley MJ, Iber C. Bronchoalveolar lavage: cytology and clinical applications. New York: Igaku-Shoin; 1991. pp.50-57.

44. Nagata N, Takayama K, Nikaido Y, et al. Comparison of alveolar septal inflammation to bronchoalveolar lavage in interstitial lung diseases. Respiration 1996; 63:94-99.

45. DeJaegher P, Demedts M. Bronchoalveolar lavage in eosinophilic pneumonia before and during corticosteroid therapy. Am Rev Respir Dis 1984; 129:631-632.

46. Claypool WD, Rogers RM, Matuschak GM. Update on the clinical diagnosis, management and pathogenesis of pulmonary alveolar proteinosis. Chest 1984; 85:550-558.

47. Burkhalter A, Silverman JF, Hopkins MBIII, et al. Bronchoalveolar lavage cytology in pulmonary alveolar proteinosis. Am J Clin Pathol 1996; 106:504-510.

48. Prakash UBS, Barham SS, Carpenter HA, et al. Pulmonary alveolar phospholipoproteinosis: experience with 34 cases and a review. Mayo Clin Proc 1987; 62:499-518.

49. Knauer-Fischer S, Ratjen F. Lipid-laden macrophages in bronchoalveolar lavage fluid as a marker for pulmonary aspiration. Pediatr Pulmonol 1999; 27:419-422.

50. Collins KA, Geisinger KR, Wagner PH, et al. The cytologic evaluation of lipid-laiden alveolar macrophages as an indicator of aspiration pneumonia in young children. Arch Pathol Lab Med 1995; 119:229-231.

51. Kim CC, Saleba K, Baughman RP, et al. Iron staining on bronchoalveolar lavage smears for detecting occult pulmonary hemorrhage: Is it reliable? Acta Cytol 1989; 33:716.

52. Ward C, Snell GI, Zheng L, et al. Endobronchial biopsy and bronchoalveolar lavage in stable lung transplant recipients and chronic rejection. Am J Respir Crit Care Med 1998; 158:84-91.

53. Tiroke AH, Bewig B, Haverich A. Bronchoalveolar lavage in lung transplantation: state of the art. Clin Transplant 1999; 13:131-157.

54. Ohori NP. Epithelial cell atypica in bronchoalveolar lavage specimens from lung transplant recipients. Am J Clin Pathol 1999; 112:204-210.

55. Fraire AE, Guntupalli KK, Greenberg SD, et al. Amiodarone pulmonary toxicity: a multidisciplinary review of current status. South Med J 1993; 86:67-77.

56. Coudert B, Bailly F, Lombard JN, et al. Amiodarone pneumonitis: bronchoalveolar lavage findings in 15 patients and review of the literature. Chest 1992; 102:1005-1012.

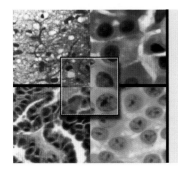

CHAPTER
16

Localized Lung Diseases

As noted in Chapter 15, a wide range of sampling methods is available for evaluation pulmonary pathology. The specific uses, limitations, and adequacy criteria for these methods have been discussed. Whereas Chapter 15 concentrated on disorders that are most commonly diffuse, with special emphasis on infectious conditions, this chapter addresses localized diseases of the lungs. Box 16-1 provides a summary of the lesions to be considered and organizes the current chapter into neoplastic and nonneoplastic conditions.

No classification of pulmonary disorders is perfect. The traditional textbooks' strict division between neoplastic and nonneoplastic conditions has been eschewed in favor of initially categorizing lesions as diffuse and localized. Each of these categories in turn contain both neoplastic and nonneoplastic conditions. Furthermore, some diseases can show either pattern; Box 16-2 summarizes some conditions that may be either localized or diffuse.

The reason for this distinction is partially clinical. The physician's approach to a lung mass is often different from that taken with patients who present with diffuse pulmonary abnormalities. The latter group is more likely to present with pulmonary symptoms, whereas many individuals with even advanced tumefactive lung conditions are asymptomatic. When incidentally discovered, a solitary lung nodule is often referred to as a *coin lesion*, reflecting its appearance on chest radiographs. The clinical differential diagnosis includes all of the entities in Box 16-3.

All cytologic sampling methods are applicable to localized pulmonary disorders. Sputum studies are often diagnostic when lung carcinoma is considered. However, three to five samples collected over several days may be required for confident diagnosis. In the current medical environment fine-needle aspiration (FNA) often provides a much more rapid and thus ultimately less expensive means of diagnosis. This can include staging by aspiration of suspected sites of metastasis, such as transcarinal lymph node FNA. Bronchoalveolar lavage (BAL) can be used for evaluation of localized lesions but is often reserved for diffuse disorders. Pulmonary artery sampling was discussed in Chapter 15 and is used exclusively for study of suspected lymphangitic carcinomatosis.

When FNA is considered, it is important to recall that the aspirating needle may pick up bits of tissue from any layer through which it passes en route to the target lesion. In the case of lung aspiration, this includes squamous cells from the skin, adipose tissue, skeletal muscle, mesothelial cells, pleural fluid components, bone, bone marrow, cartilage, pulmonary macrophages, and bronchial epithelial cells. Many of these were discussed in the previous chapter. Adipose tissue may be represented by either cohesive tissue particles with well-preserved cells or by round, clear spaces in the smear. The latter represent spilled lipid that has washed off the smear during processing through organic solvents.

If bone and cartilage are artifactually introduced to a lung sample, the radiologist performing the aspiration is usually able to inform the laboratory that the procedure was difficult. Usually, the mass has been inconveniently situated, and the needle may have contacted a rib. The presence of bone, cartilage, and adipose tissue are most misleading when a cytologic diagnosis of pulmonary hamartoma is considered.

NONNEOPLASTIC LOCALIZED DISORDERS

Noninfectious Conditions

Pulmonary Hamartoma

Hamartomas of the lung can be solitary or multiple and are more common in males. When discovered on chest radiograph, they present the usual clinical differential diagnosis of a *coin lesion* (see Box 16-3). Histologically, hamartomas consist mostly of mesenchymal tissues, and show various combination cartilage, adipose tissue, and smooth muscle. Bone is less common. Bronchial epithelium–lined clefts divide the mass into lobules. When delicate calcifications are seen on chest x-ray, they may have a characteristic lacy pattern that reflects this lobular architecture.

The only cytologic sampling method applicable to hamartomas of the lung is FNA[1] (Box 16-4). Based on the previous discussion of tissues that may be incidentally introduced into an FNA sample, it is clear that the mere presence of cartilage, adipose tissue (or clear circular spaces), or normal-appearing bronchial cells may not be sufficient for diagnosis. The most dependable finding is not well-formed

BOX   16-1

Localized Diseases of the Lung

Nonneoplastic
Noninfectious localized diseases
Hamartoma
Pulmonary infarct
Localized radiation fibrosis
Rounded atelectasis
Benign intrabronchial papillomas (transitional, squamous,
    glandular, or mixed)
Hematoma
Endometriosis
*Infectious localized diseases**
Cavitary pneumocystis†
Granulomas†
Mycetomas†
Lung abscess†
Malakoplakia
Parasitic nodules
Uncommon nonneoplastic localized diseases not unique
to the lung
Amyloidoma
Inflammatory myofibroblastic pseudotumor†
Rheumatoid nodules†
Whipple's disease†
Wegener's granulomatosis

Neoplastic
Carcinoma
Squamous cell carcinoma
• In situ
• Well differentiated
• Moderately differentiated
• Poorly differentiated
• Variants (see text)
Adenocarcinoma
• Acinar
• Papillary
• Solid
• Variants (see text)
Bronchioloalveolar carcinoma (BAC)‡ and related adenomas
• Mucinous BAC
• Nonmucinous BAC
• Sclerotic BAC
Large cell undifferentiated carcinoma
• Not otherwise specified (NOS)
• Variants (see text)

Neuroendocrine carcinoma
• Grade 1 (classical carcinoid tumor)
Peripheral spindle cell carcinoid tumor
• Grade 2 (atypical carcinoid tumor)
• Grade 3, small cell type (small cell anaplastic carcinoma)
• Grade 3, large cell type (large cell neuroendocrine
    carcinoma)
• Grade 3, mixed small and large cell types
• Carcinomas identifiable as squamous, glandular or undif-
    ferentiated, but showing neuroendocrine features by elec-
    tron microscopy or immunohistochemistry
Other mixed carcinomas showing more than one histologic
        type, including those with a neuroendocrine component
Rare pulmonary neoplasms
Sclerosing hemangioma
Clear cell ("sugar") tumor
Carcinosarcoma
Pulmonary blastoma
Fetal adenocarcinoma
Pleuropulmonary blastomas of children
Uncommon neoplasms not unique to the lung
Salivary gland-type tumors†
• Mucoepidermoid carcinoma
• Adenoid cystic carcinoma
• Others
Paraganglioma†
Granular cell tumor†
Malignant melanoma as a primary tumor†
Thymoma†
Meningioma†
Teratoma†
Intrapulmonary examples of solitary fibrous tumor†
Sarcomas of various types†
Metastatic tumors
Carcinoma
Sarcoma
Malignant melanoma
Systemic hematopoietic malignancies that may involve
the lung
Malignant lymphoma
Multiple myeloma
Leukemia

*Many of these may also be diffuse and are discussed in the previous chapter.
†The cytology of these lesions is more fully addressed in other chapters.
‡May also be diffuse (pneumonic).

cartilage but a mesenchymal matrix material resembling that seen in pleomorphic adenomas of the parotid gland. This sparsely cellular material is fibrillary and contains a few scattered, benign, spindled or stellate mesenchymal cells. It is lightly cyanophilic in Pap-stained smears and brightly metachromatic with Romanowsky methods (Figure 16-1).

If pulmonary hamartoma can be confidently recognized in an FNA sample, it is safe to forego surgical excision. In

this setting, most clinicians follow the mass radiographical-ly; its size should be stable over time.

Pulmonary Infarct
In most cases, clinical findings lead to a correct diagnosis of pulmonary infarct and cytologic samples are not obtained. However, these lesions rarely present as targets for FNA,[2] and their effects may also be encountered in sputum sam-

BOX 16-2

Pulmonary Disorders that May Be Either Localized or Diffuse

Nonneoplastic disorders
Pneumocystis carinii infections
Various fungal infections
Bacterial infections
Mycobacterial infections
Amyloidosis

Neoplastic disorders
Adenocarcinoma: localized mass or masses vs. lymphangitic carcinomatosis
Bronchioloalveolar carcinoma
Malignant lymphoma
Leukemic involvement

BOX 16-3

Pulmonary Disorders that May Present Radiographically as Incidental 'Coin' Lesions

Nonneoplastic disorders
Hamartoma
Granuloma
Pulmonary abscess
Other infectious processes
Pulmonary infarct

Neoplastic disorders
Benign neoplasm
Primary malignancy
Metastatic malignancy

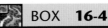

BOX 16-4

Cytomorphologic Features of Pulmonary Hamartoma

Fine-needle aspiration findings that are characteristic but not diagnostic
Adipose tissue
Round droplets of dissolved lipid
Cartilage
Bone (rarely)
Benign bronchial cells

Diagnostic fine-needle aspiration findings
Fibrillary metachromatic matrix resembling that seen in pleomorphic adenoma of the salivary glands

ples. The specimen shows a background of necrosis with macrophages containing varying amounts of hemosiderin and anthracotic pigment. Squamous metaplastic cells may be present and can show the nuclear features of repair.

If the age of the lesion is such that regeneration has supervened, one may also encounter reactive type II pneumocytes. The cytology and clinical associations of these cells were discussed in Chapter 15. If not recognized, they may lead to an incorrect diagnosis of malignancy, especially when set in a background of necrotic debris. As in other types of lung injury, their shedding is transient and should not persist more than a few weeks after the event.

Localized Radiation Fibrosis
This sequela of radiation therapy is much less common than more diffuse types of injury and has not been described in cytologic samples. Dense fibrosis would be expected to yield a sparsely cellular specimen that would probably be interpreted as nondiagnostic or even unsatisfactory. However, the histology of these lesions tells us that type II pneumocytes with reactive alterations might be obtained. In the clinical setting of a pulmonary mass in a pa-

tient who has undergone radiation therapy for treatment of a malignancy, the danger of a false-positive diagnosis could be great. Caution is in order when one encounters an atypical but sparsely cellular sample from an upper lobe lesion in a cancer patient with a history of radiation.

Rounded Atelectasis
This type of partial lung collapse presents radiographically as a pleural-based lower lobe mass that may be several centimeters in diameter. In most instances, the nidus for lung collapse appears to be an area of pleural fibrosis. In some instances, asbestos has been implicated as the ultimate pathogenesis. When the radiographic findings are not specific, FNA may be attempted. In the experience of Miller and colleagues, the sample shows pulmonary macrophages and fragments of collagenous connective tissue. Although clearly nonspecific, this combination might be useful in carefully selected cases.[3]

Intrabronchial Papillomas
In contrast with human papillomavirus (HPV)–associated laryngotracheal papillomatosis, which affects mostly children, intrabronchial papillomas are seen primarily in adults. Their epithelium may be transitional (nasal-like), squamous, glandular, or mixed.[4] These lesions are rare, and their cytologic manifestations have not been described. One might expect their cellular features to be those of the lesion's surface and not representative of the entire mass.

Histologically, reactive cytologic alterations and squamous dysplasias are common. Furthermore, carcinomas in situ and invasive malignancies may arise in papillomas. Correlation with the bronchoscopic findings indicates the presence of a papillary lesion, but precise classification should await surgical excision of the entire lesion. The authors have seen one example in which a bronchial brushing was interpreted as keratinizing squamous cell carcinoma (SCC). The excised mass showed surface keratosis and atypia, but no invasive carcinoma.

Hematoma
These may cause a radiographic picture that suggests a pulmonary neoplasm. Often, a history of trauma leads to the correct diagnosis, and cytologic sampling is not necessary.

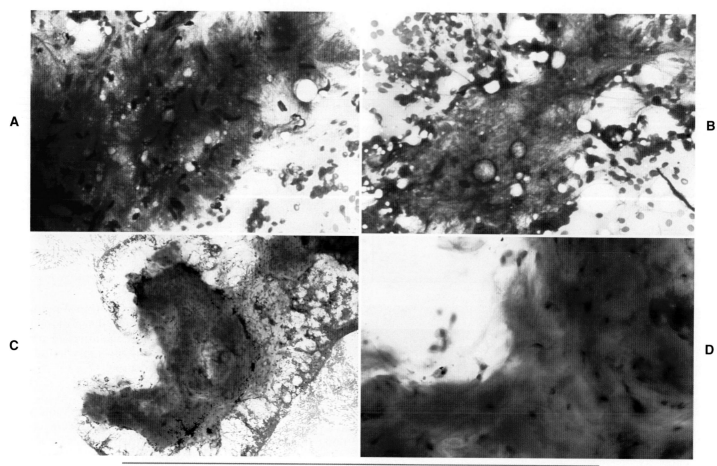

Figure 16-1 Pulmonary hamartoma. **A** and **B,** This fibrillary metachromatic matrix material that strongly resembles that of a salivary gland pleomorphic adenoma was aspirated from a small peripheral lung nodule and is diagnostic of a hamartoma. (Diff-Quik [DQ]) **C** and **D,** With the Pap stain, this material has a much more cartilaginous appearance. At higher magnification, its fibrillary structure is apparent. (Papanicolaou [Pap])

Endometriosis

The cytology of endometriosis has been described in body cavity fluids, cervicovaginal smears, urine, and FNA of various sites,[5] but publication of the first cytologic description of pulmonary involvement is pending. Sheets and clusters of small, darkly staining cells are characteristic. In some instances, both stromal and glandular cells are identified. Hemosiderin-filled macrophages are expected but may be absent.

Infectious Conditions

Box 16-1 lists several infectious disorders that may present as localized pulmonary lesions. With the exception of blastomycosis, most are more commonly diffuse and are discussed in Chapter 15. In either case, cytologic diagnosis is based on the morphologic features of the individual organisms or cytopathic effects. These are supplemented by various cultures and other tests.

Malakoplakia

Malakoplakia represents a characteristic tissue pattern in the face of an inability to kill certain types of gram-negative bacilli. Sheets of histiocytes with scattered Michaelis-Gutmann bodies are typical. The latter are laminated spheres that stain positively for calcium and iron. Electron microscopic studies show large numbers of intracytoplasmic bacilli.

This condition rarely involves the lung but can be seen in patients with or without a clear history of immunosuppression, including those with acquired immune deficiency syndrome (AIDS). It presents as an upper lobe mass that may be single or multiple and may cavitate. Such lesions can be mistaken for primary or metastatic malignancy.[6] FNA yields large numbers of foamy histiocytes. Taken alone, these are nondiagnostic, but, in the case reported by Lambert and colleagues, Michaelis-Gutman bodies were numerous, leading to the correct diagnosis.[7]

Uncommon Nonneoplastic Conditions Not Unique to the Lungs

Amyloidoma

Isolated pulmonary amyloidosis occurs primarily in either a nodular or diffuse (tracheobronchial) form. Nodular disease is often multifocal and may be bilateral. Chest radiographs usually show one or more masses that may remain stable in size for long periods of time. Most are subpleural, and larger lesions may cavitate. Dundore and colleagues indicate that nonsurgical follow-up is usually safe, once amyloidoma has been diagnosed by FNA.[8]

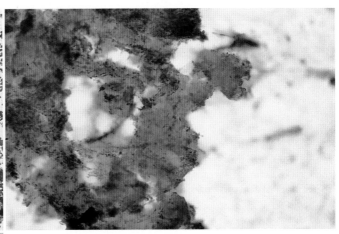

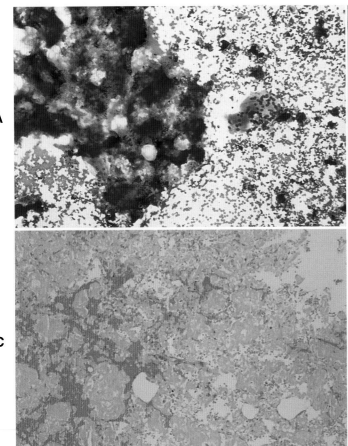

Figure 16-2 **Amyloidoma. A,** This intermediate magnification image shows large sparsely cellular fragments of amyloid in a fine-needle aspiration (FNA). A multinucleated giant cell is a common part of this type of mass. (DQ) **B,** When fixed and stained by Pap, amyloid shows this dense hyaline appearance and is essentially acellular. (Pap) **C,** Cell block sections from this FNA of an amyloidoma show the characteristic eosinophilic fluffy material. Such preparations can be used for various special stains as needed. (Hematoxylin and eosin [H&E])

Amyloid has a characteristic cytologic appearance (Figure 16-2). In Romanowsky-stained samples, it is metachromatic. Variable numbers of lymphocytes, plasma cells and foreign body-type giant cells usually accompany amyloid deposits.

Wegener's Granulomatosis

A number of clinical criteria for diagnosis of Wegener's granulomatosis (WG) have been advanced (Box 16-5). Many patients show several of these clinical features, whereas a minority present with only pulmonary hemorrhage. Furthermore, diagnosis and prognosis are currently supplemented strongly by assessment of cytoplasmic antineutrophil cytoplasmic autoantibodies (c-ANCA).

Few cases have been studied by FNA. The histologic and expected cytologic features are contrasted in Table 16-1.[9] The paired arrangement of morphologic features highlights the difficulty in reaching this diagnosis without histologic material in any but the most clinically unambiguous cases. Only in such instances, with strong supporting evidence from the clinical laboratory, does the suggestion of Kaneishi and colleagues that "The open lung biopsy . . . can be effectively replaced by FNA . . ." seem justified.[9] Once thought to be a more specific marker for WG, capillaritis has been described in a number of other conditions.[10]

In most instances the cytologic findings in WG suggest an infectious process and cultures should be instituted. Pulmonary involvement often includes multiple nodules that may simulate metastatic carcinoma. The danger of in-

TABLE 16-1

Histologic and Corresponding Cytologic Features of Wegener's Granulomatosis

Histologic Findings	Expected Corresponding Cytologic Feature
Vasculitis of muscular arteries*	Nonspecific mixed inflammation
Granulomatous vasculitis Giant cells Lymphocytes and histiocytes Eccentric arterial wall involvement	Nonspecific mixed inflammation
Confluent zones of liquefactive necrosis	Necrosis
surrounded by palisading histiocytes	Nonspecific mixed inflammation
Organizing pneumonia	Nonspecific mixed inflammation
Capillaritis†	Nonspecific mixed inflammation
Hemorrhage	Hemorrhage

*Elastic stains must often be applied to histologic sections, if this critical feature is not to be overlooked.
†This finding may be seen in several other clinical entities that are characterized by pulmonary hemorrhage. Histologically, the alveolar septa show hemorrhage, neutrophilic infiltrates, and nuclear dust.

BOX 16-5

Clinical Findings in Wegener's Granulomatosis

Pulmonary disease
Radiographic infiltrates with nodularity or cavities
Hemoptysis

Renal disease
Red blood cell (RBC) casts in the urine sediment
Free RBCs in the urine sediment

Upper aerodigestive tract disease
Oral ulcers
Nasal discharge

Multisystem
Granulomatous inflammation

appropriate diagnoses of malignancy may be heightened when highly reactive type II pneumocytes of the type discussed in the previous chapter are encountered.

NEOPLASTIC LOCALIZED DISORDERS

Carcinoma

A review of medical textbooks written early in the twentieth century indicates that carcinomas of the lung were rarely encountered at that time. The decades-long increase in incidence has been blamed on a variety of industrialization's chemicals, including asbestos and application of tar to roads. Although a link certainly exists between pulmonary carcinoma and some of these substances, the greatest statistical association is with smoking.

Many lung carcinomas are asymptomatic or masquerade as pneumonias until they reach a high stage; approximately 60% are incurable at presentation. Efforts at early detection have been based on chest radiographs and sputum cytology, often in patients at increased risk. To date, none of these programs has been successful, and all have proven to be costly.

All the sampling methods described in the previous chapter can be applied diagnosis of lung carcinoma, with the exception of pulmonary artery blood examination. Indeed, diagnosis of these neoplasms was the impetus for development of these methods. In most settings, FNA guided by tomographic scans or fluoroscopy is more common than examination of either sputum or bronchoscopic samples. Nonguided FNA can be used in some exceptional circumstances. The authors have used this method on several occasions in which a lung tumor presented with palpable chest wall mass or diffuse hepatic metastases. This type of approach provides both diagnostic and staging information in an extremely rapid fashion. Overall, transthoracic FNA has a higher diagnostic yield than bronchoscopic sampling.

Squamous Cell Carcinoma

At least some SCCs are associated with intraepithelial dysplasia or carcinoma in-situ and pass through a minimally invasive phase.[11] At one end of the cytologic spectrum are the cells described as atypical squamous metaplasia in Chapter 15. These can be seen in reactive conditions, but if persistent, may suggest a preneoplastic epithelial alteration. The degree to which persistent squamous cell atypia places an individual at increased risk for subsequent development of pulmonary carcinoma is unknown. At the other end of the cytologic spectrum are small round cells with a high nuclear to cytoplasmic (N:C) ratio, keratinized cytoplasm, and nuclear hyperchromasia. When interpreted as carcinoma in situ, some of these can be localized for resection by selective brushing of different large bronchi.[12]

Sputum cytology is the only type of investigation that could be reasonably applied to at-risk, but asymptomatic and radiographically normal patients. It can detect SCCs that are radiographically occult.[13] In one study, evaluation of 4000 male smokers over age 45 yielded seven examples of in situ or early invasive SCC.[11] Some evidence shows quantitative morphology might improve classification of abnormal cells during early tumor development.[14] In the current medical environment, it is not likely that this type of investigation will continue, and early detection will remain an unattainable goal. Intervention in the terrible and increasing toll taken by lung cancer will depend largely on smoking prevention and cessation efforts.

Most invasive SCCs are centrally located, but a significant minority are peripheral or, rarely, subpleural. Many of the peripherally located tumors are upper lobe masses with a tendency for cavitation. SCC often has a significant exophytic endobronchial component that leads to obstruction. Patients often present with an associated pneumonia. This area of infection may obscure the tumor on chest radiographs, or at least make its true size difficult to determine. Cavitation may be detected on chest x-rays. Even when extensive necrosis develops, detectable calcification is rarely noted.

SCC is classified as well, moderately, or poorly differentiated based on the extent to which the tumor cells resemble normal mature squamous cells. The most differentiated examples produce cells with keratinized cytoplasm that is sufficiently voluminous to yield a low N:C ratio. Intercellular bridges are not prominent in cytologic preparations but may be easily detected in paraffin-embedded cell blocks or other histologic material (Figure 16-3). When abundant, keratin is orangeophilic in Pap-stained material and dark blue in Romanowsky-stained preparations. Evidence of cytoplasmic maturation is more subtle in moderately differentiated examples, and, in the poorly differentiated tumors, only a few keratinized cells or intercellular bridges are identified. Box 16-6 summarizes cytologic features that indicate various levels of keratin production.

SCC that is exclusively well differentiated is less common in the lung than in head and neck sites. This observation has obvious implications for a patient found to have metastatic well differentiated SCC in FNA of a cervical lymph node. In most instances, a lung tumor is moderately differentiated with clear evidence of keratin production and some foci of highly differentiated orangeophilic cells. This may also be useful to consider when evaluating a presumed pulmonary metastasis from a primary laryngeal carcinoma.

SCC often grows in a somewhat laminated fashion. Deeper layers near the underlying stroma consist of small, clearly malignant cells with little cytoplasm. These shed

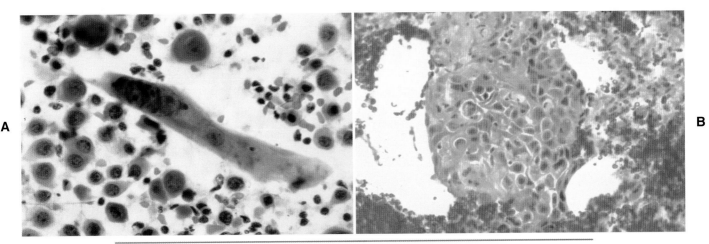

Figure 16-3 **Squamous cell carcinoma (SCC). A,** This carcinoma shows a large number of malignant cells. The large spindle-shaped cell has enough cytoplasm to make the overall nuclear cytoplasmic ratio low. The nucleus shows a combination of malignant and degenerative features with extremely coarse chromatin clumping and hyperchromasia. The smaller cells in the background also represent SCC. Each features a hyperchromatic nucleus and a small rim of cytoplasm. Squamous differentiation is manifest in the density of the cytoplasm and its very sharp cell borders. (Pap) **B,** This cell block preparation shows the typical histologic appearance of such neoplasms. These cells show extremely dense eosinophilic cytoplasm. Most cells are surrounded by a clear halo, and at higher magnification, intercellular bridges can be detected. (H&E)

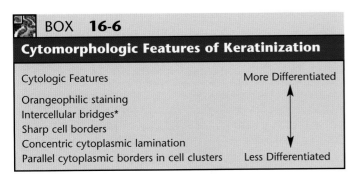

BOX **16-6**

Cytomorphologic Features of Keratinization

Cytologic Features	More Differentiated
Orangeophilic staining	↑
Intercellular bridges*	
Sharp cell borders	
Concentric cytoplasmic lamination	↓
Parallel cytoplasmic borders in cell clusters	Less Differentiated

*Best seen in cell blocks or other histologic preparations.

singly, in flat sheets, or in three-dimensional clusters. The nuclei are densely hyperchromatic but in well-preserved cells show a coarse chromatin substructure. These immature, basal-type cells show little evidence of cytoplasmic keratinization and, taken alone, resemble any other poorly differentiated non–small cell pulmonary carcinoma. In most examples, these cells are accompanied by larger, more mature cells with obvious keratinization of the type described in Box 16-6. In this laminated growth, these cells occupy more superficial layers that are further removed from the underlying stroma. These cells most often shed singly and can be visually striking, with large size, bizarre shapes and extreme orangeophilia (Figure 16-4). Table 16-2 summarizes the cytologic features of this type of carcinoma.

Some cell clusters show features intermediate between the basaloid and mature cells just described. The cytoplasm is moderate in volume and dense but usually not orangeophilic. The cells' cytoplasmic borders are sharp and distinct. When the cytoplasmic interface between cells is examined, intercellular bridges in cytologic preparations are usually not appreciated. However, evidence of keratinization can be seen in thin linear clearings between cells, as their cytoplasmic borders run parallel to one another. In many such cell clusters, some cells show a tendency toward spindling. This feature is good evidence of squamous differentiation.

A cytologic sample that contains only well-differentiated, albeit abnormal, squamous cells should be regarded with caution. Even cells with markedly abnormal shapes and dense, "India-ink spot" nuclear staining may be encountered in reactive conditions, as noted in Chapter 15. Nuclear hyperchromasia can also be a feature of degeneration, and, taken alone, does not justify a diagnosis of malignancy (Figure 16-5).

The most common difficulty in SCC diagnosis is a pattern of mature, highly keratinized cells that may be very abundant but do not show definite nuclear features of malignancy and are not associated with the smaller malignant cells described above. This problem is more common in sputum or bronchoscopy samples that may only address the tumor's more differentiated endobronchial surface. If good sampling is achieved, most FNAs are diagnostic. One must search through the large keratinized cells for occasional clusters of smaller, dark malignant cells.

Another difficulty in diagnosis of SCC is its common association with inflammatory cells. Some tumors, especially those that cavitate, can have overwhelming acute inflammation to the extent that they are mistaken for abscesses. The descriptive term *malignant abscess* has been applied to these cases and helps us keep this difficulty in mind (Figure 16-6). In other instances, keratin leads to an intense foreign body reaction. The histiocytic giant cells may lead to an erroneous diagnosis of a granulomatous lesion. This seems to be a natural error, in view of the atypical squamous metaplasia that can accompany fungal or mycobacterial infections (see Chapter 15).

The most common differential diagnostic considerations for SCC are the reactive alterations and metaplasias discussed in the preceding chapter. Cytologic diagnosis of SCC is further complicated by recognition of several variants

A   **B**

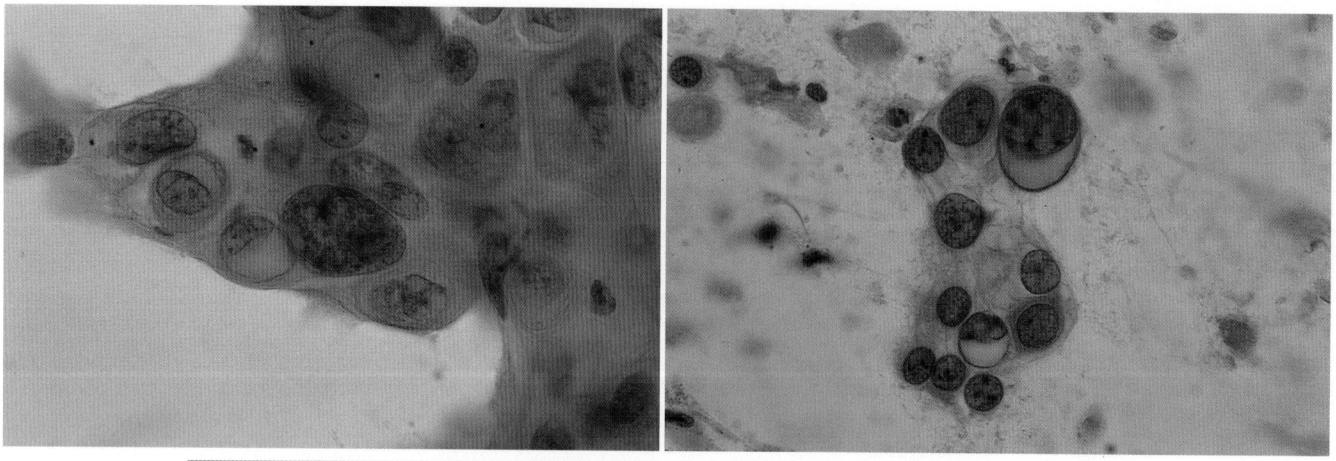

Figure 16-4 SCC. This illustrates the laminar pattern of growth with less differentiated cells in layers closer to the underlying stroma and more differentiated squamous cells in upper layers. **A,** These well-differentiated cells show hyperchromatic nuclei with prominent chromatin clumping. Their cytoplasm is dense and often shows the sharp cell borders that reflect keratin production. Occasional cells show clear cell change resulting from cytoplasmic glycogen deposition. **B,** These cells from the same SCC represent the less mature portion of the tumor. They are small with scant cytoplasm and coarsely clumped chromatin. Without features of squamous differentiation elsewhere in the preparation, these cells have no distinguishing features that would allow this carcinoma to be classified as anything but *large cell undifferentiated.* In the smear background, several rounded cyanophilic droplets represent necrotic tumor cells. (Pap)

TABLE **16-2**	CMF

Cytomorphologic Features of Well-Differentiated to Moderately Differentiated Squamous Cell Carcinoma

Immature Basal-Type Cells	More Mature Superficial Cells
Nuclear features	
Small	Variable size with some very large
Round to oval	Abnormal and bizarre shapes
Hyperchromatic	Densely hyperchromatic (India ink)
Chromatin dense or coarsely granular	May show smudgy chromatin
Cytoplasmic features	
Scant	Moderate to abundant
Cyanophilic	Orangeophilic
Borders may be indistinct (syncytial)	Dense ± concentric laminations
	Sharp borders
Cell shape	
Round to oval	Some are polygonal
	Bizarre cell shapes common

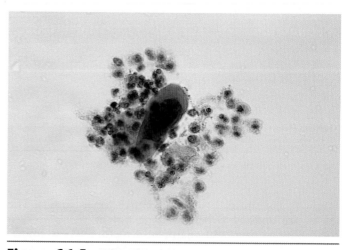

Figure 16-5 SCC. This sputum sample shows intense background inflammation and rare cells with "India-ink spot" nuclei. Squamous differentiation is manifested by extremely dense cytoplasm with sharp borders. Cells of this nature without better preserved cells showing malignant nuclear features are insufficient for an unequivocal diagnosis of carcinoma. This is especially true if these cells are present in low numbers. (Pap)

(Box 16-7). Each of these is uncommon, and few examples have been studied in cytologic samples.

First described as a tumor of the upper aerodigestive tract, basaloid SCC (B-SCC) of the lung has been recognized as an aggressive lesion, with a prognosis intermediate between those of small cell anaplastic carcinoma (SCAC; grade 3 neuroendocrine carcinoma, small cell type) and the non–small cell lung carcinomas. When case series are considered, this tumor tends to blend with fairly pure basal cell carcinomas and mixed tumors with basaloid and more prominent squamous differentiation.

Histologically, B-SCC consists of small uniform cells with hyperchromatic nuclei and inconspicuous nucleoli. These tend to be arranged in nests with peripheral nuclear palisading and do not show intercellular bridges.[15] A high mitotic rate has been described. In concert with the typical architectural and nuclear features, this finding is thought to

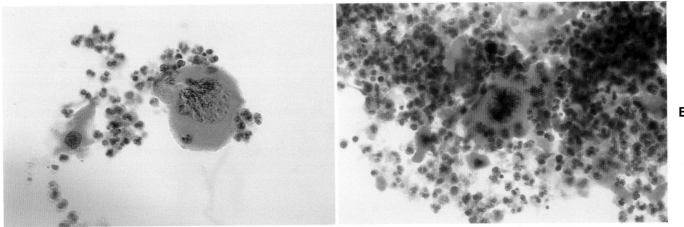

Figure 16-6   SCC. **A** and **B,** These abnormally shaped squamous cells with large nuclei, coarse chromatin clumping, and dense cytoplasm are set in a background of intense inflammation. This picture has been called *malignant abscess* and most often originates in a cavitary SCC. (Pap)

BOX   16-7

Uncommon Variants of Squamous Cell Carcinoma

Basaloid squamous cell carcinoma (B-SCC)
Small cell squamous cell carcinoma (SCC)
Spindle cell (sarcomatoid) SCC
Clear cell SCC
Endobronchial papillary SCC
Acantholytic SCC
Pseudovascular acantholytic SCC

---

be useful in separating B-SCC from poorly differentiated SCC and to maintain the integrity of this prognostically significant distinction.

The most serious differential diagnostic distinction is between B-SCC and SCAC.[16] In histologic preparations the most useful feature is abrupt formation of centrally located keratin whorls in some cell nests of B-SCC. This is unaccompanied by the single cell keratinization that can be expected in some poorly differentiated, but not basaloid, SCCs. Furthermore, SCAC can be identified by either immunohistochemical or ultrastructural evidence of neuroendocrine differentiation. This is lacking in B-SCC, although occasional cases may show minor ultrastructural evidence of glandular or squamous differentiation. Vesoulis warns that metastatic B-SCC from nonpulmonary sites can be mistaken for primary pulmonary SCAC.[17]

The small cell variant of SCC is another rare poorly differentiated form of this neoplasm.[18] Distinction from SCAC is difficult without immunohistochemical or ultrastructural demonstration of squamous features (well-developed desmosomes and tonofilaments) or neuroendocrine differentiation.

Given the relatively common diagnosis of SCAC in cytologic material with minimal or no histologic sampling and the striking similarity between this tumor and the much less common B-SCC and small cell SCC, it seems reasonable to suggest that most cases of B-SCC and small cell SCC are

mistaken for and then treated like SCAC. This rather pessimistic assessment suggests that the understanding of this tumor's cytologic and clinical features will advance only slowly.

Pulmonary carcinomas with a prominent spindle cell component are appropriately termed *sarcomatoid*. Depending on an institution's patient referral patterns, these are found to be less common than metastatic sarcomas to the lung but not nearly so rare as true pulmonary sarcomas. Many sarcomatoid carcinomas can be recognized as epithelial when foci of typical lung carcinoma are identified (Figure 16-7). These are most commonly squamous but may also be adenocarcinoma, undifferentiated large cell carcinoma, or mixtures of more than one type.[19] Immunohistochemical or ultrastructural evidence of epithelial (usually squamous) differentiation may be required for definitive diagnosis.[20]

Cytologically, sarcomatoid SCC may yield a cellular aspirate featuring spindle cells with neural, smooth muscle, or fibrous-appearing cellular features. The degree of nuclear atypia can vary widely within and between cases. Paraffin-embedded cell blocks are useful for immunostains. Furthermore, the features of squamous differentiation for which one performs ultrastructural examination often survive routine processing in paraffin so that electron microscopy can be performed using this material, if necessary.

Clear cell change is less common in SCC than in adenocarcinoma. In SCC, it is usually the result of glycogen deposition but unequivocal evidence of keratin production by tumor cells leads to the correct interpretation.

Some endobronchial papillary lesions harbor SCC that can be either in situ or invasive, as discussed previously in this chapter.

Histologically, SCC in many sites may rarely show central acantholysis in tumor cell nests. The resulting pattern resembles adenocarcinoma, in that rounded cell nests are lined by malignant cells and appear to have a central lumen. The cytology of such tumors features markedly discohesive cells with intermediate levels of cytoplasmic keratinization (sharp cell borders and lamination; see Box 16-6). This picture is most common when cervical lymph nodes with metastatic SCC from head and neck sites are aspirated but can be encountered in pulmonary material.

When the desmoplastic stroma between cell nests compresses the epithelial elements to thin strands, the tumor can acquire a pseudoangiomatous configuration. The cytology of one such case has been reported by Smith and colleagues.[21] Many of the aspirated tumor cell clusters showed an acinar configuration suggestive of adenocarcinoma. These authors

noted that the epithelial nature of the tumor was more apparent in cytologic than in histologic material.

Adenocarcinoma

Adenocarcinoma has shown an increasing prevalence in recent years, and in some parts of the world, it has become the most common type of primary lung carcinoma. Approximately two thirds of pulmonary adenocarcinoma are

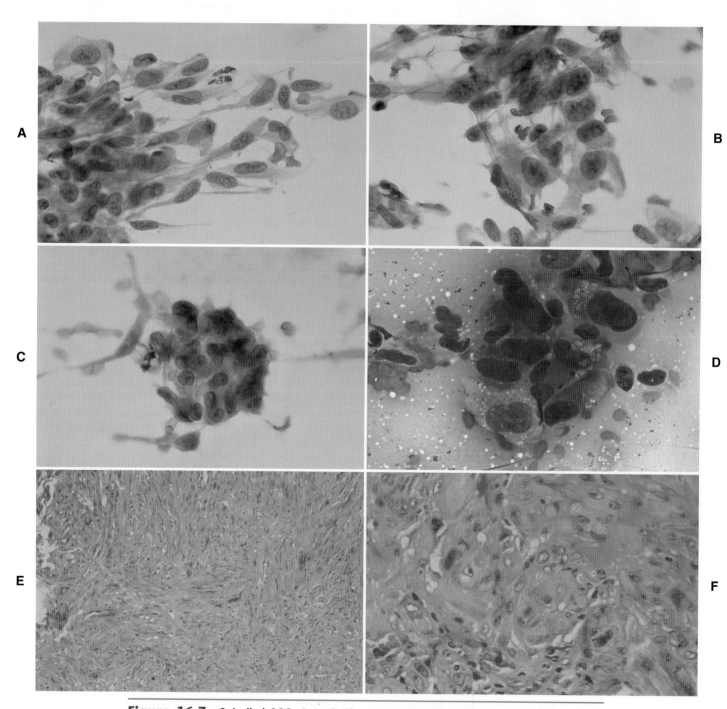

Figure 16-7   Spindled SCC. **A** to **C,** The progression through Figure 16-7, *A, B,* and *C* shows cell groups that range from purely spindled to partially polygonal to very carcinoma-like. (Pap) **D,** In the Romanowsky-stained material the cells appear more rounded and more suggestive of carcinoma than a sarcoma. (DQ) **E,** This low-magnification image shows the histology of this sarcomatoid SCC. Much of the tumor has this spindled appearance with scattered, very large hyperchromatic nuclei. (H&E) **F,** The SCC nature of this tumor is shown in poorly differentiated foci of polygonal cells such as those illustrated in this image. (H&E)

peripherally located and many of these involve the pleura. Such tumors are usually beyond the bronchoscopist's reach but can be detected in sputum or FNAs and in BAL samples. Rare examples shed copiously into the pleural space and may radiographically and cytologically suggest a diagnosis of epithelial malignant mesothelioma. Cavitation is rare in adenocarcinoma. As summarized in Table 16-3, adenocarcinoma is often associated with lung scarring but is not unique in this regard.[23]

The existence of a recognizable precursor to adenocarcinoma has been debated, and no consensus has emerged. Many cases show various degrees of hyperplasia and atypia of bronchial cells in the surrounding air spaces.[22] Given the obligatory retrospective nature of these investigations and the fact that these lesions are not amenable to cytologic sampling with subsequent follow-up, it remains difficult to demonstrate the type of relationship that exists for invasive and in situ SCC. Perhaps future molecular investigations will shed greater light on the early stages of adenocarcinoma.

Pulmonary adenocarcinoma is defined by growth as acini or papillae and by mucin production. As summarized in Box 16-8, tumors can be classified as acinar, papillary, or solid, based on the degree to which this morphologic definition is satisfied. The most differentiated examples resemble the sclerosing variant of bronchioloalveolar carcinoma. The least differentiated may show minimal evidence of

gland formation, and mucin production must be carefully sought. These factors and a host of uncommon variants indicate that pulmonary adenocarcinoma has a broad spectrum of cytologic characteristics.

The cytologic features of adenocarcinoma reflect the well, moderate, and poorly differentiated categories just outlined. They are much less successful in reproducing the architecturally based histologic categorizations of acinar, papillary, or solid growth. Box 16-9 summarizes the expected findings in moderately differentiated (and thus at least partially acinar or papillary) pulmonary AC (Figure 16-8). Some of the most important differential diagnostic problems are described in Table 16-4.

It can sometimes be difficult to distinguish a primary pulmonary adenocarcinoma from a metastatic lesion. In general, metastases tend to be multiple, whereas primary carcinomas tend to be solitary, but frequent exceptions occur. Furthermore, the lung is one of those sites from which an adenocarcinoma can lead to metastases while the primary tumor is still occult. (Others include the stomach, pancreas, and prostate.) With the exception of colonic carcinomas, metastatic adenocarcinomas usually have few, if any, specific morphologic features that point to a primary site. Historical considerations are important in these circumstances. For example, few breast carcinomas give rise to metastases before the primary tumor is detected. Immunohistochemistry can be useful. For example, an adenocarcinoma positive for hormone receptors and gross cystic disease fluid protein 15 (AP-15) usually represents metastatic breast carcinoma. AP-15 positivity can also be seen in sweat gland carcinomas, but these are not likely to be confused with breast carcinoma on clinical grounds.

Recent advances in immunohistochemistry allow us to use staining patterns with antibodies specific for cytokeratin 7 and cytokeratin 20 to determine possible sites of ori-

TABLE **16-3**	
Association of Lung Carcinomas with Scarring	
Tumor Type	**Percentage Associated with Scarring (%)**
Adenocarcinoma	72
Squamous cell carcinoma	18
Large cell undifferentiated carcinoma	10
Neuroendocrine carcinoma	0

Data from Auerbach O, Garfinkel L, Parks VR. Scar cancer of the lung: increase over a 21-year period. Cancer 1979; 43:636-642.

BOX **16-8**

Spectrum of Differentiation in Pulmonary Adenocarcinomas

Cytologic Features	More Differentiated
Highly organized growth resembling BAC	↑
Prominent acinar pattern	
Papillary growth	
Solid tumor with mucin production	
Poorly differentiated tumors that converge on the appearance of undifferentiated large cell carcinoma but have mucin production	↓
	Less Differentiated

BAC, Bronchioloalveolar carcinoma.

BOX **16-9** CMF

Cytomorphologic Features of Moderately Differentiated Pulmonary Adenocarcinoma

Cell arrangements
Single cells
Flat sheets
Three-dimensional clusters

Cytoplasmic features
Sharp cell borders are absent
Most cell borders are ill-defined with peripheral fragmentation or degeneration
Vacuoles may be present

Nuclear features
Lobulated or folded shape
Often hypochromatic
Distinct chromatin clumping and clearing
The dark nuclei of squamous cell carcinoma are not seen in the absence of degeneration
Macronucleoli
Irregular nucleolar shape

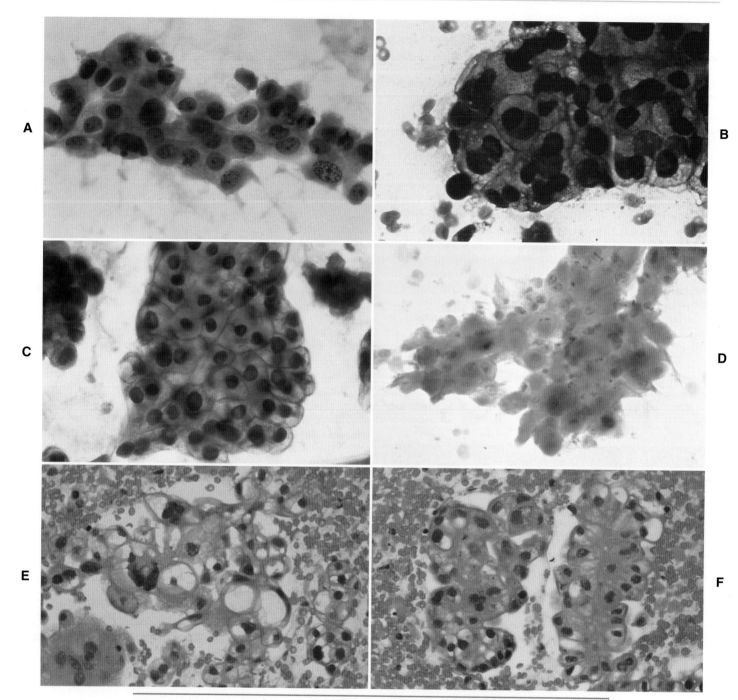

Figure 16-8 **Adenocarcinoma.** **A,** This neoplasm shows mostly flat sheets of cells. The nuclei are more pale and show less advanced chromatin clumping than is seen in SCC. The cytoplasm lacks the sharp cell borders of SCC and is much softer in appearance. (Pap) **B** and **C,** This adenocarcinoma shows a striking degree of cytoplasmic clear cell change. (**B,** DQ; **C,** Pap) **D,** This cell sheet from an aspiration smear shows that numerous cells contain a voluminous cytoplasmic droplet of mucin. (Mucicarmine [Mucin]) **E,** This cell block section from an FNA shows clear cell change similar to that noted in the smear material of Figure 16-8, *B* and *C.* (H&E) **F,** The papillary architecture of this adenocarcinoma is apparent in this cell block section from aspiration material. (H&E)

gin for a metastatic adenocarcinoma. These results are summarized in Table 16-5.[24] Positive staining for thyroid transcription factor (TTF-1) also indicates a pulmonary primary.

Box 16-10 summarizes the variants of adenocarcinoma. Each of these is rare, and most have not been described in the cytology literature. Virtually any site that can give rise to an adenocarcinoma will, on occasion, produce a tumor

with signet ring feature. Hayashi and colleagues indicated that a combination of mucin histochemistry and immunohistochemistry can be used to distinguish primary pulmonary signet ring adenocarcinoma from those examples metastatic from the gastrointestinal tract.[25]

In the vast majority of cases, a malignancy characterized by signet ring cytology is an adenocarcinoma. However, as one forms a differential diagnosis for a complex or clinically

TABLE 16-4

Differential Diagnostic Problems in Pulmonary Adenocarcinoma

Cytologic Finding	Differential Diagnostic Problem	Diagnostic Clues
Cytoplasmic eosinophilia due to degeneration	Squamous cell carcinoma (SCC)	Adenocarcinoma lacks: • Sharp cell borders • Cytoplasmic laminations • Orangeophilia • Spindled cell shapes
Nuclear pallor with minimal chromatin abnormalities	Repair atypia or other reactive conditions	Other features in Box 16-9, including single abnormal cells
Poorly differentiated cells	Poorly differentiated SCC	Adenocarcinoma lacks: • Sharp cell borders • Cytoplasmic laminations • Orangeophilia • Spindled cell shapes • India-ink spot nuclei Other features in Box 16-9
Viral inclusions mimicking large nucleoli	False-negative interpretation	Viral inclusions may feature: • Surrounding halo • Beaded chromatin • Marginated chromatin • Thickened nuclear membrane
Reactive type II pneumocytes	False-positive interpretation	This difficult problem was discussed in the previous chapter. Clinical findings may clarify the situation more than any amount of investigation at the microscope.
Adenocarcinoma cells identified correctly	Primary vs. metastatic adenocarcinoma	Clinical factors Immunohistochemistry (see text)

TABLE 16-5

Sites of Origin for Metastatic Adenocarcinomas Based on Staining for Cytokeratins 7 and 20

	Cytokeratin 7 Positive	Cytokeratin 7 Negative
Cytokeratin 20 positive	Pancreas Ovary, mucinous Transitional cell	Colon Rectum
Cytokeratin 20 negative	Lung* Breast Ovary, nonmucinous Endometrium Mesothelioma	Hepatocellular carcinoma Renal cell carcinoma Prostate

*This pattern describes pulmonary adenocarcinomas. Squamous cell carcinomas and small cell anaplastic carcinomas are usually negative for both cytokeratins 7 and 20.

BOX 16-10

Uncommon Variants of Pulmonary Adenocarcinoma

Signet ring adenocarcinoma
Mucinous adenocarcinoma
Enteric adenocarcinoma
Hepatoid adenocarcinoma
Clear cell adenocarcinoma
Choriocarcinomatous adenocarcinoma
Spindle cell (sarcomatoid) adenocarcinoma

atypical case, it is important to remember that occasional examples of malignant melanoma,[26] or even malignant lymphoma,[27] show such cells. Furthermore, malignant melanoma can show extensive stromal myxoid material that can be mistaken for mucin, leading to an erroneous diagnosis of adenocarcinoma.[28] Tsang and colleagues indicated that most examples of signet ring malignant melanoma occur as metastatic or recurrent lesions so that attention to clinical history helps avoid an incorrect interpretation. The case that they describe also showed melanin pigment, and the excised tumor was immunohistochemically positive for S-100 protein and HMB-45.

Distinctions between adenocarcinomas, some bronchioloalveolar carcinomas, and the tumors variously designated as mucinous (colloid) carcinoma or mucinous cystic lesions (benign, borderline, and malignant) are not well defined at this time.[29-31] Tumors in the latter group are rare. Generally, they are categorized on the basis of morphologic features similar to those used for mucinous neoplasms of the ovary or appendix. Examples with cytologically banal lining cells or even with microscopic foci of adenocarcinoma and mucinous dissection of surrounding tissues rarely recur and have not been reported to metastasize. One can anticipate that such tumors would present considerable difficulty in cytologic samples. The presence of abundant mucus with a few epithelial cells and histiocytes would be likely to suggest a pneumonia or bronchiectasis. Careful consideration of radiographic findings and strong assurance that the sampling needle has been accurately placed would be helpful but not diagnostic.

Metastatic carcinoma from the gastrointestinal tract is overwhelmingly more common than primary pulmonary carcinoma with enteric differentiation.[32] Hepatoid pulmonary carcinoma (large cell carcinoma with hepatoid differentiation) shares production of alpha-fetoprotein with its counterpart in the liver. Nasu and colleagues also detected des-gamma-carboxy prothrombin in the serum of the patient they reported and in the tumor cells by immunohistochemistry.[33]

Combined adenocarcinoma with choriocarcinoma, as well as human chorionic gonadotrophin (hCG) producing giant cell carcinomas have been previously reported.[34] Both these entities and primary pulmonary choriocarcinoma give readily detectable serum levels of hCG. Ikura and colleagues found that both are hemorrhagic tumors with rapidly fatal clinical progression. They suggest that distinction is difficult and probably irrelevant clinically.[35]

Clear cell carcinoma has not been described as a distinct entity in pulmonary cytology. This change is probably a nonspecific manifestation that can be the result of glycogen in SCC or mucin in adenocarcinoma. The most important differential diagnosis does not involve these two types of non–small cell lung carcinoma. Rather, the clinically relevant point is to differentiate between primary pulmonary carcinoma and a metastasis from other organs. Many sites host adenocarcinomas that may show partial or extensive clear cell change, but the most important possibility is usually renal cell carcinoma. Radiographic evaluation quickly confirms or refutes this possibility.

Spindle cell adenocarcinoma has been described, but this change is less common than in SCC.[19]

Bronchioloalveolar Carcinoma

If diagnosed using strict criteria, bronchioloalveolar carcinoma (BAC) is not a common entity. At the end of its morphologic spectrum represented by the sclerosing variant, it has considerable overlap with adenocarcinoma, and this accounts for some of the variability in frequency with which different pathologists seem to encounter it.

BAC can show any of three patterns of lung involvement. Many present as a single, usually peripheral lung mass; centrally situated examples are a minority. Other patients have multiple nodules, or even a diffuse pneumonic pattern of spread that can involve several lobes and may be bilateral. The latter patterns are much less amenable to treatment and prognostically more severe than a single peripheral nodule. Extensive disease has been treated with lung transplantation, and recurrences in the graft have been described. Occasional examples occur in children, who seem to have a better prognosis than adults.

Histologically, BAC features a growth of columnar to hobnail cells with low-grade nuclear features. These cells often grow along a preexisting scaffold of intact alveolar septa in a pattern that has been called *lepidic* (butterfly-like). However, this pattern can also be seen at the periphery of virtually any pulmonary carcinoma, including metastatic

lesions. BAC may also grow in a predominantly papillary pattern.

Nonmucinous BAC is slightly more common than the mucinous type. (Overlap between the latter and other mucus-producing pulmonary neoplasms was discussed previously in this chapter.) Mucinous and nonmucinous BAC are contrasted in Table 16-6. When the collagenous stroma and chronic inflammatory cells of nonmucinous BAC form a central scar that entraps small glandlike spaces, the tumor is designated as sclerosing BAC. As noted above, this overlaps with conventional pulmonary adenocarcinoma. However, BAC retains its relatively bland cytology. By contrast most examples of pulmonary adenocarcinoma have cells that are clearly recognized as malignant, based on traditional nuclear criteria. Necrosis and architecturally complex glandular profiles also support a diagnosis of conventional adenocarcinoma.

The cytology of BAC depends on several factors.[36-39] Only centrally located lesions are within the bronchoscopist's reach, but these are rare. As noted in Chapter 15, alveolar level cells that shed in sputum are usually degenerated and indistinguishable from macrophages. This is true for all but the most reactive type II pneumocytes. Differentiation of these cells from carcinomas was also discussed in Chapter 15; most are cytologically too atypical to suggest BAC and lead one to suspect adenocarcinoma. BAC has been encountered in BAL samples. This technique is most commonly applied to diffuse or multifocal pulmonary infiltrates so that tumors discovered by these means are usually widespread. Once the tumor cell groups are placed in the saline lavagate, they form round three-dimensional clusters (Figure 16-9). The cell arrangements seen in FNA material more closely reflect the tumor's true architectural pattern. Those with predominantly lepidic growth yield mostly flat sheets, whereas three-dimensional cell clusters originate in papillary dominant tumors. Aspirates are often highly cellular, but the nuclei are uniform and bland and may make us reticent to diagnose malignancy. Mucinous BAC also yields abundant extracellular mucus (Figure 16-10). In some aspirates of nonmucinous BAC, the tumor's papillary or lepidic growth pattern can be appreciated (Figure 16-11). Features that have been found useful in differentiating BAC from reactive lesions and conventional pulmonary adenocarcinoma are summarized in Box 16-11.

Several rare entities have been proposed as possible precursors of BAC, and variously designated papillary adenoma

TABLE 16-6	
Mucinous and Nonmucinous Bronchioloalveolar Carcinoma	
Mucinous	**Nonmucinous**
Less common	More common
May be multinodular or diffuse	Usually solitary nodule
Worse prognosis	Better prognosis
Little or no tumor stroma	Fibroinflammatory stroma
Tall columnar tumor cells	Cells more cuboidal
Little nuclear atypia	More nuclear atypia
Nucleoli not prominent	Nucleoli more prominent

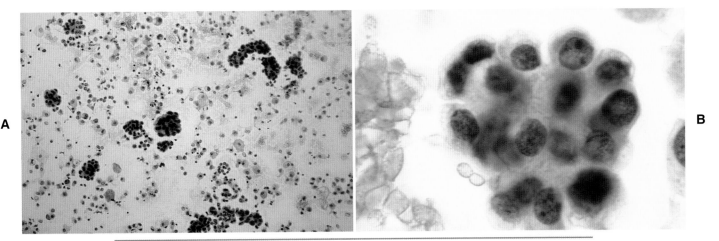

Figure 16-9 **Bronchioloalveolar carcinoma. A,** This low-magnification image shows a bronchioloalveolar carcinoma in a bronchoalveolar lavage (BAL) sample. The background consists of mostly small, free-lying, pale histiocytes. Standing out against this are several rounded three-dimensional clusters of more darkly staining cells. The epithelial nature of these clusters is highlighted by their tightly cohesive growth in three-dimensional clusters. (Pap) **B,** This high-power image of a BAL sample shows the remarkably three-dimensional nature of this cohesive cluster. The nuclei are uniform, pale staining, and show little chromatin clumping. (Pap) (**A** from Stanley MW, Henry-Stanley MJ, Iber C. Bronchoalveolar lavage: cytology and clinical applications. New York: Igaku-Shoin; 1991.)

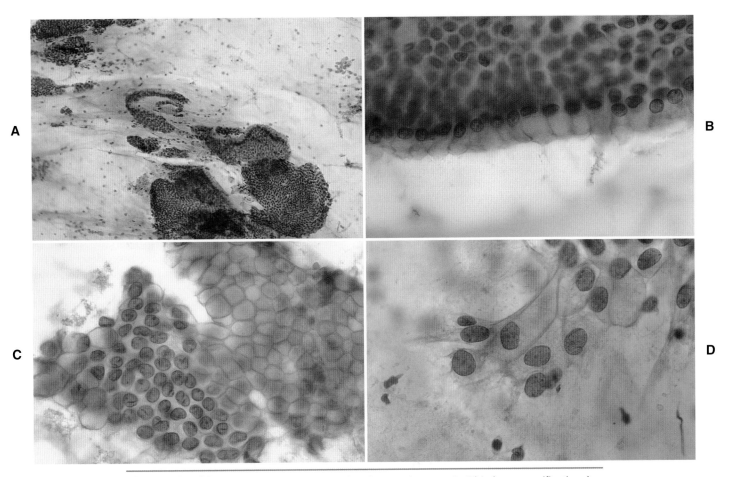

Figure 16-10 **Mucinous bronchioloalveolar carcinoma. A,** This low-magnification image shows a smear from an FNA. In this preparation, the mucin is pale staining and wispy. Large amounts of neoplastic tissue have been aspirated and are arranged almost exclusively as flat sheets. (Pap) **B,** At the edge of one of these flat sheets, the bland nuclear morphology, cellular uniformity, and abundant mucinous cytoplasm are apparent. (Pap) **C,** This flat sheet of carcinoma cells is present on two focal planes in this image. One shows the sharp, uniform, and highly organized borders of these cells. In the other plane of focus the bland nuclear morphology is highlighted. The nuclei are uniform with finely divided chromatin, some nuclear grooves, and inconspicuous nucleoli. (Pap) **D,** The bland nuclear features and background mucin of this tumor are highlighted in this high magnification image. (Pap)

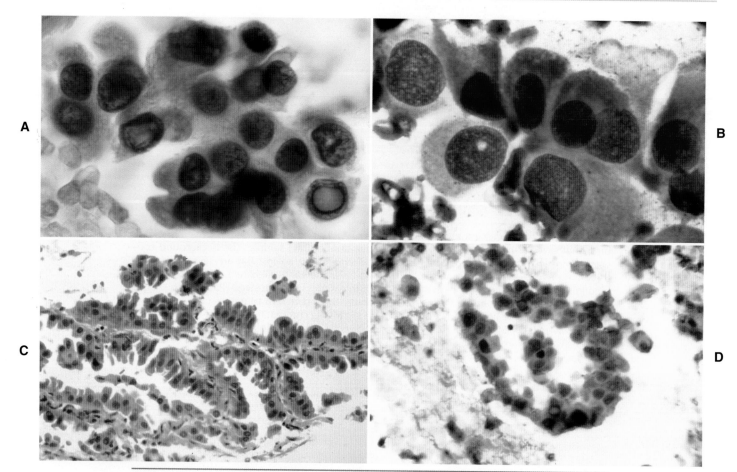

Figure 16-11 Nonmucinous bronchioloalveolar carcinoma in an FNA sample. **A** and **B,** The cells are uniform with moderate amounts of fluffy cytoplasm. Intranuclear cytoplasmic inclusions are a prominent part of this example. (**A,** Pap; **B,** DQ) **C,** This cell block section shows a papillary or lepidic growth pattern. (H&E stain) **D,** This cell block section shows intense immunostaining for the pulmonary surfactant apoprotein indicating the Clara cell differentiation of this particular bronchioloalveolar carcinoma (pulmonary surfactant apoprotein immunostain).

of type II pneumocytes, bronchioloalveolar adenoma, and alveolar adenoma. Most are small and, although not yet described in the cytology literature, can be expected to be indistinguishable from BAC.

Large Cell Undifferentiated Carcinoma

Most of the tumors of large cell undifferentiated carcinoma (LCUC) are large bulky masses that may be located centrally or peripherally. Histologically, this entity is defined as a growth of large malignant cells that lack light, microscopic evidence of glandular, squamous, or other specific differentiation. Mucicarmine staining is, by definition, uniformly negative. However, glandular features (intracytoplasmic lumen formation or microvilli) or squamous differentiation (well-developed desmosomes and tonofilament bundles) are often detected at the ultrastructural level. Other examples show neuroendocrine differentiation and are currently classified as grade 3 neuroendocrine carcinoma, large cell type (large cell neuroendocrine carcinoma). As discussed more fully in the next section, this tumor is a specific entity with prognostic significance.[40] LCUC can also be a component of a mixed tumor with grade 3 neuroendocrine carcinoma, small cell type (small cell anaplastic carcinoma).[41-42] The cytologic features of LCUC are summarized in Table 16-7.

In addition to the neuroendocrine variants mentioned previously, other types of LCUC have been described (Box 16-12). Giant cell carcinoma features large, bizarre, multinucleated tumor cells that overwhelm smaller malignant cells. This tumor often engenders a striking neutrophilic response; the presence of numerous neutrophils within the tumor cells' cytoplasm is one of the hallmarks of this entity. Morphologically identical neoplasms may arise elsewhere, including sites such as the pancreas and thyroid. These tumors may then involve the lung secondarily.

Lymphoepithelioma-like carcinoma (LEC) features a syncytial growth of large cells with pale vesicular nuclei, ill-defined cytoplasm, and prominent nucleoli.[45-47] These features are recapitulated in the FNA cytology of this tumor (Box 16-13). Small lymphocytes are distributed throughout. The relative amounts of epithelial and lymphoid cells vary over a wide range, and some lymphocyte-predominant examples may be mistaken for malignant lymphoma. It is important to exclude the presence of an occult nasopharyngeal lesion before assuming that a pulmonary tumor does not represent a metastasis. LEC is much more common in that site than in the lung and often presents at a high stage, even with nasopharyngeal disease that is difficult to detect. Multiple blind biopsies of the nasopharynx may be re-

BOX **16-11**

Cytomorphologic Features Useful in Differentiating BAC from Reactive Lesions and Conventional Pulmonary Adenocarcinoma

Favor BAC over a reactive lesion
Prominent flat sheets and three-dimensional clusters*
Tight cohesion in sheets and clusters*
Intranuclear cytoplasmic inclusions*
Multinucleated cells are not prominent*
Very uniform cellular morphology
Minimal atypia
Nucleoli not prominent

Favor BAC over conventional pulmonary adenocarcinoma
Prominent flat sheets†
Delicate nuclear chromatin†
Minimal atypia†
Nuclear grooves†
Abundant extracellular mucus†

BAC, Bronchoalveolar carcinoma.
*From Zaman SS, van Hoeven KH, Slott S, et al. Distinction between bronchioloalveolar carcinoma and hyperplastic pulmonary proliferations: a cytologic and morphometric analysis. Diagn Cytopathol 1997;16:396-401.
†Auger M, Katz RL, Johnston DA. Differentiating cytological features of bronchioloalveolar carcinoma from adenocarcinoma of the lung in fine-needle aspirations: a statistical analysis of 27 cases. Diagn Cytopathol 1997; 16:253-257.

 BOX **16-12**

Uncommon Variants of Large Cell Undifferentiated Carcinoma

Giant cell carcinoma*
Spindle cell carcinoma*
Clear cell carcinoma
Lymphoepithelioma-like carcinoma

*These two tumors are sometimes combined into the entity *pleomorphic carcinoma.*

 BOX **16-13** | CMF

Cytomorphologic Features of Lymphoepithelioma-like Carcinoma

Sheets or clusters of tumor cells
Large tumor cells
Vesicular nuclei
Prominent nucleoli
Variable numbers of small lymphocytes

TABLE **16-7** | CMF

Cytomorphologic Features of Large Cell Undifferentiated Carcinoma

Feature	Description
Background	May show necrosis
Cell size	Variable but many are large
Cell arrangements	Numerous single cells
	Small clusters or syncytia
	Large cohesive tissue particles are rare
Cytoplasm	Variable amount; may be scanty or abundant
	Lacks the density of squamous cells
	May be lacy or vacuolated
	Borders may be ill-defined
Nuclei	Variable size
	Round, oval, or lobulated
	Irregular chromatin distribution
Nucleoli	Prominent
	May be multiple
Mitotic figures	Often easily detected

quired. This tumor appears to be more common in Asian patients, in whom it is often associated with evidence of Epstein-Barr virus infection.

Neuroendocrine Carcinoma

This complex family of lesions differentiates to resemble the small population of neuroendocrine cells within the normal bronchial epithelium. These represent the pulmonary component of the diffuse neuroendocrine system that is most clearly demonstrated in the gastrointestinal tract. Increased numbers of these cells (hyperplasia) can be seen in either a diffuse (linear, intramucosal) form or as microscopic nodules. Various degrees of hyperplasia have been noted in normal epithelia, those associated with a variety of nonneoplastic conditions and epithelia near various types of neuroendocrine neoplasia.

Earlier conceptualizations of this category centered around a two level classification with carcinoid tumors (CTs) at one end and SCAC (oat cell carcinoma) at the other. CTs have characteristic gross, histologic, and clinical features discussed in the following text and a good prognosis. In all but the rare examples that present with low-stage disease, SCAC has a dismal prognosis.

This nosology has become more complex over a period of several years because a variety of additional factors have been included in the various classification schemes:
1. SCAC variants including an intermediate cell type, the spindled or fusiform cell type, and combinations have been described. In most instances, the primary impor-

tance of recognizing these variants is ensuring that all examples of SCAC receive proper treatment because this differs greatly from the clinical management of most non–small cell carcinomas.
2. Peripheral carcinoids (PCs) differ from their more common central or typical counterparts in several ways, including an even better prognosis.
3. A subset of central carcinoid tumors with a clinical course between those of typical CT and SCAC led to a cluster of criteria used to define atypical CT.

4. Large cell carcinomas with subtle architectural evidence of neuroendocrine differentiation can be clearly placed in this category by confirming immunohistochemical or ultrastructural studies. As noted previously, some investigators consider this a prognostically significant subcategory.[40]

5. Occasional carcinomas that completely lack architectural evidence of neuroendocrine differentiation on hematoxylin and eosin (H&E)–stained sections can show immunohistochemical or ultrastructural evidence of this phenotype.

As the less differentiated, or less obviously neuroendocrine, of these entities is approached, it is necessary to confirm this type of differentiation with various immunohistochemical or ultrastructural tools (Table 16-8). In those tumors without typical architectural evidence of neuroen-docrine growth, these analyses become critical. Even these evaluations may become more difficult in the more distant parts of the realm, with some cases showing only a few dense core granules or cell processes by electron microscopy. Thus, at different levels of differentiation, architectural, immunohistochemical, and ultrastructural features form the definition of NEC.

As summarized in Table 16-9[48-50] several classifications of pulmonary neuroendocrine neoplasia are extant. When discussing these lesions with clinical colleagues, it is often necessary to slip easily between several terminologies so that the relationships summarized in this table must be clearly understood. Box 16-1 reflects the authors' preference for the scheme of Dresler, Ritter, and Wick.[50] This relates each of these entities under the umbrella of neuroendocrine carcinoma and accommodates all of the variations noted above.

Despite the nosologic preference of the authors, the term *CT* is so entrenched in common usage, that *Grade 1 Neuroendocrine Carcinoma* is not likely to acquire the status of a clinical colloquialism in the near future. Most examples are not clinically, pathologically, or prognostically problematic, so this seems to us an acceptable compromise, and this comfortable terminology is used here. After all, it is not this entity that has occasioned so many revisions of the authors' thinking about neuroendocrine neoplasms over the years. Widespread use of the older terminology for CT variants (atypical CT and spindle cell CT) is also likely to continue.

CTs are, by definition, centrally located and usually present as a polypoid intrabronchial mass. They are often bilobed (dumbbell-shaped), having a second extrabronchial lobe. Symptoms can be the result of bronchial obstruction (pneumonia or lung collapse), hemorrhage, or rarely because of secretion of protein hormones (adrenocorticotrophic hormone), or serotonin production. The latter can result in carcinoid syndrome and gives positive urine studies for 5-HIAA.

CT is quite vascular and covered by an intact ciliated mucosa. Alternatively, the mucosa may show squamous metaplasia. The latter feature can lead to negative bronchial brushings and washings, despite ready bronchoscopic access to the tumor. However, examples diagnosed by sputum and bronchial brushings have been reported.[51] In such instances, the overlying mucosa is probably ulcerated. Forceps biopsy may result in dangerous degrees of hemorrhage so that transbronchial FNA is sometimes preferred. The clinical and bronchoscopic findings often alert the cytopatholo-

---

TABLE 16-8

Histologic, Ultrastructural, and Immunohistochemical Features Used to Define a Neuroendocrine Carcinoma

Type of Feature	Specific Finding
Architectural features	Rounded cell nests, trabecula, festoons
	Less well-defined nesting
	Some nesting with peripheral palisading
	Poorly formed rosettelike structures
Immunohistochemical features	
General epithelial markers	Cytokeratins
Neuroendocrine markers	Chromogranins A and B
	Synaptophysin
	Neurofilament protein
	Leu-7
	Peptide hormones*
	Serotonin
Ultrastructural features	Neurosecretory granules
	Cell processes

*Many have been described as immunohistochemically detectable in carcinoid tumors of the lung.

TABLE 16-9

Classification Schemes for Neuroendocrine Carcinoma

Historical	Carcinoid tumor Small cell carcinoma	Atypical carcinoid tumor		Small cell carcinoma
Warren and colleagues[48]	Carcinoid tumor	Well-differentiated neuroendocrine carcinoma (NEC)	Intermediately differentiated NEC	Small cell carcinoma
Travis and colleagues[49]	Carcinoid tumor	Atypical carcinoid tumor	Large cell NEC	Small cell NEC
Dresler and colleagues[50]	Grade 1 NEC	Grade 2 NEC	Grade 3 NEC, large cell type	Grade 3 NEC, Small cell type

NEC, Neuroendocrine carcinoma.

gist to the likelihood of this diagnosis. The histologic features of CT are summarized in Table 16-10 and are reflected in the cytology of this neoplasm[51-53] (Table 16-11 and Figure 16-12). The arrangement of tumor cells in nests, trabecular bars, or festoons imparts a particularly organized appearance to the histology of CT and related entities that has been termed *organoid*. Mitotic activity is generally low.

CTs that are architecturally neuroendocrine, as may be confirmed by immunohistochemical or ultrastructural evaluation, but that depart from the typical histology by showing necrosis, mitoses, and significant nuclear atypia are termed *atypical carcinoid tumors* (ACTs) (grade 2 neuroendocrine carcinoma; also designated malignant CT by some authors). The term *ACT* is likely to remain the preferred clin-

TABLE 16-10
Histologic Features of Carcinoid Tumors

Feature	Description
Architecture	
Usual	Cells arranged in rounded nests, trabecula, or festoons
Variants	Solid, glandular, rosettes, papillary, thyroid-like follicles
Vascularity	Numerous small vessels
Stromal alterations	Hyaline change, calcification, ossification, amyloid deposits
Cells	Small, round and uniform
Nuclei	Centrally placed and uniform*
Chromatin	Evenly distributed and finely stippled (salt-and-pepper)
Cytoplasm	Moderate and pale to eosinophilic (hematoxylin and eosin)†
Mucicarmine stain	Usually negative‡
Mitotic figures	Not identified or very rare
Necrosis	Absent

*Some may show large hyperchromatic atypical nuclei similar to those often encountered in endocrine adenomas. Taken alone, this finding does not justify a diagnosis of atypical carcinoid (grade 2 neuroendocrine carcinoma).
†Oncocytic variants, clear cell change, and melanin production are noted rarely.
‡Rare glandular spaces may be positive.

TABLE 16-11   CMF
Cytomorphologic Features of Typical Carcinoid Tumor (Neuroendocrine Carcinoma, Grade 1)

Feature	Description
Background	Clean, without necrosis
Cell size	Uniform
Cell shape	Round to slightly oval
	Occasional spindle cells, singly or in clusters
Cell arrangements	Single cells, loose clusters, three-dimensional groups
Cytoplasm	Scant to moderate
	Homogenous
	If detected, granularity is slight
Nuclei	Uniform, round to oval
	Finely stippled chromatin
	Often striped of cytoplasm to lie bare and single
Nucleoli	Uniformly small and distinct
Mitotic figures	Not detected
Stroma	Usually scanty or not present
	Capillary-size blood vessels covered with tumor cells

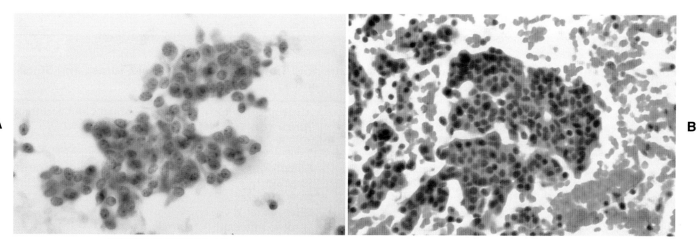

A   **B**

Figure 16-12   **Carcinoid tumor. A,** FNA material from this carcinoid tumor is highly cellular. The arrangement of these cells in small rounded clusters reflects the neuroendocrine nature of this neoplasm. The individual cells are quite uniform and show a moderate amount of cytoplasm. The nuclei feature chromatin that ranges from finely stippled to slightly more clumped (salt-and-pepper), and most cells show a single small nucleolus. (Pap) **B,** A cell block section from an FNA reinforces the nested arrangement of these small uniform cells. (H&E)

ical colloquialism for some time. The quantitative aspects of this histologic definition vary somewhat among investigators[48-50,54] (Table 16-12). CT outnumbers ACT by 9:1 or 10:1. Atypical examples tend to be larger. Most are centrally located and associated with a history of smoking.

This neoplasm is prognostically different from typical CT and should be approached clinically in a manner similar to non–small cell pulmonary carcinomas. In one investigation, the incidence of lymph node metastases at diagnosis was 70% for ACTs compared with 5% for typical CT.[54] Even in the rare event of metastases from CT, these tend to progress slowly and are compatible with prolonged survival. ACTs, in contrast, can lead to more extensive metastases and death from the tumor in up to 30% of cases.[54]

The comparative cytologies of CTs, ACTs, and SCAC (grades 1, 2 and 3 neuroendocrine carcinoma, respectively) are summarized in Table 16-13.[55,56] In most instances, ACTs are readily distinguished from CT (Figure 16-13). However, its cytologic overlap with SCAC can be confusing. In particular, examples with prominent spindling may suggest a diagnosis of SCAC designated as the spindle cell type in previous subclassifications of this tumor. The relatively large cells of ACTs may by thought to represent the intermediate cell type of SCAC. Understanding of these problems is limited at the present, and individual cases are likely to cause considerable difficulty. For now, the most clinically relevant conclusion seems to be that all stage I neuroendocrine neoplasms, regardless of whether they are ultimately CTs, ACTs, or SCAC (the latter is rare), should be surgically excised.

An occasional CT presents as a peripheral lung mass. Most of these show a proliferation of bland spindle cells, and only a few feature the rounded cells and organoid pattern of their centrally located counterparts. Most such tumors have uniform, cigar-shaped nuclei with finely granular chromatin that suggest a diagnosis of a smooth muscle tumor (Figure 16-14).

Peripheral CT is listed as a special entity (see Box 16-1), because it has uniquely excellent prognosis. Regional lymph node metastases are rare, and most of these lesions are cured by lobectomy. Fekete and colleagues report one such tumor that was followed nonsurgically without radiographic changes for more than 5 years.[57]

SCAC and oat cell carcinoma are the most commonly employed designations for grade 3 neuroendocrine carcinoma of the small cell type. Other terms that are largely meant to describe cytologic variations have been used in

---

TABLE 16-12

Histologic Definitions of Atypical Carcinoid Tumors

Reference Number	Architecture and Necrosis	Mitotic Activity	Nuclear Atypia
48	Some loss of organoid pattern Limited necrosis	>5/10 hpf	Present
49	Any necrosis	2 < mitoses > 10 hpf	Present
50	Some loss of organoid pattern Limited necrosis in centers of cell nests	5 < mitoses > 10 hpf	Present
54	Necrosis present Disorganization of nests Increased cellularity Hyperchromasia Large nucleoli	1 mitosis/ 1 or 2 hpf (average)	Pleomorphism

hpf, High power field.

TABLE 16-13

Comparison of Cytomorphologic Features of Typical Carcinoid Tumor Atypical Carcinoid Tumor and Small Cell Carcinoma (Neuroendocrine Carcinoma, Grades 1, 2, and 3)

Cytologic Feature	Carcinoid Tumor (Grade 1 NEC)	Atypical Carcinoid Tumor (Grade 2 NEC)	Small Cell Carcinoma (Grade 3 NEC)
Cell arrangements	Three-dimensional clusters High group cohesion	Small acinar clusters Palisading	Loose clusters Steaming single cells
Cell size	Small	Small	Smallest
Cell shape	Round to oval ± Spindled	Round to oval Often spindled	Round to oval ± Spindled
Cytoplasmic volume	Scant to moderate	Scant to moderate	Scant
Chromatin	Uniformly granular	Coarsely granular	Variable*
Nucleoli	Small and distinct	Prominent	Small or absent
Mitotic figures	Absent	Present	Frequent
Necrosis	Absent	Variable	May be abundant

NEC, Neuroendocrine tumor.
*See text description of small cell anaplastic carcinoma.

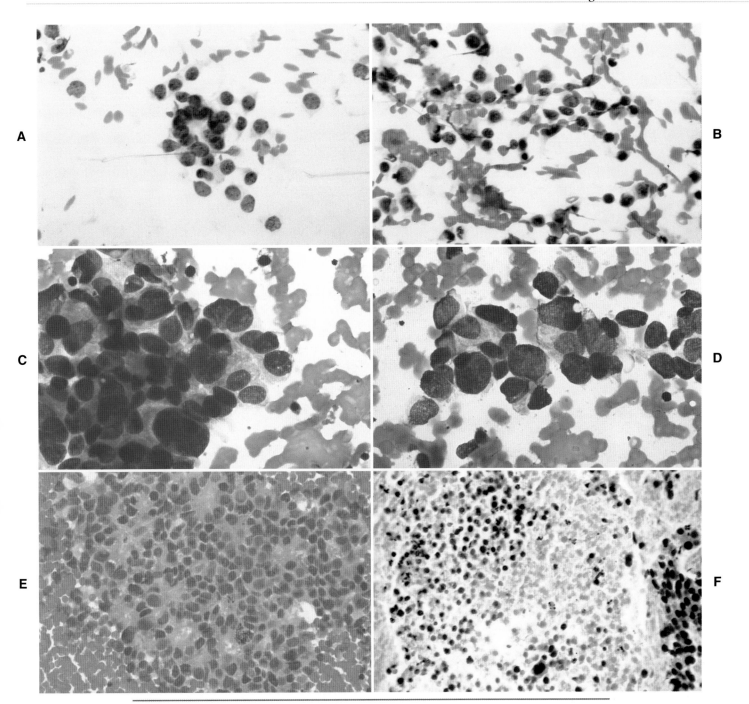

Figure 16-13 **Atypical carcinoid tumor (grade 2 neuroendocrine carcinoma). A,** The cells of this neoplasm tend to be smaller than those of a classical central carcinoid tumor. Their nuclei are more hyperchromatic, and their cytoplasm is scanty. The nested arrangement is less well-defined than in classical carcinoid tumor but reflects the tumor's neuroendocrine nature. (Pap) **B,** Another field shows mostly single cells. Individual cells show hyperchromatic nuclei and scanty cytoplasm. The cyanophilic round bodies in the smear background represent individual necrotic tumor cells. This cytologic presentation is much more reminiscent of small cell anaplastic carcinoma (grade 3 neuroendocrine carcinoma) than of typical carcinoid tumor. (Pap) **C,** In air-dried preparations the range of nuclear sizes is accentuated. This cell cluster shows a vague nesting of cells suggesting neuroendocrine differentiation. (DQ) **D,** Decreased cellular cohesion is further illustrated in this image. (DQ) **E,** This cell block preparation from FNA shows nesting and rosette formation, strongly indicating neuroendocrine differentiation. (H&E) **F,** Another field from the cell block shows the necrosis that is common in atypical carcinoid tumors. (Mucin)

Continued

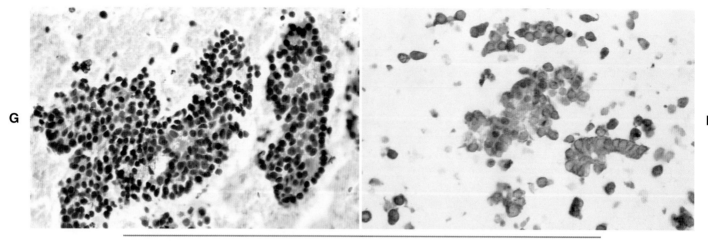

Figure 16-13, cont'd G, Another field of this atypical carcinoid tumor shows well-defined rosettes with centrally located mucicarmine-positive material. (Mucin) **H,** This immunostain for chromogranin confirms the neuroendocrine nature of atypical carcinoid tumor. (Chromogranin immunoperoxidase [Chromo])

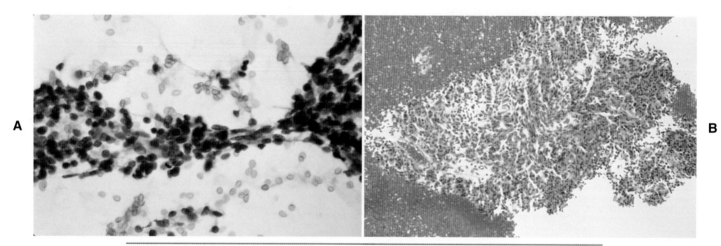

Figure 16-14 **Peripheral spindle cell carcinoid tumor. A,** This neoplasm has been sampled by FNA. Most of the cells were distinctly spindled, with uniform nuclei showing delicate chromatin. (Pap) **B,** In this field a suggestion of rosette formation can be identified.

different classification schemes over the last several decades (Table 16-14). The prognostic significance of large cell neuroendocrine carcinoma was mentioned previously.[40] The various subdivisions of SCAC (lymphocyte-like, intermediate, spindle cell, and combined) are without prognostic significance. Their importance lies in the need to recognize accurately all cases that represent any form of SCAC, a therapeutically critical category. This tumor is so unique that division of pulmonary carcinomas into small cell and non–small cell is sufficient for most clinical decision making. Most are centrally located and present with systemic dissemination. These features take surgical therapy out of the question so that chemical treatment is the typical approach. The obvious implications of these observations for cytopathology are summarized in Table 16-15. The association of SCAC with smoking is statistically so strong, that some pause to reconsider strongly the diagnosis, if a clear nonsmoking history is forthcoming.

Some examples of SCAC present with massive mediastinal lymphadenopathy with or without a pneumonic lung infiltrate. When this overshadows a central lung mass, diagnoses of malignant lymphoma or thymoma may be considered. Cytology can play an immediately decisive role in selecting the appropriate course of diagnosis and therapy.

The most common cause of superior vena cava syndrome is SCAC of the lung. (Most cases associated with other malignancies are the result of malignant lymphoma.) This oncologic emergency requires immediate treatment. Diagnosis by FNA can sanction the needed intervention, literally in a manner of minutes. The authors have seen patients in whom the massive mediastinal tumor extends superiorly to form a mass palpable in the supraclavicular fossa. This makes a target for FNA that eliminates the need for radiographic guidance and speeds the procedure greatly.

Histologically, the cells of SCAC grow in sheets that lack the organoid arrangements of lower-grade neuroendocrine

TABLE **16-14**	
Descriptive Terms Used in Classification of Small Cell Anaplastic Carcinoma (Grade 3 Neuroendocrine Carcinoma)	
Cell Type	**Tumor Classification**
Small with scant cytoplasm (20 μm cell diameter)	Oat cell Small cell Lymphocyte-like
Larger cells with more cyto-plasm (30 μm cell diameter)	Polygonal Intermediate
Spindle	Spindle Fusiform
Mixtures of small, inter-mediate and spindle cells	Combined
Mixtures of small cells and larger cells	Mixed small cell/large cell

TABLE **16-15**	
Implications for Cytologic Diagnosis of Small Cell Anaplastic Carcinoma (Grade 3 Neuroendocrine Carcinoma)	
Clinical Finding	**Implication for Cytology**
Most are centrally located	Sputum, brushings, and washings often diagnostic
Most are large	Fine-needle aspiration (FNA) is usually appropriate and diagnostic
Chemical therapy is used for small cell anaplastic carcinoma, as surgery in not indicated	1. Incorrect diagnosis of small cell anaplastic carcinoma (SCAC) as non–small cell carcinoma results in unwarranted surgery. 2. Incorrect diagnosis of non–small cell carcinoma as SCAC may deprive the patient of needed surgery. 3. Incorrect diagnosis of non–small cell carcinoma as SCAC may lead to severe complications or death resulting from unnecessary chemotherapy.*

*This situation has formed the basis for legal action against pathologists on more than one occasion.

carcinoma and are interrupted by broad zones of necrosis. A fibroinflammatory reaction is minimal or absent in most cases. Even in histologic material, the defining characteristics of this tumor are largely cytologic. When translated into cytologic preparations, these characteristics are similar to those seen in section material. The details are to some extent dependent on the type of preparation, as summarized in Table 16-16.

Earlier descriptions of linear cell arrangements featuring extreme nuclear molding, nonexistent cytoplasm, and hyperchromatic nuclei completely lacking chromatin substructure were based on degenerated cells identified in sputum samples (Figure 16-15). More contemporary sampling methods give larger numbers of cells. At least some of these show a thin rim of cytoplasm and delicate chromatin stippling. In such cells, small, blue dotlike cytoplasmic inclusions have been noted in Romanowsky-stained smears. Rounded cell clusters are more common than linear arrangements (Figure 16-16). Nuclear molding within these clusters can be minimal, as if the intact cytoplasm acts to prevent so close an approach of adjacent nuclei.

The smear background in SCAC has a characteristic "dirty" appearance that contributes strongly to the overall cytologic picture. This is partly the result of the same abundant necrosis seen in histologic preparations. Also present are single cells that, although necrotic, can be identified as tumor cells. These lie singly as dense, round cyanophilic bodies that are the same size as viable tumor cells elsewhere on the slide. These structures are often numerous. Some contain varying amounts of residual hyperchromatic nuclear debris. Any reasonably cellular sample of SCAC has these apoptotic bodies. Unless a specimen is sparsely cellular, they are virtually required for the diagnosis.

The difficult differential diagnosis of SCAC with basaloid and small cell SCC was discussed previously in this chapter. In the less differentiated tumors, immunohistochemical studies may become less diagnostic, and only ultrastructural evaluation resolves any diagnostic dilemma. As noted earlier, most examples of these rare SCC variants are probably evaluated with cytology or small biopsies and interpreted as SCAC. Thus, clinical, therapeutic, and prognostic differences among these entities remain difficult to understand.

Rare examples of SCAC are present as stage I masses and may even be peripherally located. Furthermore, the idea that any stage I neuroendocrine carcinoma should be regarded as a surgical lesion, regardless of its grade (CT, ACT, or SCAC) seems well established. Rarely, very early, even occult examples of SCAC have been detected in cytologic material.[58] Cytologic samples are also effective in diagnosing metastatic lesions and extension to the pleural space. Some patients present with massive pleural effusions so that a thoracentesis with cytologic examination may the be initial diagnostic event. Patients with this presentation have high-stage disease and a very poor prognosis. Cerebrospinal fluid may also yield a positive result.[59]

FNA can increase the detection of SCAC metastatic to the liver.[60] In many instances this tumor involves the liver in a diffuse miliary fashion with enormous numbers of tiny metastatic deposits. In this situation, radiographic guidance is sometimes not necessary for successful and safe FNA at the bedside. Blind aspiration of palpable liver lesions in this situation has been described in detail.[61]

Carcinomas histologically indistinguishable from SCAC of the lung have been described as arising in essentially every epithelium of the body. However, all extrapulmonary examples are rare, when compared with lung lesions. Thus, whenever a diagnosis of primary SCAC of any nonpulmonary site is considered, the possibility of a metastasis from an as-yet unrecognized lung tumor must receive immediate and careful attention. When a lung lesion is detected, the extrapulmonary disease is almost always recognized as a manifestation of systemic involvement.

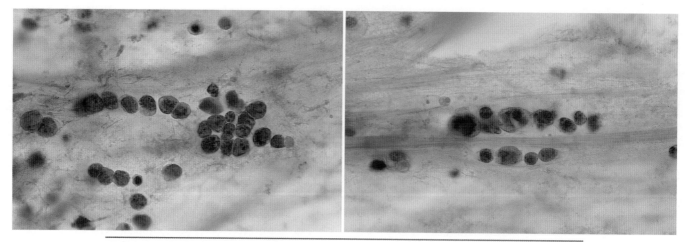

Figure 16-15 **Small cell anaplastic carcinoma.** These two images represent sputum samples. These cells are small with little if any apparent cytoplasm. Many of them lie singly or form linear files. Cells arranged in this linear fashion often appear to be caught up in a stream of mucous, giving rise to a very characteristic appearance. When the cells are arranged in a cluster, nuclei tend to mold to one another. Some of these cells show fine nuclear chromatin and occasional small nucleoli, whereas others are quite degenerated with nuclear membrane fragmentation. (Pap)

TABLE 16-16		CMF

Cytomorphologic Features of Small Cell Carcinoma (Neuroendocrine Carcinoma, Grade 3) Using Different Sampling Methods

Cytologic Feature	Less Direct Sampling*	More Direct Sampling†
Cellularity	Few cells recovered	Large numbers of cells recovered
Cell arrangements	Mostly single cells	Many single cells
	Few clusters	A few distinct clusters
	Linear groups trapped in mucus	
Damaged cells‡	Frequent	Frequent
Mitotic figures	May or may not be detected	Usually present
Necrosis	May or may not be detected	Usually present
Necrotic single cells	May or may not be detected	Almost always present
Nuclear shape	Angulated, wrinkled, spindled	Round, oval, spindled
Nuclear hyperchromasia	Marked	Slightly less intense
Nuclear molding	Very prominent	Less prominent
Chromatin	Smudgy, without detail	Finely granular
Nucleoli	Absent	Absent or tiny
Cytoplasm	Minimal to undetectable	Tiny rim; cyanophilic

*This description stems from classical studies based on sputum but may also apply to bronchial washings or other preparations that yield only cells in a relative poor state of preservation. Many of these findings represent degenerative alterations that cause the cytologic picture to depart from the more realistic picture seen in more directly obtained samples.
†Bronchial brushing and fine-needle aspirates.
‡These occur as naked nuclei in various states of preservation, or smearing, and cyanophilic cytoplasmic debris.

Carcinomas Showing More than One Histologic Type (Including Those with a Neuroendocrine Component)

The degree to which a pulmonary carcinoma shows more than one line of differentiation often depends on the level at which it is examined; at the ultrastructural level, many are mixed. However, standard epidemiologic and therapeutic concepts of lung cancer diagnosis, treatment, and prognosis are firmly grounded in light microscopic patterns. If one pattern is predominant and only minor elements of a second pattern are discovered, the tumor is classified based on the major pattern. Thus, SCC with occasional muci-carmine positive cells is still classified as SCC. A keratinized cell or focus does not detract from a diagnosis of adenocarcinoma. When both components contribute significantly to the overall pattern, a diagnosis of adenosquamous carcinoma is in order.

Other combinations of mixed carcinomas are summarized in Table 16-17. The particular combination of SCAC and LCUC is known as *mixed small cell* and *large cell carcinoma*. This combination is particularly important in that it is much less responsive to chemotherapy than pure SCAC.[62,63]

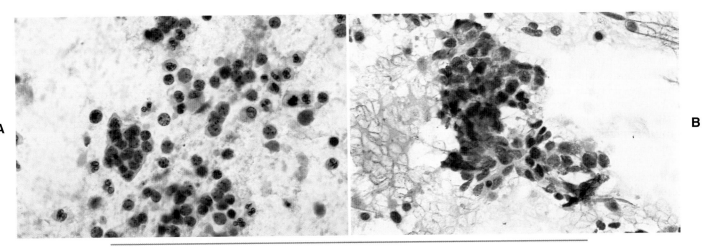

Figure 16-16 **Small cell anaplastic carcinoma. A** and **B,** This FNA has a background of necrotic debris and apoptotic individual cells. In this well-preserved material, more cytoplasm is apparent than in the sputum smears illustrated in Figure 16-15; thus, molding is less pronounced. Many of the nuclei show stippled chromatin with various degrees of clumping and occasional small nucleoli. (Pap)

TABLE 16-17

Examples of Combined-Type Lung Carcinoma

First Type of Carcinoma	Combined with . . .
Squamous cell carcinoma (SCC)*	Adenocarcinoma*
Small cell anaplastic carcinoma	SCC
	Adenocarcinoma
	Large cell undifferentiated carcinoma†

*This combination is designated adenosquamous carcinoma.
†This combination is specifically termed *mixed small cell* and *large cell carcinoma.*

TABLE 16-18 `CMF`

Cytomorphologic Features of Sclerosing Hemangioma

Feature	Description
Smear background	Blood
	Hemosiderin-filled macrophages
Smear cellularity	High cellularity*
Cell arrangements	Papillary tissue fragments
	Flat sheets of cells
Cell shape	Round to columnar
Nuclear features	Uniform
	Clear inclusions may be numerous
Nucleoli	Occasional small nucleoli
Mitoses	Not seen

*This finding is based largely on the papillary areas of the tumor. Less abundant material that may lack diagnostic features is obtained from the sclerotic or hemorrhagic areas.

Mixed carcinomas can be confusing in cytologic samples, particularly if one component is preferentially represented or if one is much more necrotic than the other. A fundamental misclassification at the critical level of small cell vs. non–small cell is not inconceivable. Yang suggested that a pseudo–small cell component can actually represent degenerated nonviable cells of what is in reality a purely non–small cell carcinoma.[62] In the experience of Fushimi and colleagues, FNA was more successful than either postbiopsy bronchial brushing or sputum in identifying both elements of mixed small cell and large cell carcinoma.[63]

Rare Pulmonary Neoplasms

Sclerosing hemangioma is a benign, usually solitary tumor that most often occurs in adult women. Despite a long-running controversy regarding the histogenesis of this neoplasm, its derivation from type II pneumocytes now seems well established. This is based on immunohistochemical staining for epithelial markers and surfactant apoprotein. The ultrastructural findings of surface microvilli and laminated cytoplasmic inclusions add strength to this concept.

Histologically, sclerosing hemangioma can be solid, papillary, or sclerotic, with varying degrees of hemorrhage, foam cell aggregation, and granulomatous reaction. Blood-filled spaces may be sufficiently prominent to suggest a vascular neoplasm. Perhaps the best known pattern is papillary, in which the pneumocyte nature of the tumor is well recognized.

When studied by FNA, these columnar cells often feature prominent intranuclear cytoplasmic inclusions and shed singly or in rounded clusters[64,65] (Table 16-18). The primary differential diagnosis is BAC, and these two may be impossible to differentiate based on cytologic and immunohistochemical findings. It is conceivable that sclerosing hemangioma could be confused with the alveolar adenomas discussed previously, but this has not been reported. Metastatic papillary carcinoma from various sites also figures in the differential diagnosis (Box 16-14).

Clear cell (sugar) tumor presents as an isolated mass on chest radiographs and can occur at any age; it is occasionally seen in children. Most are benign, but it has been suggested that those larger than 2.5 cm or showing necrosis have at least some metastatic potential.[66] The histology features sheets of polygonal cells with abundant clear cytoplasm and centrally placed bland nuclei. These are interrupted by large, thin-walled or sinusoidal blood vessels. The tumor takes its name from abundant cytoplasmic glycogen. Few cases have been described in the FNA literature[67] (Table 16-19). The most important differential diagnostic consideration is metastatic clear cell carcinoma, with renal cell carcinoma the most likely possibility. These are contrasted in Table 16-20. The other most likely differential diagnostic possibilities include clear cell alterations in a CT or a mesenchymal tumor.

The histogenesis of clear cell tumor is uncertain, but its frequent positivity with a panel of antibodies most commonly used to recognize malignant melanoma is fascinating. Fetsch and colleagues have recently extended this observation, previously based on S-100 protein and HMB-45, to include Mart-1. The latter immunoreagent decorates the melanoma antigen recognized by tumor-infiltrating lymphocytes. These authors used their observations to strengthen further the apparent relationship between the clear cell tumor, pulmonary lymphangioleiomyomatosis, and angiomyolipoma. These entities had previously been united by the common morphologic finding of perivascular epithelioid cells with varying degrees of smooth muscle differentiation and melanin production.[68]

Carcinosarcoma is a persistent term that is not commonly used today. Although most major textbooks seem to recognize this entity, the reasons for continuing to distinguish it from various types carcinoma with sarcomatoid features are unclear. Most neoplasms described as carcinosarcoma are centrally located, where they are commonly associated with an endobronchial component. A minority is peripherally situated, and a few grow with extensive pleural involvement. The latter examples may be difficult to distinguish from malignant mesothelioma. Carcinosarcoma behaves aggressively. Box 16-15 summarizes the histologic components seen in pulmonary carcinosarcoma. FNA diagnosis depends on adequate sampling of all components, and has been described in two cases.[69,70]

Pulmonary blastoma (embryoma) is a tumor of adults that takes its name from a resemblance to fetal lung tissue. It behaves in a manner similar to carcinosarcoma, and the two are probably related and may even represent different poles of the same entity. Histologically, it consists of distinct round to oval glands or cell nests that are set in a cellular stroma composed of small round or spindle-shaped cells. The glands' nuclei sit at various levels within the epithelium, depending on the extent to which they are displaced by abundant cytoplasmic glycogen. The stroma may show a variety of heterologous elements. As in carcinosarcoma, identification of both epithelial and stromal compo-

---

BOX 16-14

Cytologic Differential Diagnosis of Sclerosing Hemangioma

Bronchioloalveolar carcinoma*
Bronchial cell adenomas of various types*
Metastatic papillary carcinoma†

*These are probably indistinguishable in cytologic samples, and immunohistochemistry is noncontributory.
†Some of these may be morphologically similar to the other entities in this table. However, immunohistochemistry can be used to identify certain examples such as metastatic papillary carcinoma from the thyroid.

TABLE 16-19   CMF

Cytomorphologic Features of Clear Cell (Sugar) Tumor

Feature	Description
Smear background	Clear, without hemosiderin-filled macrophages
Smear cellularity	High cellularity
Cell arrangements	Strongly cohesive clusters and flat sheets
Cell shape	Polygonal Spindled
Nuclear features	Uniform Round to oval Finely granular chromatin
Nucleoli	Inconspicuous to absent
Cytoplasm	Ill-defined Moderate amount Clear or slightly granular
Mitoses	Not seen

TABLE 16-20

Differential Diagnosis of Clear Cell (Sugar) Tumor with Metastatic Renal Cell Carcinoma

Feature	Clear Cell Carcinoma	Renal Cell Carcinoma
Histologic features	Absence of hemorrhage Absence of necrosis Thin (sinusoidal) vessels	Hemorrhage is common Necrosis may be seen Thick-walled vessels may be seen
Cytologic features	Low nuclear grade May show spindle cells	Grade variable but may be high May show spindle cells
Special stains		
Glycogen stain	+	−
Fat stain	−	+
Immunoprofile		
EMA	−	+
Cytokeratin	−	+
S-100 protein	+	−
HMB-45	+	−
Mart-1	+	−

nents is required for diagnosis. Cosgrove and colleagues report an example studied by FNA in which both smears are cell block sections were diagnostic.[71]

Well-differentiated fetal adenocarcinoma may be thought of as a monophasic pulmonary blastoma that lacks a stromal component. The vacuolated glandular cells and frequent squamous morules combine to give this tumor a strong histologic resemblance to endometrial tissue in histologic preparations. A single case studied by FNA has been described.[72]

The pleuropulmonary blastomas of childhood can range from predominantly cystic to mostly solid, with the latter showing aggressive behavior, even in the face of aggressive therapy. Tumors of this type can arise in pleuropulmonary tissues or in the mediastinum. Histologically, an undifferentiated small round cell stroma alternates with proliferations of spindle cells. Heterologous elements of chondrosarcoma or rhabdomyosarcoma have been described, but an epithelial component is absent, unless nonneoplastic cells from a contiguous tissue are entrapped within the tumor. The latter feature and the young age of the patients distinguish pleuropulmonary blastoma of childhood from the previously discussed pulmonary blastoma. The histologic findings are recapitulated at the time of FNA.[73]

Uncommon Neoplasms Not Unique to the Lung

Most of the entities listed for this category in Box 16-1 are not only rare, but they often have not been the subject of cytopathology reports. In some instances, the FNA findings can be predicted based on available knowledge of histopathology or experience with a given entity in another body site where it is more common.

Salivary gland-type neoplasms are usually located in the large bronchi or trachea, where they probably arise from submucosal glands. All are rare, and each type is cytologically identical to its namesake in the major or minor salivary glands. Examples of the neoplasms that have been described are summarized in Table 16-21,[74-78] along with some of the differential diagnostic considerations that arise when such neoplasms are encountered in pulmonary material.

Paraganglioma, granular cell tumor, malignant melanoma, thymoma, meningioma, teratoma, and solitary fibrous tumor,[79-85] as well as sarcomas of various types[86,87] may occur rarely as primary pulmonary neoplasms. Each of these is discussed more fully in chapters devoted to their more common sites of origin (Table 16-22).

Paragangliomas in the lung usually represent metastatic disease from some other site, but apparently primary examples have been described. The differential diagnosis with CT can be difficult, or impossible, to the extent that the very existence of primary pulmonary paraganglioma has been called into question. The features favoring one over the other in histologic preparations are summarized in Table 16-23.[79] The cytology of metastatic paraganglioma has been described and is similar to that noted in other sites.[79] It can be speculated that these features might be useful in cyto-

---

BOX 16-15

Histologic Patterns of Pulmonary Carcinosarcoma

Carcinoma component*
Squamous cell carcinoma
Adenocarcinoma
Large cell undifferentiated carcinoma
Adenosquamous carcinoma
Neuroendocrine carcinoma, grade 2 or 3

Sarcoma component
Fibrosarcoma
Malignant fibrous histiocytoma
Osteosarcoma
Chondrosarcoma
Rhabdomyosarcoma

*A majority of cases show a combination of SCC and fibrosarcoma.

TABLE 16-21

Salivary Gland-Type Neoplasms that Can Occur in the Large Bronchi

Tumor Type*	Primary Differential Diagnosis	Clues to the Correct Diagnosis
Pleomorphic adenoma[74]	Hamartoma	Peripheral location of hamartoma vs. central location of adenoma
Myoepithelioma	Other spindle cell tumors	S-100 positive, EM, history†
Oncocytoma[75]	Oncocytic carcinoid tumor	NE markers, EM
Adenoid cystic carcinoma[76,77]	Basaloid squamous cell carcinoma; metastasis	Squamous differentiation; history
Low-grade mucoepidermoid carcinoma[77,78]	Benign obstructive lesions with squamous metaplasia	May be impossible in cytologic samples
High-grade mucoepidermoid carcinoma	Adenosquamous carcinoma	Some are indistinguishable
Adenocarcinoma	Adenocarcinoma of bronchial mucosa	Some are indistinguishable
Acinic cell carcinoma	Metastasis from a salivary gland tumor	Clinical history
Epithelial-myoepithelial carcinoma	Metastasis from a salivary gland tumor	Clinical history

EM, Electron microscopy; *NE,* neuroendocrine.
*Superscript numbers refer to chapter reference list.
†Most pulmonary spindle cell neoplasms represent metastases, and many will have presented previously in a different site.

logic samples, especially if paraffin-embedded cell block material is available.

Granular cell tumors occur in many body sites but for the cytopathologist are most often encountered as breast masses suitable for FNA. It is in that context that this entity is most fully discussed (see Chapter 29). Pulmonary examples have been described in bronchial brushings and in BAL fluids.[80,81] Immunostaining for S-100 protein or a traditional periodic acid Schiff (PAS) stain can support this diagnosis. Fuzesi and colleagues emphasize that primary bronchial granular cell tumor may be multiple, in a pattern that may clinically simulate metastatic carcinoma.[80] The bronchial epithelium overlying this tumor often shows squamous metaplasia that may be atypical. Just as in oral or cutaneous examples of this tumor, the degree of squamous epithelial hyperplasia may be so great as to be mistaken for SCC in a superficial biopsy. The same difficulty could arise in sputum, brushings, or washings.

In cytologic material, malignant melanoma is most often represented by FNA of a metastatic deposit, and this is certainly true for the lung[82] (Figure 16-17). Primary melanoma of bronchial origin probably exists (as it does for many other epithelia), but it must be rare and has not been described in cytologic terms. Because it is not uncommon for malignant melanoma of visceral mucosal origin to present as a metastatic lesion before the primary tumor has been detected, the diagnosis of primary bronchial melanoma should be regarded with considerable skepticism.

It is important to recall that the cytology of malignant melanoma is highly variable. Given an aspirate from a pulmonary mass, a wide range of carcinomas, sarcomas, and even hematopoietic neoplasms may enter the differential diagnosis. The well-known immunohistochemical patten of melanoma resolves most diagnostic difficulties, as long as the correct diagnosis has been entertained.

Primary pulmonary meningioma is even more rare than a metastasis from a central nervous system lesion.[83,84] Solitary fibrous tumor (fibrous mesothelioma) is usually a pleural mass but may present as primarily intraparenchymal, where it represents a reasonable target for FNA.[85] The spindle cells of this tumor are immunoreactive with antibodies to CD-34, in contrast with most of the other spindle cell masses likely to be detected in this setting.

Several benign and malignant neoplasms of mesenchymal origin occur rarely as primary pulmonary masses. This group of tumors has not been effectively addressed in cytologic terms. An interesting recent development involves identification of human herpes virus-8 in BAL fluids from patients with AIDS who have pulmonary Kaposi's sarcoma.[86,87]

Metastatic Malignancies

Metastases in the lungs may be single, large, multiple, miliary, or lymphangitic. Many tend to be multiple and bilateral. In most instances a previous diagnosis of malignancy is available, and confirmation of the clinically suspected deposit is all that is required of the cytopathologist. However, some pulmonary metastases present before the primary tumor has been identified and may require careful investigation, if inappropriate diagnosis and treatment of presumed lung carcinoma are to be avoided. This has been seen with

TABLE 16-22

Tumors that Can Occur Rarely as Primary Pulmonary Neoplasms

Tumor Type	Chapter
Paraganglioma	23 (Adrenal Gland)
Granular cell tumor	29 (Breast)
Thymoma	17 (Mediastinum)
Meningioma	14 (Direct Sampling of the Central Nervous System)
Teratoma	25 (Pelvis and Scrotum)
Solitary fibrous tumor	28 (Soft Tissue and Bone)
Sarcomas of various types	28 (Soft Tissue and Bone)

TABLE 16-23

Histopathologic Differential Diagnosis of Pulmonary Paraganglioma with Carcinoid Tumor

Histologic Finding	Paraganglioma	Carcinoid Tumor
Architecture	"Zellballen" pattern throughout	Mostly a nested pattern Rosettes Ribbons Festoons
Mucicarmine staining	Negative	Occasionally positive
Nuclear pleomorphism	Often prominent	Often minimal to absent
Stromal amyloid	May be present	May be present
Cytoplasmic melanin	May be present	May be present
Spindle cells	May be present	May be present
Immunocytochemistry		
Cytokeratin	Usually negative	Usually positive
S-100	Sustentacular cells positive	Rarely mimics paraganglioma
Chromogranin	Positive	Positive
Synaptophysin	Positive	Positive
Peptide hormones	May be present	May be present

tumors of the stomach or pancreas and less commonly with papillary thyroid carcinoma and adenoid cystic carcinoma of the head and neck. Previously mentioned in this chapter was the possibility of mistaking metastatic B-SCC for a primary lung carcinoma.[17]

One of the most deadly patterns of metastatic disease in the lung is lymphangitic carcinomatosis, in which microscopic disease fills lymphatic channels throughout the lungs. This is diagnosed in pulmonary artery samples and in BAL. Numerous carcinomas can lead to this complication, but many cases result from breast carcinoma (Figure 16-18). It is not unusual for these patients to die in a matter of weeks.

Immunohistochemistry can be of at least some use in unraveling such difficulties. Cytokeratins 7 and 20 have a role to play when various carcinomas are considered (see Table 16-5). Metastatic malignant melanoma shows nega-

tive staining for cytokeratins with positive reactions for S-100 protein, HMB-45 and MART-1 (melanoma antigen recognized by T cells[63]). Reactions for gross cystic disease fluid protein-15 (GCDFP-15) and hormone receptors may point to breast carcinoma, whereas prostatic acid phosphatase and prostate-specific antigen (PSA) immunoreactivity lead to investigation of that organ. Staining for various combinations such as placental alkaline phosphatase, α-fetoprotein, and β-hCG usually indicates a germ cell tumor, but the number of somatic carcinomas that express germ cell tumor markers seems to increase constantly.

In other instances the clinical findings may be compelling to the point that few differential diagnostic considerations need to be evaluated. For example, a man in his twenties who presents with massive hemoptysis and numerous large pulmonary nodules ("cannonballs") probably

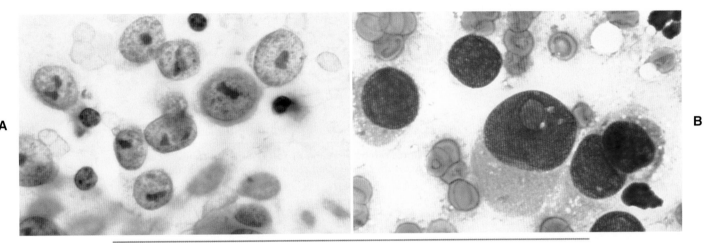

Figure 16-17 **Metastatic malignant melanoma. A,** This FNA shows loosely cohesive cells with large nuclei and prominent nucleoli. (Pap) **B,** The cells of metastatic malignant melanoma often feature eccentrically placed nuclei and may show intranuclear cytoplasmic inclusions. (DQ)

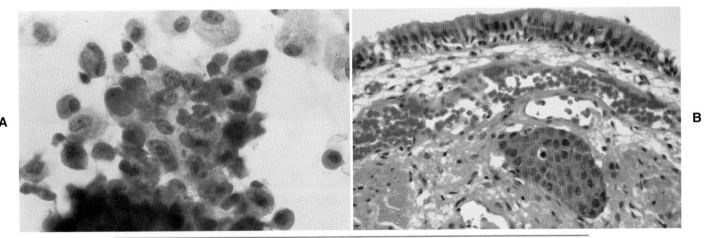

Figure 16-18 **Lymphangitic metastatic breast carcinoma. A,** This loosely cohesive cluster of malignant cells was obtained by BAL. The tumor cells show hyperchromatic nuclei and occasional nucleoli. Pulmonary macrophages present in the background show a much lower nuclear to cytoplasmic (N:C) ratio and paler nuclear staining. (Pap) **B,** This bronchoscopically obtained biopsy illustrates the histologic correlate of Figure 16-18, *A.* An unremarkable ciliated mucosa overlies submucosal soft tissues with numerous vessels. One of these is filled and distended with an aggregate of metastatic carcinoma cells. (H&E) (**B** from Stanley MW, Henry-Stanley MJ, Iber C. Bronchoalveolar lavage: cytology and clinical applications. New York: Igaku-Shoin; 1991.)

has choriocarcinoma, regardless of how innocuous his testicular physical examination may be. A urine pregnancy test provides immediate confirmation of the diagnosis.

When a sarcoma is considered, the expanding role of cytogenetic analysis in diagnosis and classification of mesenchymal neoplasms should be appreciated. Sterile aspirate material collected in a tissue culture medium is appropriate for such investigations.

Most spindle cell malignancies in the lung represent metastatic sarcomas.[88-90] These vastly outnumber primary pulmonary sarcomas and the various sarcomatoid carcinomas. In many instances, the patient has a well-established history, often with archival resection material available for review. The cytopathologist's task is usually to distinguish among metastatic sarcoma, a second malignancy, an infectious condition, or other processes. This is especially important in those cases where metastases are treated by surgical excision, such as in Wilms' tumor or childhood osteosarcoma (Figures 16-19 and 16-20). Most sarcomas lack specific immunohistochemical profiles so that history

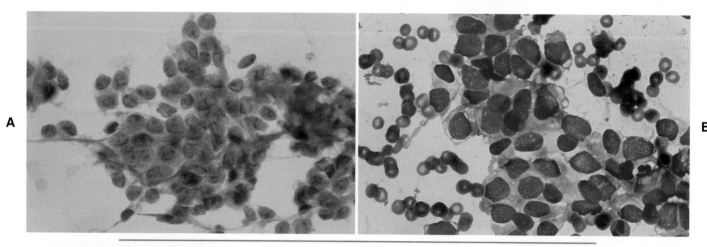

Figure 16-19 Metastatic Ewing's sarcoma. **A** and **B,** This FNA shows cohesive clusters of monotonous small cells with scanty cytoplasm, stippled chromatin, and occasional small nucleoli. (**A,** Pap; **B,** DQ)

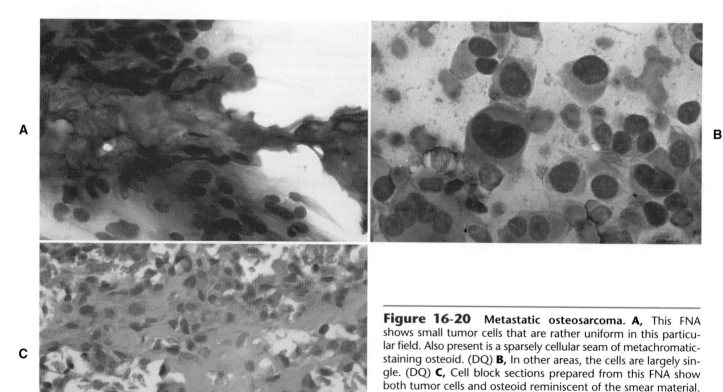

Figure 16-20 Metastatic osteosarcoma. **A,** This FNA shows small tumor cells that are rather uniform in this particular field. Also present is a sparsely cellular seam of metachromatic-staining osteoid. (DQ) **B,** In other areas, the cells are largely single. (DQ) **C,** Cell block sections prepared from this FNA show both tumor cells and osteoid reminiscent of the smear material. (H&E)

and morphology are the key diagnostic features (Figure 16-21). Confusion with fragments of normal bronchial smooth muscle obtained by brushing was discussed in Chapter 15.

Systemic Hematopoietic Malignancies that May Involve the Lung

In most patients with hematopoietic neoplasms (leukemias, malignant lymphomas, or multiple myeloma), lung cytology is directed toward finding an infectious explanation for infiltrates that evolve rapidly, as discussed in Chapter 15. Less commonly, pulmonary involvement by the primary disease or a second malignancy may be identified[91-95]

(Figures 16-22 to 16-24). Such neoplasms have been seen in bronchial brushings, bronchial washings, BALs, FNA, and pulmonary artery catheter samples.

In many instances, the patient's initial disease is well characterized before pulmonary sampling. Immunophenotypic, cytogenetic, or gene rearrangement studies can be used to confirm extension of the original condition if necessary. Also, in patients who present initially with pulmonary evidence of malignant lymphoma, these studies may be used to confirm the diagnosis. This is especially useful in low-grade lymphoid proliferations. In this regard, it is important to note that most of the lung lesions previously designated as pseudolymphoma are now considered low-grade malignancies.

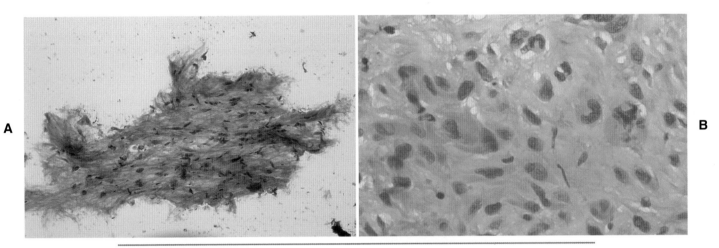

Figure 16-21   Metastatic malignant fibrous histiocytoma. A, This patient with a well-established history of sarcoma underwent bronchial brushing for evaluation of suspected metastatic disease. This cellular fragment shows a spindle cell neoplasm with varying degrees of nuclear atypia. (Pap) **B,** A simultaneously obtained transbronchial biopsy correlates well with the cytologic diagnosis. (H&E)

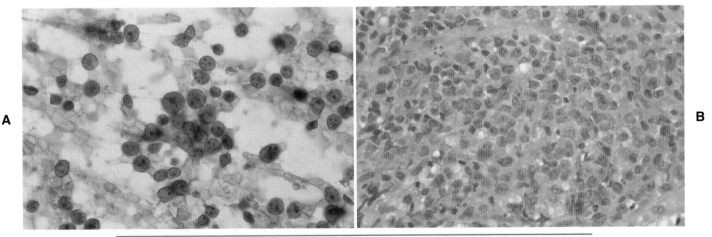

Figure 16-22   Malignant lymphoma. A, This cellular bronchial brushing shows evidence of pulmonary involvement by this patient's previously diagnosed malignant lymphoma. (Pap) **B,** The cytologic findings depicted in Figure 16-22, *A,* correlate well with the patient's previously obtained lymph node-based malignant lymphoma. (H&E)

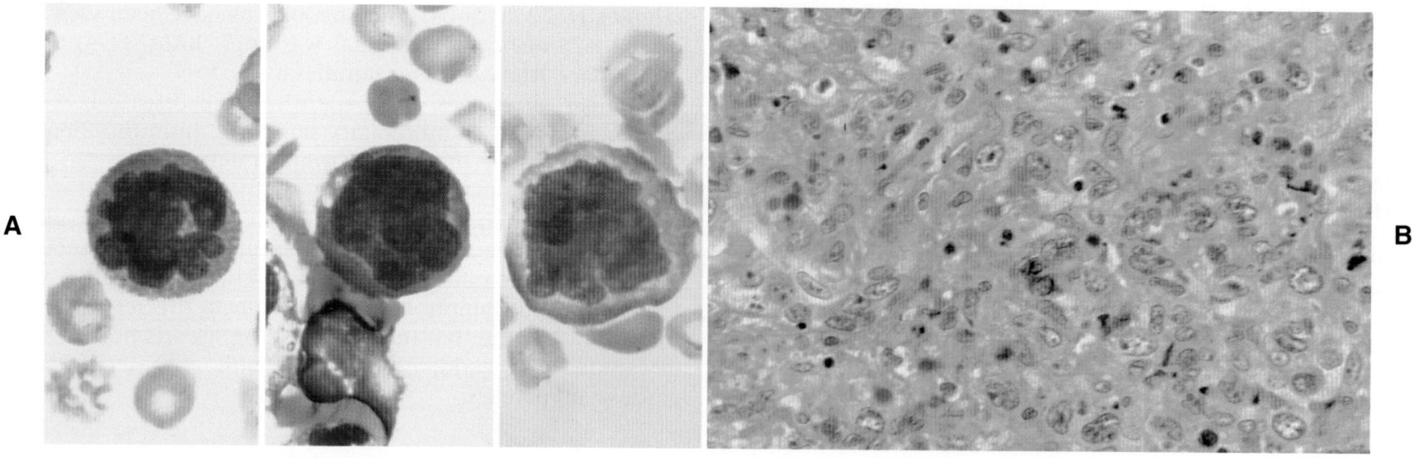

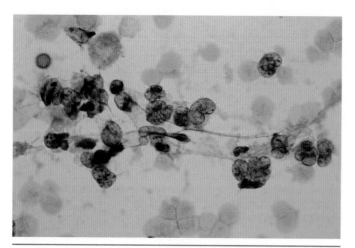

A | | | B

Figure 16-23 **Malignant lymphoma. A,** These three cells are smaller than most carcinoma cells, as measured against the red blood cells (RBCs) in the background. They feature a high N:C ratio and complexly lobulated nuclei. These cells were scattered widely through cytocentrifuge slides prepared from a BAL fluid. The patient had acquired immune deficiency syndrome (AIDS) and was being evaluated for pulmonary infiltrates of unknown etiology. (DQ) **B,** At autopsy, the presence of a pleomorphic large cell malignant lymphoma was confirmed. (H&E)

Figure 16-24 **Acute myelogenous leukemia.** In many instances, cytologic identification of a hematopoietic malignancy is readily accomplished. However, subclassification may not be straightforward without special ancillary testing. This collection of noncohesive, small cells with hyperchromatic nuclei and scanty cytoplasm represent pulmonary involvement by the patient's previously diagnosed leukemia. (Pap) An interpretation such as this should only be given after consideration of the patient's peripheral white blood cell count and differential count.

References

1. Hamper UM, Khouri NF, Stitik FP, et al. Pulmonary hamartoma: diagnosis by transthoracic needle-aspiration biopsy. Radiology 1985; 115:15-18.
2. Silverman JF, Weaver MD, Shaw R, et al. Fine needle aspiration cytology of pulmonary infarct. Acta Cytol 1985; 29:162-166.
3. Miller WT Jr, Gupta PK, Grippi MA, et al. Rounded atelectasis: diagnosis by fine-needle aspiration cytology. Diagn Cytopathol 1992; 8:617-620.
4. Flieder DB, Koss MN, Nicholson A, et al. Solitary pulmonary papillomas in adults: a clinicopathologic and in situ hybridization study of 14 cases combined with 27 cases in the literature. Am J Surg Pathol 1998; 22:1328-1342.
5. Tabbara SO, Covell JL, Abbitt PL. Diagnosis of endometriosis by fine-needle aspiration cytology. Diagn Cytopathol 1991; 7:606-610.
6. Crouch E, White V, Wright J, et al. Malakoplakia mimicking carcinoma metastatic to lung. Am J Surg Pathol 1984; 8:151-156.
7. Lambert C, Gansler T, Mansour KA, et al. Pulmonary malakoplakia diagnosed by fine needle aspiration: a case report. Acta Cytol 1997; 41:1833-1838.
8. Dundore PA, Aisner SC, Templeton PA, et al. Nodular pulmonary amyloidosis: diagnosis by fine-needle aspiration cytology and a review of the literature. Diagn Cytopathol 1993; 9:562-564.
9. Kaneishi NK, Howell LP, Russell LA, et al. Fine needle aspiration cytology of pulmonary Wegener's granulomatosis with biopsy correlation: a report of three cases. Acta Cytol 1995; 39:1094-1100.
10. Green RJ, Ruoss SJ, Kraft SA, et al. Pulmonary capillaritis and alveolar hemorrhage. Update on diagnosis and management. Chest 1996; 110:1305-1316.
11. Melamed MR, Zaman MN, Flehinger BJ, et al. Radiologically occult in situ and incipient invasive epidermoid lung cancer: detection by sputum cytology in a survey of asymptomatic cigarette smokers. Am J Surg Pathol 1977; 1:5-16.
12. Tyers GF, McGavran MH. Diagnostic and therapeutic challenges following the cytologic diagnosis of in situ carcinoma of the lung. Chest 1976; 69:33-38.
13. Matsuda M, Horai T, Doi O, et al. Diagnosis of squamous-cell carcinoma of the lung by sputum cytology: with special reference to correlation of diagnostic accuracy with size and proximal extent of resected tumor. Diagn Cytopathol 1990; 6:248-251.
14. Saito Y, Imai T, Nagamoto N, et al. A quantitative cytologic study of sputum in early squamous cell bronchogenic carcinoma. Anal Quant Cytol Histol 1988; 10:365-370.
15. Brambilla E, Moro D, Veale D, et al. Basal cell (basaloid) carcinoma of the lung: a new morphologic and phenotypic entity with separate prognostic significance. Hum Pathol 1992; 23:993-1003.
16. Dugan JM. Cytologic diagnosis of basal cell (basaloid) carcinoma of the lung: a report of two cases. Acta Cytol 1995; 39:539-542.

17. Vesoulis Z. Metastatic laryngeal basaloid squamous cell carcinoma simulating primary small cell carcinoma of the lung on fine needle aspiration lung biopsy: a case report. Acta Cytol 1998; 42:783-787.

18. Abe S, Ogura S, Nakajimi I, et al. Small-cell-type poorly differentiated squamous cell carcinoma of the lung: cytologic, immunohistochemical and nuclear DNA content analysis. Anal Quant Cytol Histol 1990; 12:73-77.

19. Matsui K, Kitagawa M, Miwa A. Lung carcinoma with spindle cell components: sixteen cases examined by immunohistochemistry. Hum Pathol 1992; 23:1289-1297.

20. Addis BF, Corrin B. Pulmonary blastoma, carcinosarcoma and spindle cell carcinoma: an immunohistochemical study of keratin intermediate filaments. J Pathol 1985; 147:291.

21. Smith AR, Raab SS, Landreneau RJ. Fine-needle aspiration cytologic features of pseudovascular adenoid squamous-cell carcinoma of the lung. Diagn Cytopathol 1999; 21:265-270.

22. Rao SK, Fraire AE. Alveolar cell hyperplasia in association with adenocarcinoma of lung. Mod Pathol 1995; 8:165-169.

23. Auerbach O, Garfinkel L, Parks VR. Scar cancer of the lung: increase over a 21-year period. Cancer 1979; 43:636-642.

24. Chu P, Wu E, Weiss LM: Cytokeratin 7 and cytokeratin 20 expression in epithelial neoplasms: a survey of 435 cases. Mod Pathol 2000; 13:962-972.

25. Hayashi H, Kitamura H, Nakatani Y, et al. Primary signet-ring cell carcinoma of the lung: histochemical and immunohistochemical characterization. Hum Pathol 1999; 30:378-383.

26. Tsang WY, Chan JK, Chow LT. Signet-ring cell melanoma mimicking adenocarcinoma: a case report. Acta Cytol 1993; 37:559-562.

27. Gilcrease MZ, Sahin M, Perri RT. Fine needle aspiration of signet-ring cell lymphoma: a case report with differential diagnostic considerations. Acta Cytol 1998; 42:1461-1467.

28. Hitchcock MG, White WL. Malicious masquerade: myxoid melanoma: seminars in Diagn Pathol 1998; 15:195-202.

29. Roux FJ, Lantuejoul S, Brambilla E. Mucinous cystadenoma of the lung. Cancer 1995; 76:1540-1544.

30. Dixon AY, Moran JF, Wesselius LJ, et al. Pulmonary mucinous cystic tumor. Case report with review of the literature. Am J Surg Pathol 1993; 17:722-728.

31. Graeme-Cook F, Mark EJ. Pulmonary mucinous cystic tumors of borderline malignancy. Hum Pathol 1991; 22: 185-190.

32. Tsao MS, Fraser RS. Primary pulmonary adenocarcinoma with enteric differentiation. Cancer 1991; 68:1754-1757.

33. Nasu M, Soma T, Fukushima H, et al. Hepatoid carcinoma of the lung with production of alpha-fetoprotein and abnormal prothrombin: an autopsy report case. Mod Pathol 1997; 10:1054-1058.

34. Adachi H, Aki T, Yohida H, et al. Combined choriocarcinoma and adenocarcinoma of the lung. Acta Pathol Jpn 1989; 39:147-152.

35. Ikura Y, Inoue T, Tsukuda H, et al. Primary choriocarcinoma and human chorionic gonadotrophin-producing giant cell carcinoma of the lung: are they independent entities? Histopathology 2000; 36:17-25.

36. Lozowski W, Hajdu SI. Cytology and immunocytochemistry of bronchioloalveolar carcinoma. Acta Cytol 1987; 31:717-725.

37. Zaman SS, van Hoeven KH, Slott S, et al. Distinction between bronchioloalveolar carcinoma and hyperplastic pulmonary proliferations: a cytologic and morphometric analysis. Diagn Cytopathol 1997; 16:396-401.

38. Auger M, Katz RL, Johnston DA. Differentiating cytological features of bronchioloalveolar carcinoma from adenocarcinoma of the lung in fine-needle aspirations: a statistical analysis of 27 cases. Diagn Cytopathol 1997; 16:253-257.

39. Saleh HA, Haapaniemi J, Khatib G, et al. Bronchioloalveolar carcinoma: diagnostic pitfalls and immunocytochemical contribution. Diagn Cytopathol 1998; 18:301-306.

40. Wick MR, Berg LC, Hertz MI. Large cell carcinoma of the lung with neuroendocrine differentiation: a comparison with large cell "undifferentiated" pulmonary tumors. Am J Clin Pathol 1992; 97:796-805.

41. Yang GC. Mixed small cell/large cell carcinoma of the lung. Report of a case with cytologic features and ultrastructural correlation. Acta Cytol 1995; 39:1175-1181.

42. Fushimi H, Kukui M, Morino H. Detection of large cell component in small cell lung carcinoma by combined cytologic and histologic examinations and its clinical implication. Cancer 1992; 70:559-605.

43. Nonomura A, Mizukami Y, Shimizu J, et al. Small giant cell carcinoma of the lung diagnosed preoperatively by transthoracic aspiration cytology: a case report. Acta Cytol 1995; 39:129-133.

44. Craig ID, Desrosiers P, Lefcoe MS. Giant-cell carcinoma of the lung: a cytologic study. Acta Cytol 1983; 27:293-298.

45. Chow LT, Chow WH, Tsui WM, et al. Fine-needle aspiration cytologic diagnosis of lymphoepithelioma-like carcinoma of the lung: report of two cases with immunohistochemical study. Am J Clin Pathol 1995; 103:35-40.

46. Chan JK, Hui PK, Tsang WY, et al. Primary lymphoepithelioma-like carcinoma of the lung: a clinicopathologic study of 11 cases. Cancer 1995; 76:413-422.

47. Chen FF, Yan JJ, Lai WW, et al. Epstein-Barr virus-associated nonsmall cell lung carcinoma: undifferentiated "lymphoepithelioma-like" carcinoma as a distinct entity with better prognosis. Cancer 1998; 82:2334-2342.

48. Warren WH, Faber LP, Gould VE. Neuroendocrine neoplasms of the lung: a clinicopathologic update. J Thorac Cardiovasc Surg 1989; 98:321-322.

49. Travis WD, Rush W, Flieder DB, et al. Survival analysis of 200 pulmonary neuroendocrine tumors with clarification of criteria for atypical carcinoid and its separation from typical carcinoid. Am J Surg Pathol 1998; 22:934-944.

50. Dresler CM, Ritter J, Wick MR, et al. Clinical-pathologic analysis of 40 patients with large cell neuroendocrine carcinoma of the lung. Ann Thorac Surg 1998; 63:180-185.

51. Nguyen GK. Cytopathology of pulmonary carcinoid tumors in sputum and bronchial brushings. Acta Cytol 1995; 39:1152-1560.

52. Mitchell ML, Parker FP. Capillaries: a cytologic feature of pulmonary carcinoid tumors. Acta Cytol 1991; 35:183-185.

53. Anderson C, Ludwig ME, O'Donnell M, et al. Fine needle aspiration cytology of pulmonary carcinoid tumors. Acta Cytol 1990; 34:505-510.

54. Arrigoni MG, Woolner LB, Bernatz PE. Atypical carcinoid tumors of the lung. J Thorac Cardiovasc Surg 1972; 64: 413-421.

55. Frierson HF Jr, Covell JL, Mills SE. Fine needle aspiration cytology of atypical carcinoid of the lung. Acta Cytol 1987; 31:471-475.

56. Jordan AG, Predmore L, Sullivan MM, et al. The cytodiagnosis of well differentiated neuroendocrine carcinoma: a distinct clinicopathologic entity. Acta Cytol 1987; 31:464.

57. Fekete PS, Cohen C, DeRose PB. Pulmonary spindle cell carcinoid. Needle aspiration biopsy, histologic and immunohistochemical findings. Acta Cytol 1990; 34:50-56.

58. Bell WR Jr, Johnston WW, Bigner SH. Cytologic diagnosis of occult small-cell undifferentiated carcinoma of the lung. Acta Cytol 1982; 26:73-77.

59. Pedersen AG, Olsen J, Nasiell M. Cerebrospinal fluid cytology diagnosis of meningeal carcinomatosis in patients with small-cell carcinoma of the lung. A study of interobserver and intraobserver variability. Acta Cytol 1986; 30:648-652.

60. Miralles TG, Gosabez F, de Lera J, et al. Percutaneous fine needle aspiration biopsy cytology of the liver for staging small cell lung carcinoma: comparison with other methods. Acta Cytol 1993; 37:499-502.

61. Stanley MW, Lowhagen T. Fine needle aspiration of palpable masses. Boston: Butterworth-Heinemann; 1993. pp. 138-141.

62. Yang GC. Mixed small cell/large cell carcinoma of the lung. Report of a case with cytologic features and ultrastructural correlation. Acta Cytol 1995; 39:1175-1181.

63. Fushimi H, Kukui M, Morino H, et al. Detection of large cell component in small cell lung carcinoma by combined cytologic and histologic examinations and its clinical implication. Cancer 1992; 70:599-605.

64. Wang SE, Nieberg RK. Fine needle aspiration cytology of sclerosing hemangioma of the lung: a mimicker of bronchioloalveolar carcinoma. Acta Cytol 1986; 30:51-54.

65. Wojcik EM, Sneige N, Lawrence DD, et al. Fine-needle aspiration cytology of sclerosing hemangioma of the lung: case report with immunohistochemical study. Diagn Cytopathol 1993; 9:304-309.

66. Gaffy MJ, Mills SE, Askin FE, et al. Clear cell tumor of the lung: a clinicopathologic, immunohistochemical and ultrastructural study of eight cases. Am J Surg Pathol 1990; 14:248.

67. Nguyen GK. Aspiration biopsy cytology of benign clear cell ("sugar") tumor of the lung. Acta Cytol 1989; 33: 511-515.

68. Fetsch PA, Fetsch JF, Marincola FM. Comparison of melanoma antigen recognized by T cells (MART-1) to HMB-45: additional evidence to support a common lineage for angiomyolipoma, lymphangiomyomatosis, and clear cell sugar tumor. Mod Pathol 1998; 11:699-703.

69. Finley JL, Silverman JF, Dabbs DJ. Fine-needle aspiration cytology of pulmonary carcinosarcoma with immunocytochemical and ultrastructural observations. Diagn Cytopathol 1988; 4:239-243.

70. Tao CW, Chen CH, Chiu MH, et al. Pulmonary carcinosarcoma: diagnostic approach by fine needle aspiration biopsy. Chung Hua I Hsueh Tsa Chih (Chin Med J) 1993; 51:235-237.

71. Cosgrove MM, Chandrasoma PT, Martin SE. Diagnosis of pulmonary blastoma by fine-needle aspiration biopsy: cytologic and immunocytochemical findings. Diagn Cytopathol 1991; 7:83-87.

72. Lee KG, Cho NH. Fine-needle aspiration cytology of pulmonary adenocarcinoma of fetal type: report of a case with immunohistochemical and ultrastructural studies. Diagn Cytopathol 1991; 7:408-414.

73. Nicol KK, Geisinger KR. The cytomorphology of pleuropulmonary blastoma. Arch Pathol Lab Med 2000; 124:416-448.

74. Ebihara Y, Fukushima N, Asakuma Y. Double primary lung cancers: with special reference to their exfoliative cytology and to the rare, malignant "mixed" tumor of the salivary-gland type. Acta Cytol 1980; 24:212-223.

75. Laforga JB, Aranda FI. Multicentric oncocytoma of the lung diagnosed by fine-needle aspiration. Diagn Cytopathol 1999; 21:51-54.

76. Pitman MB, Sherman ME, Black-Schaffer WS. The use of fine-needle aspiration in the diagnosis of metastatic pulmonary adenoid cystic carcinoma. Otolaryngol Head Neck Surg 1991; 104:441-447.

77. Segletes LA, Steffee CH, Geisinger KR. Cytology of primary pulmonary mucoepidermoid and adenoid cystic carcinoma: a report of four cases. Acta Cytol 1999; 43:1091-1097.

78. Brooks B, Baandrup U. Peripheral low-grade mucoepidermoid carcinoma of the lung: needle aspiration cytodiagnosis and histology. Cytopathology 1992; 3:259-265.

79. Stephen MR, Moffat D, Burnett RA. The cytology of bronchial brushings from a malignant paraganglioma metastasizing to the lung. Cytopathology 1999; 10:211-215.

80. Husain M, Nguyen G-K. Cytopathology of granular cell tumor of the lung. Diagn Cytopathol 2000; 23:294-295.

81. Guillou L, Gloor E, Anani PA, et al. Bronchial granular-cell tumor: report of a case with preoperative cytologic diagnosis on bronchial brushings and immunohistochemical studies. Acta Cytol 1991; 35:375-380.

82. Khoddami M. Cytologic diagnosis of metastatic malignant melanoma of the lung in sputum and bronchial washings. A case report. Acta Cytol 1993; 37:403-408.

83. Baisden BL, Hamper UM, Ali SZ. Metastatic meningioma in fine-needle aspiration (FNA) of the lung: cytomorphologic finding. Diagn Cytopathol 1999; 20:291-294.

84. Ueno M, Fujiyama J, Yamazaki I, et al. Cytology of primary pulmonary meningioma: report of the first multiple case. Acta Cytol 1998; 42:1424-1430.

85. Apple SK, Nieberg RK, Hirschowitz SL. Fine needle aspiration biopsy of solitary fibrous tumor of the pleura. A report of two cases with a discussion of diagnostic pitfalls. Acta Cytol 1997; 41:1528-1533.

86. Tamm M, Reichenberger F, McGandy CE, et al. Diagnosis of pulmonary Kaposi's sarcoma by detection of human herpes virus 8 in bronchoalveolar lavage. Am J Respir Crit Care Med 1998; 157:458-463.

87. Benfield TL, Dodt KK, Lundgren JD. Human herpes virus-8 DNA in bronchoalveolar lavage samples from patients with AIDS-associated pulmonary Kaposi's sarcoma. Scand J Infect Dis 1997; 29:13-16.

88. Kim K, Naylor B, Han IH. Fine needle aspiration cytology of sarcomas metastatic to the lung. Acta Cytol 1986; 30:688-694.

89. Logrono R, Wojtowyca MM, Wunderlich DW, et al. Fine needle aspiration cytology and core biopsy in the diagnosis of alveolar soft part sarcoma presenting with lung metastases: a case report. Acta Cytol 1999; 43:464-470.

90. Dodd LG, Chai C, McAdams HP, et al. Fine needle aspiration of osteogenic sarcoma metastatic to the lung: a report of four cases. Acta Cytol 1998; 42:754-758.

91. Rossi GA, Balbi B, Risso M, et al. Acute myelomonocytic leukemia: demonstration of pulmonary involvement by bronchoalveolar lavage. Chest 1985; 87:259-260.

92. Davis WB, Gadek JE. Detection of pulmonary lymphoma by bronchoalveolar lavage. Chest 1987; 91:787-790.

93. Kuruvilla S, Gomathy DV, Shanthi AV, et al. Primary pulmonary lymphoma: report of a case diagnosed by fine needle aspiration cytology. Acta Cytol 1994; 38:601-604.

94. Reyes CV, Jensen JA, Chinoy M. Pulmonary lymphoma in cardiac transplant patients treated with OKT3 for rejection: diagnosis by fine-needle aspiration. Diagn Cytopathol 1995; 12:32-36.

95. Betsuyaku T, Munakata M, Yamaguchi E, et al. Establishing diagnosis of pulmonary malignant lymphoma by gene rearrangement analysis of lymphocytes in bronchoalveolar lavage fluid. Am J Respir Crit Care Med 1994; 149:526-529.

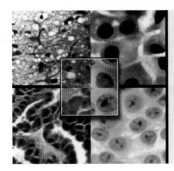

Mediastinum

CHAPTER 17

The mediastinum consists of those organs and tissues that occur within the thoracic cavity between the sternum anteriorly and the vertebral column posteriorly, between the pleural cavities laterally, and from the diaphragm up to the thoracic inlet. The mediastinum contains a wide variety of normal anatomic structures, all of which give rise to either benign or malignant tumors. The thymus and lymph nodes appear to be the most important because they are the sites of a great proportion of all primary and metastatic neoplasms. The mediastinum can be divided into several hypothetical compartments on the basis of internal and external anatomic landmarks; the system that is commonly used is based on the simple lateral chest x-ray. Although imaginary, these compartments do provide useful information in formulating differential diagnoses as specific tumors and nonneoplastic lesions show marked proclivities to occur within specific compartments. Mediastinal masses can be approached by fine-needle aspiration (FNA) biopsies with radiologic guidance and a transthoracic approach, during bronchoscopy with transbronchial aspirates, and through the esophagus with endoscopic-ultrasound guidance.[1-5] In the majority of instances, FNA biopsy provides diagnostic material in the evaluation of mediastinal mass lesions.[6] In some instances, this information is not only diagnostic but also provides crucial data to the clinician regarding staging of malignancies. In the authors' experiences, this is most common by demonstration of lymph node metastases of small cell carcinoma primary in the lung.[3]

CYSTS

Cystic masses of the mediastinum account for no more than 10% of all radiographically detected mass lesions in this body site.[7] Their cystic nature is generally apparent by a variety of radiographic procedures. These are only infrequently sampled by FNA biopsy. In general, aspiration smears are poorly cellular and may not allow a specific diagnosis.

However, it is important to recognize that a number of different histologic types of cysts[5] occasionally are aspirated.[8] The two major types of thymic cysts are developmental, or unilocular, and acquired, or multilocular.[7] The histology of the former demonstrates a cyst lining that consists of completely benign-appearing squamous epithelial cells and a fibrous wall that is generally thin and lacks an inflammatory infiltrate and cholesterol granulomas. These smears include relatively small numbers of the squamous cells that may be difficult to distinguish from mesothelial cells, as may be acquired in aspirates of pericardial cysts. Suster and Rosai have argued that the multilocular cysts of the thymus are related to cystic change within ducts derived from the branchial pouch secondary to an acquired inflammatory reaction.[9] Histologically, they may show a variety of epithelial cell types, including stratified squamous epithelium, simple columnar epithelium, or one or more layers of cuboidal epithelial cells. The walls of these cysts are thicker and include a well-developed acute and chronic inflammatory infiltrate, foci of hemorrhage and necrosis (including cholesterol granulomas), and benign lymphoid follicles. In some specimens, hyperplastic squamous epithelium is present within the fibrous wall, simulating the pattern of invasive carcinoma. Accordingly, aspiration smears from acquired thymic cysts may show a more heterogeneous cellular picture that includes a variety of benign epithelial cell types (mostly squamoid), segmented leukocytes, a spectrum of lymphoid cells, and necrotic debris. Thus, the differential diagnosis needs to include cystic varieties of thymoma that may show similar reactive inflammatory components in their wall.[10]

Bronchogenic cysts may arise in any of the mediastinal compartments as a round mass lesion that is usually asymptomatic. Histologically, these cysts may be unilocular or multilocular and are lined by respiratory type epithelium—that is, pseudostratified columnar epithelium with cilia and goblet cells. Deeper in the wall, one may find islands of mature hyaline cartilage and smooth muscle. Any of these elements could appear in aspiration samples and would be difficult or impossible to distinguish from hypocellular smears from cystic teratomas.

Enteric cysts, which occur almost exclusively within the posterior compartment, on the other hand often present with a variety of symptoms. The mucosal lining of these cysts varies from stratified squamous epithelium, columnar glandular epithelium resembling the stomach with or without parietal cells, or respiratory epithelium. The wall includes two layers of smooth muscle similar to the normal gastrointestinal tract. Any of these components may be present in FNA biopsy specimens and again would need to be distinguished from benign neoplastic elements derived from cystic teratomas.

Pericardial cysts are typically present in the middle compartment near the base of the heart and are usually asymptomatic. However, they may appear in any of the mediastinal regions. Histologically, a thin band of fibrous connective tissue is lined by a solitary layer of benign mesothelial cells. Presumably, these cells may exfoliate from the surface into the cyst fluid similar to effusions in serous cavities; an example of a pericardial cyst aspirate has been examined, which contained large numbers of obviously benign mesothelial cells.[3]

As concisely detailed by Wakely, a variety of primary mediastinal neoplasms may appear largely as a cystic lesion, radiographically and grossly.[11] These include thymoma, thymic carcinoma, germinoma, mature teratoma, non-Hodgkin's lymphoma, and Hodgkin's disease. Unless more solid portions of these neoplasms are sampled by FNA biopsy, a false-negative interpretation is likely to be rendered. Such samples would be expected to be poorly cellular and may not contain any of the neoplastic elements. Thus, whenever a neoplasm (rather than a true cyst) is suspected radiographically and clinically, extensive sampling of the mass by the needle in multiple locations is imperative.

THYMOMAS

The most common primary epithelial neoplasm to arise within the mediastinum is the thymoma.[7,10,12-20] These represent neoplasms of thymic epithelium that are associated with variable amounts of benign, nonneoplastic lymphocytes. The vast majority of thymomas arise in the anterosuperior compartments. These neoplasms may affect individuals of all ages including, rarely, children. Most, however, occur in adults with a median age of 50 years; men and women are involved with relatively equal frequency. Although many patients with thymoma are completely asymptomatic and a mass is discovered on an incidental chest film, other patients experience local manifestations of a mass lesion that include cough, chest pain, dyspnea, and the superior vena cava syndrome. Another group of patients comes to clinical attention because of an associated paraneoplastic syndrome, the most common of these being myasthenia gravis. Others include benign hematologic conditions such as pure red cell aplasia.

Thymomas have been tortured by being subject to a number of different histopathologic classification schemes over the years.[13,18,20-24,71] In the United States the most widely used system is that of Bernatz and colleagues, which divided thymoma into four major categories: (1) epithelial predominant, in which two thirds of the cross sectional histologic areas are occupied by neoplastic cells; (2) lymphocyte predominant, in which two thirds of the area is occupied by nonneoplastic lymphocytes; (3) mixed lymphoepithelial, and (4) spindle cell types.[20] It is important to emphasize immediately that for a neoplasm to be considered a thymoma, the tumor cells are bland cytologically. This is the classification that is used in diagnosing thymomas by aspiration biopsies and histologically. In 1985, Marino and Müller-Hermelink introduced an allegedly histogenetic classification.[21] Their four types of thymomas included (1) cortical, (2) predominantly cortical, (3) medullary, and (4) mixed. This was based on whether the neoplastic elements demonstrated medullary or cortical differentiation. Subsequently, these authors have added a fifth tumor: the well-differentiated thymic carcinoma.[22] Although this system has gained support in many areas, it is not generally used in the United States. Suster and Moran have proposed a classification scheme based on the degree of differentiation of the architectural and cytologic features of the neoplastic cells.[23,24] Their three categories are (1) thymoma, (2) atypical thymoma, and (3) thymic carcinoma. The authors also have stated that one can demonstrate within a single neoplasm transition among the three categories.

The authors of the latter two classification schemes have suggested that their different variants may be associated with clinically significant differences in prognosis.[21-24,72] However, the single best prognostic factor in thymomas is whether the neoplasm invades into and through its capsule. The vast majority of thymomas are completely encapsulated, readily excised at surgery, and therefore considered clinically benign neoplasms. The malignant thymoma is defined grossly and microscopically by infiltration of the tumor capsule. At surgery, this is manifested by the tumor's attachment to adjacent structures that may make the excision difficult. Although the neoplasms are cytologically indistinguishable from benign tumors, they have a worse prognosis. They may recur or even metastasize, and thus, therapy postoperatively may be dictated by the histologic demonstration of capsular invasion.[69] The less common type of malignant neoplasm derived from thymic epithelium is the thymic carcinoma.[12,22,23,25,26] These neoplasms are cytologically malignant. Many of these appear undifferentiated or demonstrate squamous differentiation. Less common variants include mucoepidermoid carcinoma and clear cell carcinoma.[26]

Aspiration smears of thymomas are moderately to highly cellular and typically demonstrate a characteristic mixed population of cells (Figures 17-1 to 17-8).[6,8,27-33] This consists

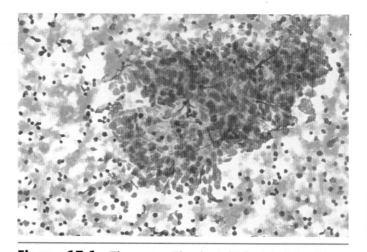

Figure 17-1 **Thymoma.** The classic biphasic cellular pattern of thymoma is present in this field. Lymphocytes not only surround but also co-mingle with the neoplastic epithelium. In this particular example, cohesion is well maintained among the uniform neoplastic epithelial cells. The latter have ovoid nuclei of homogeneous diameters, finely reticulated chromatin, and scant cytoplasm. (Diff-Quik [DQ])

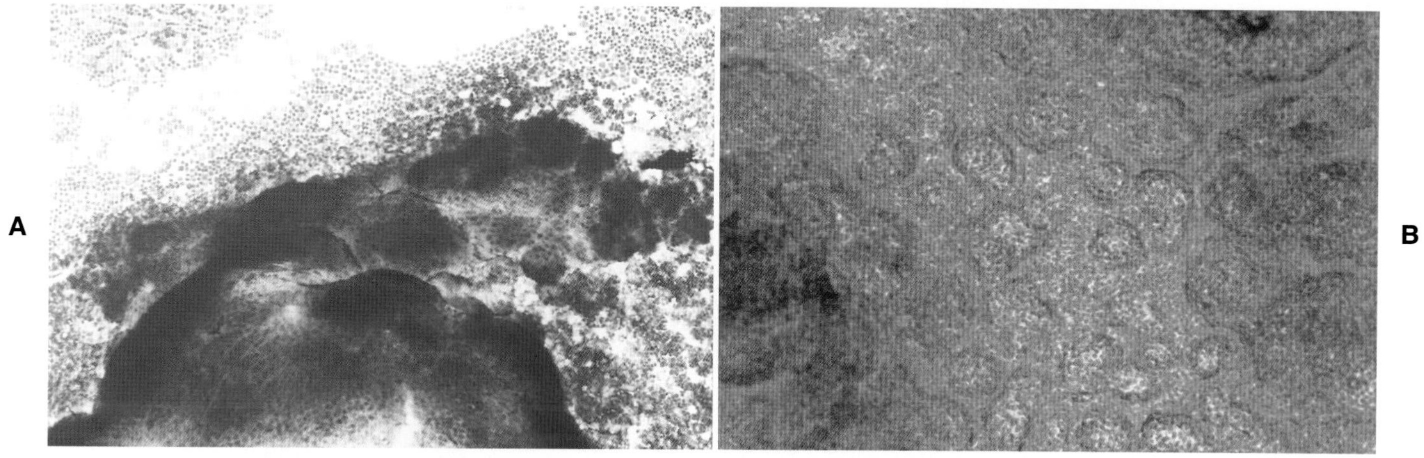

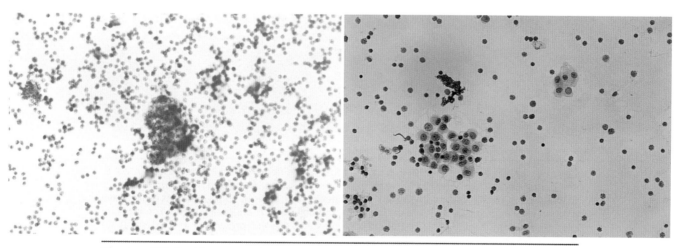

Figure 17-2 **Thymoma.** Very large cohesive fragments of neoplasm are situated within a sea of dispersed lymphocytes, most of which are small. In both **A** and **B**, the lobulated or nested appearance of the neoplastic epithelium is readily apparent. (**A,** DQ; **B,** Papanicolaou [Pap])

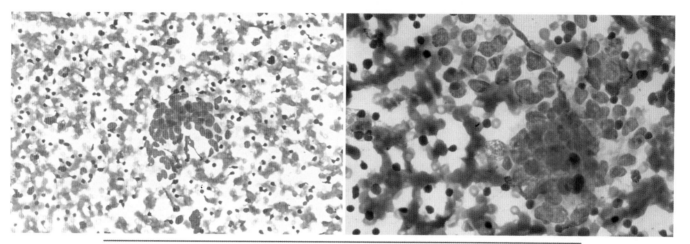

Figure 17-3 **Thymoma.** Intercellular cohesion is less well maintained in this example, as the neoplastic cells are present in smaller and less sharply delineated clusters than in Figure 17-2. Again, the interplay between the reactive lymphoid cells and the neoplastic epithelium is evident. The tumor cells have solitary slightly ovoid or round nuclei with smooth membranes, very finely reticulated uniformly dispersed chromatin, and inapparent nucleoli. Although cytoplasm is present, it is scanty, resulting in relatively high nuclear-to-cytoplasmic (N:C) ratios among the thymoma cells. (DQ)

Figure 17-4 **Thymoma.** Numerous dispersed lymphocytes are scattered about and among the neoplastic thymic epithelium. The latter are present in small flat to three-dimensional aggregates. In addition, rare individual tumor cells are also present. The tumor cells have solitary round or slightly ovoid nuclei of uniform sizes. The nuclear membranes are delicate and smooth; the chromatin is very finely granular, uniformly dispersed, and pale stained. Nucleoli are not evident. Scant to moderate volumes of cytoplasm result in relatively high N:C ratios. Note the lymphocytes that percolate among the neoplastic epithelium. (Pap)

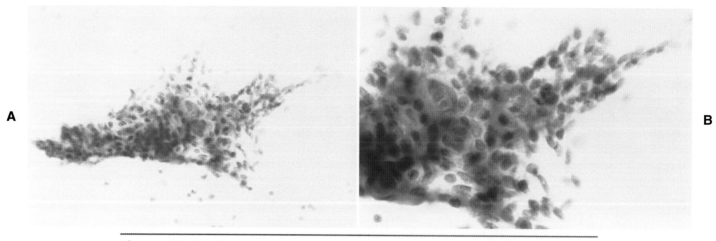

Figure 17-5 **Thymoma.** Lymphocytes are sparse in this epithelial-rich thymoma. The neoplastic cells are present in rather cohesive large fragments. **A,** The uniformity of the nuclei is apparent even at low magnification. The nuclei are not hyperchromatic and nucleoli are not evident. This is confirmed at higher magnification in **B.** Nuclear membranes are smooth and almost imperceptible. Malignant features are distinctly lacking. (Pap)

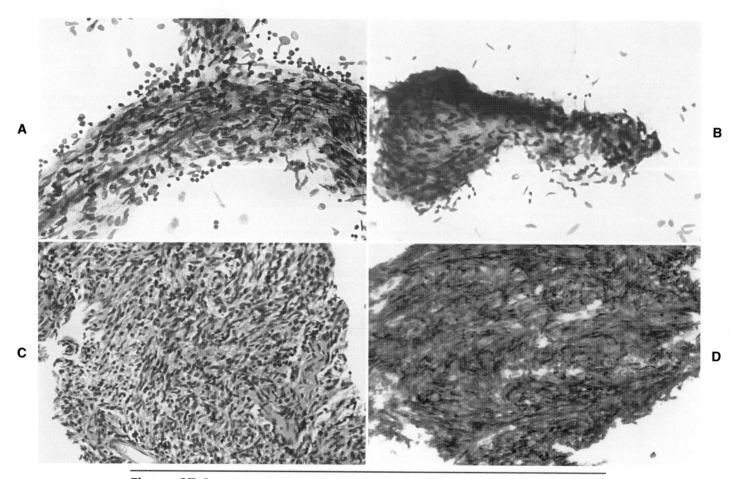

Figure 17-6 **Spindle cell thymoma. A,** Most of the neoplastic cells are present in cohesive bundles or fascicles. These cells are characterized by solitary elongated nuclei, the long axes of which often parallel one another. Some of the nuclei have straight edges, whereas others have a more wavy appearance. Cytoplasm is evident, but cell borders are poorly defined. A capillary runs through the center of this fragment. Lymphocytes are not present to any extent. (DQ) **B,** Uniform, slender, elongated nuclei characterize the neoplastic cells. The cells appear to be separated by varying amounts of some sort of matrix material. A few individual cells are also evident. (DQ) **C,** In the cell block the spindle cell contour of the neoplastic cells is accentuated. In addition, the chromatin appears to be uniformly dispersed and fairly darkly stained. Many of the cells appear to be arranged in short bundles or fascicles. A small number of lymphocytes is also evident. (Hematoxylin and eosin [H&E]) **D,** The intense and diffuse immunostaining by cytokeratin confirms the epithelial nature of these spindle shaped neoplastic cells. (H&E)

of the intimate admixture of neoplastic epithelial cells and benign lymphoid elements. The degree of intercellular cohesion in aspiration smears is variable from tumor to tumor. In some instances, large sheets and aggregates of tumor cells predominate the smears, whereas in others, the specimen is dominated by individually dispersed neoplastic cells. Many cases show admixtures of both individual and aggregated cells. The neoplastic cells vary both in size and appearance from thymoma to thymoma, but within a given neoplasm, they are usually morphologically homogeneous. In most neoplasms, thymoma cells have round to polygonal contours. Infrequently, they possess a distinctly spindled or elongated shape (see Figures 17-6 and 17-7). In the latter the tumor cells can be found in interlacing fascicles simulating a mesenchymal neoplasm in direct smears and cell blocks. Within cohesive aggregates, cell borders are usually quite distinct. The nuclei of the conventional thymoma and invasive or malignant thymoma do not possess attributes typically associated with malignancies (see Figure 17-8)—that is, nuclei are round or ovoid with delicate smooth membranes, finely dispersed and rather pale-stained chromatin, and small and inconspicuous nucleoli.

The lymphocytes often appear to infiltrate the epithelial aggregates and to surround the neoplastic cells. The vast majority of lymphocytes are small and mature-appearing. However, a spectrum of lymphoid cell maturation is seen. By immunophenotyping, these cells are T lymphocytes (Box 17-1).

No cytomorphologic means to differentiate conventional thymomas from malignant thymomas in aspiration smears is currently available.[34] As stated previously, the neoplastic cells in both have fine, even chromatin and minute nucleoli. Histologic evidence of invasion of the tumor capsule is required to identify the tumor as a malignant thymoma. Obviously, this could not be determined in a FNA biopsy (analogous to thyroid follicular neoplasms).

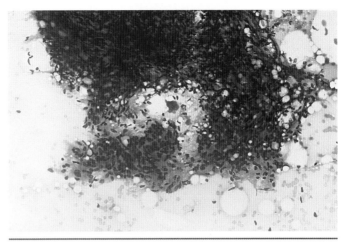

Figure 17-7 **Spindle cell thymoma.** As in Figure 17-6, most of the neoplastic cells are present within cohesive tissue fragments, often with the long axis of the nuclei paralleling one another. In addition, intercellular matrix material is evident, creating a superficial resemblance to a schwannoma. One important clue to the proper diagnosis is that this mass arose in the anterior mediastinal compartment and not the posterior one. (DQ)

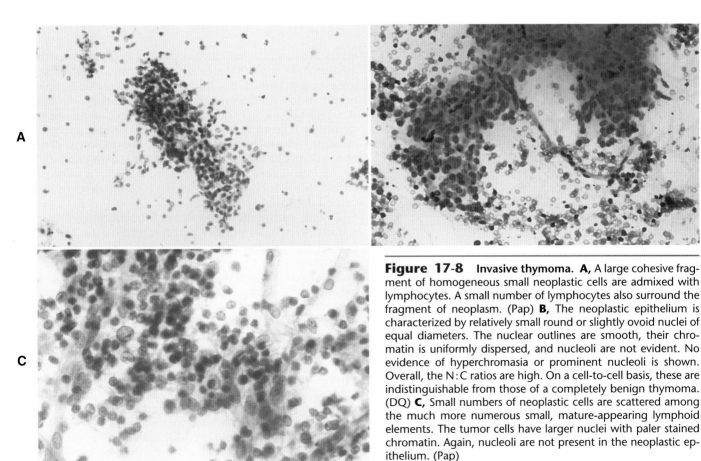

Figure 17-8 **Invasive thymoma.** **A,** A large cohesive fragment of homogeneous small neoplastic cells are admixed with lymphocytes. A small number of lymphocytes also surround the fragment of neoplasm. (Pap) **B,** The neoplastic epithelium is characterized by relatively small round or slightly ovoid nuclei of equal diameters. The nuclear outlines are smooth, their chromatin is uniformly dispersed, and nucleoli are not evident. No evidence of hyperchromasia or prominent nucleoli is shown. Overall, the N:C ratios are high. On a cell-to-cell basis, these are indistinguishable from those of a completely benign thymoma. (DQ) **C,** Small numbers of neoplastic cells are scattered among the much more numerous small, mature-appearing lymphoid elements. The tumor cells have larger nuclei with paler stained chromatin. Again, nucleoli are not present in the neoplastic epithelium. (Pap)

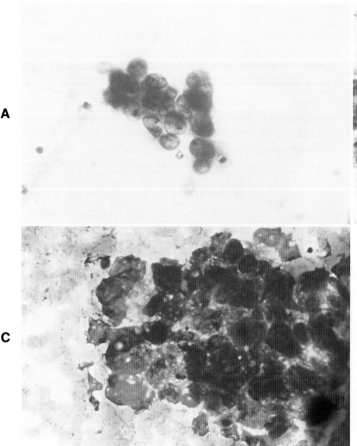

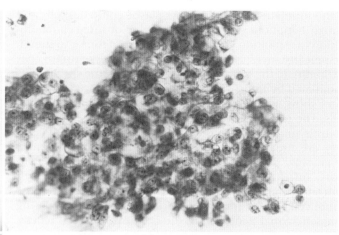

Figure 17-9 Thymic carcinomas. **A,** These obviously malignant cells have moderately sized nuclei with thick and variably contoured membranes. The chromatin is finely to coarsely granular and darkly stained. Some cells have obvious nucleoli. The cytoplasm is scanty resulting in high N:C ratios. Only rare lymphocytes are present in this field. (Pap) **B,** The cells have larger nuclei with more prominent membranes and much more distinct nucleoli. Hyperchromasia is obvious. The cells possess a greater volume of cytoplasm. No distinct differentiation is evident. (Pap) **C,** These malignant cells are characterized by large solitary nuclei with dense chromatin and scant to moderate volumes of cytoplasm. Rare cytoplasmic vacuoles are evident. In some cells, the nuclei appear peripherally located within the relatively scanty cytoplasm suggesting possible glandular differentiation. (DQ)

 BOX 17-1   CMF

Cytomorphologic Features of Thymoma

Moderate to high cellularity
Dual population of homogeneous neoplastic epithelial cells and lymphocytes
Variable intercellular cohesion among neoplastic cells
Tumor cells usually polygonal or ovoid, rarely spindled
Neoplastic nuclei have delicate membranes, bland chromatin, and small nucleoli

By contrast, thymic carcinomas are by definition composed of cytologically malignant cells (Figure 17-9).[35] Many of these will not demonstrate any evidence of specific epithelial differentiation. The malignant nuclei vary tremendously. In some, they are large and pleomorphic, with thick irregular membranes and large macronucleoli. Darkly stained chromatin and high nuclear-to-cytoplasmic (N:C) ratios are demonstrated. Infrequently, a spindle cell variant resembling a sarcoma may be encountered.

The cytomorphologic differential diagnosis of thymomas is that of lymphocyte-rich smears and thus includes malignant lymphomas, benign thymic hyperplasia, lymphoid hyperplasia of mediastinal lymph nodes, and germinomas. In addition, one might consider the possibility of a

metastasis from a well-differentiated carcinoma to either mediastinal lymph nodes or thymus (Table 17-1). In reaching a final diagnosis, it is important to integrate all clinical information with the aspiration cytomorphology and often the results of ancillary diagnostic procedures. Immunocytochemistry is probably the most helpful. With the exception of most non-Hodgkin's lymphomas, the majority of the lymphocytes in the other entities are small and mature in appearance. Sampling may prove problematic in some thymomas like the cystic type and the recently described micronodular variant.[10,19]

Thymic carcinomas engender a different differential diagnosis. It includes primary and metastatic germ cell neoplasms, particularly embryonal carcinoma, and metastatic carcinomas from other sites. The most common type of metastasis is non–small cell bronchogenic carcinoma. It may be impossible to distinguish these entities based purely on cytomorphology. In addition, immunocytochemistry may not be helpful in that cytokeratin positivity would characterize the neoplastic elements in all these tumors. Although not perfectly specific and sensitive, many thymic carcinomas are positive for CD5, and most germ cell neoplasms and metastatic carcinomas are negative.[36] The tumor cells of embryonal carcinoma may be immunopositive for placental alkaline phosphatase and α-fetoprotein. Many but not all large cell undifferentiated bronchogenic carcinomas are reactive with thyroid transcription factor 1, whereas primary thymic neoplasms would be expected to be negative.

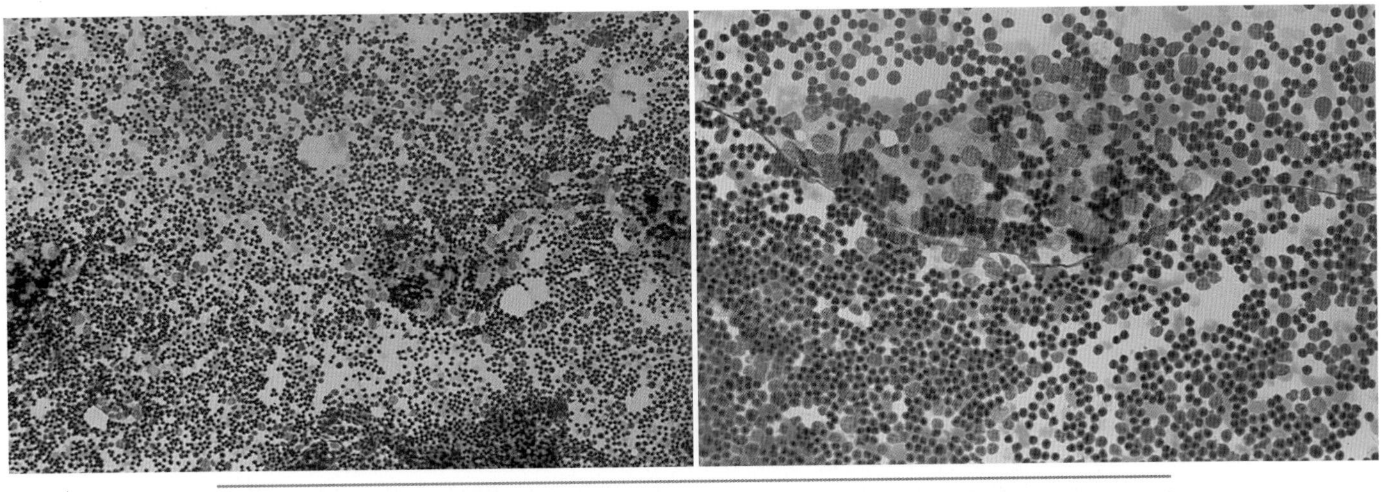

A

B

Figure 17-10 **True thymic hyperplasia. A,** Both individual and cohesive clusters of thymic epithelial cells are almost obscured by the numerous lymphocytes. The lymphoid elements are dissociated as single cells; they are dominated by small, mature-appearing lymphocytes, but larger lymphoid cells are also present. **B,** At higher magnification, the bland appearance of the thymic epithelium is evident. They have round nuclei with smooth delicate membranes, very finely reticulated uniformly dispersed chromatin, and inconspicuous nucleoli. Cytoplasm is scant to moderate and cell borders are ill defined. Lymphocytes not only surround but also infiltrate among the thymic epithelium. (DQ)

TABLE 17-1

Differential Diagnosis of Lymphocyte-Rich Aspirates

Diagnosis	Age Group	Lymphoid Cells	Tumor Cells	Immunohistochemistry
Thymoma	Middle-age adults	Small, mature	Bland nuclei, cohesion	CK+
Thymic hyperplasia	Any	Polymorphic, mostly small	—	B-cells
Non-Hodgkin's lymphoma	Children and young adults	Atypical, monomorphic	Atypical, monomorphic	LCA+
Hodgkin's disease	Children and young adults	Small, mature	Large, sparse	LeuM$_1$+
Germinoma	Young adults (males)	Small, mature	Large	CK±

CK, Cytokeratin; *LCA,* leukocyte common antigen.

THYMIC HYPERPLASIA

Thymic hyperplasia is an uncommon cause of enlargement of this organ. The two major varieties of thymic hyperplasia are follicular hyperplasia and true thymic hyperplasia.[37-42] Follicular hyperplasia is more common and typically occurs in association with myasthenia gravis; although the thymus is generally enlarged, it may not be. Histologically, well-developed lymphoid follicles with prominent germinal center formation are present within the pericapsular spaces at the periphery of the organ. Aspiration biopsies yield a polymorphous lymphoid picture with a predominance of small mature lymphocytes.[32,39] Lymphohistiocytic aggregates and tingible-body histiocytes are also found within the smears. Chhieng and colleagues have reported a case of an aspirate of follicular hyperplasia that occurred in association with a multiloculated cyst in a patient with human immunodeficiency virus (HIV). The aspiration smears morphologically resembled a thymoma.[43] By immunophenotyping, a greater proportion of aspirated lymphocytes is B cells, compared with thymoma.

The other form of hyperplasia is true thymic hyperplasia. The thymus is enlarged, but the histology recapitulates the normal gland completely. True thymic hyperplasia occurs in two major clinical scenarios. In children, it may occur as an idiopathic entity.[41] These pediatric patients may present with respiratory embarrassment and recurrent infections of the lung or are asymptomatic. The second type of true hyperplasia occurs in individuals who have experienced stressful situations including trauma or burns and patients with a variety of endocrine diseases, after the systemic administration of corticosteroids, and after the administration of cytotoxic chemotherapeutic for the therapy of a variety of malignancies (most commonly Hodgkin's disease).[32,38,42] Some have referred to this as a *rebound phenomenon,* in that the stress induces atrophy of the thymus. With removal of the stressful stimulus, a regrowth of the gland to an enlarged size occurs. Aspiration biopsies yield numerous lymphocytes, most of which are small and mature in type (Figure 17-10). However, a spectrum of lymphoid cells, including immunoblasts, is present, as are thymic epithelial cells. In several reported instances, this aspiration cytomorphology is so closely simulated by thymoma that surgery has been performed.[32,42]

In distinguishing thymoma from thymic hyperplasia in FNA biopsy, an accurate clinical history is imperative. For example, if the mass was known to develop subsequent to completion of a chemotherapy protocol or a major life-threatening stress, then hyperplasia should enter into the differential diagnosis.

 ## MALIGNANT LYMPHOMAS

The most common primary mediastinal neoplasms sampled by aspiration biopsy are malignant lymphomas.[3] Clinically, patients may present with symptoms related to the effects of a mass lesion, especially respiratory embarrassment, or invasion of adjacent structures. However, a large proportion of individuals are completely asymptomatic with the mass being discovered on a chest x-ray obtained for completely unrelated reasons. Although any form of lymphoma may secondarily involve the mediastinum, most primary lymphomas in this location represent one of three major types.[44-47] Both the large cell variant of non-Hodgkin's lymphoma and Hodgkin's disease most commonly affect young adult women, whereas teenage boys are the group most commonly involved by lymphoblastic lymphoma. The distinctions among these three forms are important because both therapies and prognoses differ. Chapter 24 provides a more detailed description of the aspiration cytomorphology of these three forms of lymphoma.[48-54]

Hodgkin's disease is the most common lymphoma primary in the mediastinum.[44] Most patients have the nodular sclerosing histologic variant. In many patients, peripheral lymph nodes, especially supraclavicular nodes, are also enlarged. The overall prognosis is excellent, with a 5-year survival rate exceeding 90%. The differential diagnosis of Hodgkin's disease includes benign lymphoid hyperplasia and thymic hyperplasia. In both of these conditions, the smears are dominated by a polymorphous lymphoid infiltrate with numerous small lymphoid cells. In addition, tingible-body macrophages and lymphohistiocytic aggregates may be well demonstrated in the smears. The key difference is the absence of Reed-Sternberg cells in both types of hyperplasia. A concerted effort must always be made to examine carefully the periphery of such smears in that a tendency exists for relatively large cells to be concentrated at the smears' edges. Fortunately, because of the Reed-Sternberg cells' large size, they can usually readily be seen at low magnification.

The differential diagnosis would also include Ki-1 positive anaplastic lymphoma, metastatic giant cell carcinomas, pleomorphic sarcomas, and primary choriocarcinoma. In the first of these entities, the appearance of the largest tumor cells may be even more bizarre than those seen in Hodgkin's disease; furthermore, the majority of the cells are not small mature lymphocytes but rather quite atypical and polymorphic. Some degree of intercellular cohesion is manifested in aspirates of choriocarcinoma, giant cell carcinoma, and most sarcomas. In addition, the number of malignant cells is usually much greater than one would expect to find in examples of Hodgkin's disease. It is important to recall that small or even moderately sized loose clusters of tumor cells may be seen in the syncytial variant.

Although they occur in the same clinical population, the large cell variants of non-Hodgkin's lymphoma should not provide morphologic difficulty in their separation. Aspiration smears are often much more highly cellular than Hodgkin's disease and are composed of relatively monomorphic atypical lymphoid cells. For the most part, the diagnosis of large cell lymphoma is straightforward, just as it is in aspiration biopsies of more peripheral lymph nodes. At times, pseudocohesion is evident as aggregates of malignant cells; such clumps could lead to confusion with epithelial neoplasms.[48] However, the vast majority of the tumor cells in smears should be individually dispersed. The large cell lymphomas primary in the mediastinum may be quite sclerotic; the dense collagen may compress the lymphoma cells, forcing them into a spindled or elongated contour.[51,52]

In children and young adults, lymphoblastic lymphoma is the most common cause of a malignant mediastinal mass. This high-grade lymphoma predominantly affects males. The vast majority of neoplasms are T-cell in type. The cytologic differential diagnosis of lymphoblastic lymphoma includes other small cell malignancies and benign lymphoid hyperplasia.[53,54] The only other small cell malignancy encountered with any frequency in the mediastinum in relatively young individuals is neuroblastoma. In contrast with lymphoblastic lymphoma, these neoplasms typically occur in the posterior compartment and involve younger patients. The cytomorphology should permit an easy distinction with the presence of true intercellular cohesion, including pseudorosette formation, variable numbers of larger neoplastic ganglion cells, and a fibrillary background[55] (Table 17-2).

 ## GERM CELL NEOPLASMS

In adults, the mediastinum is the most common site of origin of extragonadal germ cell neoplasms.[56-58] In children, the mediastinum follows the sacrococcygeal region as a site of origin for these tumors. The majority of all mediastinal

TABLE 17-2
Differential Diagnosis of Small Cell Tumors

Diagnosis	Compartment	Age	Cytology
Small cell carcinoma	Any	Adults, smokers	Molding; dark chromatin
Neuroblastoma	Posterior	Child	Delicate chromatin; rosettes; neuropil
Lymphoblastic ML	Anterosuperior	Child, young adult	No cohesion; lymphoglandular bodies

ML, Malignant lymphoma.

germ cell neoplasms are benign cystic teratomas that affect women and men with relatively equal frequency. However, among the malignant germ cell tumors, men are much more often affected than are women. Of these cancers, by far the most common is germinoma. Rarely, mediastinal germ cell malignancies arise in association with lymphoreticular (hematologic) neoplasms.

Aspiration biopsies of germinomas produce moderately to highly cellular samples that are comprised of large homogeneous tumor cells with little preservation of intercellular cohesion.[59,60] Each malignant cell is characterized by a solitary large nucleus with a thick, obvious membrane, a vesicular chromatin, and one or more large nucleoli. The cytoplasm appears to be fragile because it is often stripped away from the nuclei. Thus, a large proportion of the tumor cells have relatively scanty volumes of cytoplasm with irregular frayed edges. Stripped malignant nuclei are also present with some frequency. However, within cohesive aggregates, cellular borders are typically well defined. The cytoplasm varies from optically clear to dense and cyanophilic. The smear background characteristically appears frothy or bubbly; this is often referred to as having a *tigroid appearance.* This is related to the fragility of the glycogen-rich cytoplasm. The smears also contain numerous small mature lymphoid cells and possibly epithelioid cells and multinucleated histiocytic elements (Box 17-2).

Due to the relative lack of intercellular cohesion and the appearance of the germinoma cells themselves, the differential diagnosis includes large cell lymphoma.[6] However, the latter contains more irregularly shaped nuclei, show no evidence of true cohesion, and has numerous lymphoglandular bodies in the background. For examples of germinoma, in which cohesion is rather well maintained, thymic carcinomas, embryonal carcinomas, and carcinomas metastatic to mediastinal lymph nodes must also be considered in the differential diagnosis.[6] None of these should possess the characteristic tigroid background. The latter, although not completely pathognomonic for germinoma, is extremely suggestive of this diagnosis.

Pure nongerminomatous malignant germ cell tumors are infrequent as primary neoplasms of the mediastinum. Yolk sac tumors (endodermal sinus tumors) are more common in children than they are in adults. These high-grade neoplasms may be associated with elevations in the serum level of alpha-fetoprotein. Histologically, yolk sac tumors are composed of small malignant epithelial cells in a wide variety of architectural patterns, often associated with intercellular basement membrane–like material.[56] The cytomorphologic picture of yolk sac tumors in aspirates reflect this histologic heterogeneity. However, overall, the cells are rather uniform in appearance.[60] They typically have polygonal to somewhat elongated contours, visible and frequently vacuolated basophilic cytoplasm, and solitary nuclei with prominent or at least distinct nucleoli. With the Romanowsky stain, the extracellular matrix material is metachromatic. The neoplastic cells may be individually dispersed, present in spherical or papillary clusters, or embedded within the matrix material. The latter appears as a faint green substance with the Pap stain.

Pure embryonal carcinoma of the mediastinum is a rare primary neoplasm. These are extremely aggressive tumors that typically result in a rapid patient demise, despite modern chemotherapeutic agents. FNA biopsy yields cellular smears that are obviously malignant and epithelial.[60] Large, rather uniform carcinoma cells are displayed as spheres, syncytial sheets, and papillae (Figure 17-11). They are characterized by huge nuclei with visible membranes, dark and irregularly distributed chromatin, massive nucleoli, and

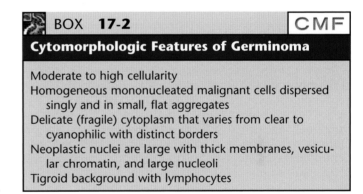

BOX 17-2 CMF

Cytomorphologic Features of Germinoma

Moderate to high cellularity
Homogeneous mononucleated malignant cells dispersed singly and in small, flat aggregates
Delicate (fragile) cytoplasm that varies from clear to cyanophilic with distinct borders
Neoplastic nuclei are large with thick membranes, vesicular chromatin, and large nucleoli
Tigroid background with lymphocytes

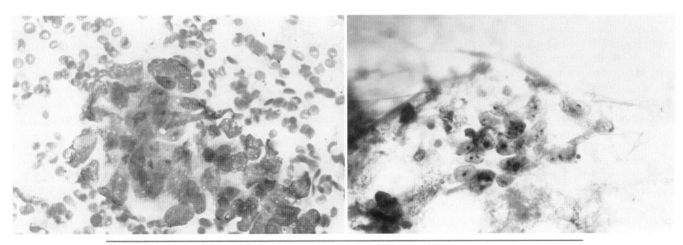

Figure 17-11 **Embryonal carcinoma.** Large, undifferentiated epithelial cells are characterized by solitary huge nuclei with smooth to irregular outlines, generally finely reticulated chromatin, and distinct nucleoli. Although most of the malignant cells have high N:C ratios, primitive acinar formation is suggested. (DQ, Pap)

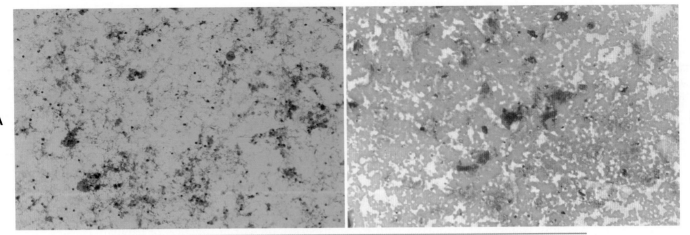

Figure 17-12   Benign cystic teratoma. **A,** This poorly cellular smear consists of rare benign nucleated squamous cells, infrequent anucleated squames, proteinaceous debris, and a sparse mixed inflammatory cell infiltrate. (Pap) **B,** Moderate numbers of anucleated squamous cells are present. (DQ)

rather high N:C ratios. Based purely on cytomorphology, they may be impossible to distinguish from metastases of other high-grade carcinomas.

Pure nongestational choriocarcinoma primary in the mediastinum is an exceedingly rare neoplasm. Essentially, all cases have occurred in young adult men. Only a solitary example of FNA biopsy of a primary mediastinal choriocarcinoma has been reported.[60] In this specimen, smear cellularity was scanty, probably the result of abundant necrosis that was seen subsequently in the mass histologically. These smears contained clearly malignant large tumor cells both individually and in relatively small cohesive aggregates. Both cytotrophoblasts and syncytiotrophoblasts were present. The nuclei had variable chromatin that spanned the spectrum from finely reticulated to dense and homogeneous. Nuclear outlines were irregular, and prominent nucleoli were evident. Tumor cell cytoplasm was moderate to voluminous and dense and amphophilic, and often possessed numerous small vacuoles. Choriocarcinoma certainly is among the most pleomorphic and anaplastic of all primary mediastinal malignancies. If the dual tumor cell population is correctly recognized, then the diagnosis is likely to be made, despite the rarity of the neoplasm. The differential diagnosis would need to include large cell undifferentiated carcinoma metastatic to the mediastinum from the lung or similar neoplasms arising in organs such as thyroid and pancreas. Patients with the latter neoplasms would likely be much older than those with a primary choriocarcinoma. By immunocytochemistry, the malignant cells are positive for human chorionic gonadotrophin. As is typically the case, tumor burden is often huge, and in such patients, a urine pregnancy test is positive.

As stated previously, the most common primary germ cell neoplasm of the mediastinum is the teratoma. Most of these are histologically mature and benign. They occur through a broad age range, although they are most common in young adults. These neoplasms may present almost as a pure cyst or mixed solid and cystic mass. Histologically, the contributions from the different germ cell layers are completely mature in their appearance. The major component of these cystic teratomas is usually unremarkable stratified squamous epithelium with keratin production. In as-

pirates, one sees mostly anucleated squamous cells, possibly mixed with viable mature squamous elements (Figure 17-12). The differential diagnosis would include a thymic cyst. The presence of cutaneous adnexal elements or other forms of mature epithelium and mesenchyme supports the diagnosis of teratoma. However, the possibility exists that these elements might be inadvertently picked up by the needle en route to the mass and have nothing to do with the tumor.

Only a small proportion of all teratomas arising within the mediastinum are histologically immature—that is, they are characterized by one or more cellular components that appear less differentiated or fetal in type. Most often, the major component in immature teratomas is neural. Immature teratomas may yield cellular samples that most commonly are dominated by small neuroblastic cells.[60] The latter are characterized by small, round hyperchromatic nuclei, inconspicuous nucleoli, and very high N:C ratios. These cells are typically situated within a fibrillary matrix material, which aids in distinguishing them from the cells of a hematopoietic malignancy. This matrix stains pinkish-gray with the Romanowsky stains and green with the Pap stain. The differential diagnosis would need to include primary mediastinal and metastatic neuroblastoma. Primary mediastinal neuroblastomas usually occur in young individuals as a posterior compartment mass that may be associated with an increase in serum catecholamine levels. Germ cell tumors, including teratomas, on the other hand, almost always arise in the anterior compartment.

NEUROENDOCRINE NEOPLASMS

Primary neuroendocrine neoplasms may arise in the thymus.[61-63] Corresponding to their ultimately aggressive clinical course, these neoplasms histologically are best characterized as an atypical or malignant carcinoid tumor, as described for the lung. Chapters 15 and 16, dedicated to this organ, detail the grading of neuroendocrine carcinomas. The majority of patients with thymic carcinoids are either identified as a result of the effects of a mass lesion or are

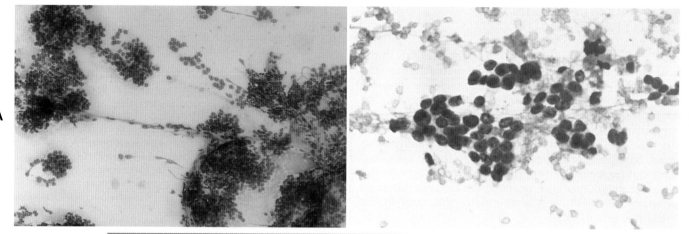

Figure 17-13 Carcinoid tumor. **A,** Large cohesive fragments of homogeneous neoplastic cells dominate the smear. Some of the aggregates appear to be intimately associated with capillaries. The tumor cells are small with solitary uniform slightly ovoid nuclei and high N:C ratios. (DQ) **B,** The chromatin is seen as homogeneous and fairly darkly stained; nucleoli are not evident. Cytoplasm is barely perceptible. However, well-developed nuclear molding is not evident. (Pap)

TABLE 17-3				
Differential Diagnosis of Spindle Cell Tumors				
Diagnosis	**Compartment**	**Cell Pattern**	**Nuclear Shape**	**Immunochemistry**
Thymoma	Anterosuperior	Bundles, sheets	Smooth	CK+
Carcinoid	Anterosuperior	Sheets, rosettes	Smooth	CK+
				SYN+
PNST	Posterior	Fascicles, palisading	Wavy	S100 protein+

PNST, Peripheral nerve sheath tumor; *CK,* cytokeratin; *SYN,* synaptophysin.
NOTE: Plus signs (+) refer to positivity.

asymptomatic, with the tumor discovered incidentally on a chest x-ray obtained for unrelated purposes. However, one third of these patients come to clinical attention because of systemic endocrine findings, which almost always are diagnosed as Cushing's syndrome. Aspiration biopsies yield moderately to highly cellular smears dominated by cohesive aggregates of small homogeneous polygonal neoplastic cells (Figure 17-13).[64,65] A minority of tumors are composed of spindle-shaped cells.[66] At low magnification, one may even appreciate a suggestion of an anastomosing trabecular pattern. With the Romanowsky stains, the chromatin is finely reticulated and evenly disbursed throughout the nucleus. With alcohol fixation and Pap staining, the chromatin appears finely granular, uniformly distributed, and darkly stained. Small nucleoli may or may not be evident. These cells have high N:C ratios and only thin rims of basophilic cytoplasm surround the round to ovoid nuclei. Within the cohesive aggregates, mild nuclear molding and rosette formation may be apparent.

Rarely, primary small cell carcinomas, morphologically indistinguishable from primary neoplasm of the lung, arise in the thymus. Their aspiration cytomorphology is indistinguishable from that of other small cell carcinomas.

NEUROGENIC NEOPLASMS

Neurogenic neoplasms account for the majority of all tumors arising within the posterior compartment.[7] The two major groups are tumors of peripheral nerve sheath origin and of neuroectodermal derivation; the former is more common. Most of these are benign schwannomas or neurofibromas. These tumors typically occur in young adults and most commonly as asymptomatic masses found on chest films. Malignant neoplasms of peripheral nerve sheath origin may also arise in this compartment; these are much more apt to present clinically as a result of the effects of a mass lesion. Neuroectodermal tumors are much more likely to be malignant and to occur in children. The latter category includes neuroblastoma, ganglioneuroblastoma, and ganglioneuroma. Both groups are amenable to diagnosis by FNA biopsy.[67]

Chapter 28 provides a detailed description of the aspiration cytomorphology of benign and malignant nerve sheath tumors. Similarly, the neuroectodermal neoplasms are described in Chapter 23. With the nerve sheath neoplasms, a rather limited differential diagnosis of primary mediastinal spindle cell neoplasms is brought forward[68] (Table 17-3).

INTRAMEDIASTINAL THYROID TISSUE

A small but significant proportion of all mass lesions in the mediastinum are intrathoracic thyroid parenchyma. The vast majority of these occur in the anterosuperior compartments as a downward extension of a cervical goiter. The vast majority of these represent benign nonneoplastic hyperplasia and/or degeneration of thyroid parenchyma. Thus, the aspiration smears contain various quantities of colloid, flat sheets of benign follicular epithelial cells, and foamy and pigmented histiocytes. Rarely, both benign and malignant neoplasms arise in intrathoracic thyroid. Their aspiration cytomorphology recapitulates that seen in the thyroid (see Chapter 26).

INTRAMEDIASTINAL PARATHYROID TISSUE

Both hyperplasia and neoplasms of parathyroid tissue occur in the anterosuperior mediastinum. Although some of these arise from ectopic mediastinal parathyroid glands, others are the result of descent from a cervical location. Most appear as a small mass near or even within the thymus. However, hypercalcemia is the herald of most lesions. Occasionally, such lesions may undergo prominent cystic change and therefore need to be distinguished from other mediastinal cysts. In this situation, the smears may be extremely poorly cellular. If suspected before the aspiration biopsy, then an aliquot of the cyst fluid can be biochemically analyzed for the levels of parathyroid hormone that should be expected to be quite high.[70]

METASTASES

The most common indication for aspiration biopsy of the mediastinum is to document the presence of metastasis. Often, this represents a secondary lesion in a patient with a previously diagnosed cancer, but in other cases, it represents the first morphologic evaluation of the neoplasm. The authors have found this to be most common with transbronchial aspirates of mediastinal lymph nodes in patients suspected of having small cell carcinoma of the lung. In a large multi-institutional study of mediastinal aspiration biopsies, Powers and colleagues found that most neoplasms represented metastases.[3] In that study, two thirds were derived from the lung, and were most commonly small cell carcinomas. The second most common site of origin was carcinoma of the breast.

References

1. Westcott JL. Percutaneous aspiration of hilar and mediastinal masses. Radiology 1981; 141:323.
2. Sterett G, Whitaker D, Shilkin KB, et al. The fine needle aspiration cytology of mediastinal lesions. Cancer 1983; 51:127.
3. Powers CN, Silverman JF, Geisinger KR, et al. Fine-needle aspiration biopsy of the mediastinum: a multiinstitutional analysis. Am J Clin Pathol 1996; 105:168.
4. Fritscher-Ravens A, Sriram PV, Babrowski C, et al. Mediastinal lymphadenopathy in patients with or without previous malignancy: EUS-FNA-based differential cytodiagnosis in 153 patients. Am J Gastroenterol 2000; 95:2278-2284.
5. Panelli F, Erickson RA, Prasad VM. Evaluation of mediastinal masses by endoscopic ultrasound and endoscopic ultrasound-guided fine needle aspiration. Am J Gastroenterol 2001; 96:401-408.
6. Geisinger KR. Differential diagnostic considerations and potential pitfalls in fine needle aspiration biopsies of the mediastinum. Diagn Cytopathol 1995; 13:436-442.
7. Wick M. The mediastinum. In: Sternberg SS, Antonioli DA, Carter D, et al, editors. Diagnostic surgical pathology. 3rd ed. Philadelphia: Lippincott Williams and Wilkins; 1999. pp.1147-1208.
8. Powers CN, Geisinger KR. Fine needle aspiration biopsy of the mediastinum: an overview. Pathol Case Rev 2001; 6:49-58.
9. Suster S, Rosai J. Multilocular thymic cyst: an acquired reactive process (a study of 18 cases). Am J Surg Pathol 1991; 15:388-398.
10. Suster S, Rosai J. Cystic thymomas: a clinicopathologic study of 10 cases. Cancer 1992; 69:92-97.
11. Wakely PJ. Thymic cysts: an association with thymic neoplasia. Pathol Case Rev 2001; 6:59-63.
12. Walker AN, Mills SE, Fechner RE. Thymomas and thymic carcinomas. Semin Diagn Pathol 1990; 7:250.
13. Kuo T-T, Lo S-K. Thymoma: a study of the pathologic classification of 71 cases with evaluation of the Müller-Hermelink system. Hum Pathol 1993; 24:776.
14. Morgenthaler IT, Brown LR, Colby TV, et al. Thymoma. Mayo Clinic Proc 1993; 68:1110.
15. Park HS, Shin DM, Lee JS, et al. Thymoma: a retrospective study of 87 cases. Cancer 1994; 73:2491.
16. Ramon Y, Cajal S, Suster S. Primary thymic epithelial neoplasms in children. Am J Surg Pathol 1991; 15:466.
17. Ho FCS, Fu KH, Lam SY, et al. Evaluation of a histogenic classification for thymic epithelial tumors. Histopathology 1994; 25:21.
18. Quintanilla-Martinez L, Wilkins EW Jr, Choi N, et al. Thymoma: histologic subclassification is an independent prognostic factor. Cancer 1994; 74:606-617.
19. Suster S, Moran CA. Micronodular thymoma with lymphoid B-cell hyperplasia. Clinicopathologic and immunohistochemical study of eighteen cases of a distinctive morphologic variant of thymic epithelial neoplasm. Am J Surg Pathol 1999; 23:955-962.
20. Bernatz PE, Harrison EG Jr, Clagett TO. Thomoma: a clinicopathologic study. J Thorac Cardiovasc Surg 1961; 42:424-444.
21. Marino M, Müller-Hermelink HK. Thymoma and thymic carcinoma: relation of thymoma epithelial cells to the cortical and medullary differentiation of thymus. Virchows Arch A Pathologic Anat Histopathol 1985; 407:119.
22. Kircher T, Schalke B, Buchwald J, et al. Well-differentiated thymic carcinoma. An organotypical low-grade carcinoma with relationship to cortical thymoma. Am J Surg Pathol 1992; 16:1153.
23. Suster S, Moran CA. Primary thymic epithelial neoplasms showing combined features of thymoma and thymic carcinoma. A clinicopathologic study of 22 cases. Am J Surg Pathol 1996; 20:1469-1480.
24. Suster S, Moran CA. Thymoma, atypical thymoma, and thymic carcinoma. A novel conceptual approach to the classification of thymic epithelial neoplasm. Am J Clin Pathol 1999; 111:826-833.

25. Snover DC, Levine GD, Rosai J. Thymic carcinoma: five distinctive histological variants. Am J Surg Pathol 1982; 6:451.
26. Ritter JH, Wick MR. Primary carcinomas of the thymus gland. Sem Diagn Pathol 1999; 16:18-31.
27. Pak HY, Yokota SB, Friedberg HA. Thymoma diagnosed by transthoracic fine needle aspiration. Acta Cytol 1982; 26:210.
28. Dahlgreen S, Sandstedt B, Sundstrom C. Fine needle aspiration cytology of thymic tumors. Acta Cytol 1983; 27:1.
29. Tao LC, Pearson FG, Cooper JD, et al. Cytopathology of thymoma. Acta Cytol 1984; 28:165.
30. Sherman ME, Black-Schaffer S. Diagnosis of thymoma by needle biopsy. Acta Cytol 1990; 34:63-68.
31. Ali SZ, Erozan YS. Thymoma: cytopathologic features and differential diagnosis of fine needle aspiration. Acta Cytol 1998; 42:845-854.
32. Shin HJ, Katz RL. Thymic neoplasia as represented by fine needle aspiration biopsy of anterior mediastinal masses: a practical approach to the differential diagnosis. Acta Cytol 1998; 42:855-864.
33. Friedman HD, Hutchison RE, Kohman LJ, et al. Thymoma mimicking thyroid papillary carcinoma: another pitfall in fine-needle aspiration. Diagn Cytopathol 1996; 17:61-63.
34. Riazmontazer N, Beydat C, Izadi B. Epithelial cytologic atypia in fine needle aspirate of an invasive thymoma: a case report. Acta Cytol 1992; 36:387.
35. Finely JL, Silverman JF, Strausbauch P, et al. Malignant thymic neoplasms: diagnosis of fine-needle aspiration biopsy with histologic, immunocytochemical, and ultrastructural confirmation. Diagn Cytopathol 1986; 2:118.
36. Kornstein JM et al. CD5 labeling in thymic carcinoma and other nonlymphoid neoplasms. Am J Clin Pathol 1998; 190:722-726.
37. Levine OD, Rosai J. Thymic hyperplasia and neoplasia: a review of current concepts. Hum Pathol 1978; 9:495.
38. Carmosino L, DiBenedetto A, Feffer S. Thymic hyperplasia following successful chemotherapy: a report of two cases and review of the literature. Cancer 1985; 56:1526-1528.
39. Riazmontazer N, Bedayat G. Aspiration cytology of an enlarged thymus presenting as a mediastinal mass: a case report. Acta Cytol 1993; 37:427-430.
40. Bangerter M, Behnisch W, Griesshammer M. Mediastinal masses diagnosed as thymus hyperplasia by fine needle aspiration cytology. Acta Cytol 2000; 44:743-747.
41. Hoerl HD, Wojtowycz M, Gallagher HA, Kurtyz DF. Cytologic diagnosis of true thymic hyperplasia by combined radiologic imaging and apsiration cytology: a case report including flow cytometric analysis. Diagn Cytopathol 2000; 23:417-421.
42. Geisinger KR, Woodruff RD, Cappellari JO. True thymic hyperplasia following cytotoxic chemotherapy: a cause of a false positive aspiration biopsy. Pathol Case Rev 2001; 6:64-67.
43. Chhieng DC, Demaria S, Yee HT, Yang GC. Multilocular thymic cyst with follicular lymphoid hyperplasia in a male infected with HIV: a case report with fine needle aspiration cytology. Acta Cytol 1999; 43:1119-1123.
44. Strickler JG, Kurtin PJ. Mediastinal lymphoma. Semin Diagn Pathol 1991; 8:2.
45. Perrone T, Frizzera G, Rosai J. Mediastinal diffuse large-cell lymphoma with sclerosis: a clinicopathologic study of 60 cases. Am J Surg Pathol 1986; 10:176.
46. Lamarre L, Jacobson JO, Alsenberg AC, et al. Primary large cell lymphoma of the mediastinum: a histologic and immunophenotypic study of 29 cases. Am J Surg Pathol 1989; 13:730.
47. Sheibani K, Nathwani BN, Winberg CD, et al. Antigenically defined subgroups of lymphoblastic lymphoma: relationship to clinical presentation and biological behavior. Cancer 1987; 60:183.
48. Geisinger KR et al. Lymph nodes. In: Geisinger KR, Silverman JF, editors. Fine needle aspiration cytology of superficial organs and body sites. New York: Churchill Livingstone; 1999.
49. Kardos TF, Vinson JH, Behm FG, et al. Hodgkin's disease: diagnosis by fine needle aspiration biopsy: analysis of cytologic criteria from a selected series. Am J Clin Pathol 1986; 86:286.
50. Moriarity A, Banks E, Block T. Cytologic criteria for subclassification of Hodgkin's disease using fine needle aspiration. Diagn Cytopathol 1998; 5:122.
51. Silverman JF, Raab SS, Park HK. Fine-needle aspiration cytology of primary large cell lymphoma of the mediastinum: cytomorphologic findings with potential pitfalls in diagnosis. Diagn Cytopathol 1993; 9:209.
52. Singh HK, Silverman JF, Powers CN, et al. Diagnostic pitfalls in fine-needle aspiration biopsy of the mediastinum. Diagn Cytopathol 1997; 17:121-126.
53. Kardos TF, Sprague RI, Wakely PE Jr, Frable WJ. Fine aspiration biopsy of lymphoblastic lymphoma and leukemia: a clinical, cytologic, and immunologic study. Cancer 1987; 60:2448.
54. Jacobs JC, Katz RL, Shabb N, et al. Fine needle aspiration of lymphoblastic lymphoma: a multiparameter approach. Acta Cytol 1992; 36:887.
55. Silverman FJ, Dabbs DJ, Ganick DJ, et al. Fine needle aspiration cytology of neuroblastoma including peripheral neuroectodermal tumor with immunocytochemical and ultrastructural confirmation. Acta Cytol 1988; 32:367.
56. Dehner LP. Germ cell tumors of the mediastinum. Semin Diagn Pathol 1990; 7:266.
57. Hoffmann OA, Gillespie DJ, Aughenbaugh GL, Grown LR. Primary mediastinal neoplasms (other than thymoma). May Clin Proc 1993; 68:880.
58. Dulmet EM, Maechiarini P, Suc B, et al. Germ cell tumors of the mediastinum: a 30-year experience. Cancer 1993; 72:1984.
59. Akhtar M, Ali MA, Hug M, et al. Fine-needle aspiration biopsy of seminoma and dysgerminoma: cytologic, histologic and electron microscopic correlations. Diagn Cytopathol 1990; 6:99.
60. Collins KA, Geisinger KK, Wakely P Jr, et al. Extragonadal germ cell tumors: a fine needle aspiration biopsy study. Diagn Cytopathol 1995; 12:223.
61. Wick MR, Rosai J. Neuroendocrine neoplasms of the mediastinum. Semin Diagn Pathol 1991; 8:35.
62. Moran CA, Suster S. Spindle-cell neuroendocrine carcinomas of the thymus (spindle-cell thymic carcinoid): a clinicopathologic and immunohistochemical study of seven cases. Mod Pathol 1999; 12:587-591.
63. Moran CA, Suster S. Neuroendocrine carcinoma of the thymus. Pathol Case Rev 2001; 6:41-48.
64. Wang D-Y, Kuo S-H, Chang D-B, et al. Fine needle aspiration cytology of thymic carcinoid tumor. Acta Cytol 1995; 39:423.
65. Nichols GL Jr, Hopkins MB 3rd, Geisinger KR. Thymic carcinoid: report of a case with diagnosis by fine needle aspiration biopsy. Acta Cytol 1997; 41:1839-1884.
66. Dusenbery D. Spindle-cell thymic carcinoid occurring in multiple endocrine neoplasia I: fine-needle aspiration findings in a case. Diagn Cytopathol 1996; 15:435-441.
67. Geisinger KR, Abdul-Karim FW. Fine needle aspiration biopsies of soft tissue tumors. In: Enzinger X, Weiss X. Soft tissue tumors. 4th ed. St. Louis: Mosby; 2001. pp.147-188.

68. Slagel DD, Powers CN, Melaragno MJ, et al. Spindle-cell lesions of the mediastinum: diagnosis by fine-needle aspiration biopsy. Diagn Cytopathol 1997; 17:167-176.

69. Johnson SB, Eng TY, Giaccone G, et al. Thomoma: update for the new millenium. Oncologist 2001; 6:239-246.

70. Abati A, Skarulis MC, Shawker T, et al. Ultrasound-guided fine-needle aspiration of parathyroid lesions: a morphological and immunocytochemical approach. Hum Pathol 1995; 26:338-343.

71. Okumura M. Ohta M, Tateyama H, et al. The World Health Organization histologic classification reflects the oncologic behavior of thymoma: a clinical study of 273 cases. Cancer 2002; 94:624-632.

72. Suster S, Moran CA. Primary thymic epithelial neoplasms: spectrum of differentiation and histological features. Sem Diagn Pathol 1999; 16:2-17.

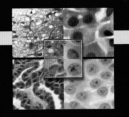

ABDOMEN

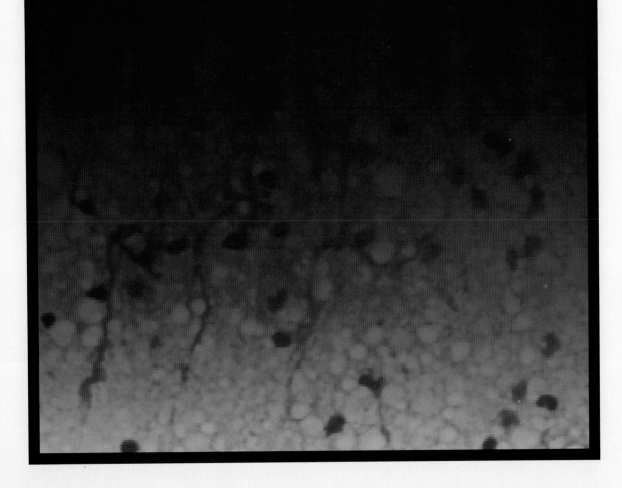

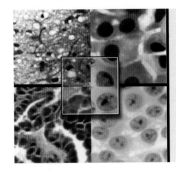

CHAPTER
18

Gastrointestinal System

The gastrointestinal (GI) tract is involved with a variety of inflammatory and neoplastic disorders that have been better described and categorized in the surgical pathology than the cytology literature. In the past, the cytomorphologic description of these GI lesions has been limited, despite the fact that most of these clinically significant diseases, with a few exceptions, involve the mucosal surface.[1-5]

With the widespread use of flexible fiberoptic endoscopy, GI pathology is now experiencing a rapid growth.[1-4] Numerous recent studies have demonstrated that endoscopically obtained tissue biopsies with concurrent cytology specimens are diagnostically complementary because performance of both procedures results in greater sensitivity and specificity than biopsy alone.[2,3] Moreover, exfoliative cytology has several advantages over tissue biopsies, based mainly on the ability of the endoscopic brush to sample epithelial cells and organisms from a wider surface area of the mucosa than the more targeted tissue biopsy.[1-7] This greater sampling of the mucosa is especially valuable in surveillance programs for patients with Barrett's esophagus and ulcerative colitis in which the dysplastic mucosa and early carcinomas may not be endoscopically distinct from the surrounding benign mucosa. Exfoliative cytology also benefits from the principle that dysplastic and malignant cells have a lower level of intercellular cohesion than normal cells, allowing the endoscopic brush procedure to selectively sample these discohesive elements. The brushing cytology procedure is often more successful for sampling neoplasms and other lesions that occur in stenotic areas of the GI and hepatobiliary tract, when compared with tissue obtained by biopsy forceps. The collection of cytology specimens is also less traumatic and less expensive than histologic examination. This may be especially valuable in large surveillance programs in which numerous endoscopic biopsies are obtained.[3,8,9] In addition, biopsy of certain types of specimens such as lymphoid lesions is prone to crush artifact; therefore, the cytologic specimen may be more diagnostic. Exfoliative cytology may have a more rapid turnaround time than is usually obtained with biopsy specimens.

Despite these advantages, cytology is currently underused in the workup of patients with GI or hepatobiliary disease. A common theme that is presented throughout this chapter is the complementary value of both cytology and histology resulting in an increased diagnostic yield.

 ## SPECIMEN COLLECTION AND PREPARATION

GI cytology has been underused in the workup of GI diseases, due in part to the lack of satisfactory methods for collecting large numbers of normal, dysplastic, and neoplastic well-preserved cells from these sites.[2,3] In the past, the primary method used to obtain samples from the upper and lower GI tracts has been lavage cytology. This procedure involves instilling large volumes of fluid (usually saline) either orally or rectally and then maneuvering the patients in various positions so that the fluid contacts the entire mucosal surface of the hollow viscus, facilitating mucosal sampling. Obviously, this procedure was not well tolerated by either patients or medical personnel, although some renewed interest exists in the performance of washing cytology in the evaluation of patients with large intestinal adenocarcinomas or endoscopically inapparent lesions. Various methodologies have been employed to concentrate the lavage cytology specimens, such as cytocentrifugation, liquid-based preparations (LBPs), cell blocks, and direct smears.

With the introduction of the flexible fiberoptic endoscope, the new diagnostic era for GI cytology began because brushing cytology could now directly sample any grossly evident mucosal abnormality. The flexible fiberoptic endoscope not only allowed the transmission of visual images of the GI tract but also had the ability to transverse the tortuous lumen of this hollow viscus. Colonoscopes are even more flexible than endoscopes, and both types of scopes can undergo retroflexion so that the endoscopists can better visualize the mucosa. Endoscopes are equipped with a channel through which biopsy forceps and cytologic brushes can be passed. The cytologic brushes are most often composed of nylon that can be either disposable or reusable following sterilization. A protected sheath prevents loss of the cellular material as the brush is removed from the endoscope. Cytologic brushing samples are most often prepared by direct smearing of the contents of the brushes on the slides. It is recommended that the cytologic brushing be obtained before taking endoscopic tissue biopsies so that the cytologic specimen is not diluted by blood.[10,11]

Salvage cytology specimens are based on the principle of retrieving and processing material that is initially present on the external surface of the biopsy forceps but was dislodged after withdrawal of the forceps through the biopsy channel. The channel is flushed with saline or a fixative. This fluid is collected in a mucous trap from which the cellular material is concentrated for processing, either as smears or a cell block. This procedure is complementary to biopsies and is believed by some to be more expeditious than doing concurrent brushing cytology.[12-14]

Transmucosal fine-needle aspiration (FNA) biopsy is a newer cytologic technique for sampling lesions located in the wall of the GI tract. It is used to sample lesions that cannot be reached by either lavage or brushing cytology due to an intact overlying mucosa. Transmucosal FNA cytology has been especially useful for diagnosing submucosal neoplasms such as carcinoid tumors and malignant lymphomas, stenotic tumors, lesions that are diffusely infiltrative, or necrotic.[15-19] As in other types of FNA biopsies, direct smears and/or cell blocks can be prepared.

Transmucosal FNA biopsy of intramural GI masses and of lesions located in adjacent organs or tissues has recently enjoyed a great flowering. This is due to the development of GI endoscopes fitted with ultrasound transducers. Endoscopic ultrasound (EUS) allows real-time visualization of the mass, its surroundings, and the aspirating needle. Accurate needle placement permits sampling of most lesions. Doppler capabilities improve identification of blood vessels so that they can be both avoided by the needle and evaluated for invasion by a malignancy. Many masses that can be localized, characterized, and sampled with EUS guidance are poorly visualized with computed tomography (CT) scans.

In addition to intramural GI tract masses, EUS has been used successfully to sample lesions in the pancreas, liver, lymph nodes, adrenal glands, lung, and retroperitoneum. Its most frequent application is sampling of pancreatic masses, and this is discussed in more detail in Chapter 21. Most upper GI tract carcinomas are initially diagnosed with mucosal biopsy. Then EUS can be used to sample regional lymph nodes and to evaluate possible vascular invasion. The staging information thus obtained is often instrumental in tailoring a patient's therapy. Positive lymph nodes or vascular invasion usual render a malignancy unresectable; these individuals can be triaged to chemotherapy or radiation treatment, without the need for exploratory surgery.

In the case of lymphadenopathy without a mucosal abnormality, EUS-guided FNA biopsy can identify granulomatous inflammation or malignant lymphoma and lead the clinical team along still other therapeutic pathways. The samples obtained are suitable for microbiologic culture or for flow cytometric immunophenotyping. Preparation of paraffin-embedded cell blocks in the manner outlined in Chapter 2 makes the aspirated material available for the full armamentarium of special stains and immunohistochemistry that characterize the modern laboratory of surgical pathology.

As noted in Chapter 2, FNA biopsy is often preferable to core biopsy because it leaves most tumor stroma behind as it extracts and concentrates a nearly pure population of ma-

lignant cells. This is especially useful in the consideration of adenocarcinomas of the pancreas and biliary tract. The volume of many such neoplasms is often made up largely of collagenous stroma. Core biopsies may be difficult to interpret, as they contain little of the diagnostic epithelial component. FNA concentrates the diagnostic component and facilitates confident interpretation.

Touch imprint cytology of tissue biopsy specimens has been used as a complementary procedure at the time of biopsy because of enhanced diagnostic yield as the cytologic preparations provide superior morphologic detail and better demonstrate organisms and have less loss of mucoid material.[20,21] Touch imprints do not compromise the histologic examination of the biopsies.

Cytologic samples obtained by brushings are most often prepared as direct smears that require rapid fixation. This is seen as a disadvantage because if immediate fixation is not accomplished, air-drying artifacts can compromise the cytologic examination. However, obtaining air-dried smears that are subsequently stained with Romanowsky type stains may circumvent this problem. These preparations are better for evaluating organisms because of their larger sizes in these types of smears. Alternatively, others have preferred to rinse the material from the brush in a preservative solution so that cytocentrifuged slides or LBPs can be prepared.[21,22] These techniques can also be applied to washing and salvage cytology specimens.[23] In most laboratories, the Pap stain is applied to alcohol-fixed material, although others have preferred Romanowsky stains or hematoxylin and eosin (H&E).[24,25] Applications of ancillary studies such as immunocytochemistry and image morphometry have been relatively limited for the evaluation of GI tract lesions.

Other abrasive sampling techniques have been employed in addition to visually directed brushing cytology. The most common of these is a balloonlike sampling device that has been used primarily to evaluate esophageal lesions. The balloon device is swallowed in its deflated state and passed into the stomach where it is then inflated and pulled back through the gastroesophageal junction, thereby sampling the entire mucosal surface. The balloon is then deflated at the level of the cricoid and removed. Cytologic specimens are prepared, either by direct smearing of the balloon on a glass slide or rinsing the balloon in saline or fixative with subsequent preparation of a sediment by using a concentration technique. The surface of the balloon is covered with various types of material to enhance its abrasive sampling of the mucosa. The balloon sampling procedure is well-accepted by patients and can be effectively and expeditiously performed by nonphysician medical professionals. This is an advantage for large surveillance programs.[26-34] Other abrasive devices have also been developed.[35]

GENERAL PRINCIPLES

In the evaluation of GI cytology specimens, both the low-power pattern of the cells and background and the high-power cell details are important. At scanning power, the overall cellularity of the smears and the degree of cellular preservation and cohesion can be evaluated. Architectural arrangements of the cells can also be assessed because this is an important factor in distinguishing benign from malignant lesions. The background smear pattern can also be examined for inflammation and necrosis. High-power cytologic detail is then used by applying classic cytologic criteria for the diagnosis of benign vs. malignant conditions, dysplasia, and reparative processes.

The authors' cytologic interpretations use the terminology of surgical pathology, and they categorically find the use of a class reporting system unacceptable. An attempt is made to be as specific as possible, again using diagnostic terminology employed in surgical pathology, although it is recognized that on occasion, a specific diagnosis cannot be rendered. If this is the case, then the report reflects the level of uncertainty, with a comment to qualify the diagnosis.

 ## COMMON PITFALLS FOR FALSE-POSITIVE DIAGNOSIS OF MALIGNANCY IN THE GASTROINTESTINAL TRACT

Epithelial Reparative Atypia

A common, major challenge in interpreting cytologic specimens obtained from any GI tract site is the separation of epithelial reparative atypia from a neoplastic process. The squamous and glandular epithelia that line the mucosa often undergo repair secondary to ulceration or inflammation. Histologic examination of this healing process is char-acterized by regenerative epithelial cells having nuclei larger than normal, often ovoid in shape, with prominent nucleoli, and possessing pale, finely granular chromatin. With glandular epithelium, cytoplasmic mucin is often decreased or absent, and the cytoplasm of the cells has an eosinophilic hue with indistinct borders. Reparative squamous epithelium has cytoplasm that is less dense and homogeneous than normal squamous cells. In both squamous and glandular epithelium, the cytoplasmic volumes may be increased and neutrophilic leukocytes can be seen in the background and within the epithelial cells. If an ulcer is present, the biopsies often reveal some fibrinopurulent exudate and occasional organisms such as bacteria and fungi.

The cytologic appearance of repair is one of the most challenging diagnostic problems in the evaluation of GI cytologic preparations (Table 18-1). The most helpful cytomorphologic feature to distinguish reparative atypia from a malignant process is the low-power arrangement of cohesive, flat sheets of cells in repair. These cohesive sheets can be small or large, but individually scattered atypical cells with intact cytoplasm are not seen or are uncommon.* Within the reparative groups, polarity is maintained, and cells appear well oriented to one another, with a characteristic streaming pattern in which all the cells and nuclei appear to be oriented in the same direction. The cells can either be of normal size or somewhat enlarged, with mild variation in nuclear and cytoplasmic size. However, an overall relative homogeneity from cell to cell contrasts with malignancy, where cells are arranged with loss of polarity and demonstrate much greater variability in size and shape.

Moving from the low-power scanning assessment of cell groups to a high-power view, cells with uniform, round-to-oval nuclear contours and finely granular, evenly distributed, pale-staining chromatin are typical of repair. Prominent nucleoli, a worrisome feature, are present, but nucleolar irregularity and thickening are not generally seen. The chromatin remains delicate and vesicular, rather than hyperchromatic and clumpy. In fact, cells with this nuclear-nucleolar dyssynchrony are characteristic of repair and constitute an extremely helpful feature for the differentiation of reparative epithelium from carcinoma. Although the nuclear to cytoplasmic (N:C) ratio may be increased, it is lower than what would be seen in the cells from most GI tract carcinomas. Mitotic figures may be appreciated and are not unexpected in a reparative process. Neutrophils may also be present, both within the epithelial groups and in the background.

Cytoplasmic vacuolization is less conspicuous, and intercellular borders remain sharply defined. The cells of repair do not appear to have blending of the cytoplasmic borders; therefore, syncytial arrangements are not present. Cellular cohesion is strictly maintained, accounting for one of the cardinal features of repair, which is the lack or paucity of atypical single cells. If atypical intact single cells are present with any degree of frequency, then the diagnosis of repair should seriously be questioned.

In the evaluation of esophagitis, reparative squamous cells can have coarsely granular chromatin and high N:C ratios. However, reparative cells lack the well-developed nuclear hyperchromasia and thickened, contorted nuclear membranes, which are features of malignancy.[2]

TABLE 18-1	CMF

Cytomorphologic Differential Diagnostic Features of Epithelial Repair Versus Malignancy in Gastrointestinal Cytology

Epithelial Repair	Gastrointestinal Malignancy
Groups of cells	Groups of cells
Rare single cells	Many intact single cells
Flat metaplastic sheets maintaining honeycomb	Syncytial arrangement pattern or
Distinct cytoplasmic borders	Variable to indistinct cytoplasmic borders
Cellular polarity maintained	Loss of polarity
Enlarged nuclei	Enlarged nuclei
Round to oval nuclei with smooth nuclear borders	Irregular nuclear borders
Uniform nuclei	Variably sized nuclei (anisonucleosis)
Vesicular and hypochromatic to mildly hyperchromatic with even chromatin distribution	Opaque to hypochromatic nuclei with irregular chromatin distribution and parachromatin clearing
Nucleoli may be prominent	Nucleoli often irregular in shape
Normal mitotic figures	Normal and abnormal mitotic figures
No diathesis unless ulceration is present	Clear background or tumor diathesis

*References 2, 3, 4, 21, 36, and 37.

In cytologic brushings of ulcers, reactive stromal cells originating from the granulation tissue at the base of the ulcer may be present in the smears. These cells are individually scattered or in loose clusters and have spindle to stellate shapes. The nuclei are usually oval to spindle, with a bland chromatin distribution, and lack prominent nucleoli.

Prior radiation and chemotherapy can cause atypical cytologic changes that could superficially simulate an esophageal malignancy. This scenario usually occurs in patients irradiated for a prior carcinoma, making this differential diagnosis even more challenging. The changes are similar to those reported in the irradiated uterine cervix or lung (see Chapter 15) and include nuclear and cytoplasmic enlargement with degenerative changes such as cytoplasmic bichromasia and vacuolization, as well as nuclear vacuolization with chromatin smudging. The irradiated cells are often arranged in a repairlike pattern. However, if the smear shows increased N:C ratios, nuclear membrane irregularity, hyperchromatic nuclei, or intact atypical single cells, the possibility exists that irradiated malignant cells rather than benign cells are present. Cells exhibiting laser effect show changes similar to irradiated benign cells including degenerative nuclear alteration.[38] Lastly, in the

evaluation of atypical cells in patients who have received irradiation, chemotherapy, or laser treatment, a definitive diagnosis of malignancy should never be made if only poorly preserved or degenerated cells are available for evaluation.[38]

ESOPHAGUS

Normal Histology and Cytology

Almost the entire length of the esophagus is lined by nonkeratinized stratified squamous epithelium with the distal 1 to 2 cm covered by a mucin-producing simple columnar epithelium.[39] The underlying lamina propria consists of loose connective tissue containing gastric cardia-like glands. These glands secrete neutral rather than acidic mucin. Goblet cells are not normally present in the esophagus or stomach.

Cytologic brushing specimens from the normal esophagus are characterized by the presence of benign superficial and intermediate squamous cells (Figure 18-1). Superficial squamous cells are polygonal and contain abundant delicate eosinophilic cytoplasm and a single central pyknotic

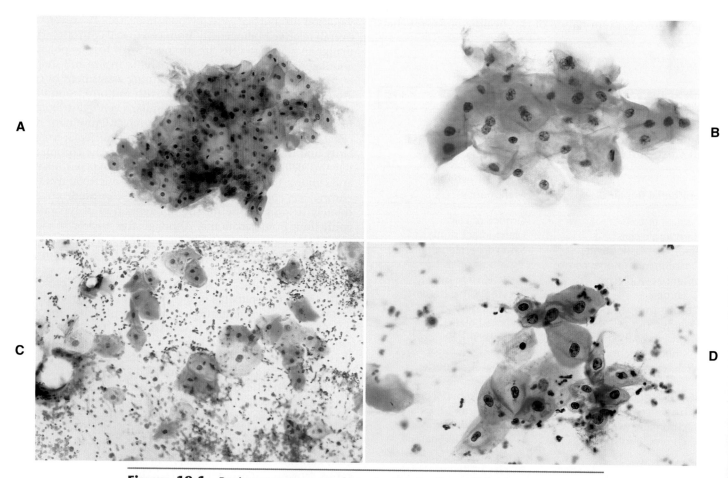

Figure 18-1 Benign squamous esophageal cells. **A,** Clump of benign squamous cells from esophageal brushing. **B,** Flat sheet of benign squamous cells having low nuclear to cytoplasmic (N:C) ratios. **C,** Brushing cytology of acute esophagitis showing benign squamous cells and neutrophils in the background. **D,** Brushing of acute esophagitis in which benign squamous cells are present, showing some reactive changes, including slight nuclear enlargement and perinuclear halos. Scattered neutrophils are present in the background. (Papanicolaou [Pap])

nucleus. Some cells may show keratohyaline granules. Intermediate cells have slightly larger nuclei with finely granular chromatin and small chromocenters; nucleoli are not evident.[28] Brushing cytology samples both superficial and intermediate squamous cells that are often arranged in large, flat sheets; small clusters; or concentric pearl-type arrangements. Scattered single cells may also be seen. Rarely, parabasal cells can be present when the brushing procedure is quite vigorous. Parabasal cells are usually individually scattered and have higher N:C ratios with round-to-oval nuclei possessing vesicular chromatin surrounded by dense cyanophilic cytoplasm.

It is not uncommon to see glandular cells in brushings of the esophagus. These originate by inadvertent sampling, either of the proximal stomach or of the glandular columnar cells present in the distal 1 to 2 cm of the esophagus. These cells are arranged in small to large, flat sheets in which the nuclei are evenly spaced with surrounding sharply defined cytoplasmic borders imparting a honeycomb pattern (Figure 18-2). The nuclei are small and round with finely granular pale-staining chromatin and inconspicuous nucleoli surrounded by delicate finely granular cytoplasm lacking large vacuoles.

Contaminants, including ciliated respiratory columnar cells, macrophages, food particles, and clumps of oral bacteria, can sometimes be present.

Infectious Esophageal Lesions

Inflammatory lesions are the most common esophageal disorders, with patients complaining of dysphagia, odynophagia, heartburn, or severe chest pain. Gastroesophageal reflux disease (GERD) is the most common cause of esophagitis. The clinical and radiologic features may suggest a specific cause, but the cytologic findings of esophagitis are usually nonspecific. The major exception is the cytologic demonstration of a causative organism.

Candidal Esophagitis

The most common cause of clinically significant infectious esophagitis is *Candida albicans*. Candidiasis is most often

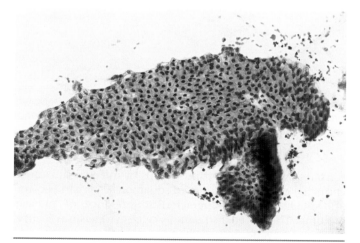

Figure 18-2 **Benign glandular cells from esophageal-gastric junction.** Flat sheet of benign glandular cells from esophageal-gastric junction. Note the honeycomb arrangement of the glandular cells. (Pap)

seen in immunosuppressed patients such as those receiving chemotherapy for either leukemia or lymphoma, irradiation for solid malignancies, or steroids and/or immunotherapy for transplantation. *Candida* organisms classically produce a pseudomembrane that is attached to the squamous mucosa. A neutrophilic infiltrate and degenerative changes of the epithelium may be present.

The diagnosis of *Candida* esophagitis is made when the characteristic pseudohyphae are recognized.[2,40] The pseudohyphae are delicate, have a magenta color in the Pap-stained smears and lack true septation (Figure 18-3). Indentations along their long axis simulates "sausage-link chains." Although more difficult to identify, the smaller, budding yeast cells are also typically present. The fungal elements can be found in the background trapped within acute inflammatory exudate, or infiltrating the squamous cell clusters. They are most readily found in inflammatory foci containing granular debris. Although a silver stain is usually not needed to identify the fungus, occasional cases occur in which pseudohyphae are few in number and the Gomori methenamine silver (GMS) stain will facilitate the identification of the few scattered fungal yeasts.

A repair-like pattern of the epithelial cells is often noted in cases of candidal esophagitis (Figure 18-4). Cytologic smears and biopsies are complementary for the evaluation of inflammatory esophageal conditions, and cytologic preparations are believed to be more sensitive for the detection of *C. albicans* than concurrently obtained biopsies because *C. albicans* organisms are typically present on the mucosal surface that is best sampled by brushing cytology.[1-3,5,41,42] Rarely, other types of fungi such as *Phycomycetes* species (mucor) can be sampled by esophageal brushing (Figure 18-5). *Filamentous leptothrix*–type organisms have also been diagnosed in esophageal brushings from patients with esophageal malignancies (Figure 18-6).

Herpetic Esophagitis

The most common type of viral esophagitis results from herpes simplex virus (HSV). Patients usually have predisposing conditions including mucosal trauma secondary to prior nasogastric intubation, malignancy (especially hematopoietic malignancies), prior chemotherapy and/or irradiation, or other immunodeficiency states such as acquired immune deficiency syndrome (AIDS).[40,43] Occasionally, however, symptomatic herpetic esophagitis occurs in otherwise healthy individuals. Herpetic esophagitis can resolve spontaneously, even in immunosuppressed patients. The classic endoscopic appearance is multiple small, shallow ulcers with punched-out edges having a predilection for involvement of the distal third of the organ. In some patients, extensive mucosal sloughing occurs, or a nonspecific inflammatory appearance is evident. The herpes virus infects the intact squamous mucosa; therefore, the edge of the ulcer should be brushed rather than the base because samples of the ulcer bed granulation tissue are nondiagnostic.

Both histologically and cytologically, the infected squamous epithelial cells may show two types of viral cytopathic nuclear changes: (1) the classic Cowdry type A eosinophilic viral inclusion that is separated from the thick nuclear membrane by a halo or clear zone or (2) a faintly basophilic homogeneous change to the chromatin. Nuclear membrane thickening—a collection of "bended necklage" chromatin clumps—may be seen. These are identical to the

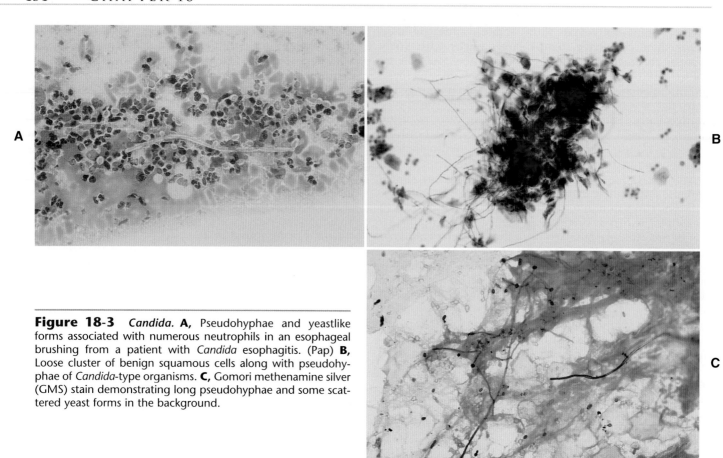

Figure 18-3 *Candida.* **A,** Pseudohyphae and yeastlike forms associated with numerous neutrophils in an esophageal brushing from a patient with *Candida* esophagitis. (Pap) **B,** Loose cluster of benign squamous cells along with pseudohyphae of *Candida*-type organisms. **C,** Gomori methenamine silver (GMS) stain demonstrating long pseudohyphae and some scattered yeast forms in the background.

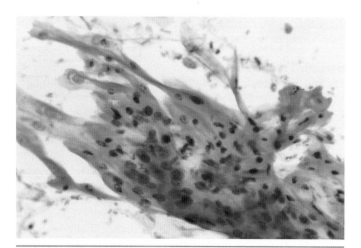

Figure 18-4 Repair, esophagus. Streaming repair pattern of esophageal squamous mucosa in patient with acute esophagitis and ulceration. (Pap)

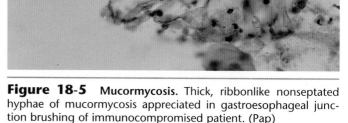

Figure 18-5 Mucormycosis. Thick, ribbonlike nonseptated hyphae of mucormycosis appreciated in gastroesophageal junction brushing of immunocompromised patient. (Pap)

alterations noted in herpetic bronchitis (Figure 18-7; see Chapter 15). In both types of virocytes, the nuclear and cytoplasmic volumes are increased, but the N:C ratios are not generally elevated. Multinucleation of the virally infected cell is also characteristic with the nuclei typically molding each other. In some cases, only a few squamous cells may be infected, requiring a careful search of the smears.

The cytomorphologic diagnosis of herpes esophagitis is based on recognition of virocytes present as individually scattered cells and/or within groups of infected squamous epithelial cells. Virally infected squamous cells can become multinucleated with characteristic presence of nuclear molding. The infected squamous cells' cytoplasm is scanty, dense, and cyanophilic. When the ulcer base is also sampled, necrotic debris, and neutrophils are seen. Reparative atypia of the epithelium can also be present.

The major differential diagnosis of herpetic esophagitis is squamous cell carcinoma. Resulting difficulties may arise

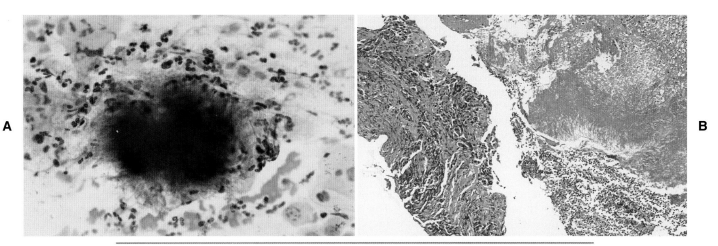

Figure 18-6 Filamentous bacteria, esophagus. **A,** Filamentous clump of actinomyces type organisms associated with adenocarcinoma of the esophagus (Papanicolaou stain). **B,** Hematoxylin and eosin (H&E) stain of filamentous organisms associated with adenocarcinoma in esophageal biopsy.

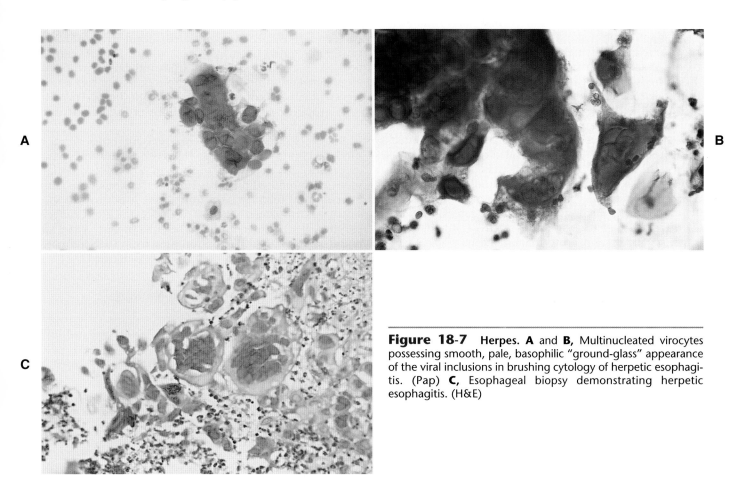

Figure 18-7 Herpes. **A** and **B,** Multinucleated virocytes possessing smooth, pale, basophilic "ground-glass" appearance of the viral inclusions in brushing cytology of herpetic esophagitis. (Pap) **C,** Esophageal biopsy demonstrating herpetic esophagitis. (H&E)

due to the irregular shapes of some virally infected cells and the potential of misinterpreting the viral inclusions for the macronucleoli of malignant cells. A helpful feature is the characteristic "ground-glass" chromatin. In virocytes, this is pale and agranular, contrasting with the fine to coarsely granular hyperchromatic chromatin of squamous cell carcinoma. In the Cowdry type A viral inclusion, a perfectly clear halo is present, whereas in cancer cells, chromatin granules are noted in the nucleus.

Although small cell carcinoma can show nuclear molding, this diagnosis should not be entertained because of the large size of the infected squamous cells and the presence of the abundant cytoplasm.[44] Radiation esophagitis can also be considered in the differential if a prior history of such treatment is evident. In radiation esophagitis, the enlarged squamous cells can also have multiple nuclei and a degenerative structureless chromatin that can simulate the homogeneous ground-glass type viral inclusions. However, they lack the typical nuclear molding, higher N:C ratios, and Cowdry type A viral inclusion bodies. HSV also shares some morphologic features with cytomegalic virus (CMV), which is discussed in the following text.

There is limited literature that discusses the cytologic diagnosis of herpetic esophagitis,[2] with some controversy as to whether endoscopic biopsies or cytology are more sensitive for the diagnosis.[1-3,5] Again, the authors believe that surgical biopsies and brushing cytology are complementary for the diagnosis.

Cytomegalovirus Esophagitis

CMV esophagitis, although rare in the general population, occurs with some frequency in patients with AIDS.[40,45] The clinical, endoscopic, and radiologic features are nonspecific. Patients present with complaints of either dysphagia or chest pain. Endoscopically, irregular ulcers are present and can be sampled by biopsy and brushing cytology. CMV infects endothelial cells, fibroblasts, and glandular elements—sites that do not readily lend themselves to surface mucosal sampling. Thus, the typical cytologic alterations are found in endothelial cells, pericytes, and stromal cells of the ulcer bed and granulation tissue. These virally infected cells have enlarged nuclei possessing a huge viral inclusion separated from the thick nuclear membrane by a clear halo (Figure 18-8). Although binucleated CMV virocytes can be found, multinucleation and ground-glass chromatin are not seen and thus allow differentiation from HSV. Some virocytes also demonstrate granular cytoplasmic inclusion bodies, another feature not seen in herpes. Important differentiating features are that HSV infects squamous cells, whereas CMV infects glandular and stromal cells. Although quite unusual, there is a report of both CMV and HSV present in the same specimen.[45]

In esophageal brushings, usually only rare CMV virocytes are present in a background of reactive epithelial cells, granulation tissue, and acute inflammation.[40,45] The virocytes are typically present as individually scattered cells showing significant nuclear and cytoplasmic enlargement. Granular cytoplasmic inclusions can also be present but are difficult to identify in cytologic material. The alcohol-fixed, Pap-stained smears demonstrate the intranuclear inclusions

to advantage, whereas air-dried Diff-Quik (DQ)–stained smears may accentuate the cytoplasmic inclusions.

In contrast with HSV, which is optimally sampled when the edge of the ulcer is brushed, identification of CMV requires that the endoscopist biopsy and brush the base of the esophageal ulcer because the virocytes are found in the underlying granulation tissue. However, the number of infected cells is often low, which requires a diligent search to identify the virocytes.

In other portions of the GI tract, CMV also infects the glandular epithelium, and thus, virocytes may be present in much greater numbers. Biopsies are believed to be more sensitive for the diagnosis of CMV esophagitis than cytology preparations, although there are reports of positive brushing cytology specimens.[1,5,45] The major cytologic differential diagnosis of CMV esophagitis is HSV esophagitis (Table 18-2).

Other Infections

Primary bacterial infections are a common cause of esophagitis, with most cases resulting from saprophytes that affect individuals who are immunosuppressed or on long-term antibiotic therapy.[40] In cytologic preparations, bacteria can usually be appreciated, although specific identification requires Gram stain and culture. Bacteria can also be seen in esophageal smears from individuals who have esophagitis resulting from other causes, and in this setting, represent either a contaminant or co-contributor. Therefore, it is recommended that the presence of bacteria be documented in the cytology report.

Besides *C. albicans,* it is unusual for other fungi to produce clinical esophagitis. However, organisms such as aspergillus can rarely be present in brushings from immunocompromised patients. Human papillomavirus (HPV) infection has recently been implicated as a cause for some squamous esophageal lesions[46,47] and cytologic features of esophageal HPV infection have been reported.[47] A rare case report of esophageal disease resulting from trichomonas in an AIDS patient has also been recently published.[48]

Radiation-Related and Chemotherapy-Related Esophagitis

Irradiation to the chest and mediastinum is a common cause for esophagitis.[49] Although patient susceptibility varies, the degree of esophagitis is usually related to the to-

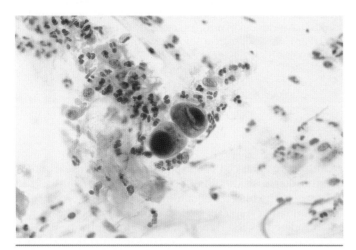

Figure 18-8 Cytomegalovirus (CMV). Esophageal brushing in which a few scattered virocytes having large intranuclear inclusions with surrounding halos consistent with CMV. (Pap)

TABLE **18-2**		
Cytologic Differential Diagnosis of Esophageal Viral Infections		
Feature	**HSV**	**CMV**
Cell type infected	Squamous	Stromal, glandular
Multinucleation	+	−
Ground-glass chromatin	+	−
Cytoplasmic inclusions	±	+

Modified from Geisinger KR, Silverman JF. Gastrointestinal cytology. In: Silverberg SG, editor. Principles and practice of surgical pathology and cytopathology. 3rd ed. New York: Churchill Livingstone; 1997. pp.1563-1593.
HSV, Herpes simplex virus; *CMV,* cytomegalovirus; +, present; −, not present; ±, may or may not be present.

tal dose of irradiation, the fraction delivered per treatment session, and the time course over which this therapy is given.[40] Cytotoxic chemotherapeutic agents can also injure the esophagus in a similar fashion, and the effects of radiation and chemotherapy may actually potentiate each other by lowering the threshold for injury.

Irradiation and chemotherapy-related esophagitis is histologically characterized by the presence of large, atypical squamous cells with increased nuclear and cytoplasmic size but maintaining relatively unremarkable N:C ratios. With irradiation, the nuclei show degenerative changes that typically impart a pale or washed-out appearance to the chromatin, and nucleoli are not enlarged. With chemotherapy, hyperchromasia and enlarged nuclei are more likely to occur. Increased mitotic activity is also present and is seen above the normal basal layer of the epithelium. Beneath the epithelium, atypical stromal cells, including endothelium have enlarged, smudged, hyperchromatic irregular nuclei, and stellate to irregularly shaped cytoplasm.

The cytomorphologic features of irradiation esophagitis recapitulate the histologic changes. These include cells showing significant nuclear and cytoplasmic enlargement but retaining relatively unremarkable N:C ratios (Figure 18-9).[2,40] Degenerative nuclear and cytoplasmic vacuolization is seen, along with nuclear membrane irregularity and multinucleation. In contrast with malignancy and viral-related changes, the chromatin maintains a finely granular appearance or is structureless and pale staining. In chemotherapy-related esophagitis, however, nucleoli can be prominent and the chromatin appears more darkly stained and coarsely granular. These worrisome features can prompt consideration of a malignant process.

The major differential feature separating chemotherapy-related changes from malignancy is the maintenance of more unremarkable N:C ratios in the former, in contrast with the high N:C ratios of malignant squamous cells. However, this is not always an easy decision, and a conservative approach is warranted. Diagnosis may be further complicated when malignant cells also show irradiation and/or chemotherapy effects. These cells, however, tend to demonstrate high N:C ratios, significant hyperchromasia, and nuclear irregularity in addition to treatment-related changes.

O'Morchoe and colleagues have reported chemotherapy-related changes of the upper GI tract from patients without esophageal carcinoma.[50] The cytologic features in squamous cells included loss of polarity within aggregates; increased N:C ratios; variability in nuclear size and shape; hyperchromasia; prominent, often multiple nucleoli; and chromatin clumping. Their findings also support the belief that chemotherapy-associated atypia, in contrast with irradiation changes, more closely simulates cancer. Therefore, a definitive diagnosis of carcinoma should always be made with caution in patients who have a known history of prior chemotherapy.

The differential diagnoses of squamous abnormalities seen in patients with therapy-associated esophagitis, chemotherapy-related changes, infection, and malignancy

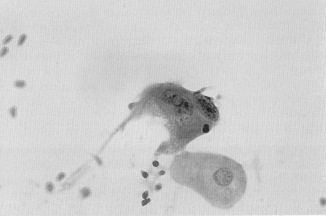

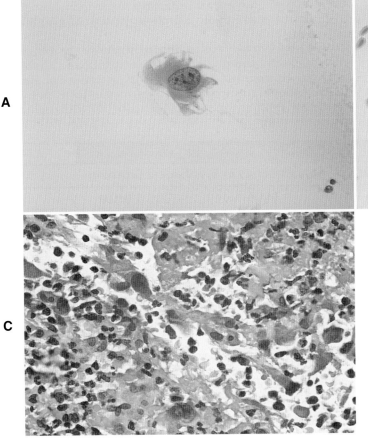

Figure 18-9 Radiation atypia. **A** and **B,** Few scattered cells from radiation atypia characterized by nuclear and cytoplasmic enlargement with low N:C ratios and degenerative changes. (Pap) **C,** H&E of biopsy of radiation atypia with surface ulceration and inflammation.

are presented in Table 18-3. Although HSV virocytes enter into the differential diagnosis of malignancy, distinguishing radiation- and chemotherapy-associated alterations from squamous cell carcinoma are usually more challenging. As mentioned above, this diagnostic problem is further accentuated when residual or recurrent malignant cells also show superimposed treatment-related changes.

Gastroesophageal Reflux Disease

Regurgitation of gastric and possibly duodenal contents through an incompetent lower esophageal sphincter results in GERD. When the esophageal squamous mucosa comes in contact with hydrochloric acid, pepsin, or bile, these substances irritate the mucosa leading to chemical (reflux) esophagitis. Endoscopically, an erythematous mucosa is appreciated, with or without erosions, in the distal portion of the esophagus. Complications of reflux esophagitis include peptic ulcers, fibrosing strictures, and Barrett's esophagitis.

Histologic examination of the squamous esophageal epithelium in patients with reflux demonstrates both inflammation and reactive epithelial changes.[50-52] Reflux can be histologically suspected when proliferative changes of the esophageal mucosa are demonstrated by basal cell hyperplasia and papillomatosis, along with superimposed degenerative changes of the epithelial cells. When an inflammatory component is present, neutrophils and/or eosinophils are seen infiltrating into the squamous mucosa. These findings are not totally specific because allergic causes and "pill effect" can cause similar changes.

Brushing cytology of reflux esophagitis has no specific cytologic features; rather the nonspecific findings of reparative epithelial changes and associated acute inflammation are seen. These cytologic alterations were discussed previously in this chapter. Although playing a prominent part in the histologic diagnosis, eosinophils have not been reported to be a prominent component of GERD in brushing cytology.[5,40] If an ulcer or erosion is present, sampling of parabasal cells and the presence of a fibrinopurulent exudate and granulation tissue from the ulcer bed may be appreciated.

Barrett's Esophagus

A major complication of reflux esophagitis that can affect 10% or more of patients with longstanding GERD is Barrett's esophagus.[53] Barrett's esophagus represents a benign metaplastic process in which the normal squamous mucosal lining is replaced by glandular epithelium in reaction to reflux. No specific clinical signs and symptoms suggest that this metaplasia has occurred, and in fact, some patients have reported a reduction in their esophagitis symptoms, following the development of metaplasia.

The historical definition of Barrett's metaplasia as simple replacement of squamous epithelium with columnar epithelium for some length of the mucosal surface has now been operatively supplemented with the requirement that intestinal metaplasia be present. This circumvents difficulties in classification of lesions that involve only small segments of mucosal surface and eliminates any need to identify the location of the original squamocolumnar junction. Furthermore, this intestinalization poses an increased risk for the subsequent development of adenocarcinoma.

Histologically, the metaplastic glandular epithelium can resemble either gastric or intestinal types of mucosa, and combinations occur. The gastric-type mucosa can be either cardia or fundic type. Goblet cells in the glandular epithelium can be recognized when large barrel-like vacuoles containing slightly basophilic cytoplasmic acidic mucin are seen within the glandular epithelium with basal displacement of the nuclei.[53,54] In some histologic types of intestinal metaplasia, a villous architecture and Paneth cells may also be present. It is critical to recognize definite Barrett's esophagus because this is believed to be the premalignant type of glandular metaplasia from which most adenocarcinomas of the esophagus arise.[54,55] The transition from Barrett's type of intestinal metaplasia to carcinoma usually requires the intermediate morphologic stage of glandular dysplasia.

Brushing cytology has an important role for the recognition of both Barrett's intestinal metaplasia and dysplasia.[40,56-59] Differential diagnostic cytologic features of glandular lesions of the upper GI are presented in Table 18-4. In brushing cytology specimens of patients with benign

TABLE 18-3   CMF

Cytomorphologic Differential Diagnosis of Squamous Cell Abnormalities in Esophageal Brushings

Feature	HSV	RT	SCCA	Repair
Chromatin	Smudged or cleared	Pale, fine granularity, even distribution	Dense or variably granular, irregular particle size and distribution	Pale, fine granularity, even distribution
Nucleoli	–	±	+	+
Nuclear inclusion body and halo	+	–	–	–
Multinucleation	+	+	±	–
Keratinization	±	±	±	–
N:C ratio	Moderately increased	Normal to slightly increased	Slightly to greatly increased	Normal to slightly increased
Intercellular cohesion	Variable	Variable	Reduced	Preserved

Modified from Geisinger KR, Silverman JF. Gastrointestinal cytology. In: Silverberg SG, editor. Principles and practice of surgical pathology and cytopathology. 3rd ed. New York: Churchill Livingstone; 1997. pp.1563-1593.
HSV, Herpes simplex virus; *RT,* radiation; *SCCA,* squamous cell carcinoma; *N:C,* nuclear to cytoplasmic; +, present; –, not present; ±, may or may not be present.

Barrett's esophagus, the smears generally contain numerous glandular cells arranged in large, flat cohesive sheets (Figure 18-10).[40,56-58] The external boundaries of these sheets of cells maintain a smooth contour, reflecting a high level of intercellular cohesion. Depending on the arrangement of the cells on the smears, the groups could either have a honeycomb or palisaded appearance because of the maintenance of normal polarity (Figure 18-11). Within the sheets and groups the nuclei are equidistance from one another with distinct intercellular borders. In contrast, when reparative atypia involving the benign Barrett's epithelium is present, the glandular groups consist of cells having a streaming pattern with all the nuclei flowing in the same direction (Figure 18-12).

The diagnosis of Barrett's is predicated on the identification of goblet cells within the glandular groupings (Figure 18-13). The goblet cells have basally placed nuclei with large, punched-out, clear cytoplasmic vacuoles. The nuclei of the glandular epithelium are uniform, maintaining round-to-oval shapes with delicate nuclear chromatin and smooth nuclear membranes. Nucleoli are generally not conspicuous, unless regenerative atypia is present. The smear background is generally clean, although inflammatory cells may be present. A discussion of dysplasia in Barrett's esophagus and adenocarcinoma in Barrett's is presented in the following text. Although ancillary studies have not been generally used in the cytologic workup of patients with Barrett's esophagus, a few studies have reported the application of villin immunohistochemistry for the diagnosis of Barrett's metaplasia and *p53* nuclear protein for surveillance of esophageal dysplasia and adenocarcinoma in the setting of Barrett's.[60,61]

Squamous Cell Carcinoma

The most common malignant neoplasm of the esophagus is squamous cell carcinoma, accounting for approximately 85% of all esophageal cancers worldwide.[62] An incidence of approximately 2.5 cases in 100,000 individuals results in approximately 12,000 cases each year in the United States. Within this country, African-American individuals are 4.5 times more likely to develop esophageal squamous cell carcinoma than whites. The male-to-female ratio is approximately 3:1 in whites and 4:1 in blacks. Squamous cell carcinoma of the esophagus in the United States is a highly lethal malignancy with 5-year survival rates of approxi-

TABLE **18-4**			CMF
Cytomorphologic Differential Diagnosis of Glandular Lesions in Barrett's Esophagus and the Stomach			
Feature	Repair	Dysplasia	Adenocarcinoma (Intestinal Type)
Cellular aggregates	Large, smooth edges, normal polarity	Small, frayed edges, altered polarity	Small, frayed edges, altered polarity
Individual cells	Rare to absent	Few	Few to many
Nuclear contours	Smooth, round to oval	Slight irregularities, elongated	Slight to prominent irregularities
Chromatin	Pale	Hyperchromatic	Hyperchromatic
Nucleoli	Large, prominent, smooth	Large	Large, angulated
N:C ratio	Normal to slightly increased	Slightly to moderately increased	Slightly to greatly increased
Background	Clean	Clean	Diathesis

Modified from Geisinger KR, Silverman JF. Gastrointestinal cytology. In: Silverberg SG, editor. Principles and practice of surgical pathology and cytopathology. 3rd ed. New York: Churchill Livingstone; 1997. pp.1563-1593.

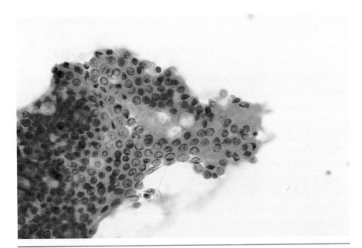

Figure 18-10 **Barrett's esophagus.** Flat sheet of glandular cells arranged in a honeycomb pattern from patient with Barrett's esophagus. This group of cells lacks the diagnostic goblet cells of intestinal metaplasia. (Pap)

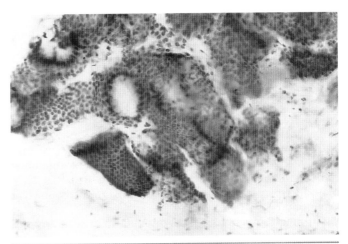

Figure 18-11 **Barrett's esophagus.** Numerous flat groups of glandular cells showing both a honeycomb and picket fence arrangement. (Pap)

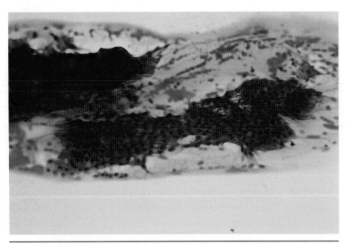

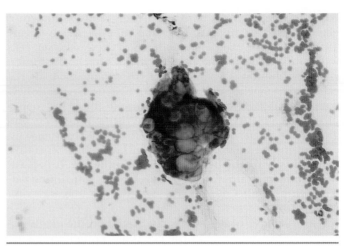

Figure 18-12 Barrett's esophagus. Brushing cytology from Barrett's esophagus in which some of the groups of glandular cells have a more streaming pattern suggesting repair. (Pap)

Figure 18-13 Barrett's esophagus. Cluster of glandular cells including goblet cells. (Pap)

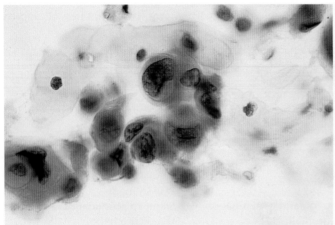

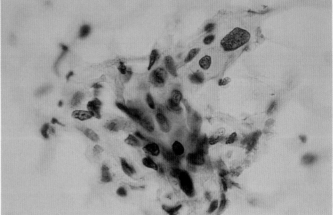

Figure 18-14 Well-differentiated squamous cell carcinoma. Loose clusters of malignant keratinized cells having dense orangeophilic cytoplasm with irregular shapes and enlarged hyperchromatic nuclei. (Pap)

mately 10%, perhaps related to the fact that these tumors are usually detected late in their course.

Worldwide variation exists in the incidence rate of squamous cell carcinoma with more than half the cases occurring in China. Even in high-incidence countries such as China, Iran, and South Africa, both high and low rates can be found, depending on regional differences. Environmental factors implicated are diets high in nitrates and nitrites, which are converted to carcinogenic nitrosamines; low dietary levels of vitamins A, C, and riboflavin; tobacco use; and alcohol abuse. Caustic injury to the mucosa occurring with lye ingestion increases the long-term risk of squamous cell carcinoma. Recently, it has been suggested that HPV may also play a role in the development of esophageal carcinoma.

Although squamous cell carcinoma can arise at any site along the esophagus, the middle portion is the most common location. A variety of different endoscopic appearances may be present, such as large polypoid masses; deep, irregular ulcers; or flat, mucosal elevations. Squamous cell

carcinoma often causes considerable stenosis of the esophagus, compromising the ability to obtain tissue biopsies of the malignancy. This produces the common and late symptom of dysphagia. It is in this setting that brushing cytology may be especially useful to make a specific diagnosis.

Three histologic grades of squamous esophageal carcinoma occur, representing a spectrum from well-differentiated carcinoma with prominent cytoplasmic keratinization and dense pyknotic nuclei to poorly differentiated squamous cell carcinoma having cells with a more finely granular chromatin, prominent nucleoli, and dense cyanophilic cytoplasm.

The brushing cytology findings in esophageal squamous cell carcinoma reflect the grade of the malignancy.[2,29,40] In well-differentiated squamous cell carcinoma, intercellular cohesion is relatively well maintained, with smears containing variably sized aggregates of large tumor cells having abundant dense cytoplasm (Figure 18-14). Cytoplasmic keratinization is optimally demonstrated with the Pap stain, with neoplastic cells demonstrating bright, orangeophilic

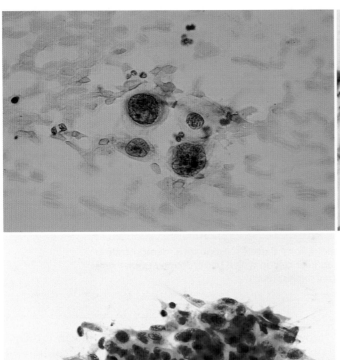

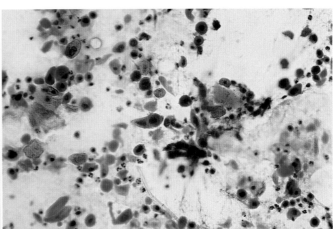

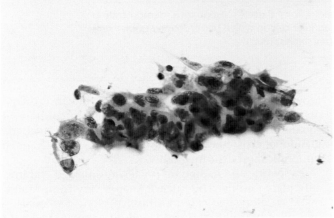

Figure 18-15 Poorly differentiated squamous cell carcinoma. Poorly differentiated squamous cell carcinoma consisting either of disassociated single cells with high N:C ratios or individually scattered bizarre spindle-shaped cells and clumps of cells showing no obvious squamous differentiation. (Pap)

cytoplasm. The nuclei are often centrally positioned and may have very sharply angulated contours. The chromatin can vary from coarsely granular and hyperchromatic to almost pyknotic in appearance. Keratin pearls may be appreciated, as well as individually scattered cells having bizarre shapes, including tadpolelike forms. Numerous anucleated keratinized squamous cells may also be present.

As the squamous cell carcinoma becomes less differentiated, discohesion increases, reflected by the presence of numerous individually scattered malignant cells (Figure 18-15). Although the cytoplasm remains dense, with sharp borders reflecting squamous differentiation, the squamous cells now have more cyanophilic cytoplasm, rather than demonstrating orangeophilia as evidence of keratinization. Although well-differentiated keratinized squamous cell carcinomas can have cells with relatively low N:C ratios, the N:C ratios significantly increase in the more poorly differentiated cancers. The chromatin varies from finely to coarsely granular, nucleoli are more apparent, and dense pyknotic nuclei are not commonly seen.

Published brushing cytology series have demonstrated diagnostic yields for all histologic types of squamous cell carcinoma as 80% to 100%, with a weighted mean yield of 92%.[3-5] Diagnostic accuracy of concomitant biopsies varies from 63% to 96%, with a weighted mean yield of 84%. When the results of both cytology and surgical biopsies are combined, the resultant combined weighted mean yield is increased to 98%, confirming the complementary value of the two diagnostic procedures. Although some series do

not histologically subdivide their esophageal carcinomas, it appears that for well-differentiated squamous cell carcinomas, the mean diagnostic yields for cytology, surgical biopsy, and both procedures are 93%, 87%, and 99%, respectively.[3,4]

In high-prevalence regions such as China, large-scale screening programs for detection of early esophageal squamous cell carcinoma and its precursors are used.[28-36] Because the only hope for increased survival is early detection, these surveillance programs are optimally in place to identify squamous dysplasias and carcinoma in situ before their evolution to invasive squamous cell carcinoma. For these surveillance programs to be successful, technically feasible abrasive techniques that are cost effective are needed. Before the implementation of the current surveillance procedures, the cytologic diagnosis of esophageal squamous cell dysplasia was rarely made,[63,64] but current reports from these high-risk populations have demonstrated the success of the screening programs.[26,28,29,34] At the present time, it does not appear that cytologic surveillance in low-incidence countries is practical, although individuals who are at higher risk for developing squamous cell carcinomas could potentially benefit from these types of programs.[32,34]

Barrett's Dysplasia and Adenocarcinoma

In the United States and other parts of the western world, a dramatic increase has occurred in the absolute and relative incidence of adenocarcinoma of the esophagus. This neo-

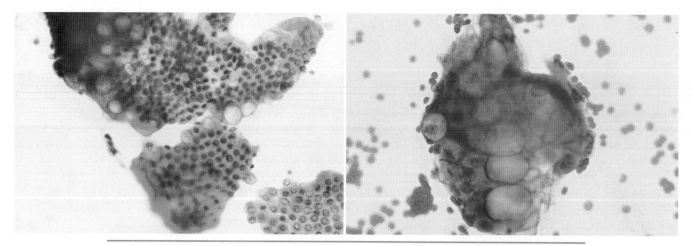

Figure 18-16 Barrett's esophagus. Brushing from Barrett's esophagus demonstrating honeycomb and picket-fence arrangements of glandular cells in which barrel-shaped goblet cells are apparent as rounded, clear, or lightly basophilic circles. (Pap)

plasm accounted for only 5% to 10% of all primary carcinomas of this organ 20 years ago, whereas today, nearly half the malignancies are adenocarcinomas with almost all arising in the background of preexisting Barrett's esophagus (Figure 18-16).[53,55,65] In contrast with squamous cell carcinoma of the esophagus, whites are affected approximately three times more often than blacks with a male-to-female ratio of 7:1 in whites and even greater gender disparity in African Americans. Adenocarcinomas almost always occur in the distal one third of the esophagus and often involve the gastroesophageal junction. Patients present with dysphagia and endoscopically have either large ulcers or fungating polypoid masses, which can significantly reduce the luminal diameter of the esophagus.

Most esophageal adenocarcinomas are well to moderately differentiated, whereas signet ring carcinomas are uncommon.[53] The most important prognostic feature of esophageal adenocarcinoma is the depth of invasion into the wall of the organ. Dysplastic Barrett's epithelium is the precursor to invasive carcinoma and is characterized by columnar-shaped epithelial cells having enlarged, oval to somewhat elongated hyperchromatic nuclei that are typically pseudostratified (Figure 18-17). The nuclei can possess large nucleoli, and N:C ratios are increased. In low-grade dysplasia, the nuclei are more basally located, whereas in high-grade dysplasia, the nuclei approach the luminal glandular border.

The cytologic diagnosis of adenocarcinoma is usually not challenging. The malignant cells are arranged individually and in loose clusters that reflect the cellular discohesion of malignancy. Although adenocarcinoma shares many cytologic features with glandular dysplasia, brushings of adenocarcinoma generally produce much greater numbers of individually scattered abnormal cells, whereas dysplasia may only have a few such cells (Figure 18-18).

In both adenocarcinoma and Barrett's dysplasia, altered polarity exists within the group, and the cells are arranged haphazardly with overlapping abnormal nuclei (Figure 18-19). The cytoplasmic borders merge, creating a syncytial pattern (Figure 18-20). A tendency exists for the dysplastic aggregates to be larger than the small, loosely cohesive

groups of adenocarcinoma. Cytoplasmic mucin is often reduced in both dysplasia and carcinoma.* In contrast with squamous cell carcinoma the dysplastic and malignant glandular cells have cytoplasm that has a pale, or amphophilic, and delicate quality.

Dysplastic and malignant nuclei are enlarged and invariably pleomorphic. The nuclear shapes vary from round or ovoid to elongated. Pseudostratified elongated nuclei are typical of both dysplasia and well-differentiated adenocarcinomas (Figure 18-21). Nuclear membranes are thickened and irregular in shape, and hyperchromasia is evident with one or more large, irregular nucleoli. In addition to the increased numbers of abnormal cells, a dirty tumor diathesis accompanies invasive adenocarcinoma.

Therefore, although dysplasia can be suspected, it cannot be absolutely differentiated from a well-differentiated adenocarcinoma in the cytology smears. Tissue biopsy is needed to make a more definitive diagnosis. Furthermore, dysplasia cannot be adequately graded by cytologic examination.

The diagnostic accuracy of cytology for esophageal adenocarcinoma ranges from 72% to 100% with a weighted mean yield of 84% in published series.[3-5,58,66] The corresponding biopsies have diagnostic accuracies from 67% to 100% with a weighted mean yield of 79%. When both cytology and biopsies are combined, the yield ranged from 88% to 100% with a combined weighted mean yield of 91%. These results confirm that although neither procedure is as good for the diagnosis of adenocarcinoma as for squamous cell carcinoma, when both cytology and biopsy are used, the diagnostic accuracy is enhanced.

Surveillance programs have also been developed to monitor patients with Barrett's esophagus.[53,55,70,71] Most of these programs have involved taking numerous endoscopically directed tissue biopsies throughout the length of the metaplastic esophageal segment. Only a few programs have also included brushing cytology. The authors believe that brush-

---

*References 2, 4, 40, 56-58, 66-69.

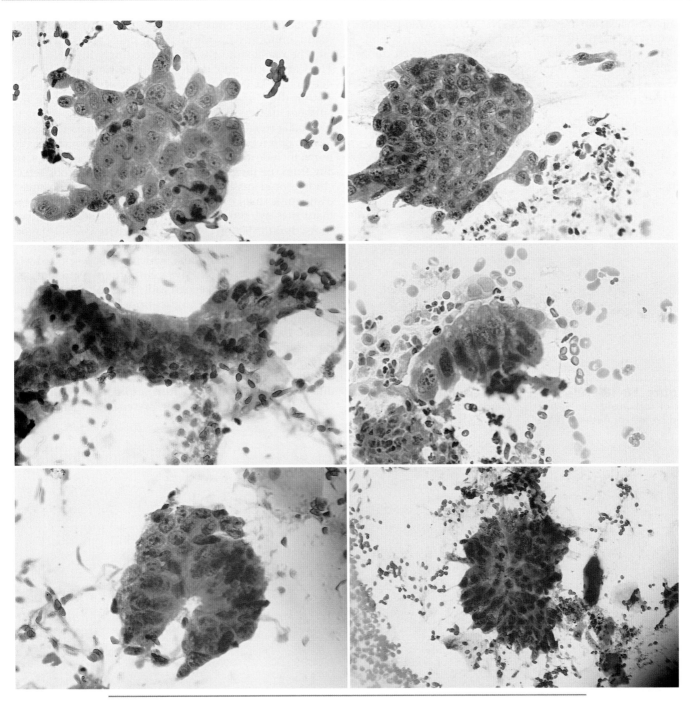

Figure 18-17 **Barrett's dysplasia.** Varying degrees of dysplasia in Barrett's esophagus are appreciated in these images. The dysplastic glandular cells demonstrate stratification of nuclei with nuclear enlargement and hyperchromasia. However, a paucity of single atypical cells is evident and mitigate against a diagnosis of invasive adenocarcinoma. (Pap)

ing cytology has considerable use in this setting because it allows for a greater sampling of the mucosal surface than the more directed surgical biopsies.[27,31] Limited experience has accumulated with blindly obtained balloon samples for the diagnosis of Barrett's esophagus.

Small Cell Carcinoma

Neuroendocrine neoplasms of the esophagus are uncommon, accounting for less than 5% of all esophageal tumors.

In contrast with other areas of the GI tract where carcinoid tumor is most often seen, this highly lethal small cell carcinoma is the more common neuroendocrine neoplasm at this site. Approximately 100 cases have been reported in the literature.[72,73] Small cell carcinoma is a malignancy of middle age or older individuals arising in the middle or distal segment of the esophagus. The patients most often present with the nonspecific clinical symptom of dysphagia. In histologic sections, the characteristic appearance of a small cell carcinoma is appreciated, including the presence of small malignant cells having very high N:C ratios, ovoid to elongated hyperchromatic nuclei, and no discernable nucleoli.

These neoplasms closely resemble their much more common pulmonary counterparts as illustrated in Chapter 16. In cytologic smears, a population of small malignant cells are present, having oval, round, or elongated nuclei that lack conspicuous nucleoli. Chromatin is hyperchromatic, uniformly distributed, and finely to coarsely granular. The malignant cells have exceedingly high N:C ratios. They are both individually scattered and present within densely packed groups, rosettelike structures, and chains. Within these aggregates, the nuclei either overlap or mold adjacent nuclei. The malignant cells are positive for low molecular weight cytokeratin and neuroendocrine markers.

The differential diagnoses of esophageal small cell carcinoma include a metastasis from a small cell carcinoma, usually from the lung, poorly differentiated squamous cell carcinoma, and malignant lymphoma. It is not possible to distinguish small cell carcinomas arising from different primary sites by conventional morphology, although thyroid transcription factor-1 (TTF-1) positivity would favor a metastasis from the lung. The differential diagnosis also includes malignant lymphoma, which can be suspected when a predominantly discohesive cell pattern is present, consisting of cells having recognizable nucleoli. Nuclear molding is not appreciated in smears from lymphoma, although occasional clusters of lymphoid cells can show overlapping nuclei. In smears from poorly differentiated squamous cell carcinoma with numerous small malignant cells, a diligent search demonstrates at least some cells showing more obvious squamous differentiation characterized by greater volumes of dense cytoplasm with sharp borders, more hyperchromatic chromatin, and the presence of well-developed nucleoli.

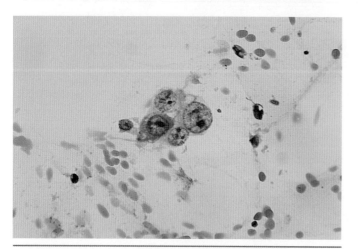

Figure 18-18   **Adenocarcinoma of esophagus.** Loose cluster of malignant cells having high nuclear-to-cytoplasmic ratios and prominent nucleoli. (Pap)

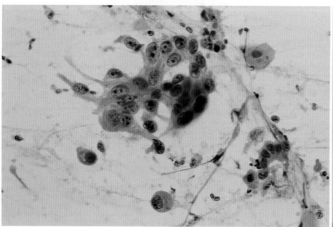

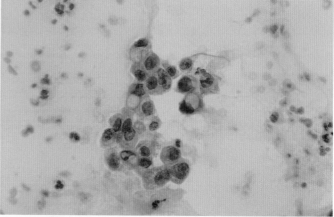

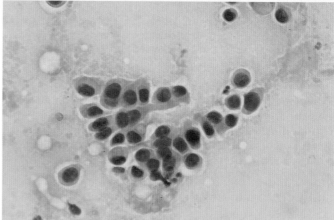

Figure 18-19   **Esophageal adenocarcinoma.** Esophageal brushings of adenocarcinoma show loose clusters of cells and individually scattered malignant cells. (Pap)

Other Esophageal Malignancies

Rarely, other primary or metastatic cancers can not only involve but also initially present clinically in the esophagus. These include malignant melanoma, hematopoietic malignancies, sarcomas, and germ cell tumors.

Both primary and metastatic malignant melanoma can have a variety of different appearances, but all tend to be characterized by a discohesive smear pattern. The size and shape of the tumor cells can vary significantly, with polygonal, spindled, or giant cell forms. Melanoma should be suspected when dispersed high-grade malignant cells with one or more large eccentrically placed nuclei showing thick membranes and huge nucleoli are identified. Mirror-image binucleated tumor cells are characteristic. The diagnosis is further supported when nuclear pseudoinclusions are found. When dark brown, coarsely or finely granular intracytoplasmic melanin pigment is present or the cytoplasm has a brownish dusky blush, the diagnosis can be made with confidence.

Melanin is often dark-green in air-dried preparations (Figure 18-22). However, if additional data are needed to confirm the rare primary melanoma of the esophagus or metastatic melanoma, application of melanocytic immunohistochemical markers such as HMB-45, MelanA, or S-100 can be useful.

The initial presentation of a malignant hematopoietic neoplasm in an esophageal cytologic specimen is quite rare. Fulp and colleagues reported three patients with acute myeloblastic leukemia involving the esophagus.[74] In all three patients, the cytologic specimens demonstrated numerous malignant leukocytes. The leukemic blasts had enlarged round nuclei, prominent nucleoli, and exceedingly high N:C ratios. Two patients demonstrated monocytoid differentiation, with more irregular nuclei and increased cytoplasm. Rarely, soft tissue sarcomas and malignant germ cell tumors have been reported in esophageal cytologic specimens.[75,76] Metastatic malignancies can also be cytologically identified.[14,77]

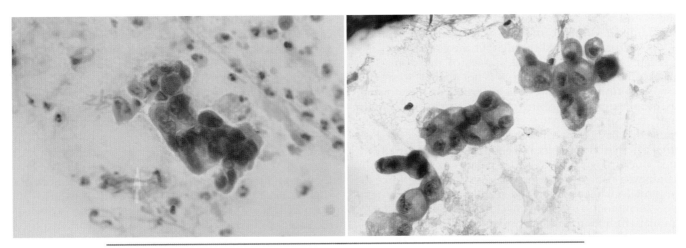

Figure 18-20 **Adenocarcinoma.** Esophageal brushings of adenocarcinoma demonstrating syncytial grouping of cells with loss of polarity. (Pap)

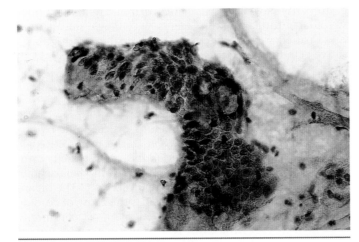

Figure 18-21 **Dysplasia.** Markedly atypical cluster seen in Barrett's esophagus in which hyperchromatic pseudostratified nuclei are present and extend to the luminal surface. Based on this field alone, it would not be possible to separate severe dysplasia in Barrett's metaplasia from an adenocarcinoma. (Pap)

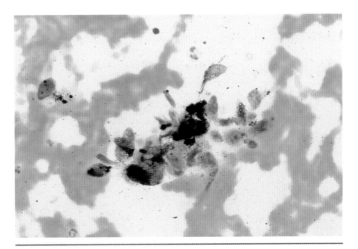

Figure 18-22 **Metastatic melanoma to esophagus.** Brushing of a metastatic malignant melanoma. Note the atypical spindle-shaped cells, many of which contain clumpy intracytoplasmic pigment. (Diff-Quik [DQ])

STOMACH

Normal Gastric Histology and Cytology

The stomach is divided into four major regions based on grossly visible landmarks. Immediately contiguous to the distal esophagus is the cardia portion that empties into the body of the stomach. The body of the stomach comprises the greatest portion of the mucosal surface. The fundus is the portion superior to an imaginary horizontal line drawn through the cardia opening. The distal portion of the stomach is divided into the antrum and pylorus; the latter is contiguous with the first segment of the duodenum. The entire mucosal surface of the stomach is lined by similar-appearing, mucous-secreting columnar cells that have small, basally oriented, round-to-oval nuclei; abundant cytoplasmic mucin; and low N:C ratios.[78] Similar cells line the gastric pits, which represent the superficial portion of the mucosa and connect to the more deeply located glands. In the cardia and antral portions of the stomach, mucus cells are also the dominant elements in the glands, whereas the fundus and body of the stomach have parietal and chief cells admixed with the mucous-secreting cells. Neuroendocrine cells are scattered throughout the glands.

Because the entire mucosal surface of the stomach is lined by similar-appearing cells, it is not possible to specify, based on brushings alone, which portion of the stomach has been sampled. Brushing cytology specimens contain large, cohesive aggregates of glandular epithelial cells arranged in flat, honeycomb sheets with sharply defined external cytoplasmic borders and equally distant, centrally located nuclei (Figure 18-23). The polarity of the nuclei is maintained with no evidence of overlapping or three-dimensional characteristics. The glandular nuclei are relatively small, round to slightly oval with pale staining, finely granular chromatin and inconspicuous nucleoli. The cytoplasm of these surface mucosal cells has a pale granular to slightly foamy appearance. When the cells are oriented on edge, they maintain a picket-fence pattern consisting of a line of columnar-shaped cells with basally placed nuclei.

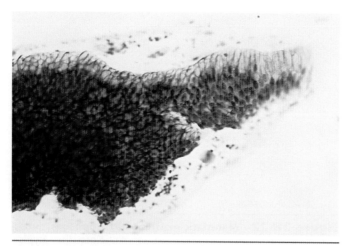

Figure 18-23 **Benign gastric mucosa.** Brushing of gastric antrum showing a flat, sheetlike grouping of glandular cells demonstrating both a honeycomb and peripheral palisading pattern. (Pap)

Individually scattered, benign glandular cells are relatively sparse in the brushings but are more commonly seen in lavage specimens and may be very numerous in aspirate samples obtained at the time of EUS.

The smear background is generally clear with only a few benign mononuclear cells and neutrophils. Intestinal metaplasia, as demonstrated by the presence of goblet cells, is not present in the normal stomach. Contaminants from the oral cavity and esophagus, especially benign squamous cells and food particles, including skeletal muscle fibers are often present.

Gastritis

Gastritis may be the result of a variety of etiologic factors, unfortunately resulting in confusing terminology and classification systems that have rather poor clinicopathologic correlation.[79] In addition, the endoscopic appearance often does not correlate with the surgical biopsy results. During the last decade, numerous studies have supported the role of *Helicobacter pylori* as the major cause of chronic gastritis and have challenged many of the older concepts of the causes of gastritis and the significance of many of the previously described histopathologic abnormalities.

Acute gastritis is secondary to a variety of etiologic factors and is a term often used to describe a nonspecific, self-limited disorder that is characterized by epigastric pain, nausea, vomiting, anorexia, and bleeding. Generally, patients experiencing episodes of acute gastritis do not undergo endoscopy. However, when the occasional patient is examined, the mucosa shows variable erythema, but brushing cytology is usually not obtained. If smears are procured, they contain neutrophils, fresh blood, and normal to slightly reactive glandular epithelial cells. Reparative glandular cells are not present unless the mucosa is eroded or ulcerated.

It is in the setting of chronic gastritis that endoscopy, biopsies, and cytologic sampling are most often obtained. Chronic gastritis is better characterized based on etiologic factors and histology, but all cases share similar cytologic features.[79] Certain clinically specific forms such as chemical gastropathy have been associated with bile reflux and nonsteroidal antiinflammatory agents.[80] Cytologic smears from these patients generally consist of normal-appearing to reactive glandular elements.

Helicobacter-Associated Gastritis and Other Organisms

During the past 15 years, numerous articles and reports have described the role of *H. pylori* as the major etiologic agent in upper GI diseases. *H. pylori* has been strongly associated with most cases of duodenitis and duodenal peptic ulcers, and to a lesser extent, gastric ulcers.[79,81-83] The organism has also been directly implicated as the cause of chronic diffuse antral or type B gastritis. Patients most commonly present with epigastric distress. Histologic examination of endoscopic biopsies from the antral mucosa characteristically show a superficial diffuse infiltrate of plasma cells, neutrophils infiltrating the epithelial elements, and deeply located lymphoid nodules and follicles. *H. pylori* organisms can be identified attached to the luminal mucosal surface or present within the overlying mucoid exudate. These gram-negative spiral bacteria can be visualized in the routine H&E-stained material and with a variety of Romanowsky stains or the Warthin-Starry silver stain.[84,85] An immunohistochemical method is also available. Although a number of other diagnostic methods are used to detect *H. pylori,* including culture, serologic tests, urease production, in-situ hybridization, and the polymerase chain reaction, the diagnosis is often made at the time of endoscopic biopsy using conventional H&E stains, along with one of the histochemical stains.[84] Cytologic preparations can enhance the diagnosis because the gastric mucosal surface is better sampled and organisms are readily identified in the smears.

Cytologic preparations from patients with *Helicobacter*-associated gastritis contain large, cohesive groups of glandular epithelial cells that can, at times, also demonstrate reparative atypia and intestinal metaplasia, along with numerous neutrophils and *Helicobacter* organisms. The epithelial cells, although demonstrating inflammatory atypia and reparative change, are recognized as benign because of the preservation of normal cellular cohesion and polarity. As illustrated previously, the presence of goblet cells interspersed among the columnar absorptive cell is diagnostic of intestinal metaplasia.

Helicobacter organisms measure from 1 to 3 μm in length and possess a curved or spiral configuration typically manifesting as an S or C shape. When present in significant numbers, bacteria can be recognized at high dry magnification without the need for oil immersion microscopy (Figure 18-24). The organisms are closely associated with glandular cells or within clumps of extracellular mucus. The long axis of the organism typically parallels the long axis of the mucous strands.[86] Occasionally, *H. pylori* appears to be within the cytoplasm of neutrophils. False-positive identification of *H. pylori* has been reported when excessively thick clumps of mucus are present.[87] The organisms are readily seen in alcohol-fixed Pap-stained smears but are more easily identified in air-dried DQ or other Romanowsky-stained smears because of their larger size in these preparations. A variety of different stains has been used on gastric brushing cytology to identify the organisms.[84] Other cocci and rod-shaped bacteria may also be found in the smears and should be differentiated from the spiral-shaped *Helicobacter.*

A number of reports have compared endoscopic brushings with biopsies for the identification of *H. pylori.*[86-90] Others compare touch imprints of biopsies with the histologic preparation.[85,91-94] A variety of stains has been used in these studies including Pap, Romanowsky, Gram, Steiner, and triple stain. Independent of which stain is used, cytologic preparations have been found to be more sensitive than histology, most likely a reflection of sampling of a greater mucosal surface area by cytology than the more directed endoscopic biopsy. Some authors have proposed that

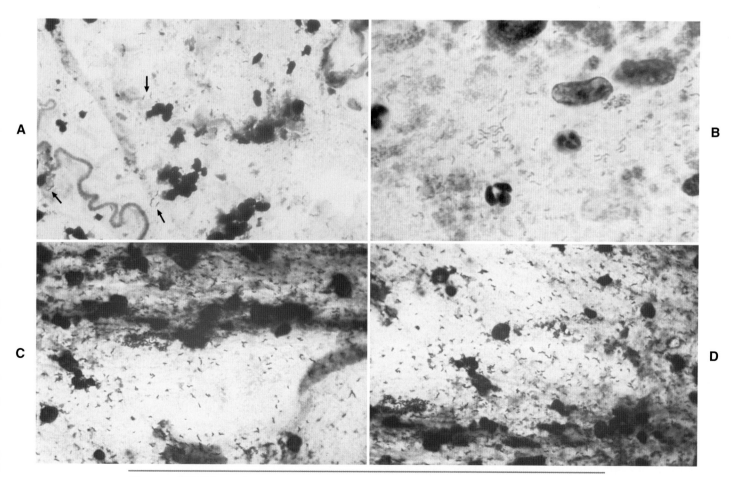

Figure 18-24   *Helicobacter.* **A** and **B,** In these Pap-stained smears, the spiral-shaped organisms of *Helicobacter* can be appreciated. **C** and **D,** In these DQ-stained smears, numerous *Helicobacter*-type organisms are identified.

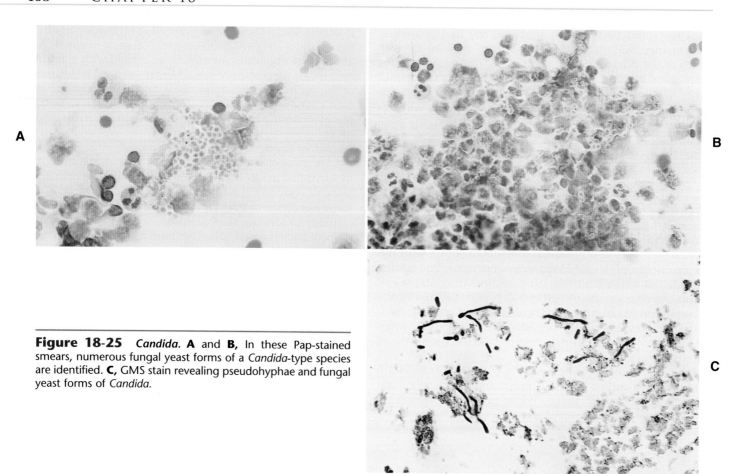

Figure 18-25   *Candida.* **A** and **B,** In these Pap-stained smears, numerous fungal yeast forms of a *Candida*-type species are identified. **C,** GMS stain revealing pseudohyphae and fungal yeast forms of *Candida.*

an attempt be made to identify *H. pylori* in smears at the time of the endoscopy, thereby prompting early initiation of appropriate therapy. The authors believe that both biopsy and brushing cytology should be used because they are complementary. In addition, because brushing samples a greater area of the mucosa than biopsies, Ching and colleagues used brushing material for the urea broth test, a biochemical colorimetric assay for *H. pylori.*[95] These authors compared urea test results using antral biopsies vs. brushing material and found that in patients with histologic evidence of *H. pylori*-associated gastritis, positive test results occurred in brushings and biopsies in 97% and 76%, respectively. A positive result was obtained within 5 minutes from the brushing material vs. 60 minutes from the biopsies.

Another advantage of cytology examination is the assessment for other organisms that can be identified in gastric brushing smears. Overlying some gastric ulcers, *Candida*-type species can be appreciated when the characteristic yeast or pseudohyphae are seen (Figure 18-25). *Candida* is probably not a true pathogen but rather represents secondary colonization of preexisting benign and malignant ulcers.

Other organisms are noted rarely. Rod-shaped and cocci-shaped bacteria are usually considered contaminants in gastric brushings. However, clusters of filamentous organisms described in both benign and malignant esophageal and gastric brushing cytology specimens are often associated with an underlying malignant tumor.[96] A rare case of mi-crofilaria diagnosed in gastric brushing cytology has been published.[97] Cytomegalovirus and various parasites have also been reported.[40,41,98] CMV virocytes are usually associated with systemic disease and are most commonly seen in patients with AIDS.

Peptic Ulcer Disease

Peptic ulcers are defined as chronic ulcerating lesions of the GI tract secondary to the enzymatic action of hydrochloric acid and pepsin. Nearly 100% of peptic ulcers occur in either the stomach or the duodenum; approximately 80% occur in the latter location. Recent evidence has linked *H. pylori* infection to the vast majority of peptic ulcers.[81] Peptic ulcers most often occur in young to middle-age adults but can be seen in all ages. Classic symptoms consist of burning epigastric pain occurring within approximately 1 hour of eating.

Endoscopic examination generally reveals a small ulcer usually measuring less than 3 cm in diameter, with round or ovoid, sharply delineated borders. The underlying scar causes puckering of the surrounding mucosa. Although characteristic, neither the radiologic nor endoscopic appearance can consistently and accurately distinguish benign from malignant ulcers. This is because many gastric adenocarcinomas present with an ulcerating defect, although this would be unusual for malignant lesions of the duodenum. Therefore, brushing of duodenal ulcers is performed much less often than is the case with gastric ulcers.

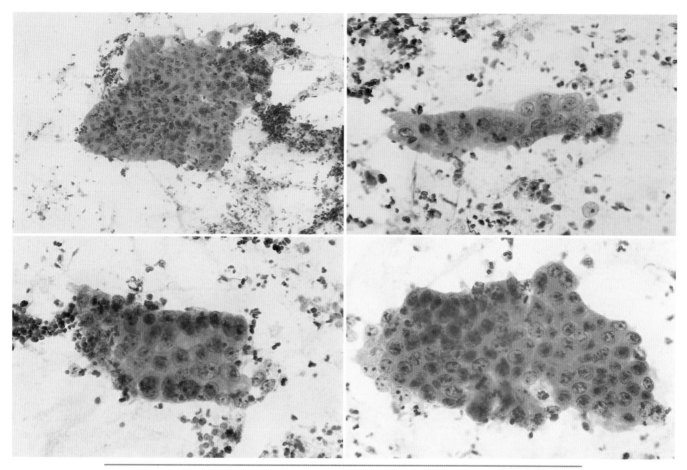

Figure 18-26 **Repair.** Brushing cytology from gastric ulcers shows cohesive groups of reactive and reparative gastric epithelial cells. Some mildly atypical features including prominent nucleoli are noted. However, maintenance of polarity and absence of atypical single cells help exclude a diagnosis of carcinoma from consideration. (Pap)

Histologic examination of the gastric ulcers reveals an ulcer bed consisting of granulation tissue with surrounding fibrosis. Overlying the ulcer bed is necrotic debris and neutrophils. At the edges of the lesion, regenerating epithelium is present.

When biopsies and brushings are taken from the interface of the intact mucosa with the ulcer, reparative glandular epithelium is procured. These cells are characterized by enlarged nuclei with prominent nucleoli but with maintenance of polarity and relative preservation of cohesion (Figures 18-26 and 18-27). Brushing cytology smears also contain numerous neutrophils and granular debris. *H. pylori* may be appreciated in the background or attached to some of the glandular cell surfaces.

The atypical epithelium can generally be distinguished from adenocarcinoma in most cases; however, occasionally, this differential diagnosis can be quite challenging.[2-4] The major criteria used to differentiate adenocarcinoma from repair have been previously outlined and presented in Table 18-1.

Some investigators do not believe that gastric brushings should be routinely employed if six or more biopsy specimens are obtained.[99-101] They would restrict the use of brushing cytology to the evaluation of huge ulcers or to difficult-to-biopsy lesions in locations such as the cardia. They also use brushing cytology in patients from whom prior biopsies were negative for carcinoma in the face of an endoscopic picture suspicious for malignancy. In contrast, these authors and other investigators believe that brushing cytology should be routinely incorporated into the evaluation of any gastric mucosal abnormality. It complements and enhances the diagnostic accuracy of biopsies with little additional cost, time, or patient discomfort.[3,102,103]

Atrophic Gastritis

Chronic atrophic gastritis connotes a progressive loss of the fundic secretory elements, accompanied by inflammatory infiltrates of lymphocytes and plasma cells. This results in a thin mucosa containing goblet cells. Because of the atrophic changes, hydrochloric acid is significantly reduced. Some patients are believed to have an autoimmune disorder resulting from the presence of circulating autoantibodies. Patients with atrophic gastritis have a statistically increased risk of developing adenocarcinoma, which is believed to evolve through glandular dysplasia.[104]

In uncomplicated atrophic gastritis, no distinctive features identify this condition in cytology specimens. The

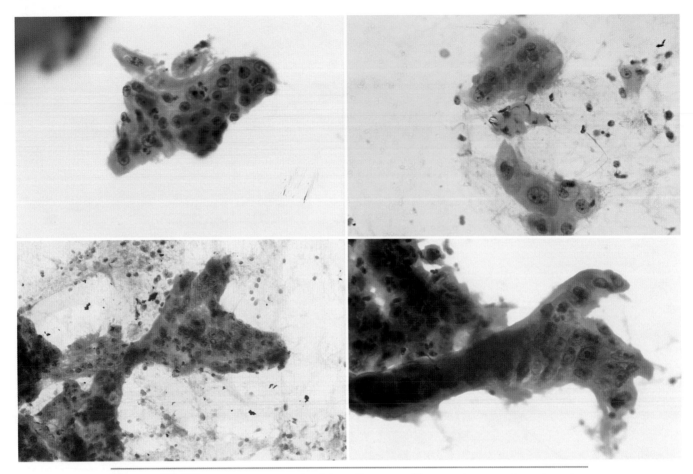

Figure 18-27   **Repair.** Reactive glandular cells arranged in a repair type pattern characterized by streaming of the nuclei, maintenance of cohesion, and no loss of polarity. Despite the prominence of nucleoli, the cells' N:C ratios remain within normal limits. (Pap)

smears contain only cohesive groups of benign glandular cells, which may include goblet cells, and mixed inflammatory cells. If dysplastic glandular epithelium is present, the cytologic findings recapitulate those seen in dysplasia from Barrett's mucosa (Figure 18-28). The dysplastic aggregates tend to be small to large with irregular jagged edges. The dysplastic nuclei are larger than normal and often have an elongated shape and possess one or more prominent nucleoli. Pseudostratified nuclei can be appreciated within the groups. The dysplastic cells have nuclei with finely to coarsely granular, hyperchromatic chromatin, and nuclear contours vary from smooth to slightly irregular. Cytoplasmic mucin is reduced or not apparent. The N:C ratios are increased, and within the groups, the nuclei are crowded and overlapping and often demonstrate molding. Similar to Barrett's esophagus, dysplastic glandular epithelium can generally be distinguished from benign repair but cannot reliably be separated from some examples of well-differentiated adenocarcinoma.[57,105] Although not absolutely diagnostic, the most significant cytologic feature present in smears from adenocarcinoma but not noted in dysplasia is a greater number of individually dispersed, intact abnormal-appearing cells. If this latter feature is appreciated with any degree of frequency, then adenocarcinoma should be strongly suggested.

Chemotherapy-Associated Atypia

As illustrated previously, marked cytologic atypia in actively regenerating cells can occur secondary to systemically administered cytotoxic cancer chemotherapy.[106] Although the gastric mucosa can manifest chemotherapy-associated atypia, it is often not sampled because of the patient's lack of gastric symptoms. Hepatic artery infusion is a relatively unusual clinical circumstance. This form of chemotherapy administration has been associated with a higher incidence of gastric mucosal defects because the hepatic artery also contributes a portion of the vascular supply to the stomach. When a higher concentration of cytotoxic drugs is delivered to the gastric mucosa, patients may develop ulcers that can simulate either conventional peptic ulcers or gastric adenocarcinoma. Brushing cytology specimens of these chemotherapy-induced ulcers can manifest significant epithelial atypia that potentially could be mistaken for adenocarcinoma.[106] The atypical epithelial cells are arranged in large, flat sheets, small clusters, and individually, but three-dimensional configurations were not appreciated in the study by Becker and colleagues.[106] The most troublesome cytologic feature was the marked increase in cytoplasmic and nuclear volumes, but the N:C ratios remained relatively low. Although one or more prominent nucleoli were present in many nuclei and occasional mononucleated to

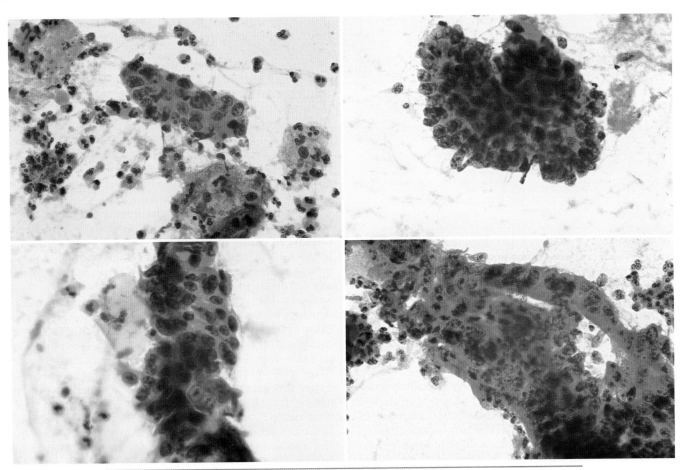

Figure 18-28   Gastric dysplasia. Dysplastic gastric glandular epithelium in which cells shows nuclear enlargement, hyperchromasia, and pseudostratification of the nuclei. The maintenance of polarity and lack of single atypical cells favors a dysplastic process rather than adenocarcinoma. (Pap)

multinucleated atypical cells were seen, the nuclear contours remained relatively smooth and the chromatin was evenly distributed. All of these features should suggest a benign diagnosis.

Polyps

The two most frequent polyps to involve the gastric mucosa are hyperplastic polyps and adenomas. Small single and multiple nonneoplastic hyperplastic polyps have only a slightly increased risk of having an associated gastric carcinoma. Histologic examination reveals elongation of the gastric pits with tentacles of delicate, smooth muscle cells extending into the lamina propria. The surface of the polyp can show erosion with secondary regenerating epithelium and acute inflammation. Brushing cytology reveals reparative glandular epithelium with associated neutrophils and necrotic debris, cytologic features indistinguishable from those obtained from the edge of a gastric ulcer. Gastric adenomas, in contrast, carry a markedly increased risk of adenocarcinoma of the stomach. Histologically and cytologically, the cells of gastric adenomas are indistinguishable from adenomas of the lower GI tract, as well as dysplastic epithelium occurring in the setting of Barrett's esophagus. In the brushing cytology specimen, the atypical glandular epithelium from an adenoma shows all the changes seen in brushings from dysplastic epithelium and occasional papillary-like fragments (Figure 18-29).

Adenocarcinoma

Gastric adenocarcinoma remains one of the most common forms of malignancy worldwide, although the incidence is declining.[104] In the United States in the 1930s, gastric carcinoma was the single most common cancer. It has been suggested that carcinomas arising from the gastric cardia differ from those occurring more distally, and despite the overall decline in incidence of gastric carcinoma, the frequency of carcinoma of the cardia is actually increasing.[104] This latter type of malignancy appears to be closely related to Barrett's mucosa-associated carcinoma, which is also increasing in frequency.[65]

Worldwide, considerable variation in the incidence and etiologic factors of gastric carcinoma is evident. Predominantly environmental, and to a lesser extent, hereditary factors have been implicated as causal agents for gastric adenocarcinoma. The incidence appears to be especially high in countries having diets with a high salt content or increased consumption of smoked meats. Other predisposing conditions include atrophic gastritis with metaplasia

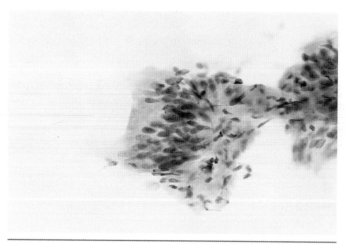

Figure 18-29 **Adenomatous polyp.** Brushing from adenomatous polyp of the stomach demonstrating elongated pseudostratified hyperchromatic nuclei. (Pap)

and prior partial gastrectomy. The latter condition predisposes patients to develop carcinoma in the gastric stump. Gastric dysplasia has been invoked as an intermediate morphologic stage that evolves into gastric carcinoma.

Adenocarcinoma of the stomach is predominantly a disease of middle-age and older adults, who unfortunately usually present with advanced disease. The symptoms of gastric adenocarcinoma are generally nonspecific, including nausea, heartburn, anorexia, weakness, and weight loss. Patients with early gastric carcinoma are often asymptomatic.

Several classification schemes are available for adenocarcinoma of the stomach, based on stage of disease, gross findings, and/or histologic type. Grossly and endoscopically, adenocarcinomas can be divided into early and advanced forms, with the early carcinomas confined to the mucosa or submucosa independent of the patient's regional lymph node status. Although uncommon in the western world, early carcinoma is often diagnosed in those countries having a high incidence and thus active surveillance programs. In Japan, approximately one third of all gastric cancers are of the early carcinoma type. Early carcinomas are generally small with a gross and endoscopic appearance of only a slightly elevated or excavated mucosa. The prognosis is considerably improved in comparison with the more advanced carcinomas, which usually appear as polypoid masses or large ulcerating lesions. The latter gross presentation may be difficult to distinguish endoscopically and radiographically from a peptic ulcer.

The two major histologic forms of gastric adenocarcinoma, as described by Lauren,[107] are the more common intestinal gland-forming variant and the less common diffuse form. The intestinal or gland-forming variant is characterized by rather well-formed glandular structures lined by malignant-appearing columnar cells. This variant is generally well to moderately differentiated, in contrast with the diffuse form. The latter lacks any glandular differentiation and is composed predominantly of small malignant cells arranged individually in small nests. These show extensive infiltration of the gastric wall associated with a surrounding desmoplastic response. Signet ring tumor cells have large cytoplasmic mucin vacuoles that eccentrically displace and

distort the malignant nucleus. The indentation of the nucleus by the large mucin vacuole often creates sharply pointed nuclear tips.

Histologically and cytologically, a diagnostic challenge is to separate malignant signet ring forms having a relatively bland appearance from benign glandular cells showing intestinal metaplasia, as well as scattered mucinophages having a coarsely vacuolated cytoplasm.

Advanced gastric adenocarcinoma has a dismal prognosis with only 15% of the patients surviving 5 years. The diffuse variant is even more aggressive. However, if early gastric carcinoma is resected, even with lymph node metastasis, the prognosis can still be excellent.

Cytologic examination of the intestinal type of adenocarcinoma recapitulates the findings described for adenocarcinoma arising in Barrett's esophagus (see Table 18-4). A hypercellular smear pattern contains loosely cohesive groups showing loss of polarity along with many individually scattered malignant cells (Figures 18-30 and 18-31). Some of the groups have prominent three-dimensional depth of focus, and their external borders are irregular because of frayed cytoplasmic membranes. Within the groups, malignant cells demonstrate crowding, overlapping, and molding with considerable variation in nuclear size and shape. High-power examination reveals large round to oval hyperchromatic nuclei with thick nuclear membranes demonstrating significant irregularity. One or more prominent nucleoli will be appreciated. The cytoplasm is fragile and has a vacuolated to granular amphophilic appearance. N:C ratios are increased. Stripped tumor cell nuclei can also be noted in the background; in some cases, this may be the predominant finding. Although the diagnosis can be suspected, one is cautioned not to make an unequivocal diagnosis of malignancy without identifying at least a few intact, isolated, obviously malignant cells. Similar to what can be found in benign peptic ulcers, the background contains granular necrotic debris and neutrophils.

In contrast with the usually straightforward cytologic diagnosis of intestinal-type adenocarcinoma, the diffuse form can be challenging. Fewer malignant cells are seen and can be easily confused with benign elements, especially if significant nuclear atypicality is not present. Signet ring carcinoma cells are notable for their ability to demonstrate considerable variability in appearance. Some cells have obvious malignant features such as hyperchromatic irregular nuclei and prominent nucleoli, whereas other cells take on a much more bland appearance. The large mucin vacuole abuts the nucleus, producing a concave nuclear configuration with sharply pointed tips and angles (Figure 18-32). The vacuole may be sharply delineated and appear either optically clear or somewhat granular and palely stained. In occasional cases, only a few scattered signet ring carcinoma cells are present and can be easily overlooked when they are individually scattered throughout the smear background. In some cases the cytologic distinction of the two major types of adenocarcinoma cannot be reliably achieved.[105]

The most challenging differential diagnosis is the separation of signet ring carcinoma from nonneoplastic mucus-producing columnar and goblet cells and from mucin-containing histiocytes (muciphages). This is especially challenging when the signet ring forms have a relatively bland appearance, although careful search of these smears

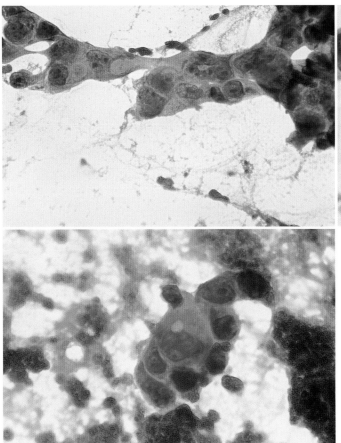

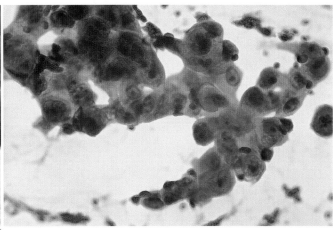

Figure 18-30 **Gastric carcinoma, intestinal type.** Brushings from gastric carcinoma demonstrating loosely cohesive groups of malignant cells with loss of polarity. The tumor cells have hyperchromatic irregular nuclei with prominent nucleoli. (Pap)

will often demonstrate a few scattered cells with obvious malignant features. Individually scattered histiocytes and benign glandular cells lack the sharply pointed nuclear tips of carcinoma. Rather, histiocytes will have a characteristic bean-shaped nucleus that is not distorted by mucin vacuoles. Signet ring cells will have N:C ratios that will be considerably higher than those seen in either benign glandular cells or histiocytes.[2] In air-dried smears, signet ring cells are accentuated by their large sizes and by metachromatic staining of the large cytoplasmic mucin droplet.

Many studies have demonstrated the greater diagnostic sensitivity and specificity of biopsies over brushing cytology for the diagnosis of gastric adenocarcinoma.[2-4] Some studies have also shown that if six or more biopsies are endoscopically obtained from most adenocarcinomas, a definitive diagnosis usually can be rendered. However, in the authors' and others' experience, endoscopic surgical biopsies and cytologic brushings are complementary. The diagnostic yields for biopsies range from 74% to 95% with a weighted mean yield of 89%; brushing cytology diagnostic yields vary from 77% to 100% with a weighted mean yield of 87%.* When both procedures are used, the combined yield increases to 88% to 100%, with a diagnostic mean yield of 96%. Transmucosal FNA biopsy may also increase the diagnostic accuracy for the diffuse type of adenocarcinomas because this procedure is better suited to sampling the involved gastric wall. Imprint cytology performed on endoscopic

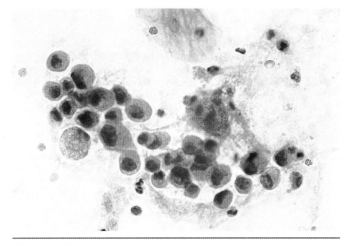

Figure 18-31 **Gastric carcinoma, intestinal type.** The presence of numerous single malignant cells helps establish the diagnosis of a gastric carcinoma. (Pap)

biopsy has also been demonstrated to increase the accuracy for diagnosing malignancy of the GI tract.[108]

Malignant Lymphoma

The most common site for extranodal non-Hodgkin's lymphoma is the GI tract with approximately one half occurring in the stomach.[109] Approximately 5% of all gastric cancers are lymphomas. Many of these lymphomas resemble

---

*References 3, 22, 24, 100, 102, 103.

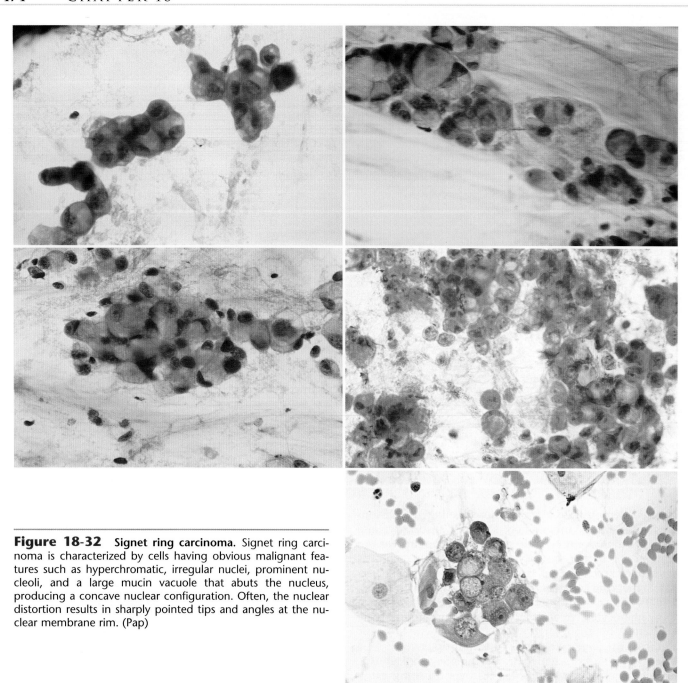

Figure 18-32   Signet ring carcinoma. Signet ring carcinoma is characterized by cells having obvious malignant features such as hyperchromatic, irregular nuclei, prominent nucleoli, and a large mucin vacuole that abuts the nucleus, producing a concave nuclear configuration. Often, the nuclear distortion results in sharply pointed tips and angles at the nuclear membrane rim. (Pap)

those seen as primary neoplasms of lymph nodes, although special types of lymphoid neoplasms are unique to sites containing mucosa-associated lymphoid tissue (MALT). Most patients with primary GI tract lymphomas are adults who present with gastric ulcers, obstruction, or bleeding. Although most examples of gastric lymphoma present with a solitary mass having focal or diffuse involvement, a few cases present as multiple polypoid lesions. When solitary, the lymphoma can present as a polypoid lesion, as a mural nodule that is ulcerated, or as a massive rugal enlargement that may be indistinguishable from the more common adenocarcinoma. Although a variety of different lymphoma types can involve the stomach, diffuse large cell type is the most common. Almost all gastric lymphomas express a B-

cell immunophenotype. In contrast, Hodgkin's disease is exceedingly rare in the GI tract.

If the overlying mucosal surface is intact, brushing cytology may not sample the diagnostic malignant lymphoid cells. However, if ulceration is present, the cytology smears can contain large numbers of individually scattered lymphoid cells having a uniformly atypical appearance (Figure 18-33). Although tumor cells may appear to be crowded or clustered when entrapped in the mucoid exudate, no evidence of true cohesion is apparent. In large cell lymphoma, the cells have a single nucleus with a thick and sometimes irregularly shaped nuclear membrane, vesicular chromatin, and one or more conspicuous nucleoli. Such cells also feature very scanty cytoplasm resulting in high N:C ratios

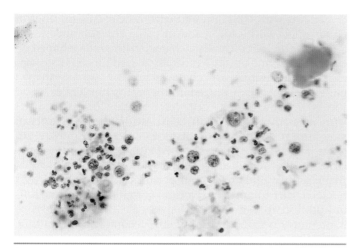

Figure 18-33 **Malignant lymphoma.** Brushing of gastric lymphoma characterized by scattered atypical lymphoid cells admixed with neutrophils. (Pap)

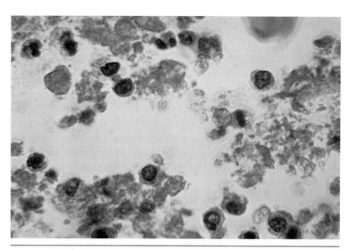

Figure 18-34 **Malignant lymphoma.** High-power view of large cell lymphoma in which individually scattered malignant cells show high N:C ratios. Note the small but prominent nucleoli in many of the cells. (Pap)

TABLE 18-5		CMF
Cytomorphologic Differential Diagnosis of Gastric Lymphoid Lesions		
Feature	**Malignant Lymphoma**	**Follicular Hyperplasia**
Lymphoid cell population	Homogeneous	Polymorphic, with small to large cells (predominance of small)
Nuclear contours	Variable, may be highly irregular	Most are round and smooth
Tingible body macrophages	Present in higher grades of malignant lymphomas	Present
Plasma cells	Infrequent, but when present, usually numerous	Often present in low numbers

Modified from Geisinger KR, Silverman JF. Gastrointestinal cytology. In: Silverberg SG, editor. Principles and practice of surgical pathology and cytopathology. 3rd ed. New York: Churchill Livingstone; 1997. pp.1563-1593.

(Figure 18-34). In small-cleaved cell lymphoma, the atypical lymphoid cells are smaller, with a greater degree of nuclear irregularity and higher N:C ratios. The chromatin is more darkly stained, and nucleoli are inconspicuous. Although a few neutrophils may be present, they do not make up a significant portion of the cellular infiltrate. Because of the bland appearance of small lymphocytes seen in small lymphocytic lymphoma and low-grade MALT-associated lymphomas, these types of lymphomas are not usually diagnosed in brushing cytology preparations.[2,110]

The cytologic differential diagnoses of GI tract lymphomas include a variety of benign and malignant entities, the majority of which is characterized by a dissociative smear pattern. The differential diagnosis includes benign lymphoid hyperplasia (Table 18-5). This diagnosis is based on the presence of a polymorphic population of lymphoid cells rather than a uniform population of atypical lymphoid cells in lymphoma. In smears from these reactive lymphoid processes, tingible body macrophages may also be present. The diffuse form of gastric adenocarcinoma also enters into the differential diagnosis because relatively small individually scattered malignant cells are present. However, the cells from diffuse adenocarcinoma possess a greater amount of cytoplasm and have eccentrically placed nuclei that are often displaced by an obvious mucin vacuole. With careful searching of the smears, a few groups of truly cohesive epithelial cells are often appreciated. Stromal tumors can also consist of individually scattered cells, but these tend to have spindled or elongated configurations, with fine, delicate chromatin and few prominent nucleoli.

Multiple gastric biopsies are more helpful than brushing cytology for making the diagnosis of lymphoma, although the two techniques are complementary. In the study of Sherman and colleagues, 15% of lymphoma cases had positive cytology smears but negative biopsies, with an overall sensitivity for cytology of 48%.[110] In their review, gastric brushing cytology for the diagnosis of lymphoma had a diagnostic rate of 15% to 83%.[110] Cabre-Fiol and Vilardell[111] also reported the value of brushing cytology, although only 21% of the primary gastric lymphomas reported by Lozowski and Hajdu[112] were correctly diagnosed in the cytology brushings. Layfield and colleagues reported the value of FNA cytology for excluding malignant lymphoma when prominent gastric folds are present endoscopically.[18] Transmural FNA biopsy can also be of value because gastric lymphoma generally has a submucosal predilection. EUS-guided FNA can provide tissue sufficient for immunophenotyping by flow cytometry.

Gastrointestinal Stromal Neoplasia

Stromal neoplasms arise in the walls of the GI tract, with the stomach being the most common site, followed by the small intestine. Although comprising only a small portion of all gastric neoplasms, they have invoked considerable interest, reflected by the numerous investigations studying their histogenesis and prognosis.[113] Although most were previously considered to be benign or malignant smooth muscle tumors, the concept of gastrointestinal stromal tumor (GIST) has evolved due to the lack of immunohistochemical staining for specific muscle markers and positive staining of the cells for CD 34 and the C-kit protooncogene (CD 117). A recent concept is that most GISTs represent tumors derived from the interstitial cell of Cajal, believed to be the GI pacemaker cell.

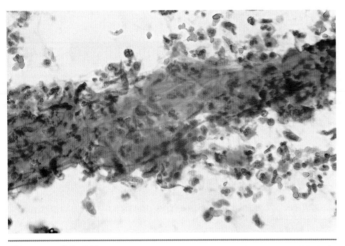

Figure 18-35 Gastrointestinal stromal tumor (GIST). Brushing of ulcerated GIST in which atypical spindle-shaped nuclei are present. (Pap)

Patients with GISTs present with nonspecific findings of either upper GI bleeding and/or pain. The submucosal location of the lesion causes a characteristic dome-shaped elevation with one or more centrally placed ulcers. Histologically, these lesions are characterized by spindle-shaped mesenchymal cells arranged in interlacing bundles or broad sheets.[113] These spindle cells have single elongated nuclei with tapered to squared-off ends. Although the cytoplasm may appear eosinophilic, this does not reflect muscle differentiation. Some tumors consist either of an entire population of epithelioid mesenchymal cells having polygonal shape with well-defined borders and centrally placed oval nuclei. Other tumors show a focal component of these cells in addition to the spindle-shaped cells. The diagnosis of malignancy is based on tumor size, pleomorphism, mitotic activity, necrosis, and the site of the neoplasm.[113,114] The behavior of some tumors is very difficult to predict.

Only a few reports have been made of the cytologic features of GISTs.[70,99,102,103,115] As mentioned earlier, if an overlying intact mucosa is present, the diagnostic cells are not sampled. However, in ulcerated areas, brushing cytology can obtain a few to moderate numbers of usually spindle-shaped cells arranged singly or in small to large clusters (Figure 18-35). When the cells are present in clusters, they may be associated with extracellular matrix material (Figure 18-36). The spindled to ovoid-shaped cells have high N:C ratios and possess single elongated nuclei often with blunt ends. The chromatin is generally finely granular and evenly distributed, and nucleoli are not prominent. The cytoplasm is cyanophilic with indistinct cell borders, causing the tumor cells to blend with each other or into the adjacent stromal matrix.

The brushing cytology of a GIST can be unrewarding because of the lack of diagnostic cells, when the overlying mucosa is intact. Even when an ulcer is present, the differential diagnosis may still include benign mesenchymal cells and granulation tissue. Most believe that the diagnostic sensitivity of brushing cytology for a gastric stromal neoplasm is low. Even when a GI stromal neoplasm is suspected in the brushing cytology specimen, it may be impossible to

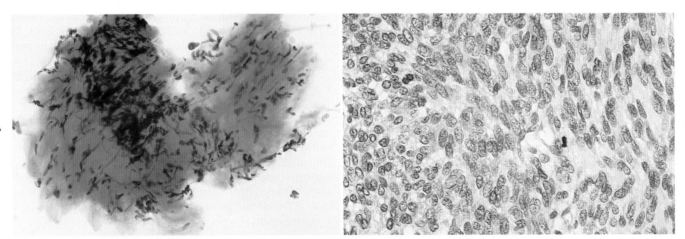

A   B

Figure 18-36 GIST. **A,** In this brushing of an ulcerated GIST, occasional loose clusters of atypical spindle-shaped cells were present, along with associated matrix. (Pap) **B,** Cell block sections of GIST aspirated with EUS guidance, demonstrated interlacing fascicles of atypical spindle-shaped cells in which occasional mitotic figures are present. The tumor cells were positive for CD34 and CD117. (H&E)

separate benign from malignant lesions because the latter assessment is based on tumor size, mitotic activity, necrosis, and the site of the neoplasm. However, some of the limitations of brushing cytology for establishing a specific diagnosis of GIST and categorizing these stromal neoplasms into benign and malignant groups are also shared by endoscopic biopsies.

With its excellent ability to access mural masses, EUS-guided FNA is currently the most efficacious approach to sampling of GISTs.[115,116] It is not uncommon to recover abundant material to the extent that when the aspirate is expressed onto a slide, numerous grossly visible tissue particles are identified. These are frequently very cohesive and remain intact after smearing. Using techniques for preparing paraffin-embedded cell blocks that were described in Chapter 2, cytopathologists routinely allocate a generous portion of the specimen for histologic study. This permits application of immunostains that improve the diagnosis in two ways. First, the immunoprofile discussed previously allows exclusion of the less common, but occasionally encountered, smooth muscle tumors. Second, confirmation of CD 117 expression leads to the chemical therapy to which many of these tumors are at least initially responsive.

Carcinoid Tumor

Neuroendocrine neoplasms are most often seen in the appendix, but they occur with some frequency throughout the entire GI tract. Most are conventional carcinoid tumors because atypical carcinoid and small cell carcinomas only rarely occur in the GI tract. Some gastric carcinoid tumors are believed to arise in the background of atrophic gastritis with associated endocrine cell hyperplasia. Gastric carcinoid tumors most often occur in adults who present with upper abdominal pain, GI bleeding, or the carcinoid syndrome. Rarely, other hormonal manifestations may occur.

Characteristically, the endoscopic and gross appearance is that of a small submucosal lesion that may show overlying ulceration. Histologic examination reveals uniform-appearing cells arranged in cords or nests. The cells show a moderate amount of granular cytoplasm, a round nucleus with evenly dispersed chromatin and inconspicuous nucleoli. In the conventional carcinoid tumor, little pleomorphism, mitotic activity, or necrosis occurs. The overlying mucosa tends to be attenuated but intact. This limits the cells' availability for cytologic brushings. Consequently, only a few cytology reports of GI tract carcinoids have been noted.[2,117] If ulceration occurs, the smears may contain scattered small to moderately sized neuroendocrine cells possessing round to oval nuclei with delicate nuclear membranes; evenly dispersed, finely to moderately granular chromatin; and small to inconspicuous nucleoli (Figure 18-37). The cytoplasm can range from slight to moderate in volume and is granular because of the numerous neuroendocrine granules. When only a thin rim of surrounding cytoplasm is present, the N:C ratios are quite high. The cells are usually individually scattered in the smears but may be present in small, loose aggregates arranged in sheets, spheres, or acini. Although the nuclei may be crowded, there is no evidence of nuclear overlapping or molding.

EUS-guided FNA can more readily sample the submucosal nodules, and one report showed its superiority to biopsy for identifying the neoplastic neuroendocrine cells.[16] It is not possible to predict the biologic behavior of carcinoid tumor based on histologic or cytologic features because this is more dependent on the site of involvement, the size of the neoplasm, and its infiltrative qualities.

The differential cytologic diagnoses include other lesions that consist of relatively small, dispersed cells including chronic inflammation, malignant lymphoma, and the diffuse type of adenocarcinoma (Table 18-6). Appreciation of any degree of intercellular cohesion would mitigate against a diagnosis of either a benign or malignant lymphoid process. Although the N:C ratios can be high in cells from carcinoid tumor, they are higher in lymphoid lesions. The presence of nucleoli and nuclear irregularity would also favor lymphoma. In the diffuse type of adenocarcinoma, the tumor cells show greater pleomorphism with prominent nucleoli and occasional cytoplasmic vacuoles. Primary and metastatic small cell carcinoma also enters into the differ-

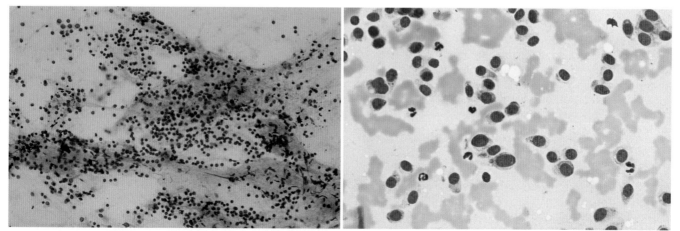

A   **B**

Figure 18-37   **Carcinoid tumor. A,** Brushing of gastric carcinoid tumor demonstrating individually scattered small uniform cells. (Pap) **B,** High-power view of gastric carcinoid in which the dissociative cells take on a plasmacytoid appearance. (DQ) (**A,** Courtesy Josh Sickel, MD, Mountain View, Calif.)

TABLE 18-6   CMF

Cytomorphologic Differential Diagnosis of Poorly Cohesive Cells in Gastric Cytology

Feature	Carcinoid Tumor	Signet Ring Adenocarcinoma	Lymphoma	Stromal Tumor
Intercellular cohesion	Variably preserved	Poorly preserved	Absent	Variably preserved
Cytoplasm	Granular	Single dominant vacuole	Scant, nondescript	Scant to moderate, spindled
Nuclear contours	Round, smooth	Variable, sharp points characteristic	Clefts, notches, indentations	Elongated
Chromatin pattern	Salt and pepper granularity	Coarse	Usually fine	Usually fine
Nucleoli	− or inconspicuous	+	+, may be multiple	±
N:C ratio	High	Moderate	High	Moderate to high

Modified from Geisinger KR, Silverman JF. Gastrointestinal cytology. In: Silverberg SG, editor. Principles and practice of surgical pathology and cytopathology. 3rd ed. New York: Churchill Livingstone; 1997. pp.1563-1593.
N:C, Nuclear to cytoplasmic; +, present; −, absent.

ential diagnosis. The cells from small cell carcinoma have more irregular, angulated nuclei with hyperchromatic chromatin; evidence of nuclear molding; and higher N:C ratios.

 ## DUODENUM

Normal Histology and Cytology

Although the adult small intestine measures more than 20 feet in length, it is only the proximal portion of the duodenum that, for all practical purposes, is ever cytologically sampled. The mucosal surface area of the duodenum is expanded by the presence of numerous villi. These are covered by tall, columnar absorptive epithelial cells having small basally oriented oval nuclei, pale fine chromatin, and small to inconspicuous nucleoli. Because of small nuclei and abundant cytoplasm, the N:C ratios are very low. The cytoplasm tends to be eosinophilic and granular. The apical surface of the absorptive cells is distinguished by having a striated border. Admixed among the absorptive cells are mucous-producing goblet cells.

Cytologic brushing or incidental sampling during EUS-guided FNA procures large, flat sheets of uniform epithelial cells arranged in honeycomb groupings. Occasionally, three-dimensional aggregates are present. When seen on end, the absorptive cells have a picket-fence arrangement, consisting of tall columnar cells with cyanophilic cytoplasm, low N:C ratios, and basally placed nuclei. The large barrel-shaped mucous vacuoles of goblet cells are also seen (Figure 18-38).

Infectious Agents

A variety of infectious agents can involve the duodenum. In immunocompromised patients, CMV can infect both glandular and stromal cells. Virocytes involving the surface epithelium, crypt lining cells, and underlying stromal elements can be present with or without ulceration. Cytologic examination of these virocytes demonstrates considerable nuclear and cytoplasmic enlargement and large basophilic nuclear inclusions separated from the thickened nuclear membranes by a wide clear halo. Cytoplasmic inclusions can also be seen. As glandular cells can be infected, more virocytes are appreciated than seen in cytology brushings of ulcerated esophageal lesions. The glandular cells can also be arranged in aggregates rather than only as individually dispersed cells throughout the smears.

As noted previously, duodenitis is nonspecific, often associated with concurrent or prior peptic ulcers associated with *Helicobacter*-type organisms. Mixed inflammatory cell infiltrates, reparative changes, and gastric surface cell metaplasia can be present. Cytologic smears resemble those obtained from *Helicobacter*-associated gastritis.

The most common pathogenic intestinal protozoan in the western world is *Giardia lamblia*, which infests individuals of all ages, although it is more common in children. Patients may be asymptomatic, serving as carriers or may develop clinical symptoms of diarrhea, which can be severe. Individuals with late-onset hypogammaglobulinemia are prone to develop severe clinical manifestations of giardiasis. Endoscopic examination reveals normal duodenal mucosa or surface flattening.

Although the diagnosis is often made by the identification of cysts in stool specimens, on occasion, duodenal biopsy and aspiration specimens are employed. The duodenal biopsies may appear unremarkable, with normal villous architecture and no appreciable increase in inflammatory cells. The only abnormality is the presence of the trophozoites of *G. lamblia*, closely opposed to the mucosal surface or lying within a mucoid exudate. In patients with hypogammaglobulinemia, prominent, diffuse nodular lymphoid hyperplasia is present, with reduction of the number of plasma cells and associated blunting of the villi.

In cytologic brushings of the duodenum, the trophozoites measure from 12 to 15 μm in maximum dimension and have a characteristic pear-shaped or, when seen on edge, a thin sickle-shaped configuration (Figure 18-39).[91,118] Two mirror-image nuclei are noted in the expanded portion of the organism, which is opposite from the tapered flagella. These nuclei are better seen in air-dried Romanowsky-stained material than the alcohol-fixed Pap-stained preparations. When trophozoites are present in large numbers, a granular green smear background may be appreciated.[91,118]

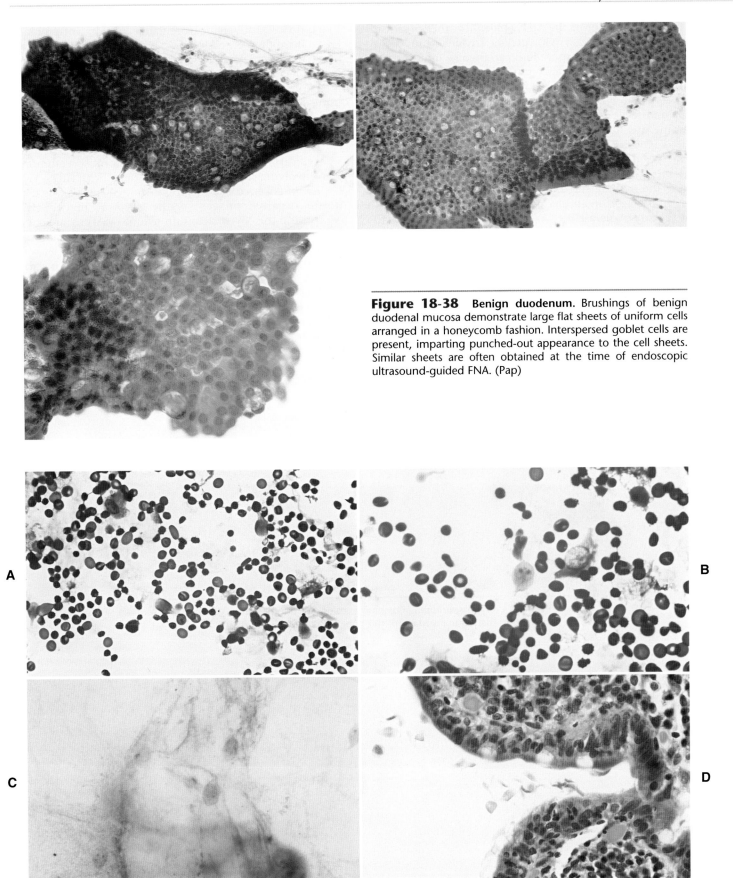

Figure 18-38 Benign duodenum. Brushings of benign duodenal mucosa demonstrate large flat sheets of uniform cells arranged in a honeycomb fashion. Interspersed goblet cells are present, imparting punched-out appearance to the cell sheets. Similar sheets are often obtained at the time of endoscopic ultrasound-guided FNA. (Pap)

Figure 18-39 *Giardia.* **A** and **B,** DQ-stained smears of duodenal brushing cytology demonstrate *Giardia* trophozoites having a characteristic pear shape. Note the mirror-image nuclei and tapered flagellum. **C,** Pap-stained smear of *Giardia* trophozoites. **D,** Concomitant biopsy demonstrating the pear- to crescent-shaped organisms. (H&E)

With the advent of the AIDS epidemic, other organisms are being encountered with greater frequency in the GI tract. Although cryptosporidium can involve immunocompetent patients, it is more commonly present in those with AIDS. The organism can infest the small and large intestines, as well as the biliary tract. Most patients present with diarrhea and fever with the symptoms more likely to be more chronic and more severe in immunosuppressed patients. The diagnosis is made by the demonstration of oocysts in stool specimens, or less commonly by mucosal biopsy. In tissue sections, these small spherical organisms are aligned along the luminal surface of the columnar epithelial cells. The number of organisms present seems to correlate with the severity of disease.[119,120] When the mucosal surface of the duodenum is brushed, cryptosporidia measuring 2 to 4 μm in diameter and having round to pyramidal shapes may be identified. They may lie freely or, more characteristically, be aligned along the luminal surface of glandular cells. With the DQ-stained smear, the organisms have a basophilic stippled appearance (Figure 18-40).[121]

Both conventional tuberculosis and atypical mycobacteria can involve the small intestine. In countries such as India, ileocecal tuberculosis remains a significant problem. Generally, however, endoscopic biopsies and brushings are nondiagnostic. Several reports document the value of transmucosal FNA cytology for the diagnosis of mycobacterial infections.[122] These authors have encountered such cases using EUS-guided FNA of various sites, including regional lymph nodes. Material sufficient for culture is usually obtained. The smears show necrotic debris, lymphocytes, and epithelioid histiocytes.

Atypical mycobacterial infection is most commonly seen involving the duodenum in patients with AIDS. With the use of air-dried DQ or Wright-stained smears, the diagnostic negative images of the atypical mycobacteria comprising the Mycobacterium avium (MAI) complex can be identified (Figure 18-41).[123] The smears contain pale macrophages having a striated pseudo-Gaucher appearance in the Pap-stained smears. In air-dried material, negative images are identified within the cytoplasm of the histiocytes and in the background. The diagnosis can be confirmed with special stains for acid-fast bacilli (AFB) or with cultures.[123] It is generally advisable to use one of the AFB stains designed to identify these weakly acid-fast organisms,

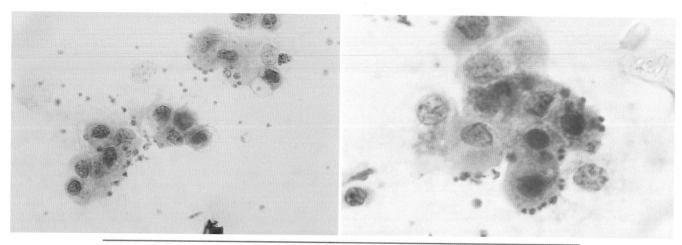

Figure 18-40 *Cryptosporidium.* Brushing cytology of duodenum in which cryptosporidia are identified along the luminal surface of the benign glandular cells. (DQ)

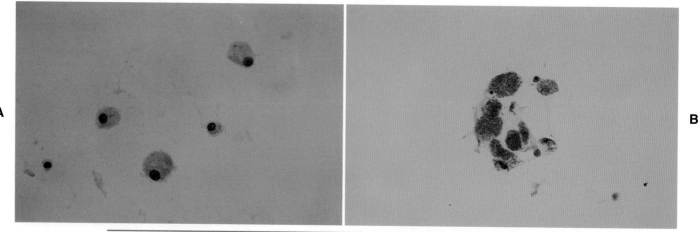

Figure 18-41 *Mycobacterium.* **A,** Brushing of atypical mycobacteria in which scattered histiocytes are present, including some containing linear striation in the cytoplasm. (Pap) **B,** Acid-fast bacilli (AFB) stain of histiocytes from duodenal brushing, demonstrating numerous acid-fast mycobacteria.

such as the Fite stain. A traditional Ziehl-Neelsen stain may not identify the organisms (see Chapter 15).

Peptic Ulcer

Despite the fact that peptic ulcers are more common in the duodenum than in the stomach, histologic and cytologic examinations are less often employed because almost all these ulcers are benign. As expected, the cytologic findings recapitulate those seen in the gastric ulcers, with the presence of flat sheets of benign glandular cells, including occasional groups showing reparative changes, and associated neutrophils and granular necrotic debris. *Helicobacter*-type organisms may also be present.

Malignancy

Malignant lymphoma, carcinoid tumor, and adenocarcinoma occur with approximately equal frequency throughout the entire length of the small intestine. The most common malignancy to involve the small intestine is malignant lymphoma, with most occurring distal to the duodenum; therefore, it is infrequently sampled by endoscopic biopsies or brushing cytology. Domizo and colleagues reported that the single most common presenting symptom was abdominal pain often related to intestinal perforation with peritonitis.[124] Other symptoms include obstruction, weight loss, diarrhea, and an abdominal mass. The majority are B-cell type, although one third of the neoplasms expressed a T-cell immunophenotype. This is a greater frequency than lymphomas occurring elsewhere in the GI tract. The B-cell neoplasms tend to be larger and occur as annular or exophytic masses in the ileum, whereas the T-cell neoplasms typically present as an ulcerating stricture or plaque in the jejunum. The T-cell tumors tend to be more high-grade, consisting of pleomorphic medium to large cell variants.[124] Cytologic findings in duodenal lymphomas resemble those seen in the stomach. Carcinoid tumors can also involve the small intestine and the cytologic features recapitulate those described for the stomach.

Although adenocarcinoma is not the most common malignancy involving the small intestine, it is the most common cancer involving the duodenum, lending itself to both endoscopic brushings and cytologic examination. Patients usually present with jaundice, anemia, or obstructive symptoms. In the duodenum, adenocarcinoma often involves the region of the ampulla of Vater, where it presents as an exophytic mass. Less commonly, adenocarcinoma can involve the distal small bowel, where it often presents as a napkin-ring growth causing obstruction. Histologically, small bowel adenocarcinomas often arise in the background of a villous adenoma. If the carcinoma is resected before lymph node metastasis, the prognosis is good. Cytologic examination of adenocarcinoma of the small bowel resembles adenocarcinomas of intestinal type of the stomach and Barrett's-associated adenocarcinoma (Figure 18-42). The smears tend to be cellular with numerous malignant cells arranged in loose clusters, aggregates, and individually.

Metastatic malignancy can involve any portion of the GI tract, although a predilection for the small bowel is evident.

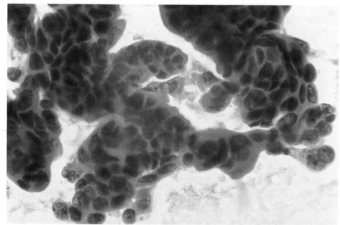

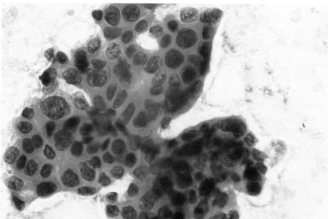

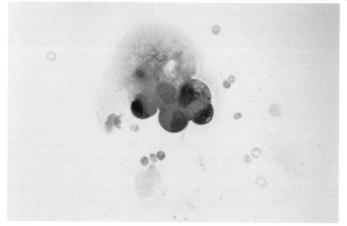

Figure 18-42 Adenocarcinoma. **A** to **C,** Loose clusters of cells consistent with adenocarcinoma. Note the three-dimensional, syncytial arrangement of the groups and loss of polarity. (Pap) *Continued*

Figure 18-42, cont'd **D** and **E,** DQ-stained smears of adenocarcinoma of the jejunum. Loose clusters of malignant cells are present along with a few individually scattered tumor cells.

The most common primaries are malignant melanoma and carcinomas of the breast, ovary, and lung.[14,77] Only a few cytology reports describe metastatic malignancies to the small bowel.[15,77]

LARGE INTESTINE

Normal Histology and Cytology

The large intestine is lined by a mucosa consisting of straight tubular crypts covered by columnar absorptive cells. The latter show eosinophilic cytoplasm and a striated luminal border that is not as well developed as that of the small bowel. In comparison with the small intestine, the goblet cells are quite numerous, both in the surface epithelium and in the crypts. Paneth cells, when present, are almost exclusively located in the most proximal right side of the normal large intestine but can be seen in any area as a response to inflammation. Cytologic brushings of benign colonic mucosa consist of large, flat monolayer sheets of cells having equidistantly placed nuclei surrounded by a moderate amount of cytoplasm and well-defined cell borders (Figure 18-43). Goblet cells, characterized by large barrel-shaped vacuoles, are numerous. The tubular profiles of intact crypts may be present.

Inflammatory Bowel Disease

Although the large intestine can be involved with a variety of acute and chronic inflammatory processes, cytologic specimens are seldom obtained from such patients. However, in patients with chronic ulcerative colitis or Crohn's disease, cytologic specimens are sometimes obtained. The major complication of ulcerative colitis, and to a lesser degree Crohn's disease, is the development of adenocarcinoma usually arising in the setting of longstanding pancolitis. Patients develop adenocarcinoma at a younger age than the general population, and these malignancies tend to be quite aggressive. A premalignant dysplastic phase may be present before adenocarcinoma develops. Because of the propensity to develop adenocarcinoma, patients with inflammatory bowel disease are typically subjected to regu-lar surveillance programs for dysplasia and early carcinomas. These examinations include periodically obtained endoscopic biopsies from multiple mucosal sites in search of any dysplastic or malignant changes. These serious pathologic conditions may not endoscopically appear to be different from immediately adjacent areas of benign reactive or inactive mucosa. Although not generally used, a few centers have incorporated brushing cytology into the surveillance programs in an effort to more extensively sample the mucosal surface.[125-128]

Because of the considerable acute inflammation and ulceration that characterize both ulcerative colitis and Crohn's disease, mucosal brushings typically show reparative glandular epithelium and inflammation. The smears consist of cohesive groups of enlarged glandular epithelial cells that have prominent nuclei with thickened membranes and macronucleoli.[32,125-127] Recognition of the low-power arrangement of these reparative cells into cohesive flat sheets with well-defined cell borders and no loss of polarity is critical (Figure 18-44). The streaming nature of the cells is also a helpful feature. Characteristically, individually scattered intact atypical cells tend to be nonexistent or few in number.

Regenerative epithelium must be differentiated from true glandular dysplasia, especially when patients with active colitis are cytologically sampled.[21,126,127] Dysplastic nuclei are larger than those seen in repair, and the chromatin tends to be more moderate to coarsely granular and hyperchromatic (Figure 18-45). Although nuclear membranes tend to be smooth, they sometimes show slight irregularity. Nucleoli may be single or multiple and large, and N:C ratios are increased. The dysplastic cells are arranged in small aggregates with obvious loss of polarity, in contrast with the maintenance of polarity seen in repair. Abnormal nuclei can be crowded or overlapping and may show molding. When the cells are arranged in groups with merging of cytoplasmic borders and loss of polarity, a syncytial pattern is appreciated. These feature frayed external cytoplasmic borders. In contrast with invasive adenocarcinoma, individually scattered atypical cells are not present in any significant numbers. However, reliably differentiating dysplasia from well-differentiated adenocarcinoma may not be possible in cytologic preparations.

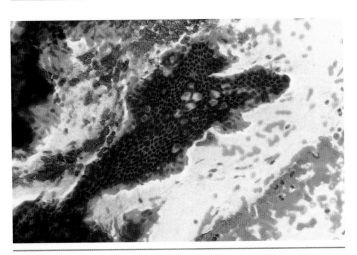

Figure 18-43 **Normal colonic mucosa.** Cytologic brushing of benign colonic mucosa characterized by a flat sheet of cells maintaining a honeycomb pattern in which interspersed goblet cells are present. (Pap)

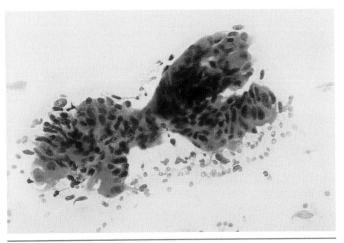

Figure 18-45 Dysplastic colonic mucosa in the setting of inflammatory bowel disease. Brushing of dysplastic colonic epithelium in a patient with ulcerative colitis. Note the stratified hyperchromatic nuclei. Single atypical cells were not appreciated. (Pap)

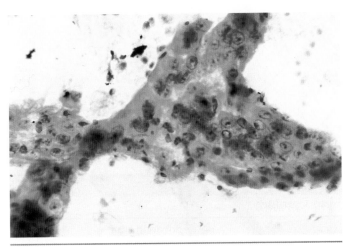

Figure 18-44 **Repair in the setting of inflammatory bowel disease.** Brushing of the edge of a colonic ulcer showing a repair pattern characterized by a sheet of streaming epithelial cells having enlarged vesicular nuclei with prominent nucleoli. Some admixed neutrophils are present. (Pap)

Adenomas and Adenocarcinoma

Brushing cytology has a limited role in colorectal cancer. Its primary purpose is to increase the diagnostic sensitivity for the detection of adenocarcinomas. The precursors to adenocarcinoma are adenomas, which can be found anywhere in the large intestine, but tend to be concentrated in the sigmoid and rectum.[129] Adenomas can have a tubular, villous, or mixed histologic pattern and may be either grossly pedunculated or sessile.[129] Smaller adenomas tend to be tubular, whereas the larger ones have a villous component. The epithelium of both tubular and villous lesions is atypical by definition. In routine histologic preparations, their tall, crowded cells stain darkly both because of nuclear enlargement with hyperchromasia and because of cytoplasmic mucin depletion. These cells are identical to those seen in dysplasia involving the colon or other GI mucosae. Thus, when adenomas are considered, descriptions of cytologic

abnormalities less than those of adenocarcinoma are without clinical significance. Furthermore, during evolution of carcinoma within a preexisting adenoma, increasing cytologic derangement is paralleled by escalating architectural complexity.

Adenomas are believed to be the precursors of the majority of colorectal carcinomas through the adenoma-carcinoma sequence; therefore, colorectal screening is done in an attempt to identify and remove the premalignant lesions. Since the incidence increases progressively between patients ages 50 and 70, screening programs are limited to adults and usually begin at age 50.

Cytologic examination of colorectal adenomas has limited value because adenomas are often endoscopically visible and amenable to complete removal. In addition, cytologic separation of the dysplastic-appearing cells of an adenoma from the well-differentiated malignant cells of adenocarcinoma is often not possible, unless there are large numbers of single abnormal glandular cells (Table 18-7). In the few cytologic reports in the literature, direct brushing of adenomas has generated cellular smears with small to large three-dimensional groups of glandular cells (Figure 18-46).[2,130,131] In those adenomas with a villous configuration, branched papillary patterns can be appreciated at low magnification. The nuclei are elongated, often with cigar-shaped contours, and possess finely to moderately hyperchromatic chromatin with one or more small nucleoli. Thabet, MacFarlane, and colleagues referred to these elements as needle cells because of their long, thin appearance.[130] The nuclei can be crowded, pseudopalisaded, or overlapped. In contrast with adenocarcinoma, individually dispersed abnormal cells tend to be absent or limited in number. However, free-lying, darkly staining, needle-shaped nuclei without cytoplasm may be numerous. These contrast with the single malignant cells with intact cytoplasm that characterize smears from adenocarcinomas.

Adenocarcinoma of the large bowel is one of the most common cancers of men and women in the United States, accounting for a significant portion of cancer-related deaths with almost 150,000 new cases diagnosed annually. Some individuals appear to have an inherited predisposi-

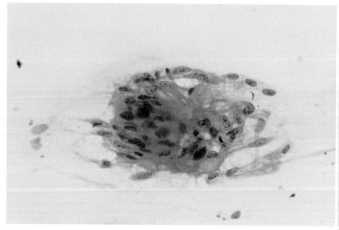

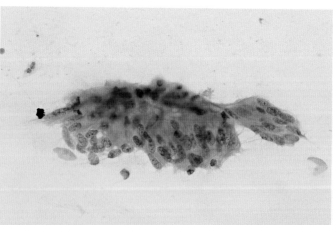

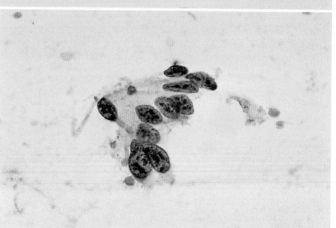

Figure 18-46 **Adenomatous polyp. A to C,** Brushing cytology of an adenomatous polyp demonstrating pseudostratified hyperchromatic nuclei. The nuclei assume elongated, thin, cigar- to needle-shaped contours. (Pap)

TABLE 18-7			CMF
Cytomorphologic Differential Diagnosis of Colonic Brushing Cytology			
Feature	**Normal**	**Adenoma**	**Adenocarcinoma**
Cellular aggregates	Large, flat, smooth edges, normal polarity	Large, three-dimensional, smooth edges, altered polarity	Small, three-dimensional, frayed edges, altered polarity
Individual cells	Few	Few	Moderate to many
Cell contours	Columnar to polygonal	Columnar (needle)	Round
Nuclei	Round, smooth, euchromatic	Elongated, hyperchromatic	Round to irregular, hyperchromatic
Nucleoli	Small, inconspicuous	Small to large	Small to large
Mucin	Abundant	Greatly reduced	Variable

Modified from Geisinger KR, Silverman JF. Gastrointestinal cytology. In: Silverberg SG, editor. Principles and practice of surgical pathology and cytopathology. 3rd ed. New York: Churchill Livingstone; 1997. pp.1563-1593.

tion for this neoplasm. This is in addition to the effects of carcinogenic dietary and environmental cofactors that include high animal fat consumption and low fiber intake. Other predisposing conditions include inflammatory bowel disease, polyposis syndromes, prior pelvic irradiation, and preexisting adenomas. Although colorectal adenocarcinoma can occur at any age, it most often involves adults in the fifth and sixth decades of life who present with rectal bleeding, anemia, obstruction, or changes in bowel habits.

More than half of the carcinomas arise in the rectosigmoid. The left-sided neoplasms classically have a napkin ring–like luminal constriction, whereas the more clinically silent right-sided lesions tend to produce large exophytic masses. Most adenocarcinomas are moderately differentiated, gland-forming tumors. If abundant extracellular mucin is present, the carcinomas are referred to as *colloid* or *mucinous carcinomas,* and this feature may be associated with a worse prognosis. The most important prognostic factors are the pathologic and clinical stages. The overall 5-year survival is approximately 50% to 55%, with those patients having tumors confined to the bowel doing relatively well and those with lymph node metastasis or disseminated disease having a poorer prognosis.

Brushing cytology is not the procedure of choice used to make a diagnosis of adenocarcinomas because many of these tumors cannot be cytologically differentiated from adenomas. However, the major use of brushing cytology is to sample malignant colonic strictures that are not amenable to forceps biopsy procedures.[25] Mortensen and colleagues evaluated a large series of patients with both malignant and benign strictures and found that endoscopic brushing cytology was more sensitive than biopsies for the detection of adenocarcinoma in this setting.[25] Although its greatest value is in the evaluation of stenotic lesions, brushing cytology has also been employed to evaluate polypoid masses that could not be removed by endoscopic polypec-

tomy.[132] In studies comparing the use of endoscopic biopsies and cytology, diagnostic yield by biopsy varied from 63% to 86% with a weighted mean yield of 73%, whereas cytology had a diagnostic range from 74% to 86% with a weighted mean yield of 79%. When both procedures were employed, the diagnostic accuracy was from 74% to 100% with a weighted mean yield of 87%. Transmucosal FNA biopsy can also increase the diagnostic yield for carcinoma.[116]

Brushing cytology of adenocarcinoma usually generates moderate to highly cellular smears consisting of numerous individually scattered malignant cells and small to large loose clusters (Figure 18-47). The aggregates are often

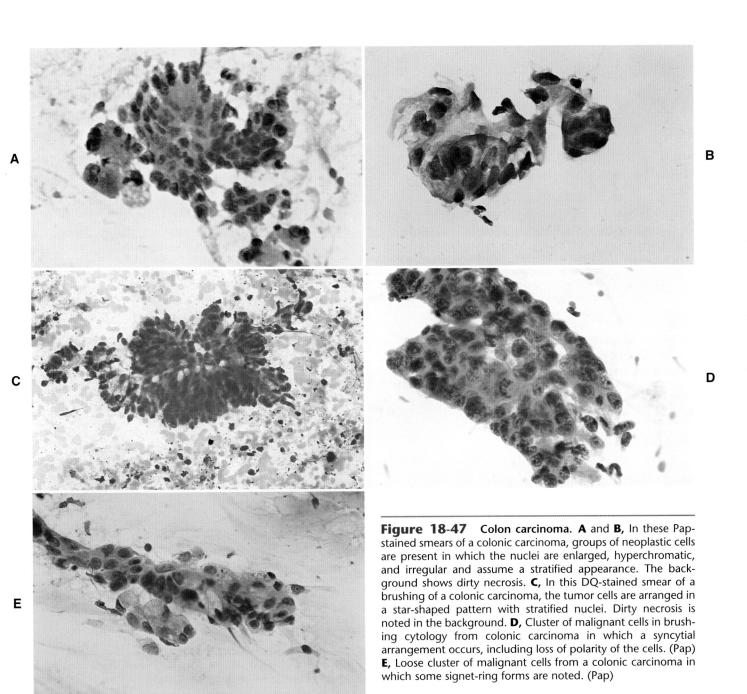

Figure 18-47   Colon carcinoma. A and **B,** In these Pap-stained smears of a colonic carcinoma, groups of neoplastic cells are present in which the nuclei are enlarged, hyperchromatic, and irregular and assume a stratified appearance. The background shows dirty necrosis. **C,** In this DQ-stained smear of a brushing of a colonic carcinoma, the tumor cells are arranged in a star-shaped pattern with stratified nuclei. Dirty necrosis is noted in the background. **D,** Cluster of malignant cells in brushing cytology from colonic carcinoma in which a syncytial arrangement occurs, including loss of polarity of the cells. (Pap) **E,** Loose cluster of malignant cells from a colonic carcinoma in which some signet-ring forms are noted. (Pap)

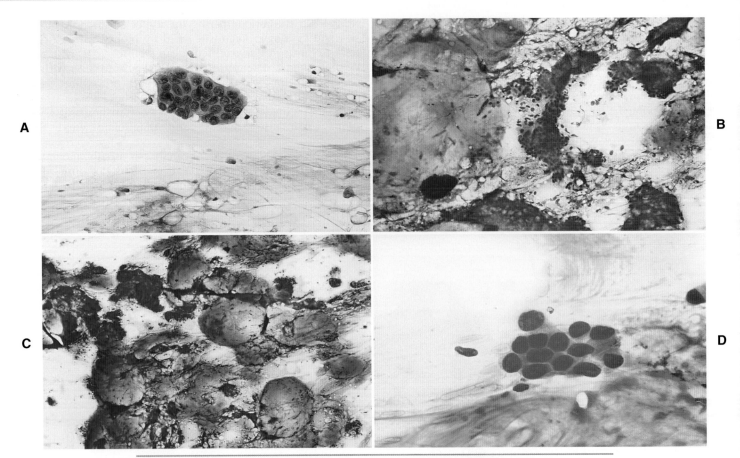

Figure 18-48   Mucinous colon carcinoma. **A,** Cluster of malignant cells in brushing of mucinous carcinoma of the colon in which stringy and fibrillary mucinous material is noted in the background. (Pap) **B, C,** and **D,** In these DQ-stained smears, abundant variably metachromatic mucinous material is noted in the background, along with neoplastic cells.

arranged in small, three-dimensional groupings and have irregular frayed borders. Many individual malignant cells having rounded shapes with large hyperchromatic nuclei and prominent nucleoli are present. A variable amount of mucin may be present (Figure 18-48).

 ANUS

Normal Histology and Cytology

The anal canal is lined by nonkeratinized stratified epithelium throughout most of its length. The proximal transitional zone has a variable mucosa, somewhat similar to the urothelium. The latter consists of epithelial cells that can be arranged in flat sheets of cuboidal or columnar cells. Cytologic smears of the normal anal canal usually consist of intermediate squamous cells, although the other cell types may be present.

Dysplastic Squamous Lesions and Malignancy

HPV-related changes, dysplasia, and carcinoma can involve the squamous mucosa of the anus.[133,134] HPV types 6 and 11 are most often associated with condyloma and low-grade dysplasia, whereas types 16 and 18 have a greater association with carcinoma and high-grade dysplasia.

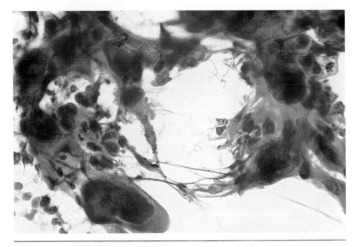

Figure 18-49   Anal squamous cell carcinoma. Brushing of squamous cell carcinoma of the anus reveals keratinized malignant cells associated with poorly differentiated cells having dense, cyanophilic cytoplasm. (Pap)

In heterosexual individuals, squamous cell carcinoma, an uncommon form of GI malignancy, is more commonly seen in women than men. However, the incidence of squamous dysplasia and carcinoma appears to be increasing in homosexual men, independent of their human immuno-

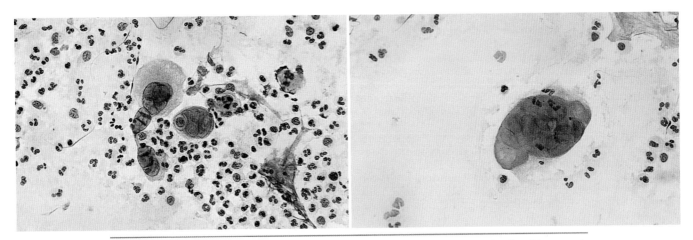

Figure 18-50   Herpes. Virocytes showing characteristic multinucleated cells with ground-glass cytoplasm and margination of the chromatin in these brushings of a perianal herpetic abscess. (Pap)

deficiency virus (HIV) status. The major risk factors for dysplasia and carcinoma in all individuals include HPV infection and anoreceptive intercourse.[133]

Concomitant with increased incidence of HPV-related lesions, dysplasia, and squamous carcinoma, the use of anal cytology has increased (Figure 18-49).[135-140] Recognition of HPV-related changes is based on the diagnostic criteria employed in the uterine cervix, although koilocytes appear to be present less commonly in anal mucosal lesions than in their cervical counterparts.[135-137] It has been suggested that additional studies are needed to establish better cytologic guidelines for diagnosis.[139,141] Sherman and colleagues have demonstrated that automated LBPs enhance the diagnostic yield for anal dysplasia compared with conventional smears.[142] Herpes has also been diagnosed with brushing cytology (Figure 18-50).

References

1. Wang HH, Jonasson JG, Ducatman BS. Brushing cytology of the upper gastrointestinal tract. Obsolete or not? Acta Cytol 1991; 35:195-198.
2. Geisinger KR, Wang HH, Ducatman BS, et al. Gastrointestinal cytology. In: Hajdu SI, editor. Values and limitations of cytologic examinations (vol. 11). Philadelphia: WB Saunders; 1991. pp. 403-441.
3. Geisinger KR. Alimentary tract (esophagus, stomach, small intestine, colon, rectum, anus, biliary tract). In: Bibbo M, editor. Comprehensive cytopathology. 2nd ed. Philadelphia: WB Saunders; 1997. pp. 413-444.
4. Geisinger KR, Silverman JF. Gastrointestinal cytology. In: Silverberg SG, editor. Principles and practice of surgical pathology and cytopathology. 3rd ed. New York: Churchill Livingstone; 1997. pp. 1563-1593.
5. Geisinger KR. Endoscopic biopsies and cytologic brushings of the esophagus are diagnostically complementary. Am J Clin Pathol 1995; 103:295-299.
6. Kobayashi S, Kasugai TR. Brushing cytology for the diagnosis of gastric cancer involving the cardia or the lower esophagus. Acta Cytol 1978; 22:155-157.
7. Chambers LA, Clark WE II. The endoscopic diagnosis of gastroesophageal malignancy: a cytologic review. Acta Cytol 1986; 30:110-114.
8. Achkar E, Carey W. The cost of surveillance for adenocarcinoma complicating Barrett's esophagus. Am J Gastroenterol 1988; 83:291-294.
9. American Society of Gastrointestinal Endoscopy. The role of endoscopy in the surveillance of premalignant conditions of the upper gastrointestinal tract: guidelines for clinical application. Gastrointest Endosc 1988; 34:185-205.
10. Keighley MRB, Thompson H, Moore J, et al. Comparison of brush cytology before or after biopsy for diagnosis for gastric carcinoma. Br J Surg 1979; 66:246-247.
11. Zargar SA, Khuroo MS, Jan GM, et al. Prospective comparison of the value of brushings before and after biopsy in the endoscopic diagnosis of gastroesophageal malignancy. Acta Cytol 1991; 35:549-552.
12. Graham DY, Spjut HJ. Salvage cytology: a new alternative fiberoptic technique. Gastrointest Endosc 1979; 25:137-139.
13. Green LK, Zachariah S, Graham DY. The use of gastric salvage cytology in the diagnosis of malignancy: a review of 731 cases. Diagn Cytopathol 1990; 6:1-4.
14. Caos A, Olson N, Willman C, Gogel HK. Endoscopic "salvage" cytology in neoplasms metastatic to the upper gastrointestinal tract. 1986; 30:32-34.
15. Abdul-Karim FW, O'Mailia JJ, Wang KP, et al. Transmucosal endoscopic needle aspiration: utility in the diagnosis of extrinsic malignant masses of the gastrointestinal tract. Diagn Cytopathol 1991; 7:92-94.
16. Benya RV, Metz DC, Hijazi YM, et al. Fine needle aspiration cytology of submucosal nodules in patients with Zollinger-Ellison syndrome. Am J Gastroenterol 1993; 88:258-265.
17. Kochhar R, Gupta SK, Malik AK, Mehta SK. Endoscopic needle aspiration biopsy. Acta Cytol 1987; 31:481-484.
18. Layfield LJ, Reichman A, Weinstein WM. Endoscopically directed fine needle aspiration biopsy of gastric and esophageal lesions. Acta Cytol 1992; 36:69-74.
19. Vilmann P, Hancke S, Henriksen FW, et al. Endoscopically guided fine needle aspiration biopsy of malignant lesions in the upper gastrointestinal tract. Endoscopy 1993; 25:523-527.
20. Young JA, Hughes HE, Lee FD. Evaluation of endoscopic brush and biopsy touch smear cytology and biopsy histology in the diagnosis of carcinoma of the lower esophagus and cardia. J Clin Pathol 1980; 33:811-814.

21. Cohen MB, Wittchow RJ, Johlin FC, et al. Comparison of cytologic features of adenocarcinoma and benign biliary strictures. Mod Pathol 1995; 8:498-502.

22. Cusso X, Mones J, Ocana J, et al. Is endoscopic gastric cytology worthwhile: an evaluation of 903 cases of carcinoma. J Clin Gastroenterol 1993; 16:336-339.

23. Bhasin DK, Kochhar R, Rajwanshi A, et al. Endoscopic suction cytology in upper gastrointestinal tract malignancy. Acta Cytol 1998; 32:452-454.

24. Shanghai Gastrointestinal Endoscopy Cooperative Group. Value of biopsy and brush cytology in the diagnosis of gastric cancer. Gut 1982; 23:774-776.

25. Mortensen NJMcC, Eltringham WK, Mountford RA, Lever JV. Direct vision brush cytology with colonoscopy: an aid to the accurate diagnosis of colonic strictures. Br J Surg 1984; 71:930-932.

26. Berry AV, Baskind AF, Hamilton DG. Cytologic screening for esophageal cancer. Acta Cytol 1981; 25:135-141.

27. Chittajallu RS, Falk GW, Richter JE, et al. Balloon cytology for the detection and surveillance of Barrett's esophagus. Gastroenterology 1995; 108:A71.

28. Shen Q, Liu SF, Dawsey SM, et al. Cytologic screening for esophageal cancer: results from 12,877 subjects from a high-risk population in China. Int J Cancer 1993; 54: 185-188.

29. Shu Y-J. The cytopathology of esophageal carcinoma: precancerous lesions and early cancer. New York: Masson; 1985.

30. Shu Y-J. Cytopathology of the esophagus: an overview of esophageal cytopathology in China. Acta Cytol 1983; 27:7-16.

31. Fennerty MB, DiTomasso J, Morales TG, et al. Screening for Barrett's esophagus by balloon cytology. Am J Gastroenterol 1995; 90:1230-1232.

32. Greenbaum E, Schreiberk, Shu Y-J, et al. Use of the esophageal balloon in the diagnosis of carcinomas of the head, neck and upper gastrointestinal tract. Acta Cytol 1984; 28:9-15.

33. Dawsey SM, Yu Y, Taylor PR, et al. Esophageal cytology and subsequent risk of cancer: a prospective follow-up study from Linxian, China. Acta Cytol 1994; 38:183-192.

34. Dowlatshahi K, Skinner DB, DeMeester TR, et al. Evaluation of brush cytology as an independent technique for detection of esophageal carcinoma. J Thorac Cardiovasc Surg 1985; 89:848-851.

35. Qin D, Zhou B. Elastic plastic tube for detecting exfoliative cancer cells in the esophagus. Acta Cytol 1992; 36: 82-86.

36. Dziura BR, Otis R, Hukill P, et al. Gastric brushing cytology: an analysis of cells from benign and malignant ulcers. Acta Cytol 1997; 21:187-190.

37. Koss LG. Diagnostic cytology and its histopathologic bases. 4th ed. (vol. 2). Philadelphia: Lippincott-Raven: 1992. pp. 1018-1081

38. Atkinson B, Silverman JF. Atlas of difficult cytologic diagnosis. Philadelphia: WB Saunders; 1998.

39. DeNardi FG, Riddell RH. The normal esophagus. Am J Surg Pathol 1991; 15:296-309.

40. Teot LA, Geisinger KR. Diagnostic esophageal cytology and its histologic basis. In: Castell DO, editor. The esophagus. 2nd ed. Boston: Little, Brown; 1995. pp. 179-204.

41. Wright RG, Augustine B, Whitfield A. *Candida* in gastroesophageal cytological and histological preparations: a comparative study. Labmedica 1987; 4:29-30.

42. Young JA, Elias E. Gastroesophageal candidiasis: diagnosis by brush cytology. J Clin Pathol 1985; 38:293-296.

43. Lightdale CJ, Wolf DJ, Marcucci BA, et al. Herpetic esophagitis in patients with cancer: antemortem diagnosis by brush cytology. 1977; 39:223-226.

44. Hoda SA, Hajdu SI. Small cell carcinoma of the esophagus: cytology and immunohistology in four cases. Acta Cytol 1992; 36:113-120.

45. Teot LA, Ducatman BS, Geisinger KR. Cytologic diagnosis for cytomegalovirus esophagitis: a report of three acquired immunodeficiency syndrome-related cases. Acta Cytol 1993; 37:93-96.

46. Winkler B, Capo Y, Reuman WA, et al. Human papilloma virus infection of the esophagus. Cancer 1985; 55:149-155.

47. deBorges FJ, Acevedo F, Miralles E, et al. Squamous papilloma of the esophagus diagnosed by cytology: report of a case with concurrent occult epidermoid carcinoma. Acta Cytol 1986; 30:487-490.

48. Borczuk AC, Hagan R, Chipty F, et al. Cytologic detection of trichomonas esophagitis in a patient with acquired immunodeficiency syndrome. Diagn Cytopathol 1998; 19:313-316.

49. Berthrong M, Fajardo LF. Radiation injury in surgical pathology II: alimentary tract. Am J Surg Pathol 1981; 5:153-178.

50. O'Morchoe PJ, Lee DC, Kozak CA. Esophageal cytology in patients receiving cytotoxic drug therapy. Acta Cytol 1983; 27:630-634.

51. Geisinger KR. Histopathology of human reflux esophagitis and experimental esophagitis in animals. In: Castell DO, editor. The esophagus. 2nd ed. Boston: Little Brown; 1995. pp. 481-503.

52. Frierson HF Jr. Histological criteria for the diagnosis of reflux esophagitis. Pathol Annu 1992; 27:87-104.

53. Haggitt RC. Barrett's esophagus, dysplasia, and adenocarcinoma. Hum Pathol 1994; 25:982-993.

54. Paull A, Trier JS, Dalton MD, et al. The histologic spectrum of Barrett's esophagus. N Engl J Med 1976; 295:476-480.

55. Haggitt RC. Adenocarcinoma in Barrett's esophagus: a new epidemic? Hum Pathol 1992; 23:475-476.

56. Geisinger KR, Teot LA, Richter JE. A comparative cytopathologic and histologic study of atypia, dysplasia and adenocarcinoma in Barrett's esophagus. Cancer 1992; 69:8-16.

57. Wang HH, Ducatman BS, Thibault S. Cytologic features of premalignant glandular lesions in the upper gastrointestinal tract. Acta Cytol 1991; 35:199-203.

58. Robey SS, Hamilton SR, Gupta PK, et al. Diagnostic value of cytopathology in Barrett's esophagus and associated carcinoma. Am J Clin Pathol 1988; 89:493-498.

59. Wang HH, Sovie S, Zeroogian JM, et al. Value of cytology in detecting intestinal metaplasia and associated dysplasia at the gastroesophageal junction. Hum Pathol 1997; 28:465-471.

60. MacLennan AJ, Orringer MB, Beer DG. Identification of intestinal-type Barrett's metaplasia by using the intestine-specific protein villin and esophageal brush cytology. Mol Carcinog 1999; 24:137-143.

61. Tsai TT, Bongiorno PF, Orringer MB, et al. Detection of *p53* nuclear protein accumulation in brushings and biopsies of Barrett's esophagus. Cancer Detection and Prevention 1997; 21(4):326-331.

62. Haddad NG, Fleischer DE. Neoplasms of the esophagus. In: Castell DO, editor. The esophagus. 2nd ed. Little, Brown: Boston; 1995. pp. 269-291.

63. Behmard S, Sadeghi A, Bagheri SA. Diagnostic accuracy of endoscopy with brushing cytology and biopsy in upper gastrointestinal lesions. Acta Cytol 1978; 22:153-154.

64. Bishop D, Lushpihan AR, Louis C. The cytology of carcinoma in situ and early invasive carcinoma of the esophagus. Acta Cytol 1977; 21:298-300.

65. Hamilton SR, Smith RRL, Cameron JL. Prevalence and characteristics of Barrett's esophagus in patients with adenocarcinoma of the esophagus or esophagogastric junction. Hum Pathol 1988; 19:942-948.

66. Shurbaji MS, Erozan YS. The cytopathologic diagnosis of esophageal adenocarcinoma. Acta Cytol 1991; 35:189-194.

67. Wang HH, Doria MI, Purohit-Buch S, et al. Barrett's esophagus: the cytology of dysplasia in comparison to benign and malignant lesions. Acta Cytol 1992; 36:60-64.

68. Robey SS, Hamilton SR, Gupta PK, Erozan YS. Diagnostic value of cytopathology in Barrett's esophagus and associated carcinoma. Am J Clin Pathol 1988; 89:493-498.

69. Belladonna JA, Hajdu SI, Bains MS, Winawer SJ. Adenocarcinoma in situ of Barrett's esophagus diagnosed by endoscopic cytology. N Engl J Med 1974; 291:895-896.

70. Robertson CS, Mayberry JF, Nicholson DA, et al. Value of endoscopic surveillance in the detection of neoplastic change in Barrett's esophagus. Br J Surg 1988; 75:760-763.

71. Reid BJ, Weinstein WM, Lewin KJ, et al. Endoscopic biopsy can detect high-grade dysplasia or early adenocarcinoma in Barrett's esophagus without grossly recognizable neoplastic lesions. Gastroenterology 1988; 94:81-90.

72. Briggs JC, Ibrahim NBN. Oat cell carcinoma of the esophagus: a clinicopathologic study of 23 cases. Histopathology 1983; 7:261-277.

73. Tenvall J, Johansson L, Albertson M. Small cell carcinoma of the esophagus: a clinical and immunohistopathologic review. Eur J Surg Oncol 1990; 16:109-115.

74. Fulp SR. Nestok BR, Powell BL, et al. Leukemic infiltration of the esophagus. Cancer 1993; 71:112-116.

75. Sapi Z, Papp I, Bodo M. Malignant fibrous histiocytoma of the esophagus: report of a case with cytologic, immunohistologic and ultrastructural studies. Acta Cytol 1992; 36:121-125.

76. Trillo AA, Accettulo LM, Yeiter TL. Choriocarcinoma of the esophagus: histologic and cytological findings: a case report. Acta Cytol 1979; 23:69-74.

77. Kadakia SC, Parker A, Canales L. Metastatic tumors to the upper gastrointestinal tract: endoscopic experience. Am J Gastroenterol 1992; 87:1418-1423.

78. Owen DA. Normal histology of the stomach. Am J Surg Pathol 1986; 10:48-61.

79. Appelman HD. Gastritis: terminology, etiology, and clinicopathological correlations: another biased view. Hum Pathol 1994; 25:1006-1019.

80. Quinn CM, Bjarnason I, Price AB. Gastritis in patients on nonsteroidal antiinflammatory drugs. Histopathology 1993; 23:341-348.

81. Graham DY, Go MF. *Helicobacter pylori:* current status. Gastroenterology 1993; 105:279-282.

82. Correa P. *Helicobacter pylori* and gastric carcinogenesis. Am J Surg Pathol 1995; 19(Suppl 1):537-543.

83. Genta RM, Hamner HW, Graham DY. Gastric lymphoid follicles in *Helicobacter pylori* infection: frequency, distribution, and response to triple therapy. Hum Pathol 1993; 24:577-583.

84. Ghoussoub RAD, Lachman MF. A triple stain for the detection of *Helicobacter pylori* in gastric brushing cytology. Acta Cytol 1997; 41:1178-1182.

85. Misra SP, Misra V, Dwivedi M, et al. Diagnosing *Helicobacter pylori* by imprint cytology: can the same biopsy specimen be used for histology? Diagn Cytopathol 1998; 18:330-332.

86. Schnadig VJ, Bigio EH, Gourley WK, et al. Identification of *Campylobacter pylori* by endoscopic brush cytology. Diagn Cytopathol 1990; 6:227-234.

87. Davenport RD. Cytologic diagnosis of *Campylobacter pylori*-associated gastritis. Acta Cytol 1990; 34:211-213.

88. Rodriguez IN, de Santamaria SJ, Rubio Mdel MA, et al. Cytologic brushing as a simple and rapid method in the diagnosis of *Helicobacter pylori* infection. Acta Cytol 1995; 39:916-919.

89. Caselli M, Trevisani L, Pazzi P, et al. Suggestions for the rapid diagnosis of *Campylobacter pylori* infection in endoscopic settings. Endoscopy 1989; 21:110-111.

90. DeFrancesco F, Nicotina PA, Picciotto M, et al. *Helicobacter pylori* in gastroduodenal diseases: rapid identification by endoscopic brush cytology. Diagn Cytopathol 1992; 9:430-433.

91. Debongnie JC, Mairesse J, Donnay M, et al. Touch cytology: a quick, simple, sensitive screening test in the diagnosis of infections of the gastrointestinal tract. Arch Pathol Lab Med 1994; 118:1115-1118.

92. Faverly D, Fameree D, Lamy V, et al. Identification of *Campylobacter pylori* in gastric biopsy smears. Acta Cytol 1990; 34:205-210.

93. Trevisani L, Sartori S, Ruina M, et al. Touch cytology: a reliable and cost-effective method for diagnosis of *Helicobacter pylori* infection. Dig Dis Sci 1997; 42:2299-2303.

94. Rey E, Carrion I, Mendoza ML, et al. Imprint cytology in the diagnosis of *Helicobacter pylori* infection. Acta Cytol 1997; 41:1144-1146.

95. Ching CK, Buxton C, Holgate C, et al. Cytological brushing urea broth test: a highly sensitive and specific test for *Helicobacter pylori* infection. Gastrointest Endosc 1991; 37:550-551.

96. Walsh D, Immins E, Dutton J. Filamentous organisms in benign and malignant gastric cytology brushes. Cytopathology 1997; 8:63-69.

97. Singh M, Mehrotra R, Shukla J, et al. Diagnosis of microfilaria in gastric brush cytology: a case report. Acta Cytol 1999; 43:853-855.

98. Strigle SM, Gal AA, Martin SE. Alimentary tract cytopathology in human immunodeficiency virus infection: a review of experience in Los Angeles. Diagn Cytopathol 1990; 6:409-420.

99. Qizilbash AH, Castelli M, Kowalski MA, et al. Endoscopic brush cytology and biopsy in the diagnosis of cancer of the upper gastrointestinal tract. Acta Cytol 1980; 24:313-318.

100. Cook IJ, de Carle DJ, Haneman B, et al. The role of brushing cytology in the diagnosis of gastric malignancy. Acta Cytol 1988; 32:461-464.

101. Kiil J, Andersen D, Jensen M. Biopsy and brush cytology in the diagnosis of gastric cancer. Scand J Gastroenterol 1979; 14:189-191.

102. Waldron R, Kerin M, Ali A, et al. Evaluation of the role of endoscopic biopsies and cytology in the detection of gastric malignancy. Br J Surg 1990; 77:62-63.

103. Moreno-Otero R, Marron C, Cantero J, et al. Endoscopic biopsy and cytology in the diagnosis of malignant gastric ulcers. Diagn Cytopathol 1989; 5:366-370.

104. Antonioli DA. Precursors of gastric carcinoma: a critical review with a brief description of early (curable) gastric cancer. Hum Pathol 1994; 25:994-1005.

105. Hustin J, Lagneaux G, Donnay M, et al. Cytologic patterns of reparative processes, true dysplasia and carcinoma of the gastric mucosa. Acta Cytol 1994; 38:730-736.

106. Becker SN, Sass MA, Petras RE, et al. Bizarre atypia in gastric brushings associated with hepatic artery infusion chemotherapy. Acta Cytol 1986; 30:347-350.

107. Lauren P. The two histological main types of gastric carcinoma: diffuse and so-called intestinal-type carcinoma. Acta Pathol Microbiol Scand [A] 1965; 64:31-49.

108. Sharma P, Misra V, Singh PA, et al. A correlative study of histology and imprint cytology in the diagnosis of gastrointestinal tract malignancies. Indian J Pathol Microbiol 1997; 40(2):139-146.

109. Isaacson PG. Gastrointestinal lymphoma. Hum Pathol 1994; 25:1020-1209.

110. Sherman ME, Anderson C, Herman LM, et al. Utility of gastric brushing in the diagnosis of malignant lymphoma. Acta Cytol 1994; 38:169-174.

111. Cabre-Fiol V, Vilardell F. Progress in the cytological diagnosis of gastric lymphoma. Cancer 1978; 41:1456-1461.

112. Lozowski W, Hajdu SI. Preoperative cytologic diagnosis of primary gastrointestinal malignant lymphoma. Acta Cytol 1984; 26:563-570.

113. Lewin KJ, Riddell RH, Weinstein WM. Mesenchymal tumors. In: Gastrointestinal pathology and its clinical implications (vol 1). New York: Igaku-Shoin; 1992. pp.284-319.

114. Koga H, Ochiai A, Nakanishi Y, et al. Reevaluation of prognostic factors in gastric leiomyosarcoma. Am J Gastroenterol 1995; 90:1307-1312.

115. Lozano MO, Rodriguez J, Algarra SM, et al. Fine-needle aspiration cytology and immunocytochemistry in the diagnosis of 24 gastrointestinal sroma tumors: a quick, reliable diagnostic method. Diagn Cytopathol 2003; 28:131-135.

116. Zargar SA, Khuroo MS, Mahajan R, et al. Endoscopic fine needle aspiration cytology in the diagnosis of gastroesophageal and colorectal malignancies. Gut 1991; 32: 745-748.

117. Lozowski W, Hajdu SI, Melamed MR. Cytomorphology of carcinoid tumors. Acta Cytol 1979; 23:360-365.

118. Marshall JB, Kelley DH, Vogele KA. Giardiasis: diagnosis by endoscopic brush cytology of the duodenum. Am J Gastroenterol 1984; 79:517-519.

119. Genta RM, Chapell CL, White AC Jr, et al. Duodenal morphology and intensity of infection in AIDS-related intestinal cryptosporidiosis. Gastroenterology 1993; 105: 1769-1775.

120. Clayton F, Heller T, Kotter DP. Variation in the enteric distribution of cryptosporidia in acquired immunodeficiency syndrome. Am J Clin Pathol 1994; 102:420-425.

121. Silverman JF, Levine J, Finley JL, et al. Small-intestinal brushing cytology in the diagnosis of cryptosporidiosis in AIDS. Diagn Cytopathol 1990; 6:193-196.

122. Strigle SM, Gal AA, Martin SE. Alimentary tract cytopathology in human immunodeficiency virus infection: a review of experience in Los Angeles. Diagn Cytopathol 1990; 6:409-420.

123. Guajardo RG, Quintana OB, Padilla PP. Negative images due to MAI infection detected in Papanicolaou-stained duodenal brushing cytology. Diagn Cytopathol 1998; 19:462-464.

124. Domizio P, Owen RA, Shepherd NA, et al. Primary lymphoma of the small intestine. A clinicopathological study of 119 cases. Am J Surg Pathol 1993; 17:429-442.

125. Galambos JT, Massey BW, Klayman MI, Kirsner JB. Exfoliative cytology in chronic ulcerative colitis. Cancer 1959; 9:152-159.

126. Melville DM, Richman PI, Shepherd NA, et al. Brush cytology of the colon and rectum in ulcerative colitis: an aid to cancer diagnosis. J Clin Pathol 1988; 41:1180-1186.

127. Festa VI, Hajdu SI, Winawer SJ. Colorectal cytology in chronic ulcerative colitis. Acta Cytol 1985; 29:262-268.

128. Granqvist S, Granberg-Ohman I, et al. Colonoscopic biopsies and cytological examination in chronic ulcerative colitis. Scand J Gastroenterol 1980; 15:283-288.

129. Geisinger KR. Pathology of colonic polyps. In: Ott DJ, Wu WC, editors. Polypoid disease of the colon: emphasis on radiologic evaluation. Baltimore: Urban and Schwarzenberg; 1986. pp. 3-30.

130. Thabet RJ, MacFarlane EWE. Cytological field patterns and nuclear morphology in the diagnosis of colon pathology. Acta Cytol 1962; 6:325-331.

131. Kannan V, Masters CB. Cytodiagnosis of colonic adenoma: morphology and clinical importance. Diagn Cytopathol 1991; 7:366-372.

132. Marshall JB, Diaz-Arias AA, Barthel SJ, et al. Prospective evaluation of optimal number of biopsy specimens and brush cytology in the diagnosis of cancer of the colorectum. Am J Gastroenterol 1993; 88:1352-1354.

133. Maden C, Coates RJ, Sherman KJ, et al. Sexual practices, sexually transmitted diseases and the incidence of anal cancer. N Engl J Med 1987; 317:973-977.

134. Duggan MA, Boras VF, Inoue M, et al. Human papillomavirus DNA determination of anal condylomata, dysplasias, and squamous carcinomas with in situ hybridization. Am J Clin Pathol 1989; 92:16-21.

135. de Ruiter A, Carter P, Katz DR, et al. A comparison between cytology and histology to detect anal intraepithelial neoplasia. Genitourin Med 1994; 70:22-25.

136. Sonnex C, Scholefield JH, Kocjan G, et al. Anal human papillomavirus infection: a comparative study of cytology, colposcopy and DNA hybridization as methods of detection. Genitourin Med 1991; 67:21-25.

137. Surawicz CM, Kirby P, Critchlow C, et al. Anal dysplasia in homosexual men: role of anoscopy and biopsy. Gastroenterology 1993; 105:658-666.

138. Palefsky JM, Holly EA, Hogeboom CJ, et al. Anal cytology as a screening tool for anal squamous intraepithelial lesions. J Acquir Immune Defic Syndr Hum Retrovirol 1997; 14:415-422.

139. Scholefield JH, Johnson J, Hitchcock A. Guidelines for anal cytology: to make cytological diagnosis and follow up much more reliable. Cytopathology 1998; 9:15-22.

140. Palefsky JM, Holly EA, Ralston ML. High incidence of anal high-grade squamous intraepithelial lesions among HIV-positive and HIV-negative homosexual and bisexual men. AIDS 1998; 12:495-503.

141. Geisinger KR. Refinements in screening strategy for identification of anal dysplasia in homosexual men. Am J Gastroenterol 1994; 89:1114-1115.

142. Sherman ME, Friedman HB, Busseniers AE, et al. Cytologic diagnosis of anal intraepithelial neoplasia using smears and Cytyc Thin-Preps. Mod Pathol 1995; 8:270-274.

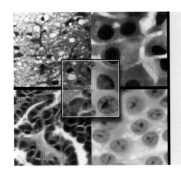

The Biliary Tract, Pancreatic Ductal System, and Ampullary Region

CHAPTER
19

By far, the most common clinical sign associated with anatomic disorders of the extrahepatic biliary ductal system is jaundice. This results from obstruction to the normal flow of the bile from the liver into the duodenum with resultant cholestasis. Jaundice is often painless and associated with pruritus.

Benign strictures of the biliary ducts are typically fibrotic narrowings that may occur as the result of a number of inflammatory disorders. These include cholecystitis, gallstones, pancreatitis, primary sclerosis cholangitis, ascending cholangitis, trauma (especially surgically induced), and papillitis. The most ominous causes of ductal obstruction are malignant neoplasms. Most of these are either cholangiocarcinomas or pancreatic adenocarcinomas.[1] Hepatocellular carcinoma is rarely responsible.[2]

Exfoliative cytology plays a key role in distinguishing these glandular cancers from the benign conditions.[2-31] Diagnostic imaging techniques are important starting points in the investigation of patients with suspected biliary tract strictures. Noninvasive imaging techniques include abdominal ultrasound and computerized tomography. Invasive procedures include upper gastrointestinal endoscopy (at times with ultrasound), endoscopic retrograde cholangiopancreatography (ERCP), and percutaneous transhepatic cholangiography (PTC). In the presence of a mass lesion, the noninvasive techniques are often sufficient to demonstrate the abnormality and to direct percutaneous fine-needle aspiration (FNA) biopsies. However, many primary neoplasms of the extrahepatic biliary ducts are small and may not be visualized by these procedures. Furthermore, many are associated with a prominent desmoplastic reaction that may prevent aspiration of a sufficient number of tumor cells. The invasive procedures have greater diagnostic yields but still do not provide either pathologic confirmation of neoplasm or its absence. The two major categories of exfoliative specimens in this situation are (1) direct cytologic examination of bile and pancreatic juice and (2) brushing smears obtained during either ERCP or PTC. Tissue biopsies for histologic examination often are not performed because of a relatively high rate of complications that may include bile leakage with peritonitis, hemorrhage, and subsequent stricturing scar formation. Overall, brushing cytology, although not without compli-

cations, is a safer procedure.[12] In addition, cytology may be less expensive than endoscopically directed tissue biopsies.[11] In the vast majority of patients, obtaining a morphologic diagnosis of an underlying cause of the biliary stricture is essential for therapeutic decision making and determining prognosis.

As reviewed by Sterrett and colleagues, the direct cytologic examination of bile for tumor cells in most series has had an unacceptably low level of diagnostic sensitivity.[4] When the bile was collected by catheterization of the ampulla of Vater, sensitivity ranged from 20% to 77%. Sensitivity varied from 34% to 73% in series that examined percutaneous bile drainage (either with a T-tube or PTC). Similar sensitivity levels have also been reported for bile obtained by catheterization during ERCP. Simsir and colleagues have also reviewed the relevant literature with exfoliative bile samples obtained by duodenal aspiration having diagnostic sensitivities ranging from 41% to 82%. Yields obtained during PTC and ERCP ranged between 30% and 76%. In their small series, Simsir and colleagues had a sensitivity of 75% when examining cytologic effluence of stents after their removal.[15] Although their sensitivity is rather high, this procedure delays the morphologic diagnosis of adenocarcinoma by several months. Mohandas and colleagues also improved diagnostic sensitivity for bile cytology by dilating the stricture before aspiration of the fluid.[10] Although false-positive cytologic interpretations have been rendered, in many series, specificity is 100%.[4,25]

A number of valid reasons have been offered for the relatively low levels of diagnostic sensitivity associated with this direct cytologic examination of bile. A large portion of all cholangiocarcinomas are well-differentiated adenocarcinomas. As a result, it may be difficult to distinguish these low-grade neoplasms from benign reactive changes resulting from inflammation. As emphasized by Peralta-Venturina and colleagues, pathologists need to be conservative in this setting because a false-positive diagnosis needs to be avoided.[3] Many of these adenocarcinomas are associated with an extensive sclerosing reaction in the surrounding stroma that prevents the exfoliation of tumor cells. This is one of the reasons that such samples typically have a low cellularity. The morphologic preservation of both benign and malignant epithelial cells is quite variable in these samples (Figures 19-1 to 19-3). The degeneration may be prominent because bile is a toxic substance. Such degenerative alterations in cells may be overinterpreted, leading to the rare false-positive result. Thus, bile samples need to be transported rapidly to and processed by the cytology laboratory. Fresh aspirates rather than bile collected in drainage bags are suitable for cytomorphologic evaluations.[4] A sizeable proportion of neoplasms causing obstruction of the bile ducts are extrinsic to the ductal system and thus may not be exposed to the mucosal surface.

The cytologic evaluation of pure pancreatic juice for identification of adenocarcinoma has shown a somewhat better diagnostic yield than bile. Reported sensitivities have ranged from 30% to 79%.[32,33] The diagnostic yield may be improved if patients receive an intravenous (IV) dose of secretin before fluid collection. Nakaizumi and colleagues reported a positive correlation between the volume of pancreatic juice collected and positive cytologic diagnoses.[32] They reported an inverse relationship between the size of the neoplasm and the rate of positive diagnoses with neoplasms less than 2 cm in diameter providing the highest yield. These authors suggested that large carcinomas may obstruct the main pancreatic duct preventing cells from being obtained.[32] Additionally, necrotic debris might also interfere with the interpretation. Although not universally agreed on, these authors also found that positive diagnoses were more common in patients whose tumors were present in the head, rather than the body or tail of the pancreas. Fewer cells were obtained from the latter sites. In their review, Nakaizumi and colleagues found reported false-positive diagnoses ranging up to nearly 9%.[32]

In an attempt to enhance diagnostic yield of pure pancreatic fluid, Kondo and colleagues evaluated the juice by both conventional cytology and molecular biology.[33] In the latter the polymerase chain reaction was used to look for mutations in the *K-ras* oncogene; it was identified in two thirds of the carcinomas that were negative by cytology. Neither healthy controls nor patients with chronic pancreatitis were positive for this mutation.

Overall, the improvements in diagnostic yields with brushing samples obtained from the biliary and pancreatic ducts are significant compared with the direct examination of bile and pancreatic juice. In their review, Sterrett and colleagues found diagnostic sensitivities varying from 18% to 60%.[4] Other authors have found somewhat similar changes: Layfield: 33% to 85%, de Peralta-Venturina: 30% to 79%, Kocjan: 33% to 85%; Geisinger: 31% to 85%, Bardales: 20% to 70%, Renshaw: 33% to 80%, Vadmal: 34% to 83%, and Ishimaru: 20% to 92%.* This last series was limited to brushings of the pancreatic duct. Most series do not report any false-positive cytologic diagnoses in brushings obtained from the biliary and pancreatic ducts. However, one series had a diagnostic specificity of only 83%.[26] In an excellently illustrated investigation, de Peralta-Venturina and colleagues compared different biliary tract specimen types for the diagnosis of carcinoma.[3] The diagnostic sensitivity for brushings obtained at either ERCP or PTC was 89%, which was better than that of direct examination of bile (50%). For brushings, the diagnostic specificity was 96% (one false positive). Diagnostic yield by ERCP was higher than that by PTC (Box 19-1).

*References 3, 13, 16, 17, 20, 21, 25, 34.

A number of excellent studies have been dedicated to the description of the cytomorphology of adenocarcinomas of brushing samples obtained during ERCP (Figures 19-4 to 19-7).† Box 19-2 contains a distillation of cytomorphologic features from the literature and the authors' personal experiences.

Several published studies have analyzed the cytomorphologic features of biliary tract brushings with statistical methods. Cohen and colleagues evaluated a series of 90 biliary tract brushings obtained at ERCP by logistic regression analysis.[9] Of the cytomorphologic features, 18 different ones were analyzed. The three that emerged as significant major criteria were (1) chromatin clumping, (2) molding of nuclei within aggregates, and (3) elevated nuclear to cytoplasmic (N:C) ratios. The diagnostic sensitivity for all three features combined was 40%, whereas the specificity was 100%. If two of the three major criteria were present, the sensitivity and specificity were 83% and 98%, respectively. The authors also identified helpful minor or secondary cytomorphologic criteria. These included enlarged nuclei, irregular nuclear contours, nuclear grooves, variability in nuclear size, and macronucleoli. These authors, however, did not evaluate the presence of individually dispersed intact abnormal epithelial cells as a marker of reduced intercellular cohesion.[9] In the authors' experience,[16,20] this is an exceedingly important criterion for separating benign from frankly malignant proliferations.[3,13] Perhaps this can be explained on the basis of specimen type; Cohen and colleagues evaluated cytospins of cells suspended from the brushes rather than direct smears. However, Vadmal and colleagues did not find isolated cells to aid in the benign vs. malignant distinction.[25] Renshaw and colleagues investi-

†References 3, 6, 7, 9, 17, 20, 21, 25, 35.

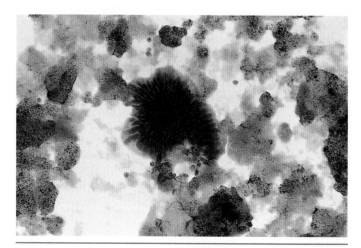

Figure 19-1 **Normal biliary ductal epithelium in direct sampling of bile.** A single cohesive cluster of highly uniform epithelial cells is centered about small to large clumps of biliary pigment material. With the Pap stain, the latter has a distinct golden-brown to green coloration. The epithelial cluster with its sharply demarcated smooth edge is a manifestation of the retention of normal intercellular cohesion. The nuclei are slightly ovoid with smooth membranes, finely granular and evenly distributed chromatin, and inapparent nucleoli. Although cytoplasm is evident, the nuclear-to-cytoplasmic ratios appear to be relatively high. Note the absence of individual, atypical epithelial cells.

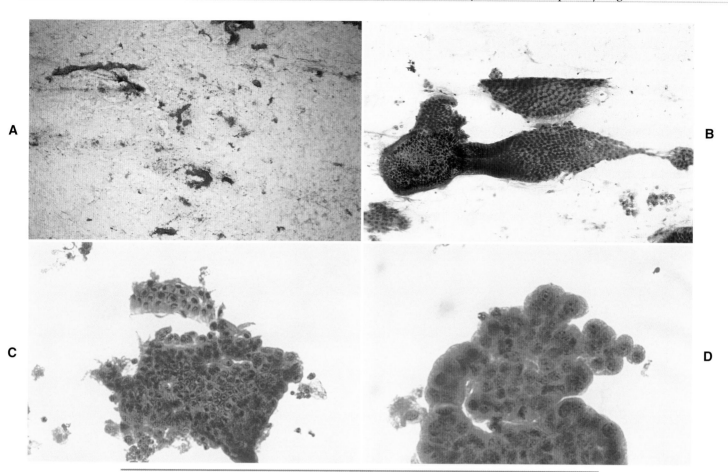

Figure 19-2 Normal biliary duct brushings. **A,** On a clean background, the typical low level of smear cellularity is apparent. Essentially all of the epithelial cells are present in small to moderately sized and generally flat sheets of ductal epithelium. The sharply defined edges and the lack of isolated cells are manifestations of the maintenance of normal cohesion. **B,** Larger sheets of normal ductal epithelium are present in this sample. In addition to the well-maintained cohesion, the retention of normal polarity is readily evident. This manifests with the distinct honeycomb appearance of the sheets—that is, the nuclei are evenly dispersed with surrounding cytoplasm and distinct cell borders. The nuclei are round, dark, and of equal diameters; note the absence of nucleoli. The smear background is lacking inflammatory elements and necrotic debris. **C,** The well-preserved intercellular cohesion and polarity are obvious. Each cell has a single round nucleus with a smooth outline; evenly dispersed, rather pale-stained chromatin; and inapparent nucleoli. A small rim of cyanophilic cytoplasm surrounds each nucleus. Cell borders are well defined. **D,** The nuclei are strikingly homogeneous from cell to cell, as are the nuclear to cytoplasmic (N:C) ratios. The chromatin is distinctly granular and uniformly distributed throughout the nucleoplasm. Intercellular borders are distinct. (Papanicolaou [Pap])

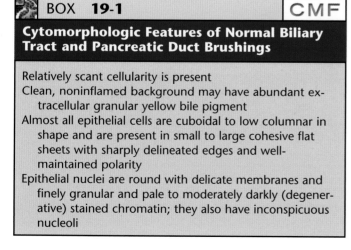

BOX **19-1**	CMF

Cytomorphologic Features of Normal Biliary Tract and Pancreatic Duct Brushings

Relatively scant cellularity is present
Clean, noninflamed background may have abundant extracellular granular yellow bile pigment
Almost all epithelial cells are cuboidal to low columnar in shape and are present in small to large cohesive flat sheets with sharply delineated edges and well-maintained polarity
Epithelial nuclei are round with delicate membranes and finely granular and pale to moderately darkly (degenerative) stained chromatin; they also have inconspicuous nucleoli

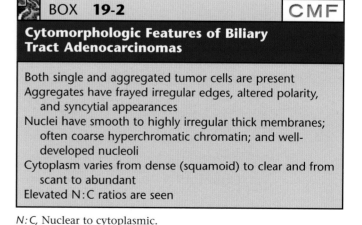

BOX **19-2**	CMF

Cytomorphologic Features of Biliary Tract Adenocarcinomas

Both single and aggregated tumor cells are present
Aggregates have frayed irregular edges, altered polarity, and syncytial appearances
Nuclei have smooth to highly irregular thick membranes; often coarse hyperchromatic chromatin; and well-developed nucleoli
Cytoplasm varies from dense (squamoid) to clear and from scant to abundant
Elevated N:C ratios are seen

N:C, Nuclear to cytoplasmic.

gated the ability to validate diagnostic sensitivity and specificity of the criteria of Nakajima and colleagues and Cohen and colleagues.[9,18,21] Using a series of 165 brushings (mostly direct smears), three morphologists evaluated each specimen independently for the criteria of these two studies and for their own criteria, which were a combination of features drawn from the work of Nakajima and Cohen and their associates. Their three features were loss of polarity, nuclear molding, and chromatin clumping. In addition, they assessed the observers' gestalt of benign vs. malignant without seeking specific individual cytomorphologic attributes. It was this last aspect, an overall evaluation of malignancy, which proved to be the single best predictor of carcinoma (sensitivity 36%, specificity 95%). Among individual cyto-

logic features, chromatin clumping had the greatest statistical strength for predicting cancer (sensitivity 36%, specificity 92%).[21] This same study by Renshaw and colleagues looked at the reproducibility of criteria among morphologists.[21] Excellent reproducibility, as measured by kappa statistics, were found for the overall assessment of malignancy and for clumping of chromatin granules.

Several authors have discussed criteria for glandular dysplasia in brushings obtained from the biliary and pancreatic ducts and its distinction from adenocarcinoma.[13,14,17] This will be mentioned later, in the discussion of adenomas of the ampullary region near the end of this chapter.

The major consideration in the differential diagnosis of carcinoma in brushings is benign reparative epithelial

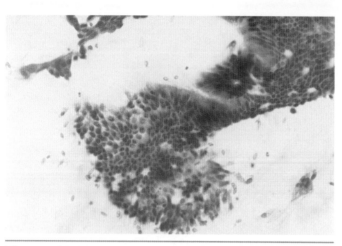

Figure 19-3 **Normal pancreatic duct brushings.** Both cohesion and polarity are well preserved in this sheet of ductal epithelial cells. This is manifested by sharply defined edges, the absence of individually dispersed, intact epithelial cells, and the even distribution of the nuclei within the sheets. The nuclei are strikingly uniform in appearance and lack nucleoli. Occasional cells manifest cytoplasmic mucin and have slightly lower N:C ratios than the majority of the epithelial elements. (Pap)

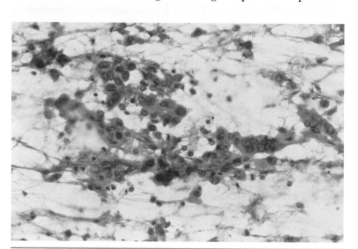

Figure 19-4 **Cholangiocarcinoma.** This relatively cellular sample is composed largely of small, loosely cohesive aggregates of malignant epithelial cells. Mild variability in nuclear size and contour is evident. The malignant nuclei are characterized by thick and, at times, irregularly shaped membranes, fine to coarse hyperchromatic chromatin, and distinct nucleoli. Altered polarity is noted by the crowding and overlapping of nuclei in some of the clusters. In addition, cohesion is reduced, as manifested by several individually dispersed malignant cells. The N:C ratios are variable but generally high. (Pap)

A

B

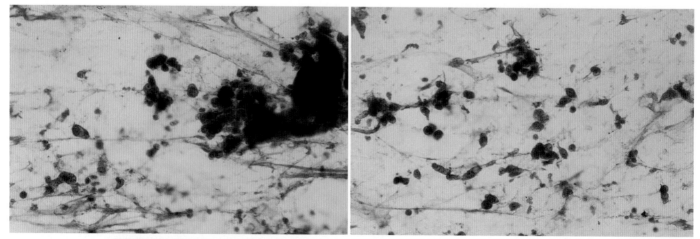

Figure 19-5 **Ductal adenocarcinoma.** In this pancreatic duct brushing, the adenocarcinoma is characterized by large hyperchromatic nuclei and reduced cohesion. The latter is witnessed by the presence of numerous individual malignant cells with intact cytoplasm and by small irregular cellular groupings. In both **A** and **B**, the N:C ratios are generally very high, although an occasional cell has more abundant cytoplasm.

atypia (Figures 19-8 and 19-9). With this in mind, it is important to recognize the appearance of normal bile duct and pancreatic duct epithelium. Normal glandular epithelium presents in the smears as monolayers of uniform cells manifesting both cohesion and polarity.[4,25] Thus, the sheets typically have sharply defined, smooth edges. Importantly, individually dispersed and intact atypical cells are extremely rare or not present. Within the sheets, the nuclei are equidistant from one another and cell borders are well defined, creating the classic honeycomb arrangement.[16,25] The epithelial cells at the borders of the groups often manifest a columnar or picket-fence configuration when seen on edge. The nuclei are homogeneous and round or ovoid with smooth delicate membranes, finely granular pale chromatin, and inconspicuous nucleoli. The smear background may contain bile pigment and crystals, some of which may be cholesterol in type.

The cytomorphologic attributes of reparative atypia (benign repair) involves epithelium closely resembling that seen elsewhere in the gastrointestinal tract in the presence of significant inflammation and/or mucosal defect[16] (Box 19-3).

Kocjan and Smith published a large study of 267 bile duct brushings and then reviewed their false-negative specimens.[17] These authors concluded that there were four major reasons for relatively low levels of diagnostic sensitivity for these preparations. The first of these was poor sampling. This has been the experience of many other workers in the field.[20,24] In fact, for Logrono and colleagues, sampling error accounted for two thirds of their false-negative specimens.[24]

Several different technical problems are associated with failure of the endoscopist to brush the appropriate portion of a stricture. These include poor visualization, extensive scarring, and the presence of a benign epithelium overlying the neoplasm. On-site evaluation of ERCP by a cytopathologist at the time may improve this accuracy.[13] The use of transmucosal FNA biopsy during ERCP may also increase diagnostic yield.[24] Another reason for false-negative results is failure to recognize special types of neoplasms, namely, mucinous and papillary tumors.[17] A third reason is the inability to diagnose accurately glandular dysplasia. Finally, failure to appreciate the significance of the smear background is considered important. The presence of an extensive inflammatory infiltrate and necrotic debris may conceal malignant cells when they are present in low numbers. Kocjan

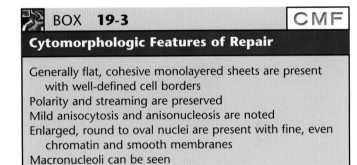

BOX 19-3 CMF

Cytomorphologic Features of Repair

Generally flat, cohesive monolayered sheets are present with well-defined cell borders
Polarity and streaming are preserved
Mild anisocytosis and anisonucleosis are noted
Enlarged, round to oval nuclei are present with fine, even chromatin and smooth membranes
Macronucleoli can be seen
Mitotic figures are present

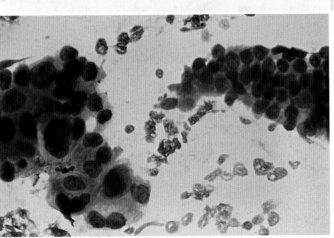
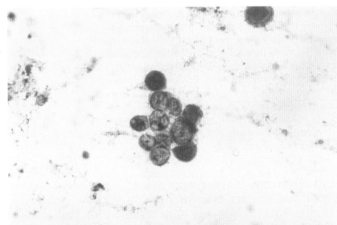
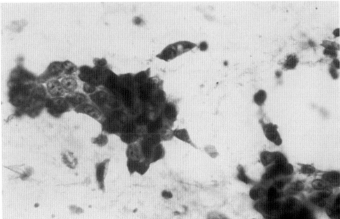

A **B** **C**

Figure 19-6 Cholangiocarcinomas. **A,** This small, irregular, and loosely cohesive cluster is composed of obviously malignant epithelial cells. The latter have thick, irregular nuclear membranes, variably granulated and darkly stained chromatin, and prominent nucleoli. Additionally, only thin rims of cytoplasm surround each nucleus. **B,** Large nucleoli and hyperchromatic chromatin are two major diagnostic criteria for carcinoma in this sample. In addition, the N:C ratios are high, cohesion is reduced with individual tumor cells, and polarity is disrupted with stratification of the malignant cells. **C,** Moderate pleomorphism and hyperchromasia are obvious in this particular example with nuclei varying in contour and size. Nucleoli are evident in many of the tumor cells. (Pap)

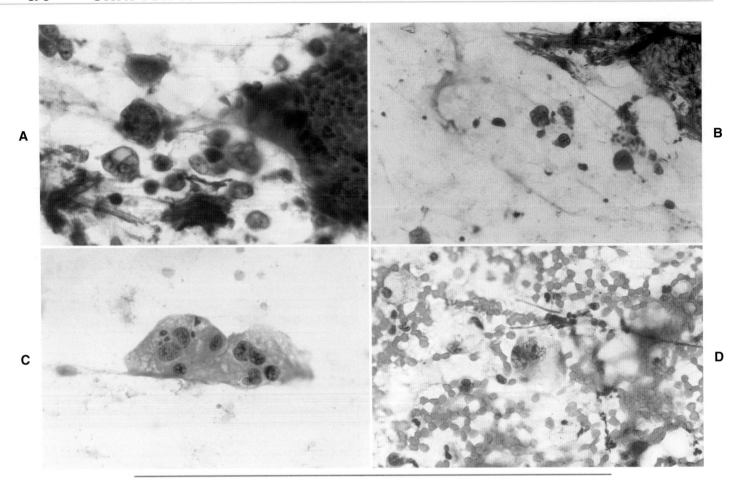

Figure 19-7 **Cholangiocarcinomas. A,** The carcinoma cells contrast sharply with the benign cells present in the flat cohesive sheet. The malignant nuclei are much larger, have thicker and more irregular membranes, and contain much more prominent nucleoli. Within these small clusters of adenocarcinoma cells, the nuclei are crowded and overlap, in contrast with the even distribution of the benign nuclei. Some of the cells have well-developed cytoplasmic secretory vacuoles. **B,** The nuclei of the individual malignant cells are irregular with variable thickness and corrugations. Nucleoli are evident and the N:C ratios are exceedingly high. **C,** Coarsely granular and darkly stained chromatin is present within large malignant nuclei. Despite the rather huge nuclear sizes, the N:C ratios are low because the cells possess abundant delicate cytoplasm. A mild variability of nuclear size and contour is evident. **D,** These two tall columnar epithelial cells are centered in this field of blood and inflammatory elements. The nuclei have irregularly distributed chromatin granules and distinct nucleoli. (Pap)

and Smith suggest that the presence of necrosis is an ominous sign and should be an indication for additional investigation if neoplastic cells are not identified.[17]

As with all testing, a negative result does not exclude disease, or in this case, tumor. The overall low levels of diagnostic yield with biliary and pancreatic cytology are well recognized. Yet little attention has been paid to the potential value of repeating the procedure with a second brushing sample to improve sensitivity. Rabinovitz and colleagues provided some evidence that this is indeed the case.[27] In addition, these authors demonstrated that the likelihood of having a cholangiocarcinoma declined to 5% after three consecutive negative brushing specimens.

Several investigative teams have attempted to enhance diagnostic sensitivity of endoscopic brushings by the use of ancillary diagnostic testing. A few groups have analyzed the value of DNA content in separating benign from malignant specimens.[36,37,49] Yeaton and colleagues reported that ploidy and the proportion of proliferating cells were both useful in

this distinction.[36] These authors used static image analysis. Ryan and Baldauf evaluated ploidy by flow cytometry.[37] During ERCP, specimens were obtained for both conventional cytology and cytometry. Both examinations had a diagnostic sensitivity of 42% for recognizing cancer. The diagnostic specificity for cytology exceeded that for flow cytometry (92% vs. 77%). When the results of both tests were combined, the diagnostic sensitivity increased to 63% but the specificity declined to 69%. When the additional expense of the ploidy determination is considered, it is believed that the measurement of DNA content, with its increased rate of false-positive interpretations, should be considered with marked caution.

Ishimaru and colleagues evaluated conventional cytology with immunostaining for p53 in pancreatic ductal brushings obtained during ERCP.[34] The diagnostic sensitivity, specificity, and accuracy of immunochemistry was equal to or better than that obtained by conventional cytology. In addition, the two techniques were somewhat

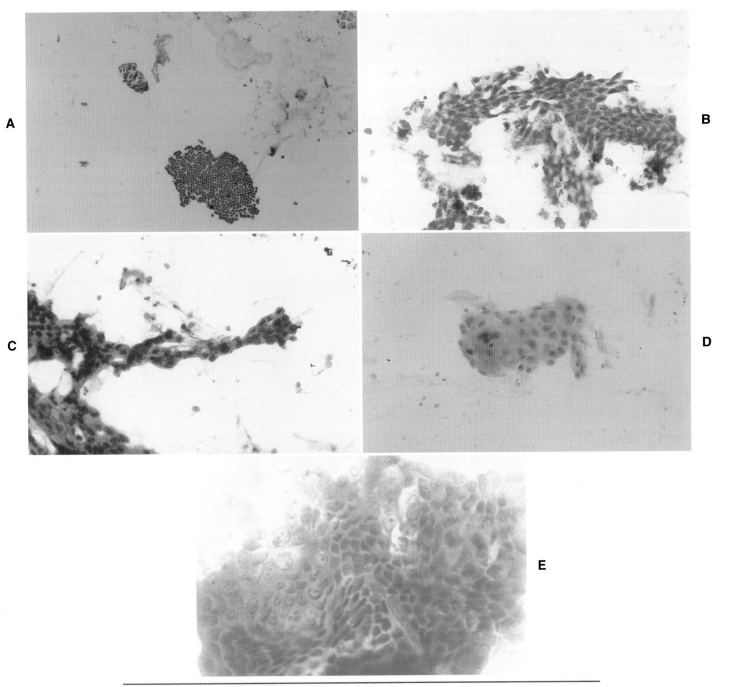

Figure 19-8   **Benign reactive (reparative) biliary ductal epithelium. A,** In this scanning lens view, two flat sheets of ductal epithelial cells are present, both of which are benign. The larger one is totally normal, whereas the smaller cluster is composed of cells showing reparative atypia. Compared with the normal cells, the latter have larger nuclei, more vesicular chromatin, distinct nucleoli, and greater volumes of cytoplasm. **B,** A streaming effect is present within this cohesive aggregate of atypical ductal epithelial cells. This is related to the fact that the long axes of the cells and their nuclei are all pointing in the same direction. Small nucleoli are apparent. Note the bile pigment in the background. **C,** Although this aggregate of epithelial cells is stretched out, intercellular cohesion is well preserved. The nuclei are larger than normal and have delicate, smooth membranes, fine, even chromatin, and small but distinct nucleoli. **D,** The classic nuclear attributes of repair are easily appreciated in this example. Nuclei are larger than normal and ovoid in contour. They have delicate but distinct membranes, vesicular chromatin, and well-developed nucleoli. Importantly, both cohesion and polarity are well maintained. **E,** Variability in nuclear size is mild to moderate in this example of repair. Each nucleus has a delicate membrane, very finely granular and pale-stained chromatin, and distinct nucleoli. Many of the latter are small but do stand out because of the pale staining of the chromatin. Cell borders are well defined, polarity is preserved, and cohesion is maintained. (Pap)

complimentary, increasing diagnostic yield slightly. No false-positive cytomorphologic or immunocytochemical results were found. Evaluation of K-ras mutations in material obtained during ERCP was evaluated by Van Laethem and colleagues.[38] Diagnostic yields improved, and no false-positive interpretations in patients with pancreatitis were made.

In a series of 57 patients, mutations of both the p53 gene and K-ras genes were assessed by Sturm and colleagues in brushings from the ducts in the head of the pancreas in surgically resected specimens.[39] These results were compared with those obtained in the corresponding tissue samples. Due to the nature of this study, it was biased toward individuals with carcinoma; only 9% of the pancreatic specimens were benign. The results from the paired samples were the same in 84% for p53 and 88% for K-ras. Several valid reasons for the discordant data were offered, including sam-

pling error and intratumor heterogeneity. In addition, in two patients, K-ras abnormalities were detected in brushings that were not present in the carcinomas. This was explained by the brushing of premalignant mucinous ductal epithelial hyperplasia. The authors concluded that such testing may not be appropriate for diagnosis in the clinical setting.

Largely based on work done in Japan, a new neoplastic entity has come to be recognized, namely, the intraductal papillary-mucinous tumor (IDPMT).[40] This lesion has a number of synonyms, including mucin-producing tumor. This neoplasm, which is clearly distinct from mucinous cystic tumors, grows principally within the ductal system and thus should be notably amenable to diagnosis by exfoliative cytology. Uehara and colleagues reported a series of 14 patients with IDPMT, 11 of which were malignant and three of which were benign.[41] Cellular material was obtained by

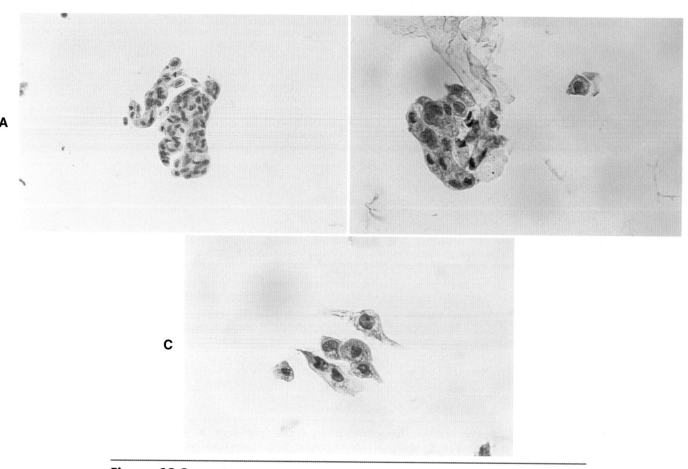

Figure 19-9   Markedly atypical benign ductal epithelial cells. In this pancreatic duct brushing, striking nuclear and cellular features are present, which may simulate well differentiated adenocarcinoma quite closely. **A,** Two cohesive aggregates of ductal epithelial cells are centered in this field, which is otherwise clean and acellular. The nuclei stand out because they are variable in contour, are hyperchromatic, and have distinct nucleoli. In addition, polarity is somewhat altered in that some of the nuclei are crowded. A few cells appear to almost detach from the aggregates. Helpful features in identifying these cells as benign include the sharply defined smooth edges of the aggregates, the absence of individually dispersed atypical cells, and the lack of truly malignant nuclear characteristics. **B,** Moderate variability in nuclear size is apparent in this one cluster of benign but markedly atypical ductal epithelial cells. In addition, a single individually dispersed benign cell is present, which has a larger than normal nucleus and a small but distinct nucleolus. **C,** Variability in nuclear contours, including jagged irregularities and hyperchromasia, is present in these cells, as are small nucleoli. Furthermore, cohesion is markedly reduced with both individual cells and very small clusters. However, elsewhere in the specimen, similar-appearing cells were present within obviously benign large flat sheets. (Pap)

collection of pancreatic juice after secretin administration. Cytology had sensitivity and specificity levels of 91% and 100%, respectively. Iwao and colleagues evaluated brushings from 15 patients with IDPMT (six with adenomas and nine with adenocarcinomas).[42] Cytomorphology was positive in 56% of the cancer cases. Immunostaining of the smears for *p53* mutations detected two additional patients with malignancies. Of the patients with adenomas, all were diagnosed as benign by cytology, and none demonstrated staining (mutations) for *p53* protein. Thus, it appears that pancreatic juice cytology may be better than brushings for diagnosing IDPMT. Finally, it should be mentioned that the eggs of the bile duct parasites may on occasion be identified in cytologic samples.[4,43]

Relative to most of the gastrointestinal tract, the duodenum is cytologically sampled rather infrequently. Normal duodenal mucosa presents in smears as flat, large monolayers of uniform glandular cells with a distinct honeycomb arrangement (Figure 19-10).[16] Occasionally, three-dimensional clusters with a possible villous configuration may be recognized. The individual cells have small, round uniform nuclei with delicate membranes, fine chromatin, and inconspicuous nucleoli. Scanty rims of cytoplasm are evident about most nuclei. When seen on end, the absorptive cells have a tall, columnar shape, cyanophilic cytoplasm, a striated luminal border, and a low N:C ratio. Goblet cells may also be seen. These are characterized by barrel-like configurations and optically clear cytoplasm.

Although benign peptic ulcers occur more often in the duodenum than in the stomach, they are histologically and cytologically sampled far less often than their gastric counterparts. In benign peptic ulcers, reparative atypia and inflammatory changes may be recognized. The cytologic repair closely resembles that described previously in the biliary tract epithelium. Key features include preservation of intercellular cohesion and polarity, and the finding of dyssynchrony between huge cytologically worrisome nucleoli and benign-appearing chromatin.[16] The major entity in the differential diagnosis is adenocarcinoma.

Adenocarcinoma is the most common malignancy arising in the duodenum.[44] Clinically, patients may manifest jaundice, anemia, or symptoms of obstruction. Within the

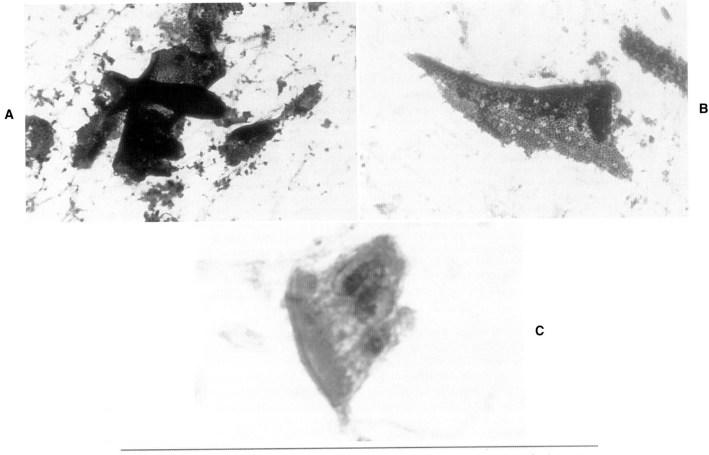

Figure 19-10 Normal duodenal mucosa. A, In this brushing smear, the cohesive aggregates of columnar epithelial cells are present in flat sheets and a three-dimensional villous projection. **B,** The edges of this large flat sheet are sharply defined and smooth. The preservation of cohesion is also witnessed by the absence of individual epithelial cells. Polarity is well maintained because the nuclei are evenly distributed within the sheet. Note the presence of scattered goblet cells, which are manifested by the more abundant and pale-stained cytoplasm. **C,** The luminal surfaces of these tall columnar cells manifest the characteristic striated border through the presence of numerous microvilli. The basally located nuclei have ovoid contours, very delicate membranes, extremely finely granular and pale-stained chromatin, and minute nucleoli. Obviously, the N:C ratios are low. (Pap)

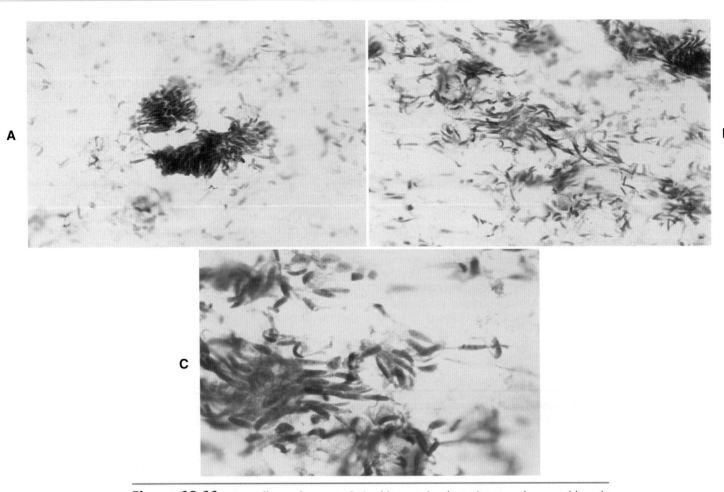

Figure 19-11   **Ampullary adenoma. A,** In this scanning lens view, two large and loosely cohesive aggregates of tumor cells are darkly stained. For the most part, this is because of the presence of large, elongated hyperchromatic nuclei within cells, which have high length-to-width ratios (needle cells). For the most part, cohesion is well maintained, but a few individual tumor cells appear to exfoliate from the surfaces of these aggregates. The smear background is clean. **B,** The needle cells are typified by elongated nuclei with evenly dispersed and darkly stained chromatin and an occasional nucleolus. Cells also have moderate volumes of cyanophilic cytoplasm, usually without evidence of mucus production. This loosely arrayed, almost storiform pattern is typical of ampullary adenomas in brushings. These have been mistaken for stromal neoplasms. **C,** At higher magnification the smooth nuclear outlines, their cigar contours, and darkly stained chromatin are readily apparent. Such needle cells are characteristic of adenomas in brushings from any portion of the gastrointestinal and biliary tracts. (Pap)

duodenum, the most common site of origin of adenocarcinoma is in the immediate vicinity of the papillae of Vater. Typically, they have an exophytic papillary endoscopic appearance. Ulcerating adenocarcinomas are uncommon in the duodenum, and thus, endoscopic sampling for histology and cytology of duodenal peptic ulcers is not often obtained. Cytomorphologically, the vast majority of duodenal adenocarcinomas resemble the intestinal variant of gastric adenocarcinoma. Thus, both small three-dimensional aggregates with irregular edges and numerous individually dispersed intact malignant cells are often present. The aggregates may have spherical and papillary configurations. Within such, the malignant nuclei are crowded, compressed, and overlapped. Most of the tumor cells have a solitary large nucleus, which varies from round to distinctly ovoid or elongated to irregular. The nuclear membranes are thick, often with obvious but minor contour irregularities. Typically, one or more nucleoli are readily apparent. The

finding of intact isolated abnormal cells is important for the diagnosis of adenocarcinoma.[16,20]

In the duodenum and especially the region of the ampulla, another glandular neoplasm needs to be considered, specifically the villous adenoma.[16,20,45,46] These tumors are typically exophytic and therefore subjected to endoscopic biopsy and brushings. Veronezi-Gurwell and colleagues described the cytomorphologic features of four ampullary adenomas.[46] The most distinctive features included what Thabet and Farlane have referred to as *needle cells.*[47] These cells are elongated, columnar epithelial elements with high length-to-width ratios (Figure 19-11). Similarly elongated nuclei maintain a generally basal orientation. These nuclei have delicate membranes, finely granular but darkly stained chromatin, and one or more distinct nucleoli. Cytoplasmic mucin is markedly reduced. In smears the cells present in variably sized and shaped aggregates and are individually dispersed. Compared with frankly malignant glandular

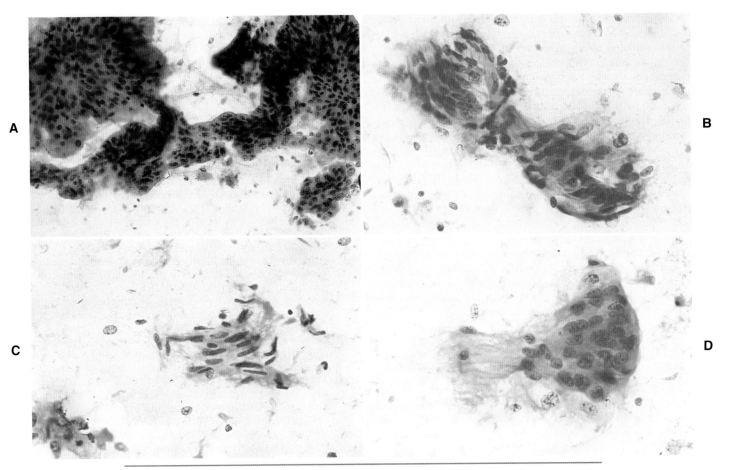

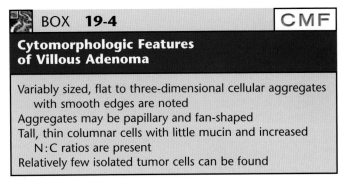

Figure 19-12 Biliary papillomatosis. **A,** A large proportion of the surface area of the smears is covered by large three-dimensional cohesive arrays of neoplastic epithelial cells. These anastomosing aggregates almost have a papillary appearance. Even at this magnification, hyperchromasia is evident, as are large and elongated nuclei. **B,** This cohesive cluster is composed of classic needle cells with elongated hyperchromatic nuclei and relatively scanty cytoplasm. Note the sharply defined smooth edge of this three-dimensional aggregate. **C,** These needle cells show mild variability in nuclear size, although all of them are quite elongated. They end in sharp to rounded tips and have evenly distributed darkly stained chromatin and inconspicuous nucleoli. For the most part, cohesion is well maintained. **D,** Some of the neoplastic cells have more rounded or ovoid nuclei with more delicate distinctly granular chromatin and minute nucleoli. Still, cohesion is well-maintained, although polarity is altered because the nuclei are crowded. (Pap)

cells, needle cells are relatively homogeneous in size and appearance, do not show coarse chromatin granularity, and possess relatively small nucleoli. In addition, within cohesive aggregates, polarity is relatively well preserved in the adenomatous epithelium.

Nine ampullary villous tumors were included in the series by Bardales and colleagues.[20] A correct diagnosis was made in three patients. Four specimens had false-negative results attributed to sampling errors in that the smears did not contain clusters of dysplastic epithelial cells. In two patients, a diagnosis of adenocarcinoma was rendered. Although this could be considered in the strictest sense a false-positive interpretation, they should not have a negative impact on patient management. Ampullary villous tumors are clearly premalignant because a large proportion evolve to adenocarcinomas. In fact, many resected adenomas are found histologically to harbor areas of frank malignancy. Thus, in patients who are surgical candidates, a diagnosis of adenoma or carcinoma should prompt a visit to the operating room.

BOX 19-4 CMF

**Cytomorphologic Features
of Villous Adenoma**

Variably sized, flat to three-dimensional cellular aggregates with smooth edges are noted
Aggregates may be papillary and fan-shaped
Tall, thin columnar cells with little mucin and increased N:C ratios are present
Relatively few isolated tumor cells can be found

N:C, Nuclear to cytoplasmic.

Although much less common, similar benign villous adenomas arise more proximally in the biliary tract and may even be multiple (papillomatosis). The cytomorphologic picture in brushings is the same (Figure 19-12 and Box 19-4).

Although complimentary, concurrently obtained endoscopic biopsies and brushings both usually demonstrate villous adenoma in this situation.[16] However, because of the greater sampling (increased surface area) by brushings, the presence of a focal adenocarcinoma within an adenoma may be more easily detected in the cytologic preparations. In general, histologic biopsy specimens in the region of the ampulla are diagnostic.[45] In this setting, however, a publication by Ponchon and colleagues is instructive.[48] These authors evaluated 69 consecutive patients thought to have benign dysfunction of the sphincter of Oddi. These individuals underwent endoscopic sphincterotomy followed 10 or more days later by biopsies. Although original biopsies were negative for tumor, three patients (4%) were found to have adenocarcinoma. The authors recommended that ampullary biopsy should be performed in all patients suspected of having sphincter dysfunction and treated by endoscopic sphincterotomy.[48] In other words, small intraampullary neoplasms may go unrecognized endoscopically and not be subjected to biopsy. In addition to biopsies, endoscopic brushings may also be of benefit in this setting.

References

1. Carriage MT, Henson DE. Liver, gallbladder, extrahepatic bile ducts and pancreas. Cancer 1995; 75:171-190.
2. Dusenburg D. Biliary stricture due to hepatocellular carcinoma: diagnosis by bile duct brushing cytology. Diagn Cytopathol 1997; 16:55-56.
3. de Peralta-Venturina MN, Wong DK, Purslow MJ, et al. Biliary tract cytology in specimens obtained by direct cholangiographic procedures: a study of 74 cases. Diagn Cytopathol 1996; 14:334-348.
4. Sterrett GF, Whitaker D, Shilkin KB. Gallbladder and extrahepatic ducts. In: Gray W, editor. Diagnostic cytpathology. Edinburgh: Churchill Livingstone; 1995. pp.403-413.
5. Kurzawinski T, Derry A, Davidson BR. Diagnostic value of cytology for biliary stricture. Br J Surg 1993; 80:414-420.
6. Rupp M, Hawathorne CM, Ehya H. Brushing cytology in biliary tract obstruction. Acta Cytol 1990; 34:221-226.
7. Howell LP, Chow H, Russell LA. Cytodiagnosis of extrahepatic biliary duct tumors from specimens obtained during cholangiography. Diagn Cytopathol 1988; 4:328-334.
8. Foutch PG. Diagnosis of cancer by cytologic methods performed during ERCP. Gastrointest Endosc 1994; 40:249-252.
9. Cohen MB, Wittchow RJ, Johlin FC, et al. Brush cytology of the extrahepatic biliary tract: comparison of cytologic features of adenocarcinoma and benign biliary strictures. Mod Pathol 1995; 8:498-502.
10. Mohandas KM, Swaroop S, Bullar SU, et al. Diagnosis of malignant obstructive jaundice by bile cytology: results improved by dilating the bile duct strictures. Gastrointest Endosc 1994; 40:150-154.
11. Savader SJ, Prescott CA, Lund GB, et al. Intraductal biliary biopsy: comparison of three techniques. J Vasc Intervene Radiol 1996; 7:743-750.
12. Ponchon T, Gagnon P, Berger F, et al. Value of endobiliary brush cytology and biopsies for diagnosis of malignant bile duct stenosis: results of a prospective study. Gastrointest Endosc 1995; 42:565-572.
13. Layfield LJ, Wax TD, Lee JG, et al. Accuracy and morphologic aspects of pancreatic and biliary duct brushings. Acta Cytol 1995; 39:11-18.
14. Lee JG, Leung JW, Baillie J, et al. Benign, dysplastic or malignant-making sense of endoscopic bile duct brush cytology: results in 149 consecutive patients. Am J Gastroenterol 1995:90:722-726.
15. Simsir A, Greenbaum E, Stevens PD, et al. Biliary stent replacement cytology. Diagn Cytopathol 1997; 16:233-237.
16. Geisinger KR. Alimentary tract (esophagus, stomach, small intestine, colon, rectum, anus, biliary tract). In: Bibbo M, editor. Comprehensive cytopathology. 2nd ed. Philadelphia: WB Saunders; 1997. pp.413-434.
17. Kocjan G, Smith AN. Bile duct brushing cytology: potential pitfalls in diagnosis. Diagn Cytopathol 1997; 16:358-363.
18. Nakajima T, Tajima Y, Sugano I, et al. Multivariate statistical analysis of bile cytology. Acta Cytol 1994; 38:51-55.
19. Gabriel M, Pawlaczyk K, Podstawski W. Use of immunohistochemical analysis of antigen expression and exfoliative cytology of biliary epithelial cells in diagnosis of mechanical jaundice. Pol Arch Med Wewn 1997; 98:400-406.
20. Bardales RH, Stanley MW, Simpson DD, et al. Diagnostic value of brush cytology in the diagnosis of duodenal biliary, and ampullary neoplasms. Am J Clin Pathol 1998; 109:540-548.
21. Renshaw AA, Madge R, Jiroutek M, et al. Bile duct brushing cytology. Statistical analysis of proposed diagnostic criteria. Am J Clin Pathol 1998; 110:635-640.
22. Cozzi G, Alasio L, Civelli E, et al. Percutaneous intraductal sampling for cyto-histologic diagnosis of biliary duct structures. Tumori 1999; 85:153-156.
23. Vandervoort J, Soetikno RM, Montes H, et al. Accuracy and complication rate of brush cytology from bile duct versus pancreatic duct. Gastrointest Endosc 1999; 43:322-327.
24. Logrono R, Kurtycz DF, Molina CP, et al. Analysis of false-negative diagnoses on endoscopic brush cytology of biliary and pancreatic duct strictures: the experience at two university hospitals. Arch Pathol Lab Med 2000; 124:387-392.
25. Vadmal MS, Byrne-Semmelmeier S, Smilari TF, et al. Biliary tract brush cytology. Acta Cytol 2000; 44:533-538.
26. Desa LA, Akosa AB, Lazzara S, et al. Cytodiagnosis in the management of extrahepatic biliary stricture. Gut 1991; 32:1188-1191.
27. Rabinovitz M, Zajko AB, Hassanein T. Diagnostic value of brush cytology in the diagnosis of bile duct carcinoma: a study of 65 patients. Hepatology 1990; 12:747-752.
28. Scudera PL, Koizumi J, Jacobson IM. Brush cytology evaluation of lesions encountered during ERCP. Gastrointest Endosc 1990; 36:281-284.
29. Foutch PG, Kerr DM, Harlan JR, et al. Endoscopic retrograde wire-guided brush cytology for diagnosis of patients with malignant obstruction of the bile duct. Am J Gastroenterol 1990; 85:791-795.
30. Foutch PG, Kerr DM, Harlan JR, et al. A prospective, controlled analysis of endoscopic cytotechniques for diagnosis of malignant biliary strictures. Am J Gastroenterol 1991; 86:577-580.
31. Ferrari AP, Lichtenstein DR, Slivka A, et al. Brush cytology during ERCP for the diagnosis of biliary and pancreatic malignancies. Gastrointest Endosc 1994; 40:140-145.
32. Nakaizumi A, Tatsuta M, Uehara H, et al. Cytologic examination of pure pancreatic juice in the diagnosis of pancreatic carcinoma. Cancer 1992; 70:2610-2614.
33. Kondo H, Sugano K, Fukayama N, et al. Detection of point mutations in the K-ras oncogene at codon 2 in pure pancreatic juice for diagnosis of pancreatic carcinoma. Cancer 1994; 73:1589-1594.
34. Ishimaru S, Itah M, Hanada K, et al. Immunocytochemical detection of p53 protein pancreatic duct brushings in patients with pancreatic carcinoma. Cancer 1996; 77:2233-2239.
35. Sawada Y, Gonda H, Hayashita Y. Combined use of brushing cytology and endoscopic retrograde pancreatography for the early detection of pancreatic cancer. Acta Cytol 1989; 33:870-874.

36. Yeaton P, Kiss R, Deviere J, et al. Use of cell image analysis in the detection of cancer from specimens obtained during endoscopic retrograde cholangiopancreatography. Am J Clin Pathol 1993; 100:497-501.

37. Ryan ME, Baldauf MC. Comparison of flow cytometry for DNA content and brush cytology for detection of malignancy in pancreaticobiliary strictures. Gastrointest Endosc 1994; 40:133-139.

38. Van Laethem JL, Vertongen P, Deviere J, et al. Detection of c-K-ras codon 12 mutations from pancreatic duct brushings int he diagnosis of pancreatic tumors. Gut 1995;36: 78-1787.

39. Sturm PD, Hruban RH, Ramsoekh TB, et al. The potential diagnostic use of K-ras codon 12 and p53 alterations in brush cytology from the pancreatic head region. J Pathol 1998; 186:247-253.

40. Shimizu M, Hirokawa M, Manabe T, et al. Cytologic findings in noninvasive intraductal papillary-mucinous carcinoma of the pancreas. A report of two cases. Acta Cytol 1999; 43:243-246.

41. Uehara H, Nakaizumi A, Iishi H, et al. Cytologic exam of pancreatic juice for differential diagnosis of benign and malignant mucin-producing tumors of the pancreas. Cancer 1994; 74:826-833.

42. Iwao T, Tsuchida A, Hanada K, et al. Immunocytochemical detection of p53 protein as an adjunct in cytologic diagnosis from pancreatic duct brushings in mucin-producing tumors of the pancreas. Cancer Cytopathol 1997; 81:163-171.

43. Papillo JL. Cytologic diagnosis of liver fluke infestation in a patient with subsequently documented cholangiocarcinoma. Acta Cytol 1989; 33:865-869.

44. Zhu L, Kim K, Domenica DR, et al. Adenocarcinoma of the duodenum and ampulla of Vater: clinicopathologic study and expression of p53, c-neu, TGF-2, CEA, and EMA. J Surg Oncol 1996; 61:100-105.

45. Komorowski RA, Beggs BK, Geenan JE, et al. Assessment of ampulla of Vater pathology: an endoscopic approach. Am J Surg Pathol 1991; 15:1188-1196.

46. Veronezi-Gurwell A, Wittchow RJ, Bottles K, et al. Cytologic features of villous adenoma of the ampullary region. Diagn Cytopathol 1996; 14:145-149.

47. Thabet RJ, Farlane EWE. Cytologic field patterns and nuclear morphology in the diagnosis of colon pathology. Acta Cytol 1962; 6:325-331.

48. Ponchon T, Aucia N, Mitchell R, et al. Biopsies of the ampullary region in patients suspected to have sphincter of Oddi dysfunction. Gastrointest Endosc 1995; 42:296-300.

49. Krisnamurthy S, Katz RL, Shumate A, et al. DNA image analysis combined with routine cytology improves diagnostic sensitivity of common bile duct brushing. Cancer Cytopathol 2001; 93:228-235.

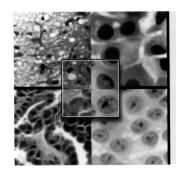

CHAPTER
20

Liver

In many medical centers the most common target of abdominal organ fine-needle aspiration (FNA) biopsy is the liver. The major indication for FNAB is the evaluation of a hepatic mass lesion. Most pathologists have been more familiar with interpreting tissue core needle biopsies of tumors involving the liver than FNA biopsy specimens. However, FNA biopsy of liver masses has become the standard procedure in the majority of hospitals; tissue core biopsy is still recommended as the procedure of choice whenever a medical (nonneoplastic) process such as viral hepatitis, drug toxicity, and/or cirrhosis is the major concern.[1] As in other sites the advantages of FNA biopsy are that the mass can be sampled in several different planes and multiple needle punctures can be performed during a single FNA biopsy procedure, which is often not done with tissue core biopsies. In addition, aspiration cytology allows for an immediate interpretation of the smears so that adequacy can be assessed, preliminary interpretation rendered, and additional material obtained for ancillary studies.[1-3] Immediate cytologic examination of touch imprints of the tissue core biopsy can also be used to assess adequacy and provide a preliminary interpretation.

The sensitivity of FNA biopsy of liver neoplasm ranges from 92% to 96%.[4-12] Although most large series of liver aspirates have stressed the role of FNA biopsy in the workup of metastatic carcinoma, an increasing number of reports demonstrate the value of FNA biopsy for the diagnosis of primary hepatocellular carcinoma (hepatoma).[1,10-20]

In the evaluation of liver aspirates, it is imperative to appreciate the cytomorphologic spectrum of benign hepatocytes. Hepatocytes vary from polygonal to round with well-defined cell borders (Figure 20-1). Typically, a moderate amount of uniform, granular dense cytoplasm is present. With the Pap stain, small eosinophilic or deeply basophilic cytoplasmic granules can be seen, and in occasional cases, bile, lipofuscin pigment, and/or lipid vacuoles are present (Figure 20-2). With the Diff-Quik (DQ) stain, bile has a green hue, whereas with the Pap, it is a golden brown (Figure 20-3). Both intracytoplasmic bile and extracellular pigmented material can be appreciated in smears.

Generally, hepatocytes possess a single centrally located round nucleus characterized by evenly distributed, finely granular chromatin and a single round prominent nucleolus. The nuclear characteristics are better visualized with the Pap stain. Benign hepatocytes demonstrate considerable variation in nuclear diameters, and hepatocytes with more than one nucleus are common (Figure 20-4). Similar to hepatocellular carcinoma, the nuclei of reactive hepatocytes are centrally positioned but in contrast have relatively low nuclear to cytoplasmic (N:C) ratios. Benign hepatocytes are generally arranged in relatively small, flat sheets consisting of 15 or fewer cells, although microtissue fragments and individually scattered hepatocytes may be present (Figure 20-5). Within the groups of hepatocytes, Kupffer and endothelial cells can be present. Both cell types have elongated, pale, finely granular nuclei with inconspicuous nucleoli and indistinct, scanty cytoplasm. When a narrow cordlike arrangement that may simulate trabeculae is present, it usually consists of only one to two layers of hepatocytes. Cell blocks and tissue core biopsies are generally better for evaluating hepatocellular architecture (Figure 20-6).[21] These specimens are also preferred when a panel of immunohistochemical studies are needed.[22] However, if the cell block is not available, many of the immunohistochemical studies can be performed on either previously stained or unstained alcohol-fixed or direct air-dried smears. Alcohol is an excellent fixative for most immunohistochemical studies.

Benign-appearing hepatocytes are present in reactive hepatocellular proliferations such as cirrhosis and benign hepatocytic neoplasms, as well as admixed in inflammatory lesions such as hepatic abscesses and granulomas. Hepatocytes are present in smears when both the inflammatory mass and the surrounding benign liver tissue are sampled. Benign hepatocytes are also present in the smears when a malignant lesion has not been accurately sampled. Importantly, the appreciation of a two-cell population of benign hepatocytes and malignant cells is a characteristic feature of most aspirates of metastatic malignancies. Other benign elements that can be seen in liver smears include bile ducts, which are usually arranged in small, flat honeycomb groups of uniform cuboidal ductal epithelial cells with central, small, round nuclei surrounded by a moderate amount of cytoplasm.

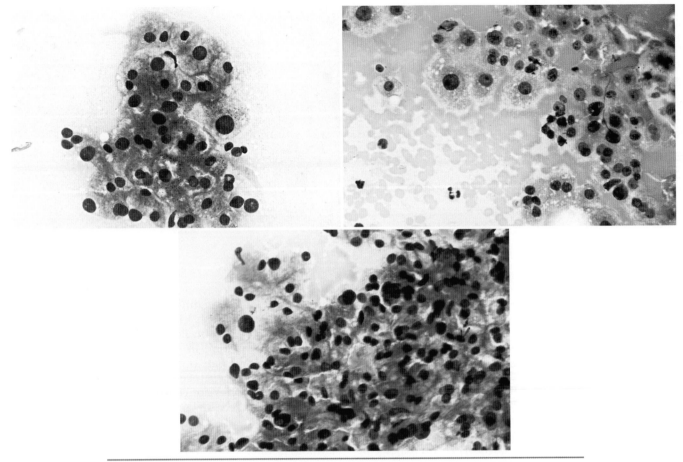

Figure 20-1   Benign liver. In these Diff-Quik-(DQ-)stained smears, polygonal to round benign hepatocytes with well-defined cell borders are present. The nuclei are centrally placed with surrounding granular cytoplasm. Varying degrees of vacuolization are related to the glycogen and fat content of the cells.

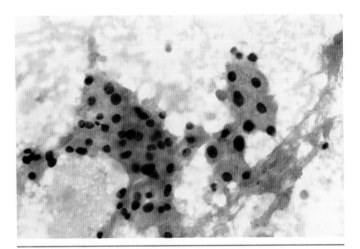

Figure 20-2   Benign liver. In this Papanicolaou-(Pap-)stained smear, the hepatocytes have uniform granular, dense cytoplasm.

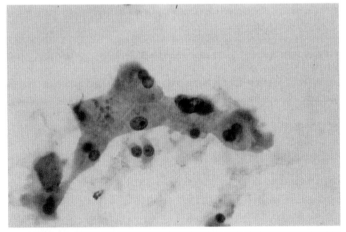

Figure 20-3   Benign liver. Bile is granular with a yellow to golden-brown color in Pap-stained smears and can be present both within the cytoplasm of the hepatocytes and in the background. Note the variability in nuclear size and an occasional binucleated hepatocyte. (From Silverman JF, Geisinger KR. Fine needle aspiration cytology of the thorax and abdomen. New York: Churchill Livingstone; 1996. p.91.)

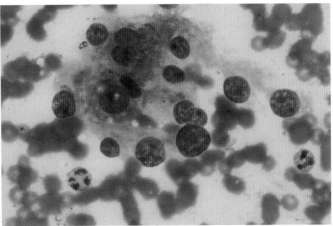

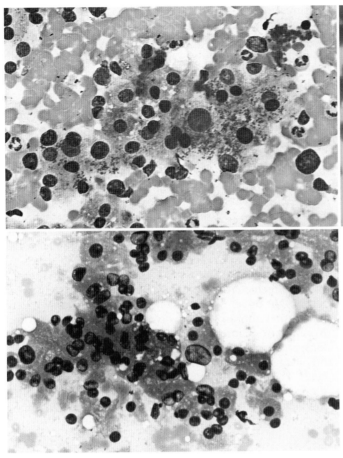

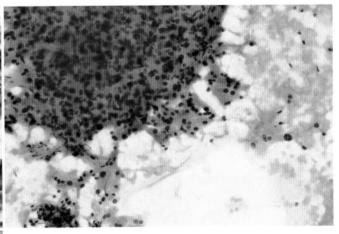

Figure 20-4   **Benign liver.** In these DQ-stained smears, reactive benign hepatocytes demonstrate variation in nuclear size but relatively low nuclear to cytoplasmic (N:C) ratios.

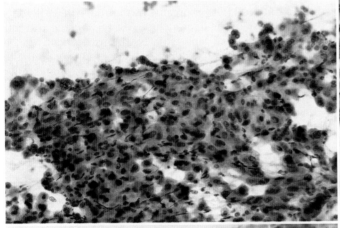

A

B

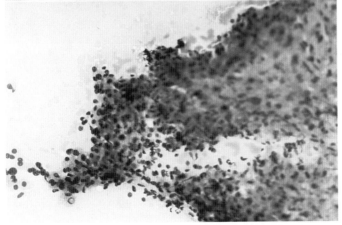

C

Figure 20-5   **Benign liver.** Microtissue fragments consist of flat sheets of benign hepatocytes with irregular, ragged borders at the periphery of the groups. (**A** and **B**, Pap; **C**, DQ)

HEPATIC ABSCESSES

Most hepatic abscesses are related to bacterial infections associated with acute cholangitis, pylephlebitis, sepsis, or trauma.[1] Patients typically have fever associated with right upper quadrant pain and point tenderness. Radiographically, one or more lesions may potentially mimic both a primary and metastatic cancer. FNA biopsy of a bacterial hepatic abscess is characterized by sheets of neutrophils, abundant granular necrotic material, and in some specimens, organisms (Figure 20-7). Although bacteria are better seen in the DQ-stained material (compared with Pap) as a result of the increased size of these structures in air-dried smears, a Gram stain confirms the presence of extracellular and intracellular bacteria and determines whether the bacteria is Gram-positive or -negative (Figure 20-8). In pyogenic abscesses, neutrophils are much more numerous than the benign hepatocytes that often show both degenerative and regenerative changes. These benign alterations may serve as a potential pitfall for a false-positive diagnosis of malignancy in aspirates of liver abscesses.[23] Degenerative

features include cytoplasmic vacuolization, pyknosis, and fragmentation of the nuclear membrane. In regeneration, the hepatocytes possess large prominent nucleoli and multiple nuclei. Conversely, a necrotic neoplasm can be potentially misinterpreted as an abscess because of the presence of extensive nuclear debris with associated neutrophilic infiltration.[23] Whenever a liver abscess is suspected, additional aspirated material should be submitted for microbiologic culture.[24] *Candida* is the most common fungus causing a hepatic fungal abscess and is recognized by the presence of pseudohyphae and/or budding yeasts. In the rare scenario of numerous eosinophils in the smears, the possibility of a trematode infection should be entertained. Clonorchiasis has been diagnosed by FNA biopsy of the liver when the ova of the *Clonorchis sinensis,* eosinophils, and Charcot-Leyden crystals were present in the liver smears.[9,25] Similar specimens associated with *Fasciola* organisms have also been seen (Figure 20-9).[1]

Hepatic amebic abscess is a relatively unusual complication of amebic enterocolitis. Patients generally present with fever, right upper quadrant pain, and a single large irregular lesion that more often involves the right hepatic lobe.[1,26] Aspirates from amebic abscesses generally do not have an extensive neutrophilic infiltrate but rather contain necrotic debris, large numbers of histiocytes, and degenerated hepatocytes. The diagnosis, however, is based on the recognition of the trophozoites of *Entamoeba histolytica.*[26,27] These trophozoites have rounded contours, abundant granular to bubbly cytoplasm, and a single round nucleus with a prominent karyosome (Figure 20-10). Often, phagocytized erythrocytes can also be appreciated within the parasites. These trophozoites need to be differentiated from benign histiocytes that have elongated to reniform-shaped nuclei with small to indistinct nucleoli. Other organisms that have been described in FNA biopsy of the liver include *Giardia lamblia*[4] and actinomyces.[28] In a case report of FNA biopsy of kala-azar, the smears contained atypical hepatocytes, groups of epithelioid histiocytes, and macrophages containing Leishman bodies.[29]

FNA biopsy can also sample granulomas in a variety of liver disorders such as granulomatous hepatitis, sarcoidosis, drug-induced and allergic reactions, and Hodgkin's disease.[30] Of course, granulomas are diagnosed when clusters

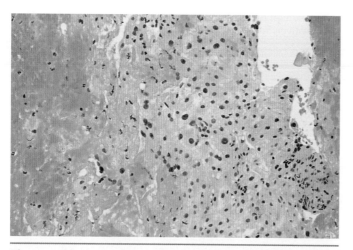

Figure 20-6 **Benign liver.** Cell block of benign liver parenchyma in which trabeculae of reactive liver cells that are two to three cell layers thick are present. (Hematoxylin and eosin [H&E])

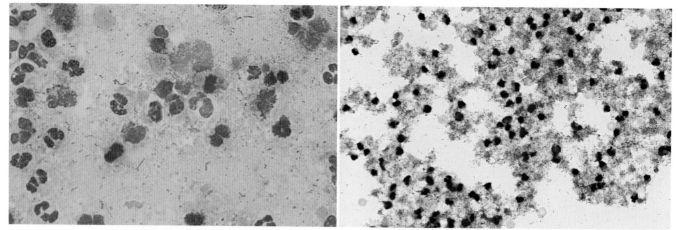

A   **B**

Figure 20-7 **Pyogenic abscess. A,** Neutrophils are present in a granular background, along with rod-shaped bacteria, in this DQ-stained smear. **B,** In this Pap-stained smear from a hepatic abscess, degenerating neutrophils and abundant granular debris are present. Because of the smaller size of the bacteria in the alcohol-fixed preparation, bacteria are not readily identified.

of epithelioid histiocytes are appreciated in the smears. The cells have elongated to bent footprint or boomerang-shaped nuclei that are usually eccentrically placed within pale cytoplasm. The nuclei have finely granular chromatin with small to indistinct nucleoli. When epithelioid cells are aggregated, merging of their indistinct cytoplasmic borders creates a syncytial arrangement. Such clusters could be confused with adenocarcinoma because both may be arranged in collections with depth of focus. This potential for a false-positive diagnosis is accentuated when the smears are over-stained. However, attention to the configuration of the epithelioid histiocytes, their delicate nuclear detail, and the maintenance of low N:C ratios should avoid an incorrect diagnosis of malignancy. Furthermore, cytoplasm dominates the periphery of granulomas, whereas malignant nuclei appear to occupy much of the external surface of the aggregates of metastatic carcinoma cells.

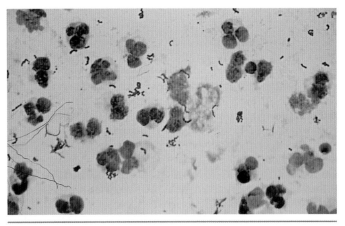

Figure 20-8 **Pyogenic abscess.** The Gram stain demonstrates the bacteria in this aspirate of a pyogenic liver abscess.

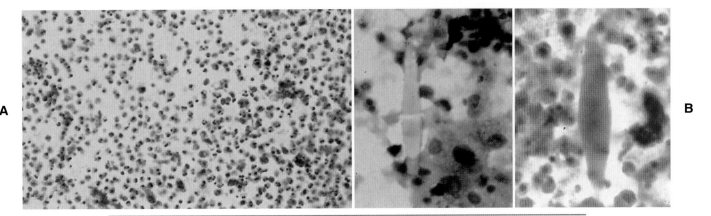

A

B

Figure 20-9 *Fasciola hepatica* and **Charcot-Leyden crystals.** Aspirate from a middle-age woman in which eosinophils and Charcot-Leyden crystals are present. The patient was serologically positive for *Fasciola hepatica,* although organisms were not found in the smears. **A,** Numerous bilobed eosinophils are present in this DQ-stained smear. **B,** In this DQ-stained smear, acellular, pale-blue, elongated, polygonal-shaped Charcot-Leyden crystals having sharply defined edges are identified, as are some scattered eosinophils. Charcot-Leyden crystals are accentuated with the periodic acid–Schiff stain (From Silverman JF, Geisinger KR. Fine needle aspiration cytology of the thorax and abdomen. New York: Churchill Livingstone; 1996. p.94.)

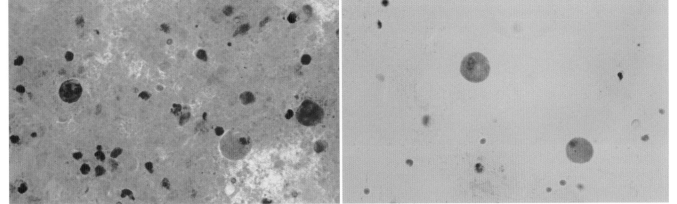

A

B

Figure 20-10 **Amebic abscess. A,** Liver aspirate in which abundant necrotic debris is seen in the background without a neutrophilic infiltrate. The diagnosis of an amebic abscess is based on the presence of trophozoites of *Entamoeba histolytica* with round contours, abundant bubbly cytoplasm and a single small, round nucleus with a prominent karyosome. The trophozoites can potentially be confused with benign histiocytes, although the latter has nuclei that are ovoid or slightly bent. In addition, nucleoli are generally not prominent in histiocytes, and therefore should not be confused with the prominent karyosome of trophozoites. (DQ) **B,** In this DQ-stained smear of an amebic abscess, two trophozoites of *Entamoeba histolytica* are identified. Also note the lack of a neutrophilic exudate.

CYSTS

Hepatic cysts can cause a clinically worrisome mass lesion. Cysts can be single or multiple; small to large; and of congenital, parasitic, or neoplastic origin. Congenital cysts represent unilocular cystic dilatation of the biliary tree and therefore are lined by a single layer of cytologically bland ductal epithelial cells that can vary from flat, cuboidal, or columnar. The surrounding liver tissue consists of either atrophic, degenerative, or regenerative hepatocytes. Aspirates of benign congenital cysts often yield a copious amount of clear fluid,[7,31,32] which is best processed in the cytology laboratory by using a fluid concentration technique. Cytocentrifugation is preferred because air-dried, DQ-stained smears can also be prepared. Cytologic examination of the fluid generally reveals proteinaceous material with scattered histiocytes and a few groups of benign epithelial cells from the cyst's lining. The histiocytic-appearing cells can be either macrophages or degenerating epithelial cells. The FNA cytology of a benign, ciliated hepatic foregut enteric cyst has been reported.[33] Diagnostic cytologic features included the presence of columnar-shaped cells with terminal bars and cilia similar to cells of a bronchogenic cyst.

Hydatid disease is caused by the tapeworm *Echinococcus granulosus*.[24] Humans serve as inadvertent hosts in whom consumed infected ova develop into embryos in the small intestine and ultimately reach the liver through the bloodstream. The right lobe of the liver is usually involved by multilayered cysts having an inner germinal layer producing brood capsules. The FNA diagnosis can be made when scoleces possessing two rows of hooklets are recognized in the smear background that also contains fragments of laminated cyst membrane (Figure 20-11) from the wall that appears as thick eosinophilic refractile bands.[24] Patients usually come to clinical attention when presenting with right upper quadrant abdominal pain or findings suggestive of biliary tract obstruction, although infrequently, they may be completely asymptomatic. It is generally be-

lieved that FNA biopsy is contraindicated because of the potential risk of inducing an anaphylactic reaction resulting from intraabdominal spillage of cyst contents by the FNA procedure.[24] However, echinococcal cysts have been aspirated without any adverse effects.

 BILIARY CYSTADENOMA

Biliary cystadenomas are rare benign neoplasms that are solitary, well-delineated, multiloculated cystic masses occasionally with calcification.[34] The vast majority of patients are women with abdominal pain and/or mass. Infrequently, cystadenomocarcinomas occur, at times appearing to arise through progressive dysplasia in a preexisting cystadenoma.[34]

Histologically, the cystadenomas are generally lined by a single layer of cytologically bland mucin-producing epithelium. The latter is usually columnar in shape and has small, basally oriented nuclei and low N:C ratios.[34] In women, the stroma beneath the epithelium is rather cellular and composed of spindle-shaped cells, providing a resemblance to ovarian or embryonic biliary stroma. In men, such stroma does not exist; rather, hyalinized connective tissue is present. If stromal invasion by tumor cells is present, then a diagnosis of cystadenocarcinoma is rendered. Others make this interpretation histologically on the basis of architecturally complex and cytologically abnormal tumor cells.

Only rarely have aspiration biopsies been reported.[35,36] The smears were moderately cellular at best and did not contain obvious background mucin. The neoplastic cells were present in small, generally flat clusters and individually. They appear small with uniform dark, round nuclei concentrated in a basal location. Cytoplasmic mucin was evident. The authors could not identify with certainty the typical cellular stroma in this aspirate from an adult woman. No signs of malignancy were present. Sampling error, however, could clearly play a role in missing such cells in an FNA biopsy sample.[36] Pinto and Kaye described an aspirate that lacked tu-

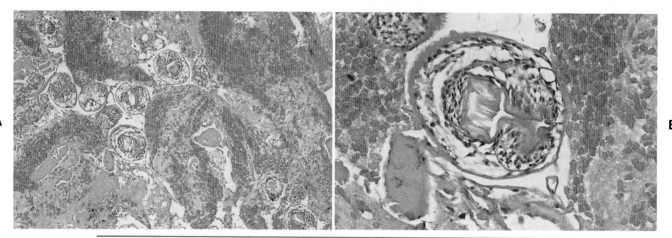

A   **B**

Figure 20-11 *Echinococcus granulosa.* A 15-year-old boy was injured during a soccer game, which led to the discovery of his asymptomatic cystic liver mass and prompted a fine-needle aspiration (FNA) biopsy. **A,** In the cell block, numerous *E. granulosus* are evident, without the presence of an associated inflammatory cell response. (H&E) **B,** At higher magnification, an inverted scolex, including hooklets, is evident (H&E). (Specimen courtesy of Dr. B. Naylor, Ann Arbor, Mich.)

mor cells but had an elevated level of carcinoembryonic antigen in the cyst fluid, distinguishing it from a simple cyst.[35]

 CIRRHOSIS

Cirrhosis is a chronic multietiologic disorder, resulting in a liver architecture that is distorted by variably sized nodules of regenerating hepatocytes surrounded by anastomosing bands of fibrous connective tissue. In the United States, chronic alcoholism is the most common etiologic factor of cirrhosis. Cirrhosis is a clinical condition that carries a relatively high mortality because of complications of portal hypertension and/or hepatic failure. Tissue core biopsy is the procedure of choice for evaluating patients with conventional cirrhosis because the architectural distortion of this entity is best recognized in the histologic specimen and is more apt to provide morphologic cues as to the underlying etiologic factors.

As hepatocellular carcinoma usually, but not always, arises in the background of cirrhosis, it is in this setting that cirrhotic patients are most often evaluated when they present with a dominant nodule.[37] Usually, the differential diagnosis is a dominant, regenerative cirrhotic nodule vs. primary hepatocellular neoplasm or less often, a metastatic malignancy.

When the dominant nodule in a cirrhotic liver assumes a relatively large size and an FNA biopsy is performed to exclude neoplasm, aspirates reveal cellularity that can vary from scant to high, which is usually a reflection of the amount of connective tissue present. A key cytologic feature for the diagnosis of cirrhotic nodule is the appreciation of the variable appearances of the liver cells in the smears.[1,7,24,32] Although the majority of the hepatocytes appear unremarkable, others usually manifest atypical features, including nuclear enlargement, binucleation, anisonucleosis, and occasionally, hyperchromasia (Figure 20-12). In fact, it is the polymorphic appearance of the hepatocytes within the same cell clusters that is characteristic of cirrhosis and an exceedingly helpful feature in distinguishing it from hepatocellular carcinoma, which is usually

characterized by a more uniform population of abnormal hepatocytes. Aspirates from patients with cirrhosis also demonstrate variable levels of cellular cohesion in the same specimen. Therefore, it is not unusual to see numerous individually dispersed, single, benign hepatocytes, along with small, flat groups of liver cells in rows or columns that are usually no greater than two cell layers thick.[1] The groups of hepatocytes have irregular to ragged external borders because of the lack of encircling sinusoidal cells (Figure 20-13). If a cell block is available and a reticulin stain is evaluated, the latter substance is usually not reduced in quantity. Other cytologic elements that may be appreciated in the smears include groups of bile duct cells, bile thrombi, fragments of fibrous connective tissue, and individually scattered necrotic cells. The bile duct cells are arranged in flat or three-dimensional groups. Occasionally, chronic inflammatory cells may be numerous. Aspirates of regenerative nodules of cirrhosis can occasionally contain cytologically atypical (dysplastic)

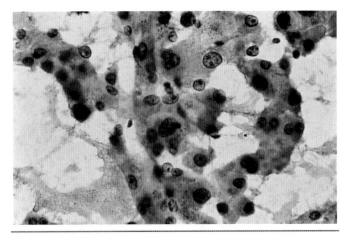

Figure 20-12 **Cirrhosis.** In this Pap-stained smear, considerable variation in nuclear size and shape of the hepatocytes with the presence of small but prominent nucleoli. (From Silverman JF, Geisinger KR. Fine needle aspiration cytology of the thorax and abdomen. New York: Churchill Livingstone; 1996. p.97.)

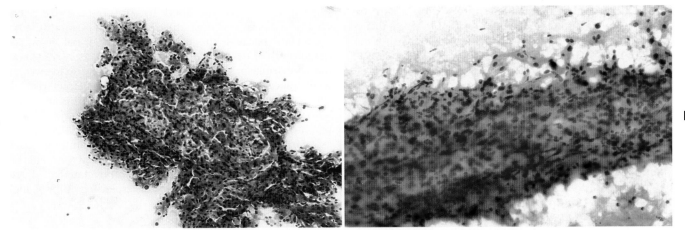

Figure 20-13 **Cirrhosis.** In aspirates of cirrhosis, the microtissue fragments have irregular borders. (**A,** DQ; **B,** Pap)

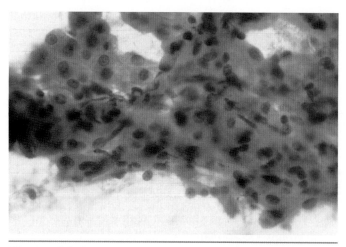

Figure 20-14   **Dysplastic liver cells.** In this aspirate of a cirrhotic nodule, considerable variation in the nuclear size of the dysplastic liver cells. A benign diagnosis is supported by the admixture of bland-appearing hepatocytes and the lack of nuclear irregularity. (DQ) (From Silverman JF, Geisinger KR. Fine needle aspiration cytology of the thorax and abdomen. New York: Churchill Livingstone; 1996. p.92.)

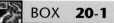

BOX 20-1   CMF
Cytomorphologic Features of Cirrhosis

Variable cellularity and cohesion is present
Hepatocytes are arranged in thin trabeculae and cords (one to two cells thick)
Hepatocytes (polymorphism) have a variable appearance.
Low N:C ratios are found
Clusters of bile duct cells are present
Chronic inflammatory cells are in variable numbers
Occasional fragment of fibrous connective tissue can be found
Scattered dysplastic (atypical) cells may be present

N:C, Nuclear to cytoplasmic.

hepatocytes, which, on an individual cell basis, may be indistinguishable from malignant cells (Figure 20-14).[1,38-40] However, these cells will be relatively infrequent and admixed with the numerous benign-appearing hepatocytes with low N:C ratios. Again, the variability in the appearance of hepatocytes is a feature in favor of cirrhosis rather than hepatocellular carcinoma (Box 20-1).

HEPATOCELLULAR CARCINOMA (HEPATOMA)

Hepatocellular carcinoma, one of the most common cancers worldwide, is the most common primary hepatic malignancy.[41,42] Hepatocellular carcinoma is especially common in China, Southeast Asia, and the sub-Saharan portion of Africa. In contrast, in the United States, less than 3000 new cases are diagnosed annually, with 90% of the patients having an underlying cirrhosis resulting from either alcoholism or hepatitis B or C infection. However, more recently in this country, many centers are witnessing an increasing number of hepatocellular carcinomas resulting from a variety of different factors such as the increasing incidence of hepatitis C infection and global travel.[43] Hepatocellular carcinoma may also develop from a number of proposed chemical carcinogens, mycotoxins, Thorotrast, α-1-antitrypsin deficiency, hemochromatosis, and long-term anabolic steroid use.

In the United States, hepatocellular carcinoma is generally a malignancy of older men who usually have nonspecific complaints of abdominal pain, right upper quadrant abdominal mass, and weight loss. Although a variety of radiologic presentations is possible, the most common is as a single large space occupying mass in the liver. Occasionally, the radiologic scans present as multiple nodules simulating a metastatic cancer or as a diffuse process. Most patients also have an elevated serum α-fetoprotein (AFP) level. In

the United States, the majority of patients survive less than 6 months.[44,45] Most patients who survive have a small single lesion that can be completely excised, allowing an adequate margin of resection. Unfortunately, most patients present with advanced large tumors that are not amenable to surgical resection. In this setting, FNA biopsy becomes an important procedure for definitive diagnosis because surgery with concomitant intraoperative surgical biopsy is not the best therapeutic and/or diagnostic option. Aspiration biopsy may also be well used to provide a rapid confirmation of tumor just before radioablation.[46]

FNA biopsy has high levels of diagnostic sensitivity and specificity for hepatocellular carcinoma.[31,32,47-49] The cytologic features of hepatocellular carcinoma have been well characterized.* Moderately-differentiated hepatocellular carcinomas are most easily diagnosed because the tumor cells demonstrate both malignant features and hepatocytic differentiation. The more challenging cases occur at both ends of the spectrum. Well-differentiated hepatocellular carcinomas have overlapping cytologic features with both benign hepatocytes and hepatocytic neoplasms, and poorly differentiated hepatocellular carcinomas are occasionally indistinguishable from high-grade metastatic carcinomas.[1]

Aspirates of well-differentiated hepatocellular carcinomas generally demonstrate a cellular specimen with cell clusters having a cohesive trabecular pattern. The thick plates of abnormal liver cells are lined by sinusoidal cells (Figure 20-15).[1] The hepatocytic nature of the cells is not difficult to appreciate because the cells resemble normal liver cells based on their cuboidal and polygonal shapes, opaque granulated cytoplasm, distinct cell borders, and one to two centrally placed nuclei. The neoplastic cells characteristically show a uniform atypia with increased N:C ratios and nuclei with slightly irregular, thickened membranes and mild hyperchromasia (Figure 20-16). In well-differentiated hepatocellular carcinoma, the cells also possess prominent nucleoli, which can be multiple and occasionally irregular in shape. Pseudoinclusions may also be appreciated, and cytoplasmic inclusions from lipid vacuoles, eosinophilic Mallory

---

*References 4, 5, 13, 17, 20, 31, 32, 38, 47, 49-56.

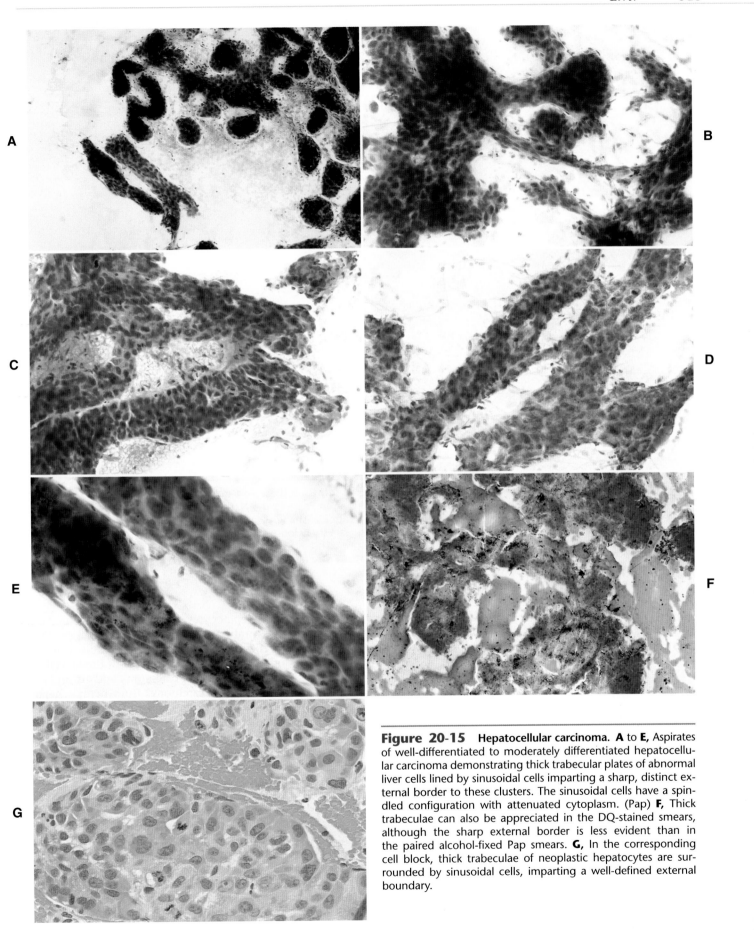

Figure 20-15 **Hepatocellular carcinoma. A** to **E,** Aspirates of well-differentiated to moderately differentiated hepatocellular carcinoma demonstrating thick trabecular plates of abnormal liver cells lined by sinusoidal cells imparting a sharp, distinct external border to these clusters. The sinusoidal cells have a spindled configuration with attenuated cytoplasm. (Pap) **F,** Thick trabeculae can also be appreciated in the DQ-stained smears, although the sharp external border is less evident than in the paired alcohol-fixed Pap smears. **G,** In the corresponding cell block, thick trabeculae of neoplastic hepatocytes are surrounded by sinusoidal cells, imparting a well-defined external boundary.

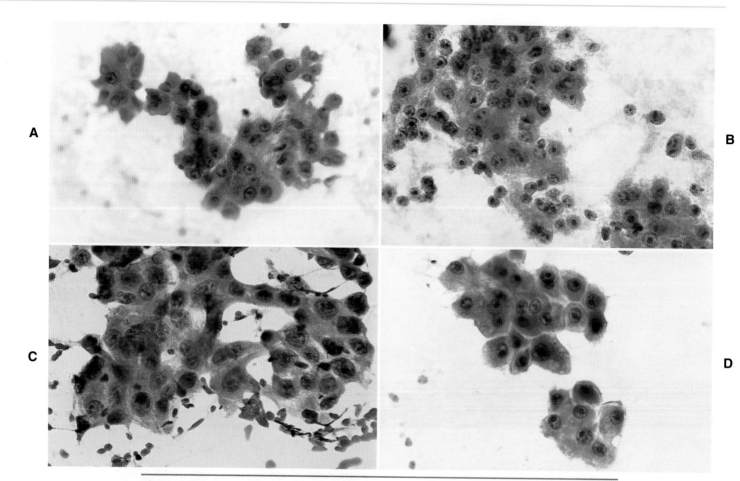

Figure 20-16   Hepatocellular carcinoma. **A** and **B,** In these Pap-stained aspirates, the neoplastic cells demonstrate uniform atypia, plus an increase in the N:C ratios. The hepatocellular nature of the cells is reflected by their cuboidal-shape, centrally placed nuclei, and granular cytoplasm. **C** and **D,** The Pap-stained smears show loose clusters of neoplastic cells in an aspirate of hepatocellular carcinoma. The tumor cells have centrally placed nuclei with surrounding granular to slightly vacuolated cytoplasm. Prominent nucleoli are also noted in many of the cells.

bodies, and basophilic globules can be present (Figure 20-17). Although bile is the most specific feature for the recognition of hepatocytic differentiation, unfortunately, it is often not evident. When bile is present, it can be appreciated as cytoplasmic granules, extracellular bile thrombi between hepatocytes or within the lumen of pseudoacini, or it can be present as extracellular pigmented material in the background (Figure 20-18 and Box 20-2).

The differential diagnosis of well-differentiated hepatocellular carcinoma includes cirrhosis and hepatocellular adenoma. In contrast with hepatocellular carcinoma, FNA biopsy of a dominant cirrhotic nodule usually shows relatively scanty cellularity resulting in part from the fibrous connective tissue present, although occasional cases can be surprisingly cellular. True trabeculae of hepatocytes are not present. The aspiration of a cirrhotic nodule demonstrates a polymorphic hepatocytic population with variable N:Cs, whereas aspirates of a hepatic adenoma consist of hepatocytes that are indistinguishable from normal surrounding benign liver tissue.

The authors believe that the most helpful diagnostic features for the recognition of hepatocellular carcinoma are

the presence of hepatocytes having uniformly increased N:C ratios, thick trabeculae, and the endothelial cells rimming the trabeculae (Figure 20-19).[1] In addition to the peripheral endothelial cells, transgressing endothelial cells are also a feature of hepatocellular carcinoma and are an aid in separating hepatocellular carcinoma from benign hepatic processes and, to a lesser extent, cholangiocarcinoma and metastatic malignancies (Figure 20-20).[55] The presence of vimentin-positive, spider-shaped Kupffer cells has been touted as a helpful cytologic finding for the diagnosis of hepatocellular carcinoma.[57] In these authors' experience, endothelium rimming of the thick trabeculae is better appreciated in the alcohol-fixed Pap preparation than the air-dried DQ preparation and is best seen in cell blocks or tissue core biopsies (Figures 20-21 and 20-22). The endothelial rimming also imparts a sharp, external border to the trabeculae, in contrast with the irregular ill-defined borders of benign liver tissue. Endothelial rimming can be confirmed by immunostaining with CD34.[56,58] The trabeculae are often arranged in a complex branching or anastomosing pattern.[1] As the histologic grade of the hepatocellular carcinoma increases, a progressive loss of cellular cohesion occurs with a

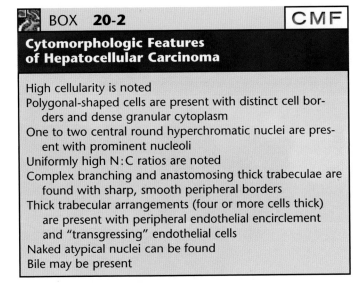

Figure 20-17 **Hepatocellular carcinoma. A,** Intranuclear inclusions are readily identified in this aspirate of hepatocellular carcinoma. (Pap) **B** to **D,** In this aspirate, many of the neoplastic hepatocytes possess intracytoplasmic globular inclusions. (DQ)

BOX 20-2   **CMF**

Cytomorphologic Features of Hepatocellular Carcinoma

High cellularity is noted

Polygonal-shaped cells are present with distinct cell borders and dense granular cytoplasm

One to two central round hyperchromatic nuclei are present with prominent nucleoli

Uniformly high N:C ratios are noted

Complex branching and anastomosing thick trabeculae are found with sharp, smooth peripheral borders

Thick trabecular arrangements (four or more cells thick) are present with peripheral endothelial encirclement and "transgressing" endothelial cells

Naked atypical nuclei can be found

Bile may be present

---

shift to greater numbers of individually dispersed malignant cells throughout the smears. In addition, the smears may contain numerous stripped (naked) malignant hepatocytic nuclei, another useful diagnostic feature for hepatocellular carcinoma.[1,16,20,50,54] Benign hepatocytes can also be present in the aspirated smears of hepatocellular carcinoma, but this results from sampling of the surrounding benign hepatic parenchyma.[1] However, the benign hepatocytes are usually not associated intimately with malignant cells but are instead present in different areas of the smears—a helpful but subtle feature to suggest the correct diagnosis.[13,17]

Although the formation of trabeculae is the most common pattern found in smears of hepatocellular carcinoma, an occasional aspirate may demonstrate prominent pseudoacinar formation by the liver cells, creating a luminal space that potentially mimics gland formation in an adenocarcinoma. A helpful cytologic feature for recognizing the hepatocellular nature of the cells is the presence of bile within the lumens of the pseudoacini, as well as the constituent cells retaining hepatocytic features such as eosinophilic granular cytoplasm with centrally placed nuclei (Figure 20-23). True glandular cells, in contrast, generally are cuboidal to columnar in appearance with pale amphophilic cytoplasm and basally oriented nuclei. However, occasional aspirates of hepatocellular carcinoma may contain a few liver cells having more peripherally located nuclei with and without vacuoles that could potentially simulate glandular cells.[13] The endothelial lining of these pseudoacini is another helpful cytologic finding to suggest the hepatocellular origin of these structures.

Due to the many overlapping cytologic features between benign and malignant hepatocytes, no single cytologic feature is diagnostic for hepatocellular carcinoma.* In an attempt to differentiate better benign from malignant hepatocytes, a number of investigators have systematically analyzed cytologic features to identify the key criteria for diagnosis. Using regression analysis, Cohen and colleagues found three statistically significant cytologic features useful for the diagnosis of hepatocellular carcinoma, including uniformly high N:C ratios, a trabecular pattern, and scattered, stripped (naked), atypical hepatocellular nuclei.[50] The authors concur that all of these features are helpful, although the presence of high N:C ratios is the pivotal cytologic feature because trabecular patterns and atypical stripped nuclei can occasionally be seen in a variety of other benign and malignant tumors (Figure 20-24). Of the latter, one example is well-differentiated neuroendocrine carcinomas. A trabeculae-like pattern can occasionally be present in aspirates of benign hepatocytic lesions but usually tends to be focal and consists of only one- to two-cell–thick cords of hepatocytic cells, rather than the wider trabeculae of hepatocellular carcinoma. Cohen and colleagues also identified several secondary cytologic features

---

*References 1, 5, 18, 19, 22, 50, 52.

for hepatocellular carcinoma including an irregular distribution of chromatin, uniformly prominent nucleoli, and multiple nucleoli.[50] These cytologic features, however, did not achieve statistical significance. Noncontributory cytologic features include hypercellular smears, cellular pleomorphism, hyperchromatic nuclei, and cells arranged in acinar grouping. Several other investigators have confirmed that uniformly high N:C ratios is an important diagnostic feature, but trabecular arrangement and/or naked hepatocytic nuclei were not statistically significant parameters.[18,23] Pittman and Szyfelbein reported that the presence of peripherally arranged endothelium around the trabeculae and transgressing (transversing) endothelium into the sheets of hepatocytes were highly sensitive and specific features of hepatocellular carcinoma that were not present in either cholangiocarcinoma or metastatic tumors.[55]

Ancillary studies for cytoplasmic antigens are generally not helpful for distinguishing benign from malignant hepatocytes. Most hepatocellular carcinomas show positive staining of the liver cells for low molecular weight cytokeratin and negative staining for high molecular weight cytokeratin. The differential cytokeratins, CK7 and CK20, are generally negative. In the differential diagnosis of hepatocellular adenoma versus hepatocellular carcinoma, im-

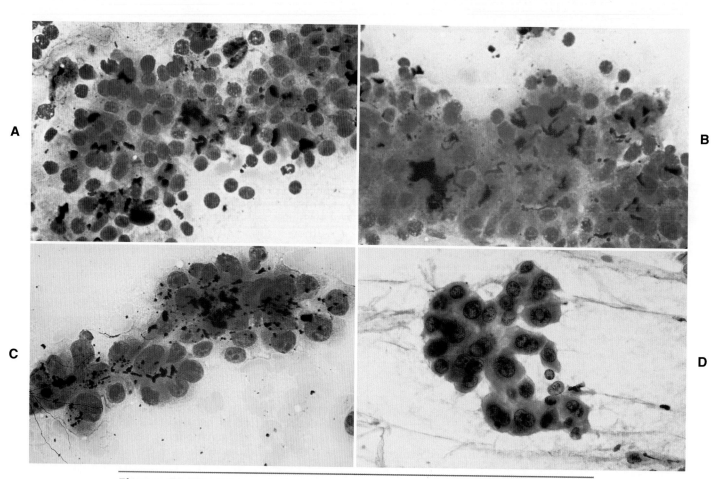

Figure 20-18 **Hepatocellular carcinoma. A, B,** and **C,** In these DQ-stained smears, blackish-green cytoplasmic staining and bile thrombi are noted. Note that the bile tends to be present in the canalicular spaces. **D,** In this Pap-stained smear, a small bile plug with a greenish hue is in the canalicular spaces between neoplastic liver cells.

munohistochemical expression of the endothelial cells for CD34 has been suggested as a useful feature pointing to carcinoma.[58] This marker is occasionally helpful, especially when applied to cell block material. However, CD34 is not specific because it also decorates occasional sinusoidal cells present in adenomas and benign hepatic parenchyma.

The use of a reticulin stain is also quite useful in distinguishing benign from malignant hepatic parenchyma. In cell blocks, most benign samples demonstrate a normal outlining of cords by reticulin.[57,59] This staining is greatly reduced in hepatocellular carcinomas. However, this is not totally specific because a reduction of reticulin is associated with infrequent examples of fatty liver and cirrhosis.

The other major differential diagnostic challenge is separating poorly differentiated hepatocellular carcinoma from metastases to the liver. Bottles and colleagues, using logistic regression analysis, found three statistically significant cytologic features for the diagnosis of hepatocellular carcinoma, including the presence of polygonal-shaped tumor cells with centrally placed nuclei, groups of neoplastic cells separated by sinusoidal capillaries, and bile pigment.[54] As noted above, the latter feature, although specific for the diagnosis of hepatocellular carcinoma, lacks sensitivity. Secondary cytologic features in their series included the presence of nuclear pseudoinclusions and endothelial cells rimming clusters of neoplastic cells.[54] Attributes considered not helpful in the separation of hepatocellular carcinoma from metastatic malignancy were the presence of granular cytoplasm, cytoplasmic vacuoles and inclusions, prominent nucleoli, and multinucleated tumor giant cells. One problem with this study was that it included melanomas, sarcomas, and lymphomas in the metastatic group. Such neoplasms are less likely to be confused with hepatocellular carcinoma than is metastatic non–small cell carcinoma.

Very recently, Salamâo and colleagues have conducted a similar study but limited the metastatic group to adenocarcinomas.[20] Five pathologists independently examined a series of 52 hepatocellular carcinomas and 56 metastatic carcinomas for 11 cytomorphologic criteria. Using multivariate regression analysis, the presence of polygonal tumor cells with central nuclei and malignant cells separated by sinusoidal capillaries accurately distinguished hepatocellular carcinoma from metastatic adenocarcinoma. True lumen formation by neoplastic cells suggested adenocarcinoma.

Poorly differentiated hepatocellular carcinomas can be subclassified into pleomorphic large cell type and small cell types.[1,38] In aspirates of the large cell pleomorphic type, some of the smaller malignant cells are usually readily rec-

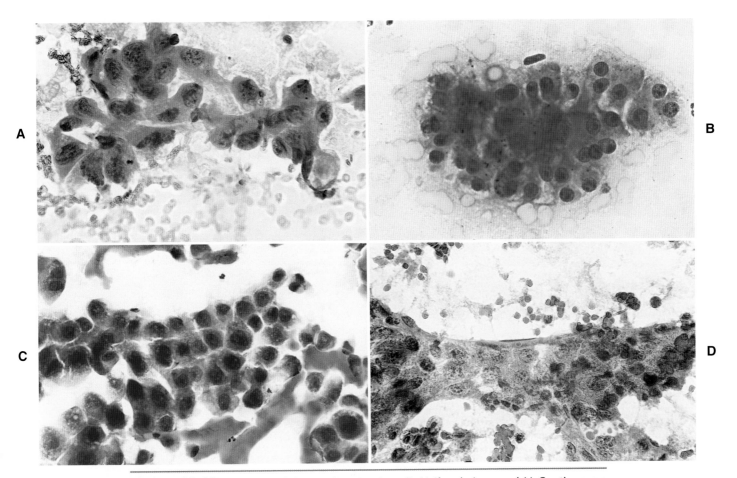

Figure 20-19 Hepatocellular carcinoma. **A** to **C,** Uniformly increased N:C ratios are a feature of hepatocellular carcinoma. (**A,** Pap; **B** and **C,** DQ) **D,** Endothelial rimming imparting a sharp border to the thick trabeculae is a feature of hepatocellular carcinoma. Also note the uniformly high N:C ratios of these atypical hepatocytes. (Pap)

ognized as hepatocytic in origin (Figure 20-25). These cells are admixed with larger tumor giant cells.[51,54] Therefore, the diagnosis of the pleomorphic type of poorly differentiated hepatocellular carcinoma is predicated on the appreciation that the smaller atypical cells are malignant rather than reactive hepatocytes. In the small cell type of hepatocellular carcinoma, numerous individually scattered, uniform-appearing malignant cells having single nuclei with high N:C ratios are seen (Figures 20-26 and 20-27).[1] The eccentrically placed nuclei with surrounding scant cyanophilic cytoplasm can simulate a metastatic small cell malignancy. Cytomorphologic features helpful for the diagnosis of hepatocellular carcinoma include the recognition of cells with smooth, round nuclei and nucleoli and surrounding granu-

lar, dense cytoplasm. The search for other larger malignant cells showing more obvious evidence of hepatocytic differentiation (usually more cytoplasm) is also helpful for the correct diagnosis of this hepatocellular carcinoma variant.

As mentioned previously, cell blocks and tissue core biopsies can be invaluable in the evaluation of hepatocellular carcinoma. Several studies have demonstrated that cell blocks and direct cytologic smears are complimentary for the diagnosis of hepatocellular carcinoma.* In histologic preparations, broad trabeculae greater than three cells thick and surrounded by an endothelial layer are more easily rec-

---

*References 10, 13, 15, 31, 47, 60-62.

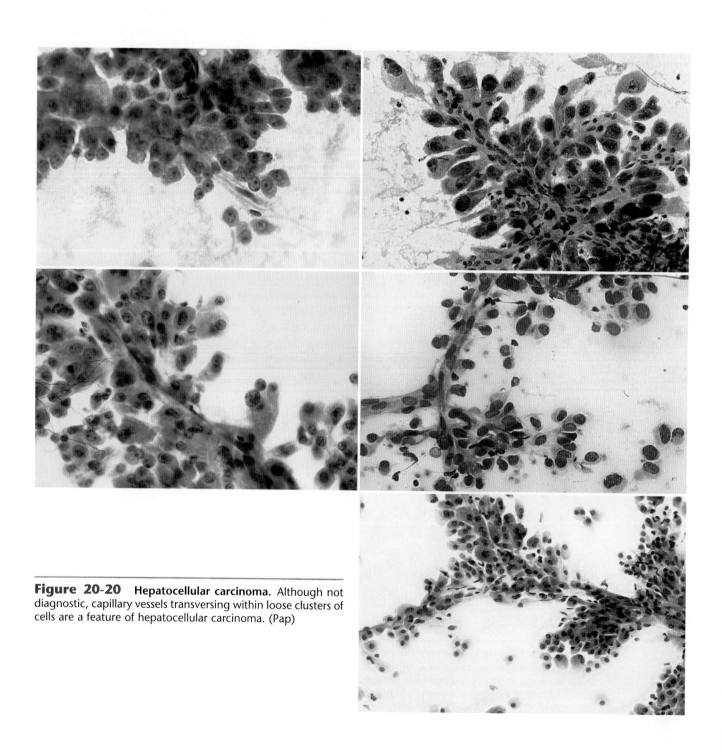

Figure 20-20   **Hepatocellular carcinoma.** Although not diagnostic, capillary vessels transversing within loose clusters of cells are a feature of hepatocellular carcinoma. (Pap)

ognized (Figure 20-28). In contrast, smear preparations may overestimate the width of the trabeculae because of thick smears. Zainol and Sumithran diagnosed 80% of the hepatocellular carcinomas based on the cytologic smears, with the cell blocks contributing to the diagnosis in the remaining cases.[47] Another advantage of using cell block or bioptic tissue core biopsies is the performance of a panel of ancillary immunohistochemical studies that serve as an aid for distinguishing hepatocellular adenomas, primary hepatocellular carcinomas, cholangiocarcinomas, and metastatic carcinomas.[1,5,55,60-65] A number of antibodies have been used to separate hepatocellular carcinoma from metastatic adenocarcinoma. One immunohistochemical marker with great use is polyclonal carcinoembryonic antigen (CEA).[63-66] In contrast to metastatic adenocarcinomas, which usually show diffuse cytoplasmic and membranous staining for polyclonal CEA, hepatocellular carcinoma demonstrates a characteristic canalicular staining pattern (Figure 20-29). This staining pattern is not seen with monoclonal CEA. Although adenocarcinomas can stain with both low and/or high molecular weight cytokeratin (e.g., CAM 5.2 and AE1 and AE3), the cells from hepatocellular carcinoma generally react only with the low molecular weight cytokeratin (i.e., CAM 5.2). In addition, the high and low molecular weight cytokeratin cocktail (AE1/3) decorates benign and malignant bile duct epithelium but not benign or malignant he-

patocytes. The differential cytokeratins CK7 and CK20 do not usually react with either benign or malignant hepatocytes, whereas a variety of metastatic lesions often stain for one or both of these markers, depending on the cell lineage and site of cancer. Although epithelial membrane antigen

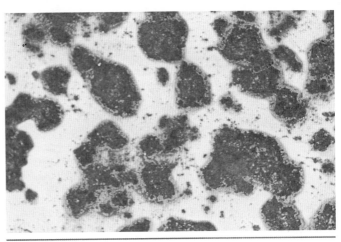

Figure 20-21 **Hepatocellular carcinoma.** In this hypercellular aspirate, the thick trabeculae demonstrate peripheral endothelial rimming, but this feature in general is better appreciated in Pap-stained smears. (DQ)

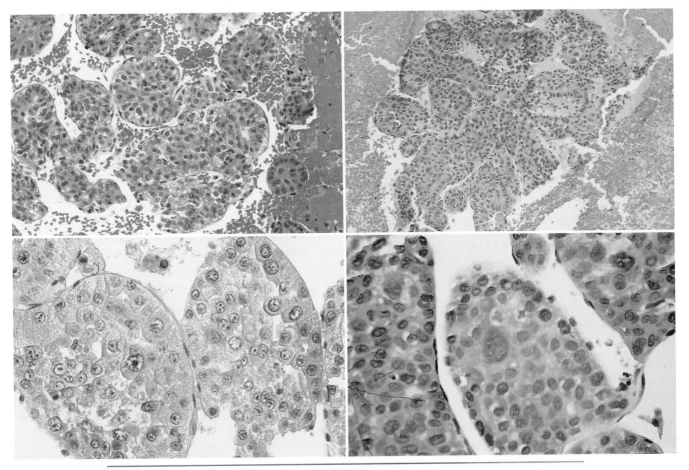

Figure 20-22 **Hepatocellular carcinoma.** Cell blocks from aspirates of hepatocellular carcinoma readily demonstrate the peripheral endothelial rimming of neoplastic trabeculae in hepatocellular carcinoma. The trabeculae are broad and consist of uniformly atypical cells in which variation occurs in nuclear size and shape. (H&E)

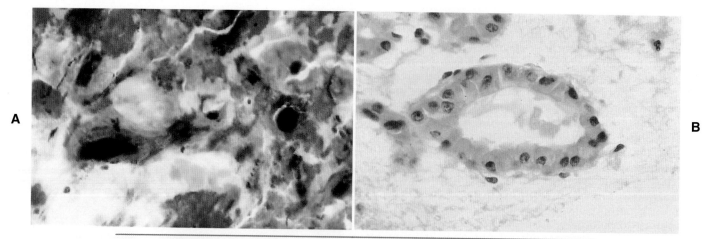

Figure 20-23 **Hepatocellular carcinoma. A,** In this aspirate, blackish-green bile plugs are present in canalicular spaces, creating a pseudoacinar pattern in this DQ-stained smear. **B,** In this cell block of hepatocellular carcinoma, the neoplastic cells are arranged in a pseudoacinar pattern with yellowish-green bile in the lumen. Although pseudoacini can simulate neoplastic glands, the presence of centrally positioned nuclei and the peripheral endothelial lining are features in keeping with hepatocytic origin. (H&E) (From Silverman JF, Geisinger KR. Fine needle aspiration cytology of the thorax and abdomen. New York: Churchill Livingstone; 1996. p.101.)

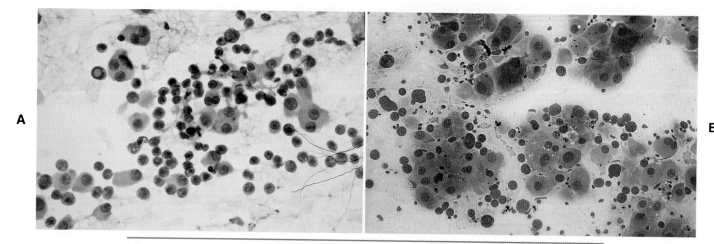

Figure 20-24 **Hepatocellular carcinoma. A,** The presence of numerous stripped hepatocytic nuclei is a feature in some aspirates of hepatocellular carcinoma. (Pap) **B,** In this DQ-stained smear of hepatocellular carcinoma, scattered, stripped nuclei are present, in addition to the numerous intact neoplastic liver cells.

(EMA) immunohistochemical staining is generally negative, occasional cases of hepatocellular carcinoma show positive staining for this marker. Serum levels for AFP are often elevated in hepatocellular carcinoma, but in the authors' experience, immunohistochemical expression for this antigen often is not seen. The literature, however, reports AFP positivity in hepatocellular carcinoma in the range of approximately 45% to 58% of the cases.[4,52,66] This marker, however, is not specific because germ cell tumors can also be AFP positive. Hepatocyte Paraffin-1 (Hep Par-1) is another new, relatively sensitive and specific marker for hepatocellular carcinoma.[67,68] Immunohistochemical studies for the surface antigen of hepatitis B virus is also highly specific, but insensitive.[66]

Electron microscopy (EM) can also be employed when a poorly differentiated liver malignancy is encountered.[14,48,69,70] Ultrastructural examination of hepatocellular carcinoma reveals cells having an organelle-rich cytoplasm with characteristic small intracellular lumens lined by blunt villi corresponding to the bile canaliculi.[69,70] Intracytoplasmic smooth and rough endoplasmic reticulum, glycogen, lipid, and bile are also demonstrated. Ultrastructural examination of metastatic adenocarcinomas and cholangiocarcinomas reveals intracytoplasmic or large intercellular lumens lined by microvilli with well-defined internal structures. Site-specific features may also be present such as mucous vacuoles, neurosecretory granules, well-developed bundles of intermediate filaments, and/or melanosomes.

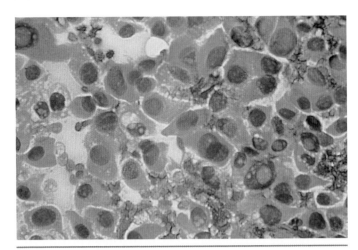

Figure 20-25 Hepatocellular carcinoma. In this aspirate, reduction in cohesion occurred, with numerous individually scattered, large pleomorphic neoplastic hepatocytes, including some with prominent intranuclear inclusions. (Pap)

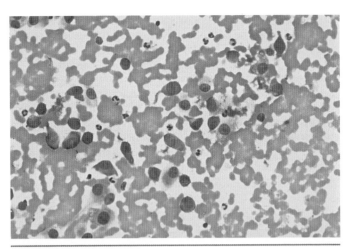

Figure 20-27 Hepatocellular carcinoma, small cell variant. A prominent loss of intercellular cohesion manifests as numerous individually scattered cells with high N:C ratios with a slight amount of cytoplasm. (DQ)

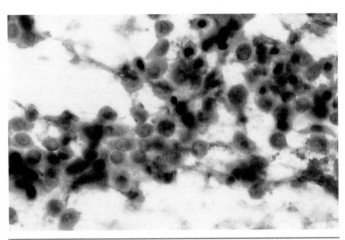

Figure 20-26 Hepatocellular carcinoma, small cell variant. In this aspirate of a small cell variant of hepatocellular carcinoma, loosely clustered and individually scattered, small malignant hepatocytes are seen that potentially could be confused with cells from a metastatic small cell carcinoma. However, the cells lack the nuclear molding of a metastatic small cell carcinoma. In addition, a greater amount of cytoplasm is present, and the presence of a few small but discernible nucleoli should discourage a diagnosis of a metastatic small cell carcinoma. (Pap) (From Silverman JF, Geisinger KR. Fine needle aspiration cytology of the thorax and abdomen. New York: Churchill Livingstone; 1996. p.107.)

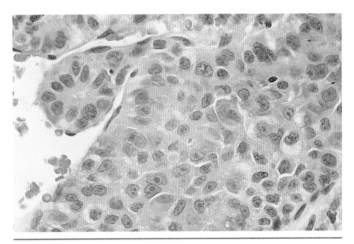

Figure 20-28 Hepatocellular carcinoma. In this cell block from an aspirate of hepatocellular carcinoma, thick trabeculae consisting of abnormal hepatocytes are present along with evidence of endothelial rimming. (H&E)

 ## OTHER MORPHOLOGIC VARIANTS OF HEPATOCELLULAR CARCINOMA

Fibrolamellar Hepatocellular Carcinoma and Small Cell, Clear Cell, and Mixed Carcinoma Types

Other recognized but uncommon morphologic variants of hepatocellular carcinoma exist. Fibrolamellar hepatocellular carcinoma, which is seen more often in younger adults with nearly equal male-to-female ratios, is usually not associated with an underlying cirrhosis.[71] Fibrolamellar hepatocellular carcinoma may have a better prognosis than

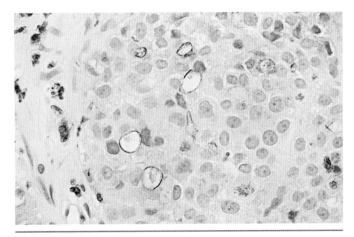

Figure 20-29 Hepatocellular carcinoma, polyclonal carcinoma embryonic antigen (CEA). This immunohistochemical stain for polyclonal CEA reveals the characteristic canalicular staining pattern of hepatocellular carcinoma in this cell block from an aspirate of hepatocellular carcinoma. In contrast, metastatic adenocarcinoma demonstrates diffuse cytoplasmic staining of the neoplastic cells.

conventional hepatocellular carcinoma, especially if the malignancy can be completely resected. Furthermore, these patients generally fare better after a liver transplant than do patients with conventional hepatocellular carcinomas.[72,73] Histologically, fibrolamellar hepatocellular carcinoma is characterized by a population of large neoplastic hepatocytes possessing abundant granular eosinophilic cytoplasm and huge nuclei with prominent nucleoli. Intracytoplasmic pale and/or hyaline globules may be present. Ultrastructurally, numerous mitochondria are present, imparting an oncocytic, granular quality to the cytoplasm. The lamellar component of the malignancy results from stacked bundles of collagen fibers.

In the aspiration smears the diagnosis is made when very large atypical hepatocytes with abundant granular cytoplasm, one or more round uniform large nuclei with prominent nucleoli, and fragments of fibrous connective tissue are present (Figures 20-30 to 20-32).[1,71,74-77] Aspirates of fibrolamellar carcinoma also demonstrate considerable cellular discohesion, in contrast with the generally well-formed trabeculae seen in aspirates of conventional hepatocellular carcinoma. This finding and the presence of neoplastic cells having surprisingly low N:C ratios because of the abundant cytoplasm can serve as potential pitfalls for a false-negative diagnosis of benign reactive hepatocytes. It is only when one appreciates that the tumor cells with low N:C ratios are considerably larger than benign hepatocytes that the correct diagnosis is made (see Figure 20-32).[71,74-77] Bile pigment may not be a feature in the smears, but intracytoplasmic and stripped extracellular pale bodies may be noted (Box 20-3).

Clear cell hepatocellular carcinoma is a histologic subtype that can be potentially confused with a variety of metastatic clear-cell malignancies to the liver such as those arising in the kidney, ovary, and adrenal gland.[78] This variant of hepatocellular carcinoma clinically behaves in a similar fashion to conventional hepatocellular carcinoma. The aspirates contain atypical cells with abundant, diffusely homogeneous and/or vacuolated optically clear cytoplasm

---

BOX 20-3   CMF

Cytomorphologic Features of Fibrolamellar Carcinoma

Moderate cellularity is found
Very large polygonal cells have abundant granular cytoplasm
Low N:C ratios are noted
Pale cytoplasmic inclusions may be present
One to two central round nuclei are found
Variable cohesion occurs, and individual single cells may predominant
Fragments of layered-appearing collagen are present

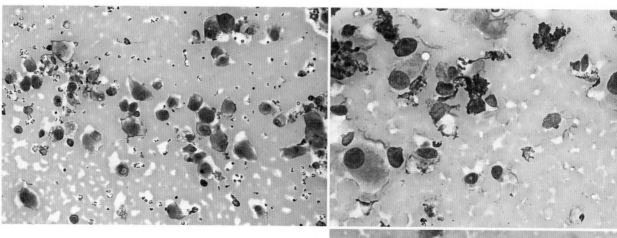

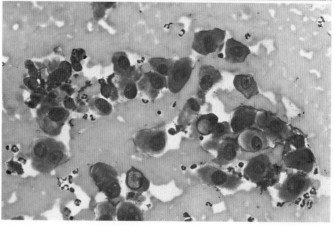

Figure 20-30 **Fibrolamellar carcinoma.** In these DQ-stained smears from a fibrolamellar carcinoma, considerable cellular discohesion is present. The large size of the neoplastic hepatocytes can be appreciated when compared with the background inflammatory and red blood cells.

with well-defined cell borders (Figure 20-33).[79-81] Intercellular cohesion of the cells may also be decreased. Similarly, the small cell variant of hepatocellular carcinoma consists of neoplastic hepatocytes having a relatively small size due to the scant amount of cytoplasm. Accordingly, the N:C ratio is markedly elevated. However, in contrast with metastatic small cell carcinoma, nucleoli are appreciated (Figure 20-34). In addition a helpful diagnostic feature for both these variants is the appreciation of more conventionally appearing cells of hepatocellular carcinoma in the smears (Figure 20-35). Ancillary studies such as EM demonstrate the ultrastructural features of hepatocellular differentiation,[81] and positive staining for α-1-antitrypsin has also been used as a diagnostic aid for making the correct diagnosis.[79] Recently, a clear cell variant of fibrolamellar carcinoma has been described.[82] Neoplastic cells were either oncocytic or had clear cytoplasm. By EM, the latter resulted from swollen, degenerated mitochondria.

Rarely, primary malignant hepatic neoplasms may show both hepatocellular and glandular differentia-

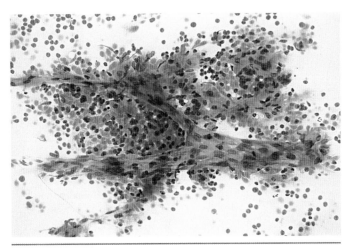

Figure 20-31 **Fibrolamellar carcinoma.** In addition to the neoplastic liver cells, stacked columns of fibroblastic cells corresponding to the so-called fibrolamellar component are present in this aspirate. (DQ)

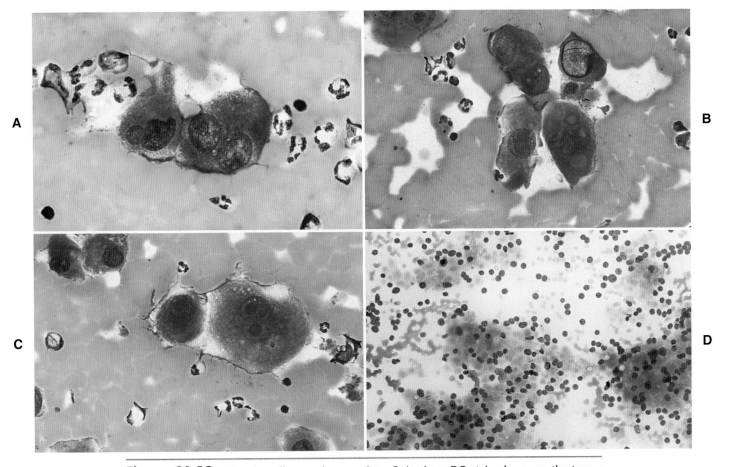

Figure 20-32 **Fibrolamellar carcinoma. A** to **C,** In these DQ-stained smears, the tumor cells of the fibrolamellar variant of hepatocellular carcinoma have a deceptively bland appearance resulting from their relatively low N:C ratios. However, the neoplastic nature of the cells is appreciated by the recognition of the significantly larger size of these atypical hepatocytes as compared with benign liver cells. **D,** In this DQ-stained smear, scattered pale bodies are noted within the intact hepatocytes and in the background. Also present are numerous stripped hepatocytic nuclei.

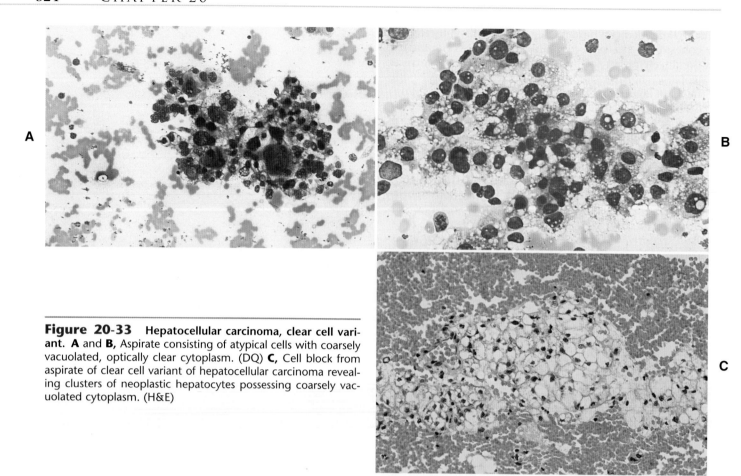

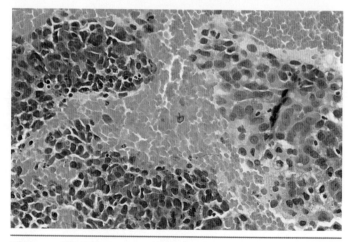

Figure 20-33   Hepatocellular carcinoma, clear cell variant. **A** and **B,** Aspirate consisting of atypical cells with coarsely vacuolated, optically clear cytoplasm. (DQ) **C,** Cell block from aspirate of clear cell variant of hepatocellular carcinoma revealing clusters of neoplastic hepatocytes possessing coarsely vacuolated cytoplasm. (H&E)

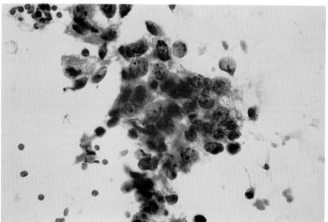

Figure 20-34   Hepatocellular carcinoma, small cell variant. Aspirate of small cell variant of hepatocellular carcinoma consisting of loose clusters of neoplastic small cells having very high N:C ratios. These small neoplastic cells could potentially be confused with a metastatic small cell carcinoma. A helpful diagnostic feature is the presence of cells with readily discernible nucleoli in the small cell variant of hepatocellular carcinoma. In contrast, nucleoli are not present in metastatic small cell carcinoma. (Pap)

Figure 20-35   Hepatocellular carcinoma, small cell variant. In this aspirate of small cell variant of hepatocellular carcinoma, two clusters of neoplastic small hepatocytes are seen with a cluster of more conventional-appearing hepatocellular carcinoma consisting of larger atypical cells with abundant granular cytoplasm. (Pap)

tion.[83,84] These primary combined carcinomas behave more like conventional hepatocellular carcinoma; therefore, it is important to recognize this variant and not confuse it with metastatic adenocarcinoma or cholangiocarcinoma. In the FNA smears, malignant cells showing both hepatocellular and glandular differentiation are present,

along with transitions between the two cell types (Figure 20-36).[85] The hepatocytic cells show eosinophilic granular cytoplasm with centrally placed nuclei and bile, whereas the glandular cells have eccentrically placed oval to irregular nuclei with vacuolated wispy cytoplasm that may be mucin positive. Immunohistochemical studies demon-

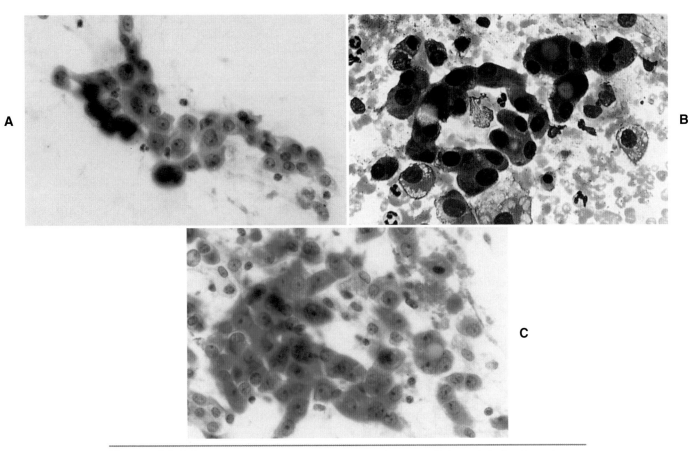

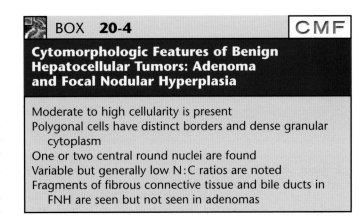

Figure 20-36   **Mixed carcinoma. A,** In this mixed hepatocellular and cholangiocarcinoma, the malignant cells in this field are consistent with malignant hepatocytes because of the polygonal contours; well-defined cellular borders; granular opaque cytoplasm; and round, centrally positioned nuclei. An endothelial coating is not evident. (Pap) **B,** In this field, some of the tumor cells have large cytoplasmic vacuoles that displace the nucleus to one pole of the cell. Other tumor cells have eccentrically placed nuclei without cytoplasmic vacuoles. These features represent glandular differentiation in a mixed carcinoma. These cytoplasmic vacuoles were positive for mucicarmine in the cell block of this specimen. (DQ) **C,** In this field, the juxtaposition and possible transition between hepatocytic and glandular cells are present. (Pap) (From Silverman JF, Geisinger KR. Fine needle aspiration cytology of the thorax and abdomen. New York: Churchill Livingstone; 1996. p.112.)

strate the specific features of both hepatocellular and glandular differentiation.[85]

 BENIGN HEPATOCELLULAR TUMORS

Although relatively uncommon, benign hepatocellular adenoma and focal nodular hyperplasia (FNH) should always be considered in the differential when a hepatic mass is aspirated.[40,86] The clinical history can be critical in making the correct diagnosis because adenomas are seen largely in adult females taking oral contraceptives. Although most patients are asymptomatic, occasionally, adenomas become clinically evident because of hemorrhage within the neoplasm. Rarely, hepatocellular adenomas have been reported in adult men using exogenous anabolic steroids and have also been described in children. Adenomas vary in size, generally occurring as a single mass lesion (Box 20-4).

FNH is also seen predominantly in adult women, although it occurs with relatively greater frequency in men and children. FNH is most often discovered as an inciden-

BOX   20-4   CMF

Cytomorphologic Features of Benign Hepatocellular Tumors: Adenoma and Focal Nodular Hyperplasia

Moderate to high cellularity is present
Polygonal cells have distinct borders and dense granular cytoplasm
One or two central round nuclei are found
Variable but generally low N:C ratios are noted
Fragments of fibrous connective tissue and bile ducts in FNH are seen but not seen in adenomas

FNH, Focal nodular hyperplasia.

tal finding and does not have the strong association with oral contraceptive use. Histologically, both adenomas and FNH consist of benign-appearing hepatocytes. However, FNH contains thick-walled blood vessels and bile ducts in a centrally located scar, whereas delicate thin-walled blood vessels are present between the thin trabeculae of adenomas. Adenomas also lack bile ducts and/or portal tracts. In the aspirated smears, a specific diagnosis of either FNH or adenoma cannot be made because both contain an identical cellular population of unremarkable-appearing hepatocytes (Figures 20-37 and 20-38).[87] Most of the liver cells have centrally placed round nuclei with even, nuclear contours, finely granular chromatin, and small nucleoli with surrounding granular cytoplasm that may contain lipid vacuoles, resulting in low N:C ratios. Only when adenoma or FNH are clinically or radiologically suspected and the needle placement is fairly certain can the case be considered *normal-appearing hepatocytes*, consistent with either FNH or adenoma. Obviously, the normal-appearing hepatocytes could also represent inadvertent sampling of benign hepatic tissue surrounding other types of hepatocellular lesions including primary or metastatic malignancies. Therefore, if no clinical support is evident for the diagnosis of FNH or adenoma and the placement of the needle is uncertain or unknown, the case is considered to be benign hepatocytes with an appropriate comment to detail the uncertainty of the diagnosis. It is apparent that in all of these types of cases, the need for clinical correlation is crucial and confirms the principal that radiologists and pathologists must work closely together. The authors recommend, if possible, that pathologists personally witness the placement of the computed tomography (CT) or ultrasound-guided needle biopsy. Finally, to challenge the cytopathologist even further, Tao has described the presence of dysplastic ap-

pearing hepatocytes in aspirates from a small series of adenomas.[88] The presence of dysplastic liver cells in this setting could potentially serve as a source for a misdiagnosis of either cirrhosis or a well-differentiated hepatocellular carcinoma. However, the lack of a uniform population of these atypical hepatocytes would again favor a benign diagnosis.

 METASTASIS

The liver is the second most common abdominal site for metastatic cancer after the lymph nodes. Metastatic carcinoma to the liver is far more common than primary hepatic malignancies, accounting for approximately 95% of all malignant hepatic neoplasms. Adenocarcinoma from a variety of sites, including the gastrointestinal tract, pancreas, breast, and lung, is the most common histologic type. Other common metastatic malignant tumors include small cell carcinoma of the lung, melanoma, and gastrointestinal and pancreatic neuroendocrine tumors. Metastatic squamous cell carcinomas are relatively uncommon in FNA biopsy of the liver; when they occur, they most often arise from the esophagus and lung. Adenocarcinoma of the colorectum is the most common malignancy to metastasize to the liver.[1] Metastatic tumors to the liver most often present with multiple nodules, although single metastatic deposits can also be found. With conventional cytology, most metastatic adenocarcinomas do not have specific features to suggest the

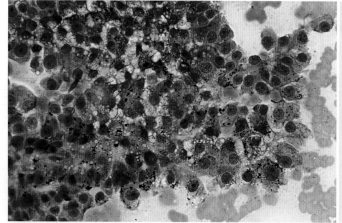

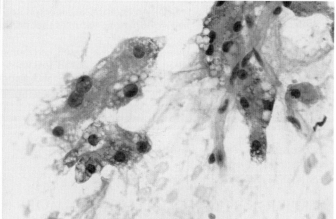

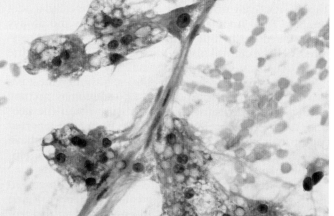

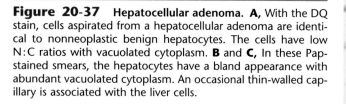

Figure 20-37 **Hepatocellular adenoma. A,** With the DQ stain, cells aspirated from a hepatocellular adenoma are identical to nonneoplastic benign hepatocytes. The cells have low N:C ratios with vacuolated cytoplasm. **B** and **C,** In these Pap-stained smears, the hepatocytes have a bland appearance with abundant vacuolated cytoplasm. An occasional thin-walled capillary is associated with the liver cells.

primary site. However, metastatic colorectal carcinoma often produces a characteristic cytologic pattern of cohesive groups of tumor cells demonstrating peripheral palisading of elongated cigar-shaped nuclei associated with dirty background necrosis (Figure 20-39). The latter results from the presence of intact and degenerating neutrophils, necrotic tumor cells, and granular necrotic debris. Mucin vacuoles may occasionally be seen in the malignant cells, as well as abundant extracellular mucin (Figure 20-40). When a signet ring adenocarcinoma pattern is recognized, a primary lesion in the stomach or breast (lobular type) should be suggested (Figure 20-41). Metastatic pleomorphic giant cell carcinomas can arise from a variety of different sites, including the lung, thyroid, and pancreas, although the latter is the most common primary origin of this type of malignancy to involve the liver. Whenever a pleomorphic giant cell or spindle cell neoplasm is encountered, the possibility of metastatic melanoma should always be considered. Spindle cell malignancies should also invoke the possibility of a metastatic sar-

coma, often of gastrointestinal origin. Metastatic small cell malignancies can be seen in both pediatric and adult populations. The differential diagnosis of small cell malignancies includes metastatic, well-differentiated neuroendocrine carcinomas, small cell carcinoma, small, round cell tumors of childhood, small cell variant of melanoma, and lymphoma (Figure 20-42 to 20-45).[89-92]

After the recognition that a potential metastatic malignancy of unknown primary site at the time of immediate interpretation may exist, a request for additional specimens such as a cell block or bioptic tissue core biopsy to facilitate ancillary studies is strongly recommended. These types of specimens better allow a panel of immunohistochemical stains to be performed, which is often exceedingly helpful in not only confirming the metastatic origin of the malignancy but also in identifying the specific cell lineage and possible primary site. An immunohistochemical panel for adenocarcinomas should include differential cytokeratins such as cytokeratins (CK) 7 and 20, epithelial membrane

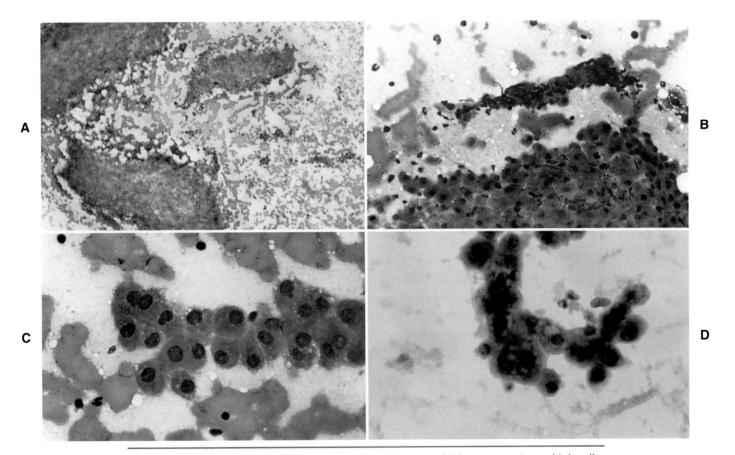

Figure 20-38   Focal nodular hyperplasia (FNH). **A,** In this low-power view, a high cellularity of the aspirate is present. Most of the hepatocytes are arranged in large cohesive aggregates, along with a few small clusters and individual hepatocytes. (DQ) **B,** A large sheet of benign-appearing hepatocytes is present, along with a fragment of collagenized stroma, which possibly represents sampling of a connective tissue septae separating nodules within the mass. However, bile duct structures are not present within this fragment. (DQ) **C** and **D,** The hepatocytes from FNH are indistinguishable from normal liver cells. The cells have polygonal contours; sharply defined cellular borders; granular dense cytoplasm; and central, round nuclei without discernible nucleoli. Lipid vacuoles are present in the cytoplasm of a few of the cells. Most importantly, the N:C ratios are uniformly low. (**C,** DQ; **D,** Pap) (From Silverman JF, Geisinger KR. Fine needle aspiration cytology of the thorax and abdomen. New York: Churchill Livingstone; 1996. p.114.)

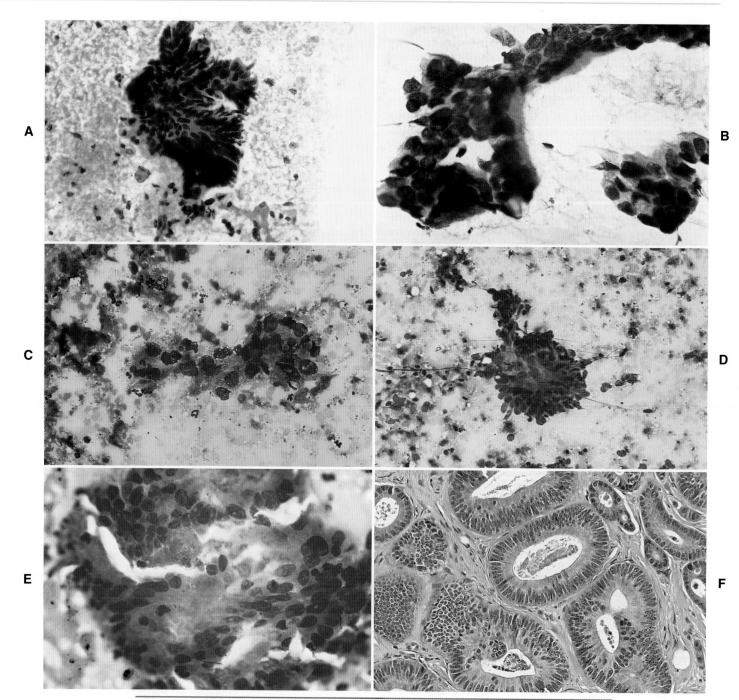

Figure 20-39 **Metastatic colon carcinoma. A** and **B,** In these Pap-stained smears, metastatic colon adenocarcinoma to the liver can be suspected because of the characteristic appearance of the neoplastic glands and presence of background dirty necrosis. The tumor cells have hyperchromatic, pseudostratified, oval to elongated nuclei, and high N:C ratios. **C** to **E,** In these DQ-stained smears, loose clusters of more cuboidal-shaped neoplastic cells from an aspirate of metastatic colon carcinoma are noted. In addition, the characteristic dirty necrosis in the background is present, consisting of granular debris and neutrophils. **F,** Cell block from metastatic colonic carcinoma to the liver demonstrating neoplastic glands having pseudostratified elongated nuclei with granular necrotic debris within the lumen of the neoplastic glands. (H&E)

antigen (usually negative in hepatocellular carcinoma and often positive in metastatic adenocarcinoma), polyclonal CEA (diffuse cytoplasmic positivity in metastatic adenocarcinoma and canalicular staining pattern in hepatocellular carcinoma), and selected other site-specific and cell lineage

antibodies such as thyroid transcription factor 1 (positive in lung and thyroid cancers but generally negative in other types of malignancies). The workup of melanoma includes immunoperoxidase stains for S-100, HMB-45, and MelanA. The immunohistochemical evaluation of small cell malig-

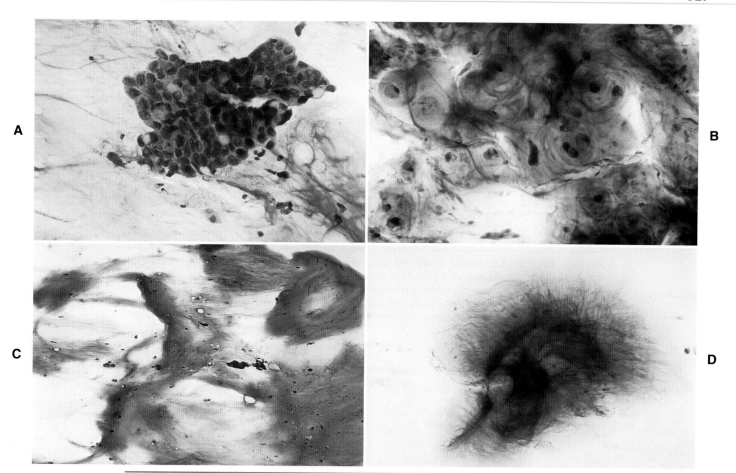

Figure 20-40 Metastatic colon carcinoma. **A,** In this Pap-stained smear, a cluster of metastatic colon cancer is present in which some of the cells have intracytoplasmic mucin vacuoles. Also note the slight amount of extracellular fibrillary mucin material nearby. **B,** In this metastatic colon cancer, neoplastic cells are embedded in abundant extracellular mucinous material consistent with features of colloid (mucinous) carcinoma. (Pap) **C,** In this Pap-stained smear of a liver aspirate, a mucinous colon cancer should be suspected when abundant extracellular mucinous material is identified. Although not present in this field, neoplastic cells were present nearby. **D,** Extracellular vascularized mucinous material is evident in an aspirate of metastatic colon cancer to the liver. Vascularized clumps of mucin are another clue that a malignancy is present. (DQ)

nancies in the pediatric age group includes markers such as neuron-specific enolase (NSE), synaptophysin, low molecular weight cytokeratin, actin, leukocyte common antigen, and CD99. In the adult population, other neuroendocrine markers such as chromogranin can also be used for the study of carcinoids and islet cell tumors. Specific hematopoietic markers can be used to confirm the diagnosis of lymphoma, and sarcomas can be identified from the usual lack of staining for epithelial markers and positive staining for vimentin, CD34, c-kit, and other more specific mesenchymal markers, depending on the type of sarcoma. Some metastatic tumors such as prostate and thyroid have specific immunologic markers to suggest the correct primary site. Another helpful morphologic feature in distinguishing metastatic malignant tumor from poorly differentiated hepatocellular carcinoma is the appreciation of a bimorphic smear pattern consisting of benign hepatocytes and a second population of metastatic malignant cells. However, this finding is not specific because it is possible that when a small malignant mass is aspirated, the surrounding benign liver tissue may also be sampled.

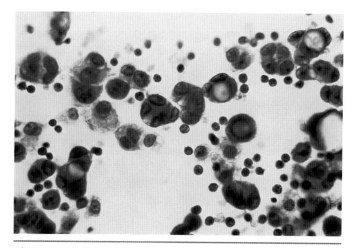

Figure 20-41 Metastatic signet ring carcinoma. The dissociative pattern of the tumor cells along with the coarse cytoplasmic vacuoles, including some with a targetoid pattern characterized by centrally placed inspissated mucinous material in this DQ-stained smear are typical.

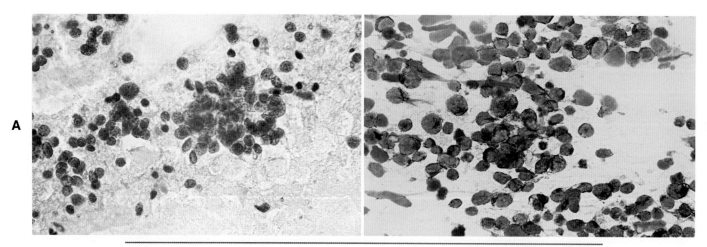

Figure 20-42 **Metastatic small cell carcinoma. A,** This is characterized by clusters of small neoplastic cells having very high N:C ratios, along with individually scattered cells. **B,** Immunoperoxidase stains for low molecular weight cytokeratin (CAM 5.2) were performed on one of the smears. It shows positive staining. Besides neuroendocrine markers, immunohistochemical staining for low molecular weight cytokeratin is helpful in the workup of metastatic small cell malignancies.

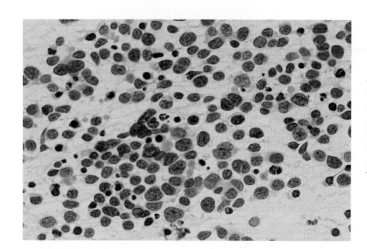

Figure 20-43 **Metastatic small cell carcinoma.** In this aspirate of metastatic small cell carcinoma of the lung involving the liver, the malignant cells have a predominantly discohesive pattern that could be readily confused with a malignant lymphoma. The nuclear features of small cell carcinoma and the lack of numerous cytoplasmic fragments in the background (lymphoglandular bodies) should strongly favor a metastatic small cell carcinoma rather than lymphoma. (Pap)

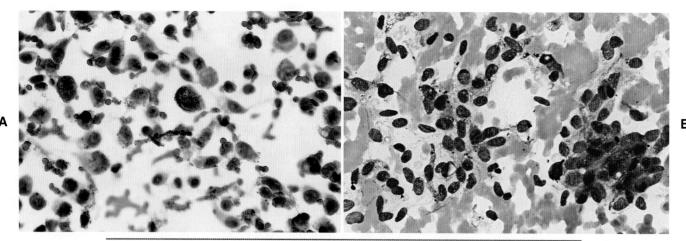

Figure 20-44 **Metastatic malignant melanoma. A,** Helpful cytologic features for the diagnosis of metastatic melanoma are the dissociative pattern, polygonal to spindle-shaped cells, prominent nucleoli, intranuclear inclusions, and/or the presence of intracytoplasmic melanin pigment. (Pap) **B,** In this DQ-stained smear, the melanoma cells have a more spindled configuration. A rare intranuclear inclusion and some fine cytoplasmic pigment are seen.

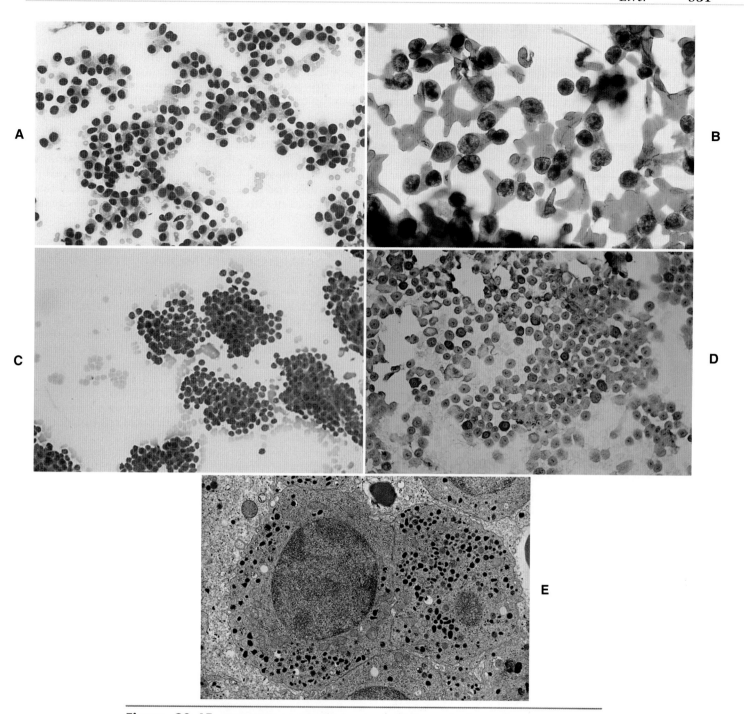

Figure 20-45 **Metastatic carcinoid tumor. A,** This sample demonstrates a dissociative smear pattern of uniform cells having a slightly plasmacytoid appearance with eccentrically placed nuclei and granular cytoplasm. Abortive rosette formation is noted. (DQ) **B,** In this Pap-stained smear, the neoplastic cells are individually scattered and are characterized by eccentrically placed nuclei with a granular salt-and-pepper type chromatin and associated granular cytoplasm. **C,** Occasionally, metastatic carcinoid tumor can consist of cohesive groups of cells simulating a metastatic adenocarcinoma. Close attention to the neuroendocrine cytologic features and ancillary studies can establish the correct diagnosis. (DQ) **D,** Positive immunohistochemical staining of the cells for gastrin in this case helped confirm the presence of a metastatic gastrin-producing carcinoid tumor to the liver. **E,** Ultrastructural examination of cells obtained from this liver aspirate shows numerous neuroendocrine granules.

CHOLANGIOCARCINOMA

Cholangiocarcinoma is a relatively uncommon primary adenocarcinoma of the liver that arises from the intrahepatic bile ducts.[93,94] It is very uncommon in children but does represent the second most common primary hepatic malignant tumors in adults, after hepatocellular carcinoma. The risk factors for cholangiocarcinoma include congenital cystic liver disease, chronic inflammatory bowel disease (especially ulcerative colitis), exposure to thorium dioxide, and parasitic trematode infections such as *Clonorchis* organisms.[1] In contrast with hepatocellular carcinoma, no gender predilection or association with pre-existing cirrhosis or viral infections is evident. However, similar to hepatocellular carcinoma, the prognosis is dismal.

In smears, cholangiocarcinoma consists of a neoplastic population of glandular cells. Not surprisingly, the differential diagnosis includes metastatic adenocarcinoma from a variety of sites such as the colon, stomach, and pancreas. Although not specific, a helpful cytomorphologic pattern to suggest the diagnosis of a cholangiocarcinoma is aspiration of a single mass lesion generating relatively hypocellular smears resulting from a high stroma to tumor cell ratio secondary to desmoplastic fibrosis. The malignant glandular cells present are also found in a relatively clean smear background (Figure 20-46).[1] In contrast, aspirates of metastatic colorectal carcinoma usually are more cellular and are associated with a dirty smear background. The neoplastic cells of cholangiocarcinoma often demonstrate ancillary features of adenocarcinoma, such as positive staining for cytoplasmic mucin and diffuse immunohistochemical cytoplasmic positivity for both high and low molecular weight cytokeratin, EMA, and CEA. In contrast, hepatocellular carcinoma's canalicular staining pattern for polyclonal CEA is not appreciated. Cholangiocarcinomas often coexpress CK 7 and 20, in contrast with the usual CK 20–positive and CK 7–negative staining of colorectal carcinomas, and negativity for both by hepatocellular carcinomas (Box 20-5).

SMALL CELL TUMORS

Small cell neoplasms can be appreciated in FNA biopsy of both adult and pediatric patients.[89-92] In children, the most common small cell malignant tumors to involve the liver are primary hepatoblastoma, metastatic neuroblastoma, and lymphoreticular neoplasms.[89,90] In adults, primary poorly differentiated hepatocellular carcinoma and metastatic small cell carcinoma of the lung, islet cell tumor, carcinoid tumor, lobular carcinoma of the breast, ovarian granulosa cell tumor, and malignant lymphoma can present with a small cell pattern. Metastatic small cell carcinoma of the lung is by far the most common. Contributing to the diagnosis is a long history of cigarette smoking in an adult patient with a hilar pulmonary mass appreciated in the chest x-ray. However, rarely, extrapulmonary metastatic small cell carcinomas to the liver can be sampled by FNA biopsy.[89] As an example, a small FNA series of metastatic small cell carcinomas of the gastrointestinal tract to the liver has been reported.[92]

The characteristic cytomorphologic features of metastatic small cell carcinoma include malignant cells with high N:C ratios, the characteristic evenly distributed, salt-and-pepper type chromatin, and the lack of obvious nucleoli. Nuclear molding and DNA streaking are additional cytologic features. The tumor cells may also show a strikingly

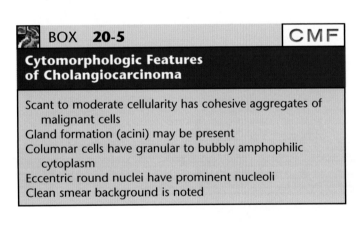

BOX 20-5   CMF

Cytomorphologic Features of Cholangiocarcinoma

Scant to moderate cellularity has cohesive aggregates of malignant cells
Gland formation (acini) may be present
Columnar cells have granular to bubbly amphophilic cytoplasm
Eccentric round nuclei have prominent nucleoli
Clean smear background is noted

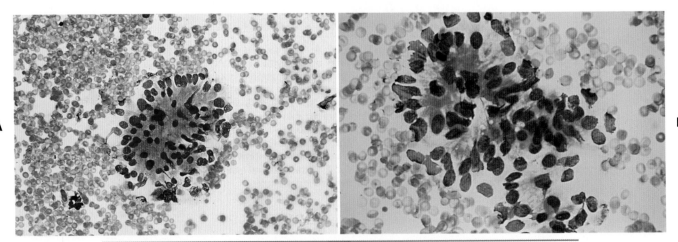

Figure 20-46 **Cholangiocarcinoma.** In these DQ-stained smears from an aspirate of cholangiocarcinoma, glands consist of neoplastic cells with elongated hyperchromatic nuclei. In contrast with metastatic colonic carcinoma, the smear background is clean.

discohesive cell pattern that potentially could be confused with malignant lymphoma (see Figure 20-43). Although occasionally present, appreciable numbers of lymphoglandular bodies, a feature of lymphoma, are not seen.

The cytomorphology of metastatic carcinoid and islet cell tumors is identical, consisting of a uniform population of relatively small cells with slight to moderate granular cytoplasm usually arranged in a dissociative fashion. Occasionally, neuroendocrine cells may be arranged in acinar groupings and tight clusters that could potentially simulate groups of cells from metastatic adenocarcinoma. In other instances, an anastomosing cord arrangement is prominent and may superficially resemble hepatoma. The nuclei show the prototypical salt-and-pepper neuroendocrine type chromatin distribution. A helpful cytologic feature is the plasmacytoid appearance of the cells in the DQ preparation resulting from the eccentrically placed nuclei and peripheral basophilic staining of the cytoplasm. Stripped nuclei and vascular fragments can also be seen in the background.[1] Ancillary studies may be helpful, including the ultrastructural demonstration of numerous dense core neurosecretory type cytoplasmic granules and/or positive immunohistochemical staining for neuroendocrine markers such as NSE, synaptophysin, chromogranin, and a perinuclear dotlike pattern with low molecular weight cytokeratin (CAM 5.2).

Metastatic medullary carcinoma of the thyroid is another neuroendocrine malignancy that also consists of numerous small- to medium-size malignant cells with high N:C ratios and at times abundant granular magenta-staining cytoplasm in the DQ smears. In addition to immunocytochemical positivity for neuroendocrine markers, the diagnosis is confirmed by positive staining for calcitonin; occasionally, CEA positivity can be demonstrated.[95] Metastatic lobular carcinoma of the breast generally presents with cohesive groups of small neoplastic cells having solitary round nuclei possessing finely granular chromatin, small nucleoli, and small intracytoplasmic mucin-containing vacuoles. An occasional, helpful cytologic feature is the linear arrangement of the cells without prominent nuclear molding. Immunohistochemical studies for gross cystic fluid protein-15, as well as estrogen and progesterone receptors may be of value, if the primary breast cancer was also positive for these hormonal markers. Metastatic ovarian granulosa cell tumor consists of a uniform population of small cells with high N:C ratios and nuclei demonstrating a characteristic longitudinal nuclear groove.[96] The chromatin is generally finely granular with usually inconspicuous nucleoli. The diagnosis can be confirmed with immunoperoxidase stains for inhibin.[96] Malignant melanoma should always be considered in the differential because a small cell variant exists and nuclear grooves have also been described.[91,97]

Lymphoid malignancies are characterized by numerous individually scattered malignant cells with high N:C ratios, round to highly irregular nuclear contours, and prominent to inconspicuous nucleoli.[98,99] A helpful cytologic feature is the appreciation of scattered small cytoplasmic fragments referred to as lymphoglandular bodies in the background of DQ-stained smears, although they can also be found in alcohol-fixed Pap preparations. The cytologic features are discussed in detail in Chapter 24. Cavanna and colleagues has reported the simultaneous sampling of a malignant lymphoma and a hepatocellular carcinoma in a FNA biopsy.[100]

 # HEPATOBLASTOMA

Hepatoblastoma is the most common primary hepatocellular malignancy in the pediatric age group and usually can be distinguished from hepatocellular carcinoma based on clinical and cytologic findings.[1,101-105] Generally, the patients are less than 4 years of age, and cirrhosis is not present. The tumor cells may resemble either fetal or embryonal hepatocytes, and a mesenchymal-like component and evidence of extramedullary hematopoiesis can be present.[1,101-105] A small cell-undifferentiated component has been described as associated with a worse prognosis.[106] In the smears, a hypercellular population with uniform-appearing malignant cells is present, arranged individually and in trabeculae, acini, and aggregates.[1,101-105,107] The hepatocellular differentiation is manifested by cells with solitary centrally placed nuclei surrounded by granular cytoplasm (Figure 20-47). Nucleoli may be prominent or inconspicuous. The amount of cytoplasm can vary from scant to moderate, depending on whether the cells are embryonal or fetal in appearance, respectively. Occasionally, cells are arranged in anastomosing trabeculae and stripped tumor nuclei may be appreciated—features that are typical of primary hepatocellular malignancies. The better-differentiated fetal cells have more abundant cytoplasm, compared with the more primitive embryonal cells with high N:C ratios with scanty basophilic, nongranular cytoplasm (Figure 20-48). Although relatively uncommon, fragments of fibrous connective tissue, primitive hematopoietic elements, or osteoid may be present (Figure 20-49).[101-105] In contrast with conventional hepatocellular carcinoma, considerably less pleomorphism of the tumor cells is present, and giant tumor cells are generally not seen.[1] Ancillary studies can be helpful because the embryonal and fetal types of tumor cells are positive for low molecular weight cytokeratin and negative for other immunohistochemical markers that can be present in other small, round cell pediatric malignancies. Ultrastructural examination reveals evidence of hepatocellular differentiation.[105] Other primary pediatric neoplasms that could be sampled include hemangioendothelioma, angiosarcoma, malignant rhabdoid tumor, mesenchymal hamartoma, and embryonal (undifferentiated) sarcoma of the liver.[108-112] Vascular neoplasms demonstrate positive immunohistochemical staining for endothelial markers, including factor VIII, CD31, and CD34, while embryonal sarcoma shows myofibroblastic differentiation of the malignant cells.[109-111] Although quite uncommon, hepatocellular carcinoma may also occur in children (Box 20-6).

BOX 20-6 **CMF**

Cytomorphologic Features of Hepatoblastoma

High cellularity and uniform cell population is present
Small to medium-size, round to polygonal-shaped cells are noted
Single, round hyperchromatic nuclei with or without prominent nucleoli are present
Moderate to very high N:C ratios are noted
Cells are arranged in trabeculae, acini, cords, and/or individually
Hematopoietic elements may be present
Mesenchymal elements (e.g., osteoid) may be present

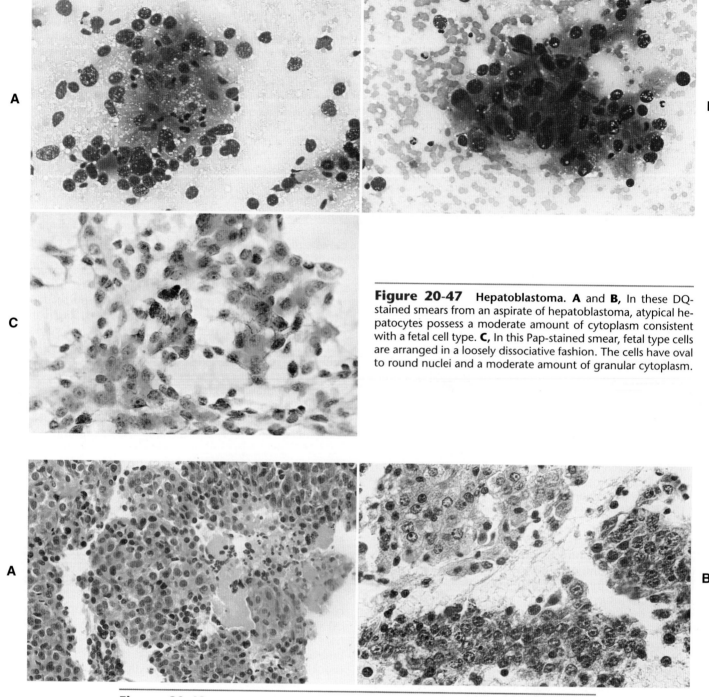

Figure 20-47 Hepatoblastoma. **A** and **B,** In these DQ-stained smears from an aspirate of hepatoblastoma, atypical hepatocytes possess a moderate amount of cytoplasm consistent with a fetal cell type. **C,** In this Pap-stained smear, fetal type cells are arranged in a loosely dissociative fashion. The cells have oval to round nuclei and a moderate amount of granular cytoplasm.

Figure 20-48 Hepatoblastoma. **A,** In this cell block from an aspirate of hepatoblastoma, an embryonal epithelial component has been sampled, characterized by small neoplastic cells having high N:C ratios, admixed with other cells having more abundant eosinophilic granular cytoplasm consistent with fetal cell type differentiation. In addition, some amorphous eosinophilic material is seen, possibly representing osteoid. (H&E) **B,** In this cell block, larger fetal type cells are contrasted with more primitive, smaller embryonal cells having higher N:C ratios. (H&E)

MALIGNANT LYMPHOMA

A few reports of FNA cytology of malignant lymphoma involve the liver.[98,99] The majority of lymphomas involving the liver are of large cell type, characterized by cellular smears populated by atypical large malignant lymphoid cells in a dissociative smear pattern with numerous lymphoglandular bodies in the background. Ancillary studies are helpful in confirming the diagnosis, with most cases demonstrating a B-cell immunophenotype either by immunohistochemistry or flow cytometry.[98] Although most of

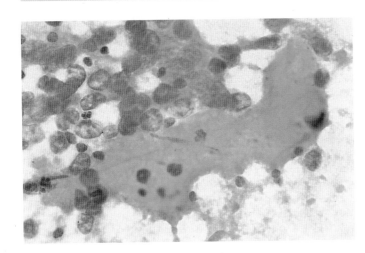

Figure 20-49 **Hepatoblastoma.** In this Pap preparation, the neoplastic hepatocytes are associated with eosinophilic amorphous osteoid.

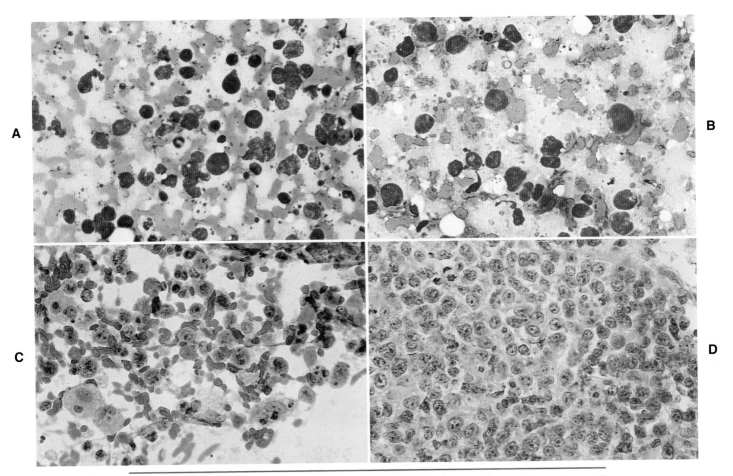

Figure 20-50 **Lymphoma.** **A** and **B,** In these DQ-stained smears from a primary large cell lymphoma of the liver, neoplastic lymphoid cells are present in a dissociative fashion with cytoplasmic fragments (lymphoglandular bodies) in the background. **C,** In the Pap preparation, nuclear detail is better seen including the appreciation of small nucleoli in this aspirate of lymphoma involving the liver. **D,** In the H&E-stained cell block, a loose noncohesive fragment of neoplastic lymphoid cells is present in an aspirate of large cell lymphoma involving the liver.

these cases represent liver involvement in disseminated systemic disease, primary hepatic lymphomas have also been diagnosed by FNA biopsy (Figure 20-50).[99] FNA of myeloproliferative disorders involving the liver has been reported.[113] Application of DQ and other Romanowsky-type stains is especially helpful in diagnosing lymphoid and myeloproliferative disorders in aspiration cytology. Separation of lymphoid from myeloid precursors and recognition of megakaryocytes are enhanced in the Romanowsky-stained smears.

STROMAL NEOPLASMS

Hemangioma, the most common neoplasm of the liver, is most often found incidentally during surgery or radiologic imaging of the abdomen. Hemangiomas are usually small and solitary but occasionally may attain a large size or appear as multiple lesions. As the radiographic appearance is usually diagnostic and a potential to bleed is common, these lesions are seldom aspirated. However, occasionally, FNA biopsies are performed either to confirm or exclude the possibility of a hepatic hemangioma, usually in the workup of metastatic disease in a patient with a known extrahepatic malignancy. Unfortunately, the FNA diagnosis of hemangioma is a diagnosis of exclusion because the aspirate is generally not diagnostic due to the dilution of the smears by blood.[114] A few scattered endothelial cells having elongated nuclei, and scanty cytoplasm may be present, but this is seldom diagnostic. The suspicion of a hemangioma may be supported based not only on the radiologic findings, but also a nondiagnostic aspirate of bloody smears with a few scattered endothelial cells. However, the smear preparations by themselves are considered inadequate or insufficient for definite diagnosis.

Angiosarcoma, although uncommon, is the most common primary sarcoma of the liver. This malignancy has been associated with environmental exposure to thorium dioxide, arsenic, polyvinyl chloride, and anabolic steroids.[1,115] Most patients are middle-age or older men with abdominal pain and/or a palpable mass. Angiosarcomas are highly aggressive tumors, with most deaths attributed to hepatic failure, massive hemorrhage, or metastatic disease. The cytologic features of angiosarcoma are variable consisting of smear patterns that can be highly cellular or markedly diluted with blood.[116,117] The malignant endothelial cells may vary from spindle to polygonal in shape, although one contour often predominates in a given specimen. The N:C ratios are variable, nuclei are generally single and hyperchromatic, and nucleoli can be prominent or indistinct. The tumor cells may be arranged in a number of different patterns, including vasoformative-appearing structures or solid aggregates and papillary structures (Figure 20-51).

The most common sarcomas involving the liver encountered in the FNA experiences of these authors are leiomyosarcoma and gastrointestinal stromal sarcomas, which are most often metastatic from an infradiaphragmatic primary.[118-120] The two tumors demonstrate essentially identi-

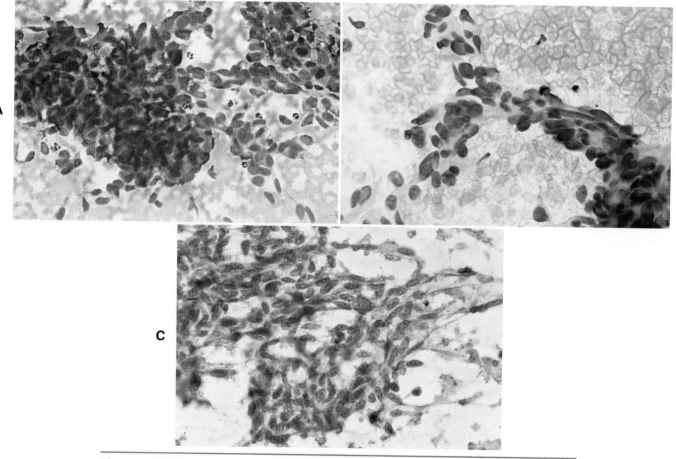

Figure 20-51   Angiosarcoma. **A,** This primary angiosarcoma of the liver consists of solid to papillary-type clusters of spindle-shaped cells plus individually scattered spindle-shaped cells in the background (DQ). **B,** In the Pap-stained smears, the tufted appearance of the neoplastic cells is seen. **C,** The neoplastic cells have a spindled configuration and are loosely arranged. The differential diagnosis might include metastatic spindle cell lesions to the liver. Immunohistochemical studies, including positive staining of the neoplastic cells for Factor VIII, CD31, and/or CD34 would confirm the vascular nature of the malignancy.

cal cytomorphologic attributes. Primary leiomyosarcomas may be expected to be more frequently encountered because of their increased incidence in acquired immunodeficiency syndrome (AIDS) and their predilection to occur in unusual sites such as the liver in this disorder.[119] FNA cytology of aspirated leiomyosarcomas is variable with most cases, showing a moderate level of cellularity with varying degrees of intracellular cohesion.[119] The individually scattered cells and the cells in microtissue fragments vary from spindle shape to epithelioid. Most of the cases examined consisted of spindle-shape cells with solitary hyperchromatic oval to elongated nuclei with characteristic blunt cigar-shape ends (Figures 20-52 and 20-53). Occasionally, perinuclear vacuoles can also be seen. The spindle cells in the groups have a tendency to demonstrate blending of the cytoplasm, and cellular pleomorphism is usually not evident. When epithelioid leiomyosarcomas or gastrointestinal stromal tumor (GIST) is encountered, the differential diagnosis includes metastatic adenocarcinomas resulting from the round to polygonal appearance of these epithelioid malignant mesenchymal cells.[118,121,122]

In the pediatric population the rare undifferentiated or embryonal sarcoma is the most common type of primary mesenchymal malignancy.[108-110] Histologically, these large, often fatal tumors have malignant cells in a myxoid background with areas of hemorrhage and necrosis. FNA biopsy of embryonal sarcoma of the liver consists of moderately cellular smears in which scattered neoplastic cells are set in a myxoid matrix.[108-110] The tumor cells vary from spindle to round, possessing solitary hyperchromatic nuclei and high N:C ratios. The FNA biopsy differential diagnosis of primary metastatic spindle cell neoplasms in adults and children are presented in Tables 20-1 and 20-2.

MISCELLANEOUS LESIONS

A variety of miscellaneous space-occupying, mass-producing lesions can involve the liver. On occasion, foci of steatosis can present as a focal lesion, rather than having the usual diffuse involvement of the liver.[123] The aspirated smears contain benign-appearing hepatocytes with one or more prominent intracytoplasmic lipid vacuoles.[124] Aspirates of amyloid deposits in the liver contain acellular, amorphous, metachromatically staining material with the DQ stain, which can be confirmed as amyloid with Congo

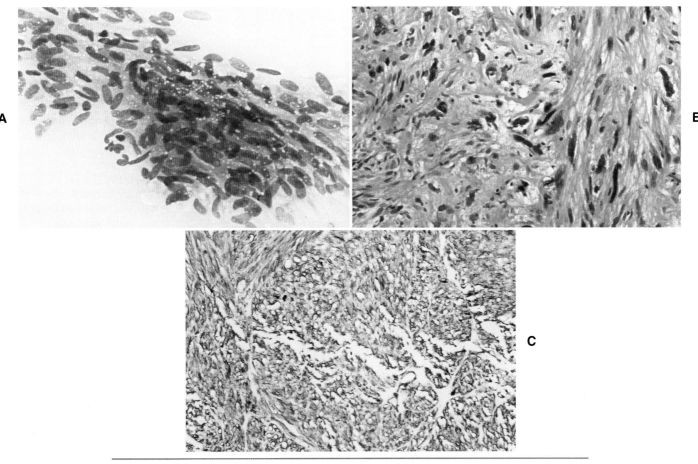

Figure 20-52   **Metastatic leiomyosarcoma. A,** Loose clusters of large atypical spindle cells, including many having so-called cigar-shaped nuclei. (Pap) **B,** The cell block demonstrates interlacing fascicles of atypical spindle cells, including some having very bizarre hyperchromatic nuclei. (H&E) **C,** An immunohistochemical stain for muscle-specific actin (HHF-35) intensely decorates the neoplastic cells.

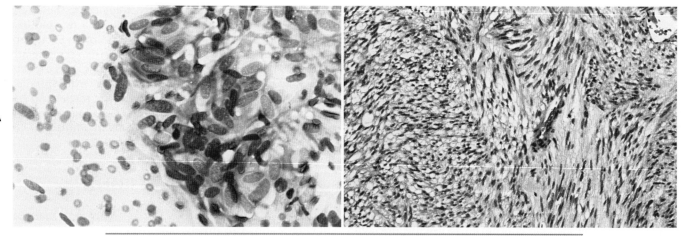

Figure 20-53 Gastrointestinal stromal tumor (GIST). **A,** Metastatic GIST consisting of a loose cluster of uniform spindle-shaped cells with wispy cytoplasmic processes. A few stripped nuclei are also present. (DQ) **B,** Primary GIST of stomach consisting of interlacing fascicles of uniform spindle-shaped cells. (H&E)

TABLE 20-1

Differential Diagnosis of Hepatic Spindle Cell Neoplasms in Adults

Diagnosis	Cytology	Immunohistochemistry	Electron Microscopy
Benign			
Leiomyoma	Differential probably not possible	Same as LS +Desmin, MSA	Same as LS
Fibroma	Same as LS		Same as fibrosarcoma
Malignant			
GIST	Spindle and/or epithelioid cells	+CD34, CD117	Noncontributory
LS	Single spindle cells with bipolar cytoplasmic process, fragments with overlapping nuclei	+Desmin, MSA	Basal lamina, microfilaments with dense bodies, pinocytotic vesicles, nuclear contractions
Fibrosarcoma	Same as LS	−Desmin, MSA	Abundant RER, type I collagen around cells
Malignant schwannoma	Malignant spindle cells often with multinucleated giant cells	+S-100, −Desmin, MSA	Long, thin, intertwining cell processes; long space collagen
Malignant fibrous histiocytoma	Pleomorphic multinucleated giant cells and malignant spindle cells	−Desmin, ± MSA, +α-1-antitrypsin, +α-1-antichymotrypsin	Facultative histiocytic cells with primary and secondary lysosomes
Sarcomatoid HCC	Admixed malignant polygonal epithelial cells, ± giant cells, and spindle cells	−α-fetoprotein, +cytokeratin	Desmosomes, Mallory's hyaline
Cholangiocarcinoma with spindle cells	Admixed malignant glandular cells	+Cytokeratin, +CEA, +mucin	Desmosomes, mucin granules
Kaposi's sarcoma	Vascular slits in tissue fragments	± MSA, desmin, Ulex europeus, factor VIII, CD31, CD34	Numerous erythrophagolysosomes

Modified from Smith MB, Silverman JF, Raab SS, et al. Fine-needle aspiration cytology of hepatic leiomyosarcoma. Diagn Cytopathol 1994; 11:321-327.

LS, Leiomyosarcoma; *MSA,* muscle-specific actin; *GIST,* gastrointestinal stromal tumor; *RER,* rough endoplasmic reticulum; *HCC,* hepatocellular carcinoma; *CEA,* carcinoembryonic antigen.

TABLE 20-2

Differential Diagnosis of Hepatic Spindle Cell Neoplasms in Children

Diagnosis	Cytology	Immunohistochemistry	Electron Microscopy
Benign			
Inflammatory pseudotumor	Spindle cells with numerous neutrophils, histiocytes, lymphocytes, and plasma cells	−Desmin, myoglobin +/− alk	Dilated RER, some cells with few filaments and dense bodies
Infantile hemangioen-dothelioma	Not reported	+Factor VIII, Ulex europeus, CD31, CD34	Vascular lumina, right junctions, marginal folds, basal lamina, and Weibel-Palade bodies
Mesenchymal hamartoma	Not reported	−Desmin, myoglobin	Spindle cells (fibroblasts), same as fibrosarcoma
Malignant			
Undifferentiated (embryonal) sarcoma	Single cells, some multinucleated giant cells in a myxoid background	−Desmin, myoglobin; PAS diastase-resistant globules (+α-1-antitrypsin, +α-antichymotrypsin)	Dilated RER, variable numbers of lipid-laden vacuoles, few microfilaments with dense bodies

Modified from Smith MB, Silverman JF, Raab SS, et al. Fine-needle aspiration cytology of hepatic leiomyosarcoma. Diagn Cytopathol 1994; 11:321-327.
RER, Rough endoplasmic reticulum.

red stain with polarization.[125,126] Angiomyolipoma, a benign tumor more common to the kidney, occasionally occurs in the liver and can be diagnosed by FNA biopsy.[127,128] The smears or cell block show the diagnostic features of an admixture of thick-walled vessels, adipose tissue, and smooth muscle. The smooth muscle cells can occasionally have an atypical spindle cell and/or epithelioid appearance, which can potentially lead to an incorrect diagnosis of either sarcoma or carcinoma.[129] Ancillary studies can be quite helpful in confirming the diagnosis because cells from angiomyolipoma usually show positive staining for muscle-specific actin and HMB-45.[127,129] Other rare conditions presenting as hepatic masses and diagnosed by FNA biopsy include inflammatory pseudotumor, primary endodermal sinus tumor, and familial hemophagocytic syndromes.[130-132]

References

1. Silverman JF, Geisinger KR. FNA of thorax and abdomen. New York: Churchill Livingstone; 1996. pp.89-134.
2. Silverman JF, Finley JL, O'Brien KF, et al. Diagnostic accuracy and role of immediate interpretation of fine needle aspiration biopsy specimens from various sites. Acta Cytol 1989; 33:791-796.
3. Silverman JF, Frable W. The use of the Diff-Quik stain in the immediate interpretation of fine-needle aspiration biopsies. Diagn Cytopathol 1990; 6:366-369.
4. Frias-Hidvegi D. Guides to clinical aspiration biopsy: liver and pancreas. New York: Igaku-Shoin; 1988.
5. Kung ITM, Chan SK, Fung KH. Fine-needle aspiration in hepatocellular carcinoma: combined cytologic and histologic approach. Cancer 1991; 67:673-680.
6. Lundqvist A. Fine-needle aspiration biopsy of the liver. Acta Med Scand 1971; 520:1-28.
7. Nguyen G-K. Fine needle aspiration biopsy cytology of hepatic tumors in adults. Pathol Annu 1986; 21:321-349.
8. Suen KC. Diagnosis of primary hepatic neoplasms by fine-needle aspiration cytology. Diagn Cytopathol 1986; 2:99-109.
9. Tao L-C. Liver and pancreas. In: Bibbo M, editor. Comprehensive cytopathology. Philadelphia: WB Saunders; 1991. pp.822-859.
10. Stewart CJ, Coldewey J, Stewart IS. Comparison of fine needle aspiration cytology and needle core biopsy in the diagnosis of radiologically detected abdominal lesions. J Clin Pathol 2002; 55:93-97.
11. Hertz G, Reddy VB, Green L, et al. Fine-needle aspiration biopsy of the liver: a multicenter study of 602 radiologically guided FNA. Diagn Cytopathol 2000; 23:326-328.
12. Guo Z, Kurtycz DFI, Salem R, et al. Radiologically guided percutaneous fine-needle asiration biopsy of the liver: retrospective study of 119 cases evaluating diagnostic effectiveness and clinical complications. Diagn Cytopathol 2002; 26:283-289.
13. Wee A, Nilsson B, Chan-Wilde C, et al. Fine needle aspiration biopsy of hepatocellular carcinoma. Some unusual features. Acta Cytol 1991; 35:661-670.
14. Ali MA, Akhtar M, Mattingly RC. Morphologic spectrum of hepatocellular carcinoma in fine needle aspiration biopsies. Acta Cytol 1986; 30:294-302.
15. Noguchi S, Yamamoto R, Tatauta M, et al. Cell features and patterns in fine-needle aspirates of hepatocellular carcinoma. Cancer 1986; 38:321-328.
16. Pedio G, Landolt U, Zobeli L, et al. Fine needle aspiration of the liver: significance of hepatocytic naked nuclei in the diagnosis of hepatocellular carcinoma. Acta Cytol 1988; 32:437-442.
17. Greene C-A, Suen KC. Some cytologic features of hepatocellular carcinoma as seen in fine needle aspirates. Acta Cytol 1984; 28:713-718.
18. Sole M, Calvet X, Cuberes T, et al. Value and limitations of cytologic criteria for the diagnosis of hepatocellular carcinoma by fine needle aspiration biopsy. Acta Cytol 1993; 37:309-326.

19. Granados R, Aramburu JA, Murillo N, et al. Fine-needle aspiration biopsy of liver masses: diagnostic value and reproducibility of cytological criteria. Diagn Cytopathol 2001; 25:365-375.

20. Salamão DR, Clayton AC, Keeney GL, et al. Reproducibility of proposed cytologic criteria to discriminate hepatocellular carcinoma from metastatic adenocarcinoma in fine needle aspiration. Acta Cytol 2001; 45:857.

21. Cardesa A. Value and limitations of cytologic criteria for the diagnosis of hepatocellular carcinoma by fine needle aspiration biopsy. Acta Cytol 1993; 37:309-326.

22. Silverman JF, Geisinger KR. Ancillary studies in FNA of the liver and pancreas. Diagn Cytopathol 1995; 13: 396-410.

23. Wee A, Nilsson B, Yap I, Chong S-M. Aspiration cytology of liver abscesses: with an emphasis on diagnostic pitfalls. Acta Cytol 1995; 39:453-462.

24. Silverman JF. Infectious and inflammatory diseases and other non-neoplastic disorders. New York: Igaku-Shoin; 1991. pp.245-257.

25. Tao L-C. Transabdominal fine-needle aspiration biopsy. New York: Igaku-Shoin; 1990.

26. Walsh TJ, Berkman W, Brown NL, et al. Cytopathologic diagnosis of extracolonic amebiasis. Acta Cytol 1983; 27:671-675.

27. Bhambhani S, Kashyap H. Amoebias? Diagnosis of aspiration and exfoliative cytology. Cytopathology 2001; 12:328-333.

28. Shurbaji MS, Gupta PK, Newman MM. Hepatic actinomycosis diagnosed by fine needle aspiration: a case report. Acta Cytol 1987; 31:751-755.

29. Kumar PV, Omrani GH, Saberfirouzi M, et al. Kala-azar: liver fine needle aspiration findings in 23 cases presenting with a fever of unknown origin. Acta Cytol 1996; 40: 263-268.

30. Stormby N, Akerman M. Aspiration cytology in the diagnosis of granulomatous liver lesions. Acta Cytol 1973; 17:200-204.

31. Whitlach S, Nunez C, Pitlik DA. Fine needle aspiration biopsy of the liver. Acta Cytol 1984; 28:719-725.

32. Bottles K, Cohen MB. An approach to fine-needle aspiration biopsy diagnosis by hepatic masses. Diagn Cytopathol 1991; 7:204-210.

33. Zaman SS, Langer JE, Gupta PK. Ciliated hepatic foregut cyst: report of a case with findings on fine needle aspiration. Acta Cytol 1995; 39:781-784.

34. Devaney K, Goodman ZD, Ishak KG. Hepatobiliary cystadenoma and cystadenoma-carcinoma: a light microscopic and immunohistochemical study of 70 patients. Am J Surg Pathol 1994; 18:1078-1091.

35. Pinto MM, Kaye AD. Fine needle aspiration of cystic liver lesions: cytologic examination and carcinoembryonic antigen assay of cyst contents. Acta Cytol 1989; 33: 852-856.

36. Del Poggio P, Jamoletti C, Forloni B, et al. Malignant transformation of biliary cystadenoma: a difficult diagnosis. Dig Liv Dis 2000; 32:733-736.

37. Bralet MP, Regimbeau JM, Pineau P, et al. Hepatocellular carcinoma occurring in nonfibrotic liver: epidemiologic and histopathologic analysis of 80 French cases. Hepatology 2000; 32:200-204.

38. Tao LC, Ho CS, McLoughlin MJ, et al. Cytologic diagnosis of hepatocellular carcinoma by fine-needle aspiration biopsy. Cancer 1984; 53:547-552.

39. Berman JJ, McNeill RE. Cirrhosis with atypia: a potential pitfall in the interpretation of liver aspirates. Acta Cytol 1988; 32:11-14.

40. International Working Party. Terminology of nodular hepatocellular lesions. Hepatology 1995; 22:983-993.

41. Bisceglie AM, Rustgi VK, Hoofnagle JH, et al. Hepatocellular carcinoma. Ann Intern Med 1988; 108:390-401.

42. Colombo M. Hepatocellular carcinoma. J Hepatol 1992; 15:225-236.

43. Rullier A, Trimoulet P, Urbaniak R, et al. Immunohistochemical detection of HCV in cirrhosis, dysplastic nodules, and hepatocellular carcinomas with parallel-tissue quantitative RT-PCR. Mod Pathol 2001; 14:496-505.

44. Falkson G, Canaan A, Schutt AJ, et al. Prognostic factors for survival in hepatocellular carcinoma. Cancer Res 1988; 48:7314-7318.

45. Barbara L, Benzi G, Gaini S, et al. Natural history of small untreated hepatocellular carcinoma in cirrhosis: a multivariate analysis of prognostic factors of tumor growth rate and patient survival. Hepatology 1992; 16:132-137.

46. Moreland WS, Zagoria RJ, Geisinger KR. Use of fine needle aspiration biopsy in radiofrequency ablation. Acta Cytol 2002; 46:819-822.

47. Zainol H, Sumithran E. Combined cytological and histological diagnosis of hepatocellular carcinoma in ultrasonically guided fine needle biopsy specimens. Histopathology 1993; 22:581-586.

48. Pinto MM, Avila NA, Heller CI, Criscuolo EM. Fine needle aspiration of the liver. Acta Cytol 1988; 32:15-21.

49. Sbolli G, Fornari F, Civardi G, et al. Role of ultrasound guided fine needle aspiration biopsy in the diagnosis of hepatocellular carcinoma. Gut 1990; 31:1303-1305.

50. Cohen MB, Haber MM, Holly EA, et al. Cytologic criteria to distinguish hepatocellular carcinoma from non-neoplastic liver. Am J Clin Pathol 1991; 95:125-130.

51. Wee A, Nilsson B, Tan LKA, et al. Fine needle aspiration biopsy of hepatocellular carcinoma. Diagnostic dilemma at the ends of the spectrum. Acta Cytol 1994; 38:347-354.

52. Goellner JR, Salamão DR. Hepatocellular carcinoma: needle biopsy findings in 74 cases. Acta Cytol 1994; 38:800.

53. Pisharodi LR, Lavoie R, Bedrossian CWM. Differential diagnostic dilemmas in malignant fine-needle aspirates of liver: a practical approach to final diagnosis. Diagn Cytopathol 1995; 12:364-371.

54. Bottles K, Cohen MB, Holly EA, et al. A step-wise logistic regression analysis of hepatocellular carcinoma: an aspiration biopsy study. Cancer 1988; 62:558-563.

55. Pitman MB, Szyfelbein WM. Significance of endothelium in the fine-needle aspiration biopsy diagnosis of hepatocellular carcinoma. Diagn Cytopathol 1995; 12:208-214.

56. de Boer BW, Segal A, Frost FA, et al. Cytodiagnosis of well-differentiated hepatocellular carcinoma: can indeterminate diagnoses be reduced? Cancer 1999; 87:270-277.

57. Wu HHJ, Tao LC, Cramer HM. Vimentin-positive spider-shaped Kupffer cells: a new clue to cytologic diagnosis of primary and metastatic hepatocellular carcinoma by fine-needle aspiration biopsy. Am J Clin Pathol 1996; 106: 517-521.

58. de Boer WB. Segol A, Frost FA, et al. Can CD34 discriminate between benign and malignant hepatocytic lesions in fine needle aspirates and thin core biopsies? Cancer Cytopathol 2000; 90:273-278.

59. Bergman S, Graeme-Cook F, Pitman MB. The usefulness of the reticulin stain in the differential diagnosis of liver nodules in fine-needle aspiration biopsy cell block preparations. Mod Pathol 1997; 10:1258-1264.

60. Axe SR, Erozan YS, Ermatinger SV. Fine-needle aspiration of the liver: a comparison of smear and rinse preparations in the detection of cancer. Am J Clin Pathol 1986; 86: 281-285.

61. Bell DA, Carr CP, Szyfelbein WM. Fine needle aspiration cytology of focal liver lesions. Results obtained with examination of both cytologic and histologic preparations. Acta Cytol 1986; 30:397-402.

62. Sangalli G, Livraghi T, Giordano F. Fine needle biopsy of hepatocellular carcinoma: improvement in diagnosis by microhistology. Gastroenterology 1989; 96:524-526.

63. Wong MA, Yazdi HM. Hepatocellular carcinoma versus carcinoma metastatic to liver: value of stains for carcinoembryonic antigen and naphthylamidase in fine needle aspiration biopsy material. Acta Cytol 1990; 34: 192-196.

64. Wolber RA, Greene CA, Dapris BA. Polyclonal carcinoembryonic antigen staining in cytologic differential diagnosis of primary and metastatic malignancies. Acta Cytol 1991; 35:215-220.

65. Carrozza MJ, Calafati SA, Edmonds PR. Immunocytochemical localization of polyclonal carcinoembryonic antigen in hepatocellular carcinoma. Acta Cytol 1991; 35:221-224.

66. Bedrossian CWM, Davila RM, Merenda G. Immunocytochemical evaluation of liver fine-needle aspirations. Arch Pathol Lab Med 1989; 113:1225-1230.

67. Zimmerman RL, Burke MA, Young NA, et al. Diagnostic value of hepatocyte paraffin 1 antibody to discriminate hepatocellular carcinoma from metastatic carcinoma in fine-needle aspiration biopsies of the liver. Cancer Cytopathol 2001; 93:288-291.

68. Siddiqui MT, Saboorian MH, Gokaslan ST, et al. Diagnostic utility of the Heplar 1 antibody to differentiate hepatocellular carcinoma from metastatic carcinoma in fine-needle aspiration samples. Cancer Cytopathol 2002; 96:49-52.

69. Neill JSA, Silverman JF. The role of ultrastructural examination in fine needle aspiration biopsy of liver neoplasms. Acta Cytol 1992; 36:621.

70. Ordonez NG, MacKay B. Ultrastructure of liver cell and bile duct carcinoma: Ultrastruct Pathol 1983; 5:201-241.

71. Davenport RD. Cytologic diagnosis of fibrolamellar carcinoma of the liver by fine-needle aspiration. Diagn Cytopathol 1990; 6:275-279.

72. El-Gazzaz G, Wong W, El-Hadary MK, et al. Outcome of liver resection and transplantation for fibrolamellar hepatocellular carcinoma. Transpl Int 2000; 13(Suppl):1:S406-409.

73. Usatoff V, Isla AM, Habib NA. Liver resection in advanced hepatocellular carcinoma. Hepatogastroenterology 2001; 48:46-50.

74. Suen KC, Magee JF, Halparin LS, et al. Fine needle aspiration cytology of fibrolamellar hepatocellular carcinoma. Acta Cytol 1985; 20:867-872.

75. Gupta SK, Das DK, Rajwanshi A, et al. Cytology of hepatocellular carcinoma. Diagn Cytopathol 1986; 2:290-294.

76. Perez-Guillermo M, Masgrau NA, Garcia-Solano J, et al. Cytologic aspect of fibrolamellar hepatocellular carcinoma in fine-needle aspirates. Diagn Cytopathol 1999; 21:180-187.

77. Sarode VR, Castellani R, Post A. Fine-needle aspiration cytology and differential diagnoses of fibrolamellar hepatocellular carcinoma metastatic to the mediastinum: a case report. Diagn Cytopathol 2002; 26:95-98.

78. Hughes JH, Jensen CS, Donnelly AD, et al. The role of fine-needle aspiration cytology in the evaluation of metastatic clear cell tumors. Cancer 1999; 87:380-389.

79. Donat EE, Anderson V, Tao L-C. Cytodiagnosis of clear cell hepatocellular carcinoma: a case report. Acta Cytol 1991; 35:671-675.

80. Gupta RK, AlAnsari AG, Fauck R. Aspiration cytodiagnosis of clear cell hepatocellular carcinoma in an elderly woman: a case report. Acta Cytol 1994; 38:467-469.

81. Singh HK, Silverman JF, Geisinger KR. Fine-needle aspiration cytomorphology of clear-cell hepatocellular carcinoma. Diagn Cytopathol 1997; 17:306-310.

82. Cheuk W, Chan JK. Clear cell variant of fibrolamellar carcinoma of the liver. Arch Pathol Lab Med 2001; 125:1235-1238.

83. Goodman ZD, Ishak KG, Langloss JM, et al. Combined hepatocellular-cholangiocarcinoma: a histologic and immunohistochemical study. Cancer 1985; 55:124-135.

84. Jarnagin WR, Weber S, Tickoo SK, et al. Combined hepatocellular and cholangiocarcinoma. Cancer 2002; 94:2040-2046.

85. Kilpatrick SE, Geisinger KR, Loggie BW, et al. Fine needle aspiration biopsy cytomorphology of combined hepatocellular-cholangiocarcinoma. Acta Cytol 1993; 37:943-947.

86. Saul SH. Neoplasms of the liver. In: Sternberg SS, editor. Diagnostic surgical pathology. Philadelphia: Lippincott-Raven; 1989. pp.1162-1166.

87. Ruschenburg I, Drose M. Fine-needle aspiration cytology of focal nodular hyperplasia of the liver. Acta Cytol 1989; 33:857-860.

88. Tao L-C. Are oral contraceptive-associated liver cell adenomas premalignant? Acta Cytol 1992; 36:338-344.

89. Silverman JF, Geisinger K, Dabbs DJ, et al. FNA cytology of small cell neoplasms of the liver. Pathol Case Review 1999; 4(4):182-186.

90. Geisinger K, Silverman J, Wakely P Jr. Pediatric cytopathology. Chicago: ASCP Press; 1994. pp.293-302.

91. Pisharodi LR, Bedrossian C. Diagnosis and differential diagnosis of small-cell lesions of the liver. Diagn Cytopathol 1998; 19:29-32.

92. Dabbs DJ, Silverman JF, Raab SS, et al. The role of immunocytochemistry for the FNA diagnosis of neoplasms involving the liver. Pathol Case Review 1999; 4(4): 176-181.

93. Nakajima T, Kondo Y. Well differentiated cholangiocarcinoma: diagnostic significance of morphologic and immunohistochemical parameters. Am J Surg Pathol 1989; 13:569-573.

94. Byrnes V, Afdhal N. Cholangiocarcinoma of the hepatic hilum (Klatskin tumor). Curr Treat Options Gastroenterol 2002; 5:87-94.

95. Gomez-Fernandez C, Kraemer HJ, et al. Metastatic medullary thyroid carcinoma in liver diagnosis by aspiration cytology. Diagn Cytopathol 1994; 11:277-280.

96. Ali SZ. Metastatic granulosa-cell tumor in the liver: cytopathologic findings and staining with inhibin. Diagn Cytopathol 1998; 19:293-297.

97. Rollins SD, Berardo MD. Presence of nuclear grooves in the cytology of malignant melanoma. Diagn Cytopathol 1998; 19:309-312.

98. Collins KA, Geisinger KR, Raab S, et al. Fine needle aspiration biopsy of hepatic lymphomas: cytomorphology and ancillary studies. Acta Cytol 1996; 40:257-262.

99. Rappaport KM, DiGiuseppe JA, Busseniers AE. Primary hepatic lymphoma: report of two cases diagnosed by fine-needle aspiration. Diagn Cytopathol 1995; 13:142-145.

100. Cavanna L, Civardi G, Fomari F, et al. Simultaneous relapse of liver cell carcinoma and non-Hodgkin's lymphoma in the liver: report of a case with diagnosis by ultrasonically guided fine needle aspiration biopsy. Acta Cytol 1994; 38:451-454.

101. Bhatia A, Mehrotra P. Fine needle aspiration cytology in a case of hepatoblastoma. Acta Cytol 1986; 30:439-441.

102. Wakely PE Jr, Silverman JF, Geisinger KR, et al. Fine needle aspiration biopsy cytology of hepatoblastoma. Mod Pathol 1990; 3:688-693.

103. Kaw YT, Hansen K. Fine needle aspiration cytology of undifferentiated small cell ("anaplastic") hepatoblastoma: a case report. Acta Cytol 1993; 37:216-220.

104. Sola-Perez J, Perez-Guillermo M, Bernal AB, et al. Hepatoblastoma: an attempt to apply histologic classification to aspirates obtained by fine needle aspiration cytology. Acta Cytol 1994; 38:175-182.

105. Cangiarella J, Greco MA, Waisman J. Hepatoblastoma: report of a case with cytologic, histologic and ultrastructural findings. Acta Cytol 1993; 38:455-458.

106. Haas JG, Feusner JH, Finegold MJ. Small cell undifferentiated histology in hepatoblastoma may be unfavorable. Cancer 2001; 92:3130-3134.

107. Ersoz C, Zorludemir U, Tanyeli A, et al. Fine-needle aspiration cytology of hepatoblastoma: a report of two cases. Acta Cytol 1998; 42:799-802.

108. Sola-Perez J, Perez-Guillermo M, Gimenez-Bascunana A, et al. Cytopathology of undifferentiated (embryonal) sarcoma of the liver. Diagn Cytopathol 1995; 13:44-51.

109. Pieterse AS, Smith M, Smith LA, et al. Embryonal (undifferentiated) sarcoma of the liver: fine-needle aspiration cytology and ultrastructural findings. Arch Pathol Lab Med 1985; 109:677-680.

110. Keating S, Taylor GP. Undifferentiated (embryonal) sarcoma of the liver: ultrastructural and immunohistochemical similarities with malignant fibrous histiocytoma. Hum Pathol 1985; 16:693-699.

111. Parham DM, Kelly DR, Donnelly WH, et al. Immunohistochemical and ultrastructural spectrum of hepatic sarcomas of childhood: evidence of a common histogenesis. Mod Pathol 1991; 4:648-653.

112. al-Rikabi AC, Buckai A, al-Sumayer S, et al. Fine needle aspiration cytology of mesenchymal hamartoma of the liver: a case report. Acta Cytol 2000; 44:449-453.

113. Raab SS, Silverman JF, McLeod DL, Geisinger KR. Fine-needle aspiration cytology of extramedullary hematopoiesis (myeloid metaplasia). Diagn Cytopathol 1993; 9:522-526.

114. Layfield LI, Mooney EE, Dodd LG. Not by blood alone: diagnosis of hemangiomas by fine-needle aspiration. Diagn Cytopathol 1998; 19:250-254.

115. Selby DM, Stocker JT, Ishak KG. Angiosarcoma of the liver in childhood: a clinicopathologic and follow-up study of 10 cases. Pediatr Pathol 1992; 12:485-498.

116. Abele JS, Miller TR. Cytology of well-differentiated and poorly differentiated hemangiosarcoma in fine needle aspirates. Acta Cytol 1982; 26:341-348.

117. Saleh HA, Tao LC. Hepatic angiosarcoma: aspiration biopsy cytology and immunocytochemical contribution. Diagn Cytopathol 1998; 18:208-211.

118. Park EA, Kim, JS, Ham EK. Fine-needle aspiration cytology of gastric epithelioid leiomyosarcoma metastasized to the liver: a case report. Acta Cytol 1997; 41:1801-1806.

119. Smith MB, Silverman JF, Raab SS, et al. Fine-needle aspiration cytology of hepatic leiomyosarcoma. Diagn Cytopathol 1994; 11:321-327.

120. Guy CD, Yuan S, Ballo MS. Spindle-cell lesions of the liver: diagnosis by fine-needle aspiration biopsy. Diagn Cytopathol 2001; 25:94-100.

121. Nguyen GK. Cytopathologic aspects of leiomyoblastoma in fine needle aspiration biopsy: report of two cases. Acta Cytol 1983; 27:173-177.

122. LaGrange W. Fine needle aspiration biopsy of myxoid variant of malignant leiomyoblastoma metastatic to the liver. Acta Cytol 1988; 32:443-446.

123. Brawer MK, Austin GE, Lewin KJ. Focal fatty change of the liver, a hitherto poorly described entity. Gastroenterology 1980; 78:247-252.

124. Layfield JL. Focal fatty changes of the liver: cytologic findings in a radiographic mimic of metastases. Diagn Cytopathol 1994; 11:385-389.

125. Bose S, Kapila K, Verma K. Amyloidosis of the liver diagnosed by fine needle aspiration cytology. Acta Cytol 1989; 33:935-936.

126. Srinivasan R, Nijhawan R, Gautam U, et al. Potassium permanganate resistant amyloid in fine-needle aspirate of the liver. Diagn Cytopathol 1994; 10:383-384.

127. Ma TWF, Tse MK, Tsui WMS, et al. Fine needle aspiration diagnosis of angiomyolipoma of the liver using a cell block with immunohistochemical study. Acta Cytol 1994; 38:257-260.

128. Nazer MA, Ali MA. Fine-needle aspiration cytology of hepatic angiomyolipoma: case report with histological, immunohistochemical and electron microscopic findings. Ann Saudi Med 2002; 21:230-233.

129. Cibas ES, Goss GA, Kulke MH, et al. Malignant epithelioid angiomyolipoma (sarcoma ex angiomyolipoma) of the kidney: a case report and review of the literature. Am J Surg Pathol 2001; 25:121-126.

130. Lupovitch A, Chen R, Mishra S. Inflammatory pseudotumor of the liver: report of the fine needle aspiration cytologic findings in a case initially misdiagnosed as malignant. Acta Cytol 1989; 33:259-262.

131. Wakely PE Jr, Krummel TM, Johnson DE. Yolk sac tumor of the liver. Mod Pathol 1991; 4:121-125.

132. Silverman JF, Singh HK, Joshi VV, et al. Cytomorphology of familial hemophagocytic syndrome (FHS). Diagn Cytopathol 1993; 9:404-410.

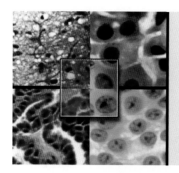

Pancreas, Extrahepatic Bile Ducts, and Gallbladder

CHAPTER
21

PANCREAS

Percutaneous, intraoperative, and endoscopic ultrasound-(EUS-)guided fine-needle aspirations (FNAs) are increasingly being used for the evaluation of solid, cystic, and inflammatory lesions of the pancreas.[1-9] The increased popularity of pancreatic FNA biopsy is the result of excellent diagnostic accuracy.[10-20] Frozen sections of core or wedge biopsies can be very difficult to interpret and may be associated with complications. Furthermore, frozen section diagnosis of pancreatic carcinoma has a high false-negative rate because of the extensive desmoplastic fibrosis and necrosis often associated with these malignancies. Sampling of the associated pancreatitis secondary to the carcinoma's obstruction of pancreatic ducts can also be confusing.[21,22] False-positive frozen section diagnoses related to atypia associated with inflammation are also notorious. Large core needle biopsies and wedge resection may lead to pancreatitis and peritonitis resulting from the leakage of exocrine enzymes and bile.[23] FNA biopsy of the pancreas, although better tolerated, is not totally without complications, with rare reports of the procedure causing needle tract seeding, fistula formation, and ascites.[23-28] However, percutaneous and intraoperative FNA biopsy of the pancreas used at the time of surgery appears to be safer than biopsies for frozen section, while maintaining a high diagnostic accuracy.[8,15] FNA biopsy can also be an effective procedure for the diagnosis of inflammatory pancreatic lesions that do not warrant a surgical procedure. Diagnostic issues related specifically to EUS-guided FNA were introduced in Chapter 18 and will be explained more fully near the end of this chapter.

It is important for the cytopathologist to recognize the benign ductal and acinar pancreatic epithelial elements in aspirates from the normal pancreas. Pancreatic ductal cells are arranged in characteristic large flat sheets with evenly spaced, round to oval nuclei and pale cytoplasm with distinct borders. Overall, such sheets have a honeycomb pattern (Figure 21-1). Nuclear contour irregularity, grooves, and nucleoli are generally not seen. Acinar cells are arranged in cohesive aggregates, consisting of cells with basally placed, small, uniform, round nuclei with finely granular chromatin and inconspicuous nucleoli surrounded by moderate amounts of granular cytoplasm. Islet cells are usually difficult to appreciate in aspirates of the normal

pancreas (Figure 21-2).[3,29] However, in some aspirates islets can be identified as loose, disorganized collections of small, round, uniform nuclei associated with variable amounts of pale, wispy cytoplasm. It is likely that these structures do not survive the process of smear preparation without considerable damage. Thus, using EUS-guided FNA samples, these authors have noted that even those smears with abundant ductal and acinar tissue rarely show identifiable islets. This chapter discusses the variety of nonneoplastic pancreatic lesions, as well as benign and malignant neoplasms that can be encountered in pancreatic aspirates.

Cystic Pancreatic Lesions

Cystic mass lesions of the pancreas can be congenital, retention, pseudocysts, parasitic, or cystic neoplasms.[30-47] The pseudocyst is the most common of these, usually resulting from postinflammatory conditions, trauma, surgery, or an unknown origin. The most common cause of pseudocyst in the United States is episodes of severe acute pancreatitis resulting from alcoholic injury. All pseudocysts, despite their etiologic factors, share an underlying pathogenesis of pancreatic enzyme release into the pancreatic parenchyma, resulting in proteolytic and lipolytic digestion of the tissue. Most pseudocysts occur within the lesser omental bursa. Pseudocysts have a luminal surface consisting of granulation tissue with surrounding fibrosis and lack, by definition, an epithelial lining.[33]

FNA of pseudocysts yields turbid fluid containing amorphous debris, calcified fragments, a few inflammatory cells, and mononucleated or multinucleated histiocytes (Figure 21-3 and Box 21-1).[1,2,10,17] Aspirates from the wall of the pseudocyst often contain fibroblasts and granulation tissue, characterized by scattered loosely cohesive groups and dispersed elongated-to-plump spindle-shaped cells. In older, inactive pseudocysts, granulation tissue may not be encountered, and the smears are very sparsely cellular.

Biochemical analysis of the pseudocyst fluid content reveals elevated amylase levels, in contrast with cystic carcinomas that have elevated levels of carcinoembryonic antigen (CEA).[34-39] Some medical centers perform biochemical analysis for these two markers when pancreatic cyst fluid is encountered.[39] Aspirates of pancreatic abscesses, in contrast, do not demonstrate either elevated amylase or CEA

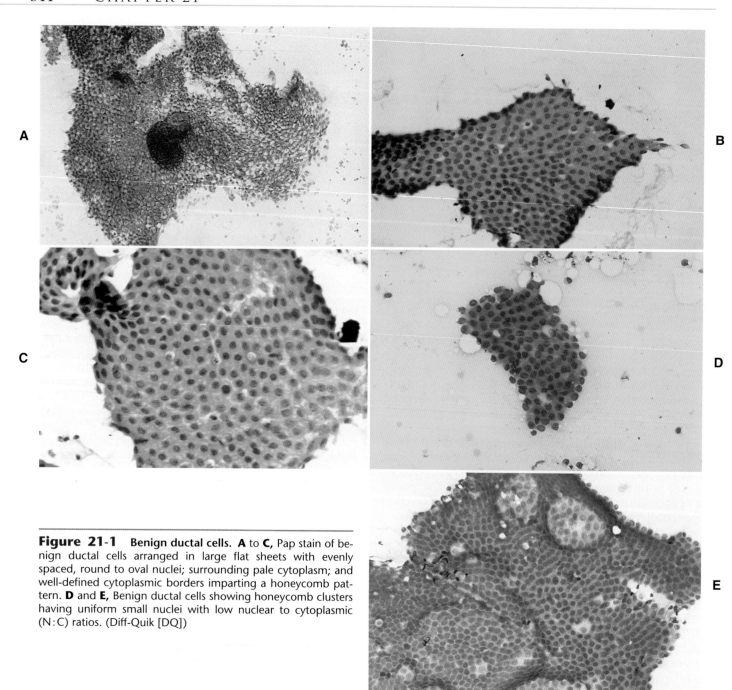

Figure 21-1   Benign ductal cells. **A** to **C,** Pap stain of benign ductal cells arranged in large flat sheets with evenly spaced, round to oval nuclei; surrounding pale cytoplasm; and well-defined cytoplasmic borders imparting a honeycomb pattern. **D** and **E,** Benign ductal cells showing honeycomb clusters having uniform small nuclei with low nuclear to cytoplasmic (N : C) ratios. (Diff-Quik [DQ])

levels. The cytologic smears of an abscess consists of neutrophils and granular debris in the background. Bacteria occasionally are seen and are better visualized in a Diff-Quik (DQ)–stained preparation. Gram stain and culture of the aspirated abscess render a more specific diagnosis.

Other unusual types of benign cystic lesions include the lymphoepithelial cyst and the dermoid cyst of the pancreas.[40-43] This pattern is familiar from sites where such lesions are more common, including the parotid gland. Aspirates of lymphoepithelial lesion consist of a mixture of mature squamous epithelial cells with and without nuclei, foamy histiocytes, lymphocytes, and cholesterol crystals.[40-43] The dermoid cyst may yield an indistinguishable picture. Malignant primary pancreatic neoplasms can present radiographically and grossly as a cystic mass. These are dis-

cussed in detail later in this chapter.[43-47] A benign epithelial cyst of the pancreas may accompany polycystic kidney disease. The aspirate will be paucicellular, consisting of a few small, flat, honeycomb clusters of epithelial cells (Figure 21-4).

Pancreatitis

Acute pancreatitis can result from a variety of underlying conditions, but the most common causes are obstruction of the pancreatic duct by gallstones and alcohol abuse.[48] An FNA biopsy is usually not performed on patients suspected to have acute pancreatitis because the diagnosis is often based on the characteristic clinical and radiologic findings, as well as laboratory tests demonstrating elevated serum

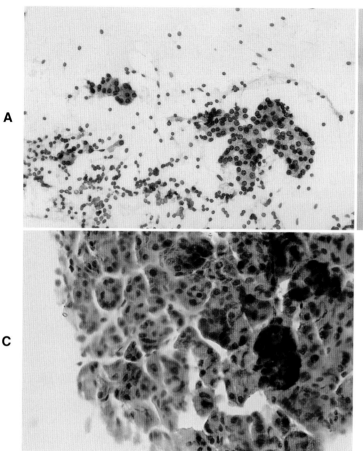

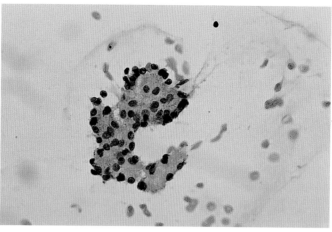

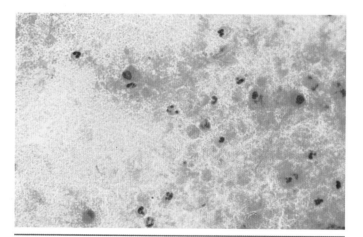

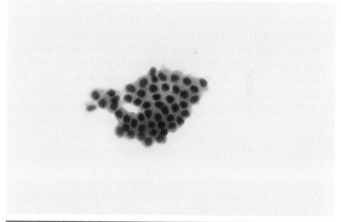

Figure 21-2 Benign acinar cells. **A** and **B,** Acinar cells are arranged in cohesive lobular clusters with small, basally placed, round nuclei and a moderate amount of granular cytoplasm. (Papanicolaou [Pap]) **C,** In this cell block from a pancreatic aspirate, the benign acinar cells maintain a lobulated pattern with basally placed nuclei and granular cytoplasm. (Hematoxylin and eosin [H&E])

Figure 21-3 Pseudocyst. Aspirate consisting predominantly of amorphous background debris with a few scattered neutrophils. (Pap)

Figure 21-4 Benign cyst. A small, flat, honeycomb cluster of benign epithelial cells is present in this aspirate of a pancreatic cyst from a patient with polycystic renal disease. (Pap)

BOX 21-1 CMF

Cytomorphologic Features of Pancreatic Pseudocyst

Scanty smear cellularity with only a few or no epithelial cells
Acute and chronic inflammatory cells, histiocytes
Granulation tissue
Background debris, calcium salts

---

levels of amylase and lipase. However, acute pancreatitis can occasionally present as a mass lesion.[49] Furthermore, both benign and malignant pancreatic neoplasms can cause obstruction of the pancreatic duct with subsequent development of an associated pancreatitis.[50] In both of these settings, a potential for a false-negative or false-positive diagnosis of malignancy exists. In an aspirate of a pancreatic neoplasm that inadvertently samples the surrounding acutely inflamed parenchyma rather than the tumor, a potential for a false-negative diagnosis exists. Conversely, an FNA biopsy of a mass related to acute pancreatitis may oc-

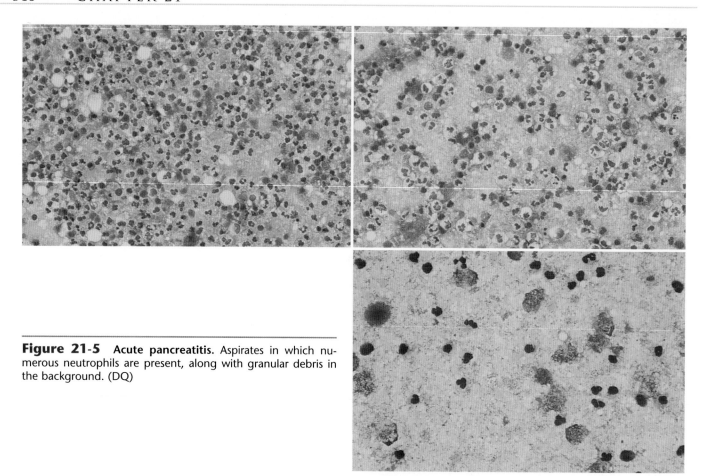

Figure 21-5 **Acute pancreatitis.** Aspirates in which numerous neutrophils are present, along with granular debris in the background. (DQ)

casionally demonstrate a significant degree of inflammatory atypia that could be misdiagnosed as a malignancy.

In any aspirate of acute pancreatitis, the smears are generally very cellular, with a predominance of intact and degenerating neutrophils (Figure 21-5 and Box 21-2). The smears contain abundant necrotic debris imparting a "dirty" appearance to the background. Pancreatic acinar cells can show varying degrees of degenerative change and inflammatory atypia but maintain their cohesive lobulated arrangement (Figure 21-6). The nuclear chromatin can vary from finely granular to pyknotic. Occasional groups of ductal cells are also present in the smears and are arranged in a flat, honeycomb pattern (Figure 21-7). Inflammatory atypia and regenerative and reparative changes of the ductal cells could also potentially contribute to a false-positive diagnosis of malignancy in aspirates of acute pancreatitis. Therefore, it is strongly recommended that a conservative approach be used whenever a prominent acute inflammatory cell infiltrate is present. A definite unequivocal diagnosis of pancreatic carcinoma should never be rendered if diagnostic criteria of malignancy are not present. A detailed discussion of the important differential diagnostic features of inflammatory atypia and pancreatic carcinoma is presented in the section of this chapter on Pancreatic Adenocarcinoma.

Chronic pancreatitis usually follows multiple episodes of acute pancreatitis, although it is not unusual for the prior episodes of acute pancreatitis to have been clinically silent. In contrast with acute pancreatitis, aspirates of chronic pancreatitis generally show a limited number of epithelial cells resulting from the fibrous replacement of the exocrine

---

BOX 21-2   CMF

Cytomorphologic Features of Acute Pancreatitis

Moderate to high smear cellularity consisting predominantly of inflammatory cells with a "dirty" smear background
Numerous neutrophils often with degenerative features
Acinar cells with variable degenerative changes
Low numbers of ductal cells with possible reparative and inflammatory atypia
Fat necrosis with granular debris and foam cells

---

parenchyma (Box 21-3). Numerous scattered acute and chronic inflammatory cells, calcified and granular debris, and fragments of fibroconnective tissue may often be seen (Figure 21-8). Acinar cells maintain their lobular arrangement, and a few scattered groups of ductal cells having a honeycomb appearance are found.

In chronic pancreatitis, prominent reparative and inflammatory atypia can be present, but in contrast with malignancy, a paucity or only a few individually scattered, single atypical cells are present. The inflammatory epithelial atypia in the ductal cells is characterized by nuclear enlargement with some nucleolar prominence. However, the epithelial atypia is usually less than what is seen in aspirates of acute pancreatitis. Fat necrosis can also be appreciated in some aspirations of pancreatitis (Figure 21-9).

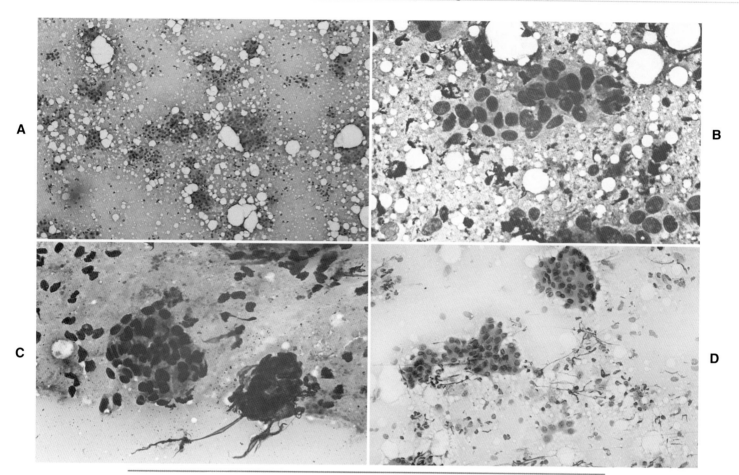

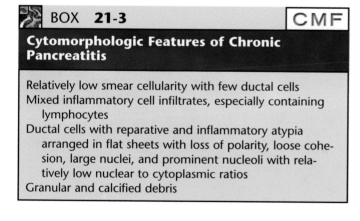

Figure 21-6 **Acute pancreatitis with inflammatory atypia. A** to **C,** Aspirate showing a moderate degree of cellularity in which the pancreatic acinar cells demonstrate inflammatory atypia characterized by slight variation in nuclear size and nuclear overlapping. A conservative approach is warranted whenever numerous neutrophils are present in the background. (DQ) **D,** In this Pap-stained smear from an aspirate of acute pancreatitis, clusters of acinar cells are present, demonstrating nuclear overlapping. Numerous neutrophils are also present in the background.

BOX 21-3 **CMF**

Cytomorphologic Features of Chronic Pancreatitis

Relatively low smear cellularity with few ductal cells

Mixed inflammatory cell infiltrates, especially containing lymphocytes

Ductal cells with reparative and inflammatory atypia arranged in flat sheets with loss of polarity, loose cohesion, large nuclei, and prominent nucleoli with relatively low nuclear to cytoplasmic ratios

Granular and calcified debris

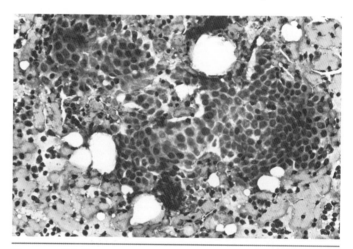

Figure 21-7 **Acute pancreatitis.** In this aspirate, flat sheets of ductal cells are present, along with numerous inflammatory cells, not only in the background, but also within the epithelial groups. (DQ)

The dense fibrosis of long-standing chronic pancreatitis can lead to very scanty aspiration samples. Evidence for this disorder can be limited to a few small fragments of parenchyma in which residual acini are widely separated by fibrous tissue. This contrasts with the normal pancreas, in which connective tissue between the acini is minimal or imperceptible. The metachromasia of extracellular matrix makes this fibrous tissue very easy to identify in air-dried smear material. It is also readily apparent in cell block sections.

A further difficulty with chronic pancreatitis is that by EUS it can either obscure mass lesions that might also be present or can itself appear tumefactive. Given nonspecific clinical findings related to pancreatitis, an equivocal sonographic picture and a sparsely cellular aspirate showing be-

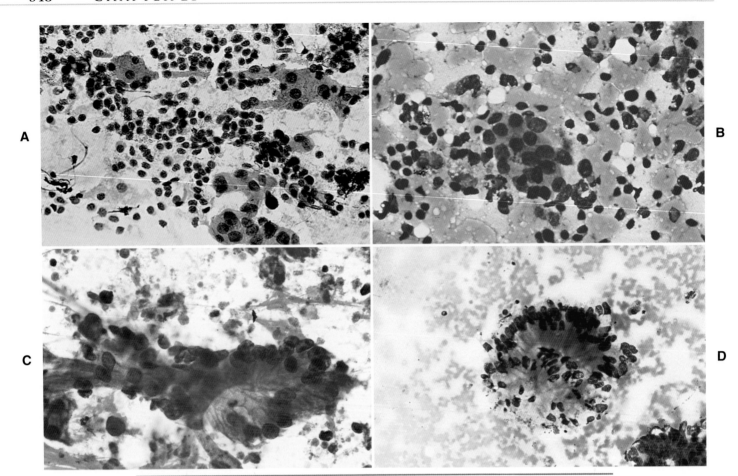

Figure 21-8   Chronic pancreatitis. **A,** In this aspirate, three small clusters of mildly atypical ductal cells are present, along with numerous lymphocytes. (Pap) **B,** Aspirate of chronic pancreatitis revealing a rare cluster of mildly atypical acinar cells showing focal nuclear overlapping. Numerous lymphocytes are present in the background. (DQ) **C,** Aspirate of chronic pancreatitis in which the rare cluster of ductal cells maintains a honeycomb pattern, although some atypical features are present, including slight variation in nuclear size and nuclear overlapping. Numerous lymphocytes are present in the background. (DQ) **D,** Aspirate of chronic pancreatitis showing a cohesive cluster of ductal cells. (DQ)

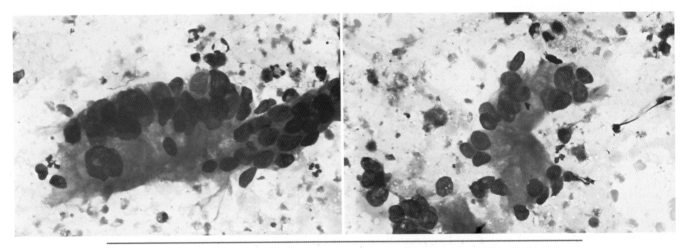

Figure 21-9   Fat necrosis. Aspirate of pancreatitis in which there is evidence of fat necrosis, as well as atypical epithelial cell clusters. (DQ)

nign (albeit abnormal) parenchyma, the ultimate diagnosis of pancreatitis is frequently not in the hands of the cytopathologist. The cytopathologist's primary contribution in such cases is to examine multiple EUS-guided aspirate samples and to pronounce them free of malignancy. Decisions regarding the extent of sampling and the final clinicopathologic correlation remain for the clinical team. These authors feel that the assistance of the cytopathologist in this situation is most effective when he or she is present at the time of EUS, is aware of the clinical dilemma, and offers immediate feedback by rapid interpretation of each sample.

Chronic pancreatitis with acinar atrophy often leaves behind extensive fibrous tissue in which numerous islets appear enlarged and crowded. Given the previously discussed limitations in islet sampling during most aspirations, cytopathologists may find themselves ill-prepared to interpret large numbers of islet cells and tissue fragments. This has been a cause of false-positive pancreatic cytology.

Pancreatic Adenocarcinoma

Adenocarcinoma of the pancreas is a common malignancy, representing approximately 3% of all cancers and 5% of cancer mortality.[51,52] An increasing incidence of pancreatic carcinoma has occurred over the past 50 years in the United States. Ductal adenocarcinoma is the most common type of pancreatic carcinoma, accounting for more than 75% of all exocrine carcinomas. Pancreatic adenocarcinoma is a malignancy of adult men and women, having an extremely aggressive course with reported survival rates of less than 5%. The majority of patients usually succumb within 12 to 16 months of diagnosis.[53] Cigarette smoking and diets high in fat have been implicated as etiologic factors for the development of pancreatic carcinoma, although it is still controversial whether chronic pancreatitis predisposes to malignancy. Long-standing diabetes, alcohol use, and caffeine use are not currently believed to be etiologic factors for the development of pancreatic carcinoma.[54]

The clinical presentation of pancreatic carcinoma is dependent on the location of the malignancy. Neoplasms located in the head of the pancreas often cause obstructive symptoms early in the patient's course. Tumors of the body and tail remain clinically silent with late presentation. Most patients also have abdominal pain and demonstrate weight loss.

The FNA cytologic diagnosis of ductal pancreatic carcinoma is usually not difficult because the smears are highly cellular. Most aspirates show atypical cells arranged in large sheets, small aggregates, and singly (Figure 21-10 and Box 21-4).[1-3] A definite diagnosis of pancreatic carcinoma should not be made when the smear is paucicellular or contains only a few individually scattered atypical epithelial cells. The prohibition on diagnosing carcinoma in the setting of appreciable acute inflammation was noted previously.

The atypical cells of pancreatic carcinoma demonstrate anisonucleosis and nuclear pleomorphism with few to many of the ductal cells having large irregular nuclei and prominent nucleoli (Figure 21-11). As the ductal carcinoma becomes more poorly differentiated, greater discohesion, with many more individually scattered malignant cells, is present, and cell clusters become more disorganized (Figure 21-12).

BOX 21-4 | CMF

Cytomorphologic Features of Ductal Adenocarcinoma

High smear cellularity with reduced cohesion and single scattered atypical cells
Altered polarity within groups and syncytial arrangement
Nuclear and cellular enlargement
Hyperchromatic, irregularly distributed chromatin
Irregular nuclear contours including grooves
Prominent nucleoli
Anisonucleosis
Relatively normal to increased nuclear to cytoplasmic ratios
Tumor diathesis

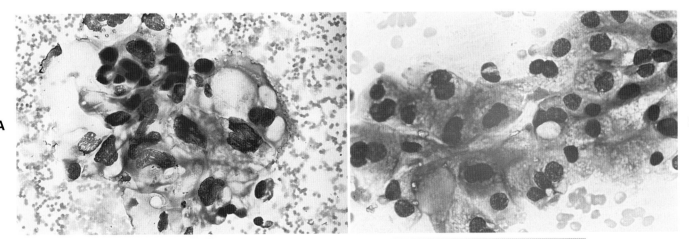

Figure 21-10 **Ductal carcinoma. A,** Pancreatic ductal carcinoma demonstrating a large sheet of malignant cells. (Pap) **B,** Smear of pancreatic carcinoma showing a large, flat sheet of malignant cells. (DQ)

In contrast with benign ductal cells, the carcinoma cells show both nuclear and cytoplasmic enlargement with increased nuclear to cytoplasmic (N:C) ratios (Figure 21-13). The latter feature, however, may not be seen in all cases, and occasional aspirates consist of atypical cells having relatively normal to only slightly increased N:C ratios (Figure 21-14). Other malignant features include loss of polarity within the groups and nuclear crowding and overlapping, which tend to be accentuated as the tumor becomes more poorly differentiated. The cell borders generally become indistinct, imparting a syncytial arrangement of the cells (Figure 21-15).

A frequent diagnostic challenge is the aspirate from a well-differentiated ductal carcinoma that contains large flat sheets of cells that maintain a highly organized honeycomb pattern (Figure 21-16). A false-negative diagnosis can be avoided when one appreciates that the cells demonstrate some variation in nuclear size within the groups and evidence of nuclear irregularity and grooving (Figure 21-17). These atypical features need to be recognized in more than a rare cell, before a definitive diagnosis of malignancy is made. If this is only an isolated feature, then a qualified diagnosis needs to be rendered reflecting the diagnostic uncertainty. As the grade of the malignancy increases, greater loss of polarity with increasing nuclear overlapping and molding is present. Greater numbers of dispersed malignant cells are also appreciated.

Although the diagnosis is most often straightforward, diagnostic challenges include the separation of benign ductal cells showing inflammatory atypia and regenerative/reparative changes in the setting of pancreatitis from an aspirate of well-differentiated adenocarcinoma. Some investigators

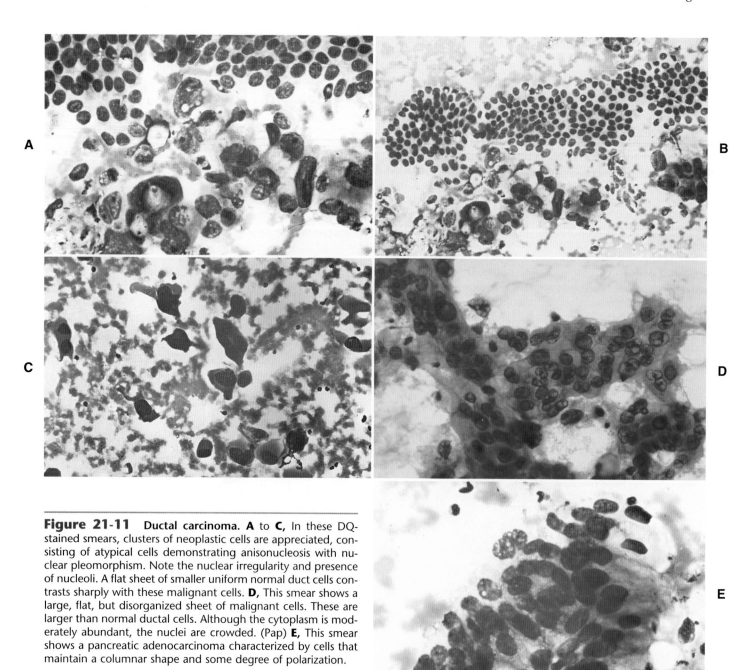

Figure 21-11 Ductal carcinoma. **A** to **C,** In these DQ-stained smears, clusters of neoplastic cells are appreciated, consisting of atypical cells demonstrating anisonucleosis with nuclear pleomorphism. Note the nuclear irregularity and presence of nucleoli. A flat sheet of smaller uniform normal duct cells contrasts sharply with these malignant cells. **D,** This smear shows a large, flat, but disorganized sheet of malignant cells. These are larger than normal ductal cells. Although the cytoplasm is moderately abundant, the nuclei are crowded. (Pap) **E,** This smear shows a pancreatic adenocarcinoma characterized by cells that maintain a columnar shape and some degree of polarization.

have found that the most helpful cytologic features of malignancy in both Pap and Romanowsky-stained smears include the presence of large nuclei that are at least two times the size of normal ductal cells, nuclear molding, and variability in nuclear size defined by cells having nuclei at least

three times the size of other atypical ductal cells within the same epithelial group (Figure 21-18). Cohen and colleagues, using these three cytomorphologic features, reported a diagnostic sensitivity and specificity of 98% and 100%, respectively, for pancreatic adenocarcinoma.[14] However, only one half of their cases of pancreatic carcinoma demonstrated all three features. In Cohen's series, benign aspirates lacked cells possessing nuclear grooves, pseudoinclusions, and macronucleoli. These cytologic features, however, were not demonstrated by carcinomas with sufficient frequency to be statistically significant.[14]

Using a similar statistical approach, Robins and colleagues, however, found that irregular nuclear contours, irregularly distributed chromatin, and crowding with overlapping of nuclei were the three most important cytologic features for the diagnosis of ductal carcinoma.[15] Additional minor cytologic features useful for the diagnosis of malignancy included nuclear enlargement, increased numbers of mitotic figures, background necrosis, and individually scattered atypical epithelial cells. If an aspirate contained two or three of the major criteria or one major and three minor features, the diagnostic sensitivity and specificity for pancreatic carcinoma were 90% and 100%, respectively.[15]

The major cytologic criteria separating ductal carcinoma from inflammatory atypia in pancreatic aspirates are de-

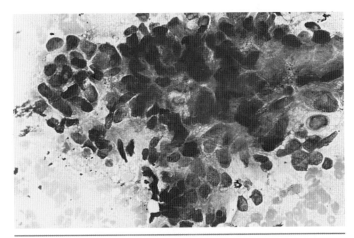

Figure 21-12 **Ductal carcinoma.** As pancreatic carcinoma becomes more poorly differentiated, the cell clusters become more disorganized. (DQ)

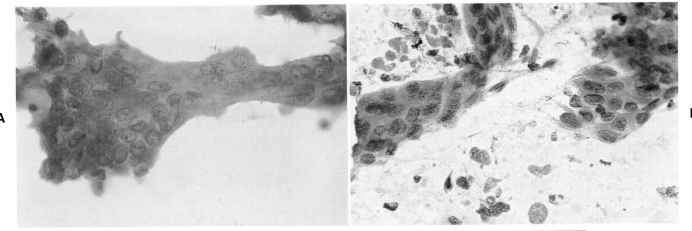

A B

Figure 21-13 **Ductal carcinoma.** **A** and **B,** In the DQ-stained smears, ductal carcinoma cells demonstrate increased nuclear size and N:C ratios.

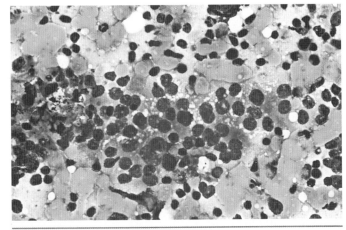

Figure 21-14 **Ductal carcinoma.** Some carcinomas show cells with only a mild elevation in N:C ratio. (DQ)

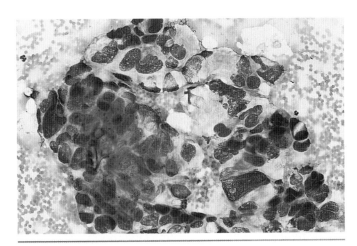

Figure 21-15 **Ductal carcinoma.** Aspirate in which the tumor cells show considerable nuclear crowding and overlapping. (DQ)

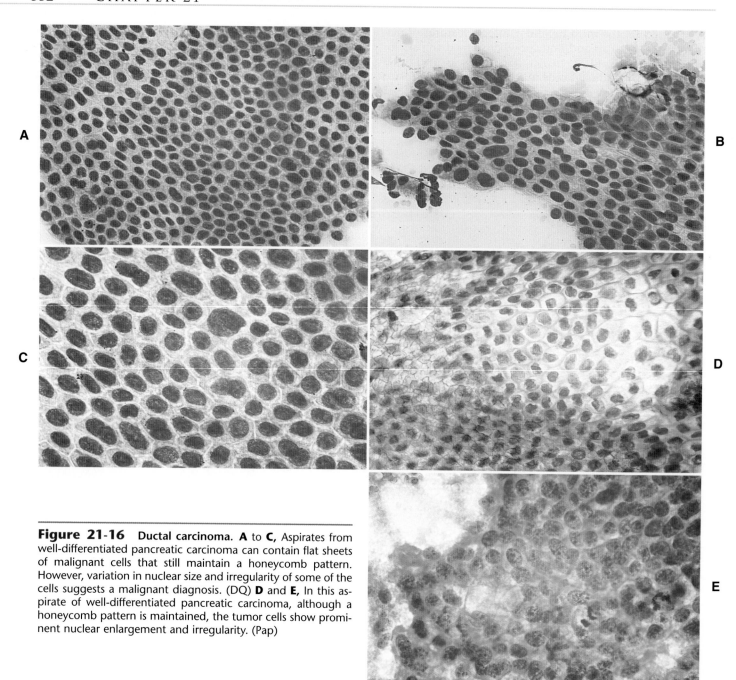

Figure 21-16 Ductal carcinoma. A to C, Aspirates from well-differentiated pancreatic carcinoma can contain flat sheets of malignant cells that still maintain a honeycomb pattern. However, variation in nuclear size and irregularity of some of the cells suggests a malignant diagnosis. (DQ) **D** and **E,** In this aspirate of well-differentiated pancreatic carcinoma, although a honeycomb pattern is maintained, the tumor cells show prominent nuclear enlargement and irregularity. (Pap)

tailed in Table 21-1. Most helpful cytologic features of acute pancreatitis are cells arranged almost exclusively in tightly cohesive monolayer sheets with a paucity of isolated single atypical cells. Inflammatory atypia of benign nuclei may be reflected by nuclear enlargement, but generally, the N:C ratios are not obviously increased. Nucleoli may be prominent but are single and smooth. In addition, the diagnostic threshold for adenocarcinoma needs to be elevated whenever neutrophils are present in the smears and especially when they are seen infiltrating the epithelial cell groups. Conversely, aspirates of well-differentiated adenocarcinoma can occasionally consist of some cellular groups arranged in a flat honeycomb pattern mimicking normal-appearing ductal cells, but nuclei are generally larger than normal

ductal cells and show a greater degree of variation in size and membrane irregularity. If the smears are carefully examined, more than a rare single abnormal glandular cell is evident.

It is well known that fresh cells shrink during fixation but swell during air-drying. The former tends to minimize and the latter to accentuate differences in size among various cell populations. In these authors' experiences, one of the most helpful features in recognizing flat sheets of well-differentiated cells as malignant is the striking range of cell and nuclear sizes within a single group. This is exaggerated in air-dried material, and these authors find that this greatly facilitates interpretation. Furthermore, this is most apparent in the lowest-grade cases. These are tumors that have

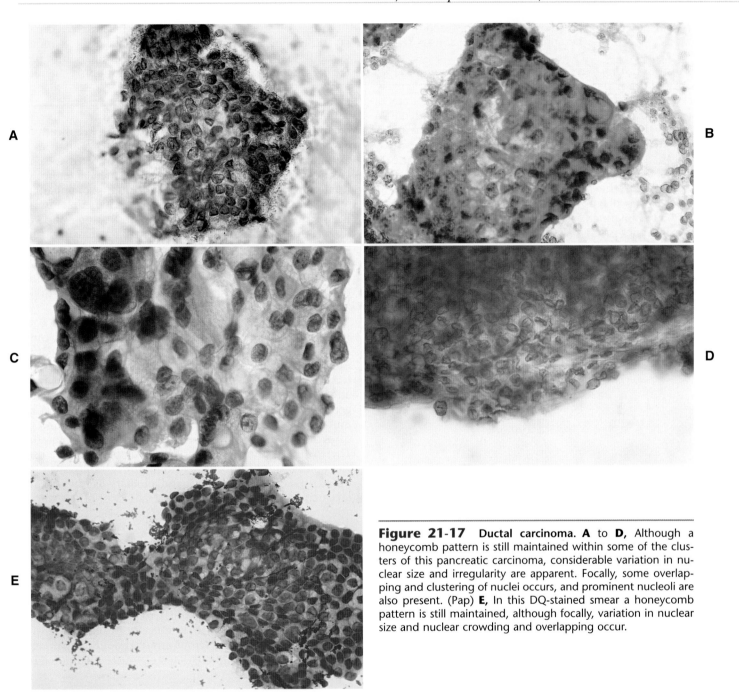

Figure 21-17 **Ductal carcinoma. A** to **D,** Although a honeycomb pattern is still maintained within some of the clusters of this pancreatic carcinoma, considerable variation in nuclear size and irregularity are apparent. Focally, some overlapping and clustering of nuclei occurs, and prominent nucleoli are also present. (Pap) **E,** In this DQ-stained smear a honeycomb pattern is still maintained, although focally, variation in nuclear size and nuclear crowding and overlapping occur.

minimal expression of malignant nuclear features; most cells show pale nuclei with rounded contours and thin smooth membranes. Thus, nuclear size variability emerges as a critical diagnostic finding.

This variation in size is also helpful in the comparison of low-grade carcinoma cells to either normal pancreatic ductal cells or to normal GI lumenal cells. As discussed more fully in the following text, the latter often heavily contaminate EUS-guided FNA samples. In air-dried preparations the often remarkable size difference between the normal cells and the carcinoma cells can be striking. In these authors' experiences, this—combined with the rapidity and ease of preparing DQ-stained smears—greatly facilitates rapid onsite interpretation of EUS samples.

Another diagnostic challenge is the accurate diagnosis of occasional mucin-producing variants of well-differentiated adenocarcinoma that could potentially be confused with benign ductal cells (Figure 21-19). Aspirates from this variant of pancreatic carcinoma occasionally consists of superficially bland-appearing cells having relatively low N:C ratios resulting from the abundant intracytoplasmic mucin. However, nuclear irregularity, including nuclear grooving, is present. Mucinous cystadenocarcinomas also have elevated CEA levels in the aspirated cyst fluid and background necrotic material and extracellular mucin.[34-38,47,55]

Occasional squamous differentiation (Figure 21-20) or papillary groupings can be present in aspirates of pancreatic cancer (Figure 21-21). Desmoplastic stromal reaction to the tumor cells can also be appreciated in the smears (Figure 21-22).

Although most centers employ percutaneous FNA biopsy of the pancreas for the workup of pancreatic mass, recent reports describe the use and diagnostic accuracy of intraoperative FNA biopsy[19,20,56-59,73-75] and EUS-guided FNA biopsy.[5,7] In a review of nine series of intraoperative FNA biopsy consisting of 274 patients, the diagnostic sensitivity of the procedure ranged from 73% to 100%, and the diagnostic specificity was 100% with no false-positive diagnoses.[59] In another report of 92 intraoperative pancreatic aspirates, the diagnostic sensitivity and specificity were 100%.[58] In a manner similar to that noted previously, Yang and colleagues[58] found that nuclear size and variability appreciated in the DQ-stained smears were the most helpful cytologic features separating pancreatitis from ductal adenocarcinoma. EUS-guided FNA biopsy of pancreatic masses has also been found to be an accurate diagnostic procedure.[4,5]

Immunohistochemistry can find utility in selected pancreatic lesions,[1,2] whereas most other ancillary techniques currently have only a limited role in the evaluation of pancreatic carcinoma.[60-67] Serologic and immunohistochemical analysis for CA-19 has also been employed for the diagnosis of pancreatic carcinoma but lack specificity.[67] *p53* Tumor suppressor gene mutation has been demonstrated in pancreatic carcinoma and may have prognostic implications. Several studies apply flow cytometry or image analysis of aspiration smears for the evaluation of DNA ploidy of pancreatic carcinoma.[61-62] As expected, most ductal adenocarcinomas are aneuploid. However, surprisingly, some pancreatic adenocarcinomas may be diploid, and aneuploidy has been seen in benign pancreatic aspirates. Bottger and colleagues found that the DNA content of pancreatic carcinoma was the second most important prognostic parameter following the type of surgical procedure employed.[63] Although these studies may infer some prognostic information, DNA analysis has a minimal role in the FNA workup of pancreatic carcinoma at the present time.

Oncogenes and tumor suppressive genes have also been studied in pancreatic carcinomas, with most ductal carcinomas demonstrating a *K-ras* oncogene mutation. Using the polymerase chain reaction, this oncogene has been detected in aspiration specimens,[64-66] whereas benign pancreatic lesions have not been shown to express the *K-ras* oncogene. The authors have previously demonstrated *K-ras* mutations in pleomorphic giant cell carcinoma and in osteoclast-like giant cell tumor using aspirated material. Therefore, this molecular marker could potentially be used to improve the diagnostic sensitivity of FNA biopsy.[67] The differential diagnostic clinical and ancillary features of ductal carcinoma are contrasted with a variety of other pancreatic neoplasms in Tables 21-2 and 21-3.

Pleomorphic Giant Cell Carcinoma

Pleomorphic giant cell carcinoma (PGCC), also known as *anaplastic carcinoma of the pancreas,* is a highly aggressive pancreatic tumor accounting for approximately 2% of pancreatic malignancies.[52,68,69] Similar to the usual pancreatic carcinoma, most patients are middle-age or older men who present with nonspecific symptoms of abdominal pain and weight loss. Not all patients have obstructive jaundice be-

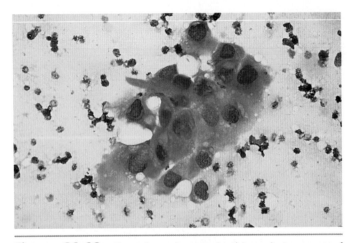

Figure 21-18 Ductal carcinoma. In this aspirate, some of the clusters simulate a repair-type pattern characterized by flat sheets having a streaming pattern of cells with relatively low N:C ratios. However, note the huge size of the nuclei compared with the red blood cells (RBCs) in the background. In other areas of the smears, individually scattered tumor cells were appreciated. (DQ)

TABLE 21-1		
Comparison of Cytomorphologic Features of Benign and Malignant Pancreatic Aspirates		
Feature	**Benign Inflammatory Atypia and Repair**	**Adenocarcinoma**
Cellularity	Low-moderate	Moderate-high
Epithelial aggregates	Flat, loose monolayers	Tight to loose three-dimensional
Polarity	Generally maintained	Altered
Isolated cells (reduced cohesion)	Rare	May be numerous
Nuclear enlargement	Present	Present
Nuclear contours	Smooth to slightly irregular	Smooth to very irregular
Macronucleoli	Rare; when present, regular	Frequent, often irregular
Nuclear to cytoplasmic ratios	Normal to slightly increased	Normal to increased
Necrotic debris	May be present	May be present

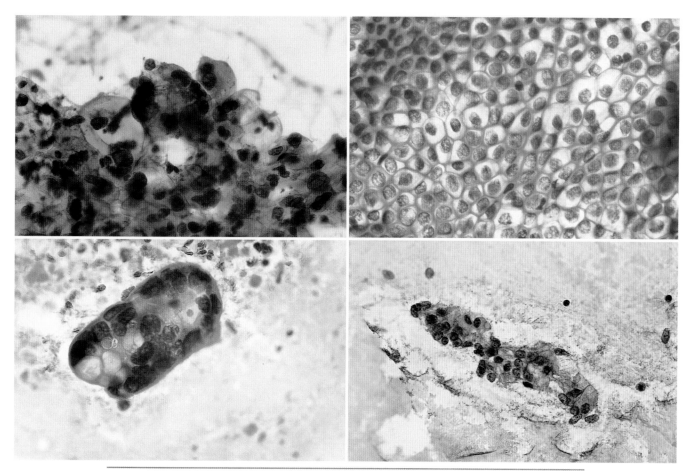

Figure 21-19 Mucin-producing adenocarcinoma. In this Pap-stained smear from an aspirate of mucin-producing well-differentiated adenocarcinoma, some of the tumor cells maintain relatively low N:C ratios. However, nuclear irregularity and some variation in nuclear size are present.

A

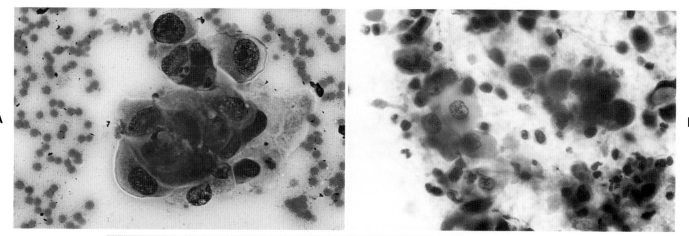

B

Figure 21-20 Poorly differentiated ductal carcinoma with squamous differentiation. **A,** In this DQ-stained smear of a poorly differentiated pancreatic carcinoma, some of the tumor cells show squamous differentiation characterized by more opaque dense cytoplasm with sharp cytoplasmic borders. **B,** In the Pap-stained smears, besides numerous individually dispersed tumor cells, loose clusters demonstrating squamous differentiation, characterized by eosinophilic opaque cytoplasm and sharp cytoplasmic borders, are present.

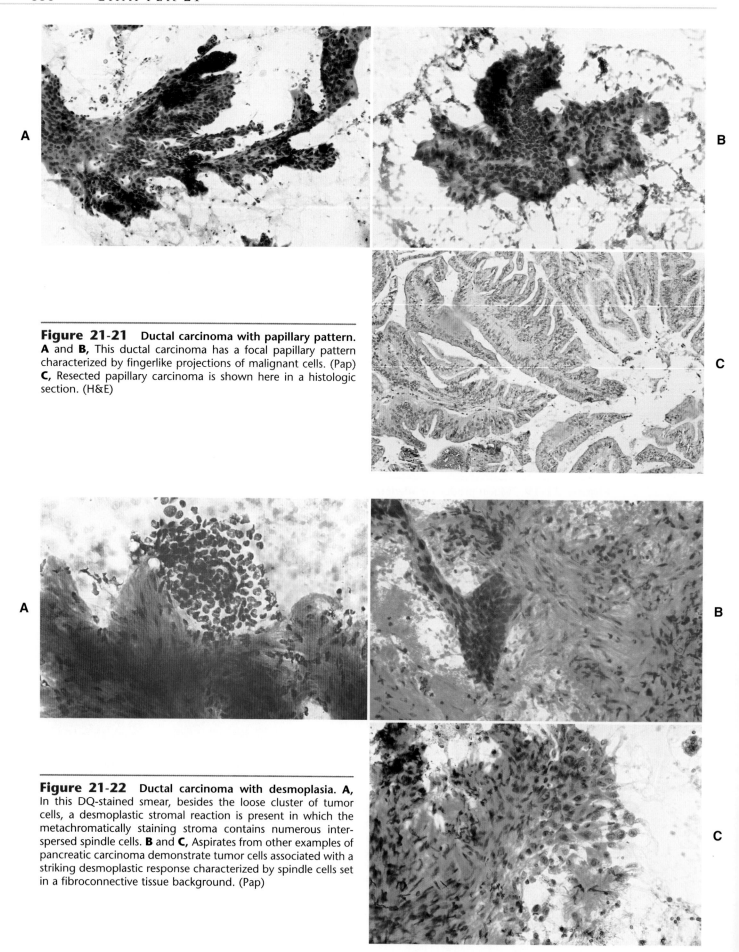

Figure 21-21 Ductal carcinoma with papillary pattern. **A** and **B,** This ductal carcinoma has a focal papillary pattern characterized by fingerlike projections of malignant cells. (Pap) **C,** Resected papillary carcinoma is shown here in a histologic section. (H&E)

Figure 21-22 Ductal carcinoma with desmoplasia. **A,** In this DQ-stained smear, besides the loose cluster of tumor cells, a desmoplastic stromal reaction is present in which the metachromatically staining stroma contains numerous interspersed spindle cells. **B** and **C,** Aspirates from other examples of pancreatic carcinoma demonstrate tumor cells associated with a striking desmoplastic response characterized by spindle cells set in a fibroconnective tissue background. (Pap)

TABLE	21-2

Pancreatic Neoplasms: Clinical Settings

Tumor Type	Age	Gender	Location	Clinical Features	Site	Prognosis	Putative Origin
Ductal cancer	Adult, middle age to elderly	1:1	Anywhere, head majority	Abdominal and back pain, jaundice, weight loss	Variable	Dismal; <2% 5-year survival	Ductal progenitor cells
ICT	Adult > child; 28-78; mean: 56.7	10F:6M	Body and tail	Hormonal syndromes; insulinomas; Z-E		Metastases common	Islets of Langerhans
PGCC	Adult 42-82; mean: 67	1F:4M	Body and tail	Mimics ductal carcinoma	Large	Metastases common; very poor	Sarcomatoid transformation
PCT	Adolescent and young adult	F>M		Long history, mimics pseudocyst		Intermediate; low malignant potential	Unknown
MCA	Middle age	F>M	Body and tail			Intermediate	Ductal cells
OGCT	Mean: 60	F>M	Head		Large	Poor	Controversial
PBT	Children; all ages		Anywhere		Large		Uncertain

Modified from Silverman JF, Geisinger KR. FNA of thorax and abdomen. New York: Churchill Livingstone; 1996. pp.135-170; Geisinger KR, Silverman JF. Fine-needle aspiration cytology of uncommon primary pancreatic neoplasms: a personal experience and review of the literature. In: Schmidt WA, editor. Cytopathology annual. Baltimore: Williams & Wilkins; 1991. pp. 1-23.

ICT, Islet cell tumor; *F,* female; *M,* male; *Z-E,* Zollinger-Ellison syndrome; *PGCC,* pleomorphic giant cell carcinoma; *PCT,* papillary-cystic tumor; *MCA,* mucinous cystadenocarcinoma; *OGCT,* osteoclastic giant cell tumor; *PBT,* pancreatoblastoma.

TABLE 21-3
Pancreatic Neoplasms: Ancillary Studies

Tumor Type	TEM	CK	EMA	V	NSE	CEA	Lysoz	A1AT	A1ACT	CGR
Ductal cancer	Junctions, microvilli, tonofilaments	+	+	≥	−	±, usually +	−	−	−	−
ICT	NSGs	±	−		+	−	−	−	−	+
PGCC	See text	±	±	+	−	±	−	−	−	−
PCT (1)	See text	−	±	±	±	±	±	±	±	−
MCA		+	+	−		+	−	−	−	−
OGCT		−	−	+		−	−	+	+	−
PBT (1)	NSGs	+	±	−	+	±	−	+	+	±

Modified from Modified from Silverman JF, Geisinger KR. FNA of thorax and abdomen. New York: Churchill Livingstone; 1996. pp.135-170; Geisinger KR, Silverman JF. Fine-needle aspiration cytology of uncommon primary pancreatic neoplasms: a personal experience and review of the literature. In: Schmidt WA, editor. Cytopathology annual. Baltimore: Williams & Wilkins; 1991. pp. 1-23.
TEM, Transmission electron microscopy; *CK,* cytokeratin; *EMA,* epithelial membrane antigen; *V,* vimentin; *NSE,* neuron specific enolase; *CEA,* carcinoembryonic antigen polyclonal antibodies (all others are monoclonal); *Lysoz,* lysozyme; *AIAT,* α-1-antripysin; *A1ACT,* α₁-antichymotrypsin; *CGR,* chromogranin; *ICT,* islet cell tumor; *NSGs,* neurosecretory-type granules; *PGCC,* pleomorphic giant cell carcinoma; *PCT,* papillary-cystic tumor; *MCA,* mucinous cystadenocarcinoma; *OGCT,* osteoclastic giant cell tumor; *PBT,* pancreatoblastoma; +, positive immunostaining; −, negative; ±, variable.

BOX 21-5 · CMF
Cytomorphologic Features of Pleomorphic Giant Cell Carcinoma (Anaplastic Carcinoma)

Highly cellular smears with predominance of individual tumor cells

Marked pleomorphism, including giant cells, both mono- and multinucleated and oval to spindle-shaped tumor cells

Large irregular nuclei with coarsely granular hyperchromatic chromatin and one or more huge nucleoli

Rhabdoid phenotype (i.e., hyaline globules) may be present in the cytoplasm

Cytophagocytosis of neutrophils

Background of necrotic debris and many neutrophils

---

cause this malignant tumor has a tendency to more often arise in the body and tail of the pancreas. The prognosis of PGCC is dismal, with almost all patients succumbing within 6 months of diagnosis.[69]

FNA of PGCC of the pancreas yields cellular smears in which a striking discohesion of the cells is reflected by numerous singly dispersed pleomorphic malignant cells (Box 21-5). Cellular and nuclear pleomorphism are apparent, with round, polygonal, spindled, or multinucleated tumor giant cells (Figure 21-23). The presence of multinucleated tumor giant cells and malignant spindle cells imparts a sarcomatoid appearance to the aspirate. Nuclei tend to be large and irregular with coarse hyperchromatic chromatin and one or more prominent irregular nucleoli. Smaller, more conventional-appearing malignant cells can also be present.

Another distinctive feature of PGCC is phagocytosis of neutrophils by the giant tumor cells (Figure 21-24). Almost all cases show a prominent tumor diathesis with scattered inflammatory cells in the background (see Figure 21-24). Some aspirates demonstrate neoplastic cells expressing a rhabdoid phenotype, characterized by round hyaline-appearing inclusions in the cytoplasm and nuclei with single large nucleoli (Figure 21-25). If numerous three-dimensional cohesive clusters of malignant cells are present or if mucin can be demonstrated, these malignant tumors are classified as poorly differentiated adenocarcinoma rather than PGCC. However, a minor component of cohesive malignant cells does not detract from the diagnosis of PGCC. Because of the sarcomatoid appearance of the cells, the differential diagnosis includes secondary involvement of the pancreas by other poorly differentiated malignancies such as a sarcoma invading from the retroperitoneum, as well as metastatic extrapancreatic pleomorphic carcinoma and malignant melanoma.[1,2,16]

On strictly cytologic grounds, it may be impossible to distinguish a PGCC from a high-grade sarcoma because both may consist of pleomorphic giant or spindle cells. Prominent cytophagocytosis and neutrophilic exudate in the background would favor a PGCC, as would immunohistochemical demonstration of cytokeratin positivity.[69] However, similar to sarcoma, PCGG is often positive for vimentin.[69] Metastatic malignant melanoma should be suspected when nuclear pseudoinclusions are seen, and the diagnosis is supported when intracytoplasmic melanin granules are demonstrated. In amelanotic cases, ancillary studies for melanocytic differentiation such as S-100 protein, HMB-45, and MelanA would be diagnostic. Ultrastructural demonstration of intracytoplasmic melanosomes and premelanosomes is reserved for the most difficult cases. For completeness sake, primary retroperitoneal or metastatic nonseminomatous germ cell tumors such as choriocarcinoma could also be considered, although this possibility is rarely encountered.[70] Germ cell tumors show some cytologic features to suggest epithelial differentiation, plus placental alkaline phosphatase (PLAP) positivity. Choriocarcinomas are positive for human chorionic gonadotrophin (HCG), and the patient will have a positive urine pregnancy test. Finally, the arbitrary distinction between a poorly differentiated ductal carcinoma and PGCC of the pancreas is predicated on the greater tendency for poorly differentiated adenocarcinoma to have intracytoplasmic mucin or cells arranged in clusters. This contrasts with the prominence of individually dispersed cells in PGCC.[1,16]

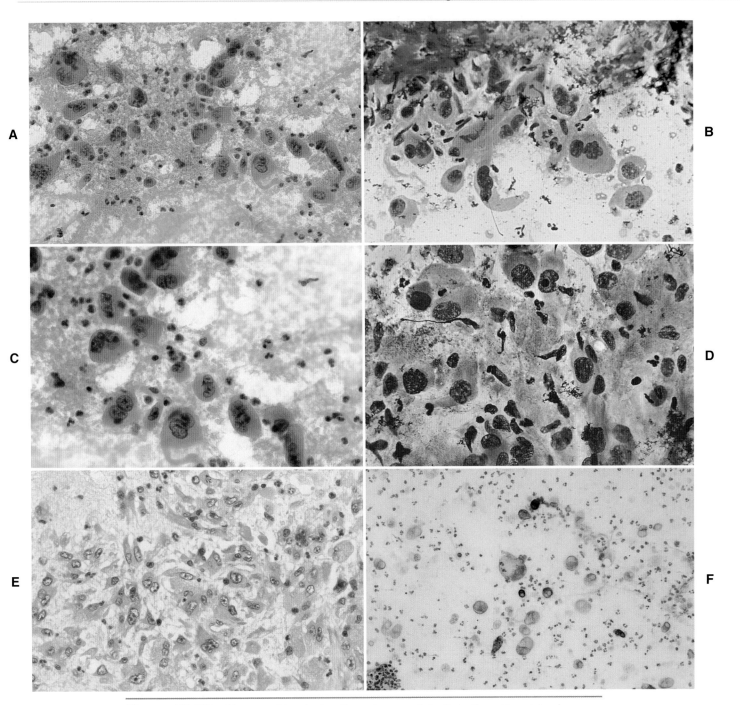

Figure 21-23 **Pleomorphic giant cell carcinoma.** **A** to **C,** In these Pap-stained smears, the characteristic feature of a pleomorphic giant cell carcinoma of the pancreas are appreciated, including both malignant multinucleated and spindle-shaped tumor cells arranged in a dissociative fashion. **D,** This DQ-stained smear of a pleomorphic giant cell carcinoma of the pancreas reveals numerous individually scattered tumor cells, including some that are multinucleated with huge nucleoli. **E,** Cell block section from an aspirate of pleomorphic giant cell carcinoma. (H&E) **F,** Cytokeratin immunohistochemical stain decorates the scattered malignant cells.

Osteoclast-Like Giant Cell Tumors

Osteoclast-like giant cell tumor (OGCT) is another exceedingly rare pancreatic malignancy that is a histologic and cytologic "look-alike" for the common giant cell tumor of bone.[71,72] In the authors' report of OGCT of the pancreas, the median age of patients was 60 years with a slight female predominance.[73] The patient's clinical signs and symptoms are no different than those in con-

ventional ductal adenocarcinoma, and like PGCC and conventional ductal carcinomas, the prognosis is poor with an average survival of less than 1 year from diagnosis. Only a few FNA cytologic reports of OGCT are in the literature.[73-76]

In the case the authors encountered, the smears were hypercellular and consisted of numerous mononucleated neoplastic cells arranged in a dissociative fashion. These all feature oval nuclei with smooth delicate nuclear membranes, finely granular evenly distributed chromatin, and small nucleoli. Most cells show a rim of eosinophilic granular cytoplasm (Figure 21-26 and Box 21-6).[73] The diagnostic cytologic feature is the presence of the distinctive osteoclast-like tumor cells scattered throughout the smears (Figure 21-27).

These large cells have 10 to 20 centrally placed, overlapping nuclei with moderate amounts of granular cytoplasm. The osteoclast-like tumor cells have nuclei identical to the smaller mononucleated tumor cells. Epithelial differentiation, defined either cytologically or immunohistochemically, has usually not been demonstrated. In the case examined here, the tumor cells were intensely positive for vimentin.[73]

Metastasis to the Pancreas

Both clinically and radiographically, metastatic malignancies to the pancreas and peripancreatic lymph nodes can closely mimic a primary pancreatic malignancy.[77,78] In the authors' FNA series reporting metastatic malignancies to the pancreas, 11% of 176 malignant pancreatic aspirates represented metastatic or systemic disease, including seven non-Hodgkin's lymphomas, two Hodgkin's lymphomas, six small cell carcinomas, three squamous cell carcinomas, and one hepatocellular carcinoma.[77] Importantly, in six of the 11 cases, the pancreatic mass was the initial presentation of the extrapancreatic malignancy. Therefore, identification of a metastatic lesion and separation from a pancreatic primary are crucial to avoid an unnecessary Whipple's procedure and ensure that appropriate chemotherapy/radiation is implemented.[77]

Cytologic features that lead the cytopathologist to suspect a metastatic malignancy include an unusual cytomorpho-

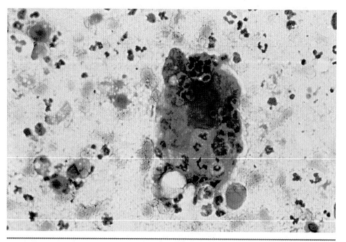

Figure 21-24 **Pleomorphic giant cell carcinoma.** Phagocytosis of neutrophils by giant tumor cells is a feature seen in some examples of pleomorphic giant cell carcinoma of the pancreas. (DQ)

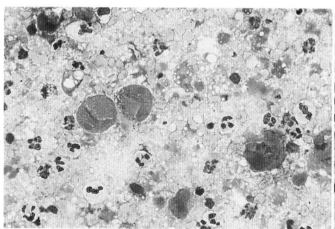

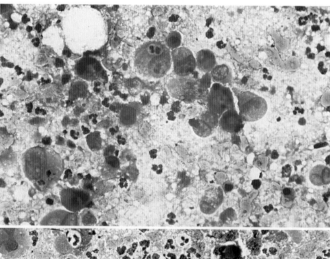

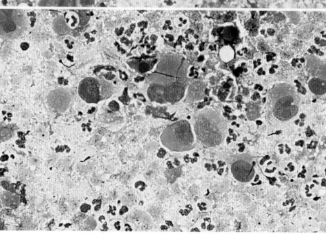

Figure 21-25 **Pleomorphic giant cell carcinoma.** In these DQ-stained smears, numerous individually scattered, bizarre tumor cells are present, including many demonstrating a rhabdoid phenotype characterized by round, hyaline-appearing cytoplasmic inclusions and huge nucleoli. Necrosis is prominent in the background.

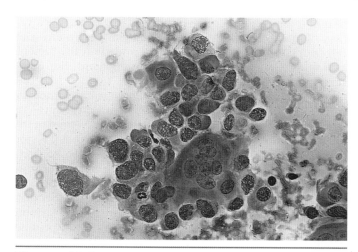

Figure 21-26 **Osteoclastic giant cell tumor.** This DQ-stained smear of an osteoclastic-like giant cell tumor of the pancreas shows numerous mononuclear neoplastic cells arranged in a dissociative fashion. The tumor cells have oval nuclei with smooth nuclear membranes and small nucleoli. A single multinucleated osteoclastic-type cell is also present.

logic appearance that is not typical of a primary pancreatic cancer. Examples include a small cell malignancy or a lymphomatous population. Small cell carcinoma should be suspected when small malignant cells with high N:C ratios with nuclear molding and the characteristic nuclear fea-

---

BOX 21-6 **CMF**

Cytomorphologic Features of Osteoclast-Like Giant Cell Tumor

Mononucleated polygonal to cuboidal-shaped cells, with some aggregated but most dissociated

Uniform round to ovoid nuclei with fine, even chromatin and small but distinct nucleoli

Eosinophilic, generally scanty cytoplasm

Scattered multinucleated osteoclast-like giant cells with central clustered nuclei that resemble nuclei of smaller tumor cells and a moderate amount of cytoplasm

Well-defined nucleoli

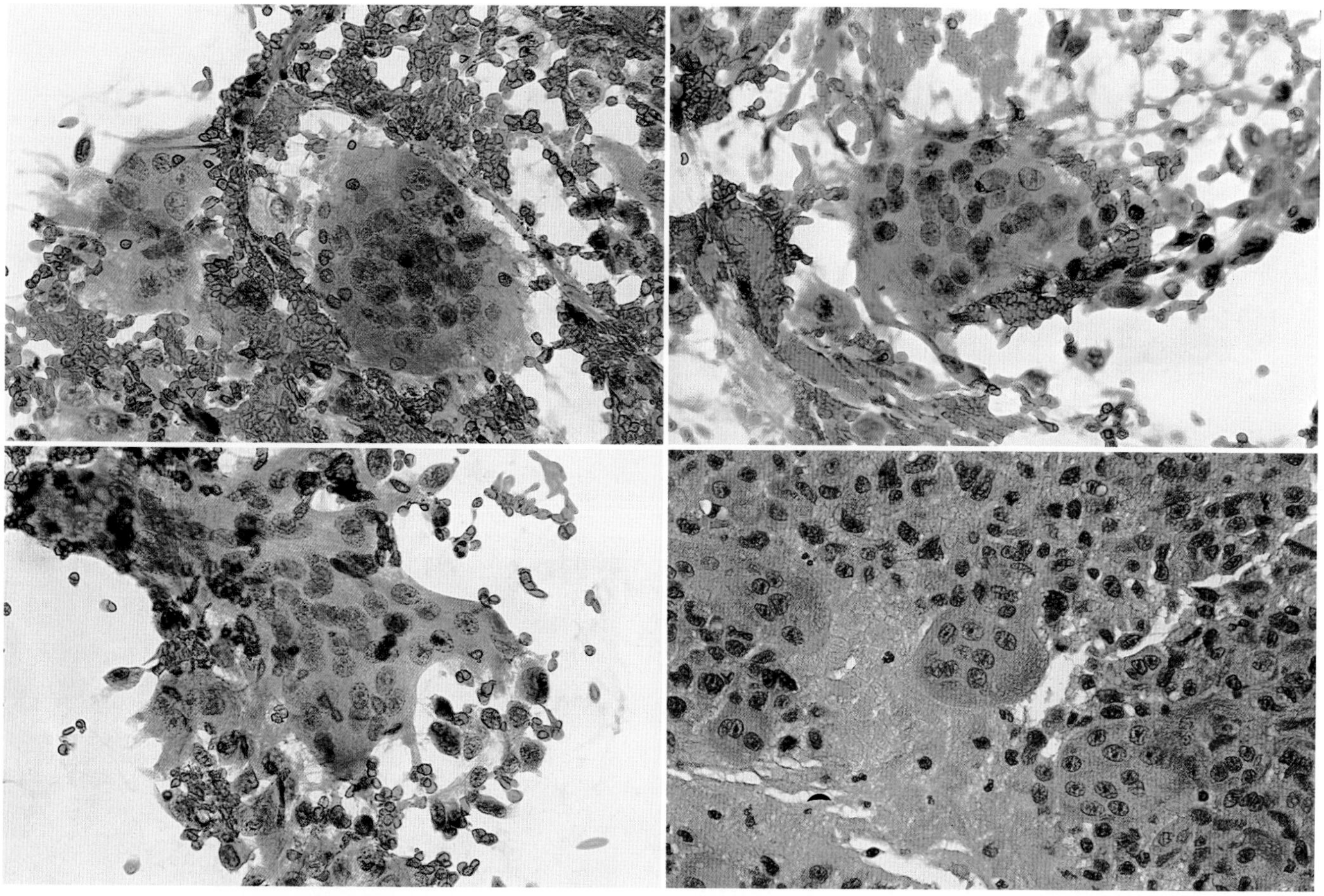

Figure 21-27 Osteoclastic giant cell tumor. **A** to **C,** Aspirate of osteoclastic giant cell tumor of the pancreas in which numerous scattered osteoclastic-like tumor cells are present, along with a few mononuclear tumor cells. (Pap) **D,** Cell block sections from this aspirate of osteoclastic giant cell tumor of the pancreas demonstrating the multinucleated osteoclastic-like tumor cells and mononuclear malignant cells. (H&E)

tures are identified (Figure 21-28). A dissociative smear pattern of small atypical lymphoid-appearing cells and lymphoglandular bodies should raise the possibility of malignant lymphoma (Figure 21-29).

If the metastasis is from an extrapancreatic adenocarcinoma, then the possibility of an extrapancreatic primary may not be raised unless suggested by the clinical history. Even sarcoma can metastasize to the pancreas, as demonstrated by a case report describing a metastatic cardiac rhabdomyosarcoma to the pancreas diagnosed by FNA biopsy.[79] This case again demonstrates that in addition to the cytologic features, ancillary immunohistochemical studies and careful evaluation of clinical findings can prove useful in making a correct diagnosis.

Islet Cell Neoplasms

Less than 10% of all clinically apparent pancreatic neoplasms are islet cell neoplasms. These tumors have generated considerable interest due to the production and secretion of a number of peptide hormones that can cause a variety of interesting clinical syndromes. However, many islet cell neoplasms are hormonally silent and clinically present as a mass. Generally, a single mass is apparent, but occasional patients have multiple pancreatic tumors. Islet cell neoplasms are the most common pancreatic tumor in childhood, although the majority of patients are adults.[1,2,16]

Most islet cell neoplasms behave either in a benign or indolent fashion, but many investigators believe that it is not possible to predict the biologic behavior based on conventional histologic and cytologic features.[16] The type of hormone produced and whether one or more hormones are present may shed some prognostic information because insulin-producing tumors behave in a more benign fashion than neuroendocrine neoplasms producing other peptide products.

In all aspirates of islet cell neoplasms, the smears are moderately cellular to hypercellular and contain a uniform population of small to medium-size cells. These mostly free-lying cells show round to oval shapes; some

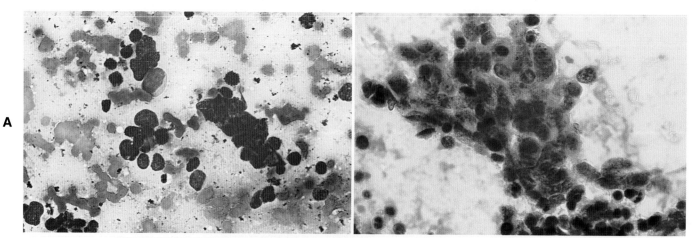

Figure 21-28 **Metastatic small cell carcinoma.** Metastatic small cell carcinoma of the lung to the pancreas characterized by small malignant cells with high N:C ratios and nuclear molding. (**A**, DQ; **B**, Pap)

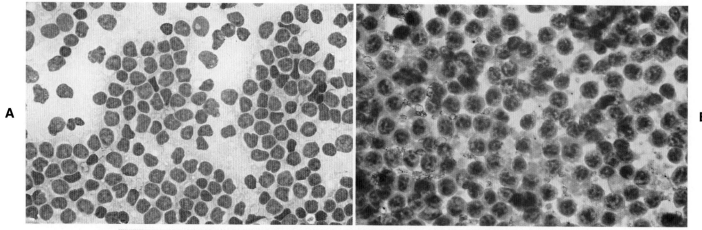

Figure 21-29 **Lymphoma.** Aspirate of large cell lymphoma involving the pancreas in which individually scattered atypical lymphoid cells are present. (**A**, DQ; **B**, Pap)

loose clusters or aggregates can be present (Figure 21-30 and Box 21-7).[1,2,80,81] However, FNA biopsy of some islet cell neoplasms are dominated by large aggregates and relatively few single tumor cells (Figure 21-31). The tumor cells generally possess a single round nucleus having the characteristic salt-and-pepper chromatin distribution. Occasionally, binucleated cells can also be seen.[82] Characteristically, nucleoli are inconspicuous or small. If nucleoli are seen with any prominence or frequency, the diagnosis of islet cell neoplasm should be seriously questioned. The nuclei of the cells are generally eccentrically placed, with a moderate amount of surrounding amphophilic to basophilic cytoplasm that can vary from opaque to more granular. In Romanowsky-stained smears, the cells have a characteristic plasmacytoid appearance but lack a paranuclear hof typical of plasma cells. A plasmacytoid appearance of the cells is a helpful feature for making a correct diagnosis. The cells often take on an on-

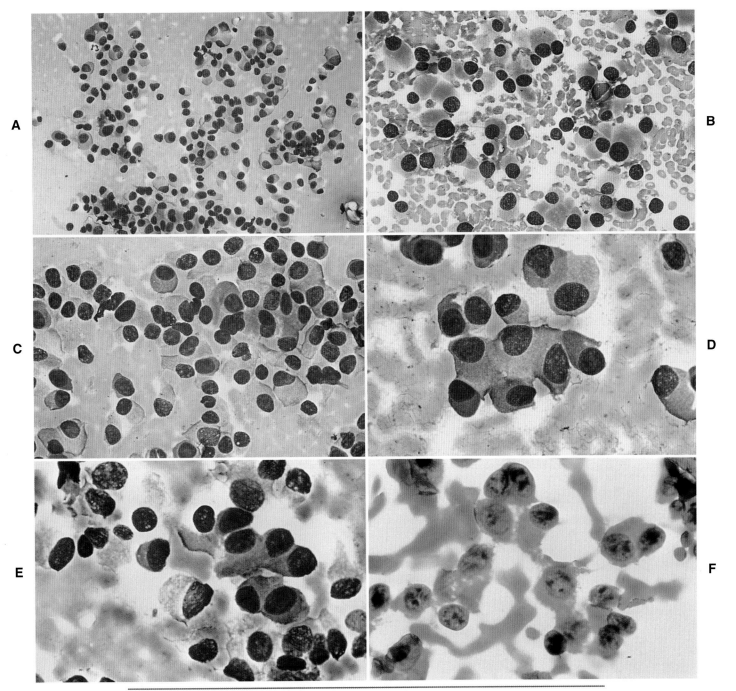

Figure 21-30 Islet cell tumor. Aspirates demonstrating a moderately cellular smear pattern consisting of a uniform population of small to medium-size cells having eccentrically placed nuclei with granular cytoplasm. The nuclei show the characteristic salt-and-pepper chromatin pattern with a lack of prominent nucleoli. (**A** to **E**, DQ; **F**, Pap)

Cytomorphologic Features of Islet Cell Neoplasms

Moderate to very cellular smears with a monotonous population of uniform, small cells

Discohesive cell pattern with many single cells and loose clusters

Cells with small, round to oval nuclei having even finely to moderately granular chromatin and lack of prominent nucleoli

Fragile, scant to moderate basophilic, granular to dense cytoplasm

Eccentrically placed nuclei with plasmacytoid appearance in Diff-Quik–stained material

Granular smear background with stripped nuclei

Vascularized fragments may be present

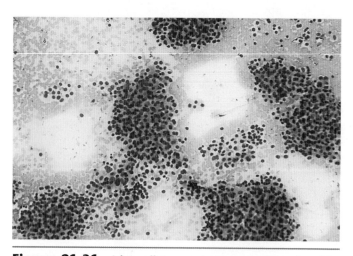

Figure 21-31   Islet cell tumor. Low-power view of an islet cell tumor aspirate in which the smears are dominated by large clusters of neoplastic islet cells. (DQ)

cocytic appearance because of an increased amount of granular eosinophilic cytoplasm (Figure 21-32).[83] This cytologic feature may even suggest consideration of an acinar cell tumor or even a poorly differentiated metastatic hepatocellular carcinoma.[82] However, ancillary studies can confirm the neuroendocrine nature of the tumor.

Alternatively, the cytoplasm of the neuroendocrine cells can be quite fragile, resulting in a smear pattern consisting of numerous stripped nuclei (Figure 21-33).[1,2] When this pattern is seen, the smear background also contains abundant granular material resulting from the spillage of cytoplasmic contents. Fragments of delicate vascular tissue may also be seen in the background or within groups of tumor cells in a manner similar to pulmonary carcinoid tumors. When a stripped nuclear pattern is present, a potential pitfall is to misinterpret the nuclei as either representing lymphocytes or a small cell carcinoma. Occasionally, the neoplastic islet cells can also be arranged in solid sheets, ribbons, and acini. It is in this setting, that the differential diagnosis includes adenocarcinoma, acinar cell carcinoma, or even normal pancreatic tissue.

Features distinguishing a well-differentiated adenocarcinoma from an islet cell neoplasm are primarily based on the nuclear characteristics of adenocarcinoma, such as the presence of cells having larger, more pleomorphic-appearing nuclei with prominent nucleoli and clusters of cells demonstrating depth of focus with tight intercellular cohesion. Acinar cell carcinoma, which is discussed in the following text, can resemble an islet cell tumor because of their similar cell size and cytoplasmic granularity. However, aspirates of acinar cell carcinoma consist of cells arranged in lobular groupings and showing coarsely clumped chromatin with easily identified nucleoli.[84] Case reports of pancreatic neoplasms demonstrating overlapping cytologic features of an islet cell neoplasm and acinar cell carcinoma have been published.[85,86]

Ancillary studies performed on the aspirated material can be quite useful in confirming an islet cell neoplasm.[1,2,16] As noted throughout this book, cell block preparations are preferred over direct smears because they better allow for a panel

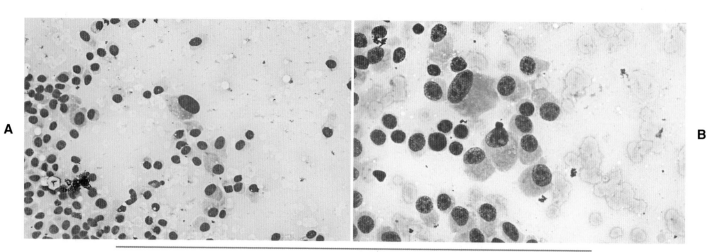

A   B

Figure 21-32   Islet cell tumor with oncocytic appearance. Aspirate in which some of the neoplastic cells have a more abundant granular eosinophilic cytoplasm imparting an oncocytic appearance. (**A,** Pap; **B,** DQ)

of immunohistochemical markers to be employed and reduce background staining that may be more prominent in direct smears. Although uncommonly used today, ultrastructural examination of the aspirated material reveals cells containing numerous neuroendocrine-type dense core granules.[87,88]

Because of the plasmacytoid appearance of islet cell neoplasms in the DQ preparation, a potential exists to confuse the rare extramedullary plasmacytoma involving the pancreas with an islet cell neoplasm. Dodd and colleagues reported two such cases.[89] Features helpful for diagnosis of plasmacytoma are the clumped "clock-face" chromatin pattern and the presence of a cytoplasmic perinuclear hof in plasma cells. Immunohistochemical staining of plasmacytomas demonstrates light chain restriction and negative staining for low molecular weight cytokeratin (CAM 5.2), as well as negative staining for neuroendocrine markers such as neuron specific enolase, synaptophysin, and chromogranin.[89] However, they are often positive for epithelial membrane antigen (EMA), a potential trap.

Islet cell neoplasms demonstrate cytomorphologic features identical to those of a carcinoid tumor; therefore, the proper classification of the neoplasm is based on the site of origin of the neuroendocrine neoplasm. However, rare tumors of the pancreas have been designated as carcinoid tumors, based on positive staining for serotonin or a clinical history of carcinoid syndrome. Pancreatic carcinoid tumor is believed to have a better prognosis than primary islet cell neoplasms.[89]

Most investigators believe that the clinical behavior of an islet cell neoplasm cannot be predicted based on the cytomorphologic appearance of the cells. However, Tao has suggested that certain cytologic features may predict a more aggressive behavior. These include the presence of huge nucleoli, nuclear pleomorphism, multinucleated tumor giant cells, increased mitotic activity, and a tumor diathesis.[4] Tao believes that if four of these five features are present in an aspirate, the neoplasm will most likely behave in a more aggressive fashion.

Islet cell neoplasms could potentially be confused with islet cell hyperplasia.[17,90,91] This problem was discussed previously during the consideration of chronic pancreatitis.

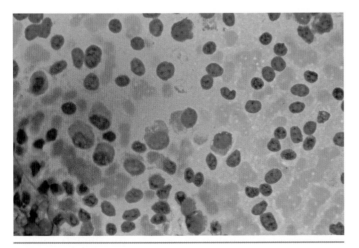

Figure 21-33 Islet cell tumor. Numerous stripped nuclei are noted in this aspirate of an islet cell tumor, along with a granular smear background. (Pap)

Papillary-Cystic Tumor

Papillary-cystic tumor of the pancreas has been known by a variety of names, including solid and papillary epithelial neoplasm and solid pseudopapillary tumor of the pancreas. This is a relatively uncommon pancreatic neoplasm, the frequency of which may be overestimated because of the number of published reports.

This neoplasm occurs almost exclusively in adolescent and young adult women, although a few examples have been seen in men.[92,93] Surgical resection is almost universally curative, although a few reports have been made of a lethal outcome when a delay in diagnosis occurs or when the neoplasm is not completely resected, leading to a protracted course.[94] Rarely has metastatic disease been documented after a long clinical course.[94]

Although the neoplasm has a radiographically and grossly cystic appearance, the papillary structures are believed to represent pseudopapillations resulting from degeneration and necrosis in solid portions of the neoplasm. The neoplastic cells are relatively small and uniform; each has a single ovoid nucleus with pale chromatin, and an inconspicuous nucleolus. Occasional cells show a longitudinal nuclear groove.[1,2] Cytoplasmic and extracytoplasmic hyaline globules may also be seen. The tumor cells tend to be arranged along a scaffolding of fibroconnective tissue, imparting a papillary pattern.

The FNA biopsy recapitulates the histologic findings with the presence of delicate, branching papillary fronds consisting of fibrovascular stalks lined by one or more layers of uniform tumor cells. Also present are small scattered clusters and singly dispersed, similar-appearing epithelial cells (Figure 21-34 and Box 21-8).[96-103] The epithelial cells have a uniform appearance with round to oval nuclei and only a moderate to scant amount of cytoplasm, contributing to N:C ratios (Figure 21-35). The chromatin is evenly dispersed, homogeneous, and finely granular. Occasional nuclei demonstrate the characteristic delicate longitudinal nuclear grooves or folds (Figure 21-36).[1,2,94] Granular debris, foam cells, cholesterol clefts, multinucleated histiocytes, and mucoid globular material may be present in the background. When the latter features predominate in an aspirate from a cystic lesion, a misdiagnosis of a pseudocyst can be made, especially if the diagnostic epithelial cells are absent or few in number. Therefore, if this occurs in an aspirate of a cystic lesion from an adolescent or young adult female, repeat aspirates should be requested in an attempt to identify diagnostic papillary groupings or epithelial cells. Amylase levels are elevated in a pseudocyst but are normal fluid from a papillary cystic tumor.[35-39,55]

The histogenesis of papillary-cystic tumors is uncertain, although most believe that it is a tumor of either endocrine or exocrine origin.[92,93] Ancillary studies have been performed to confirm the diagnosis, with demonstration of immunohistochemical positivity of the cells for vimentin and negative staining for cytokeratin.[92-94] This very helpful immunoprofile contrasts sharply the tumor's epithelial aura. Although reports of neuron-specific enolase positivity of the epithelial cells have been recorded, other more specific neuroendocrine markers have been negative. Only rarely have dense core neurosecretory granules been ultrastructurally demonstrated in cells from papillary-cystic tumor of the pancreas. Immunoreactivity for α_1-antitrypsin and ultrastructural evidence of zymogen-like granules have been

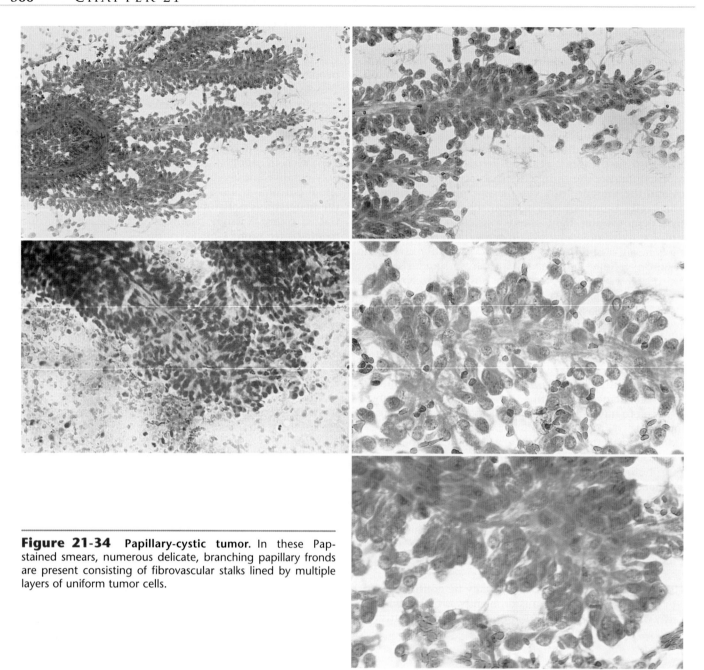

Figure 21-34 Papillary-cystic tumor. In these Pap-stained smears, numerous delicate, branching papillary fronds are present consisting of fibrovascular stalks lined by multiple layers of uniform tumor cells.

BOX   21-8   CMF

Cytomorphologic Features of Papillary-Cystic Tumor

Cellular smears with numerous individual cells and small aggregates
Straight to branched papillary structures with fibroconnective tissue cores lined by one or more layers of neoplastic epithelial cells
Uniform oval nuclei with finely granular pale chromatin, delicate nuclear membranes, and occasional longitudinal nuclear grooves
Necrotic debris, histiocytes in background
Intracytoplasmic and extracellular eosinophilic globules may be present

described, suggesting a possible acinar origin for this neoplasm, but these findings are not specific.[1,2]

In the differential diagnosis of papillary-cystic tumor of the pancreas, an islet cell neoplasm needs to be excluded. Overlapping cytologic features of these two neoplasms are present because both have cells of similar size, granular cytoplasm and nuclei that lack prominent nucleoli. Both neoplasms can also occur in young patients. However, the cytologic features of the two neoplasms differ. Islet cell tumors have cells with more coarsely granular nuclear chromatin, rather than the delicate pale nuclei of cells from papillary-cystic tumor. Cells from an islet cell neoplasm have a plasmacytoid appearance in the DQ preparation (related to more basophilic cytoplasm), a finding not seen in papillary-cystic tumor. Nuclear grooves or folds are a feature of papillary-cystic tumor and are not encountered in islet cell tumors. Papillary structures are an unexpected architectural

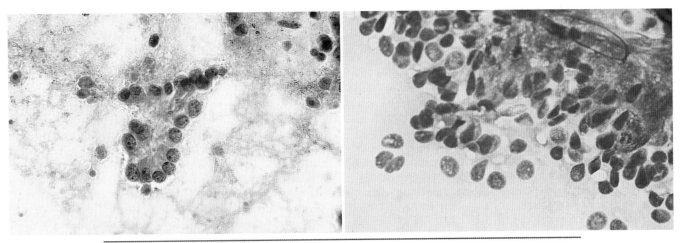

Figure 21-35 **Papillary-cystic tumor. A,** Aspirate consisting of oval-shaped cells with scant to moderate amount of cytoplasm. (Pap) **B,** Aspirate of papillary cystic tumor reveals a papillary frond in which some loosely cohesive epithelial cells are present, having a uniform appearance with high N:C ratios. (DQ)

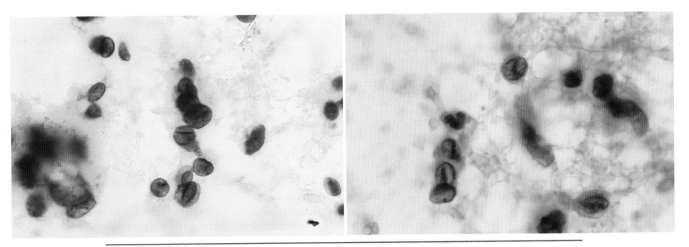

Figure 21-36 **Papillary-cystic tumor.** The cells from a papillary cystic tumor of the pancreas have evenly dispersed, granular to powdery cytoplasm and nuclei possessing longitudinal nuclear grooves or folds. (Pap)

feature of islet cell neoplasms. The radiographic evidence of a cystic component of the neoplasm would favor a papillary-cystic tumor, although cystic islet cell tumors do occur.

Lastly, a single papillary-cystic tumor pursued a aggressive course after multiple surgical biopsies and radiation treatment.[94] Aspirates of the metastatic mesenteric deposits in this case revealed cells showing a greater degree of nuclear pleomorphism than typically seen in papillary cystic tumor. Also, nuclear grooves were quite rare.[94] Multinuclear tumor giant cells were also present, and papillary structures were not prominent.

Mucinous Cystic Neoplasms and Related Conditions

Mucinous cystic neoplasms occur predominantly in middle-age women, although they can also occur in older adults.[44,45,104,105] They most often arise in the tail of the pancreas but may occur in the body and head. Typically, a large multiloculated cystic lesion is radiographically and grossly

appreciated. Although some pathologists classify these neoplasms into either benign cystadenomas and malignant cystadenocarcinomas, all of these neoplasms should be considered to be of potentially low-grade malignancy. If they are extensively sampled, a transition from histologically benign to cytologically and architecturally malignant areas can often be demonstrated.[30] An important histologic feature of mucinous cystic neoplasms is the presence of stroma composed of compactly arranged basophilic spindle cells. This closely resembles the normal ovarian stroma and is characteristic of mucinous cystic neoplasms of the pancreas. It is not recovered in aspirates.

Aspirates are generally moderately cellular because of the abundant extracellular mucinous material (Box 21-9).[1,2] The smears may consist exclusively of benign-appearing mucinous cells with no definite evidence of malignancy (Figure 21-37). However, when abundant extracellular mucinous material is found in the background, a mucinous cystic neoplasm should be suspected. The extracellular mucin has a typical stringy appearance in contrast with necrotic debris, which has a granular quality. Mucin stains metachromatically with DQ and other Romanowsky stains, and demonstrates a fibrillary quality with the Pap stain (Figure 21-38). The neoplastic cells are arranged in three-dimensional clusters, flat honeycomb sheets, or singly.

A wide spectrum of neoplastic cells may be present, from relatively bland and benign-appearing to cytologically malignant.[47] The benign-appearing cells have relatively low N:C ratios because of abundant intracytoplasmic mucinous material. Their nuclei are uniformly round to oval, with delicate membranes, evenly distributed chromatin, and small nucleoli. Even when these innocuous cytologic features are appreciated, the cytopathologist needs to suggest that a mucinous cystic neoplasm is present with a recommendation to resect the lesion, if clinically possible. Obvious malignant-appearing cells are identified when nuclei with thick, irregular membranes, clumpy chromatin, parachromatin clearing, and prominent nucleoli are seen. The malignant tumor cells can be arranged in three-dimensional clusters having a syncytial pattern, in addition to the honeycomb or picket-fence arrangement seen in the better-differentiated tumors. These cells also have a moderate to abundant amount of foamy vacuolated cytoplasm, which is mucin positive. Signet ring–like malignant cells can also be seen. A mucin stain such as mucicarmine or alcian blue (pH 2.5) confirms the presence of both intracellular and extracellular mucinous material.

The differential diagnosis of mucinous cystic neoplasm includes other benign and malignant cystic pancreatic lesions. Aspirates of pseudocysts have abundant granular necrotic material, rather than the stringy-appearing extracellular mucinous material. Furthermore, neutrophils and histiocytes are present, often to the exclusion of epithelial cells. If an aspirate of a pseudocyst samples the surrounding benign pancreatic parenchyma, these cells could be confused with the bland-appearing cells of a mucinous cystic neoplasm. However, abundant intracytoplasmic and extracellular mucin is not a feature of the normal pancreatic parenchyma.

The differential diagnosis also includes the more aggressive mucin-producing ductal adenocarcinoma undergoing necrosis with subsequent cystic change. In contrast with mucinous cystic neoplasm, the aspirates from the ductal carcinoma demonstrating mucinous differentiation are usually much more cellular and contain obviously malignant cells. It is reasonable to expect that some examples of mu-

cinous cystic neoplasm will be cytologically indistinguishable from some ductal adenocarcinomas with cystic alterations. However, the degree of cystic change as assessed radiographically or ultrasonographically will usually be greater in the mucinous cystic lesions.

Also in the differential diagnosis of mucinous cystic neoplasm is the intraductal papillary mucinous neoplasm (IPMN). IPMN is a neoplasm of the exocrine pancreas that features one or more areas of duct dilatation with intraductal papillary projections covered by a mucinous epithelium.[47,104-106] These tumors are most common in older men, in whom they tend to be located in the pancreatic head. Most previously published reports specifically discussing the cytologic findings of IPMN are limited by the small numbers of cases, varying sampling methods, or sampling limited to bench aspirates of surgical specimens. The recent apparent increase in the frequency with which IPMN is recognized is directly attributable to the previously mentioned flowering of EUS. The current classification of IPMN (World Health Organization [WHO], 2000) divides these lesions based on the degree of intraductal epithelial dysplasia as follows:[105]

1. Intraductal papillary mucinous adenoma
2. Intraductal papillary mucinous borderline tumor
3. Intraductal papillary mucinous carcinoma, with or without invasion

IPMN may show cytologic features indistinguishable from a cystic mucinous neoplasm (Figure 21-39). However, flat sheets dominate in mucinous cystic tumors, whereas papillary structures may be recovered from IPMN (Figure 21-40). Even with optimum sampling conditions, several issues impede cytologic diagnosis of IPMN, and include the following:

- IPMN is an uncommon lesion, but its true incidence is uncertain.
- It is without specific clinical findings and is usually encountered during evaluation of otherwise unexplained recurring pancreatitis.
- The cytologist's approach is complicated by the existence of cytologically benign lesions, as well as cytologically malignant examples.
- Malignant cases may be either exclusively intraductal or invasive.

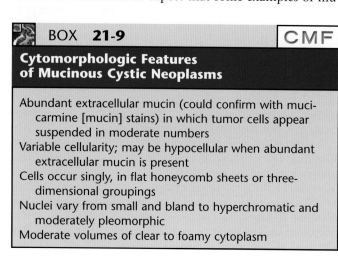

BOX 21-9 CMF

Cytomorphologic Features of Mucinous Cystic Neoplasms

Abundant extracellular mucin (could confirm with mucicarmine [mucin] stains) in which tumor cells appear suspended in moderate numbers

Variable cellularity; may be hypocellular when abundant extracellular mucin is present

Cells occur singly, in flat honeycomb sheets or three-dimensional groupings

Nuclei vary from small and bland to hyperchromatic and moderately pleomorphic

Moderate volumes of clear to foamy cytoplasm

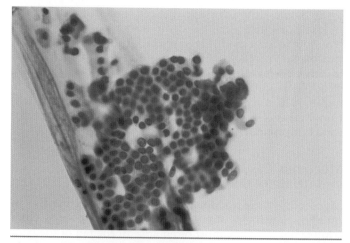

Figure 21-37 Mucinous cystic neoplasm. Aspirate consisting of innocuous-appearing cells arranged in a honeycomb pattern with some background stringy, mucinous material. (Pap)

- Many of the patients are older, often with comorbid conditions, and do not undergo confirmatory surgical excision of lesions that are clinically, sonographically, and cytologically suspected to represent IPMN.
- Specific cytologic findings do not exist, in that many examples studied by FNA are mucinous but otherwise nondescript.
- Many FNA samples are paucicellular.

Distinguishing among mucinous cystic neoplasm, mucinous ductal adenocarcinoma, and the more cytologically ominous examples of IPMN may not always be feasible based on FNA samples. The EUS findings can be very helpful in that of these three lesions, only IPMN can be shown to communicate with the duct system. However, duct dilatation due to obstruction by an extraductal mass may be confusing. In some examples, EUS will also show papillary intraductal projections.

In these authors' experiences, diagnosis of IPMN ultimately rests on a combination of findings to which the laboratory contributes only one part. A lesion that is clinically and sonographically typical of this entity will usually have FNA finding that are consistent with the diagnosis. As noted

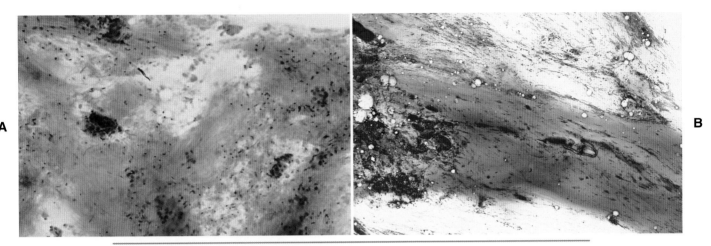

Figure 21-38 **Mucinous cystic neoplasm.** Low-power image of an aspirate of mucinous cystic neoplasm in which small clusters of bland cells are associated with abundant extracellular mucinous material. (**A,** Mucicarmine [mucin]; **B,** DQ)

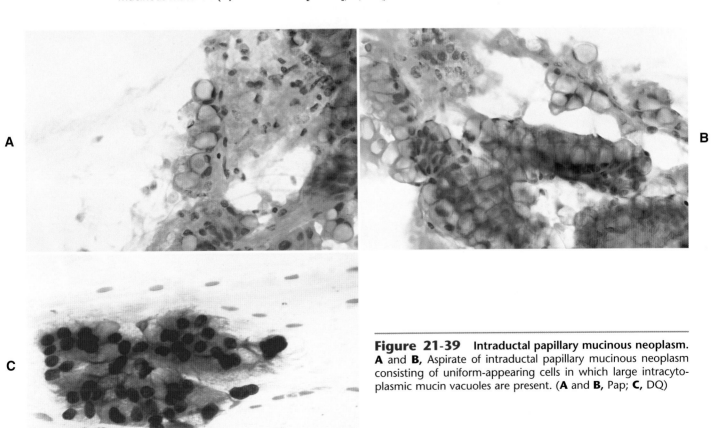

Figure 21-39 **Intraductal papillary mucinous neoplasm.** **A** and **B,** Aspirate of intraductal papillary mucinous neoplasm consisting of uniform-appearing cells in which large intracytoplasmic mucin vacuoles are present. (**A** and **B,** Pap; **C,** DQ)

previously, surgical confirmation is often not forthcoming. This has led us to suggest that the cytology of IPMN is only one part of a new triple test similar to the combination of clinical, imaging, and cytologic findings synthesized for accurate diagnosis of palpable breast lesions.[104] Biochemical analysis of aspirated material from mucinous cystic neoplasm reveals high CEA levels and negative studies for amylase.[35-38,55] In contrast, analysis of aspirated fluid from pseudocysts demonstrates elevated amylase and no CEA.

Serous Cystadenoma

Serous cystadenoma, also known as *microcystic adenoma* and *glycogen-rich cystadenoma,* is a benign, usually large pancreatic neoplasm often discovered incidentally at the time of surgery or during the workup of a patient with abdominal symptoms. Radiologically, this cystic lesion has a characteristic multiloculated Swiss cheese–like appearance. It can occur anywhere in the pancreas. This neoplasm is more common in women and in older individuals. The patient is cured by surgical resection of the cystic mass.

Only a few isolated reports of FNA cytology of microcystic adenoma have been noted.[16,31,32,107-111] The aspirate smears consist of a uniform population of cuboidal to polygonal cells with bland oval to round nuclei having inconspicuous nucleoli. Cytoplasm is scanty, causing a high N:C ratio. A helpful cytologic appearance of this neoplasm is the frequent arrangement of cells in cohesive flat sheets, somewhat reminiscent of groups of mesothelial cells (Figure 21-41).[108,109]

The diagnosis can be confirmed by the demonstration of abundant intracytoplasmic glycogen with a digested periodic acid-Schiff (PAS) stain. The tumor cells are positive for low molecular weight cytokeratins, as well as epithelial membrane antigen and negative for CEA and neuroendocrine markers.[110,111] Ultrastructural examination reveals glycogen-rich cells possessing a few lipid vacuoles and secretory granules. The apical portion of the cells is covered by microvilli and the cells are surrounded by a well-formed basal lamina.[110,111]

The differential diagnosis of microcystic adenoma in FNA cytology includes inadvertent sampling of benign mesothelial cells and other entities that are considered in the workup of cystic lesions such as pseudocysts, mucinous cystic neoplasm, and IPMN. Smears from microcystic adenomas are usually sparsely populated by tumor cells that lack nuclear grooves and are not arranged in papillary

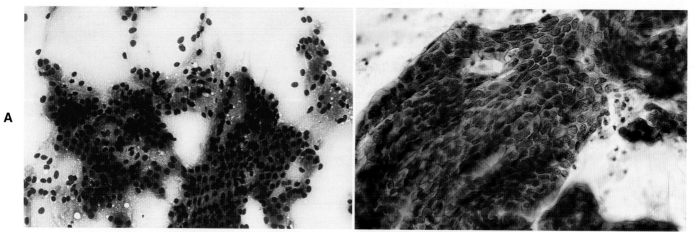

Figure 21-40 Intraductal papillary mucinous neoplasm. Papillary clusters from an aspirate of intraductal papillary mucinous neoplasm. The tumor cells have a uniform appearance with some maintenance of a honeycomb pattern. (**A,** DQ; **B,** Pap)

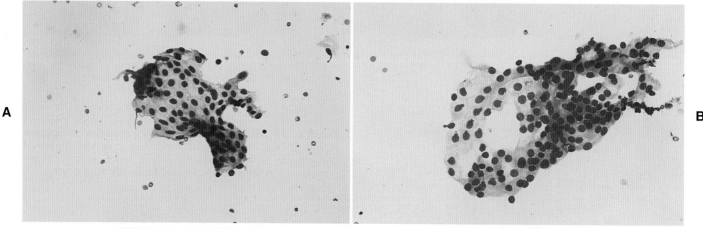

Figure 21-41 Serous cystadenoma. Aspirate consisting of cohesive, flat sheets of cells having bland, oval to round nuclei. (DQ)

fragments. However, one FNA report of serous cystadenoma with papillary features notes that the potential exists to confuse this lesion with IPMN.[134] The presence of epithelial cells and the paucity of neutrophils should exclude pseudocysts. The lack of both intracytoplasmic and extracytoplasmic mucinous material would exclude a mucinous cystic neoplasm from consideration. These authors have had the opportunity to evaluate a number EUS-guided aspirates from lesions thought clinically and sonographically to represent microcystic adenomas. In the majority of these studies, no epithelial cells were obtained. Although almost serous cystadenomas behave in a benign fashion, rare reports of a malignant variant have been made.[107] The malignant behavior cannot be predicted based either on the cytologic or histologic appearance of this cystic neoplasm.

Pancreatoblastoma

This rare childhood pancreatic malignancy generally has a favorable course, although occasional patients expire because of extensive local recurrence or metastatic disease.[112-115,135] Pancreatoblastomas are usually large tumors arising in any portion of the pancreas.

An FNA case of pancreatoblastoma was previously reported in a 4-year-old boy who presented with a large retroperitoneal mass.[115] The aspirate smears were hypercellular and consisted of numerous oval to cuboidal cells possessing a moderate amount of granular cytoplasm (Box 21-10). Triangular, elongated to spindle-shaped cells were also present, along with a population of smaller blastema-like cells showing higher N:C ratios (Figure 21-42). The cells were arranged in loose clusters and singly. The nuclei were hyperchromatic with evenly dispersed, granular chromatin and small nucleoli surrounded by a moderate amount of granular to foamy cytoplasm. Some acinar and ductal arrangements were also seen.

BOX 21-10 | CMF

Cytomorphologic Features of Pancreatoblastoma

Variable cell contours with cuboidal, columnar, triangular, and spindled shapes
Smaller cells with higher nuclear to cytoplasmic ratios
Granular cytoplasm
Oval to round vesicular nuclei with nucleoli
Cellular stromal fragments

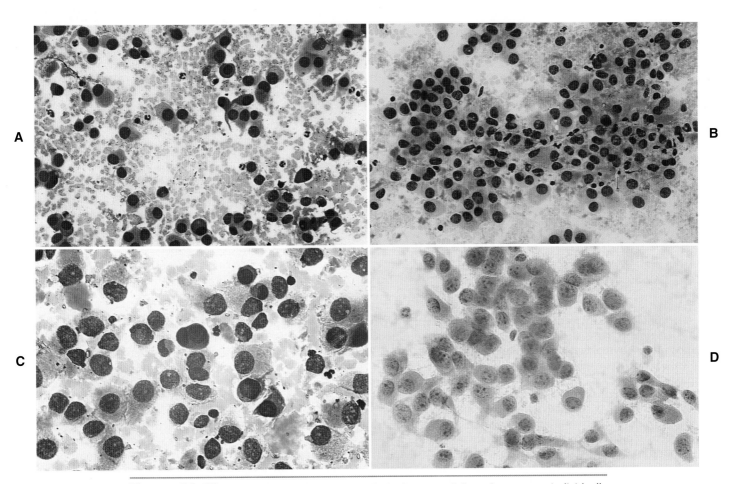

Figure 21-42 Pancreatoblastoma. **A** to **C,** Aspirate consisting of numerous individually scattered, oval to cuboidal cells having a slight to moderate amount of granular cytoplasm. (DQ) **D,** Loose cluster and individually scattered cells in an aspirate of pancreatoblastoma. The tumor cells have mildly hyperchromatic nuclei with granular chromatin surrounded by a moderate amount of granular cytoplasm. (Pap)

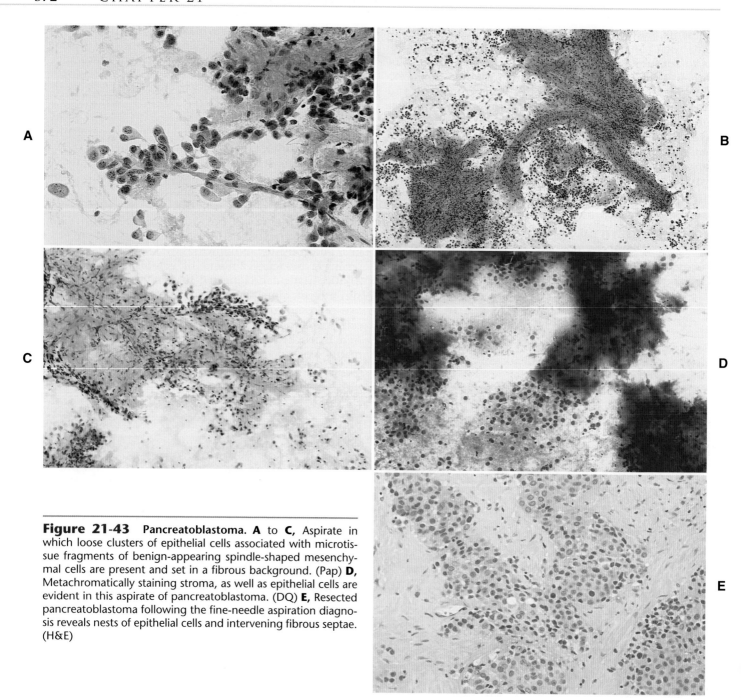

Figure 21-43 Pancreatoblastoma. **A** to **C,** Aspirate in which loose clusters of epithelial cells associated with microtissue fragments of benign-appearing spindle-shaped mesenchymal cells are present and set in a fibrous background. (Pap) **D,** Metachromatically staining stroma, as well as epithelial cells are evident in this aspirate of pancreatoblastoma. (DQ) **E,** Resected pancreatoblastoma following the fine-needle aspiration diagnosis reveals nests of epithelial cells and intervening fibrous septae. (H&E)

A helpful diagnostic feature is the presence of connective tissue fragments consisting of benign-appearing spindle-shaped mesenchymal cells and sometimes surrounded by an external layer of neoplastic epithelial cells (Figure 21-43). Immunohistochemical studies performed on the aspirated material revealed positive staining of the epithelial cells for cytokeratins (AE1/AE3), CEA, neuron-specific enolase, and α_1-antitrypsin. Ultrastructural examination demonstrated large electron dense granules in the range of 400 to 600 nm, corresponding to zymogen granules and smaller dense neuroendocrine type granules in the range of 100 to 200 nm. These findings support the blastemal origin of these cells, as they express bidirectional acinar and neuroendocrine differentiation. Rare single cells demonstrated both neuroendocrine and acinar granules, although an admixture of two dif-

ferent cell types was more prominent. In contrast with papillary-cystic tumor, which occurs in older children and adolescents, nuclear grooves were not demonstrated and the cells were not arranged in papillary fragments.

Acinar Cell Carcinoma

Acinar cell carcinoma is a rare pancreatic malignancy representing less than 1% of all pancreatic cancers. It also has a poor prognosis.[52,53,116-125] Occasional patients may present with arthropathies and widespread subcutaneous fat necrosis resulting from the release of pancreatic proteolytic enzymes (metastatic fat necrosis).[118]

Histologically, the malignant cells are arranged in solid sheets, trabecula, or acini and possess a moderate amount

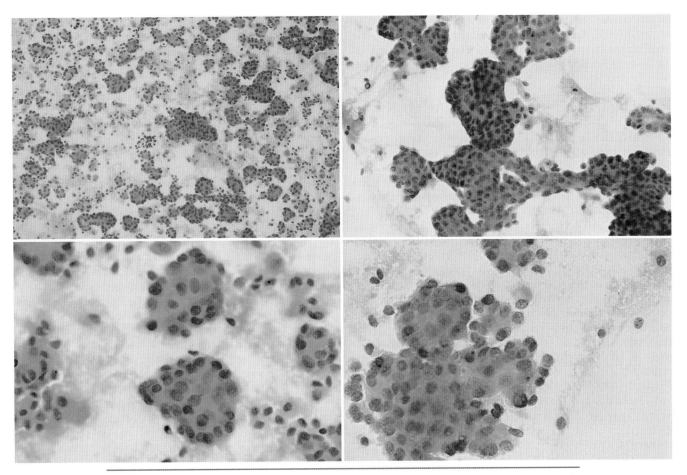

Figure 21-44 **Acinar cell tumor.** Aspirate demonstrating a hypercellular smear pattern in which the tumor cells are arranged in a lobular pattern. High-power image shows hyperchromasia of the nuclei with clumpy chromatin and small nucleoli. The tumor cells possess a granular cytoplasm. (Pap)

of densely granulated cytoplasm with a single basally placed round nucleus showing coarse chromatin and a well-developed nucleolus.

Limited literature considers FNA cytology of acinar cell carcinoma. Most reports describe a hypercellular smear with clusters of large uniform cells maintaining the lobulated arrangement of benign pancreatic acinar parenchyma (Figure 21-44 and Box 21-11).[1,2,121,123] However, in contrast with benign acinar cells, the malignant cells have more prominent nucleoli and coarser chromatin. Nuclei vary from round to irregular and are often centrally placed, in contrast with the eccentrically located nuclei of islet cell tumors. The latter entity might enter into the differential diagnosis because of similarity in cell size and presence of granular cytoplasm. However, the granularity of acinar cell carcinoma is the result of numerous zymogen granules that can be highlighted with the digested PAS stain. In a recent surgical pathology report of acinar cell carcinoma of the pancreas, positive immunohistochemical staining of the malignant cells for trypsin (100%), lipase (77%), chymotrypsin (38%), and amylase (31%) was reported.[116] A minor neuroendocrine component was also demonstrated with immunohistochemical reactivity to chromogranin and specific islet cell hormones in approximately 40% of cases. Ultrastructural examination has demonstrated exocrine features with numerous intracytoplasmic zymogen-

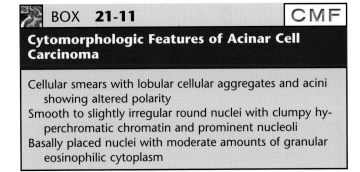

BOX 21-11 **CMF**

Cytomorphologic Features of Acinar Cell Carcinoma

Cellular smears with lobular cellular aggregates and acini showing altered polarity
Smooth to slightly irregular round nuclei with clumpy hyperchromatic chromatin and prominent nucleoli
Basally placed nuclei with moderate amounts of granular eosinophilic cytoplasm

like granules.[119] Pleomorphic, membrane-bound inclusions containing filaments were also noted and were touted as a useful ultrastructural feature for the diagnosis of acinar cell carcinoma. These structures are not seen in either islet cell tumors or carcinoid tumors.[119]

Ductal adenocarcinoma should be considered in the differential diagnosis, although the lobulated pattern and cytoplasmic granularity of acinar cell carcinoma would not be an expected feature. Aspirates of normal acinar tissue maintain a lobulated architecture, with basally placed nuclei. In contrast with the malignant features of acinar cell carcinoma, normal acinar cells will have lower N:C ratios and lack the coarse chromatin and prominent nucleoli seen in the carcinomas. Generally, aspirates of normal pancreatic acinar tissue are paucicellular, in contrast with the hypercellularity of an acinar cell malignancy.

 ## BILE DUCTS AND GALLBLADDER

FNA biopsy can be used to diagnosis ampullary, extrahepatic, biliary, and gallbladder lesions with good results.[124-133] The aspiration procedure can be performed percutaneously, intraoperatively, at the time of percutaneous transhepatic catheterization, or during endoscopic retrograde cholangiopancreatography (ERCP).

Earnhardt and colleagues reported 17 of 18 carcinomas of the ampulla and extrahepatic biliary tree diagnosed by intraoperative FNA biopsy.[122] Karstrup reported ultrasound-guided FNA biopsy of seven patients with cholangiocarcinoma located at the junction of the hepatic ducts (Klatskin tumor).[124] In the workup of obstructive jaundice, FNA biopsy at the time of percutaneous transhepatic catheterization[127] or ERCP has been performed in the evaluation of biliary strictures.[128] In one series, positive FNA biopsy occurred in 16 of 26 patients (61.5%), in contrast with concomitant brushing cytology that was positive in only two of 24 patients (8.3%).[128] One patient had a negative FNA but positive brushing cytology for cholangiocarcinoma. These findings support the idea that endoscopic brushing and FNA cytology are complementary studies for the evaluation of biliary strictures.

Zargar and colleagues[129] and Das and colleagues[133] have reported their experiences with ultrasound-guided FNA of the gallbladder. Together, they studied more than 160 patients. As expected, adenocarcinoma was the most common malignancy, followed by squamous cell carcinoma and adenosquamous carcinoma. Round cell malignancies accounted for less than 5% of the neoplasms. Complications reported after this procedure include mild pain and one instance of bile peritonitis.[129,130,133]

Hales and Miller reported a case of xanthogranulomatous cholecystitis diagnosed by aspiration cytology.[131] The intraoperative FNA biopsy revealed numerous foamy xanthoma-type histiocytes arranged in clusters and associated with capillaries, multinucleated giant cells, and benign epithelial cells. The differential diagnosis includes other histiocytic lesions that could potentially involve the gallbladder such as cholesterolosis and, rarely, malakoplakia. The authors cautioned that xanthogranulomatous cholecystitis should be a diagnosis of exclusion because it can represent changes resulting from cystic duct obstruction by carcinoma.

 ## ISSUES RELATED TO ENDOSCOPIC ULTRASOUND–GUIDED FINE-NEEDLE ASPIRATION

General features of EUS-guided FNA were introduced in Chapter 18. The most frequent use of this method is diagnosis of pancreatic masses, and the majority of these represent adenocarcinoma. Many of the patients will have adenopathy that can also be a target for FNA. Thus, either FNA showing positive lymph nodes or ultrasonographic demonstration of vascular invasion constitutes staging in-

formation that will allow the patient to avoid surgical exploration. These authors have seen many patients in whom the diagnosis of pancreatic malignancy is clinically obvious and for whom a confirmatory FNA provides clear prognostic information.

It is the practice of these authors to attend all EUS procedures at which an FNA is planned. Thoughtful coordination with the clinical team means that the cytopathologist arrives only when a sample is to be obtained, thus minimizing time spent in the endoscopy suite. Cytopathologists regard this service in much the same way they think of offering frozen sections during operative procedures or of seeing patients for pathologist-performed FNAs. Current reimbursement schedules make this a reasonable activity from a productivity point of view.

The techniques described in Chapter 2 are used to extract or concentrate aspirated tissues. Especially in the case of carcinomas, abundant tissue is often obtained and high-quality smears that facilitate rapid examination can be prepared. For rapid interpretations, the DQ stain is applied to air-dried smears. As noted in the section on Pancreatic Adenocarcinoma, many lower-grade malignancies are easier to recognize with this type of preparation because air-drying accentuates variations in nuclear size. This feature is one of the most useful cytologic characteristics of these well-differentiated neoplasms.

The cytopathologist begins by expressing the aspirated material onto a glass slide, which is often more of a temporary work surface than an object ultimately destined for microscopy. As illustrated in Chapter 2, tissue particles or small clots are removed and placed on a new slide. Often, a small smear is made of this concentrated material and is ideal for rapid review; the cytopathologist strives to avoid the need to screen an entire slide (in the manner of a conventional Pap test preparation) in the setting of rapid interpretation.

Another goal that is frequently achieved is splitting of the sample so that both a dried and a fixed slide can be prepared from each pass. This technique was described in Chapter 2, as were methods for preparation of formalin-fixed material suitable for embedding in paraffin. In many instances, part of a bloody sample may be left to clot on the original slide. This can then be easily placed in formalin. Even a mucoid aspirate can be gently placed in formalin, as fixation will lead to coagulation that renders the material more firm and cohesive. Preparation of cell blocks makes aspirates available to the full range of testing offered by the modern laboratory of surgical pathology.

In many instances, on-site interpretation rapidly results in an unequivocal diagnosis of carcinoma. In other cases the specimen can be triaged to cultures in microbiology or to flow cytometric immunophenotyping of lymphoid cells. At other times, the cytopathologist can reliably say that "diagnostic" tissue has been obtained but that further evaluation will be required for classification of the neoplasm. This usually means that immunohistochemistry will be performed on paraffin-embedded material. The impressions gained from on-site interpretation of smears can be used to emphasize collection of samples in formalin. These authors regard the need for special testing or cell blocks as a valid reason to request that additional passes be performed.

Cytologic interpretation of EUS-guided FNA material is almost always complicated by the presence of normal mucosal cells or fragments and lumenal mucus. Intermediate-type esophageal squamous cells are virtually always encountered but usually do not cause diagnostic difficulties.

Glandular cells from the gastric or duodenal surface can be confused with the cells of a low-grade neoplastic process. These are often removed as large flat sheets, a low-magnification feature that can mimic aspirates of pancreatic adenocarcinoma. However, most aspirations of the pancreas are performed across the duodenal wall. Mucosal fragments from this area exhibit a honeycomb sheet of small, uniform, darkly staining cells. These sheets are interrupted at regular intervals by pale goblet cells. This regular pattern of "holes" in the cell sheet is very useful in the identification of normal duodenal mucosa. In trying to apply this criterion during evaluation of small glandular cells that could represent IPMN or a low-grade mucinous cystic neoplasm, it is reasonable to inquire of the endoscopist whether the aspiration has been performed through the gastric wall or the duodenal wall. The use of air-dried smears also facilitates differentiation of low-grade adenocarcinoma from contaminating mucosa; air-drying maximizes the differences in cell size and nuclear size that distinguish these benign and malignant epithelia. These differences are often readily apparent at low magnification, further facilitating rapid interpretation.

Mucus is virtually always encountered. The distinction between normal lumenal mucus and the secretions of a neoplasm must be based on something other than its mere identification through the microscope. In the case of intermediate or high-grade carcinomas and of GIST or other nonepithelial lesions, this issue does not arise. Asking the endoscopist about the clinical and ultrasonographic findings may similarly indicate that a low-grade, mucin-producing neoplasm is an unlikely consideration. Occasional cases remain in which low-grade glandular cells and background mucus make it difficult to confidently diagnose a low-grade neoplasm. The extent to which molecular testing or immunohistochemistry will improve this situation remains to be investigated. In these authors' experiences, many of these aspirates are sparsely cellular and may not be suitable for ancillary testing.

The normal lumenal mucus of the upper GI tract is thin and watery and is often green or yellow. As discussed in this chapter, many aspirates of mucinous neoplasms yield very different material. Especially in the case of IPMN, non-bloody samples show extremely thick, clear, glistening mucus that is completely different from normal lumenal mucus. Grossly, this most closely resembles the material recovered when mucinous breast carcinomas are aspirated, and it is completely at variance with the appearance of normal lumenal material as the authors have seen in hundreds of examples. Simply seeing mucus on a slide prepared elsewhere by another individual deprives the cytologist of this interesting and useful finding.

References

1. Silverman JF, Geisinger KR. FNA of thorax and abdomen. New York: Churchill Livingstone; 1996. pp. 135-170.
2. Silverman JF, Geisinger KR. Fine needle aspiration cytology of the liver and pancreas. In: Silverberg SG, editor. Principles and practice of surgical pathology and cytopathology. 3rd ed. New York: Churchill Livingstone; 1997. pp. 1968-1996.
3. Teot LA, Geisinger KR. Fine needle aspiration of the liver and pancreas. In: Atkinson BF, Silverman JF, editors. Atlas of difficult diagnosis in cytopathology. Philadelphia: WB Saunders; 1998. pp. 330-339.
4. Tao L-K. Transabdominal fine needle aspiration biopsy. Igaku-Shoin: New York; 1990.
5. Suits J, Frazee R, Erickson RA. Endoscopic ultrasound and fine needle aspiration for the evaluation of pancreatic masses. Arch Surg 1999; 134:639-643.
6. Gloor B, Todd KE, Reber HA. Diagnostic workup of patients with suspected pancreatic carcinoma. Cancer 1997; 79:1780-1786.
7. Chang KJ, Nguyen P, Erickson RA, et al. The clinical utility of endoscopic ultrasound-guided fine-needle aspiration in the diagnosis and staging of pancreatic carcinoma. Gastrointest Endosc 1997; 45:387-393.
8. Saez A, Catala I, Brossa R, et al. Intraoperative fine needle aspiration cytology of pancreatic lesions: a study of 90 cases. Acta Cytol 1995; 39:485-488.
9. Hastrup J, Thommesen P, Frederiksen P. Pancreatitis and pancreatic carcinoma, diagnosed by preoperative fine needle aspiration biopsy. Acta Cytol 1997; 21:731-734.
10. Tao LC, Ho CS, McLoughlin MJ, et al. Percutaneous fine needle aspiration biopsy of the pancreas: cytodiagnosis of pancreatic carcinoma. Acta Cytol 1978; 22:215-220.
11. Mitchell MI, Carney CN. Cytologic criteria for the diagnosis of pancreatic carcinoma. Am J Clin Pathol 1985; 83:171-176.
12. Pinto MM, Avila NA, Criscuola EM. Fine-needle aspiration of the pancreas: a five year experience. Acta Cytol 1988; 32:39-42.
13. Mitchell ML, Bittner CA, Willis JS, et al. Fine-needle aspiration cytology of the pancreas: a retrospective study of 73 cases. Acta Cytol 1988; 32:447-451.
14. Cohen MB, Egerter DP, Holly EA, et al. Pancreatic carcinoma: regression analysis to identify improved cytologic criteria. Diagn Cytopathol 1991; 7:341-345.
15. Robins DB, Katz RL, Evans DB, et al. Fine-needle aspiration of the pancreas. In quest of accuracy. Acta Cytol 1995; 39:1-10.
16. Geisinger KR, Silverman JF. Fine-needle aspiration cytology of uncommon primary pancreatic neoplasms: a personal experience and review of the literature. In: Schmidt WA, editor. Cytopathology annual. Baltimore: Williams & Wilkins; 1991. pp. 1-23.
17. Nguyen G-K. Percutaneous fine-needle aspiration cytology of the pancreas. Pathol Annu 1985; 22:163.
18. Akosa AB, Desa LA, Phillips I, et al. Aspiration cytodiagnosis of pancreatic endocrine tumors. Cytopathology 1994; 5:369-379.
19. Saez A, Catala I, Brossa R, et al. Intraoperative fine-needle aspiration cytology of pancreatic lesions: a study of 90 cases. Acta Cytol 1995; 39:485-488.
20. Blandamura S, Costantin G, Nitti D, et al. Intraoperative cytology of pancreatic masses: a 10-year experience. Acta Cytol 1995; 39:23-27.
21. Hyland C, Kheir SM, Kashlan MB. Frozen section diagnosis of pancreatic carcinoma: a prospective study of 64 biopsies. Am J Surg Pathol 1981; 5:179-191.
22. Lightwood R, Reber HA, Way LW. The risk and accuracy of pancreatic biopsy. Am J Surg 1976; 132:189-194.
23. Ferrucci JT Jr, Wittenberg J, Margolies MN, et al. Malignant seeding of the tract after thin-needle aspiration biopsy. Radiology 1979; 130:345-346.
24. Rashleigh-Belcher HJC, Russell RCG, et al. Cutaneous seeding of pancreatic carcinoma by fine-needle aspiration biopsy. Br J Radiol 1986; 59:182-183.

25. Rosenbaum DA, Frost DB. Fine-needle aspiration biopsy of the pancreas complicated by pancreatic ascites. Cancer 1990; 65:2537-2538.

26. Bergenfeldt M, Genell S, Lindholm K, et al. Needle-tract seeding after percutaneous fine-needle biopsy of pancreatic carcinoma. Acta Chir Scand 1988; 154:77-79.

27. Fornari F, Civardi G, Cavanna L, et al. Complications of ultrasonically guided fine-needle abdominal biopsy. Results of a multicenter Italian study and review of the literature. Scand J Gastroenterol 1989; 24:949-955.

28. Simms MH, Tindall N, Allan RN. Pancreatic fistula following operative fine-needle aspiration. Br J Surg 1982; 69:548.

29. Herzberg AJ, Raso DS, Silverman JF. Color atlas of normal cytology. New York: Churchill Livingstone; 1999. pp. 180-189.

30. Warshaw AL, Compton CC, Lewandrowski K, et al. Cystic tumors of the pancreas: new clinical, radiologic, and pathologic observations in 67 patients. Ann Surg 1990; 212:432-443.

31. Young NA, Villani MA, Khoury P, et al. Differential diagnosis of cystic neoplasms of the pancreas by fine-needle aspiration. Arch Pathol Lab Med 1991; 115:571-577.

32. Laucirica R, Schwartz MR, Ramzy I. Fine-needle aspiration of pancreatic cystic epithelial neoplasms. Acta Cytol 1992; 36:881-886.

33. Oertel JE, Heffess CS, Oertel YC. Pancreas. In: Sternberg SS, editor. Diagnostic surgical pathology. Philadelphia: Lippincott-Raven; 1989. p. 1075.

34. Tatsuta M, Yamanoto R, Yanamamura H, et al. Cytologic examination and CEA measurement in aspirated pancreatic material collected by percutaneous fine-needle aspiration biopsy under ultrasonic guidance for the diagnosis of pancreatic carcinoma. Cancer 1983; 52:693-698.

35. Pinto MM, Kaye AD, Brogan DA, Criscuolo EH. Diagnosis of cystic lesions of the pancreas: a biochemical and cytologic analysis of material obtained utilizing radiographic or intraoperative technique. Diagn Cytopathol 1986; 2:40-45.

36. Pinto MM, Meriano FV. Diagnosis of cystic pancreatic lesions by cytologic examination and carcinoembryonic antigen and amylase assays of cysts contents. Acta Cytol 1991; 35:456-463.

37. Lewandrowski KB, Warshaw AL, Compton CC, et al. Variability in cystic fluid carcinoembryonic antigen level, fluid viscosity, amylase content, and cytologic findings among multiple loculi of a pancreatic mucinous cystic neoplasm. Am J Clin Pathol 1993; 100:425-427.

38. Lewandrowski K, Southern J, Pins M, et al. Cyst fluid analysis in the differential diagnosis of pancreatic cysts: a comparison of pseudocysts, serous cystadenomas, mucinous cystic neoplasms, and mucinous cystadenocarcinoma. Ann Surg 1993; 217:41-47.

39. Centeno BA, Pitman MB. Fine needle aspiration biopsy of the pancreas. Boston: Butterworth-Heinemann; 1999.

40. Cappellari JO. Fine-needle aspiration cytology of a pancreatic lymphoepithelial cyst. Diagn Cytopathol 1993; 9:77-81.

41. Mockli GC, Stein RM. Cystic lymphoepithelial lesion of the pancreas. Arch Pathol Lab Med 1990; 114:85-87.

42. Mandavilli SR, Port J, Ali SZ. Lymphoepithelial cyst (LEC) of the pancreas: cytomorphology and differential diagnosis on fine-needle aspiration (FNA). Diagn Cytopathol 1999; 20:371-374.

43. Liu J, Shin HJC, Rubenchik I, et al. Cytologic features of lymphoepithelial cyst of the pancreas: two preoperatively diagnosed cases based on fine-needle aspiration. Diagn Cytopathol 1999; 21:346-350.

44. Jones EC, Suen KC, Grant DR, et al. Fine-needle aspiration cytology of neoplastic cysts of the pancreas. Diagn Cytopathol 1987; 3:238-243.

45. Gupta RK, Scally J, Steward RJ. Mucinous cystadenocarcinoma of the pancreas: diagnosis of fine needle aspiration cytology. Diagn Cyotpathol 1989; 5:408-411.

46. Emmert GM, Bentra C. Fine-needle aspiration biopsy of mucinous cystic neoplasm of the pancreas: a case study. Diagn Cytopathol 1986; 2:69-71.

47. Dodd LG, Farrell TA, Layfield LJ. Mucinous cystic tumor of the pancreatic analysis of FNA characteristics with an emphasis on the spectrum of malignancy associated features. Diagn Cytopathol 1995; 12:113-119.

48. Steinberg W, Tenner S. Acute pancreatitis. N Engl J Med 1994; 330:1198-1210.

49. Jorda M, Essenfeld G, Garcia E, et al. The value of fine-needle cytology in the diagnosis of inflammatory pancreatic masses. Diagn Cytopathol 1992; 8:65-67.

50. Lin A, Feller ER. Pancreatic carcinoma as a cause of unexplained pain: report of ten cases. Ann Intern Med 1990; 113:166-167.

51. Warshaw AL, Fernandez-Del Castillo C. Pancreatic carcinoma. N Eng J Med 1992; 326:455-465.

52. Carriaga MT, Henson DE. Liver, gallbladder, extrahepatic bile ducts, and pancreas. Cancer 1995; 75:171-190.

53. Cubilla AL, Fitzgerald PJ. Classification of pancreatic cancer (nonendocrine). Mayo Clin Proc 1979; 54:449-458.

54. Gullo L, Pezzilli R, Morselli-Labate AM. Diabetes and the risk of pancreatic cancer. N Engl J Med 1994; 331:81-84.

55. Yu HC, Shetty J. Mucinous cystic neoplasm of the pancreas with high carcinoembryonic antigen. Arch Pathol Lab Med 1985; 109:375-377.

56. Parsons L Jr, Palmer CH. How accurate is fine-needle biopsy in malignant neoplasia of the pancreas. Arch Surg 1989; 124:681-683.

57. Edoute Y, Lemberg S, Malberger E. Preoperative and intraoperative fine-needle aspiration cytology of pancreatic lesions. Am J Gastroenterol 1991; 86:1015-1019.

58. Yang GC, Slott S, LiVolsi VA, et al. Rapid assessment of Diff-Quik-stained pancreatic aspirates: a retrospective study of 40 intraoperative fine-needle aspiration consultations, with measurement of nuclear size of look-alike small tissue fragments by image analysis. Acta Cytol 1994; 38:37-42.

59. Edoute Y, Lemberg S, Malberger E. Preoperative and intraoperative fine-needle aspiration cytology of pancreatic lesions. Am J Gastroenterol 1991; 86:1015-1019.

60. Allison DC, Bose KK, Hruban RH, et al. What's new in general surgery: pancreatic cancer cell DNA content correlates with long-term survival after pancreatoduodenectomy. Ann Surg 1990; 214:648-656.

61. Bose KK, Allison DC, Hruban RH, et al. A comparison of flow cytometric and absorption cytometric DNA values as prognostic indicators for pancreatic carcinoma. Cancer 1993; 71:691-700.

62. Porschen R, Remy U, Bevers G, et al. Prognostic significance of DNA ploidy in adenocarcinoma of the pancreas. Cancer 1993; 71:3846-3850.

63. Bottger TC, Storkey S, Wellek S, et al. Factors influencing survival after resection of pancreatic cancer: a DNA analysis and a histomorphologic study. Cancer 1994; 73:63-73.

64. Shibata D, Almoguera C, Forrester K, et al. Detection of K-ras mutations in fine-needle aspirates from human pancreatic carcinomas. Cancer Res 1990; 50:1279-1283.

65. Mora J, Puig P, Boadas J, et al. K-ras gene mutations in the diagnosis of fine-needle aspirates of pancreatic masses: prospective study using two techniques with different detection limits. Clin Chem 1998; 44:2243-2248.

66. Pinto MM, Emanuel JR, Chaturvedi V, Costa J. K-ras mutations and the carcinoembryonic antigen level in fine needle aspirates of the pancreas. Acta Cytol 1997; 41: 427-434.

67. Loy TS, Sharp SC, Andershock CJ, et al. The distribution of CA 19-9 in adenocarcinoma and transitional cell carcinoma. An immunohistochemical study of 527 cases. Am J Clin Pathol 1993; 99:726-728.

68. Pinto MM, Monteiro NL, Tizol DM. Fine needle aspiration of pleomorphic giant cell carcinoma of the pancreas: case report with ultrastructural observations. Acta Cytol 1986; 30:430-434.

69. Silverman JF, Dabbs DJ, Finley JL, et al. Fine-needle aspiration biopsy of pleomorphic (giant cell) carcinoma of the pancreas: cytologic, immunocytochemical, and ultrastructural findings. Am J Clin Pathol 1988; 89:714-720.

70. Collins KA, Geisinger KR, Wakely PE Jr, et al. Extragonadal germ cell tumors: a fine-needle aspiration biopsy study. Diagn Cytopathol 1995; 12:223-229.

71. Rosai J. Carcinoma of pancreas simulating giant cell tumor of bone electron-microscopic evidence of acinar cell origin. Cancer 1968; 22:333-334.

72. Jeffrey I, Crow J, Willis BL. Osteoclast-type giant cell tumor of the pancreas. J Clin Pathol 1983; 36:1165-1170.

73. Silverman JF, Finley JL, MacDonald KG Jr. Fine-needle aspiration cytology of osteoclastic giant-cell tumor of the pancreas. Diagn Cytopathol 1990; 6:336.

74. Walts AE. Osteoclast-type giant cell tumor of the pancreas. Acta Cytol 1983; 37:500-504.

75. Manci EA, Gardner LL, Pollock WJ, Dowling EA. Osteoclastic giant cell tumor of the pancreas: aspiration cytology, light microscopic, and ultrastructural with review of the literature. Diagn Cytopathol 1985; 1:105.

76. Silverman JF, Finley JL, Berns L, et al. Significance of giant cells in fine-needle aspiration biopsies of benign and malignant lesions of the pancreas. Diagn Cytopathol 1989; 5:388-391.

77. Benning TL, Silverman JF, Berns LA, Geisinger KR. Fine needle aspiration of metastatic and hematologic malignancies clinically mimicking pancreatic carcinoma. Acta Cytol 1992; 36:471-476.

78. Carson HJ, Green LK, Casteli MJ, et al. Utilization of fine-needle aspiration biopsy in the diagnosis of metastatic tumors to the pancreas. Diagn Cytopathol 1995; 12:8-13.

79. Khalbuss WE, Gherson J, Zaman M. Pancreatic metastasis of cardiac rhabdomyosarcoma diagnosed by fine needle aspiration: a case report. Acta Cytol 1999; 43:447-451.

80. Banner BF, Myrent KL, Memoli VA, Gould VE. Neuroendocrine carcinoma of the pancreas diagnosed by aspiration cytology. Acta Cytol 1985; 29:442-448.

81. Hsiu JG, D'Amato NA, Sperling MH, et al. Malignant islet-cell tumor of the pancreas diagnosed by fine needle aspiration biopsy: a case report. Acta Cytol 1985; 29:576-579.

82. Collins BT, Cramer HM. Fine-needle aspiration cytology of islet cell tumors. Diagn Cytopathol 1996; 15:37-45.

83. Pacchioni D, Papotti M, Macri L, et al. Pancreatic oncocytic endocrine tumors: cytologic features of two cases. Acta Cytol 1996; 40:742-746.

84. Labate AM, Zakowski MF. Cytologic features of acinar and islet cell tumors. Acta Cytol 1994; 38:858.

85. Nguyen-Ho P, Nguyen G-K, Jewell LD. Oncocytic neuroendocrine carcinoma of the pancreas. Acta Cytol 1994; 38:611-613.

86. Villaneuva RR, Nguyen-Ho P. Nguyen G-K. Needle aspiration cytology of acinar-cell carcinoma of the pancreas: report of a case with diagnostic pitfalls and unusual ultrastructural findings. Diagn Cytopathol 1994; 10:362-364.

87. Shaw JA, Vance RP, Geisinger KR, Marshall RB. Islet cell neoplasms: a fine needle aspiration cytology study with immunocytochemical correlations. Am J Clin Pathol 1990; 94:142-149.

88. Al-Kaisi N, Weaver MG, Abdul-Karim FW, Siegler E. Fine needle aspiration cytology of neuroendocrine tumors of the pancreas: a cytologic, immunocytochemical and electron microscopic study. Acta Cytol 1992; 36:655-660.

89. Dodd LG, Evans DB, Symmans F, et al. Fine-needle aspiration of pancreatic extramedullary plasmacytoma: possible confusion with islet cell tumor. Diagn Cytopathol 1994; 10:371-375.

90. Nguyen G-K, Rayani NA. Hyperplastic and neoplastic endocrine cells of the pancreas in aspiration biopsy. Diagn Cytopathol 1986; 2:204-211.

91. Gala I, Atkinson B, Nocosia RF, et al. Fine-needle aspiration cytology of idiopathic pancreatic islet cell adenosis. Diagn Cytopathol 1993; 9:453-456.

92. Pettinato G, Manivel JC, Ravetto C, et al. Papillary cystic tumor of the pancreas: a clinicopathologic study of 20 cases with cytologic, immunohistochemical, ultrastructural, and flow cytometric observations, and a few of the literature. Am J Clin Pathol 1992; 98:478-488.

93. Lieber MR, Lack EE, Roberts JR Jr, et al. Solid and papillary epithelial neoplasm of the pancreas: an ultrastructural and immunocytochemical study of six cases. Am J Surg Pathol 1987; 11:85-93.

94. Cappellari JO, Geisinger KR, Albertson DA, et al. Malignant papillary cystic tumor of the pancreas. Cancer 1990; 66:193-198.

95. Bondeson L, Bondeson A-G, Genell S, et al. Aspiration cytology of a rare solid and papillary epithelial neoplasm of the pancreas: light and electron microscopic study of a case. Acta Cytol 1994; 28:605-609.

96. Bose S, Kapila K, Verma K. Amyloidosis of the liver diagnosed by fine needle aspiration cytology. Acta Cytol 1989; 33:935-936.

97. Chen KTK, Workman RD, Efird TA, Cheng AC. Fine needle aspiration cytology diagnosis of papillary tumor of the pancreas. Acta Cytol 1986; 30:523-527.

98. Naresh KN, Borges AM, Chinoy RF, et al. Solid and papillary epithelial neoplasms of the pancreas: diagnosis by fine needle aspiration cytology in four cases. Acta Cytol 1995; 39:489-493.

99. Wilson MB, Adams DB, Garen PD, et al. Aspiration cytologic, ultrastructural, and DNA cytometric findings of solid and papillary tumor of the pancreas. Cancer 1992; 69:2235-2243.

100. Skarda JS, Honick AB, Gibbins CS, et al. Papillary-cystic tumor of the pancreas in a young woman: fine-needle aspiration cytology, ultrastructural and DNA analysis. Diagn Cytopathol 1994; 10:20-24.

101. Greenberg ML, Rennie Y, Grierson JM, et al. Solid and papillary epithelial tumor of the pancreas: cytologic case study with ultrastructural and flow cytometric evaluation. Diagn Cytopathol 1993; 9:541-546.

102. Katz LBK, Ehya H. Aspiration cytology of papillary cystic neoplasm of the pancreas. Am J Clin Pathol 1990; 94: 328-333.

103. Mendonca ME, Bivar-Weinholtz J, Soares J. Fine needle aspiration cytology of a solid and papillary epithelial neoplasm of the pancreas. Acta Cytol 1991; 35:258-260.

104. Stelow EB, Bardales RH, Stanley MW, et al. Intraductal finding and limitations of cytology samples obtained by endoscopic ultrasound–guided fine needle aspiration, *Am J Clin Pathol* (in press).

105. Longnedus DS, Hruban RH, Adler G, et al. Intraductal papillary mucinous neoplasm of the pancreas. In: Hamilton SR, Aaltonen LA, editors. Pathology and genetics of tumors of the digestive system. Lyon, France: IARC Press; 2000. pp. 237-240.

106. Nagai E, Ueki T, Chijiiwa K, et al. Intraductal papillary mucinous neoplasms of the pancreas associated with so-called "mucinous ductal ectasia": histochemical and immunohistochemical analysis of 29 cases. Am J Surg Pathol 1995; 19:576-589.

107. George DH, Murphy F, Michalski R, Ulmer BG. Serous cystadenocarcinoma of the pancreas: a new entity?: case report. Am J Surg Pathol 1989; 13:61-66.

108. Hittmair A, Pernthaler H, Totsch M, et al. Preoperative fine needle aspiration cytology of a microcystic adenoma of the pancreas. Acta Cytol 1991; 35:546-548.

109. Nguyen G-K, Vogelsang PJ. Microcystic adenoma of the pancreas: a report of two cases with fine needle aspiration cytology and differential diagnosis. Acta Cytol 1993; 37:908-912.

110. Shorten SD, Hart WR, Petras RE. Microcystic adenomas (serous cystadenomas) of pancreas: a clinicopathologic investigation of eight cases with immunohistochemical and ultrastructural studies. Am J Surg Pathol 1986; 10:365-372.

111. Alpert LC, Truong LD, Bossart MI, Spjut HJ. Microcystic adenoma (serous cystadenoma) of the pancreas: a study of 14 cases with immunohistochemical and electron-microscopic correlation. Am J Surg Pathol 1988; 12:251-263.

112. Morohoshi T, Kanda M, Horie A, et al. Immunocytochemical markers of uncommon pancreatic tumors: acinar cell carcinoma, pancreatoblastoma, and solid cystic (papillary-cystic) tumor. Cancer 1987; 59:739-747.

113. Buchino JJ, Castello FM, Nagaraj HS. Pancreatoblastoma: a histochemical and ultrastructural analysis. Cancer 1984; 53:963-969.

114. Polosaari D, Clayton F. Seaman J. Pancreatoblastoma in an adult. Arch Pathol Lab Med 1986; 110:650-652.

115. Silverman JF, Holbrook CT, Pories WJ, et al. Fine needle aspiration cytology of pancreatoblastoma with immunocytochemical and ultrastructural studies. Acta Cytol 1990; 34:632-652.

116. Klimstra DS, Heffess CS, Oertel JE, Rosai J. Acinar cell carcinoma of the pancreas: a clinicopathologic study of 28 cases. Am J Surg Pathol 1992; 16:815-837.

117. Klimstra DS, Rosai J, Heffess CS. Mixed acinar-endocrine carcinomas of the pancreas. Am J Surg Pathol 1994; 18:765-778.

118. Ishihara A, Sandra T, Takanari H, et al. Elastase-1-secreting acinar cell carcinoma of the pancreas. A cytologic, electron microscopic and histochemical study. Acta Cytol 1989; 33:157-163.

119. Tucker JA, Shelburne JD, Benning TL, et al. Filamentous inclusions in acinar cell carcinoma of the pancreas. Ultrastruct Pathol 1994; 18:279-286.

120. Dekker A, Lloyd JC. Fine-needle aspiration biopsy in ampullary and pancreatic carcinoma. Arch Surg 1979; 114:592-596.

121. Labate AM, Zakowski MF. Cytologic features of acinar and islet cell tumors. Acta Cytol 1994; 38:858.

122. Earnhardt RC, McQuone SJ, Minasi JS, et al. Intraoperative fine needle aspiration of pancreatic and extrahepatic biliary masses. Surg Gynecol Obstet 1993; 177:147-152.

123. Villaneuva RR, Nguyen-Ho P, Nguyen G-K. Needle aspiration cytology of acinar-cell carcinoma of the pancreas: report of a case with diagnostic pitfalls and unusual ultrastructural findings. Diagn Cytopathol 1994; 10:362-364.

124. Karstrup S. Ultrasound diagnosis of cholangiocarcinoma at the confluence of the hepatic ducts (Klatskin tumors). Br J Radiol 1988; 61:987-990.

125. Klimstra DS, Heffess CS, Oertel JE, Rosai J. Acinar cell carcinoma of the pancreas: a clinicopathologic study of 28 cases. Am J Surg Pathol 1992; 16:815-837.

126. Bondestam S, Jansson S-E, Taavitsainen M, et al. Ultrasound guided fine-needle biopsy of mass lesions affecting the hepatobiliary tract. Acta Radiol Diagn 1981; 22:549-551.

127. Kuroda C, Yoshioka H, Tokunaga K, et al. Fine-needle aspiration biopsy via percutaneous transhepatic catheterization: technique and clinical results. Gastrointest Radiol 1986; 11:81-84.

128. Howell DA, Beveridge RP, Bosco J, Jones M. Endoscopic needle aspiration biopsy at ERCP in the diagnosis of biliary strictures. Gastrointest Endosc 1992; 38:531-535.

129. Zargar SA, Khuroo MS, Mahajan R, et al. US-guided fine-needle aspiration biopsy of gallbladder masses. Radiology 1991; 179:275-278.

130. Herbetko J, Fache JS. Diagnostic fine-needle puncture of the gallbladder. Radiology 1991; 180:586.

131. Hales MS, Miller TR. Diagnosis of xanthogranulomatous cholecystitis by fine needle aspiration biopsy: a case report. Acta Cytol 1987; 31:493-496.

132. Swobodnik W, Hagert N, Janowitz P, et al. Diagnostic fine-needle puncture of the gallbladder with US guidance. Radiology 1991; 178:755-758.

133. Das DK, Tripathi RP, Bhambhani S, et al. Ultrasound-guided fine-needle aspiration cytology diagnosis of gallbladder lesions: a study of 82 cases. Diagn Cytopathol 1998; 4:258-264.

134. Rampy BA, Waxman I, Xiao S-Y, et al. Serous cystadenoma of the pancreas with papillary features: a diagnostic pitfall on fine-needle aspiration biopsy. Arch Pathol Lab Med 2001; 125:1591-1594.

135. Henke AC, Kelley CM, Jensen CS, Timmerman TG. Fine-needle aspiration cytology of pancreatoblastoma. Diagn Cytopathol 2001; 25:118-121.

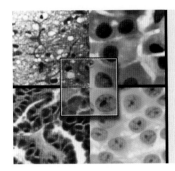

Kidney

CHAPTER
22

UTILITY OF RENAL FINE-NEEDLE ASPIRATION

As recently as 1998, the indications for image-guided (computed tomography [CT] or ultrasound) renal fine-needle aspiration (FNA) were for the suspected consideration of metastatic disease to the kidney, lymphoma, renal infarcts, or focal pyelonephritis.[1] By and large, the treatment for imaged mass lesions suspected for neoplasia was surgical, with FNA only indicated if medical problems in a patient with suspected renal carcinoma precluded surgery.[1] Over the last several years, much has been learned about the natural history and appropriate reclassification of kidney tumors based on cytogenetic abnormalities; thus, the treatment options for renal neoplasms have been altered accordingly. Kidney-sparing surgery for benign and low-grade malignancies has increasingly become an adopted approach. For many solid lesions, treatment depends on characteristic imaging findings obviating the need for FNA. The same is true with benign appearing cysts, which require only periodic follow-up. However, in combination with the widespread use of imaging and the discovery of smaller renal lesions, the practice of image-guided renal FNA has assumed a role of increasing importance with regard to potential operative approaches. Nephron-sparing surgery can be used with confidence for small lesions that are found to be potentially benign or of low nuclear grade on cytology. There are, however, institutional variations on this philosophy.

Over the last 10 years a growing trend toward the use of kidney-sparing surgery for renal tumors has surfaced[2,3] (Box 22-1). Although initially employed for patients with multiple renal lesions, impaired renal function, or a solitary kidney, studies have shown excellent long-term results with regard to tumor control and renal function, particularly for smaller lesions in appropriate candidate patients.[2] Thus, the role of partial nephrectomy for patients with a normal contralateral kidney has become increasingly realized, although the surgery can be longer and more complex (as with laparoscopic procedures).[2] Patient survival is affected by tumor stage, symptoms, laterality, and size.[3] A recently published study with 10-year follow-up of patients with renal cell carcinoma treated with partial nephrectomy revealed that patients whose tumors were greater in size than 4 cm were significantly more likely to die of disease than those with tumors less than 4 cm in size. Using the Cox proportional hazards model for multivariate analysis, the risk of death increased by 20% for each incremental 1-cm increase in size.[3]

Current indications for renal FNA include those mentioned previously, as well as the distinction between possible benign and malignant lesions, low- and high-grade renal epithelial neoplasms, diagnosis of transitional cell carcinoma (as ureterectomy is required), confirmation of renal primary in patients with inoperable and metastatic disease, evacuation of cysts, and the diagnosis and monitoring of Wilms' tumor. No special pretreatment regimen needs to be followed before a renal FNA, although aspirin use is precluded for the prior 10 days and preprocedural blood tests for patients on anticoagulant therapy are recommended.[1]

During the procedure, the patient should be in the prone position, and the needle (18 to 20 gauge) should be positioned to enter the kidney below the twelfth rib, as a preventative measure to avoid pneumothorax.[1] The postprocedural protocol usually involves patient observation for one to two hours.

The complications of renal FNA are few and usually involve only transient hematuria, although postprocedural infection is possible. There are rare reports of tumor needle track seeding and postprocedural hemorrhage requiring nephrectomy.[4-6]

The reported accuracy of renal FNA is highly variable, from 73% to 94%.[7-14] Up to 30% are reported as nondiagnostic with repeated aspirates remaining nondiagnostic in 40%.[8-10] It has been theorized that this accuracy rate will actually diminish as radiologists aspirate fewer typical benign cystic lesions. Accuracy rates may also be diminished by cytopathologists' lack of familiarity with distinct cytologic features of the benign and malignant renal lesions.[7] This is complicated by overlapping cytomorphologic features, particularly in epithelial lesions.

In general, the final diagnosis of any kidney tumor must wait for the histology. Kidney tumors are notorious for having various histologic components that must all be viewed carefully before a final diagnostic assessment. The same can also be said for nuclear grading of kidney carcinoma. However, cytologic assessments and nuclear grading of renal FNAs have been shown to be successful, yielding important diagnostic information in experienced hands. The correlation coefficient for cytologic assessment and biopsy histology for renal cell carcinomas has been shown to be 0.87. Although successfully separating low (1-2) from high (3-4) nuclear grade (0.92), the renal FNA correlation coefficient was only 0.36 for the Fuhrman nuclear grading in general.[15] A recent retrospective analysis revealed the sensitivity of renal FNA to be 92%, with a specificity of 91.9%, a positive predictive value of 89.9%, a negative predictive value of 94%, and an efficacy of 92.2%.[16]

A large study of 108 adult renal masses evaluated by FNA surveyed the effectiveness of renal FNA.[17] Diagnostic categories utilized for this study were *unsatisfactory, renal abscess, benign cystic lesion, suspicious for malignancy,* and *malignant lesion.* Immediate assessments of sample cellularity

---

BOX 22-1

Indications for Elective Partial Nephrectomy

Unilateral renal involvement
Unifocal disease
Tumor less than 4 cm

TABLE 22-1

Proposed Criteria for Adequacy of Renal FNA Samples of Solid Lesions

	General Features	Cytologic Features
Unsatisfactory	• Mesenchymal and/or normal renal tissue elements only • Blood and/or necrotic debris only • Technically poor sample	• Containing only a few cells or cell clusters, the etiology of which cannot be determined with certainty
Satisfactory	• Technically satisfactory • Representative cellularity	• Adequate number of well preserved cells that are not of normal renal parenchyma and that are interpretable as falling into a diagnostic category

Modified from Truong LD, Todd TD, Dhurandhar B, et al. Fine-needle aspiration of renal masses in adults: analysis of results and diagnostic problems in 108 cases. Diagn Cytopathol 1999; 20: 339-349.

---

and adequacy on this group of FNAs were performed at the time of aspiration. Tumor typing was attempted within the malignant group. Histologic or long-term follow-up was attempted in all cases and consisted of cell block (55%) and/or subsequent histology (35%). The spectrum of cytologic diagnoses was *unsatisfactory (16%), abscess (4%), benign cyst (28%) suspicious (10%),* and *malignant (42%).* All unsatisfactory samples were from solid lesions, representing 20% of the solid lesion aspirates. Follow-up in 10 of 17 cases revealed renal and nonrenal primary malignancies in nine and xanthogranulomatous pyelonephritis (XP) in one. Erroneous diagnoses were rendered in two of the samples interpreted as benign cyst—one was a cystic renal cell carcinoma, and one was acquired cystic kidney. Retrospective review of cytologic material in these samples did not yield features beyond that of benign cyst. Of the cases diagnosed as suspicious (N = 11), follow-up revealed six primary renal epithelial malignancies, four cystic lesions (benign and acquired), and one angiomyolipoma. Review revealed the presence of atypical cells on all samples that were either sparse, misinterpreted, or reactive in etiology. The cytologic diagnosis of malignancy was correct (with follow-up) in all of the cases interpreted as malignant, with cytologic classification of tumor type correct in 44 of 46 cases (96%). Difficulty in distinguishing renal cell carcinomas from transitional cell carcinoma resulted in the two diagnostic misinterpretations (one each).[17]

This large study also evaluated adequacy issues for renal FNA, which had thus far not been established (Table 22-1). For a solid lesion, a technically acceptable and representative smear consisted of a large number of well-preserved cells that were not considered to be of normal parenchymal origin. A cystic lesion sample was considered satisfactory if aspiration yielded fluid with no minimum requirements of cellularity[17] (Table 22-2).

One review questioned the utility of renal FNA in lesions less than 5 cm in diameter. In this cytology/histology correlative series of 25 patients, all of whom had renal cell carcinoma, only 10 FNAs were considered diagnostic. Ten samples were suspicious for carcinoma, whereas six were di-

---

TABLE 22-2

Proposed Criteria for Adequacy of Renal Fine-Needle Aspiration Samples of Cystic Lesions

	General Features	Cytologic Features
Unsatisfactory	• Mesenchymal and/or normal renal tissue elements only • Blood only	
Satisfactory	• Fluid (clear, bloody, or cloudy, regardless of cellularity)	• Targeted cystic lesion successfully sampled • Minimum cellularity not required

Modified from Truong LD, Todd TD, Dhurandhar B, et al: Fine-needle aspiration of renal masses in adults: analysis of results and diagnostic problems in 108 cases. Diagn Cytopathol 1999; 20:339-349.

agnosed as negative. Thus, pathologist or sampling errors in this group led to an erroneous negative diagnosis in 24% of cases. Correlation of cytologic Fuhrman nuclear grade was in agreement with histology in 80% of cases diagnosed as malignant.[18] Although the surgery was not adversely affected, subcapsular hematomas developed postprocedurally in 40% of patients in this series.[18]

NORMAL RENAL ELEMENTS ON FINE-NEEDLE ASPIRATION CYTOLOGY

On architectural and ultrastructural levels, the kidney is quite a complex organ. However, to the cytopathologist, the normal elements that require recognition are limited to the glomerulus and tubular systems. Once familiar with the appearance of these normal, benign elements, the potential pitfall of mistaking any of these elements for a neoplastic process is minimized (Table 22-3). It is also helpful in a renal FNA to compare the cytology of malignant vs. benign elements within the same case, particularly in the same microscopic field, for the obvious contrasts.

As most renal FNAs are performed for cortical lesions, it is the cortical elements that are most commonly seen in FNAs (Figures 22-1 to 22-4). The background of a normal renal cortex FNA will be sprinkled with the stripped round nuclei of the proximal convoluted tubular cells (PCTC; see Figure 22-2). Intact PCTC may appear singly, in small groups, in tubular structures, and, most commonly, in small, flat sheets. Their cytoplasm is voluminous and granular. Distinct cytoplasmic borders may or may not be present. These cells must

TABLE **22-3**
Potential Erroneous Neoplastic Interpretation for Normal Renal Elements

Normal Structure	Potential Erroneous Neoplastic Interpretation
Proximal tubular cells	Oncocytoma
Proximal tubular cells	Conventional low-grade renal cell carcinoma with granular cytoplasm
Distal convoluted tubular cells	Papillary renal cell carcinoma
Glomeruli	Papillary renal cell carcinoma
Glomeruli	Renal primary vascular tumor

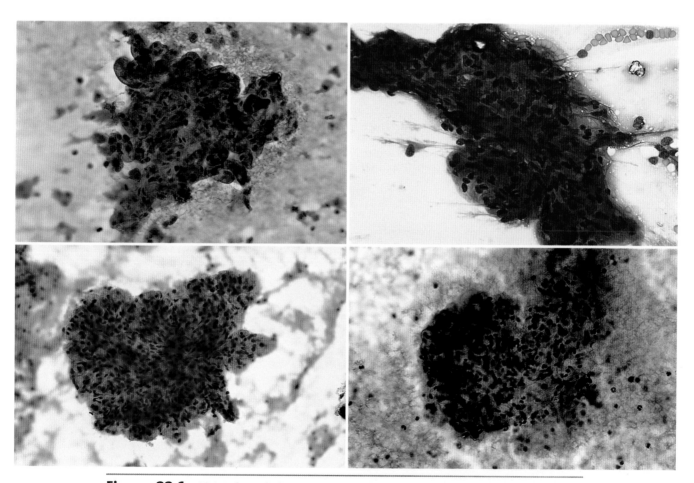

Figure 22-1 **Normal renal glomeruli.** The glomeruli are compact, rounded densely cellular structures, which are composed of a complex network of thin-walled capillaries. The endothelial cells may have elongated, oval, bean-shaped, or boomerang-shaped nuclei and indistinct cell borders. Around the edges, lumina containing red blood cells (RBCs) may be seen. At times, because of smearing artifact, glomeruli may be mistaken for tumor cell aggregates, particularly those with a papillary architecture. (Papanicolaou [Pap], Diff-Quik [DQ])

be distinguished from those of oncocytoma (which usually do not show the excessive cytoplasmic fragility) and well-differentiated conventional/clear cell renal cell carcinoma with granular cytoplasm. The sheets of bland-appearing cells in conventional renal cell carcinoma are much larger, and usually the nuclei show at least mild atypia. These cells may also be mistaken for benign hepatocytes.

The cells of the distal convoluted tubules and loops of Henle may appear similar to those of the proximal convoluted tubule, except that the cytoplasm is not granular and is less voluminous; thus, their nuclear to cytoplasmic (N:C)

ratios are higher (see Figures 22-3 and 22-4). No distinct cytoplasmic borders are evident. At times, these cells appear in small sheets, as single cells, or as intact tubular structures. The cytoplasm may show dense green cytoplasmic granules, presumably due to lipofuscin. As the nuclei of papillary renal cell carcinomas are often of low nuclear grade and may also show cytoplasmic hemosiderin pigment, these benign cells may be mistakenly identified as such. The benign tubular cells lack malignant nuclear features.

The glomeruli appear as compact, rounded, densely cellular structures, which on closer inspection are composed of

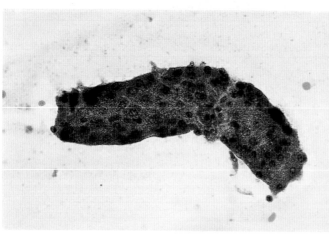

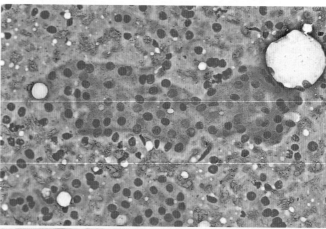

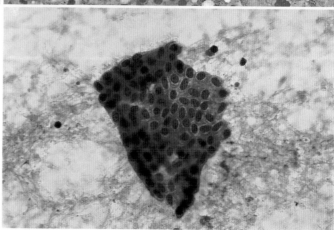

Figure 22-2 Proximal convoluted tubule cells. These appear singly; in small groups; in tubular structures; and in small, flat sheets. Their cytoplasm is voluminous and granular. Distinct cytoplasmic borders may or may not be seen. (Pap, DQ)

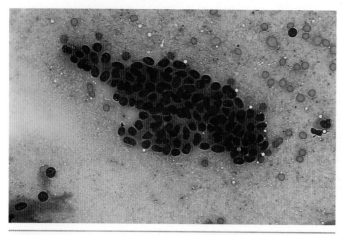

Figure 22-3 Distal convoluted tubule cells. These appear similar to those of the proximal convoluted tubule, except that the cytoplasm is not granular and is less voluminous. No distinct cytoplasmic borders are present. These cells are in a small sheet. (DQ)

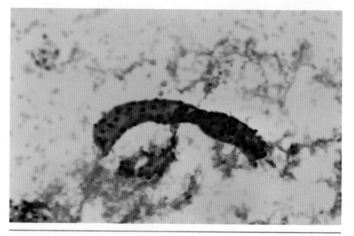

Figure 22-4 Tubular segment from the loop of Henle. This thin, three-dimensional tubule from the loop of Henle shows small, round nuclei in a three-dimensional matrix of cytoplasm without distinct cellular borders. (Pap)

a complex network of thin-walled capillaries (see Figure 22-1). The endothelial cells may have elongated, oval, bean-shaped, or boomerang-shaped nuclei and indistinct cell borders. Around the edges, lumina containing red blood cells (RBCs) may be seen. At times, due to smearing artifact, glomeruli may be mistaken for tumor cell aggregates, particularly those with a papillary architecture. Because of the rounded low-power appearance of glomeruli and the oval-to bean-shaped endothelial nuclei, glomeruli can also be mistaken for granulomata.

BENIGN NONNEOPLASTIC CONDITIONS

Cystic Lesions

It is estimated that about 50% of the population age 50 and older have some form of renal cysts. Simple, unilocular renal cysts are frequently diagnosed on imaging and are eas-ily confirmed with cytology. By and large, simple unilocu-lar cysts are the most common types discovered (Figures 22-5 and 22-6). However, cysts displaying imaging features of multilocularity, mural nodules, a thickened or calcified cyst wall, or high-density/heterogeneous cyst contents are considered atypical and require sampling (Figures 22-7 and 22-8). These complex, multiloculated cysts are becoming more frequently recognized and sampled and represent a unique set of diagnostic challenges due to potential sampling errors and reactive or neoplastic atypia of the epithelial lining cells.[19]

The most common cytologic feature of benign cysts are macrophages, which may be abundant. In smears, these appear as single cells with bland nuclei and abundant, uniformly vacuolated cytoplasm, with or without granularity and hemosiderin. In many instances, the macrophages appear as both single cells and in variably sized cohesive aggregates that may simulate neoplasia. Overall, histiocytic nuclei are less perfectly round, and the N:C ratios are lower than in epithelial cells. To differentiate these cells from neo-

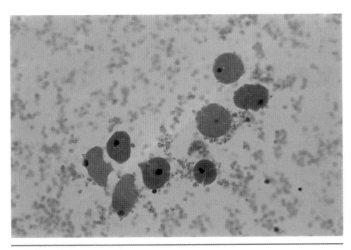

Figure 22-5 Benign renal cyst. These granular macrophages with round, bland nuclei are floating in a background of lysed RBCs. (Pap)

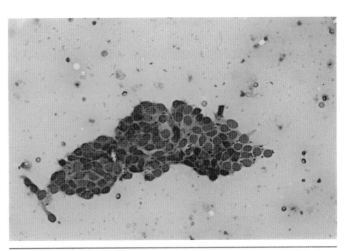

Figure 22-6 Benign renal cyst. This monolayer sheet of benign cyst lining cells/renal tubular epithelium was aspirated from a renal cyst. The background contains debris and RBCs. (DQ)

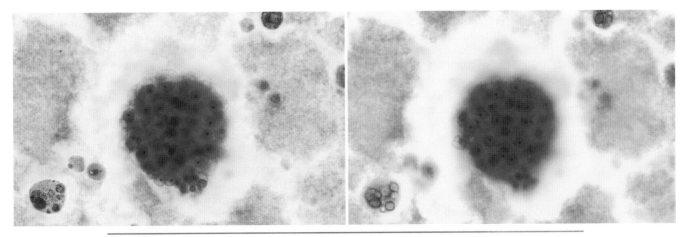

Figure 22-7 Atypical renal cyst. Simulation of focusing up and down on these atypical cells reveals these three-dimensional clusters of cells to have prominent nucleoli with adjacent nuclear clearing and abundant clear cytoplasm. Hemosiderin-laden macrophages are present. (Pap)

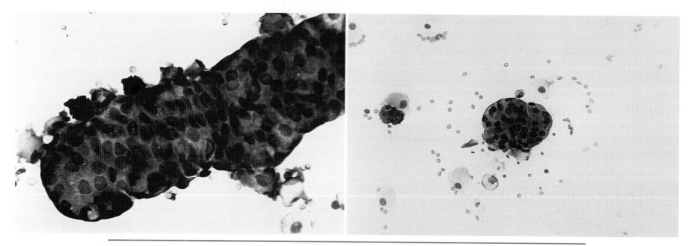

Figure 22-8   **Atypical renal cyst, suspicious for malignancy.** Bland, smooth-contoured papillary clusters of epithelial cells are present with scanty granular cytoplasm admixed with macrophages. (DQ)

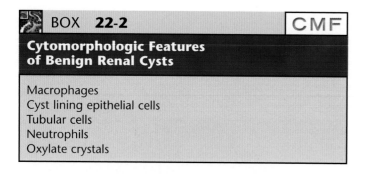

BOX 22-2   CMF

Cytomorphologic Features of Benign Renal Cysts

Macrophages
Cyst lining epithelial cells
Tubular cells
Neutrophils
Oxylate crystals

plastic renal cell carcinoma cells, immunocytochemistry would demonstrate the macrophages to be negative with cytokeratins and positive with macrophage markers (e.g., CD68)[19] (Box 22-2 and Table 22-4).

Renal tubular cells, which may also be abundant, were found to be most numerous in the cyst walls rather than in the cyst fluid.[19] These cells are most commonly proximal tubular cells, and appear as orderly two-dimensional aggregates of cells with abundant granular cytoplasm and round nuclei containing small nucleoli. They can also be seen as naked nuclei.[19] Cyst lining cells have a distinct appearance, usually seen as rare two-dimensional clusters with granular cytoplasm and poorly defined cell borders. The aggregates are mostly of less than 10 cells each.[19] Neutrophils, oxalate crystals, spindled cyst lining cells, calcified debris, and Liesegang rings may also be seen but are seen less often. Liesegang rings are lamellated concretions commonly found in chronic cystic lesions that are inflamed, fibrotic, necrotic, or hemorrhagic.[20] They resemble corpora amylacea. In many instances, however, the cyst fluid may be acellular.[19]

Oxalate Crystals

Clearly not all renal lesions with cystic components are benign. In a recent study of 41 renal cyst aspirates, Todd and colleagues described three patterns of cyst cytology that suggested potential malignancy in their series of cyst aspirates[19] (see Figures 22-7 and 22-8). The first pattern was that of a cyst with a typical radiographic benign appearance, but cytologically there were a large number of renal tubular epithelial cells, which could be mistaken for neoplastic cells. Knowledge of the cytologic spectrum of benign renal tubular elements should permit one to avoid the erroneous misinterpretation of potential neoplasia in this instance.[19] The second pattern, which was the most common and was noted in acquired and congenital polycystic disease and cystic nephroma, was the presence of three-dimensional epithelial cell clusters with abundant cytoplasm that was granular or vacuolated, with atypical nuclear features. The nuclei were large, hyperchromatic and had irregular contours. Macrophages were present in variable numbers but necrosis was absent.[19] The third pattern recognized in this series of cystic lesions was characterized by a prominent number of bland, smooth, contoured papillary clusters of epithelial cells with scanty granular cytoplasm admixed with macrophages. The follow-up on the cases with this pattern revealed cystic papillary renal cell carcinoma and clear cell renal cell carcinoma with a papillary component.[19]

In Todd and colleagues' series the cystic lesions that were diagnosed as malignant were interpreted as showing cytologic features typical of renal cell carcinoma. The cyst fluids were cellular, containing large, irregular, three-dimensional cell clusters and single cells with abundant vacuolated or reticulated cytoplasm without obvious nuclear atypia. Many naked nuclei were present in the background.[19]

Importantly, this series emphasized that the gross appearance of aspirated fluid is not a diagnostic indicator; cystic fluid may be clear, bloody, or cloudy from benign or malignant lesions.[19]

Xanthogranulomatous Pyelonephritis

XP is an uncommon subacute to chronic inflammatory disease of the kidney that may radiologically, grossly, and cytologically simulate renal cell carcinoma (Figure 22-9). It occurs more commonly in women and presents as multiple mass lesions that often extend into the perinephric fat. The clinical picture may be similar to renal cell carcinoma, with flank pain, hematuria, weight loss, and an abdominal mass lesion. The cause is usually obstruction with a secondary

TABLE 22-4
General Cytologic Approach to Renal Epithelial Cells, Benign Renal Cysts, and Renal Neoplasms

Diagnosis	Cellularity	Necrotic Background	Patterns	Naked Nuclei	N:C Ratio	Nuclear Features	Cytoplasmic Features	Comments
Renal tubular cells	Low to moderate	(−)	Variably small-sized clusters; rare single cells, may be two-dimensional	Rare to abundant	Low	Regular, round, oriented, small nucleoli in PCTC	Well-defined cell borders with homogenous cytoplasm	
Benign cyst lining cells	Low	(−)	No single cells; small, three-dimensional clusters; may be mixed with tubular cells	(−)	Intermediate	Mildly atypical	Granular cytoplasm; ill-defined cell borders	
Renal cell carcinoma	High or moderate	Frequent	Abundant, large three-dimensional clusters or flat sheets; many single cells; may be mixed with benign tubular cells	Abundant	Low	Variable, dependent on tumor type	Variable, dependent on tumor type	(See discussions of tumor types in text.)

Modified from Truong LD, Todd TD, Dhurandhar B, et al. Fine-needle aspiration of renal masses in adults: analysis of results and diagnostic problems in 108 cases. Diagn Cytopathol 1999; 20:339-349.

N:C, Nuclear to cytoplasmic; *PCTC,* proximal convoluted tubular cells.

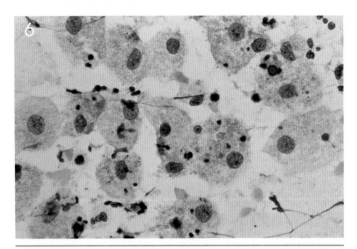

Figure 22-9 Xanthogranulomatous pyelonephritis. Numerous foamy macrophages are present that show abundant cytoplasm; low nuclear to cytoplasmic (N:C) ratios; bland, uniform, round nuclei with prominent nucleoli. Scattered lymphocytes are in the background. (Pap)

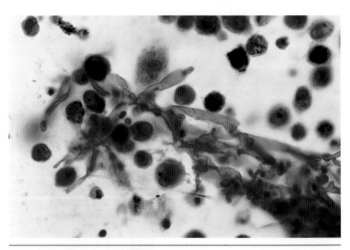

Figure 22-10 Renal abscess with mucormycosis. Abundant foamy macrophages are in the background of this renal abscess containing ribbonlike strands of mucormycosis. (Pap)

bacterial infection (typically resulting from *Proteus mirabilis* or *Escherichia coli*), although the urine may be sterile. XP often is associated with obstructive lithiasis or an obstructive renal cell carcinoma.[21,22]

The histology of XP is unique in that multiple nodules, which grossly have a characteristic yellow to orange color, are composed of a mixed inflammatory infiltrate of acute, chronic, and granulomatous (histiocytic and giant cell) etiologies. The histiocytes, which are numerous, often have foamy or eosinophilic cytoplasm, which gives the cells an epithelioid appearance. Cholesterol clefts may be present, and the background is composed of a proliferation of fibrous tissue that may be largely spindle cells.[23] The spindle cell component may be mistaken for sarcomatous change in a renal cell carcinoma. Fat necrosis may be present when XP extends beyond the renal capsule.[21]

The aspiration cytology of XP can be easily mistaken for renal cell carcinoma. The histiocytes have foamy or eosinophilic cytoplasm with round nuclei and distinct nucleoli. Importantly, the N:C ratios of XP cells are almost always lower than in renal cell carcinoma. The stroma is that of a granulation-type tissue in XP, whereas in renal cell carcinoma, it is a delicate, extensive vascular network to which the cells adhere. The multinucleated giant cells that are common in XP can be a hint to the correct diagnosis, although this is a rare finding. The immunohistochemical distinction between the histiocytes of XP and similar-appearing cells of renal cell carcinoma is identical to that in distinguishing benign clusters of macrophages in renal cysts from cells of renal carcinoma in a cyst—that is, the cells in XP mark as macrophages: *cytokeratin negative* and *CD68 (KP-1) positive*.[21]

Renal Abscess

Hematogenous spread of infectious agents to the kidney in immunocompromised hosts may give rise to a renal abscess (Figure 22-10). The FNAs of these lesions usually show abundant acute or chronic inflammatory cells with a necrotic background. Renal tubular cells may be present.

Special studies may reveal the underlying organism. Alternatively, submission of material for microbiologic evaluation may be imperative.

CLASSIFICATION OF RENAL EPITHELIAL NEOPLASMS

Renal neoplasms are relatively uncommon, comprising only 3% of all malignancies. Aside from the rare urothelial malignancies arising from the renal pelvis, they are largely epithelial neoplasms originating from the renal tubular epithelium. More frequent in males than females, the traditional clinical presentation of flank pain and hematuria has been replaced in many cases by early detection through current imaging techniques before the commencement of symptoms. Growth of these tumors is usually through the capsule into adjacent soft tissue, along the renal vein, and into the inferior vena cava. Usual sites of metastatic disease beyond the local lymph nodes are the lungs, liver, bone, brain, and distant lymph nodes.[24] Metastases to unusual locations such as skin have also been reported.[25]

Staging of these neoplasms involves both imaging and pathologic investigations. The diagnosis of a primary renal epithelial malignancy may obligate resection of the entire kidney along with Gerota's fascia, perinephric fat, renal vein, and adjacent lymph nodes. The recent restaging of renal neoplasms confined to the kidney and up to 7 cm in diameter in the tumor-node-metastasis (TNM) staging system as pT1 has downgraded the stage of many of these patients who would previously have been considered pT2.[24] This restaging format has been shown to correlate strongly with patient survival ($p < 0.0001$).[26,27]

Recent advances in the understanding of the cytogenetics of renal epithelial tumors coupled with classic morphology and the known natural evolution of these neoplasms has led to a 1997 revised histologic nomenclature used for this text[28,29] (Table 22-5). Benign parenchymal neoplasms are divided into metanephric adenoma, metanephric adenofibroma, papillary renal cell adenoma, and renal oncocy-

TABLE 22-5

Heidelberg/Union Internationale Contre le Cancer/American Joint Committee on Cancer Classification of Renal Neoplasms

Current Nomenclature	Genetic Abnormalities	Previous Designation	Comments
Malignant neoplasms			
Common/ conventional/ clear cell* Renal cell carcinoma	• 3p deletions • Mutations of VHL gene • Deletions of 6q, 8p,9p, 14q†	Clear cell carcinoma	• 5% show sarcomatoid change • 70% to 75% of renal carcinomas
Papillary renal cell carcinoma	• Trisomies of 3q, 7, 8, 12, 16, 17, and 20 • Loss of Y[61]	Chromophil (papillary) renal cell carcinoma	• 10% to 15% of renal carcinomas
Chromophobe renal cell carcinoma	• Monosomy of 1, 2, 6, 10, 13, 17, and 21 • Hypodiploid DNA[65]	Chromophobe Typical Eosinophil	• 5% of renal carcinomas • Hale's colloidal iron positive • Cytoplasmic microvesicles by EM
Collecting duct carcinoma	• Losses of 1, 6, 14, 15, and 22 • Deletions 8p and 13q[45]	Same	• <1% of renal carcinomas • Variant is medullary carcinoma, associated with sickle cell trait • Mucin and Ulex Europaeus positivity
Renal cell carcinoma, unclassified			• 4% to 5 % of renal carcinomas • Composite histology • Largely sarcomatoid elements
Benign neoplasms			
Metanephric adenoma	• Tumor suppressor gene at 2p13-21‡	Same	• Possibly related to papillary renal neoplasms
Metanephric adenofibroma	• Diploid histograms[34]		
Papillary renal cell adenoma	• Trisomy of 7 and 17 • Loss of Y[61]	Cortical adenoma	• Most incidental at autopsy • Most common neoplasm of renal tubular epithelium • <5 mm
Renal oncocytoma	• Losses of Y and 1 • Translocation at 11q13 • Loss of 14 and t(14)	Same	• 5% of renal tubular neoplasms • Abundant mitochondria by EM

From Kovacs G, Akhtar M, Beckwith BJ, et al: The Heidelberg classification of renal cell tumours. J Pathol 1997; 183:131-133; Storkel S, Eble JN, Adlakha K, et al: Classification of renal cell carcinoma: workgroup no. 1. Cancer 1997; 80(5):987-989; Reuter VE, Presti JC: Contemporary approach to the classification of renal epithelial tumors. Semin Oncol 2000; 27:124-137.
EM, Electron microscopy.
*Designation not condoned by the Heidelberg system, which considers this a specific genetic/histologic diagnostic category.
†Kovacs G. Molecular cytogenetics of renal cell tumors. Adv Cancer Res 1993; 62:89-124.
‡Pesti T, Sukosd F, Jones EC, et al. Mapping a tumor suppressor gene to chromosome 2p13 in metanephric adenoma by microsatellite allelotyping. Hum Pathol 2001; 32(1)101-104.

toma. Malignant parenchymal neoplasms are classified as common/conventional renal cell carcinoma, papillary renal cell carcinoma, chromophobe renal cell carcinoma, collecting duct carcinoma with its variant medullary carcinoma, and unclassified renal cell carcinoma.[28,29]

This modern classification of renal cell carcinoma has important prognostic significance.[30] In a recent study of 186 patients nephrectomized for similar-size renal carcinomas, it was shown that significant differences in clinical behavior were noted between the neoplasms of different histology. Patients with conventional renal cell carcinoma were found to have metastases 37% of the time at diagnosis, as compared with 16% of patients with papillary and 8% of patients with chromophobe renal cell carcinoma. Patients with conventional renal cell carcinoma were also more commonly found to have renal vein invasion than did patients with papillary renal cell carcinoma. Consequently, the survival of patients with chromophobe and papillary renal cell carcinoma was significantly better than that of patients with conventional renal cell carcinoma.[30]

Using this new classification, a recent study evaluated the patterns of metastases of the major subtypes of renal cell carcinoma. Although renal cell carcinoma has been shown to metastasize widely, in this series a pattern emerged: pulmonary metastases were much more likely to be due to clear cell renal cell carcinoma than papillary renal cell carcinoma. Chromophobe carcinoma, if metastatic, was most likely to metastasize to the liver.[31]

IMMUYNOCYTOCHEMISTRY OF KIDNEY TUMORS

Technical Considerations

When possible, for all renal lesions the evaluation of alcohol-fixed Papanicolaou (Pap-)stained smears; air-dried Diff-Quik (DQ) smears; and formalin-fixed, hematoxylin and eosin (H&E)–stained cell block material is optimal, as each preparation highlights certain cytoplasmic or nuclear features that offer clues to the correct diagnosis (Box 22-3). Nevertheless, the application of immunocytochemistry for the differential diagnosis of primary renal neoplasms is playing an ever-increasing role. Where applicable, the use of specific antibodies is discussed with each of the diagnostic entities. However, certain technical considerations need to be taken into account when attempting to perform immunocytochemistry on any renal FNA sample. This is true for immunocytochemistry on cell blocks, smears, monolayer preparations, or cytospins.

During the immunocytochemistry procedure, the kidney (similar to liver, brain, adrenal, and parathyroid tissues) may bind avidin, biotinylated horseradish peroxidase, or other biotin/avidin system components without prior addition of a biotinylated antibody. This nonspecific binding may be due to endogenous biotin or biotin-binding proteins, lectins, or nonspecific binding substances present in the kidney tissue. This uptake may yield a high background and false-positive staining, which precludes accurate interpretation of immunocytochemistry studies. This is often accentuated for antibodies that require heat-induced epitope retrieval pretreatment methods. When using the avidin biotin complex immunocytochemistry method, pretreatment of the tissue with avidin, followed by a biotin block (to block the remaining biotin binding sites on the avidin) before the addition of the primary antibody, may be of benefit in decreasing this nonspecific background staining[32,33] (Figures 22-11 and 22-12).

BENIGN RENAL NEOPLASMS

Metanephric Adenoma

The first large series of metanephric adenomas appeared in the surgical pathology literature in 1995.[34,35] It was noted that this was primarily a benign neoplasm that occurred in young adults (mean age of 40) with a female preponderance (2:1). The age range, however, is from childhood to old age (5 to 83). Although considered a benign tumor, rare reports of metastases have been made.[36]

Although most of these lesions are discovered incidentally, symptomatology, including pain, hematuria, and polycythemia have been described. The mean size of the tumors is 5 cm with a reported range of 0.3 cm to 15 cm.

BOX 22-3

Optimal Preparation of Renal Fine-Needle Aspiration Material for Cytologic Examination

Alcohol-fixed Pap-stained smears; +/− cytospins
Air-dried DQ-stained smears; +/− cytospins
Formalin fixed H&E-stained cell block; may be used for architectural evaluation; immunocytochemistry
Monolayer preparation (prep) (diagnostic value not established)

Pap, Papanicolaou; *DQ,* Diff-Quik; *H&E,* hematoxylin and eosin.

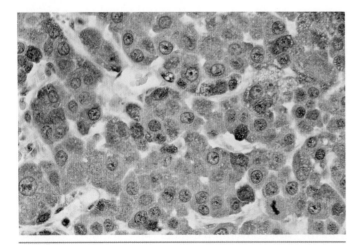

Figure 22-11 Negative control without biotin block. Cell block of carcinoma with high background resulting from endogenous biotin. The background staining in this material makes interpretation of immunocytochemical stains essentially impossible. (Hematoxylin and eosin [H&E], di-amino-benzidene [DAB])

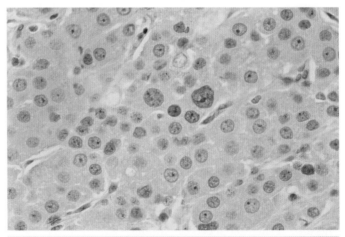

Figure 22-12 Negative control with biotin block. Biotin block on the same cell block of carcinoma in Figure 22-11 removes a majority of the nonspecific background staining, yielding the sample amenable to immunocytochemical staining and interpretation. (H&E, DAB)

Radiographically, these lesions are more commonly calcified than other renal neoplasms.[34,35]

These lesions are histologically similar to the metanephric hamartomatous component of nephroblastomatosis. Blastema is not present. Small oval epithelial cells with little cytoplasm form closely packed tubules that merge with solid nests of similar cells. They can, in some cases, form glomeruloid, papillary, and polypoid formations. Many show evidence of scarring and calcification. Although these are considered benign neoplasms, the challenge is not to mistake one for a papillary renal cell carcinoma or an epithelial Wilms' tumor.[34,35] Immunocytochemistry findings show no consistent pattern of reactivity aside from vimentin and cytokeratin staining, and epithelial membrane antigen (EMA) negativity in some of the cases.[34,37]

Reports of the cytology of metanephric adenoma are sparse[37,38] (Box 22-4). The FNAs in these rare reports have shown tightly packed clusters and papillae of small cells with overlapping nuclei arranged in tubular and rosette structures. The cells have scant cytoplasm; round, uniform nuclei; and fine, delicate chromatin. When arranged in aggregates, the cells appear to have finely granular cytoplasm. Single tumor cells and poorly formed sheets may be dispersed in the background. The cells were without pleomorphism, mitoses, or necrosis. Although the diagnosis of metanephric adenoma may be suggested on cytology, other possibilities, particularly papillary renal cell carcinoma and adult Wilms' tumor need to be excluded.[37,38] Papillary renal cell carcinoma should show diffuse cytokeratin 7 and EMA immunoreactivity.[39]

Metanephric Adenofibroma

An extremely rare variant of metanephric adenoma is metanephric adenofibroma. The histology is characterized by bland epithelial elements as described above for metanephric adenoma, interspersed in a spindled fibroblastic stroma that is cytologically similar to the spindle cells in congenital mesoblastic nephroma.[40] One can anticipate that the cytologic features would be a mixture of the two aforementioned elements, albeit in varying proportions, depending on the individual lesion.

Papillary Adenoma

Formerly called *cortical adenomas,* these incidental neoplasms histologically resemble low-grade papillary renal cell carcinoma. Their definition includes a size restriction, and therefore, they can be no larger than 5 mm. Histologically, they are composed of bland tubulopapillary structures, which may or may not have xanthoma cells and psammoma bodies. The epithelial cells are small, with round, uniform, bland nuclei. Mitotic activity is rare.[41] Their clinical and cytogenetic relationships to papillary carcinoma remain controversial. At the time of the writing of this book, there are no reports on the cytology of this lesion.[29]

Renal Oncocytoma

Renal oncocytoma, a benign group of neoplasms with a characteristic imaging and histologic appearance, comprises approximately 4% of renal neoplasms in adults, with a 2:1 male:female ratio. However, oncocytoma has been described rarely in children.[42] Multifocal, bilateral, and diffuse involvement of the kidney have also been described.[43]

Surprisingly, oncocytoma was originally described only 25 years ago.[44] Although initially believed to develop from the proximal tubules of the kidney, they are now thought to originate from the intercalated cells of the collecting duct epithelium.[45,46] The diagnosis may be suspected on imaging due to the spoke-wheel pattern of feeding vessels, central scarring, sharp demarcation, and density similar to surrounding renal parenchyma. Partial nephrectomy or enucleation has been advocated as curative.[46]

Histologically the tumor cells have abundant eosinophilic granular cytoplasm (ultrastructurally filled with mitochondria). The oncocytes are arranged in well-defined nests peripherally, and centrally are separated by fibrous tissue that forms the central scar. Although any cellular pleomorphism is considered degenerative in origin, the presence of mitoses is not tolerated. Thus, any renal tumor morphologically resembling an oncocytoma with mitotic activity should not be put into this diagnostic category. Hemorrhage and cystic change may be seen, however. By histochemistry, the cells are Hale's colloidal iron negative, which is an important discriminator of this lesion from the similar appearing chromophobe carcinoma (previously called *eosinophilic variant of chromophobe carcinoma*). Previous reports documenting rare malignant oncocytomas are most likely misdiagnosed examples of the latter.[23] The cells of oncocytoma are immunoreactive for EMA and negative for vimentin.[47]

In cytology, as in histology, necrosis and mitotic activity should not be present in renal oncocytoma (Figure 22-13 and Box 22-5). In smears, the large cells with abundant granular eosinophilic cytoplasm and distinct cellular outlines can appear singly, in clusters or in sheets. They should not exhibit an increase in the N:C ratio due to the voluminous cytoplasm. The cytoplasmic integrity is usually maintained, thus, stripped nuclei are not a common feature. The nuclei are conspicuously round, the appearance of the nucleoli may vary from inconspicuous to prominent and brightly eosinophilic. Multinucleation and atypia may be

---

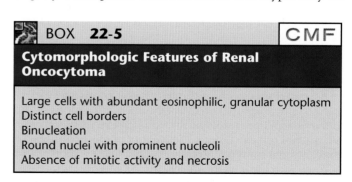

BOX 22-4   CMF

Cytomorphologic Features of Metanephric Adenoma

Small, uniform cells in tight, papillae-like clusters; in loose sheets; and singly
Uniform normochromatic nuclei +/− small nucleoli
Absence of necrosis, pleomorphism, and mitoses

BOX 22-5   CMF

Cytomorphologic Features of Renal Oncocytoma

Large cells with abundant eosinophilic, granular cytoplasm
Distinct cell borders
Binucleation
Round nuclei with prominent nucleoli
Absence of mitotic activity and necrosis

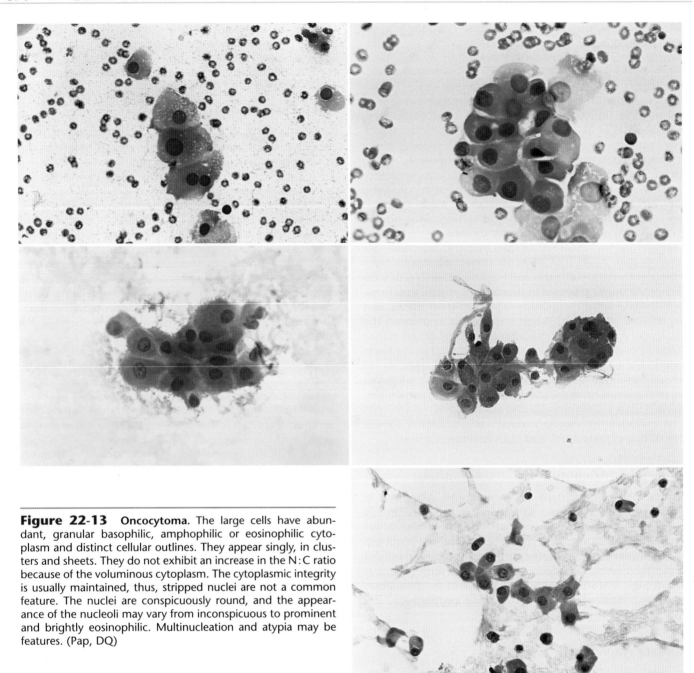

Figure 22-13 Oncocytoma. The large cells have abundant, granular basophilic, amphophilic or eosinophilic cytoplasm and distinct cellular outlines. They appear singly, in clusters and sheets. They do not exhibit an increase in the N:C ratio because of the voluminous cytoplasm. The cytoplasmic integrity is usually maintained, thus, stripped nuclei are not a common feature. The nuclei are conspicuously round, and the appearance of the nucleoli may vary from inconspicuous to prominent and brightly eosinophilic. Multinucleation and atypia may be features. (Pap, DQ)

features. If, however, other cytoplasmic features such as cytoplasmic vacuolization or perinuclear clearing are noted, one must beware of misdiagnosing a conventional or chromophobe renal cell carcinoma as an oncocytoma. Oncocytoma is immunoreactive with low molecular weight cytokeratin and is negative for vimentin, in contrast with conventional renal cell carcinoma, which should be immunoreactive with both.[23,47-49]

As stated previously, although the diagnosis of oncocytoma can be suggested on cytology, oncocytic lesions of the kidney should be histologically sampled extensively to rule out a renal cell carcinoma, particularly of chromophobe or conventional subtypes. Because kidney sparing surgery can be used successfully for oncocytoma, it is recommended that even with a presumptive FNA diagnosis of oncocy-

toma, a frozen section should be performed at the time of surgery to ensure appropriate surgical approach.[42,50] Alternatively, a less specific aspiration diagnosis (e.g., oncocytoid renal neoplasm) could be rendered, with a differential diagnostic list and recommendation offered for an intraoperative frozen section. A recent study has suggested, however, that the diagnosis of renal oncocytoma can be reliably distinguished on FNA from conventional, papillary, and chromophobe carcinoma through a combination of morphology and immunocytochemistry, as described above, using a combination of Hale's colloidal iron, vimentin, and cytokeratin, with electron microscopy providing additional information to confirm the diagnosis.[47] This approach may be imperative in patients with bilateral renal masses or impaired renal function.[47]

GRADING OF RENAL CELL CARCINOMA

The nuclear grading (Fuhrman Grading System) of renal neoplasms should be performed on conventional/clear cell renal cell carcinoma and papillary renal cell carcinoma on cell block sections[51] (Table 22-6). It is also currently recommended to use nuclear grading for chromophobe renal cell carcinoma for the purposes of ongoing clinicopathologic studies. Nuclear grading should not be used for oncocytoma or other benign renal neoplasms.[52] The final nuclear grading of the variants of renal cell carcinoma is best performed on the worst histologic appearing area of the tumor, along with an accompanying measurement of the size of the tumor exhibiting the highest grade. However, it can be performed preliminarily on the FNA cell block with the knowledge that it may be upgraded based on the final histology.

A strong correlation exists between cytologic and histologic nuclear grading of renal cell carcinoma.[53] Although the current recommendation calls to combine Fuhrman nuclear grades 1 and 2 for the creation of a three-grade system, the variations on this practice are largely institutional.[52] Sarcomatous components, which can be present in any of the renal epithelial neoplasms, mandate a high grade designation.

CONVENTIONAL/CLEAR CELL RENAL CELL CARCINOMA

Although in the new classification of renal cell carcinoma, low-grade papillary neoplasms less than 0.5 cm can be classified as papillary renal adenoma; solid clear tumors of any size should be classified as carcinoma.[52]

Clear cell renal cell carcinoma accounts for 70% to 75% of all renal cell carcinomas and has a strong genetic basis in deletions of 3p and mutations of the von Hippel-Lindau gene.[101] Clear cell renal cell carcinoma is theorized to emanate from the proximal tubules; thus, at times the cytologic distinction between benign proximal tubular cells and low-grade clear cell renal cell carcinoma can be difficult[45] (Boxes 22-6 and 22-7).

Although clear cell renal cell carcinoma can grow to great sizes, recent advances in imaging techniques have led to earlier diagnoses and the detection of smaller tumors. The neoplasms are known for their marked heterogeneity in histologic pattern, nuclear grade, and cytoplasmic characteristics, both inter- and intralesional (see Box 22-6). Typically, the solid component is composed of a complex network of thin-walled vascular channels that surround and separate the tumor cells into irregular nests. The tumor cells have a large volume of clear cytoplasm (periodic acid-Schiff [PAS] positive for glycogen and mucicarmine negative for mucin). It may, however, be variably granular in portions of the tumor. Hemorrhage, necrosis, and a prominent cystic component are common. Additional patterns within the solid areas are microcystic, tubular, sarcomatoid, and papillary, with the latter potentially resulting in an erroneous classification of a clear cell renal cell carcinoma as a papillary renal cell carcinoma, a genetically unrelated tumor.[23]

Low-grade nuclear morphology on histologic sections is characterized by round nuclear contours with invisible or

---

TABLE	22-6

Fuhrman Nuclear Grading System for Renal Cell Carcinoma

Fuhrman Grade	Description
1	Round, small ($<10\ \mu$) nuclei Hyperchromatic nuclei Inconspicuous nucleoli
2	Nuclei ($15\ \mu$) Open chromatin pattern Nucleoli not visible at $\times 10$ but visible at higher magnifications
3	Large nuclei ($20\ \mu$) Open chromatin pattern Prominent nucleoli visible at $\times 10$
4	Bizarre, pleomorphic, multilobated nuclei

From Fuhrman SA, Lasky LC, Limas C. Prognostic significance of morphologic parameters in renal cell carcinoma. Am J Surg Pathol 1982; 6:655-663.

BOX	22-6	CMF

Cytomorphologic Features of Conventional/Clear Cell Renal Cell Carcinoma

Smears of variable cellularity; may have hemorrhagic or necrotic background

Large, round cells with abundant vacuolated or granular cytoplasm

Indistinct cytoplasmic outlines

Frequent tumor cell aggregates surrounding thin-walled blood vessels associated with basement membrane–like material

Low N:C ratios

Round nuclei with prominent eosinophilic nucleoli (grade 2 and above)

Eccentric nucleus may have appearance of being pushed out of the cytoplasm

Nuclear grooves, rounded lobulations, and cytoplasmic pseudoinclusions

N:C, Nuclear to cytoplasmic.

BOX	22-7

Differential Diagnosis of Conventional/Clear Cell Renal Cell Carcinoma

Chromophobe renal cell carcinoma
Oncocytoma
Papillary renal cell carcinoma
Metastatic clear cell carcinoma
Benign adrenal cortex cells
Adrenal cortical neoplasm
Benign hepatic cells (right kidney FNA)
Benign proximal tubular elements

FNA, Fine-needle aspiration.

small nucleoli. In grade 1 lesions the nuclei are actually mildly hyperchromatic. As nuclear grade increases to grade 2 or 3, the nuclei enlarge and become hypochromatic with increasing size and prominence of the round central (single or multiple), brightly eosinophilic nucleolus. In grade 4 tumors the nuclear contours show a rounded, lobulated outline. Nuclear grooves and pseudoinclusions may be seen. As previously stated, the nuclear grade is determined by the most atypical cells within the sections.[23]

As in other cytologic preparations, the nuclear details are best viewed with alcohol-fixed Pap-stained material, whereas the cytoplasmic and stromal features are better viewed on the air-dried DQ-stained material (Figures 22-14 to 22-22). FNA of clear cell renal cell carcinoma may yield highly cellular aspirates with varying amounts of tumor cells and ac-

companying stromal components. Thus, a common finding is aggregated tumor cells adjacent to thin-walled capillaries with admixed stromal components. Basement membrane material, which stains strongly magenta-colored in DQ, is often a prominent feature of these tumor-vascular aggregates. In rare cases, round globules of this magenta-staining basement membrane can be seen intracellularly, giving an appearance similar to Mott cells. Although these globules are not described well in the cytology literature, they have been previously described as *glassy hyaline globules* in the surgical pathology literature and have been noted in clear cell renal cell carcinoma and to a lesser extent in papillary renal cell carcinoma. They are supposedly not seen in chromophobe renal cell carcinoma or oncocytoma.[54] The vacuoles in the abundant cytoplasm vary in size and uniformity of distribu-

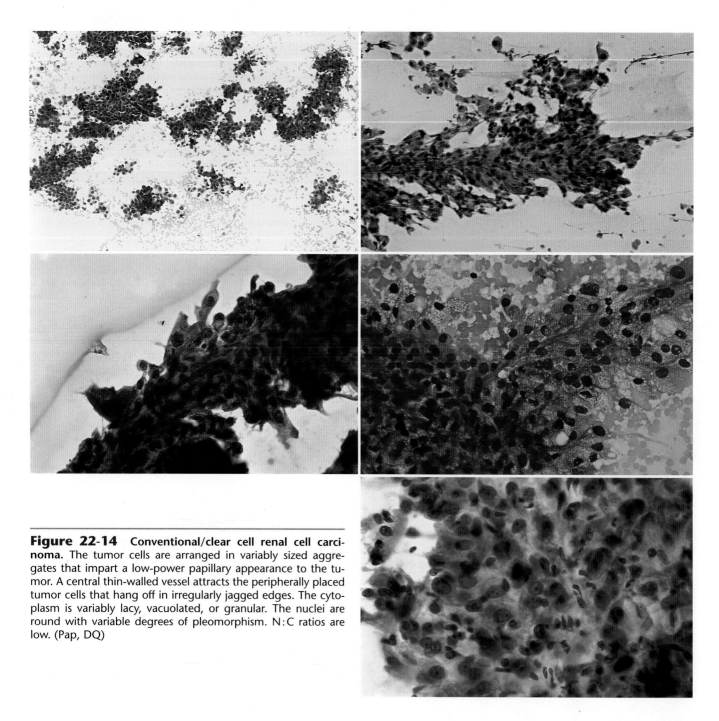

Figure 22-14 **Conventional/clear cell renal cell carcinoma.** The tumor cells are arranged in variably sized aggregates that impart a low-power papillary appearance to the tumor. A central thin-walled vessel attracts the peripherally placed tumor cells that hang off in irregularly jagged edges. The cytoplasm is variably lacy, vacuolated, or granular. The nuclei are round with variable degrees of pleomorphism. N:C ratios are low. (Pap, DQ)

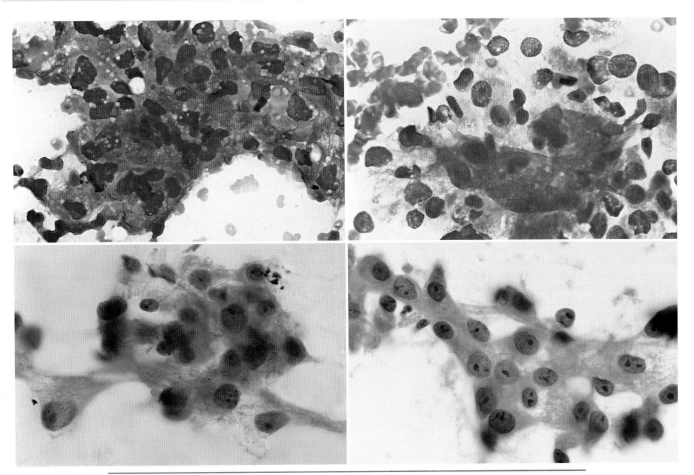

Figure 22-15 **Conventional/clear cell renal cell carcinoma.** Magenta-staining basement membrane–like material is evident in between some of the cells. The cytoplasm is variably lacy, vacuolated, or granular. The cells have indistinct cytoplasmic borders with rounded to spindled, elongated shapes. Nuclei are rounded, but can be irregularly lobulated. Nucleoli may be prominent. N : C ratios are low. (DQ, Pap)

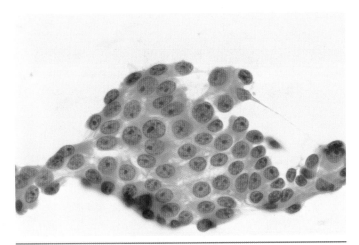

Figure 22-16 **Conventional/clear cell renal cell carcinoma.** This fine-needle aspiration (FNA) of a chest wall mass of metastatic renal cell carcinoma shows a flat sheet of benign-appearing low-grade tumor cells. These cells, particularly when present in a renal FNA, may simulate benign sheets of renal tubular cells. The prominent nucleoli that are present assist with the correct classification, as does, in this sheet, the increased N : C ratios. (Pap)

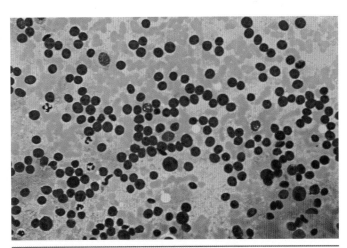

Figure 22-17 **Conventional/clear cell renal cell carcinoma.** Extreme cytoplasmic fragility may give rise to aspirates or areas of aspirates that are composed of largely stripped nuclei. The rounded shape of the nuclei and the prominent nucleoli may simulate adrenal cortical carcinoma. Aspirates of renal cell carcinoma, however, do not contain the lipid-vacuolated background appearance of aspirates of adrenal cortical carcinomas. (DQ)

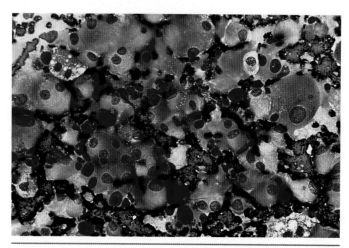

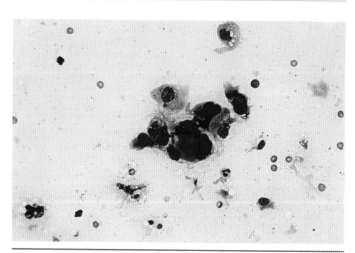

Figure 22-18 Conventional/clear cell renal cell carcinoma. The population of tumor cells can appear as single cells rather than clusters or sheets. These cells have largely abundant granular cytoplasm with eccentric rounded nuclei and, at times, prominent macronucleoli. This pattern can also closely simulate adrenal cortical carcinoma. (DQ)

Figure 22-19 Conventional/clear cell renal cell carcinoma. This small cluster of tumor cells shows intermediate-grade nuclei with vacuolated and granular cytoplasm. Within the cytoplasm of several of the cells are globules of dense magenta-staining material (glassy hyaline globules), which can be a prominent feature of some cases. (DQ)

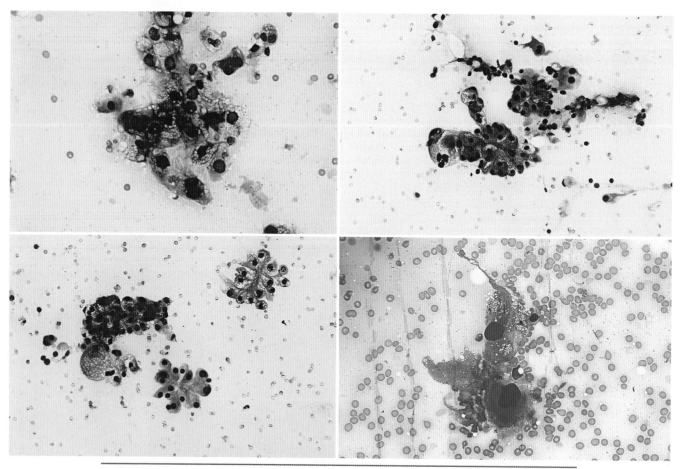

Figure 22-20 Conventional/clear cell renal cell carcinoma. These figures show a spectrum of morphology of nonvascularized aggregates of tumor cells. Clusters can be large and irregular or small and papillary-like. Cytoplasm and nuclear morphology are variable.

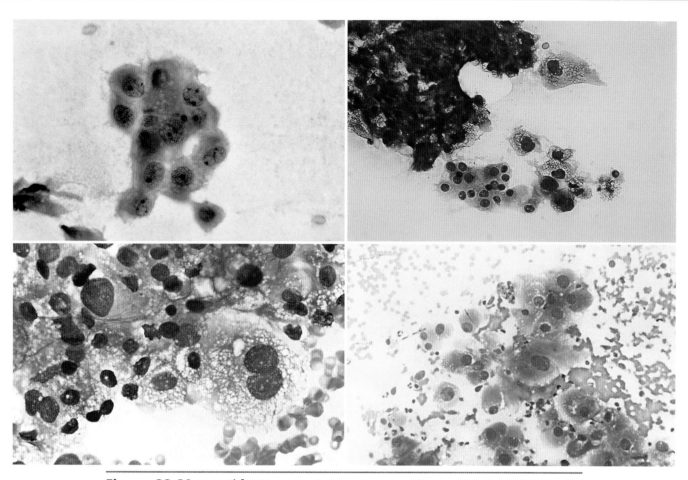

Figure 22-20, cont'd An aggregate of normal-appearing renal tubular epithelium adjacent to tumor cells. (Pap, DQ)

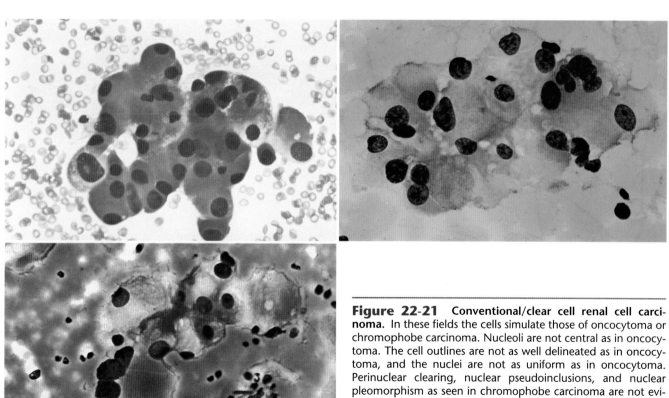

Figure 22-21 Conventional/clear cell renal cell carcinoma. In these fields the cells simulate those of oncocytoma or chromophobe carcinoma. Nucleoli are not central as in oncocytoma. The cell outlines are not as well delineated as in oncocytoma, and the nuclei are not as uniform as in oncocytoma. Perinuclear clearing, nuclear pseudoinclusions, and nuclear pleomorphism as seen in chromophobe carcinoma are not evident. (DQ)

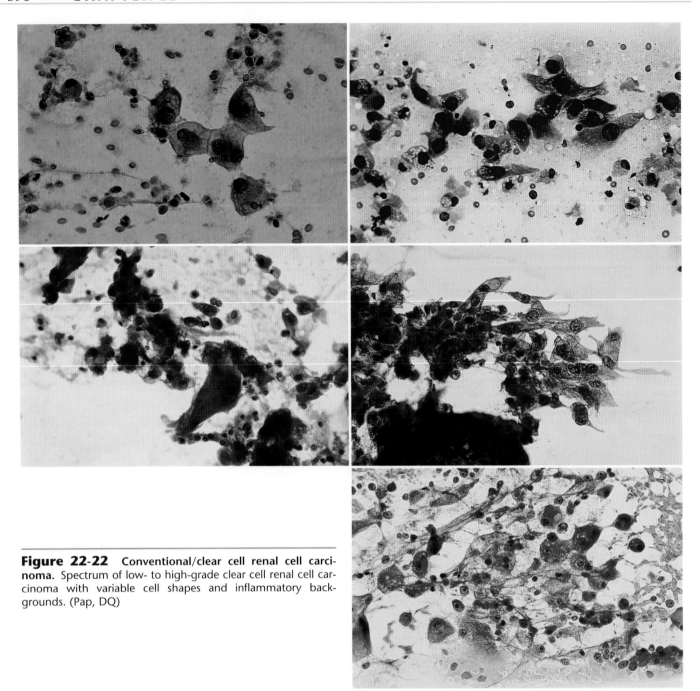

Figure 22-22 Conventional/clear cell renal cell carcinoma. Spectrum of low- to high-grade clear cell renal cell carcinoma with variable cell shapes and inflammatory backgrounds. (Pap, DQ)

tion. Some clear cell renal cell carcinoma instead have neoplastic cells with eosinophilic and distinctly granular cytoplasm. Other neoplasms are composed of variable admixtures of the two cell types. Papillary aggregates are allowable but cannot comprise the entire population of the sample. Cytoplasmic borders are often indistinguishable, a feature that is important in the distinction of clear cell renal cell carcinoma from chromophobe renal cell carcinoma, in which cytoplasmic borders are sharp.

The smear background appearance of clear cell renal cell carcinoma can be highly variable; it may be necrotic or highly hemorrhagic. Smears may appear to have a low or nonexistent cellular population, thus, the cell block may be imperative for the viewing of tissue fragments trapped in the blood. Due to the friability of the cytoplasm, stripped

nuclei are a common finding. Although intact single cells may be seen, the cells are usually in small clusters or variably sized sheets. When the cells appear in flat sheets, it may be impossible to distinguish low nuclear grade clear cell renal cell carcinoma from benign proximal tubular cells. A helpful clue is that normal tubular cells are usually seen singly or in small groups, not in the large groups characteristic of clear cell renal cell carcinoma.[7] At the time of this writing, no conventional special studies can be used for this determination. A single report of the use of microdissection of cells from a DQ preparation and subsequent polymerase chain reaction for genetic abnormalities (loss of heterozygosity) of the von Hippel Lindau gene shows how this technique can be used successfully to make this distinction.[55] In clear cell renal cell carcinoma, the neoplastic but benign-appearing cells in the flat sheets should have the classic genetic abnormalities as would be expected in clear cell renal cell carcinoma rather than normal DNA. This type of testing has not yet reached mainstream status.

The flat sheet appearance of low-grade tumor cells can also be a problem in metastatic clear cell renal cell carcinoma lesions where they can be confused with sheets of mesothelial cells. For that distinction, mesothelial markers such as HBME-1 and calretinin should be used to demonstrate immunoreactivity in the mesothelial cells that would not be present in the tumor cells.[56]

Nuclear appearance is as described above for histology with a few enhancements made accessible by the cytologic preparations. In general, the nuclei are round, grooved, or irregular, but rounded contours are maintained. The level of nuclear chromasia coincides with the grade. Interestingly, grade I lesions show round nuclei with slight hyperchromasia, no nucleoli, and little nuclear detail. As the grade progressively increases, the nuclei appear clearer with conspicuous bright red nucleoli becoming evident and fine chromatin stippling adjacent to the areas of clearing. Although in the low nuclear grade lesions nuclear size is consistently small, with the higher-grade lesions, nuclear size can be highly variable and is often large. Abundant cytoplasm is maintained so the N:C ratios should remain low. The nucleus is often eccentric and can give the appearance of being pushed out of the cytoplasm. As previously stated, nuclear grading should be done on the most atypical cells on the cell block. Sarcomatoid cells with spindled cytoplasm and high-grade nuclei may be variably present.

Differential Diagnosis

Metastatic clear cell carcinoma should always be in the differential of clear cell renal cell carcinoma if the patient has a dominant mass in another organ known to support a primary of clear cell morphology (e.g., lung, ovary) (Box 22-8; see Box 22-7). In this scenario, the site of the primary is most likely determined by the clinical evaluation because no studies can determine the cause of a clear cell carcinoma in general use.

A recently described immunohistochemical stain, vinculin, has been determined to stain the collecting duct system of normal kidney and renal neoplasms derived from the collecting duct system (e.g., oncocytoma, chromophobe renal cell carcinoma, collecting duct carcinoma, and some cases of papillary and purely sarcomatoid renal cell carcinoma).[102] Although this initial study was performed on surgical pathology material, this raises the interesting possibility of using antivinculin in aspirates as an additional ancillary study to help subtype the variants of renal cell carcinoma because clear cell renal cell carcinoma should be nonimmunoreactive with this antibody.

The distinction between clear cell renal cell carcinoma and papillary renal cell carcinoma is based on the abundance of papillary structures, cytoplasmic hemosiderin, psammoma bodies, and nuclear grooves. These features are highly characteristic of papillary renal cell carcinoma and are not present to any extent in clear cell renal cell carcinoma. Thus, the absence of these features in low- or high-grade neoplasms may make the cytologic distinction between these two entities impossible, unless aspirated material is cytogenetically analyzed.[7]

Chromophobe renal cell carcinoma may come into the differential diagnosis of clear cell renal cell carcinoma. In general, the cells of clear cell renal cell carcinoma have more uniform nuclear size and roundness than those of chromophobe renal cell carcinoma. Other morphologic features favoring clear cell renal cell carcinoma include large prominent nucleoli, preservation of intercellular cohesion, and basement membrane matrix material. Conversely, attributes arguing for chromophobe renal cell carcinoma include individually scattered bizarre neoplastic cells, irregular nuclear contours, nuclear pseudoinclusions, and perinuclear cytoplasmic clearing (halos). Using ancillary studies, Hales' colloidal iron is negative in clear cell renal cell carcinoma and positive in chromophobe renal cell carcinoma. Cytokeratin 18 should be positive in chromophobe renal cell carcinoma and vimentin should be negative, the opposite of which are expected in clear cell renal cell carcinoma.

Benign and malignant adrenal cortical cells can appear morphologically identical to the cells of clear cell renal cell carcinoma. The background of stripped round nuclei is common to both. In fact, it may be impossible to distinguish these different populations of cells based on morphology alone. Some cases of benign or malignant adrenal cortical cells may show a foamy lipid background on the smears, which is unexpected in clear cell renal cell carcinoma. This can be a helpful distinguishing feature. A recent morphologic analysis of this problem concluded that the presence of cells in sheets with central, thin-walled vascular cores, significant anisonucleosis, crushed spindle cell fragments, eccentric nuclei, and the absence of cytoplasmic vacuolizations favor the diagnosis of adrenal cortical carcinoma.[57] Using immunocytochemistry, clear cell renal cell carcinoma is immunoreactive with anti-EMA, whereas adrenal cortical cells and adrenal cortical neoplasms are not. A more recently described immunocytochemical solution to this problem is the use of antibodies to α-Inhibin and MelanA, both of which are immunoreactive in normal and neoplastic adrenal cortical tissues and are nonreactive in clear cell renal cell carcinoma[58,59] (Figure 22-23).

The distinction of clear cell renal cell carcinoma from hepatocellular carcinoma may be difficult in terms of ruling out a metastatic clear cell renal cell carcinoma in a diseased liver (Figure 22-24). In this scenario a history of a single mass and a history of preexisting liver disease (e.g., chronic he-

---

BOX 22-8

Special Studies Characteristics of Conventional/Clear Cell Renal Cell Carcinoma

PAS positive for glycogen
Mucicarmine negative for mucin
Low molecular weight cytokeratin positive
Vimentin positive
EMA positivity variable
CEA negative
Deletion of 3p
Vinculin negative
Cytoplasmic glassy hyaline globules

PAS, Periodic acid-Schiff; *EMA*, epithelial membrane antigen; *CEA*, carcinoembryonic antigen.

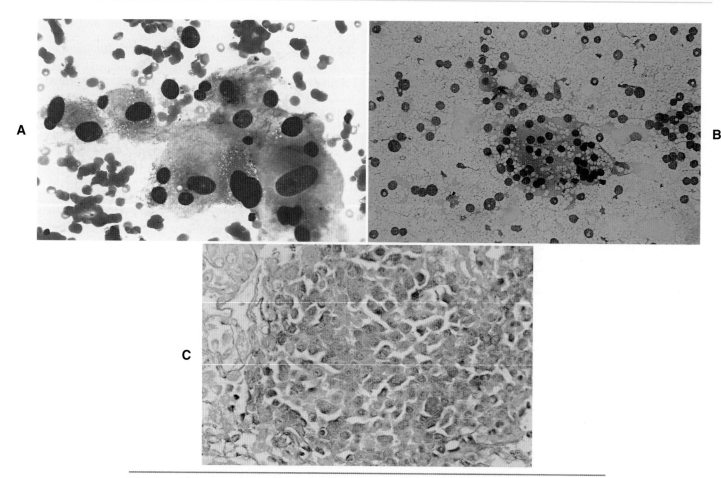

Figure 22-23   Adrenocortical carcinoma. The morphology of adrenocortical carcinoma can simulate that of conventional renal cell carcinoma and can be indistinguishable on morphology alone. **A,** These cells have rounded nuclei and abundant cytoplasm that may be vacuolated. **B,** Lipid background that is characteristic of adrenocortical carcinoma and is not seen in renal carcinoma. **C,** Cell block of adrenocortical carcinoma that is staining positively with the immunocytochemical stain for α-Inhibin, which is negative in conventional renal cell carcinoma. (DQ, H&E, DAB)

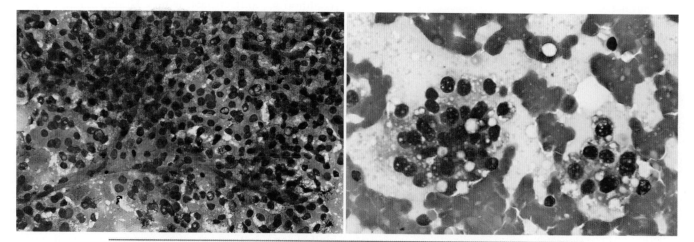

Figure 22-24   Hepatocellular carcinoma. In the distinction of metastatic renal cell carcinoma to the liver, the distinction of hepatocellular carcinoma from renal cell carcinoma may be difficult. The cells appear as aggregates around vascular centers. Cells in these samples have vacuolated cytoplasm and round nuclei. Cytoplasmic intranuclear pseudoinclusions are more common in hepatocellular carcinoma. (DQ)

patitis) are most suggestive of a primary hepatic etiology. Markers such as carcinoembryonic antigen (CEA) and α-fetoprotein would also be positive in primary liver carcinoma and negative in metastatic clear cell renal cell carcinoma. Conversely, the presence of multiple lesions and the absence of a history of previous liver disease and negative immunohistochemistry for the above markers would favor the diagnosis of metastatic clear cell renal cell carcinoma.

The presence of benign hepatic cells should always be a consideration in an FNA of the right kidney. As hepatic cells often have granulated cytoplasm and round nuclei with prominent nucleoli, it is possible to confuse these cells with those of granular cells in a clear cell renal cell carcinoma. Generally, hepatic cells have better defined cellular outlines and more evenly dispersed cytoplasmic granules.[7] Another distinguishing feature is the presence of cytoplasmic iron in the liver cells.

The distinction between clear cell renal cell carcinoma and oncocytoma is discussed in the section in this chapter on Oncocytoma.

PAPILLARY RENAL CELL CARCINOMA

Papillary renal cell carcinoma, which accounts for 10% to 15% of renal carcinomas, has previously been referred to as *chromophil renal cell carcinoma* and *tubulopapillary renal cell carcinoma*.[29] The cell of origin is theorized to be the distal convoluted tubule.[45] The histologic diagnosis of papillary renal cell carcinoma is fulfilled when at least 50% of the tumor is comprised of true papillae (i.e., fibrovascular cores lined by, in this case, malignant epithelial cells). Tubular and solid patterns are part of the histologic spectrum of papillary renal cell carcinoma.[60] Conversely, areas of papillary architecture may be present in other renal epithelial malignancies such as clear cell renal cell carcinoma (usually less than 5% of tumor), and may predominate in collecting duct carcinomas.[7,60] As with clear cell renal cell carcinoma, papillary renal cell carcinoma has a distinct set of genetic abnormalities that are strongly associated with the diagnosis: trisomies of 3q, 7, 8, 12, 16, 17, and 20 and also the loss of Y.[61] It is also known for its propensity to be multifocal within the same or both kidneys and for its association with papillary adenomas.[62]

A recent study of 105 papillary renal cell carcinoma divided these neoplasms into two distinct histologic types that correlate with clinical and immunohistochemical findings.[60] Type 1 papillary renal cell carcinomas are composed of generally short papillae covered by one or two layers of small epithelial cells with scanty, pale or clear cytoplasm. Similar cells line tubular structures when present. Many of the papillae are edematous, giving an almost cystlike appearance. Glomeruloid papillary structures may be numerous. Necrosis and hemorrhage are prominent features, as are aggregates of foamy macrophages within sheets of tumor cells or within the cores of papillae. Inflammation is often present, as are psammoma bodies (48%).[60]

In type 2 papillary renal cell carcinoma, the papillae are covered by cells with abundant eosinophilic cytoplasm that are arranged in a stratified or pseudostratified manner. Edema of papillae is not prominent, with dense fibrous cores being more common. Necrosis, hemorrhage, and inflammation are frequent, with multinucleated giant cells present.

Foamy macrophages are rarely present within papillae and are more commonly adjacent to areas of necrosis.[60]

In this study, the proportion of type 1 to type 2 tumors was almost 2:1. Sarcomatoid differentiation was found in a small subset of both types. In general, the nuclear grades were higher in the type 2 neoplasms than in the type 1. Immunohistochemical staining for cytokeratin 7, said to be specific for papillary renal cell carcinoma, was present in a majority of the type 1 lesions and was absent in the majority of type 2 lesions. All tumors were nonimmunoreactive with Ulex Europaeus, a marker said to be specific for collecting duct carcinoma that also has a papillary architecture.[60] According to this study, tumors with type 1 histology had a smaller size, a lower TNM stage, and a lower nuclear grade than type 2 lesions. Type 2 tumors seemed to occur with more frequency in patients younger than age 40.[60] To date, the authors are unaware of any study attempting to subclassify these tumors into types 1 and 2 based on aspiration specimens.

Histologically, the cells of papillary renal cell carcinoma have sparse or abundant clear or granular eosinophilic cytoplasm. The cytoplasm may contain hemosiderin granules. True papillary structures are surrounded by tumor cells. The nuclei are rounded and are of variable size and contours determined by grade. Nuclear grooves or pseudoinclusions may be seen. Foamy macrophages may be numerous.

As would be expected, the papillary architecture lends itself to facile identification on FNA, where the fibrovascular cores can be easily recognized in cell block and smear material (Box 22-9; Figures 22-25 to 22-30). In smears, however, the papillary architecture often manifests as round spherules. Relatively few isolated malignant cells may be present. Macrophages may distend the papillae. As in histologic sections, the presence of a true fibrovascular core distinguishes true papillae from pseudopapillae, which may be composed totally of epithelial cells or epithelial cells surrounding a fibrous stalk. Although nuclear appearance varies with grade, they are usually bland and may show grooves. The cells may have abundant intracytoplasmic hemosiderin, and psammoma bodies may be found. Single cells are not abundant.

Differential Diagnosis

The distinction of papillary renal cell carcinoma from clear cell renal cell carcinoma is based on the abundance of true

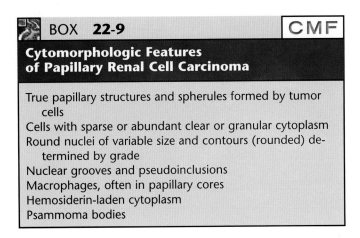

BOX 22-9 CMF

Cytomorphologic Features of Papillary Renal Cell Carcinoma

True papillary structures and spherules formed by tumor cells

Cells with sparse or abundant clear or granular cytoplasm

Round nuclei of variable size and contours (rounded) determined by grade

Nuclear grooves and pseudoinclusions

Macrophages, often in papillary cores

Hemosiderin-laden cytoplasm

Psammoma bodies

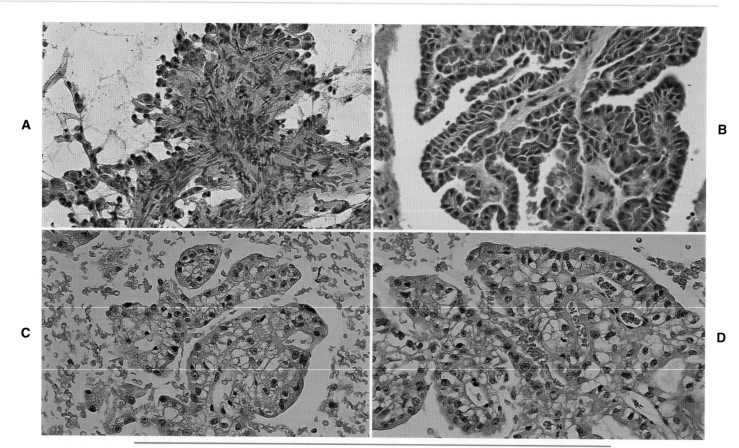

Figure 22-25 **Papillary renal cell carcinoma.** Cell blocks may be an imperative component of renal FNAs in terms of discernment of papillary architecture. This smear **(A)** and cell blocks **(B, C, D)** reveal fibrovascular cores surrounded by small cells with round nuclei and either eosinophilic or clear cytoplasm. (H&E)

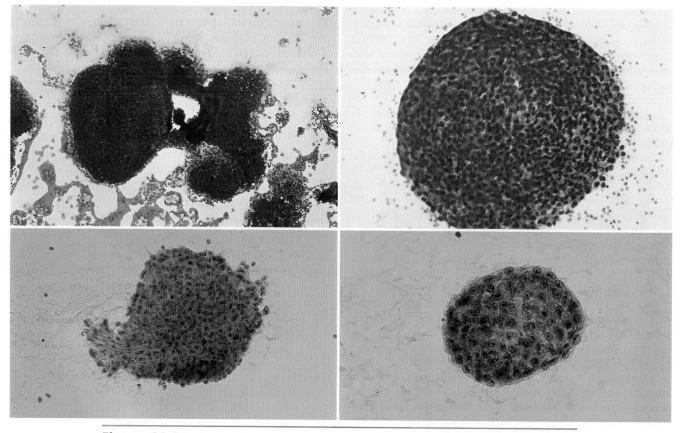

Figure 22-26 **Papillary renal cell carcinoma.** Spherules characteristic of papillary renal cell carcinoma. Note the relative uniformity of the nuclei and the clean background. (DQ, Pap)

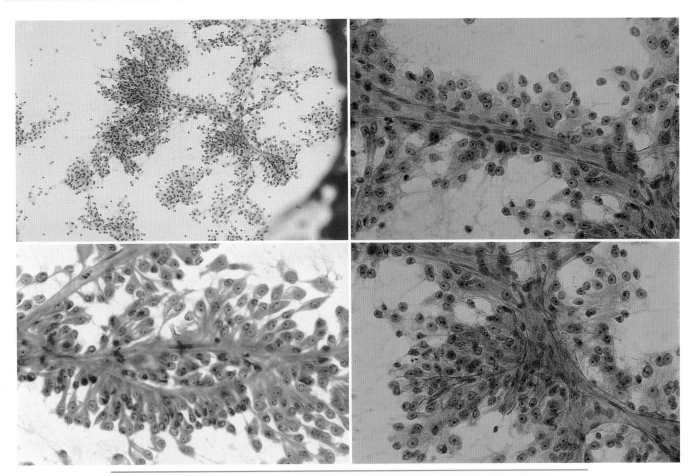

Figure 22-27 **Papillary renal cell carcinoma.** Papillary architecture noted on smears. The cells have abundant, clear cytoplasm with round nuclei and prominent nucleoli. The central fibrovascular core is prominent. Only a few single cells are noted in the background, and nuclear grooves are sparse. (Pap)

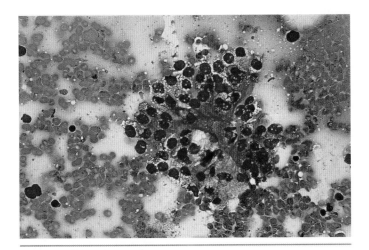

Figure 22-28 **Papillary renal cell carcinoma.** A papillary cluster of cells with basement membrane–like material and abundant vacuolated cytoplasm from a papillary renal cell carcinoma; simulates a conventional renal cell carcinoma. (DQ)

papillary structures, cytoplasmic hemosiderin, psammoma bodies and nuclear grooves (Box 22-10). These features are highly characteristic of papillary renal cell carcinoma and are not present to any extent in clear cell renal cell carcinoma. Consequently the absence of these features in low-

> **BOX 22-10**
>
> **Special Studies: Characteristics of Papillary Renal Cell Carcinoma**
>
> Cytokeratin 7 immunoreactivity variable
> Vimentin immunoreactivity variable
> Ulex Europaeus negative
> High molecular weigh keratin 34BE12 negative
> AE1/AE3 positive
> EMA positive
> Trisomies of 3q, 7, 8, 12, 16, 17 and 20; loss of Y

EMA, Epithelial membrane antigen.

or high-grade neoplasms may make the cytologic distinction between these two entities impossible.[7] A recent study evaluating the cytologic distinction between papillary renal cell carcinoma and other subtypes of renal cell carcinoma found the presence of foamy macrophages and intracytoplasmic hemosiderin to be the two most sensitive and specific markers for papillary renal cell carcinoma of both high- and low-grade types.[63]

Some collecting duct carcinomas may architecturally simulate papillary renal cell carcinoma due to its papillary

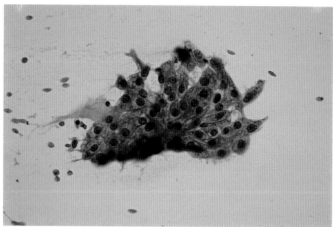

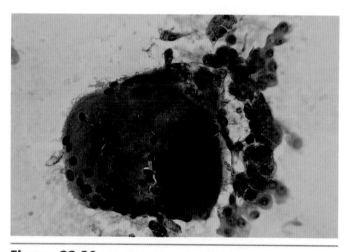

Figure 22-29 Papillary renal cell carcinoma. Sheets of papillary carcinoma cells with well-defined cell borders and bland nuclei. Some cells have pigmented (hemosiderin) cytoplasm. (DQ, Pap)

Figure 22-30 Papillary renal cell carcinoma. Multinucleated giant cell adjacent to cells of a papillary renal cell carcinoma. The tumor cells have sparse cytoplasm; round, uniform nuclei; and prominent nucleoli. (Pap)

architecture. In this differential diagnosis, the papillary renal cell carcinoma will be nonimmunoreactive for Ulex Europaeus and keratin 34BE12, whereas collecting duct carcinoma should be immunoreactive for both.

Although bland tumor cells may appear indistinguishable from benign distal tubular cells, papillary architecture should be evident elsewhere on the specimen in papillary renal cell carcinoma.

Metastatic neoplasms with papillary architecture always come into the differential of these tumors. As with all lesions of the kidney, an extensive radiologic workup determining where the patient's predominant disease is located is of the utmost importance. Likewise, ruling out metastases from particular sites in certain instances may be facilitated through the use of immunocytochemistry or molecular studies for the detection of the characteristic trisomies and losses associated with papillary renal cell carcinoma.

CHROMOPHOBE RENAL CELL CARCINOMA

Chromophobe renal cell carcinoma represents 5% of all renal cell carcinomas and has a prognosis in between that of renal oncocytoma and clear cell renal cell carcinoma. The cellular origin of chromophobe renal cell carcinoma is considered to be the intercalated cells of the collecting duct.[64] Numerous chromosomal losses, which are distinct from clear cell renal cell carcinoma and papillary renal cell carcinoma and unique (among renal neoplasms) to chromophobe renal cell carcinoma (monosomies of 1, 2, 6, 10 , 13, 17, 21 and allelic losses at 1p, 2p, 6p, 10p, 13q, 17p and 21q), have been described.[65] As with oncocytoma, partial nephrectomy can be considered in the surgical treatment.

The histology of chromophobe renal cell carcinoma is characteristic. Hemorrhage and necrosis are not usually features. Cells are arranged in trabeculae. The cells are round to polygonal, and the cytoplasm varies from variably fluffy to granular. When the granular eosinophilic morphology predominates, the diagnostic subcategory of eosinophilic chromophobe carcinoma applies. The cells have abundant cytoplasm with distinct cell borders. A prominent area of perinuclear clearing corresponding on the ultrastructural level to abundant minute perinuclear oval vesicles gives the cells a characteristic "fried-egg" appearance. The nuclei are distinctive in that they are hyperchromatic and highly variable in size with prominent nuclear membrane irregularities and small or indistinct nucleoli. Binucleation may be common. Large bizarre forms may be seen scattered indi-

vidually throughout the tumor; these are the cells most likely to have prominent nuclear pseudoinclusions. The cytoplasm is diffusely positive with Hale's colloidal iron.[66,67]

The aspiration cytology appearance of chromophobe renal cell carcinoma is thought to be sufficiently distinctive for rendering confident diagnoses (Box 22-11; Figures 22-31 and 22-32). Aspirates are generally cellular with the large round to polygonal cells arranged singly and in small

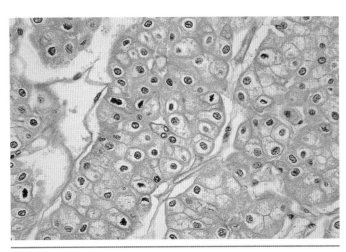

Figure 22-31 **Chromophobe carcinoma.** Cell block of FNA of chromophobe carcinoma. Cells appear in cords and exhibit the characteristic raisinoid appearance of the nuclei with perinuclear clearing. Abundant eosinophilic cytoplasm and well-delineated cytoplasmic outlines are present. (H&E)

BOX 22-11 CMF

Cytomorphologic Features of Chromophobe Renal Cell Carcinoma

Cells present singly and in small clusters
Round, oval to polygonal large cells with well-defined borders
Pleomorphism may be significant
Variegated-appearing cytoplasm (i.e., fluffy, vacuolated, or granular)
Large, hyperchromatic nuclei
Nuclear membrane irregularities
Nuclear grooves and pseudoinclusions
Frequent binucleation
Small but not prominent nucleoli
Perinuclear clearing in at least some cells

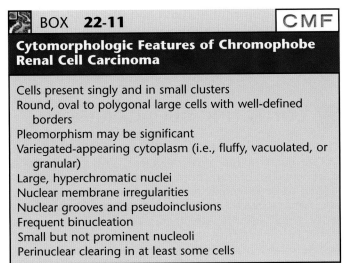

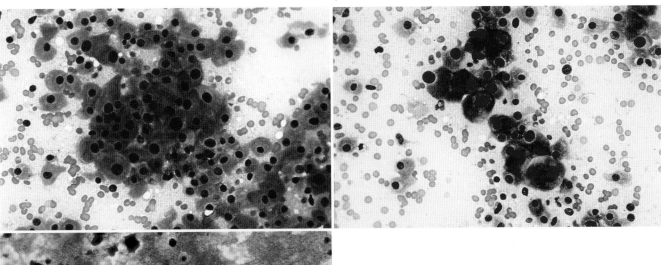

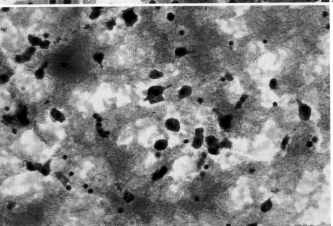

Figure 22-32 **Chromophobe carcinoma.** Cellular aspirates with large round to polygonal cells arranged singly and in small groups. The cells have sharply defined cytoplasmic borders. The cytoplasm exhibits varying degrees of granularity and vacuolization. Binucleation is present. Many of the cells exhibit a subtle but present perinuclear area of clearing visible on both Pap and DQ stain. Scattered, bizarre, pleomorphic cells with single or multiple nucleoli may be seen. No pseudoinclusions are seen in these fields. (DQ, Pap)

groups. The cells maintain their sharply defined cytoplasmic borders and appear less cohesive than those of clear cell renal cell carcinoma. The cytoplasm may exhibit varying degrees of granularity, vacuolization, or "fluffiness." Nuclei are often central and show noticeable hyperchromasia, significant size variability and irregular outlines, giving the nuclei a "raisinoid" appearance. Binucleation is a frequent occurrence. Granter and colleagues noted that when the cells have their characteristic area of perinuclear clearing on cytology, which is best seen in cell block sections, they resemble koilocytes.[66] Scattered bizarre pleomorphic cells with single or multiple nucleoli may be seen. Chromophobe renal cell carcinoma is characteristic for having cells that have quite a spectrum of morphology within a given lesion.

The eosinophilic variant of chromophobe renal cell carcinoma tends to have cells with more uniformly granular cytoplasm; however, cells with fluffy cytoplasm are usually present, although they comprise a minority. Cytoplasmic integrity is maintained, thus, stripped nuclei are not prominent.

Differential Diagnosis

The differential diagnosis of chromophobe renal cell carcinoma most commonly involves oncocytoma. In fact, it is conventional wisdom that the cases of reported malignant oncocytomas are actually misdiagnosed chromophobe renal cell carcinoma.[66] Both tumors may have isolated cells with abundant, granular cytoplasm and binucleation. However, the cytoplasm in oncocytomas is more often homogeneous without the fluffiness of chromophobe renal cell carcinoma. No perinuclear halos, pseudoinclusions, nuclear membrane irregularities, or significant nuclear hyperchromasia are present in oncocytoma. In addition, chromophobe renal cell carcinoma exhibits more of a spectrum of cells with large, bizarre pleomorphic forms, whereas in oncocytoma the cells have a more uniform appearance. Small but prominent nucleoli are more commonly seen in oncocytoma. Cells from both neoplasms, when taken in isolation, may be identical. If a diagnosis cannot be reached on morphologic grounds alone, the Hale's colloidal iron stain or electron microscopy (EM) can be used as the ultimate discriminator[66-68] (Box 22-12).

Clear cell renal cell carcinoma also comes into the differential diagnosis of chromophobe renal cell carcinoma. The cells of clear cell renal cell carcinoma have more uniform nuclear size and roundness than those of chromophobe renal cell carcinoma. Other morphologic attributes favoring clear cell renal cell carcinoma include higher nuclear grades, prominent nucleoli, and preservation of cohesion. Features pointing to chromophobe renal cell carcinoma are marked nuclear irregularities, pseudoinclusions, distinct cell borders, and perinuclear halos. Hales' colloidal iron is negative in clear cell renal cell carcinoma.

Chromophobe renal cell carcinoma has been shown to metastasize to the liver, in which case distinguishing it from hepatocellular carcinoma becomes an issue. Although both neoplasms have large cells with abundant eosinophilic cytoplasm, hepatocellular carcinoma has prominent nucleoli, more uniform cytoplasmic granularity, and possibly bile. Also in hepatocellular carcinoma the cells appear in large groups and sinusoids lined by endothelial cells.

The large, atypical eosinophilic cells seen in angiomyolipoma can also be confused with chromophobe renal cell carcinoma. In this case, the cells of angiomyolipoma are positive for HMB45 and smooth muscle markers.

 ## COLLECTING DUCT CARCINOMA

The cells of origin of collecting duct carcinoma are the collecting ducts of the renal medulla.[45] This highly malignant neoplasm has only been recently described and is considered to be extremely rare.[45] Clinically, these neoplasms are characterized by a medullary location and hypovascularity. Some authors state that many tumors with tubulopapillary architecture that should be considered unclassified have been placed erroneously into this category.[45] The genetic abnormalities that have been reported in several small series are distinct from those of papillary renal cell carcinoma and clear cell renal cell carcinoma, involving losses of 1, 6, 14, 15, and 22 and deletions of 8p, 13q.[45] This highly aggressive neoplasm usually is seen in younger patients (mean age of 34 to 45) who often present with metastatic disease at the time of diagnosis, and usually die within 24 months.[45,69,70]

These tumors may extend into the renal cortex but originate in the medulla. They may be solid or cystic, hemorrhagic, and necrotic. The histology is characterized by tumor cells forming tubules and papillae in a desmoplastic stroma often accompanied by dysplasia, in situ neoplasia, and frank carcinoma of the adjacent ducts.[45,69] The tumor cells have variably staining cytoplasm with prominent nucleoli in high-grade nuclei. Spindle cell change may be present. Foamy macrophages are not present in the papillae or in sheets as would be seen in papillary renal cell carcinoma; however, other inflammatory cells may be abundant.[45] The presence of psammoma bodies is variable. The immunohistochemical profile is distinct for immunoreactivity with CEA and Ulex Europaeus. High molecular weight cytokeratin and peanut lectin agglutinin may be positive. Many of the tumors are also mucicarmine positive.[45,69]

As these tumors manifest a histologic spectrum, the cytologic appearance can be variable[70-73] (Box 22-13; Figure 22-33). The cells are round to oval with small to moderate amounts of well-defined cytoplasm with variable degrees of vacuolization and well-defined borders. The cells are present individually, in small clusters, as tubular structures, and in cohesive groups that may have a papillary configuration. The eccentrically placed nuclei are moderately pleomorphic, hyperchromatic, and large with prominent central nucleoli

---

BOX   22-12

Ancillary Studies for Chromophobe Renal Cell Carcinoma

Hale's colloidal iron positive
Cytoplasmic oval perinuclear microvesicles on electron microscopy
Cytokeratin 18 positive
Vimentin negative
Distinct cytogenetic abnormalities: monosomy of 1, 2, 6, 10, 13, 17, 21; hypodiploid DNA

that may be multiple and show areas of chromatin clearing. Nuclear contours are irregular.[70-73] Stromal collagen and an admixture of normal cells may also be appreciated.[73] The cytology was thought to be distinct from other variants of renal cell carcinoma in that it appeared more similar to conventional adenocarcinomas of nonrenal sources.[71]

Differential Diagnosis

The differential diagnosis of collecting duct carcinoma includes papillary renal cell carcinoma, transitional cell carcinoma of the renal pelvis, and metastatic adenocarcinoma.

Although both papillary renal cell carcinoma and collecting duct carcinoma can have a papillary architecture, the distinction between collecting duct carcinoma and papillary renal cell carcinoma can usually be made because papillary renal cell carcinomas are usually of low nuclear grade as opposed to collecting duct carcinomas, which are usually of high nuclear grade. Foamy macrophages should not be present in collecting duct carcinoma, although they may be numerous in papillary renal cell carcinoma. Ulex Europaeus, which is positive in collecting duct carcinoma, is negative in papillary renal cell carcinoma, as is mucicarmine staining (Box 22-14).

The distinction between collecting duct carcinoma and metastatic adenocarcinoma depends on the cytologic and immunocytochemical profile of the primary tumor in ques-

---

BOX 22-13   CMF

Cytomorphologic Features of Collecting Duct Renal Cell Carcinoma

Cells may be dispersed in small groups, tubules, or papillary structures
Round to oval cells with well-defined cytoplasmic boundaries
Small to moderate amounts of cytoplasm with variable vacuolization
Irregular nuclear contours
Nuclei eccentric
Significant nuclear pleomorphism
Prominent central single or multiple nucleoli
Variable stromal or normal ductal components in aspirate

BOX 22-14

Ancillary Studies for Collecting Duct Carcinoma

Positive for CEA
Positive for Ulex Europaeus
Positive for high molecular weight cytokeratin
Positive for peanut lectin agglutinin
Mucicarmine positive
Chromosomal losses of 1, 6, 14, 15, 22; deletions of 8p, 13q

CEA, Carcinoembryonic antigen.

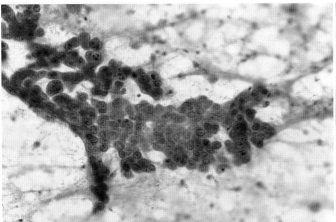

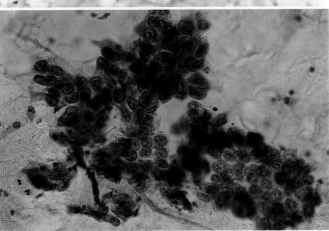

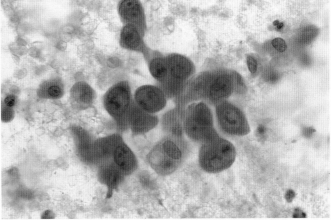

Figure 22-33 **Collecting duct carcinoma.** The cells are round to oval with small to moderate amounts of well-defined cytoplasm with variable degrees of vacuolization and focally well-defined borders. The cells are present in sheets, in small clusters, as tubular structures, and in cohesive groups that have a papillary configuration. The nuclei are eccentrically placed with prominent nucleoli and chromatin clearing. Nuclear contours are irregular. (H&E)

tion. Of note is the unique immunoreactivity of collecting duct carcinoma with Ulex Europaeus, which is unusual in other adenocarcinomas.

The cytologic appearance of transitional cell (urothelial) carcinoma depends largely on the grade. The low-grade variants appear similar to normal urothelial cells, although they may be present in papillary formations that may cause confusion. The nuclei in low-grade transitional cell carcinoma are bland, unlike the high-grade nuclei of collecting duct carcinoma. Also, the cells of transitional cell carcinoma are more commonly in multilayered sheets, a pattern distinct from collecting duct carcinoma.[71] High-grade transitional cell carcinoma, although it shares similar nuclear features with collecting duct carcinoma (e.g., eccentric nuclei with prominent nucleoli), usually has dense cytoplasm, although vacuolization may occur with glandular differentiation.

RENAL MEDULLARY CARCINOMA

Renal medullary carcinoma, a highly malignant tumor distinct from but seemingly related to collecting duct carcinoma, was first described in 1995. The cell of origin is thought to be the distal portion of the collecting ducts. As the name implies, the tumor occurs in the renal medullary region. This neoplasm has the distinction of occurring predominantly in young African Americans with sickle cell trait and occurs more often in males, unlike collecting duct carcinoma. As with collecting duct carcinoma, patients usually present with metastatic disease. Unfortunately, the mean survival in the original series was only 15 weeks from the time of diagnosis.[103]

These tumors share morphologic similarities with collecting duct carcinoma in that the nuclei are invariably high grade and the cells are arranged in tubules. Cells may also be seen in solid nests, and a growth pattern similar to that of yolk sac tumors may be seen. The stroma is desmoplastic and infiltrated by acute inflammatory cells.[45]

Only several cytologic descriptions of this entity are available[74,75] (Figure 22-34). In FNA cytology of the primary masses, the smears were moderately cellular, showing tumor cells both singly and in small, loose clusters. The cells showed solitary, hyperchromatic nuclei, central nucleoli, and high N:C ratios. Large cells with abundant cytoplasm, large nuclei, and irregular nuclear contours were also seen. A minority of the tumor cells showed coarse, cytoplasmic granules and vacuoles. In the two FNA cases, one showed a necrotic background with occasional inflammatory cells and benign stromal fragments, and the other did not. The differential diagnosis was of a Wilms' tumor, metastatic renal cell carcinoma, or a germ cell neoplasm, particularly because these were young African-American males (one with hemoglobin SC disease and the other with sickle cell trait).[74] Renal medullary carcinoma is also described in the urine and cervical cytology of an 18-year-old African-American female with sickle cell trait.[75] In the cervicovaginal smear, cells were present in tight, three-dimensional balls with a clean background. In the urine, which showed extensive blood and necrotic debris, the malignant cells were present singly and in groups. No true papillary frag-

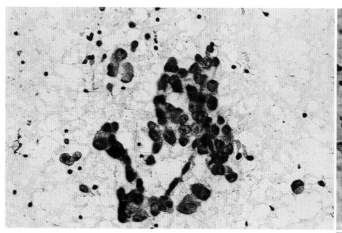

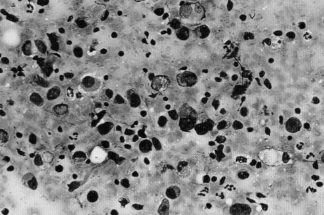

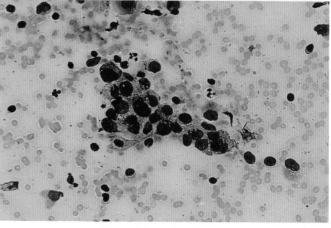

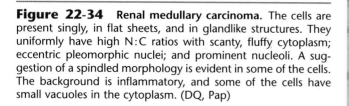

Figure 22-34 **Renal medullary carcinoma.** The cells are present singly, in flat sheets, and in glandlike structures. They uniformly have high N:C ratios with scanty, fluffy cytoplasm; eccentric pleomorphic nuclei; and prominent nucleoli. A suggestion of a spindled morphology is evident in some of the cells. The background is inflammatory, and some of the cells have small vacuoles in the cytoplasm. (DQ, Pap)

ments with fibrovascular cores were noted. The cytoplasm was granular and dense with well-delineated borders. High N:C ratios, nuclear pleomorphism, and irregular nuclear borders were prominent features. Some of the cells exhibited eccentricity of the nucleus. Prominent single or multiple nucleoli were present, and the chromatin showed irregular clumping.[75]

SARCOMATOID CHANGE IN RENAL CELL CARCINOMA

Sarcomatoid change can occur in any one of the subtypes of renal cell carcinoma and in transitional cell carcinoma of the renal pelvis. Thus, it is no longer considered a distinct diagnostic entity. Sarcomatoid change signifies a manifestation of high-grade carcinoma of the type of tumor from which it arose.[29] When no epithelial components can be seen, the tumor should be assigned to the *renal cell carcinoma, unclassified* category, as described in the following section.

In 1993, when the diagnostic category of *sarcomatoid renal cell carcinoma* was still in popular use, a cytologic study was published.[76] The cytologic findings of this study can be used to describe the features previously considered sarcomatoid change (Figure 22-35). The spindle cell component of these lesions was characterized by elongated cells present singly, in large clusters, or in an MFH-like or fibrosarcomatous pattern. The cytoplasm was scant to moderate. The degree of nuclear pleomorphism was variable but was most

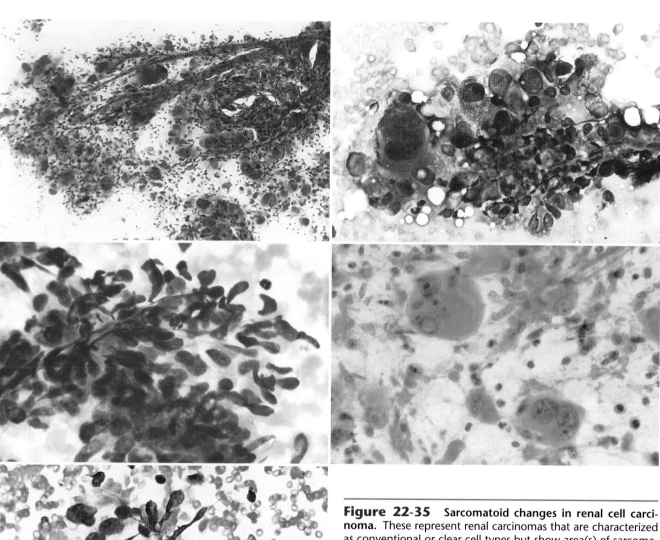

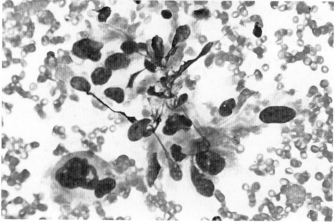

Figure 22-35 **Sarcomatoid changes in renal cell carcinoma.** These represent renal carcinomas that are characterized as conventional or clear cell types but show area(s) of sarcomatoid change. The spindle cell component of these lesions is characterized by elongated cells present singly, in large clusters, or in an malignant fibrous histiocytoma (MFH-)like or fibrosarcomatous pattern. The amount of cytoplasm is variable. The degree of nuclear pleomorphism is variable but is most marked in the malignant giant cells associated with the MFH-like pattern. In certain areas the malignant spindled cells are arranged in fascicles. (DQ, Pap)

marked in the malignant giant cells associated with the MFH-like pattern. In areas the malignant spindled cells were arranged in fascicles. In general, the chromatin pattern was fine and nucleoli were prominent.[76]

The subcharacterization of a tumor with sarcomatoid change should not be based on the sarcomatoid change, but rather on the epithelial component with which it is admixed. As such, the information provided in the previous sections should aid in the tumor classification. The presence of sarcomatoid change should be mentioned in the cytology report with the caveat that the tumor, regardless of its diagnostic category, should be considered high grade.[29]

RENAL CELL CARCINOMA, UNCLASSIFIED

The currently utilized renal carcinoma classification set forth by the Union Internationale Contre le Cancer and the American Joint Committee on Cancer contains the designation of *renal cell carcinoma, unclassified* (RCCU)[29]:

> . . . RCCU is a diagnostic category to which renal carcinomas should be assigned when they do not fit readily into one of the other categories . . . .

This group, which cannot be morphologically classified based on our current knowledge, may contribute to 4% to 7% of renal tumors and due to its heterogeneity cannot be further defined[29,45] (Box 22-15).

Tumors that fit into this category may include sarcomatoid tumors without an obvious epithelial component, tumors with composite histology/cytology, and neoplasms with mixtures of epithelial and stromal elements.[29] Other authors have stated that in practice this category is usually invoked in instances when the distinction cannot be made between two known, well-defined variants of renal cell carcinoma due to mixed or nebulous morphologic/histologic features. This usually involves the distinction of clear cell renal cell carcinoma with pseudopapillary areas from papillary renal cell carcinoma and distinguishing chromophobe renal cell carcinoma from oncocytoma or clear cell renal cell carcinoma.[45] As no defined histologic appearances are known for these tumors, the same criteria should apply for the use of this category in cytology samples.

BOX   22-15

Main Uses of the Category: Renal Cell Carcinoma, Unclassified

Tumor does not fit into one of accepted diagnostic categories
Sarcomatoid tumors without obvious epithelial component
Tumors of mixed epithelial and stromal elements
Tumors with composite histology/cytology
When the distinction cannot be made between two known, well-defined variants of renal cell carcinoma

---

TUMORS METASTATIC TO THE KIDNEY

As with any solid organ, the kidney may harbor metastatic malignancies that are amenable to diagnosis through FNA and that need to be distinguished from primary renal neoplasms. A recently published study reviewed a series of renal FNAs over a 9-year period and reported that 21% of the renal FNAs diagnosed as malignant were due to metastatic disease.[77] Overall, the incidence of metastatic neoplasms in renal FNA was 11%. Of these patients, 89% had a previous history of neoplasia elsewhere, an important clinical factor necessary for arriving at the correct diagnostic assessment. The origins of the metastatic tumors in patients with previously known primaries were: lung (39%); lymphoma (29%); hepatocellular carcinoma (11%); and one case each of breast, pancreatic, and cervical cancer. In the remaining 11% of patients with no prior history of malignancy, the diagnoses of metastatic adenocarcinoma (two cases) and squamous carcinoma (one case) were made; however, the primary sites remained undetected.[77]

In this group of patients, the single most important piece of information that must be relayed to the cytopathologist is the patient's previous history of malignancy. Of the above-mentioned diagnostic categories, in the absence of history, the diagnosis of hepatocellular carcinoma must be distinguished from oncocytoma, clear cell renal cell carcinoma, and chromophobe renal cell carcinoma. The high-grade adenocarcinomas need to be distinguished from collecting duct carcinoma because this is probably the renal tumor with nuclear and cytoplasmic morphology most closely resembling metastatic high-grade adenocarcinoma.

RENAL PELVIS

Transitional Cell/Urothelial Carcinoma

Transitional cell carcinoma (TCC) or urothelial carcinoma of the renal pelvis is strongly associated with toxin exposure (e.g., aromatic amines, phenacetin abuse, ionizing radiation, cigarette smoking, etc.), similar to the known associations with bladder cancer. Although adenocarcinomas, squamous carcinomas (associated with thorotrast exposure), and small cell carcinomas occur in a small percentage of renal pelvic tumors, the most common malignancy of the renal pelvis by far is transitional cell carcinoma (85% to 90%).[23,78] The histology and tendency for multifocality of TCC of the renal pelvis is similar to those TCCs that develop in the bladder (with flat and papillary architecture). Renal pelvic TCCs that are amenable to FNA are usually exophytic and papillary, presenting as mass lesions with ureteral obstruction and hydronephrosis.[23] In large tumors, however, the boundaries between primary pelvic and parenchymal lesions may be difficult to assess; thus, TCC should always be in the differential diagnosis of mass lesions of the kidney which may partially involve the renal pelvis.

In a review of FNA of TCC of the renal pelvis, it was stated that in a 5-year period, 14% of kidney neoplasms were TCCs of the renal pelvis, with the diagnosis made by various combinations of FNA and exfoliative cytology.[78] For optimal diagnostic results of urinary cytology in this scenario, urine must be obtained by catheterization of the ureter. Through this method, the accuracy of the cytologic diagnosis correlates with tumor stage and grade.[78] Unfortunately, the voided urine cytology samples in TCC of the renal pelvis are not reliable for the detection of this type of neoplasia.

As the grade of the lesion varies, so does the cytologic appearance (Figure 22-36 and Box 22-16). The cells have an epithelioid appearance and well-defined cytoplasmic outlines.[79] Low-grade tumors, which are usually papillary, show cells shed in sheets or in a papillary or palisading arrangement. The smear background is usually clean. The cytoplasm may be variable, but is usually dense and eosinophilic in appearance and may appear squamoid in areas. Cell shape and size is irregular. The nuclei show slight enlargement and hyperchromasia, with granular chromatin and inconspicuous nucleoli.[78] High-grade lesions may show variable amounts of hemorrhage and necrosis, with increased N:C ratios, significant nuclear hyperchromasia with coarsely irregular chromatin, irregular nuclear contours, and various degrees of vacuolization and squamous differentiation of the cytoplasm. The cells may be spindled and have a sarcomatoid appearance. In high-grade lesions the cells are much more likely to appear singly or in loose clusters.[78]

Differential Diagnosis

Although the cytology of low-grade TCC is fairly distinct, the cytologic morphology of high-grade lesions, particularly if the cells maintain any degree of papillary morphology, may resemble that of collecting duct carcinoma. The cytologic appearance of transitional cell carcinoma depends largely on the grade of the tumor in question. The low-grade variants appear similar to normal urothelial cells, although they can be present in papillary formations, which may cause confusion. The nuclei in low-grade transitional

---

BOX 22-16 | **CMF**

Cytomorphologic Features of Transitional Cell Carcinoma of the Renal Pelvis

Cells appear singly and in small groups in high-grade tumors

Cells shed in sheets and papillary formations in low-grade tumors

High N:C ratios in high-grade tumors

Low N:C ratios in low-grade tumors

Cytologic appearance varies with the grade of the neoplasm

Cytoplasm dense and variably eosinophilic but may appear squamoid or vacuolated in high-grade tumors

Cytoplasmic boundaries are well defined

Cell size and shape are variable but may have polygonal features

Increased nuclear size and hyperchromasia with higher-grade tumors

Cells may appear spindled and sarcomatoid in high-grade tumors

Nucleoli inconspicuous in low-grade tumors

Prominent nucleoli in high-grade tumors

N:C, Nuclear to cytoplasmic.

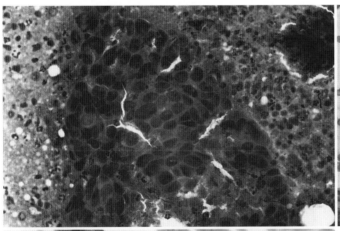

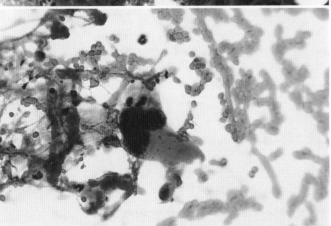

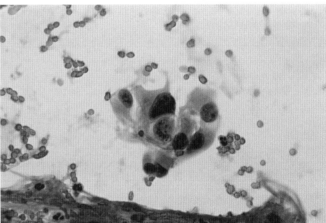

Figure 22-36 **Transitional cell carcinoma of the renal pelvis.** These aspirate samples show malignant urothelial cells present singly, in sheets, and in small groups. The cells have dense cytoplasm, irregular hyperchromatic nuclei, irregular nuclear contours, and focal nucleoli. (DQ, Pap)

cell carcinoma are bland, unlike the high-grade nuclei of collecting duct carcinoma. Also, the cells of transitional cell carcinoma are more commonly in multilayered sheets, a pattern distinct from collecting duct carcinoma.[71] High-grade TCC, although it shares similar nuclear features with collecting duct carcinoma (i.e., eccentric nuclei with prominent nucleoli), usually has dense cytoplasm, although vacuolization may occur with glandular differentiation.

The immunohistochemical profile of collecting duct carcinoma is distinct from TCC showing immunoreactivity for CEA, Ulex Europaeus, and peanut lectin agglutinin. Collecting duct carcinoma can also be mucicarmine positive.

NONEPITHELIAL NEOPLASMS OF THE KIDNEY: BENIGN MESENCHYMAL

Angiomyolipoma

Angiomyolipomas are benign neoplasms composed of a mixture of adipose tissue, smooth muscle cells, and thick-walled blood vessels. These tumors have a curious association with lymphangioleiomyoma(tosis) and clear cell "sugar" tumor by virtue of the staining of tumor constituent cells with not only muscle markers but also the melanocytic markers HMB45 and MART-1/MelanA.[80] Angiomyolipomas have a genetic association with tuberous

sclerosis, with more than half of these patients developing angiomyolipomas by the median age of 25. Cases not associated with tuberous sclerosis occur in an older age group (median age of 45).[23]

Histologically, the three components of the tumor (adipose tissue, smooth muscle cells, and thick-walled blood vessels) vary in proportion. Accordingly, the cytologic appearance is reflected likewise (Box 22-17; Figure 22-37). Although the thick-walled vessels may not be apparent in the FNA smears, they may be visible in the cell block section.[81] The smooth muscle components may be highly pleomorphic. In general, the smooth muscle cells have an epithelioid morphology with highly inconsistent degrees of nuclear atypia, which may be profound. The adipose tissue appears normal. Typically, the FNA shows vascularized tissue fragments composed of smooth muscle and adipose tissue elements.[82,83] The smooth muscle cells are positive for smooth muscle markers and HMB45 and variable with MART-1/ MelanA.[80]

Differential Diagnosis

The most important factor regarding the differential diagnosis of angiomyolipomas in renal neoplasms is to actually consider the diagnosis of angiomyolipoma (Box 22-18). Cytopathologists are conditioned to think predominantly of renal epithelial neoplasms, thus, potentially hindering diagnostic accuracy. The vascular and adipose components of angiomyolipomas can potentially be thought of as normal perirenal tissue, with the neoplastic smooth muscle cells viewed in isolation. When this occurs, the most likely diag-

---

BOX   22-17   CMF

Cytomorphologic Features of Angiomyolipoma

Triphasic components of fat, smooth muscle cells and thick-walled vessels in vascularized tissue fragments
Thick-walled vessels best seen in cell block
Tissue components are inconsistent in proportion
Epithelioid or spindled smooth muscle cells with variable atypia
Adipose tissue normal in appearance

BOX   22-18

Other Benign Mesenchymal Neoplasms Found in the Kidney

Leiomyoma
Hemangioma
Lipoma
Lymphangioma

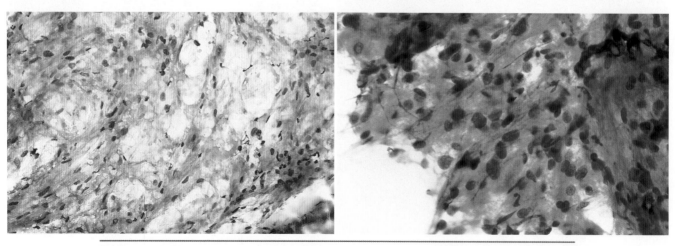

Figure 22-37   **Angiomyolipoma.** These FNAs show vascularized tissue fragments composed of smooth muscle and adipose tissue elements. The nuclei of the smooth muscle cells show a moderate degree of variability. (DQ, Pap)

nostic considerations would be a sarcoma or sarcomatoid differentiation within a renal cell carcinoma. The degree of cytologic atypia should be less pronounced in angiomyolipomas, and the immunoreactivity of angiomyolipomas for HMB45 and other melanocytic markers should make the correct diagnosis possible if it is considered. The adipose tissue component of angiomyolipomas could also possibly be misinterpreted as a primary low-grade retroperitoneal liposarcoma. Once again, noticing the triphasic components with epithelioid smooth muscle cells and the thick-walled blood vessels of the tumor should make the correct diagnosis possible[84] (Box 22-19).

NONEPITHELIAL NEOPLASMS OF THE KIDNEY: MALIGNANT MESENCHYMAL

Although primary sarcomas of the kidney are exceedingly rare (less than 1% of primary renal neoplasms), leiomyosarcoma comprises about half of the known cases[85-87] (Box 22-20). The cytology of leiomyosarcoma and other sarcomas involving the kidney are identical to those found in the soft tissue and are addressed in Chapter 28 (Figures 22-38 to 22-40).

The differential diagnosis of primary renal sarcomas includes the differentiation from the more common sarcomatoid change in an epithelial neoplasm of the kidney. Distinguishing features would be the presence of an epithelial (nonspindle cell) component, which would lead to a diagnosis of a subtype of renal cell carcinoma. Although immunocytochemical stains for vimentin would be positive in a sarcoma and most subtypes of renal cell carcinoma, the presence of low or high molecular weight cytokeratin would rule out a primary sarcoma and suggest a sarcomatoid component of renal cell carcinoma. As with sarcomas elsewhere in the body, smooth muscle markers would indicate a smooth muscle sarcoma. CD31, CD34, Factor 8, and Ulex Europaeus would indicate a vascular etiology for the sarcoma. Likewise, skeletal muscle differentiation markers would indicate a possible rhabdomyosarcoma. A difficult distinction may be that of a low-grade liposarcoma from an angiomyolipoma. The presence of thick-walled vessels and epithelioid smooth muscle cells that are immunoreactive with HMB45 and other melanoma markers would lead to the correct diagnosis of angiomyolipoma.

RENAL INVOLVEMENT WITH LYMPHOMA

Renal involvement with malignant lymphoma is not uncommon and is a serious potential diagnostic pitfall for the cytopathologist as the treatment for malignant lymphoma

---

BOX 22-19

Ancillary Studies in Angiomyolipoma: Smooth Muscle Cells

Positive for muscle markers (e.g., desmin, smooth
   muscle actin)
Positive for melanocytic markers (HMB45,
   MART-1/Melan A)
Negative for S-100

BOX 22-20

Malignant Mesenchymal Neoplasms Most Commonly Found in the Kidney

Leiomyosarcoma
Angiosarcoma
Liposarcoma
Rhabdomyosarcoma
Malignant fibrous histiocytoma

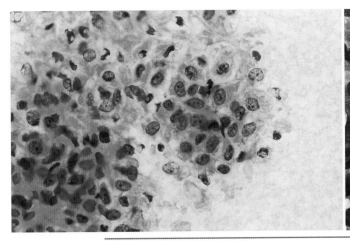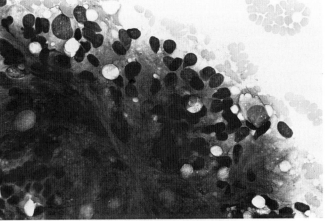

Figure 22-38 **Leiomyosarcoma of the kidney.** The cells are in aggregates and around blood vessels. The epithelioid appearance, prominent nucleoli, fluffy cytoplasm, and magenta-staining matrix may make the distinction of this from a primary renal carcinoma difficult. (DQ, Pap)

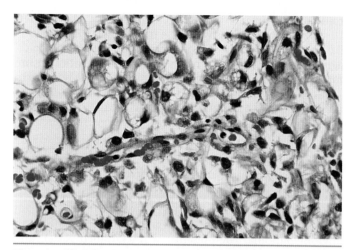

Figure 22-39 Liposarcoma. Atypical adipose cells with the characteristic thin-walled vascular channels. (H&E)

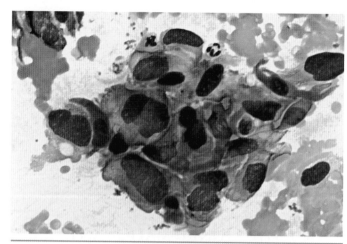

Figure 22-40 Sarcoma of the kidney. These large, highly pleomorphic cells are from a sarcoma of the kidney that was not further classifiable. (DQ)

 BOX **22-21**

Types of Malignant Lymphoma Involving the Kidney

Secondary renal lymphoma
Primary renal lymphoma
Renal intravascular lymphomatosis
Posttransplant lymphoma

BOX **22-22**

Differential Diagnosis of Most Common Malignant Pediatric Renal Neoplasms

Wilms' tumor
Clear cell sarcoma
Malignant rhabdoid tumor
Mesoblastic nephroma

is medical and not surgical (Box 22-21). Thus, a wrong diagnosis can lead to an unnecessary nephrectomy. A recent study involving a series of 19 patients revealed 10 secondary lymphomas, eight primary lymphomas, and one posttransplant lymphoma.[88] In this series, one case was misdiagnosed as transitional cell carcinoma. The final diagnoses were 18 B-cell lymphomas and one T-cell lymphoma. The cytologic features of these cases were significant for an admixture of renal tubular elements and lymphoid cell clusters reminiscent of epithelial cell aggregates (eight of 19 cases). The background cells were characteristically those of the various subtypes of malignant lymphoma. The one case originally misdiagnosed as transitional cell carcinoma displayed numerous aggregates of epithelioid spindled cells, which were misinterpreted as being epithelial in nature. However, retrospective review revealed the atypical lymphoid cells to be present in the background.[88] Lymphoglandular bodies in the smear background may provide a hint of the true nature of the neoplastic cells. This could easily be confirmed by the appropriate immunocytochemical reactions for lymphoid cells.

 ## RENAL NEOPLASMS IN CHILDREN

One large review examined a series of 27 renal aspirates in the pediatric population (Box 22-22). The aspirates were from 16 cases of Wilms' tumor, one anaplastic Wilms' tumor, two clear cell sarcomas of the kidney, two malignant rhabdoid tumors of the kidney, and six congenital mesoblastic nephromas.[89] In 94% of Wilms' tumors the stromal component was evident, with the epithelial component present in 76%. All cases showed the blastemal component (100%). Necrosis was present in 65% of the cases.[89] Samples from malignant rhabdoid tumors were very cellular, with the distinguishing characteristic of prominent eosinophilic nucleoli. Cells from clear cell sarcoma of the kidney were arranged in small, individual clusters with fragile cytoplasm. In congenital mesoblastic nephroma, the cells were spindled and very cohesive. A definite tumor type was rendered on 25 of the 27 cases (93%) of renal tumors, which is actually better than in adults.[89]

Wilms' Tumor

Wilms' tumor, or nephroblastoma, is a pediatric renal neoplasm with an incidence of 7.6 cases per million children per year and a very high cure rate. It has moved increasingly into the realm of the cytopathologist as preoperative chemotherapy has become the standard of care. This type of treatment is utilized because of extreme tumor friability and spillage with the potential for metastatic disease resulting from surgery. FNA is, however, contraindicated in patients with what is clinically considered resectable pediatric Wilms' tumor. Falling cytologically into the category of pediatric small, round blue cell tumors, the accurate recognition of Wilms' tumor in FNA is possible due to a unique feature of this tumor—that is, it is a neoplasm composed of multiple components that are usually present in most cases.[89] However, samples consisting solely of blastemal or

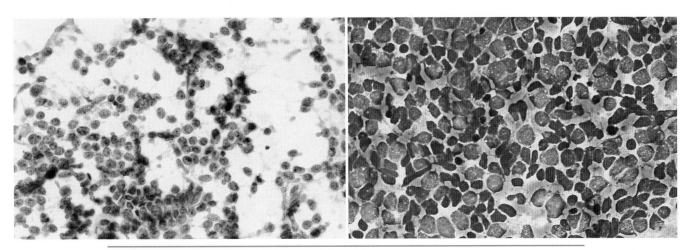

Figure 22-41 **Wilms' tumor, blastemal component.** These aspirates show diffusely dispersed small cells with scant cytoplasm; solitary, dark nuclei; and high N:C ratios. Some nuclear molding is present. The chromatin pattern is fine. Chromocenters are seen on the Pap stain. (Pap, DQ)

TABLE 22-7	CMF
Cytomorphologic Features of Wilms' Tumor	

Cytomorphologic Component	Cytomorphologic Description
Blastemal cells	Small cells with solitary, dark nuclei High N:C ratios because of scant cytoplasm
Stromal component	Closely knit, short-spindled cells Branching tissue fragments that contain capillaries and a myxoid or collagenous matrix Differentiation into smooth or skeletal muscle may be evident
Epithelial component	Glandlike arrangement of blastemal cells with central lumens Palisading or picket-fencing Cells with moderate amounts of cytoplasm, central nuclei, fine chromatin, and inconspicuous nucleoli in small groups, sheets, or fragments that may be attached to the stromal fragments Cells arranged in loose clusters or as complex branching formations

N:C, Nuclear to cytoplasmic.

tubular components (monophasic variants) should still be considered to be Wilms' tumor.[90] As with other renal neoplasms, the preparation of DQ, Pap-stained, and cell block material is important for the recognition of all cellular components (Table 22-7; Figures 22-41 to 22-43).

The *blastemal* cells usually form the majority of the cellular population, and are present either as diffuse sheets, small clusters, or individually. The clusters may surround or be incorporated within fragments of stroma. Nuclear molding can be seen. As would be expected, the cells are small and round with extremely scanty and fragile cytoplasm. Thus, bare nuclei may be numerous. Cytoplasm is basophilic and may have small vacuoles. The cytoplasm is best viewed on DQ-stained samples. The nucleoli are usually inconspicuous, with the chromatin pattern being fine and evenly distributed with several chromocenters. Occasional cells are arranged in rosettelike structures, probably representing early epithelial differentiation.[91]

The *stromal* component, although present in most cases, may actually be the predominant component. This is evident by closely knit, short-spindled cells in branching tissue fragments, which contain capillaries and a myxoid or collagenous matrix. Differentiation into smooth or skeletal muscle (or other mesenchymal tissue) may be evident in the stromal component. Rhabdomyoblastic differentiation may be seen.[91]

The *epithelial* component can be seen admixed with the blastemal and/or stromal components. Epithelial differentiation is evidenced by a glandular arrangement of primitive cells with a true central lumen. Similarly, palisading or picket-fencing may be seen.[91] Epithelial differentiation may also be evidenced by cells with moderate amounts of cytoplasm, central nuclei, fine chromatin, and inconspicuous nucleoli arranged in small groups, sheets, or tissue fragments, which may be attached to the stromal fragments.[91]

The background of the smears may consist of magenta-staining material on DQ stain. In some cases, it may simulate chondroid or myxoid matrix. Necrosis may or may not be present.[91]

Anaplasia in higher stage Wilms' tumor is important to recognize because it is associated with aggressive behavior and decreased survival, thus, more potent therapy is indicated. In these cases, the cytology exhibits marked enlargement of the tumor cell nuclei of at least three times that of adjacent similar type cells. Atypical mitotic figures and hyperchromasia is also variably present. Multinucleation may be seen, and it is important not to confuse multinucleation with nuclear enlargement.[90,92] Overdiagnosis of anaplasia may be associated with thick sections, poor fixation, DNA-smearing artifact, calcification, and basophilic extracellular mucin material simulating large nuclei. Anaplasia may also be underdiagnosed due to sampling error.[90,92] If

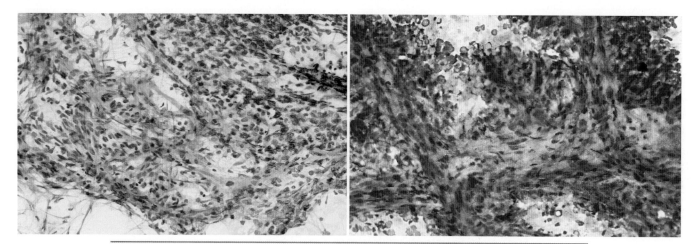

Figure 22-42 **Wilms' tumor, stromal component.** Tightly knit, short-spindled cells are in branching tissue fragments that contain capillaries and a myxoid or collagenous matrix. (Pap, DQ)

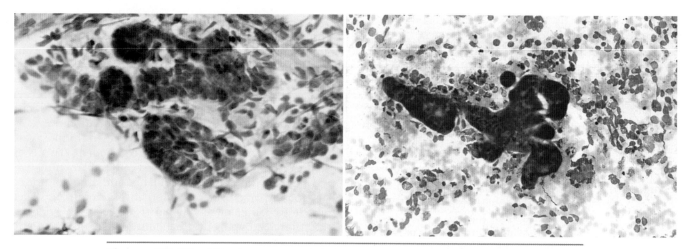

Figure 22-43 **Wilms' tumor, epithelial component.** The epithelial component is admixed with the blastemal and stromal components. Glandular arrangements of primitive cells are seen with a true central lumen. Palisading and picket-fencing is noted. (DQ, Pap)

anaplasia is detected in an FNA, it should always be stated in the report.

The differential diagnosis of Wilms' tumor includes other small, round blue cell tumors that occur in the region of the kidney, particularly neuroblastoma. Features supporting a diagnosis of Wilms' tumor include true lumen formation by epithelial tubules, triphasic differentiation, and myxoid matrix. By contrast, pseudorosettes with a fibrillar matrix centrally, neoplastic ganglion cells, and a fibrillated neuropil background are in keeping with neuroblastoma. The latter should be positive for neuron-specific enolase (NSE) and negative for cytokeratin; the reverse pattern may be evident in Wilms' tumor. Lymphoma, especially of the Burkitt's type, may occur in the kidney of children. Aspirates are characterized by a monomorphic population of dispersed cells without evidence of an organized arrangement or background matrix material. Additionally, lymphoglandular bodies are present and the tumor cells are leukocyte common antigen (LCA) positive. Rhabdomyosarcoma does not manifest epithelial differentiation. Some neoplasms are quite primitive, but others show large nucleoli and greater pleomorphism, including multinucleated tumor giant cells, which are unexpected in Wilms' tumor. By immunocytochemistry, different muscle markers are expressed in rhabdomyosarcoma. However, myogenous differentiation may also be seen in Wilms' tumor. A malignant rhabdoid tumor can be ruled out based on its monophasic population and the tendency for the cells of a malignant rhabdoid tumor to appear in sheets.[23]

The distinction between Wilms' tumor and clear cell sarcoma is important. Typically, Wilms' tumor is triphasic with evidence of epithelial (tubular/glomeruloid) and mesenchymal elements in combination with a blastemal component. In clear cell sarcoma the cells comprise a monotonous population. The cells of clear cell sarcoma have a moderate amount of pale amphophilic cytoplasm, best visualized on DQ stain, whereas the blastemal cells of Wilms' tumor have sparse cytoplasm. The nuclei of clear cell sarcoma are slightly larger than those of Wilms' tumor, and the cells of clear cell sarcoma may be arranged in a striking perivascular pattern. Nuclear grooving may or may not be a prominent feature of clear cell sarcoma.[93,94]

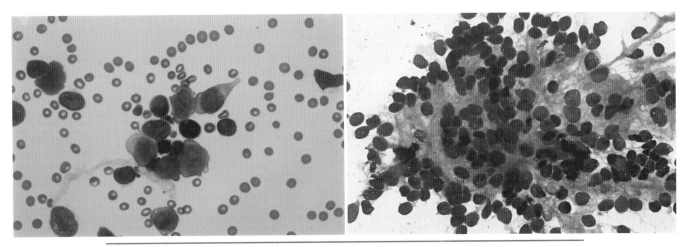

Figure 22-44 **Clear cell sarcoma of kidney.** These show the rounded nature of the malignant cells. The nuclei are round with focal nuclear pseudoinclusions, and scant cytoplasm. Abundant myxoid matrix that the cells are forming is present. (DQ)

Clear Cell Sarcoma

Clear cell sarcoma of the kidney has been referred to as *undifferentiated sarcoma* and *bone-metastasizing sarcoma of the kidney.*

The cytology of clear cell sarcoma, as in most other renal neoplasms, is best appreciated on DQ stains (Figure 22-44). The smears are cellular with the cells arranged both in dispersed and perivascular patterns. The cells have scant to abundant pale blue cytoplasm and large eccentric nuclei. The nuclear shapes are round-, oval-, pear-, or bean-shaped. They may or may not have deep nuclear grooves imparting a lobulated appearance. Nucleoli are inconspicuous. The chromatin pattern is fine with areas of chromatin condensation. The cells may be present in a loose myxoid matrix.[93,94]

Rhabdoid Tumor

This tumor, although most likely of primitive epithelial derivation, has an appearance similar to immature skeletal muscle. It is a rare tumor representing only 2% of pediatric renal neoplasms.[41] These occur predominantly in patients under age 2 with a male predominance and are highly aggressive with a mortality rate within 1 year of diagnosis.[41]

The cytology is conspicuous for the abundance of large, homogeneous, highly atypical cells with abundant eosinophilic cytoplasm and well-defined cell borders. The cells are relatively uniform and are present singly and in small groups. The nuclei are large, eccentric, and possess chromatin clearing around a large macronucleolus. Mitotic activity and necrosis are frequent. The cells are immunoreactive with both vimentin and cytokeratin.[95]

Congenital Mesoblastic Nephroma

Mesoblastic nephroma is a renal tumor associated with infancy but has been reported on occasion in adults.[96] In adults, the clinical and radiologic findings simulate those of renal cell carcinoma. Due to its rarity, the cytologic findings are limited to a few case reports.[97-100]

The cytology has been characterized as being of variable cellularity with cells appearing as naked spindle cells arranged singly or in tight, cohesive fragments simulating mesenchymal tissue. The nuclei are round to oval with small nucleoli and smooth contours. The cytoplasm is dense and stains homogeneously. The background has been described as clean or as having a mucoid fibrillar material. The matrix stains magenta on DQ.[97-100]

Normal renal elements that are trapped within the growing tumor may also be seen and may possibly lead to a misinterpretation of Wilms' tumor. In adults, the differential diagnosis would include sarcomatoid differentiation in renal cell carcinoma.

References

1. Banner MP. Uroradiology. In: Mitchell CW, editor. Radiologic interventions. 1st ed. Baltimore: Williams and Wilkins; 1998.
2. Van Poppel H, Bamelis B, Oyen R, et al. Partial nephrectomy for renal cell carcinoma can achieve long-term tumor control. J Urol 1996; 160(3 Pt 1):674-678.
3. Fergany AF, Hafez KS, Novick AC, et al. Long-term results of nephron sparing surgery for localized renal cell carcinoma: 10-year followup. J Urol 2000; 163:442.
4. von Shreeb T, Arner O, Skousted G, et al. Renal adenocarcinoma: is there a risk of spreading tumor cells in diagnostic puncture. Scand J Urol Nephrol 1967; 1:270-276.
5. Shenoy PD, Lakhkar BN, Ghosh MK, et al. Cutaneous seeding of renal carcinoma by Chiba needle aspiration biopsy: case report. Acta Radiol 1991; 32:50-52.
6. Slywotzky C, Maya M. Needle tract seeding of transitional cell carcinomas following fine needle aspiration of a renal mass. Abdom Imaging 1994; 19:174-176.
7. Renshaw AA, Granter SR, Cibas ES. Fine-needle aspiration of the adult kidney. Cancer 1997; 81(2):71-88.
8. Murphy WM, Zambroni BR, Emerson LD, et al. Aspiration biopsy of the kidney. Cancer 1985; 56:200-205.
9. Cristallini EG, Paganelli C, Bolis GB. Role of fine needle aspiration biopsy cytology of the kidney and adrenal. Diagn Cytopathol 1991; 7:32-35.
10. Nguyen GK. Percutaneous fine needle aspiration biopsy cytology of the kidney and adrenal. Pathol Annu 1987; 22(1):163-191.

11. Helm CW, Burwood RJ, Harrison NW, et al. Aspiration cytology of solid renal tumors. J Urol 1983; 55:249-253.

12. Juul N, Torp-Pederson S, Gronvall S, et al. Ultrasonically guided fine needle aspiration biopsy of renal masses. J Urol 1985; 133:579-581.

13. Dekmezian RH, Charnsangavej C, Rava P, et al. Fine needle aspiration of kidney tumors in 105 patients: a cytologic and histologic correlation. Acta Cytol 1985; 29:931 (Abstract).

14. Pilotta S, Rilke F, Alasio L, et al. The role of fine needle aspiration in the assessment of renal masses. Acta Cytol 1988; 32:1-10.

15. Daniel L, Barriol D, Lechevallier E, et al. Diagnostic value of percutaneous biopsy of the renal masses. Ann Pathol 2000; 20(2):119-123.

16. Zardawi IM. Renal fine needle aspiration cytology. Acta Cytol 1999; 43:184-190.

17. Truong LD, Todd TD, Dhurandhar B, et al. Fine-needle aspiration of renal masses in adults: analysis of results and diagnostic problems in 108 cases. Diagn Cytopathol 1999; 20:339-349.

18. Campbell SC, Novick AC, Herts B, et al. Prospective evaluation of fine needle aspiration of small, solid renal masses: accuracy and morbidity. Urology 1997; 50(1):25-29.

19. Todd TD, Dhurandhar B, Mody D, et al. Fine-needle aspiration of cystic lesions of the kidney. Morphologic spectrum and diagnostic problems in 41 cases. Am J Clin Pathol 1999; 111:317-328.

20. Pavot DR, Atkins KA, Powers CN. Liesegang rings in a submental mass: fine needle aspiration with histologic correlation. Diagn Cytopathol 2001; 25:331-333.

21. Tamboli P, Ro JY, Amin MB, et al. Benign tumors and tumor-like lesions of the adult kidney. II. Benign mesenchymal and mixed neoplasms, and tumor-like lesions. Adv Anat Pathol 2000; 7(1):47-66.

22. Goodman N, Curry T, Russell T. Xanthogranulomatous pyelonephritis (XGP): a local disease with systemic manifestations, report of 23 patients and review of the literature. Medicine 1979; 58:171-181.

23. Grignon DJ, Staerkel GA. Surgical diseases of the kidney. In: Silverberg SG, DeLellis RA, Frable WJ, editors. Principles and practice of surgical pathology and cytopathology. 3rd ed., vol. 3. New York: Churchill Livingstone; 1997. pp. 2135-2184.

24. Fleming ID, Cooper JS, Henson DE, et al. AJCC cancer staging handbook. 5th ed. Philadelphia: Lippincott-Raven; 1998. pp. 215-222.

25. Koga S, Tsuda S, Nishikido M, et al. Renal cell carcinoma metastatic to the skin. Anticancer Res 2000; 20(3B):1939-1940.

26. Moch H, Gasser T, Amin MB, et al. Prognostic utility of the recently recommended histologic classification and revised TNM staging system of renal cell carcinoma: a Swiss experience with 588 tumors. Cancer 2000; 89(3):604-614.

27. Gettman MT, Blute ML, Spotts B, et al. Pathologic staging of renal cell carcinoma: significance of tumor classification with the 1997 TNM staging system. Cancer 2001; 91(2):354-361.

28. Kovacs G, Akhtar M, Beckwith BJ, et al. The Heidelberg classification of renal cell tumours. J Pathol 1997; 183:131-133.

29. Storkel S, Eble JN, Adlakha K, et al. Classification of renal cell carcinoma: workgroup no. 1. Cancer 1997; 80(5):987-989.

30. Ljungberg B, Alamdari FI, Stenling R, et al. Prognostic significance of the Heidelberg classification of renal cell carcinoma. Eur Urol 1999; 36(6):565-569.

31. Renshaw AA, Richie JP. Subtypes of renal cell carcinoma: different onset and sites of metastatic disease. Am J Clin Pathol 1999; 111:539-543.

32. Vector Laboratories. Blocking kit product specifications package insert. Burlingame, Calif: Vector; 1997.

33. Rodriguez-Soto J, Warnke R, Rouse R. Endogenous avidin-binding activity in paraffin-embedded tissue revealed after microwave treatment. Appl Immunohistochem 1997; 5(1):59-62.

34. Jones EC, Pins M, Dickersin GR, et al. Metanephric adenoma of the kidney. A clinicopathological, immunohistochemical, flow cytometric, cytogenetic, and electron microscopic study of seven cases. Am J Surg Pathol 1995; 19(6):615-626.

35. Davis CJ, Barton JH, Sesterhenn IA, et al. Metanephric adenoma: clinicopathological study of fifty patients. Am J Surg Pathol 1995; 19(10):1101-1114.

36. Renshaw AA, Freyer DR, Hammers YA. Metastatic metanephric adenoma in a child. Am J Surg Pathol 2000; 24(4):570-574.

37. Renshaw AA, Maurici D, Fletcher JA. Cytologic and fluorescence in situ hybridization (FISH) examination of metanephric adenoma. Diagn Cytopathol 1997; 16:107-111.

38. Xu X, Acs G, Yu GH, et al. Aspiration cytology of metanephric adenoma of the kidney. Diagn Cytopathol 2000; 22(5):330-331.

39. Pins MR, Jones EC, Martul EV, et al. Metanephric adenoma-like tumors of the kidney: report of three malignancies with emphasis on discriminating features. Arch Pathol Lab Med 1999; 123:415-420.

40. Shek TWH, Luk ISC, Peh WCG, et al. Metanephric adenofibroma: report of a case and review of the literature. Am J Surg Pathol 1999; 23(6):727-733.

41. Murphy WM, Beckwith JB, Farrow GM. Tumors of the kidney, bladder, and related urinary structures. Atlas of tumor pathology. 3rd series, Fascicle 11. Washington, DC: Armed Forces Institute of Pathology; 1994.

42. Ciftci AO, Talim B, Senocak ME, et al. Renal oncocytoma: diagnostic and therapeutic aspects. J Pediatr Surg 2000; 35(9):1396-1398.

43. Tickoo SK, Reuter VE, Amin MB, et al. Renal oncocytosis: a morphologic study of 14 cases. Am J Surg Pathol 1999; 23(9):1094-1101.

44. Klein MJ, Valensi QJ. Proximal tubular adenomas of the kidney with so-called oncocytic features. Cancer 1976; 38:906-913.

45. Reuter VE, Presti JC. Contemporary approach to the classification of renal epithelial tumors. Semin Oncol 2000; 27:124-137.

46. Muzzonigro G, Minardi D, Azizi B, et al. Renal oncocytoma: pathological evaluation and clinical implications. Arch Ital Urol Androl 1996; 68(2):107-113.

47. Liu J, Fanning CV. Can renal oncocytomas be distinguished from renal cell carcinoma on fine-needle aspiration specimens? Cancer Cytopathol 2001; 93:390-397.

48. Nguyen GK, Amy RW, Tsang S. Fine needle aspiration biopsy cytology of renal oncocytoma. Acta Cytol 1985; 29(1):33-36.

49. Alanen KA, Tyrkko JE, Nurmi MJ. Aspiration biopsy cytology of renal oncocytoma. Acta Cytol 1985; 29(5):859-862.

50. Licht MR. Renal adenoma and oncocytoma. Semin Urol Oncol 1995; 13(4):262-266.

51. Fuhrman SA, Lasky LC, Limas C. Prognostic significance of morphologic parameters in renal cell carcinoma. Am J Surg Pathol 1982; 6:655-663.

52. Medeiros LJ, Jones EC, Aizawa S, et al. Grading of renal cell carcinoma: workgroup no. 2. Cancer 1997; 80(5):990-991.

53. Al Nazer M, Mourad WA. Successful grading of renal-cell carcinoma in fine-needle aspirates. Diagn Cytopathol 2000; 22(4):223-226.

54. Hes O, Michal M, Sulc M, et al. Glassy hyaline globules in granular cell carcinoma, chromophobe cell carcinoma, and oncocytoma of the kidney. Ann Diagn Pathol 1998; 2(1):12-18.

55. Beaty MW, Zhuang Z, Park WS, et al. Fine-needle aspiration of metastatic clear cell carcinoma of the kidney: employment of microdissection and the polymerase chain reaction as a potential diagnostic tool. Cancer 1997; 81(3):180-186.

56. Fetsch PA, Simsir A, Abati A. Comparison of antibodies to HBME-1 and calretinin for the detection of mesothelial cells in effusion cytology. Diagn Cytopathol 2001; 25(3):158-161.

57. Sharma S, Singh R, Verma K. Cytomorphology of adrenocortical carcinoma and comparison with renal cell carcinoma. Acta Cytol 1997; 41(2):385-392.

58. Fetsch PA, Powers CN, Zakowski MF, et al. Anti-alpha-inhibin: marker of choice for the consistent distinction between adrenocortical carcinoma and renal cell carcinoma in fine-needle aspirations. Cancer 1999; 87(3):168-172.

59. Renshaw AA, Granter SR. A comparison of A103 and inhibin reactivity in adrenal cortical tumors: distinction from hepatocellular carcinoma and renal tumors. Mod Pathol 1998; 11(12):1160-1164.

60. Delahunt B, Eble JN. Papillary renal cell carcinoma: a clinicopathologic and immunohistochemical study of 105 tumors. Mod Pathol 1997; 10(6):537-544.

61. Kovacs G, Emanuel A, Neumann HP, et al. Cytogenetics of renal cell carcinomas associated with von Hippel-Lindau disease. Genes Chromosomes Cancer 1991; 3(4):256-262.

62. Renshaw AA, Corless CL. Papillary renal cell carcinoma: histology and immunohistochemistry. Am J Surg Pathol 1995; 19(7):842-849.

63. Granter SR, Perez-Atayde AR, Renshaw AA. Cytologic analysis of papillary renal cell carcinoma. Cancer 1998; 84(5):303-308.

64. Storkel S, Steart PV, Drenckhahn D, et al. The human chromophobe cell renal carcinoma: its probable relation to intercalated cells of the collecting duct. Virchows Arch B Cell Pathol Incl Mol Pathol 1989; 56:237-245.

65. Speicher MR, Schoell B, du Manoir S, et al. Specific loss of chromosomes 1, 2, 6, 10, 13, 17, and 21 in chromophobe renal cell carcinomas revealed by comparative genomic hybridization. Am J Pathol 1994; 145(2):356-364.

66. Granter SR, Renshaw AA. Fine-needle aspiration of chromophobe renal cell carcinoma. Analysis of six cases. Cancer 1997; 81(2):122-128.

67. Wiatrowska BA, Zakowski MF. Fine-needle aspiration biopsy of chromophobe renal cell carcinoma and oncocytoma: comparison of cytomorphologic features. Cancer 1999; 87:161-167.

68. Tickoo SK, Amin MB. Discriminant nuclear features of renal oncocytoma and chromophobe renal cell carcinoma: analysis of their potential utility in the differential diagnosis. Am J Clin Pathol 1998; 110:782-787.

69. Kennedy SM, Merino MJ, Linehan WM, et al. Collecting duct carcinoma of the kidney. Hum Pathol 1990; 21:449-456.

70. Caraway NP, Wojcik EM, Katz RL, et al. Cytologic findings of collecting duct carcinoma of the kidney. Diagn Cytopathol 1995; 3:304-309.

71. Layfield LJ. Fine-needle aspiration biopsy of renal collecting duct carcinoma. Diagn Cytopathol 1994; 11(1):74-78.

72. Ono K, Nishino E, Nakamine H. Renal collecting duct carcinoma: report of a case with cytologic findings on fine needle aspiration. Acta Cytol 2000; 44(3):380-384.

73. Garcia-Bonafe M, De Torres I, Tarragona J. Renal collecting duct carcinoma. Diagn Cytopathol 1997; 16(2):180-181.

74. Nicol KK, Sutton BC, Iskandar SS, et al. Fine needle aspiration of renal medullary neoplasms: three cases involving young non-caucasian males. Cancer Cytopathol (in press).

75. Larson DM, Gilstad CW, Manson GW, et al. Renal medullary carcinoma: report of a case with positive urinary cytology. Diagn Cytopathol 1998; 18(4):276-279.

76. Auger M, Katz RL, Sella A, et al. Fine-needle aspiration cytology of sarcomatoid renal cell carcinoma: a morphologic and immunocytochemical study of 15 cases. Diagn Cytopathol 1993; 9:46-51.

77. Gattuso P, Ramzy I, Truong LD, et al. Utilization of fine-needle aspiration in the diagnosis of metastatic tumors to the kidney. Diagn Cytopathol 1999; 21:35-38.

78. Santamaria M, Jauregui I, Urtasun F, et al. Fine needle aspiration biopsy in urothelial carcinoma of the renal pelvis. Acta Cytol 1995; 39:443-448.

79. Hayes MMM, Jones EC, Verma AK, et al. Transitional cell carcinoma of the renal pelvis metastatic to the metacarpal: a case report correlating cytologic and histologic findings. Acta Cytol 1992; 36(6):946-950.

80. Fetsch PA, Fetsch JF, Marincola FM, et al. Comparison of melanoma antigen recognized by T cells (MART-1) to HMB-45: additional evidence to support a common lineage for angiomyolipoma, lymphangiomyomatosis, and clear cell "sugar" tumor. Mod Pathol 1998; 11(8):699-703.

81. Kwok-Fai T, Tse MK, Tsui WMS, et al. Fine needle aspiration diagnosis of angiomyolipoma of the liver using a cell block with immunohistochemical study. Acta Cytol 1994; 38:257-260.

82. Glentoj A, Partoft S. Ultrasound-guided percutaneous aspiration of renal angiomyolipoma: report of two cases diagnosed by cytology. Acta Cytol 1984; 28:265.

83. Nguyen G-K. Aspiration biopsy cytology of renal angiomyolipoma. Acta Cytol 1984; 261.

84. Wadih GE, Raab SS, Silverman JF. Fine needle aspiration cytology of renal and retroperitoneal angiomyolipoma: cytologic findings and clinicopathologic pitfalls in diagnosis. Acta Cytol 1995; 39:945.

85. Farrow GM, Harrison EG JR, Utz DC, et al. Sarcomas and sarcomatoid and mixed malignant tumors of the kidney in adults (I). Cancer 1968; 22:545-550.

86. Srinivas V, Sogani PC, Hajdu SI, et al. Sarcomas of the kidney. J Urol 1984; 132:13.

87. Vogelzang NJ, Fremgen AM, Guinan PD, et al. Primary renal sarcoma in adults. Cancer 1993; 71:804-810.

88. Truong LD, Caraway N, Ngo T, et al. Renal lymphoma: the diagnostic and therapeutic roles of fine-needle aspiration. Am J Clin Pathol 2001; 115:18-31.

89. Sharifah NA. Fine needle aspiration cytology characteristics of renal tumors in children. Pathology 1994; 26(4):359-364.

90. Geisinger KR, Silverman JF, Wakely PE, et al. Pediatric cytopathology. In: Johnston WW, editor. ASCP theory and practice of cytopathology 4. Chicago: American Society of Clinical Pathologists; 1994. pp. 293-354.

91. Hazarika D, Narasimhamurthy KN, Rao CR, et al. Fine needle aspiration cytology of Wilms' tumor: a study of 17 cases. Acta Cytol 1994; 38(3):355-360.

92. Zuppan CW, Beckwith JB, Luckey DW. Anaplasia in unilateral Wilms' tumor: a report from the National Wilms' Tumor Study pathology center. Hum Pathol 1988; 19: 1199-1209.

93. Srinivasan R, Nijhawan R, Dey P, et al. Fine needle aspiration cytology of clear cell sarcoma of the kidney and its distinction from Wilms' tumor. Acta Cytol 1997; 41(3): 950-951.

94. Krishnamurthy S, Bharadwaj R. Fine needle aspiration cytology of clear cell sarcoma of the kidney. A case report. Acta Cytol 1998; 42(6):1444-1446.

95. Wick MR, Cherwitz DL, Manivel JC, et al. Immunohistochemical findings in tumors of the kidney. In: Eble JN, editor. Tumors and tumor-like conditions of the kidneys and ureters. New York: Churchill Livingstone; 1991. pp. 207-247.

96. Truong LD, Williams R, Ngo T, et al. Adult mesoblastic nephroma: expansion of the morphologic spectrum and review of literature. Am J Surg Pathol 1998; 22(7):827-839.

97. Kumar N, Jain S. Aspiration cytology of mesoblastic nephroma in an adult: diagnostic dilemma. Diagn Cytopathol 2000; 23(2):124-126.

98. Drut R. Cytologic characteristics of congenital mesoblastic nephroma in fine-needle aspiration cytology: a case report. Diagn Cytopathol 1992; 8(4):374-376.

99. Dey P, Srinivasan R, Nijhawan R, et al. Fine needle aspiration cytology of mesoblastic nephroma: a case report. Acta Cytol 1992; 36(3):404-406.

100. Kaw YT. Cytologic findings in congenital mesoblastic nephroma: a case report. Acta Cytol 1994; 38(2):235-240.

101. Gnarra JR, Tory K, Weng Y, et al. Mutations of the VHL tumor suppressor gene in renal carcinoma. Nat Genet 1994; 7:85-90.

102. Kuroda N, Naruse K, Miyazaki E, et al. Vinculin: its possible use as a marker of normal collecting ducts and renal neoplasms with collecting duct system phenotype. Mod Pathol 2000; 13(10):1109-1114.

103. Davis CJ, Mostofi FK, Sesterhenn IA. Renal medullary carcinoma: the seventh sickle cell nephropathy. Am J Surg Pathol 1995; 19(1):1-11.

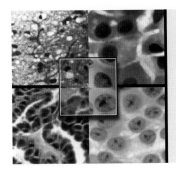

Adrenal Gland

The prevalence of adrenal masses has been estimated to be up to 4% with computed tomography (CT) examination[1] and 7% at autopsy.[2] Incidental adrenal masses (incidentaloma) are being discovered with increasing frequency due to the widespread application of noninvasive, high-resolution radiologic imaging techniques. The etiologic factors of these adrenal incidentalomas encompass a wide range of pathologic conditions of benign and malignant entities, including primary and metastatic cancers.

The diagnostic workup of adrenal incidentalomas is both controversial and variable. The multidisciplinary approach of hormonal screening, radiologic evaluation, and scintigraphy appears to be the mainstay of contemporary evaluation of these masses in many centers.[1-3] Many authorities have advocated a noninvasive management of these lesions: most adrenal incidentalomas are nonhypersecretory and benign.

Generally, if an adrenal mass is hyperfunctioning and/or large (greater than 6 cm), surgery is in order. With this approach, fine-needle aspiration (FNA) is mainly reserved for masses suspected to represent metastases extra-adrenal primaries.[1] Others have advocated that FNA should be the procedure of choice for the initial diagnosis of almost all adrenal masses.[4-7]

Whether FNA remains a major component of the adrenal nodule workup or is used in a more selective fashion, pathologists need to be familiar with the cytologic appearances of adrenal lesions to allow for an accurate diagnosis.

NORMAL ADRENAL GLAND

The right adrenal gland is pyramidal in shape, whereas the left is more elongated or round.[8-10] The normal cortex of the adult adrenal measures 1 to 2 mm in width, maintaining a cortex-to-medulla ratio of approximately 10:1.[8] The average combined weight of the adrenal glands varies throughout life and is influenced by aging and stress. In adults, the combined weight ranges from approximately 4 to 8 g.

In the adult, three zones can be histologically appreciated in the well-developed cortex. The thin and discontinuous zona glomerulosa, consisting of lipid-filled cells arranged in lobular clusters, is responsible for mineralocorticoid production, comprises approximately 10% to 15% of the cortex, and overlies the larger zona fasciculata, which is the site of glucocorticoid production (Figure 23-1). The zona fasciculata consists of abundant lipid-rich cells arranged in radial cords and columns (Figure 23-2). The inner zone of the cortex is the zona reticularis, the site of sex steroid production, and consists of smaller, compact, lipid-depleted cells containing lipofuscin pigment (Figure 23-3). The medulla is concentrated in the head and body of the adrenal gland and consists of scattered chromaffin cells (Figure 23-4).

Adrenocortical nodularity measuring from 1 to 3 mm in size is not uncommon in the adult adrenal and can form partially or completely circumscribed surface projections.[8]

FNA biopsy of the normal adrenal gland procures small clusters and cords of uniform cells with polygonal contours and centrally located, round to oval nuclei.[11-14] The adrenal cells from the zona glomerulosa and fasciculata are lipid rich, which is cytologically reflected by cytoplasm that is clear and foamy with delicate, frayed cytoplasmic membranes (Figure 23-5). In contrast, cells from the zona reticularis have a compact cyanophilic cytoplasm containing finely granular, golden brown, lipofuscin pigment with the Pap stain (Figure 23-6). Inadvertent sampling of hepatocytes is possible in aspirates of the right adrenal gland because of the proximity of the adrenal gland to the overlying liver (Figure 23-7). Moreover, liver cells can be potentially misinterpreted as adrenal cells because of their often similar vacuolated appearance, central nuclei, and pigment.[11,12] Conversely, accessory adrenocortical tissue can be found in the region of the celiac axis and can involve the liver as adrenohepatic fusions or the kidney as subcapsular foci. Other sites of adrenocortical heterotopia have been described but have been rarely reported in the FNA literature.

BENIGN ADRENAL CYSTS

Adrenal cysts are uncommon lesions that occur predominantly in middle-aged adults. It is estimated that they are found in two to six cases per 10,000 autopsies.[12] Cysts can be categorized into epithelial, parasitic, endothelial, or hemorrhagic groups.[15] The endothelial cyst is the most common type, followed by benign or malignant pseudocysts.

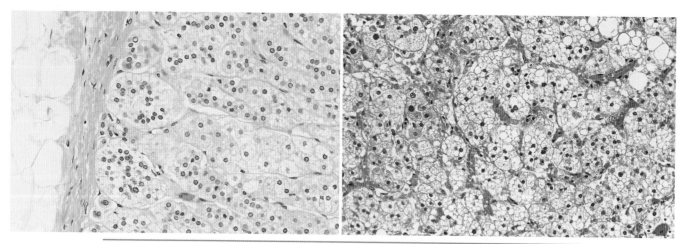

Figure 23-1   Benign adrenal tissue. Histologic examination of the zona glomerulosa reveals lipid-filled cells arranged in lobular clusters. (Hematoxylin and eosin [H&E])

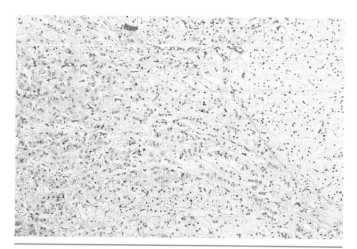

Figure 23-2   Benign adrenal tissue. Histologic examination of the zona fasciculata reveals lipid-rich cells arranged in radial cords and columns. (H&E)

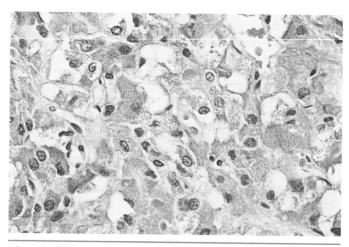

Figure 23-4   Benign adrenal tissue. Histologic examination of the medullary portion of the adrenal gland consists of chromocytes having granular pigmented cytoplasm. (H&E)

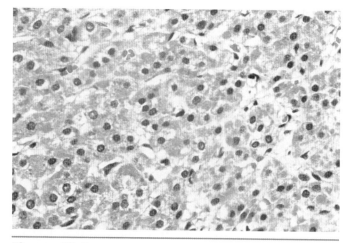

Figure 23-3   Benign adrenal tissue. Histologic examination of the zona reticularis reveals compact lipid-depleted cells containing abundant lipofuscin pigment. (H&E)

Pseudocysts, by definition, lack an epithelial lining and occur as a sequela to hemorrhage.[12] Occasionally, these cysts undergo FNA examination when they present as large lesions (measuring up to 30 cm in maximum dimension). With large cysts, the FNA procedure becomes not only diagnostic but often therapeutic, with removal of cyst fluid. The aspirates can be clear, turbid, or bloody. Endothelial cells may be present, arranged individually or in loose clusters, and are characterized by elongated shapes with round to oval nuclei. Inflammatory cells and hemosiderin-laden macrophages are often present.[12,15,16]

 INFECTIOUS DISEASES

Infectious lesions vary with age. Bacterial abscesses occur predominantly in children and fungal and mycobacterial infections occur largely in adults (Figure 23-8).[9] Worldwide, tuberculosis still remains the most common cause of Addison's disease (i.e., adrenal cortical hypofunctioning),

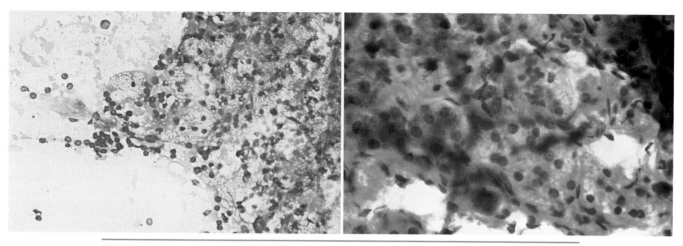

Figure 23-5 Benign adrenal tissue. Fine-needle aspiration (FNA) of zona glomerulosa from benign adrenal gland consists of lobulated clusters of lipid-rich cells having clear, pale, foamy cytoplasm with delicate frayed cytoplasmic membranes. (Diff-Quik [DQ])

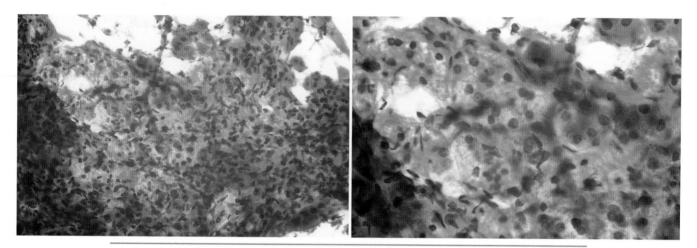

Figure 23-6 Benign adrenal tissue. FNA of benign adrenal cortex, revealing pale cells from zona fasciculata and pigmented cells from zona reticularis. (Papanicolaou [Pap])

especially in underdeveloped counties.[8] The most common cause of Addison's disease in the industrialized West is chronic idiopathic or autoimmune adrenocortical insufficiency.[8] The aspiration findings of adrenal tuberculosis are identical to aspirates of necrotizing granulomas from other sites. These cytologic features include the presence of epithelioid histiocytes and lymphocytes scattered in a background of caseous necrotic debris. However, Tao has commented that epithelioid cells and multinucleated giant cells are not as commonly seen in adrenal tuberculosis as they are in other locations.[13]

A variety of fungal infections can also cause Addison's disease. Histoplasma capsulatum is the most common fungus, but Addison's disease can also be the result of North and South American blastomycosis, coccidioidomycosis, and cryptococcosis (Figure 23-9).[8] Similar to tuberculosis, fungal infections usually cause bilateral adrenal involvement. FNA cytology and the applications of special stains or the smears demonstrate the fungi in a background of caseous necrosis and/or granulomatous inflammation. A

granulomatous response is usually diminished in patients immunosuppressed with steroids. There are a few cytologic reports of adrenal histoplasmosis and cryptococcosis that discuss diagnosis by FNA biopsy.[16-20]

In acquired immunodeficiency syndrome (AIDS), cytomegalovirus (CMV) is the most common adrenotropic infection.[8] Herpes simplex and varicella-zoster adrenalitis have also been described in the surgical pathology literature, but FNA biopsy has not been reported as a diagnostic procedure for these adrenal viral infections.

NODULAR AND HYPERPLASTIC ADRENAL GLAND

Adrenocortical nodularity is not an uncommon finding, especially in older individuals. The nodules can measure up to 5 mm in maximum dimension and are almost never associated with clinical evidence of hypercorticalism. They are usually unilateral and solitary, although occasionally,

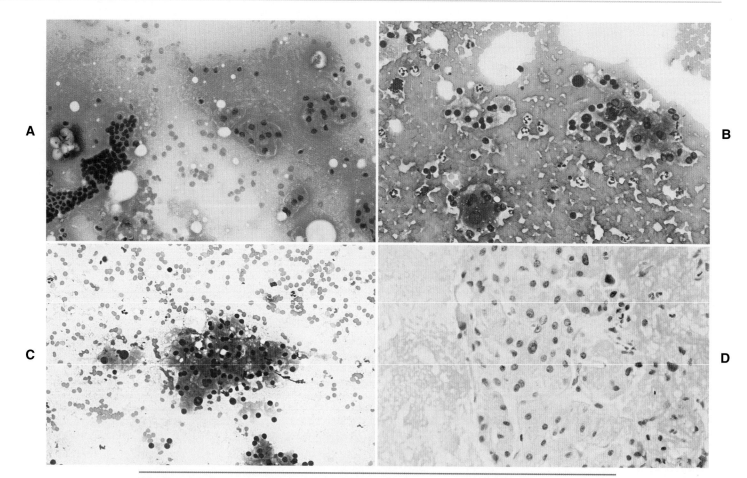

Figure 23-7 **Hepatocytes. A,** Inadvertent sampling of hepatocytes in an aspirate of the right adrenal gland reveals clusters of polygonal-shaped liver cells having vacuolated cytoplasm with centrally placed nuclei, along with a group of bile duct epithelium. (Pap) **B** and **C,** Clusters of liver cells with granular to pale cytoplasm. (DQ). **D,** Benign liver tissue in an aspirate of the right adrenal gland demonstrating anisonucleosis and binucleation with nuclei having prominent nucleoli. This could be a potential pitfall for a misdiagnosis of malignancy if the hepatocellular origin of the cells is not recognized. (DQ)

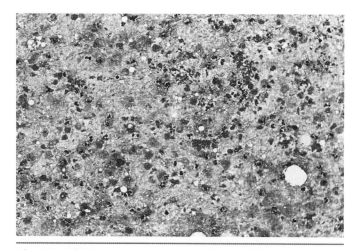

Figure 23-8 **Adrenal abscess.** FNA consisting of neutrophils with necrotic debris in the background. (Pap)

they can be bilateral and rarely be multiple on one side.[8] These nodules are believed to be a hyperplastic rather than a true neoplastic (e.g., adenoma) process.[8]

With the advent of high-resolution radiologic CT imaging, incidental adrenal nodules are being discovered with increasing frequency.[1-3] Adrenal scintigraphy has demonstrated that these are not hyperfunctioning in the absence of clinical evidence of hypercorticalism.[8] These small adrenocortical nodules are usually 3 cm or less in size, having a smooth, well-defined shape and a relatively low density with CT scan.[8] The evaluation of these adrenocortical nodules, as mentioned above, is controversial. Several algorithmic approaches have been proposed for these adrenal incidentalomas. They are based on: the imaging characteristic of the nodule, the size of the mass, the presence of hypercorticalism, or whether an adrenal metastasis needs to be confirmed or excluded in a patient with a known or suspected extra-adrenal malignancy.[8]

The size of an adrenal mass is often used as a decision threshold for surgery. General consensus is that adrenal

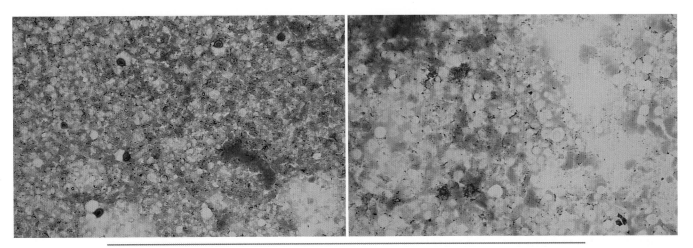

Figure 23-9 *Cryptococcus.* FNA of adrenal crytococcus infection showing numerous scattered yeast forms with surrounding halos and necrotic background. (DQ)

masses greater than 6 cm need to be surgically removed.[1] The management of smaller lesions varies with the institution with some recommending surgery for nodules ranging from 2.5 to 5 cm (usually in the 3 to 4 cm range).[1] This approach seems reasonable because the risk of malignancy is greater with increasing size; however, benign lesions are still more common among masses greater than 6 cm and malignant lesions measuring less than 2.5 cm may occur.[1] Therefore, although some authors have advocated size as a discriminating feature to avoid doing FNA, the overlapping of size of benign and malignant lesions is a strong argument for including FNA biopsy as a diagnostic procedure in the workup of these adrenal nodules.[7]

Other components of the algorithms to suggest a benign lesion include a normal scintigraphy uptake in a patient with no clinical signs of malignancy.

Hyperplasia of the adrenal cortex is almost always bilateral, diffuse, and nodular consisting of either micronodules measuring under 1 cm or macronodules greater than 1 cm.[10] Patients with adrenocortical hyperplasia may be symptomatic with excess cortical secretion (Cushing's syndrome), hyperaldosteronism, virilization, or feminization, or may suffer no symptoms at all.

FNA cytology of adrenocortical nodules and hyperplastic lesions recapitulates the findings of normal adrenal glands, including the presence of vacuolated adrenocortical cells—many with frayed cytoplasmic borders (Figure 23-10 and Box 23-1). Stripped nuclei arranged individually or in loose clusters are often found in a background that consists of frothy lipid material. This is best appreciated in the air-dried DQ preparation (Figure 23-11). When the aspirates from an adrenocortical nodule are cellular and consist of stripped nuclei, a potential pitfall exists for misinterpreting these cells as a metastatic small cell carcinoma. This potential for misdiagnosis is accentuated in the alcohol-fixed Pap preparation that dissolves out the diagnostically helpful, bubbly lipid material in the background (Figure 23-12). Therefore, air-dried DQ smears aid in the diagnosis. The cytopathologist can appreciate that the stripped nuclei are round and overlapping with small nucleoli, in contrast to small cell carcinoma that has the nuclear molding and angularity, evenly distributed salt and pepper chromatin, and

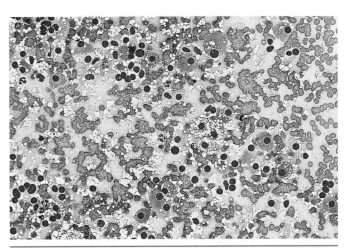

Figure 23-10 **Adrenocortical nodule.** FNA revealing numerous vacuolated adrenocortical cells including many with frayed cytoplasmic borders. (DQ)

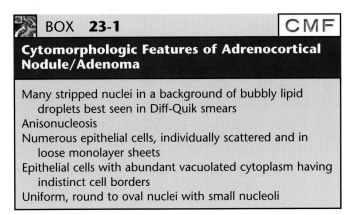

BOX 23-1 CMF

Cytomorphologic Features of Adrenocortical Nodule/Adenoma

Many stripped nuclei in a background of bubbly lipid droplets best seen in Diff-Quik smears
Anisonucleosis
Numerous epithelial cells, individually scattered and in loose monolayer sheets
Epithelial cells with abundant vacuolated cytoplasm having indistinct cell borders
Uniform, round to oval nuclei with small nucleoli

a lack of nucleoli. In addition to the frothy lipid background material and the stripped discohesive nuclei, the presence of large cohesive fragments of adrenal cells with transversing endothelial cells is another feature reported to be a cytologic feature of a benign adrenocortical nodule.[21]

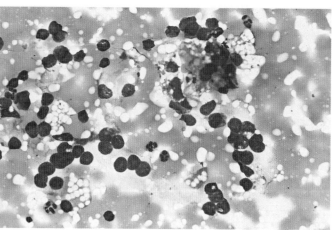

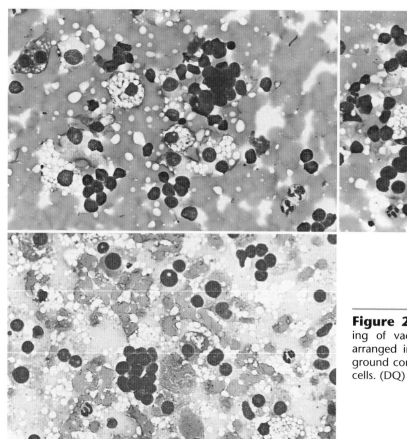

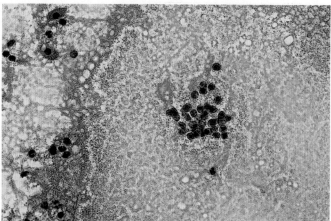

Figure 23-11 **Adrenocortical nodule.** Aspirate consisting of vacuolated adrenocortical cells and stripped nuclei arranged individually and in loose clusters. The smear background contains frothy lipid material, admixed with red blood cells. (DQ)

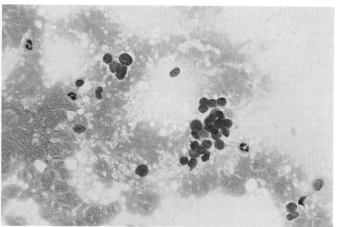

Figure 23-12 **Adrenocortical nodule.** Overlapping clusters of stripped nuclei in an aspirate from an adrenocortical nodule that could potentially be misdiagnosed as metastatic small cell carcinoma. The presence of bubbly lipid material in the background, which is often a diagnostic aid in air-dried DQ preparations, has been dissolved out in these alcohol-fixed Pap-stained smears. (Pap)

ADRENAL MYELOLIPOMA

Myelolipoma occurs most often in the adrenal gland but can be found in a variety of extraadrenal sites.[8] Approximately one half of the patients present with abdominal/flank pain, hematuria, palpable mass, hyperten-

sion, or rarely, spontaneous retroperitoneal hemorrhage.[8] Adrenal myelolipomas are most commonly seen in older adults with an equal sex distribution. Occasionally, adrenal myelolipomas can be huge, measuring up to 34 cm in maximum dimension and weighing up to 5900 grams.[22] Conversely, they can be small and found incidentally at the

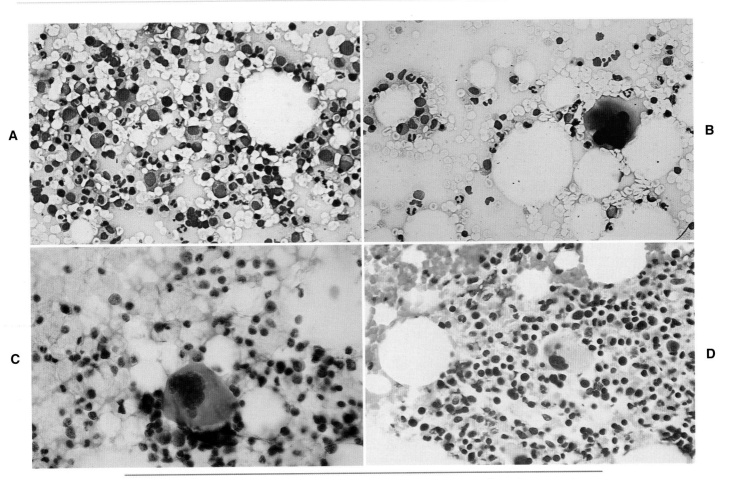

Figure 23-13 **Myelolipoma.** FNA consisting of hematopoietic cells such as megakaryocytes, mature and immature myeloid cells, and some erythroid precursors with interspersed fat. (**A** and **B,** DQ; **C,** Pap; **D,** cell block) (Courtesy Paul Wakely, MD, Ohio State University School of Medicine, Columbus, Ohio.)

time of autopsy.[8] With the advent of use of sophisticated radiologic imaging, it is not surprising that adrenal myelolipomas have been detected more often. This is also reflected by the increasing incidence of FNA reports.[5,6,23-28]

The diagnostic aspiration cytologic features include the presence of mature and immature hematopoietic elements, including myeloid and erythroid cells, lymphocytes, and megakaryocytes admixed with mature adipose tissue (Figure 23-13 and Box 23-2). These elements occasionally prompt a differential diagnosis that includes well-differentiated liposarcoma, renal angiomyolipoma, and extramedullary hematopoiesis.[6,11,28] Attention to the location of the aspirate, appreciation of admixed adrenocortical cells, and the lack of a concomitant systemic hematopoietic condition should eliminate extramedullary hematopoiesis from consideration. Adrenal myelolipoma also lacks the vascular and smooth muscle components of angiomyolipoma or the lipoblasts of well-differentiated liposarcoma.

ADRENOCORTICAL ADENOMA

Adrenocortical adenoma is a benign neoplasm accompanied by an endocrine syndrome due to excess secretions of one or more of the three major classes of steroids produced

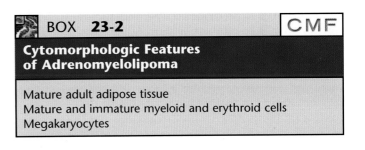

BOX 23-2 **CMF**

Cytomorphologic Features of Adrenomyelolipoma

Mature adult adipose tissue
Mature and immature myeloid and erythroid cells
Megakaryocytes

by the adrenal cortex.[8] It is morphologically impossible to distinguish adrenocortical adenoma from their nonhyperfunctioning counterpart, the benign adrenocortical nodule. Adrenocortical adenomas may be associated with hyperaldosteronism (Conn's syndrome), adrenocorticoid excess (Cushing's syndrome), or virilization and/or feminization. Benign adrenocortical neoplasms with virilization and/or feminization are relatively uncommon and should prompt the suspicion that an adrenocortical malignancy is present.[8]

The cytologic findings of aspirates from adrenocortical adenomas are exactly the same as from adrenocortical nodules (see Box 23-1). The smears are cellular consisting of uniform epithelial cells with vacuolated cytoplasm including frayed cytoplasmic borders, plus numerous stripped,

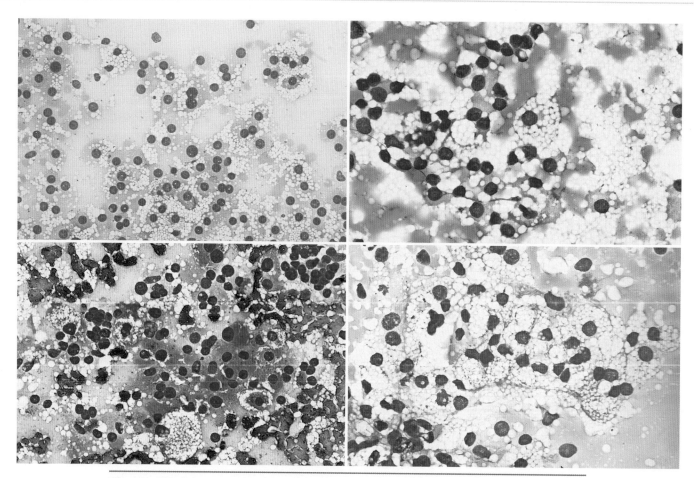

Figure 23-14 **Adrenocortical adenoma.** Aspirates consisting of uniform polygonal to cuboidal shaped cells with coarsely vacuolated cytoplasm and frayed cytoplasmic borders. (DQ)

discohesive nuclei (Figure 23-14). The nuclei can be individually scattered or clustered and overlapping, which results in a ball-like morular pattern. Adrenocortical cell nuclei possess small nucleoli and have round, smooth nuclear membranes. Again, a potential pitfall can occur by misinterpreting the stripped adrenocortical nuclei for metastatic small cell carcinoma (Figure 23-15). The lack of salt-and-pepper chromatin (better appreciated with the Pap stain), nuclear molding, and nuclear irregularity and the presence of small nucleoli should suggest the correct diagnosis. Again, an accurate diagnosis is also aided when one appreciates the abundant, frothy lipid background in the air-dried smears, a feature that can be lost if one relies strictly on alcohol-fixed Pap preparations. Adrenal adenomas often demonstrate anisonucleosis, a feature present in many aspirates of endocrine lesions, but nuclear pleomorphism should not be seen. Mitotic figures and necrotic debris are also absent.

Unusual adrenocortical neoplasms can occur that have unique cytoplasmic tinctorial qualities. FNA cytology of a "black" adenoma contains cells originating from the zona reticularis, and therefore, the cells possess abundant cytoplasmic lipofuscin granules.[8,9] These cells also have compact eosinophilic cytoplasm in addition to the lipofuscin pigment. Oncocytic adrenocortical neoplasms are rare tumors in which the cells have abundant granular eosinophilic cy-

toplasm. As expected, electron microscopy reveals numerous mitochondria.[8]

In addition to misinterpreting stripped adrenocortical nuclei as metastatic small cell carcinoma, other potential diagnostic pitfalls exist when interpreting FNA cytology of adrenocortical nodules and adenomas, especially when one is unaware of associated clinical and radiologic findings. As mentioned above, normal adrenocortical cells share the same cytologic features with cells from benign adrenocortical nodules and adenomas.[2] It is therefore essential for the cytopathologist to review the CT or ultrasound findings and correlate them with the cytologic features.[29] In FNA biopsy of the right adrenal gland, inadvertent sampling of benign hepatocytes from the nearby overlying liver can occur, as mentioned above.[11,12] In general, liver cells are larger and more polygonal in shape with opaque granular cytoplasm, well-defined cell borders, and occasional intracytoplasmic bile pigment. Nuclei tend to be centrally positioned, and nucleoli are more prominent than those seen in adrenocortical cells. Although fat can be present in hepatocytes, it is usually present as large distinct intracytoplasmic vacuoles in hepatocytes, in contrast with the microvesicular pale, frothy, indistinct vacuoles of adrenocortical cells. Recognition of bile ductular epithelium is another helpful feature to suggest inadvertent sampling of the liver in a right adrenal aspirate. Lastly, as is discussed in the follow-

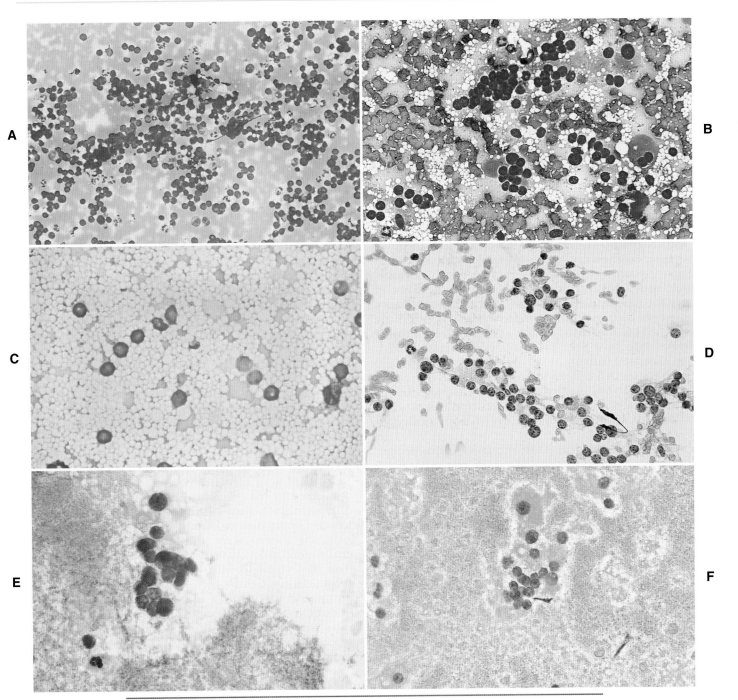

Figure 23-15 Adrenocortical adenoma. A to C, Aspirates consisting of clusters and individually scattered stripped adrenocortical nuclei that potentially could be misinterpreted as a metastatic small cell carcinoma. (DQ) **D to F,** Loose clusters of stripped adrenocortical nuclei along with a few intact cells. Note the lack of bubbly, frothy lipid material in the background in this alcohol-fixed Pap preparation.

ing section, aspirates of some well-differentiated adrenocortical carcinomas can be cytologically similar to adrenocortical nodules or adenomas. This is not surprising because a well-known diagnostic challenge in surgical pathology is the separation of adrenocortical adenoma from well-differentiated adrenocortical carcinoma. This challenging diagnostic scenario is discussed in the following section.

 ## ADRENOCORTICAL CARCINOMA

Adrenocortical carcinoma occurs most often in the fourth and fifth decades, with a second minor incidence peak in the first decade. Adrenocortical carcinoma is an uncommon malignancy with an incidence of only one or two cases per million population and a slight female predominance.[8-10]

Variable clinical presentations include abdominal and/or flank pain, palpable mass, fatigue, weight loss, and an intermittent low-grade fever. Conversely, because of its retroperitoneal location, the signs and symptoms of a mass may be obscured or delayed until the tumor becomes quite large. Adrenocortical carcinoma may be functional with a pure endocrine syndrome such as Cushing's syndrome or cause a mixed syndrome presentation, although aldosteronism is uncommon.[8] Conversely, adrenocortical carcinoma may not be associated with a functional syndrome. Adrenocortical carcinoma is an aggressive malignancy with 50% to 90% of patients dying, usually within the first 2 years of diagnosis, although occasional patients may be long-term survivors.[8]

One of the more challenging areas in surgical pathology is the diagnostic separation of adrenocortical adenoma from adrenocortical carcinoma. No single or combined histologic or nonhistologic parameters can predict biologic behavior with total accuracy,[8] since except for evidence of metastatic disease, diagnostic features that can definitively distinguish adenoma from adrenocortical carcinoma are lacking.[12] This is reflected by the plethora of classification schemes that have been proposed to distinguish benign from malignant adrenocortical neoplasms. Medeiros and Weiss have stressed histologic findings, whereas others also include clinical data in the evaluation of these adrenocortical neoplasms.[30] As mentioned previously, tumor size is a useful predictor for separating benign from malignant adrenocortical neoplasms, but is not definitive. Although most large lesions are malignant and small lesions benign, considerable variability is evident. Lack and colleagues[10] have suggested that any adrenocortical neoplasm in excess of 100 g should be considered a carcinoma. Medeiros and Weiss[30] suggest that the presence of three or more of the following histologic features can predict malignant behavior: high nuclear grade; mitotic rate greater than 5 per 50 high-power fields, atypical mitotic figures, eosinophilic tumor cell cytoplasm, diffuse architecture, necrosis, or invasion of veins, sinusoids, or the capsule. Many authorities believe that the mitotic rate may be the single most important criterion in separating benign from malignant adrenocortical neoplasms.[30] Unfortunately, accurate assessment of mitotic rate is not possible in FNA cytology nor is the evaluation for the presence of venous, sinusoidal, or capsular invasion.[12]

Adrenocortical carcinoma typically presents as a large, bulky, nodular neoplasm with the average weight ranging from 510 to 1200 g and an average size of 12 cm to more than 16 cm.[8] Within the carcinoma, foci of necrosis, hemorrhage, and cystic change may be present. Histologically, adrenocortical carcinoma may have varying patterns including trabecular, alveolar, or diffuse with the neoplastic cells separated by delicate vascular channels lined by a single layer of endothelial cells.[10] Nuclear pleomorphism can be extensive and mitotic activity brisk with numerous atypical mitotic figures.[8]

FNA cytology of adrenocortical carcinoma varies, reflecting the histologic features (Box 23-3).[11] In general, aspirates of adrenocortical carcinoma are hypercellular with numerous discohesive single cells and occasional groups of malignant cells. Nuclei are pleomorphic with contour irregularity, coarse irregular chromatin, and prominent nucleoli. The presence of anisonucleosis is not necessarily a specific feature for malignancy, as this finding can also be seen in adenomas. The presence of nuclear irregularity and coarse chromatin are good indicators that an adrenocortical carcinoma has been sampled. The cytoplasm varies from eosinophilic to clear and vacuolated. In well-differentiated adrenocortical carcinomas, more intracytoplasmic lipid is encountered, and therefore, a potential exists to confuse well-differentiated adrenocortical carcinoma with an adrenocortical adenoma (Figure 23-16).[31] Features favoring adrenocortical carcinoma include larger tumor size with the presence of hyperchromatic pleomorphic nuclei and occasional mitotic figures (Figure 23-17).[11] Adrenocortical carcinoma can also demonstrate nuclear pseudoinclusions and intracytoplasmic hyaline globules.[8] As adrenocortical carcinoma becomes more poorly differentiated, the cytoplasm appears more granular and eosinophilic.[11,12] The most poorly differentiated adrenocortical carcinomas can have a sarcomatoid appearance, which could prompt a differential diagnosis that includes other spindle cell lesions that can involve the adrenal glands such as pheochromocytoma, sarcoma, and metastatic malignancies (Figure 23-18).[29] The authors have previously reported the types of spindle cell malignancies that can involve the adrenal gland, based on their FNA biopsy experience.[32,33] Three adrenal spindle cell malignancies were encountered, including a high-grade adrenocortical carcinoma, pheochromocytoma, and metastatic cutaneous desmoplastic melanoma (Figure 23-19). Ancillary studies performed on the aspirated material were helpful in arriving at a correct diagnosis (Figure 23-20).[33]

In addition to adenoma, other neoplasms that could be considered in the differential diagnosis include renal cell carcinoma and hepatocellular carcinoma.[34] Attention to the location of the tumor and standard cytomorphologic criteria, along with ancillary studies, can usually resolve these challenging cases. Aspirates of renal cell carcinoma also have dispersed cells with vacuolated cytoplasm, although the nuclei tend to be more rounded with less pleomorphism and the vacuoles more punched out and coarse. Cells of hepatocellular carcinoma are typically arranged in thick trabeculae with sinusoidal rimming by endothelial cells. The clear cell variant of hepatocellular carcinoma could pose a distinct problem. However, adrenocortical carcinoma is typically negative for cytokeratin, whereas both

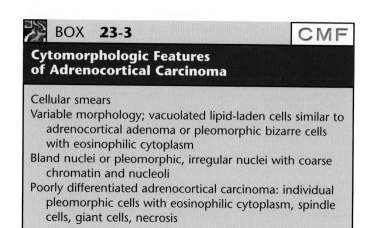

BOX 23-3   CMF

Cytomorphologic Features of Adrenocortical Carcinoma

Cellular smears
Variable morphology; vacuolated lipid-laden cells similar to adrenocortical adenoma or pleomorphic bizarre cells with eosinophilic cytoplasm
Bland nuclei or pleomorphic, irregular nuclei with coarse chromatin and nucleoli
Poorly differentiated adrenocortical carcinoma: individual pleomorphic cells with eosinophilic cytoplasm, spindle cells, giant cells, necrosis

hepatocellular carcinoma and renal cell carcinoma are low molecular weight cytokeratin positive. With the recent application of heat-induced epitope retrieval, some adrenocortical carcinomas have demonstrated positivity for low molecular weight cytokeratin (CAM 5.2). Epithelial membrane antigen positivity in renal cell carcinoma, canalicular staining for polyclonal carcinoembryonic antigen (CEA) in hepatocellular carcinoma, as well as inhibin and Melan-A positivity in adrenal neoplasms can be helpful in the differential diagnosis. Other immunohistochemical studies that can aid in the differential diagnosis of poorly differentiated and/or clear cell malignancies that could be confused with adrenocortical carcinoma have been done.

 PHEOCHROMOCYTOMA

Pheochromocytoma is an uncommon neoplasm derived from the chromatin cells of the medullary portion of the adrenal gland. It has an average annual incidence between 1.6 to 2.6 cases per million.[10] The peak age of diagnosis in some series is in the fifth decade, but malignancy can occur in any age group.[8] More than 90% of the cases are sporadic with the remaining patients having a familial history resulting from one of the multiple endocrine neoplasia (MEN) syndromes. When familial cases occur, pheochro-

mocytomas occur at an earlier age. MEN syndrome type 2A (Sipple syndrome) includes pheochromocytoma, medullary carcinoma of the thyroid, and parathyroid hyperplasia. MEN type 2B includes pheochromocytoma, medullary thyroid cancer, ganglioneuromatosis of the gastrointestinal

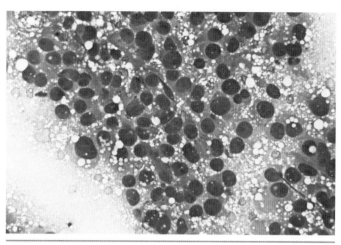

Figure 23-16 Well-differentiated adrenocortical carcinoma. Aspirate containing numerous neoplastic cells with vacuolated cytoplasm. (DQ)

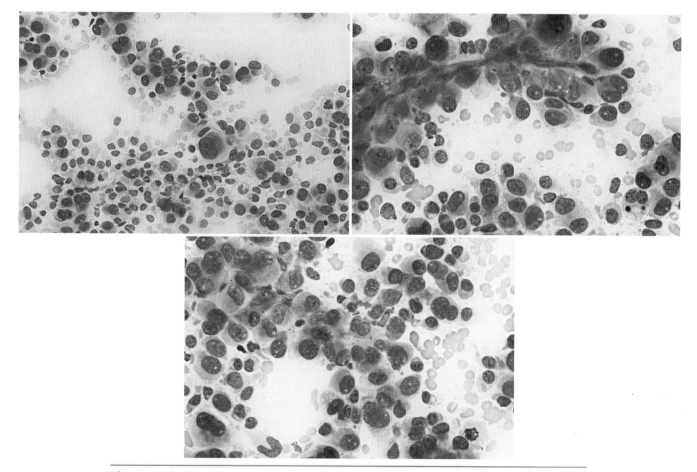

Figure 23-17 Adrenocortical carcinoma. Aspirates consisting of atypical cells showing considerable variation in nuclear size and shape. (DQ)

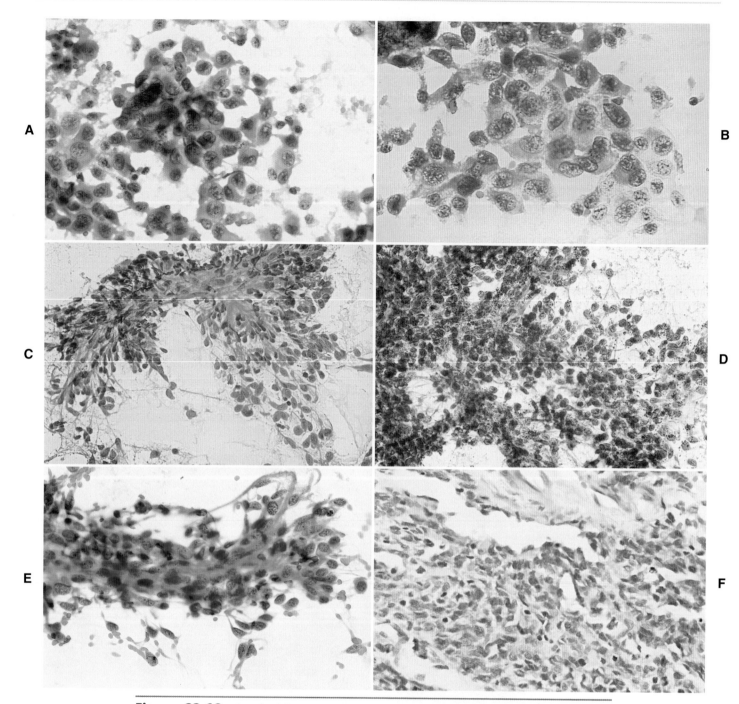

Figure 23-18 **Poorly differentiated adrenocortical carcinoma. A-E,** Aspirate consisting of loose clusters and individually scattered cells having dense to granular cytoplasm. (Pap) Aspirate of poorly differentiated adrenocortical carcinoma having a sarcomatoid appearance characterized by loose clusters of spindled cells having high nuclear-to-cytoplasmic (N:C) ratios. (Pap) **F,** Resected sarcomatoid adrenal cortical carcinoma consisting of malignant spindle-shaped cells. (H&E)

tract, multiple mucosal neuromas, and connective tissue defects imparting a Marfanoid habitus.[8]

Although clinically unsuspected or underdiagnosed examples of pheochromocytoma occur at surgery or autopsy in more than one third of the cases, the prevalence of clinically suspected cases has increased because of greater clinical awareness and the application of sophisticated radiologic imaging techniques and biochemical studies.[12] Patients can be symptomatic from the secretion of excessive amounts of catecholamines and present with paroxysmal hypertension, sweating, and palpitations. Increased levels of urinary or plasma vanillylmandelic acid (VMA) and catecholamines occur in approximately 90% of patients, although as many as 20% of tumors may be nonfunctional. Pheochromocytoma

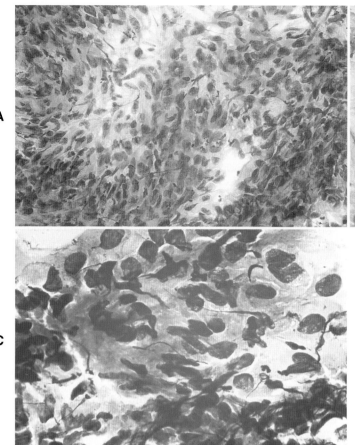

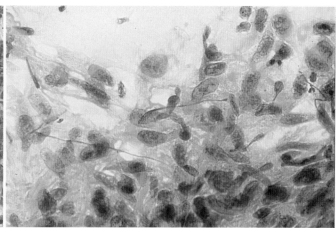

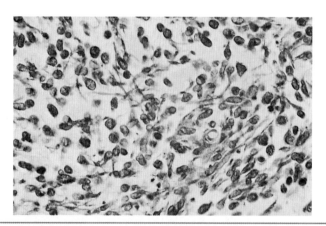

Figure 23-19 **Metastatic malignant melanoma.** FNA of metastatic cutaneous desmoplastic malignant melanoma to the adrenal gland. The neoplastic polygonal to spindle-shaped cells could be confused with both sarcomatoid adrenocortical carcinoma and pheochromocytoma. (**A** and **B,** Pap; **C,** DQ)

is known as the 10% tumor with approximately 10% of the neoplasms bilateral, 10% extraadrenal, 10% malignant, and 10% occurring in children. However, in the sporadic setting in adults, 95% of pheochromocytomas are solitary, 5% bilateral, and 5% to 10% extraadrenal, in contrast with the familial setting where more than 50% of the patients have bilateral tumors.[8]

Sporadic pheochromocytomas typically present as solitary masses measuring from 3 to 5 cm in maximum dimension and weighing an average of 100 g, although a wide range in weight occurs.[10,11] A variety of histologic patterns may occur, including anastomosing trabecular cords, diffuse or solid, and an alveolar or nested pattern with interspersed vascularized fibroconnective tissue. When the alveolar or nested pattern is well developed, a "zellballen" arrangement is seen, reminiscent of head and neck paragangliomas. The tumor cells are generally polygonal in shape with a moderate amount of pale to granular, generally basophilic cytoplasm[11,12]; however, the cytoplasm may be eosinophilic to amphophilic. Eccentrically placed nuclei are set in a cytoplasm that is ill defined with frayed borders. Nuclei can be bland, but often nuclear pleomorphism is striking. Occasional tumor cells may have a granular eosinophilic oncocytoid appearance. Other tumor cells may be spindle shaped with elongated nuclei having a coarse chromatin distribution. Occasionally, cells from pheochromocytoma can resemble large ganglion cells with eccentrically placed single or multiple vesicular nuclei, a distinct

Figure 23-20 **Adrenocortical carcinoma, sarcomatoid type.** FNA of sarcomatoid type of adrenocortical carcinoma having numerous cells with spindled shapes. The tumor cells were cytokeratin negative but vimentin positive. (Immunoperoxidase) (From Silverman JF, Geisinger KR. Fine needle aspiration cytology of the thorax and abdomen. New York: Churchill-Livingstone; 1996. pp.206.)

nuclear membrane, prominent nucleoli, and tapering cell processes with intracytoplasmic basophilic granular material reminiscent of Nissl substance. Occasional cytoplasmic vacuoles may serve as a potential pitfall for confusing a pheochromocytoma with an adrenocortical neoplasm.

Nuclear pseudoinclusions and intracytoplasmic hyaline globules may be present.[10]

Immunohistochemical studies demonstrate positive staining of the tumor cells for synaptophysin, chromogranin, neuron-specific enolase, and other neuroendocrine markers.[10] S-100 highlights the spindled- to stellate-shaped sustentacular cells surrounding the pheochromocytoma cells arranged in the alveolar zellballen pattern. Ultrastructural examination reveals diagnostic neurosecretory granules. Norepinephrine granules typically have a prominent eccentric space between the electron-dense core and surrounding limiting membranes, whereas epinephrine granules possess a narrow uniform halo around the cores.[10] Rarely, pigmented pheochromocytomas have been described in which the tumor cells contain abundant granular intracytoplasmic pigment.[8]

Aspiration cytology of pheochromocytoma generally produces hypercellular smears in which the cells are arranged predominantly in a discohesive fashion or in loose groups (Box 23-4).[11,12,35,36] The tumor cells may show considerable variation in cell size and shape. Cell contours vary from polygonal and spindled to highly pleomorphic (Figures 23-21, 23-22, and 23-23). Occasional cases consist of cells that resemble aspirates from carcinoid or an islet cell tumor. Rarely, the aspirate can contain ganglion-type cells (Figure 23-24) or cells resembling a spindle cell malignancy (Figure 23-25). Pheochromocytomas nuclei can be bland with evenly distributed chromatin or can demonstrate anisonucleosis and/or pleomorphism, including giant tumor cells having hyperchromatic nuclei with prominent nucleoli. Occasional nuclear pseudoinclusions can be seen. A helpful diagnostic feature is the presence of abundant but poorly defined granular cytoplasm that takes on a fine red granularity with Romanowsky stain. Because of the fragile cytoplasm, these red granules may also be dispersed in the background. Application of immunohistochemistry on cytologic material can be confirmed with positive staining of the tumor cells for neuroendocrine markers.

Potential diagnostic pitfalls include mistaking a pheochromocytoma for other poorly differentiated malignancies, including sarcomatoid renal cell carcinoma, adrenocortical carcinoma, or even a retroperitoneal sarcoma when bizarre spindle and/or giant cells are present in the smears (Figure 23-26). Cytologic features suggesting the correct diagnosis include the presence of polygonal to carcinoidal to spindle-shaped cells with granular cytoplasm. Applications of immunohistochemical studies and/or electron microscopy help resolve these challenging cases (Figure 23-27).

Lastly, it has been reported that FNA biopsy of a pheochromocytoma carries a potential complication of initiating a catecholamine crisis,[4,10,37] or uncontrollable hemorrhage with fatal consequences.[10] Although suspecting a pheochromocytoma has been regarded as a contraindication for FNA biopsy, it has been the authors' and others'[9] experience that this complication occurs only rarely. Casola and colleagues suggest that pheochromocytoma can be diagnosed by FNA biopsy, but the radiologist must be ready to institute emergency treatment in the event of a hypertensive crisis.[4]

 ## METASTATIC TUMORS

By anatomic site, the adrenal gland is the fourth most common extranodal location of metastatic carcinoma after lung, liver, and bone.[10] Adrenal metastasis have been documented in 9% to 20% of cancer patients at autopsy, with lung and breast cancer the most common primary malignancies. Metastases are usually unilateral but can be bilateral in up to 40% of cases. Rare tumor-to-tumor metastases to a pheochromocytoma or adrenocortical adenoma have been reported. With the application of sophisticated imaging techniques in the evaluations of patients with malignancy, more adrenal masses are being discovered. Accordingly, an increasing number of adrenal metastases that are diagnosed with FNA biopsy have been seen. With adrenal FNA biopsies, nearly one half of the aspirates represent metastatic cancer to the adrenal gland.[32] This was similar to the M.D. Anderson Cancer Center (Houston, Tex.) experience, in which more than 40% of adrenal aspirates represented metastatic malignancies.[11,16] The metastatic cancer that is most likely to involve the adrenal gland is the lung, followed by kidney and melano-

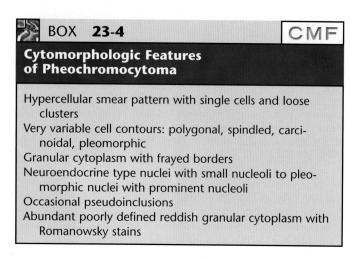

BOX 23-4   **CMF**

Cytomorphologic Features of Pheochromocytoma

Hypercellular smear pattern with single cells and loose clusters
Very variable cell contours: polygonal, spindled, carcinoidal, pleomorphic
Granular cytoplasm with frayed borders
Neuroendocrine type nuclei with small nucleoli to pleomorphic nuclei with prominent nucleoli
Occasional pseudoinclusions
Abundant poorly defined reddish granular cytoplasm with Romanowsky stains

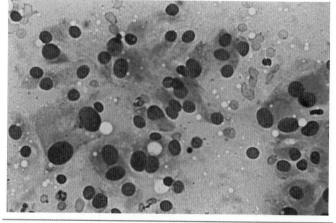

Figure 23-21   **Pheochromocytoma.** Tumor cells show considerable variation in size and shape. (DQ)

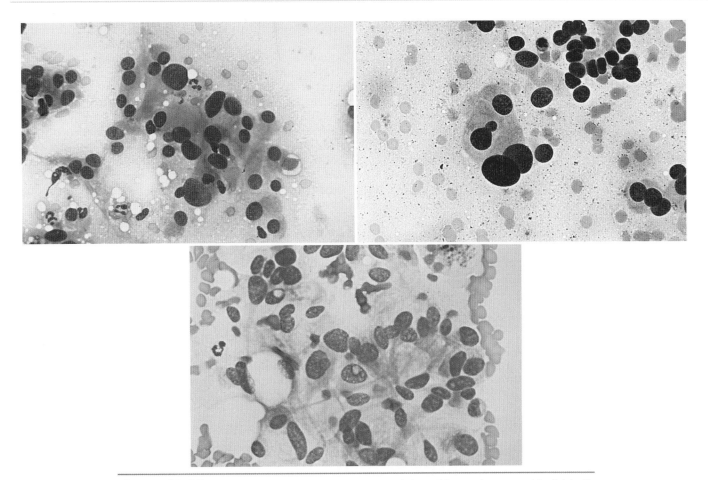

Figure 23-22 **Pheochromocytoma.** Aspirate consisting of loose clusters and individually scattered polygonal-shaped cells in which there is considerable anisonucleosis. (DQ)

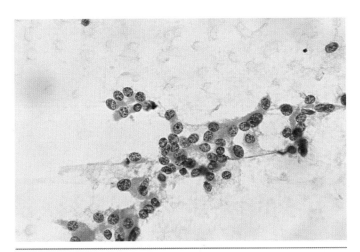

Figure 23-23 **Pheochromocytoma, carcinoidal type cells.** Aspirate of pheochromocytoma having a carcinoidal pattern consisting of loose clusters and individually scattered cuboidal-shaped cells with high N:C ratios and granular cytoplasm. (Pap)

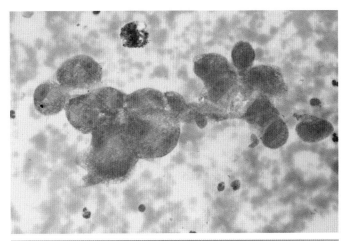

Figure 23-24 **Pheochromocytoma, ganglion type cells.** Aspirate of pheochromocytoma with ganglion type cells having large size with abundant granular cytoplasm. (Pap)

ma (Figure 23-28). Adrenal involvement by renal cell carcinoma has also been reported in approximately 60% of radical nephrectomies and 90% of patients at autopsy. This is an especially challenging diagnostic scenario because renal cell carcinoma could readily be confused with

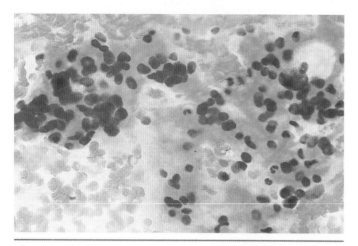

Figure 23-25 **Pheochromocytoma, small cells.** Aspirate of pheochromocytoma with clusters of cells with high N:C ratios resembling a small cell malignancy. (Pap)

adrenocortical neoplasms as discussed previously. However, a panel of immunohistochemical studies can usually aid in making the correct diagnosis.

Generally, the diagnosis of metastatic malignancy to the adrenal glands is not challenging. However, Mitchell and colleagues reported that a pulmonary adenocarcinoma metastatic to the adrenal gland mimicked benign adrenocortical epithelium.[38] Ancillary studies, including differential cytokeratins 7 and 20 for the workup of metastatic adenocarcinoma, and thyroid transcription factor-1 (TTF-1), can be extremely helpful to suggest the primary site. Lung, breast, and cancers of ovarian/endometrial origin are often positive for cytokeratin 7, whereas colon carcinomas are usually positive for only cytokeratin 20 in most cases. In contrast, adrenocortical carcinomas are generally negative for cytokeratin 7 and 20 but positive for inhibin and Melan-A.[38]

Another unusual neoplasm that may involve the adrenal gland as part of widespread systemic disease is malignant lymphoma (Figure 23-29).[39] Diagnostic cytologic features are the lymphoid appearance of the atypical cells and the presence of numerous lymphoglandular bodies in the background. In addition, primary adrenal lymphomas have also been described.[39] Other unusual adrenal malignancies reported include primary malignant melanoma and a variety

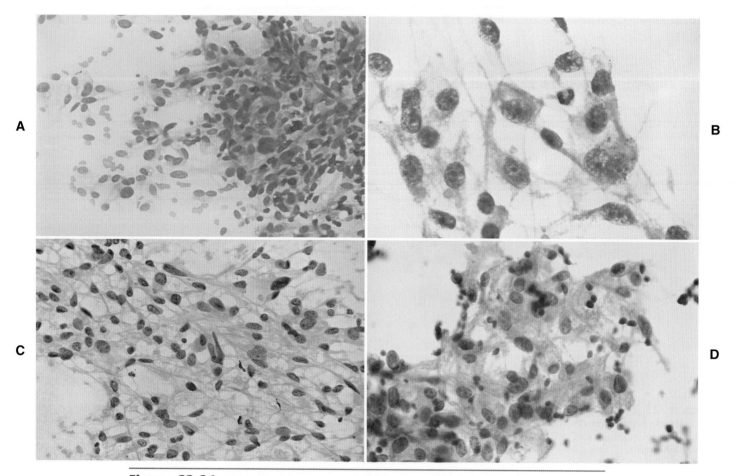

Figure 23-26 **Pheochromocytoma, spindle cells.** Aspirates from pheochromocytoma having a spindled configuration that could be confused with other poorly differentiated spindle cell malignancies such as sarcomatoid renal cell carcinoma, adrenocortical carcinoma, metastatic melanoma, or sarcoma. A helpful diagnostic feature for pheochromocytoma is the granular quality to the cytoplasm. (**A,** DQ; **B** to **D,** Pap)

of benign and malignant soft tissue type tumors (Figure 23-30).[8,40,41]

NEUROBLASTOMA

Neuroblastoma is the prototypical small round cell tumor of childhood.[42,43] It is the third most common malignancy of the pediatric age group when central nervous system tumors and the more common lymphoreticular tumors are excluded.[12] Most patients with neuroblastoma are diagnosed before age 5 with approximately 50% clinically presenting before age 2.[42,43] Neuroblastoma is the most common malignancy of the neonate with both congenital and fetal cases reported.[33] Although neuroblastoma can arise from any site containing sympathetic neural tissue, the retroperitoneum and adrenal lesions are most commonly seen.[42,43] Age and stage at diagnosis are the two most significant prognostic factors for patients with neuroblastoma. Unfortunately, approximately one third of patients present with metastasis to regional lymph nodes, liver, bones, and lungs at the time of diagnosis.

Histologic grade has a lesser impact on prognosis, although the Shimada classification stresses that the presence of stromal development, cellular differentiation, and the presence of mitotic-karyorrhectic cells expressed as an index (MKI) have prognostic implications.[44] Specifically, a more favorable prognosis correlates with the presence of a stromal-rich matrix, low MKI, or an increased number of differentiating tumor cells. Children under age 1 also have a better prognosis. Adrenal neuroblastoma has a less favorable course than its extraadrenal counterpart. In contrast with many other pediatric small round cell malignancies, neuroblastoma has not shown an improved clinical survival with applications of contemporary chemotherapeutic regimens. It is therefore critical for the pathologist to make

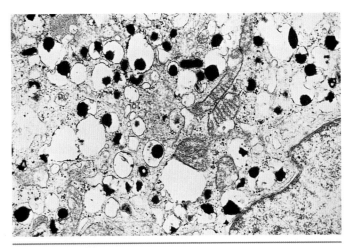

Figure 23-27 **Pheochromocytoma, electron microscopy (EM).** EM performed on aspirate of pheochromocytoma revealing numerous neurosecretory type granules.

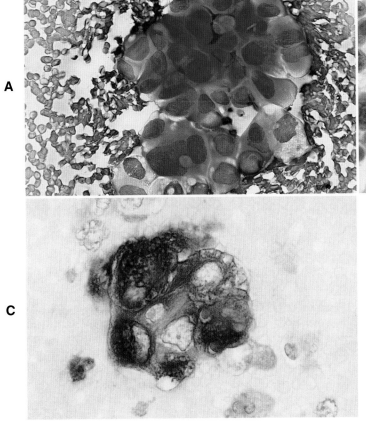

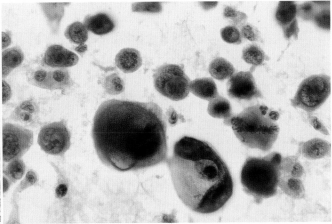

Figure 23-28 **Metastatic lung cancer. A,** Aspirates of metastatic lung cancer to adrenal gland demonstrating a cluster of neoplastic cells with pleomorphic nuclei. (DQ) **B,** Individually scattered pleomorphic cells including tumor giant cells in an aspirate of metastatic bronchogenic cancer to the adrenal gland. (Pap) **C,** Diffuse cytoplasmic carcinoembryonic antigen (CEA) staining of malignant cells from a metastatic lung cancer to adrenal gland. (Immunoperoxidase)

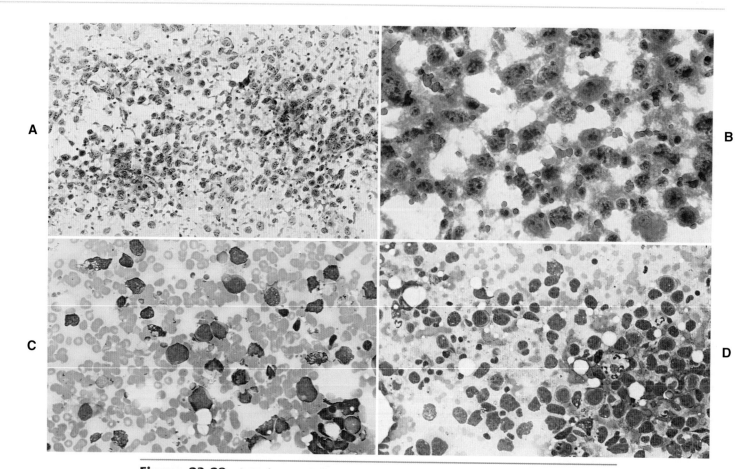

Figure 23-29 Lymphoma. Aspirate of lymphomatous involvement of adrenal gland as part of widespread systemic disease. Note the individually scattered atypical lymphoid cells. (**A** and **B,** Pap; **C** and **D,** DQ)

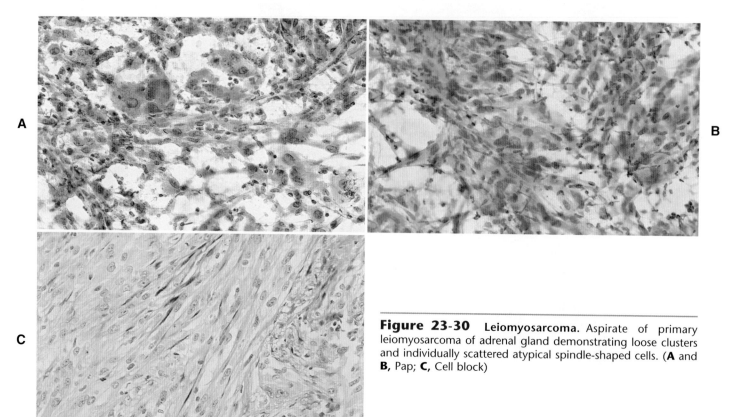

Figure 23-30 Leiomyosarcoma. Aspirate of primary leiomyosarcoma of adrenal gland demonstrating loose clusters and individually scattered atypical spindle-shaped cells. (**A** and **B,** Pap; **C,** Cell block)

an accurate diagnosis of neuroblastoma and differentiate this malignancy from others considered in the rubric of small round cell malignancies of childhood. Other prognostic factors that have been demonstrated in neuroblastoma include the *N-myc* oncogene amplication, which is associated with a more aggressive and advanced clinical course. A diploid DNA pattern also represents an adverse prognostic factor.

Grossly, adrenal neuroblastoma usually presents as a circumscribed mass with a smooth external surface or occasionally as a huge multinodular tumor. Extensive necrosis with cystic degeneration and dystrophic calcification can be present.[8] Histologically, the neuroblastic cells are arranged diffusely or in nests separated by thin fibrovascular septae. A vague lobular pattern can be discerned, although other areas may show a more diffuse or solid appearance. The neuroblastic cells have high nuclear to cytoplasmic (N:C) ratios and are often set in a pale staining fibrillar matrix. By the authors' definition, neuroblastoma is composed predominantly (greater than 50%) of neuroblasts with neuropil, in contrast with ganglioneuroma composed exclusively of mature ganglion cells, neurites accompanied by Schwann cells, and fibrous tissue.[45] Ganglioneuroblastoma consists predominantly of ganglioneuromatous elements constituting greater than 50% of the tumor and a relatively small neuroblastic component. The neuroblastic cells of neuroblastoma have a nucleus with the classic salt-and-pepper, evenly dispersed chromatin pattern, whereas the ganglion cells of ganglioneuroma and ganglioneuroblastoma have much larger vesicular nuclei with prominent nucleoli and abundant distinct cytoplasm with Nissl substance.

In aspirates of neuroblastoma, the smears are hypercellular with both numerous individually scattered small cells and cohesive aggregates (Figure 23-31 and Box 23-5).[9,44-47] The cells have high N:C ratios. The neuroblastic cell nuclei vary from oval to slightly irregular, have a finely granular, evenly dispersed salt-and-pepper chromatin pattern, and inconspicuous or no nucleoli (Figure 23-32). Within the co-

hesive groups, nuclear molding is demonstrated, and occasional Homer-Wright rosettes are seen (Figure 23-33). Some of the dispersed neuroblastic cells and those arranged in loose clusters may have wispy unipolar cellular processes. An extremely helpful cytologic feature for the diagnosis of neuroblastoma is the appreciation of the background fibrillary matrix referred to as *neuropil,* which is seen both in the Diff-Quik (DQ) and Pap-stained material (Figure 23-34). Other cytologic features that occasionally can be present in the smears include necrotic debris, mitotic figures, and dystrophic calcification. Neoplastic ganglion cells are much larger than the neuroblastic cells and have huge nuclei with prominent nucleoli (Figure 23-35). The chromatin is coarsely granular and a moderate amount of cytoplasm is present. Ganglioneuromas have, in addition to the ganglion cells, admixed spindle-shaped, Schwann cells with associated collagen matrix (Figure 23-36). In some aspirates of neuroblastoma, occasional differentiating neuroblastic cells

---

BOX 23-5   CMF

Cytomorphologic Features of Neuroblastoma

Hypercellular smears with occasional cohesive clusters and numerous individually scattered cells

Nuclear molding often present

Neuroblastic cells with high nuclear to cytoplasmic ratios and oval to slightly irregular nuclei with finely dispersed chromatin and inconspicuous nucleoli

Occasionally, neuroblastic cells with delicate unipolar processes can be present

Background fibrillary neuropil and Homer-Wright rosettes can be seen

When present, ganglion cells are larger binucleated to multinucleated cells with prominent nucleoli and abundant coarsely granular cytoplasm

---

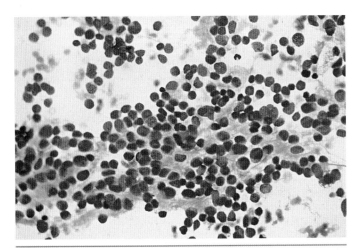

Figure 23-31 Neuroblastoma. Aspirate consisting of numerous individually scattered small cells with very high nuclear-to-cytoplasmic ratios. (Pap)

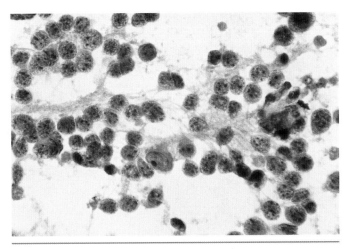

Figure 23-32 Neuroblastoma. Aspirate consisting of numerous individually scattered cells having granular evenly dispersed salt and pepper chromatin with inconspicuous to no nucleoli. A few of the tumor cells show wispy unipolar cellular processes. (Pap)

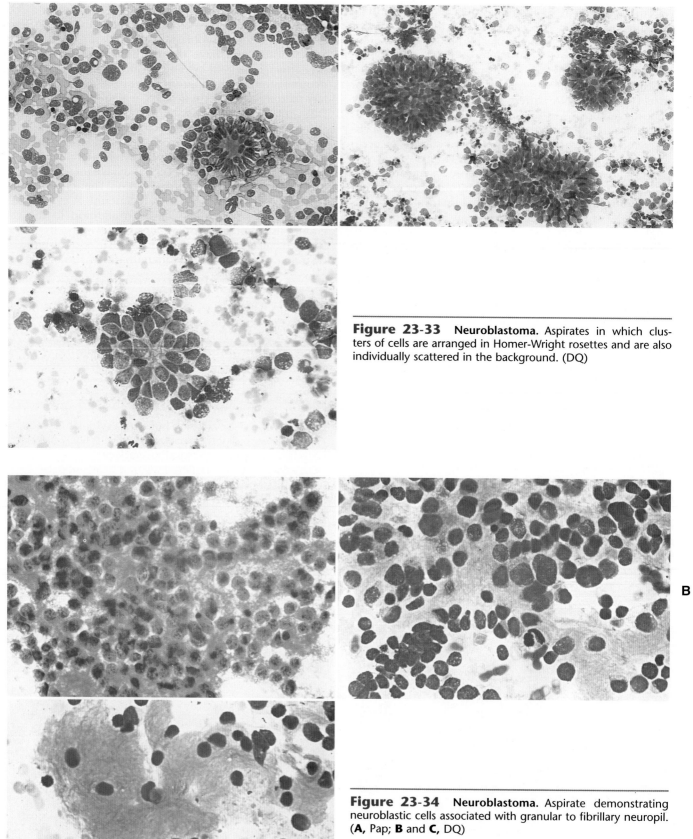

Figure 23-33 **Neuroblastoma.** Aspirates in which clusters of cells are arranged in Homer-Wright rosettes and are also individually scattered in the background. (DQ)

Figure 23-34 **Neuroblastoma.** Aspirate demonstrating neuroblastic cells associated with granular to fibrillary neuropil. (**A**, Pap; **B** and **C**, DQ)

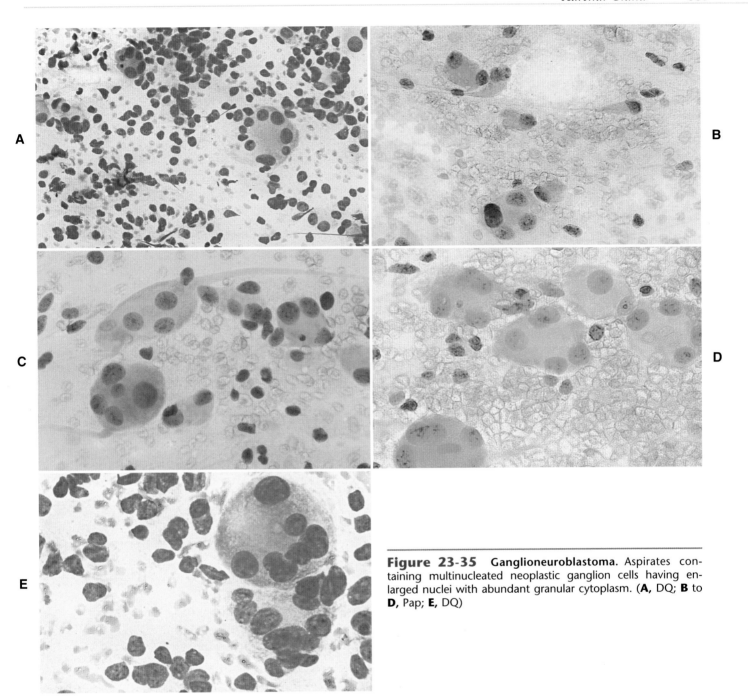

Figure 23-35 Ganglioneuroblastoma. Aspirates containing multinucleated neoplastic ganglion cells having enlarged nuclei with abundant granular cytoplasm. (**A,** DQ; **B** to **D,** Pap; **E,** DQ)

can be present, having a greater amount of cytoplasm and possessing a more vesicular chromatin pattern.

In addition to the morphologic features, ancillary studies are often essential in the workup of small round cell tumors.[45-60] Ultrastructural features of neuroblastoma include intracytoplasmic small, dense-core neurosecretory-type granules and abundant dendritic processes containing microtubules.[56-59] Immunohistochemical studies supportive of the diagnosis of neuroblastoma include positive staining of the cells for neuron-specific enolase and/or neurofilament proteins and microtubule-associated proteins (MAPs) such as MAP-2.

A potential exists to misdiagnose neuroblastoma as another pediatric small round cell tumor such as lymphoma (e.g., lymphoblastic and Burkitt's lymphoma), Wilms' tumor, and rhabdomyosarcoma.[45,57] Aspirates of lymphomas consist of atypical lymphoid cells in which numerous lymphoglandular bodies in the background are appreciated in both the air-dried DQ and alcohol-fixed Pap smears. Because of the larger size of the cytoplasmic fragments in air-dried DQ-stained smears, this preparation accentuates their presence. Aspirates of lymphoblastic lymphoma, which characteristically presents in cervical and mediastinal lymph nodes, have cells with oval to convoluted nuclei with delicate dispersed nuclear chromatin, inconspicuous nucleoli, and a scant amount of surrounding cytoplasm. Burkitt's lymphoma, which can often present as an intraabdominal mass, yields lymphoid cells of intermediate size,

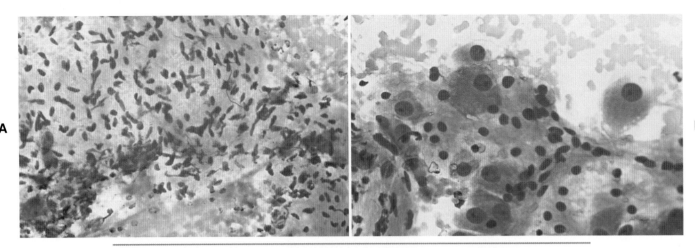

Figure 23-36   **Ganglioneuroma. A,** Aspirates from ganglioneuroma in which the neuromatous component consists of spindle-shaped, Schwann cells associated with a collagen matrix. (DQ) **B,** The ganglion cells in an aspirate from ganglioneuroma are multinucleated with a voluminous granular cytoplasm and enlarged nuclei with nucleoli. (DQ)

TABLE 23-1

Cytologic Features of Small Round Cell Tumors of Childhood

Cytologic Features	PNET	NB	ES	BL	LL	RMS	WT
Nuclear molding	+	+	±	−	−	−	±
Nucleoli	−	−	−	+(2-5)	−	+	−
Ganglion cells	−	±	−	−	−	−	−
Myxoid matrix	−	−	−	−	−	+	−
Cytoplasmic vacuoles	+	−	+(glycogen)	+(lipid)	−	−	−
Cytoplasmic tags	±	±	±	−	−	+	−
Horner-Wright rosettes	±rare	+	±rare	−	−	−	−
Tubules	−	−	−	−	−	−	+
Lymphoglandular bodies	−	−	−	+	+	−	−
Macrophages	±	±	−	+	+	−	−
Neuropil	−	+	−	−	−	−	−
Fibrous matrix	−	−	−	−	−	−	+
Spindle-shaped cells	−	−	−	−	−	+	±
Tadpole or ribbon-shaped cells	−	−	−	−	−	+	±
Dense cytoplasm	−	−	−	−	−	+	±
Karyorrhectic cells	−	+	−	+	+	−	−
Tigroid background	−	−	−	−	−	±	−

Modified from Silverman JF, Geisinger KR. Fine needle aspiration cytology of the thorax and abdomen. New York: Churchill-Livingstone; 1996. p.215; Silverman JF, Berns LA, Holbrook CT, et al. Fine-needle aspiration of primitive neuroectodermal tumors (PNET): a report of three cases. Acta Cytol 1992; 36:541.
PNET, Primitive neuroectodermal tumor; *NB,* neuroblastoma; *ES,* Ewing sarcoma; *BL,* Burkitt's lymphoma; *LL,* lymphoblastic lymphoma; *RMS,* rhabdomyosarcoma; *WT,* Wilms' tumor; +, frequently present or prominent; ±, may be present (rare) or inconspicuous; −, absent.

having nuclei with finely to moderately granular chromatin, two to five nucleoli, and basophilic cytoplasm with lipid-laden vacuoles in the aspirate.

Although not specific, scattered histiocytes can also be present throughout the smears, imparting a "starry sky" appearance to the background. Aspiration of Wilms' tumor (nephroblastoma) typically demonstrates the classic triphasic cytologic findings of primitive blastemal type cells, epithelial cells arranged as tubules or glomeruloid groupings, and spindled cells. When a monophasic blastemal pattern is present, a much greater potential exists to confuse this malignancy with neuroblastoma. Electron microscopy and

immunohistochemical studies help in differentiating these small round cell malignancies of childhood.[56-59] Intraabdominal desmoplastic small round cell tumor is a malignancy consisting of small round, oval, and spindled-shaped cells set in a desmoplastic fibrotic stroma. Characteristically, the primitive tumor cells demonstrate multidirectional immunohistochemical differentiation with staining for neuron specific enolase (NSE), desmin, and cytokeratin.[60] The tumor cells may occasionally show positivity for CD99, which does not occur in neuroblastoma. Cytogenetic and molecular diagnostic features help in differentiating the small round cell tumors that occur in the abdomen. The

TABLE 23-2

Ancillary Studies in the Fine-Needle Aspiration Workup of Small Round Cell Malignancies in Childhood

Cytologic Diagnosis	Electron Microscopy	Immunohistochemistry	Cytogenetics
Neuroblastoma	Relatively frequent DCG and prominent microtubules and cell processes than with PNET	NSE-S-100, Schwann cells, NF	Chromosome 1 deletion, short arm
PNET	Rare DCG Glycogen possible	NSE, vimentin, NF, β-microglobulin, CD99	11:22 translocation
Ewing sarcoma	Glycogen, cell junctions Fine, even chromatin CD99	Vimentin 11:22 translocation	
Burkitt's lymphoma	No specific EM features; cytoplasmic lipid vacuoles	LCA, B-cell phenotype	8:14 translocation
Lymphoblastic lymphoma	No specific EM features	LCA, B- or T-cell phenotype (usually T)	
Rhabdomyosarcoma	Myosin filaments, aberrant sarcomeres	Actin, myoglobin, desmin, Myo-Dq, myogenin	2:13 translocation in alveolar rhabdomyosarcoma

Modified from Silverman JF, Geisinger KR. Fine needle aspiration cytology of the thorax and abdomen. New York: Churchill-Livingstone; 1996. p.214; Silverman JF, Berns LA, Holbrook CT, et al. Fine-needle aspiration of primitive neuroectodermal tumors (PNET): a report of three cases. Acta Cytol 1992; 36:541.
DCG, Dense-core granules; *PNET,* primitive neuroectodermal tumor; *EM,* electron microscopy; *LCA,* leukocyte common antigen; *NSE,* neuron-specific enolase; *NF,* neurofilament.

cytologic and ancillary differential features of the small round cell tumors of childhood are presented in Tables 23-1 and 23-2.[9,61]

References

1. Barzon L, Boscaro M. Diagnosis and management of adrenal incidentalomas. J Urol 2000;163:398-407.
2. Lee JE, Evans DB, Hickey RC, et al. Unknown primary cancer presenting as an adrenal mass: frequency and implications for diagnostic evaluation of adrenal incidentalomas. Surgery 1998; 124:1115-1122.
3. Dwamena BA, Kloos RT, Fendrick M, et al. Diagnostic evaluation of the adrenal incidentaloma: decision and cost-effectiveness analyses. J Nucl Med 1998; 39:707-712.
4. Casola G, Nicolet V, van Sonnenberg E, et al. Unsuspected pheochromocytoma: risk of blood-pressure alterations during percutaneous adrenal biopsy. Radiology 1986; 159:733.
5. deBlois G, DeMay RM. Adrenal myelolipoma diagnosis by computed-tomography-guided fine-needle aspiration. Cancer 1985; 55:848.
6. Dunphy CH. Computed tomography-guided fine needle aspiration biopsy of adrenal myelolipoma: case report and review of the literature. Acta Cytol 1991; 35:353.
7. Saboorian MH, Katz RL, Charnsangavej C. Fine needle aspiration cytology of primary and metastatic lesions of the adrenal gland: a series of 188 biopsies with radiologic correlation. Acta Cytol 1995; 39:843-851.
8. Lack EE. Principles and practice of surgical pathology and cytopathology: the adrenal gland. New York: Churchill-Livingstone; 1997. pp. 2751-2799.
9. Silverman JF, Geisinger KR. Fine needle aspiration cytology of the thorax and abdomen. New York: Churchill-Livingstone; 1996. pp.197-217.
10. Lack EE, Travis WD, Oertel JE. Adrenal cortical nodules, hyperplasia, and hyperfunction. In Lack EE, editor. Pathology of the adrenal glands. New York: Churchill-Livingstone; 1990. p.75.
11. Katz RL. Kidney, adrenal, and retroperitoneum. In Bibbo M, editor. Comprehensive cytopathology. Philadelphia: WB Saunders; 1991. p.771.
12. Silverman JF, Katz R. FNA of the adrenal gland. In Schmidt WA, editor. Cytopathology annual. Baltimore: Williams and Wilkins; 1994. p.149.
13. Tao L-C. Primary lesions of the adrenals. In Tao L-C, editor. Transabdominal fine-needle aspiration biopsy. New York: Igaku-Shoin; 1990. p.218.
14. Herzberg AJ, Raso DS, Silverman JF. Color atlas of normal cytology. New York: Churchill-Livingstone; 1999. pp.190-196.
15. Laforga JBM, Bordallo A, Aranda FI. Vascular adrenal pseudocyst: cytologic and immunohistochemical study. Diagn Cytopathol 2000; 22:110-112.
16. Katz RL, Patel S, Mackay B, et al. Fine needle aspiration cytology of the adrenal gland. Acta Cytol 1984; 28:269.
17. Anderson CA, Pi WC, Weiss LM. Disseminated histoplasmosis diagnosed by fine needle aspiration biopsy of the adrenal gland: a case report. Acta Cytol 1989; 33:337.
18. Valente PT, Calafati SA. Diagnosis of disseminated histoplasmosis by fine needle aspiration of the adrenal gland. Acta Cytol 1989; 33:341.
19. Powers CN, Rupp GM, Maygarden SJ, et al. Fine-needle aspiration cytology of adrenal cryptococcosis: a case report. Diagn Cytopathol 1991; 7:88.
20. Deodhare S, Sapp M. Adrenal histoplasmosis: diagnosis by fine-needle aspiration biopsy. Diagn Cytopathol 1997; 17:42-44.
21. Wu HHJ, Cramer HM, Kho J, et al. Fine needle aspiration cytology of benign adrenal cortical nodules: a comparison of cytologic findings with those of primary and metastatic adrenal malignancies. Acta Cytol 1998; 42:1352-1358.
22. Hruban RH, Bhagavan BS, Epstein JI. Massive retroperitoneal angiomyolipoma. Am J Clin Pathol 1989; 92:805.
23. Galli L, Gaboardi F. Adrenal myelolipoma: report of diagnosis by fine needle aspiration. J Urol 1986; 136:655.

24. Gould JD, Mitty HA, Pertsemlidis D, et al. Adrenal myelolipoma: diagnosis by fine-needle aspiration. AJR 1987; 148:921.

25. Katsuta K, Nakabayashi H, Kuroda Y, et al. Adrenal myelolipoma: preoperative diagnosis by fine-needle aspiration cytology. Diagn Cytopathol 1989; 5:298.

26. Katz RL, Shirkhoda A. Diagnostic approach to incidental adrenal nodules in the cancer patient: results of a clinical, radiologic, and fine-needle aspiration study. Cancer 1985; 55:1995.

27. Pinto MM. Fine needle aspiration of myelolipoma of the adrenal gland. Report of a case with computed tomography. Acta Cytol 1985; 29:863.

28. Settakorn J, Sirivanichai C, Rangdaeng S, et al. Fine-needle aspiration cytology of adrenal myelolipoma: case report and review of the literature. Diagn Cytopathol 1999; 21:409-412.

29. Suen KC. Guides to clinical aspiration biopsy. In Kline T, editor. Retroperitoneum and intestine. New York: Igaku-Shoin; 1987. p.183.

30. Medeiros LJ, Weiss LM. New developments in the pathologic diagnosis of adrenal cortical neoplasms: a review. Am J Clin Pathol 1992; 97:73.

31. Chan JKC, Tsang WYW. Endocrine malignancies that may mimic benign lesions. Semin Diagn Pathol 1995; 12:45.

32. Wadih GE, Nance KV, Silverman JF. Fine-needle aspiration cytology of the adrenal gland: fifty biopsies in 48 patients. Arch Pathol Lab Med 1992; 116:841.

33. Nance KV, McLeod DL, Silverman JF. Fine-needle aspiration cytology of spindle cell neoplasms of the adrenal gland. Diagn Cytopathol 1992; 8:235.

34. Dusenberry D, Dekker A. Needle biopsy of the adrenal gland: a retrospective review of 54 cases. Diagn Cytopathol 1996; 14:126-134.

35. Shidham VB, Galindo LM. Pheochromocytoma. Cytologic findings on intraoperative scrape smears in five cases. Acta Cytol 1994; 43:207-213.

36. Deodhare S, Chalvardjian A, Lata A, et al. Adrenal pheochromocytoma mimicking small cell carcinoma on fine needle aspiration biopsy: a case report. Acta Cytol 1996; 40:1003-1006.

37. McCorkell SJ, Niles NL. Fine-needle aspiration of catecholamine-producing adrenal masses: a possibly fatal mistake. AJR 1985; 145:113.

38. Mitchell ML, Ryan FP, Jr, Shermer RW. Pulmonary adenocarcinoma metastatic to the adrenal gland mimicking normal adrenal cortical epithelium on fine needle aspiration. Acta Cytol 1985; 29:994.

39. Cavanna L, Civardi G, Vallisa D, et al. Primary adrenal non-Hodgkin's lymphoma associated with autoimmune hemolytic anemia: a case diagnosed by ultrasound-guided fine needle biopsy. Ann Ital Med Int 1999; 14:298-301.

40. McCutcheon J, Irvine A, Derias NW. Metastatic liposarcoma in the adrenal gland: report of two cases diagnosed by fine-needle aspiration. Diagn Cytopathol 1995; 13:330-332.

41. Hameed A, Coleman RL. Fine-needle aspiration cytology of primary granulosa cell tumor of the adrenal gland: a case report. Diagn Cytopathol 2000; 22:107-109.

42. Triche TJ, Askin FB. Neuroblastoma and the differential diagnosis of small-, round-, blue-cell tumors. Hum Pathol 1983; 14:569.

43. Triche TJ, Askin FB, Kissane JM. Neuroblastoma, Ewing's sarcoma, and the differential diagnosis of small-, round-, blue-cell tumors. In Finegold MJ, editor. Pathology of neoplasia in children and adolescents, vol 18. Philadelphia: WB Saunders; 1986. p.145.

44. Shimada H, Chatten J, Newton WA, Jr, et al. Histopathologic prognostic factors in neuroblastic tumors: definition of subtypes of ganglioneuroblastoma and age-linked classification of neuroblastomas. J Natl Cancer Inst 1984; 73:405.

45. Geisinger KR, Silverman JF, Wakely PE. Pediatric cytopathology. Chicago: American Society of Clinical Pathologists; 1994. pp.307-312.

46. Joshi VV, Silverman JF, Altshuler G, et al. Pathology of neuroblastic tumors: a report from the Pediatric Oncology Group I: systematization of primary pathologic features. Hum Pathol 1993; 24:493.

47. Silverman JF, Dabbs DJ, Ganick DJ, et al. Fine needle aspiration cytology of neuroblastoma, including peripheral neuroectodermal tumor, with immunocytochemical and ultrastructural confirmation. Acta Cytol 1988;32:367.

48. Ganick DJ, Silverman JH, Holbook CT, et al. Clinical utility of the fine needle aspiration in the diagnosis and management of neuroblastoma. Med Pediatr Oncol 1988; 16:101.

49. De Chadarevian JP, Vekemans M, Seemayer TA. Reciprocal translocation in small cell sarcomas. N Engl J Med 1984; 322:1702.

50. Maletz N, McMorrow LE, Greco A, Wolman S. Ewing's sarcoma: pathology tissue culture and cytogenetics. Cancer 1986; 58:252.

51. Whang-Peng J, Triche TJ, Knutsen T, et al. Chromosome translocation in peripheral neuroepithelioma. N Engl J Med 1984; 311:584.

52. Tsokos M, Linnoila RI, Chandra RS, et al. Neuron-specific enolase in the diagnosis of neuroblastoma and other small, round cell tumors of childhood. Hum Pathol 1984; 15:575.

53. Look AT, Hayes FA, Nitschke R, et al. Cellular DNA content as a predictor of response to chemotherapy in infants with unresectable neuroblastoma. N Engl J Med 1984; 15:575.

54. Shimada H, Seeger R, Joshi V, et al. Histopathology and N-myc gene in advanced neuroblastomas: a report from the Children's Cancer Study Group (CGSG). Pediatr Pathol 1988; 8:671.

55. Gurley AM, Silverman JF, Wiley JE, et al. The utility of ancillary studies in pediatric FNA cytology. Diagn Cytopathol 1992; 8:137.

56. Strausbach PH, Neill JSA, Benning TL, et al. Applications of electron microscopy in fine-needle aspiration cytology. In Smith WA, editor. Cytopathology annual. Baltimore: Williams and Wilkins. p.173.

57. Silverman JF, Joshi VV. Fine-needle aspiration biopsy of small round cell tumors of childhood: cytomorphologic features and the role of ancillary studies. Diagn Cytopathol 1994; 10:245.

58. Silverman JF, Berns LA, Holbrook CT, et al. Fine-needle aspiration of primitive neuroectodermal tumors (PNET). A report of three cases. Acta Cytol 1992; 36:541.

59. Joshi VV, Silverman JF. Pathology of neuroblastic tumors. Semin Diagn Pathol 1994; 11:107.

60. Akhtar M, Ali MA, Sabbah R, et al. Small round cell tumor with divergent differentiation: cytologic, histologic, and ultrastructural findings. Diagn Cytopathol 1994; 11:159.

61. Silverman JF, Berns LA, Holbrook CT, et al. Fine-needle aspiration of primitive neuroectodermal tumors (PNET): a report of three cases. Acta Cytol 1992; 36:541.

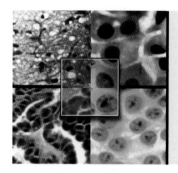

Lymph Nodes and Spleen

CHAPTER
24

Together, the lymph nodes and the spleen constitute much of the body's secondary lymphoreticular tissues. Accordingly, their various cellular components are actively involved in many infections and other antigen-presenting conditions such as sarcoidosis and autoimmune disorders. The majority of malignant lymphomas arise in or secondarily affect these organs, which may also often be infiltrated by the malignant cells of most forms of the leukemias. Their parenchyma may be variably replaced by benign histiocytic cells in storage diseases resulting from inborn errors of metabolism. Of course, they may be involved by metastases from almost any type of nonlymphoreticular cancer. All of these different pathologic conditions may enlarge lymph nodes and the spleen to the point that they are clinically apparent. Consequently, they comprise targets for fine-needle aspiration (FNA) biopsies.

 ## LYMPH NODES

In both adults and children, lymphadenopathy can be the result of a myriad of causes and represents a common clinical problem, the consequences of which range from negligible to very serious and fatal. In conjunction with a good clinical history and physical examination, FNA biopsy of enlarged nodes often supplies sufficient information to allow the clinician to triage the patient and decide among careful observation, treatment with antibiotics, the initiation of anticancer therapy, and staging of malignant neoplasms, or to pursue a lymph node biopsy with histologic examination.[1-11] Thus, FNA biopsy cytomorphology, at times with ancillary diagnostic procedures, advances clinical management in a rapid, cost-effective, and safe manner.

One important clinical question is whether the lymphadenopathy is localized or generalized. In general, a localized process favors a benign diagnosis, whereas malignancy, especially the non-Hodgkin's lymphomas, is more likely to present with generalized lymph node enlargement.[1] The palpatory quality of the node provides data that may be diagnostically useful. For example, a localized rapidly enlarging node with tender, erythematous, and swollen surrounding tissues favors a reactive, probably infectious, process (Table 24-1).

A benign nonspecific or reactive hyperplasia of lymphoid tissue is one of the most common causes of lymphadenopathy. Infectious etiologic factors that may be recognized include pyogenic bacteria, mycobacteria,[11-17] fungi,[11,17] cat-scratch disease,[18,19] toxoplasmosis,[20-24] and infectious mononucleosis.[25,26] Other nonneoplastic conditions include sarcoidosis,[27] Rosai-Dorfman disease,[28-30] and Kikuchi's disease.[31] Metastatic neoplasms, especially carcinomas and melanomas, are another common source of enlarged lymph nodes.[1-3,5,11,32,33] Finally, primary malignant lymphomas represent an additional important cause of lymphadenopathy. It is this last group that represents the most controversial aspect of FNA biopsy diagnosis.[34-39] Most investigators agree that metastatic malignancies and specific infections can be identified in FNA biopsies in the majority of cases. It is the distinction between reactive hyperplasias and the malignant lymphomas that presents the greatest challenge. It is this situation in which the ancillary diagnostic tests are most useful.

Sample Collection

Ideally, a lymph node FNA biopsy should be assessed on site to ensure adequate cellularity and to consider the possibility of a lymphoid proliferation. If an aspirate is suspicious for lymphoma, an additional sample is drawn for flow cytometry and put in a buffered saline or cell culture solution. Additional material should also be obtained to make a cell block in case immunostaining is required for nonhematopoietic antigens. Similarly, if an infection is suspected, additional material may be obtained for culture.

General Cytomorphologic Attributes

As with FNA biopsies of all body sites, a systematic assessment of the specimen is essential to achieve the correct diagnosis. This includes evaluation of the overall smear cellularity, the pattern of arrangement of cells, the predominant cell type, and the nature of any material in the smear background.

Primary lymphoid proliferations, both benign and malignant, produce moderate to highly cellular smears with marked dispersal of cells (Figure 24-1). An exception to this dispersed, dissociative picture is the presence of lympho-histiocytic aggregates, which are derived from germinal centers and consist of irregular syncytial clusters of variably sized lymphocytes, histiocytes, and dendritic reticulum cells (Figure 24-2).[1,11,40] Most metastatic neoplasms, however, include tissue fragments as evidence of true intercellular cohesion in the smears; one common exception is melanoma (Figures 24-3 and 24-4). A consistent background component of aspirates of both benign and malignant lymphoid proliferations is the lymphoglandular body, which represents pale, irregular fragments of lymphoid cytoplasm that are sheared away from the cell during the aspiration procedure (Figure 24-5).[1] Other background elements may include mucus, foreign material, and necrotic debris. Determining the predominant cell type is useful in distinguishing benign from malignant lymphoid lesions; in most benign lymphoid abnormalities, small mature-appearing lymphocytes dominate.

Ancillary Techniques

Flow Cytometry

Flow cytometric analysis is a valuable diagnostic aid when assessing hematologic malignancies.[41] The use of flow cytometry for cell surface phenotyping complements cytomorphologic assessment when evaluating the involvement of lymph nodes for non-Hodgkin's lymphoma, particularly in cases of nonlarge cell types. Flow cytometry is a useful adjunct in the diagnosis of B-cell non-Hodgkin's lymphomas.[42] It may also be used to verify T-cell populations with aberrant antigen expression, as seen in many T-cell neoplasms, but is essentially useless in Hodgkin's disease.[43] This use is especially true with the Revised European and

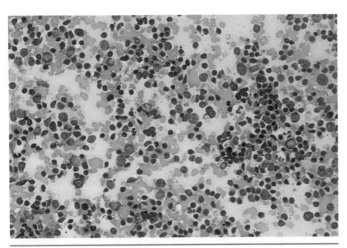

Figure 24-1 Follicular hyperplasia. Most hyperplastic lymph nodes yield highly cellular samples with a dissociative pattern—that is, the vast majority of the lymphoid cells are scattered or isolated as single cells. Regardless of the size of the lymphocytes, they typically possess a single round nucleus and a very high nuclear to cytoplasmic (N:C) ratio. Note the prominent spectrum of nuclear sizes with a predominance of small mature-appearing lymphoid cells. (Diff-Quik [DQ])

TABLE 24-1	
Correlates of Clinical Examination of Node	
Qualities	**Disease**
Firm, rubbery, uniform, nontender	Lymphoma
Firm, rubbery, uniform, tender	Acute leukemia
Firm, tender, asymmetric, matted	Suppurative lymphadenitis
Firm to soft, matted, nontender	Chronic infection
Rock hard, nontender	Metastatic carcinoma
Soft, nontender	Necrotic or keratinized metastatic carcinoma

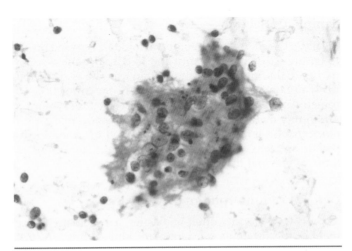

Figure 24-2 Follicular hyperplasia. Germinal centers yield loosely cohesive aggregates of lymphocytes and histiocytic cells in smears. Cell borders are indistinct and thus the lymphohistiocytic aggregates have a syncytial appearance. Much of the periphery of the aggregate appears to be represented by cytoplasm. (Papanicolaou [Pap])

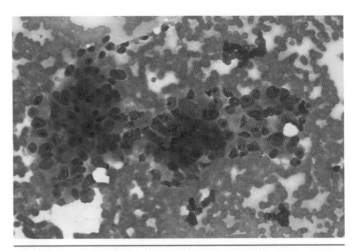

Figure 24-3 Metastatic prostatic adenocarcinoma. This lymph node aspirate was dominated by cohesive flat to three-dimensional aggregates of malignant epithelial cells. The cohesive nature of these neoplastic elements is characteristic of most metastases recognized in nodal aspirates. In this example, note the distinct acinar arrangement of the cells and the prominent nucleoli. (DQ)

American Lymphoma classification (Table 24-2).[44-46] A growing number of practitioners combine flow cytometry for immunophenotyping with cytomorphology in FNA biopsy of nodes.[44-54] Other labs use immunocytochemistry to provide similar data.[34,37-39]

Molecular Techniques

Material obtained by FNA biopsy can be used in assays for gene rearrangements using DNA or RNA probes. Southern blot analysis, dot blot, polymerase chain reaction, and *in situ* hybridization can be used.[55-58] Clonal rearrangements of genes for heavy and light immunoglobulin chains and T-cell receptors are supportive of the diagnosis of non-Hodgkin's lymphomas, as are oncogene rearrangements such as the *bcl-2* gene in follicular lymphomas.[59] A clonal population can be demonstrated even though neoplastic lymphoid cells are mixed with reactive cells. Nucleic acid from microorganisms such as herpes simplex, cytomegalovirus (CMV), and *Pneumocystis carinii* can be identified in aspirated material by *in situ* hybridization.

Cytogenetics

Specific chromosomal translocations can be sought in aspirated material to confirm a diagnosis of Burkitt's lymphoma, small cleaved cell lymphoma, or anaplastic large cell lymphoma, or to type leukemias.[60]

General Approach for Immunophenotyping Lymph Nodes

Currently, no standard panel exists for analyzing lymphoid neoplasms by flow cytometry. Depending on one's clinical and morphologic suspicions, the panel may include markers for B-cells (surface immunoglobulin [SIg], CD19, CD20, CD79a), T-cells (CD3, CD4, CD8), and nonlymphoid cells (CD14, CD45). The complete lymphoid panel consists of CD19 vs. CD5, CD10 vs. CD23, CD20 vs. Kappa, CD20 vs. Lambda, CD2 vs. HLA-DR, CD7 vs. CD3, and CD4 vs. CD8. In many cases a CD45 vs. CD14 is included, as is using 7-actinomycin D to gate out dead and dying cells in all tubes.[61] Assessing the immunologic status of cells can include the presence or absence of monoclonality, antigen or light scatter aberrancy, population excesses, and reactive changes.[62-67] The CD19 vs. CD5 study is a good example. It is used to gauge the number of normal B-cells and T-cells, because CD19 is a pan-B marker and CD5 is associated with T-cells. In certain non-Hodgkin's lymphomas, dual expression of CD19 and CD5 is evident. Determining the intensity of antigen expression on the surface is helpful in subclassifying the type of lymphoma. Thus, the antigen aberrancy helps confirm the presence of a lymphoma and subclassify it.

FNA biopsies produce a variable yield of cells. As a general rule, at least 100,000 cells are needed for flow cytometry. This number permits a limited panel of antibodies such as CD5 vs. CD19, CD20 vs. Kappa, and CD20 vs. Lambda. This provides both B-cell and T-cell sums. Usually this panel can detect the presence of a B-cell non-Hodgkin's lymphoma, but it does not further classify the lymphoma.

Normal Immunophenotype

Normal lymph nodes contain areas where circulating T-cells predominate but during an immune response these can become sites of B-cell proliferation. In addition to the predominant lymphoid cells, lymph nodes also contain histiocytes and connective tissue elements, which are typically not tested. However, these cells, especially the histiocytes, may produce false-positive results through nonspecific binding of the monoclonal antibodies. In a resting node, T-cells predominate (60% T-cells and 40% B-cells); this T-cell compartment is made up of two major types of cells.

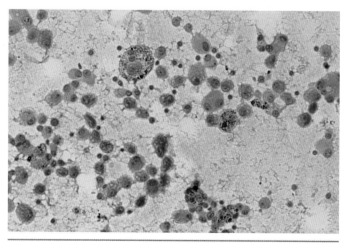

Figure 24-4 **Metastatic melanoma.** In lymph node aspirates, melanoma classically presents with a dissociative pattern of individual neoplastic cells. In this particular example, they are scattered among the smaller lymphocytes. Melanoma cells are characterized by one or more round and often eccentric nuclei, many of which possess prominent nucleoli. Melanin pigment is present within the cytoplasm of some of the neoplastic elements. (Pap)

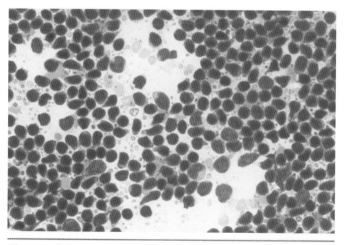

Figure 24-5 **Follicular hyperplasia.** Scattered among the associated benign lymphocytes are lymphoglandular bodies. These represent fragments of lymphoid cell cytoplasm that are torn away from the cell during the preparation of the aspiration smears. They vary in size but have the same staining qualities as the cytoplasm persisting about the nuclei. Note the range in nuclear diameters with a predominance of small lymphocytes. (DQ)

TABLE 24-2

Classification Systems of Non-Hodgkin's Lymphomas

REAL Classification	Kiel Classification	Working Formulation
B-cell neoplasms		
Low-grade non-Hodgkin's lymphoma		
Chronic lymphocytic	Chronic lymphocytic	A. Small lymphocytic consistent with chronic lymphocytic lymphoma
Prolymphocytic	Prolymphocytic	
Hairy cell leukemia	Hairy cell leukemia	
Plasmacytoid B-cell	Lymphoplasmacytoid	A. Small lymphocytic, plasmacytoid
Lymphoplasmacytic lymphoma	Lymphoplasmacytic	
Plasmacytoma/myeloma	Plasmacytic	
Mantle cell lymphoma	Centrocytic	
Monocytoid and marginal zone	Nodal marginal zone lymphomas	
Extranodal marginal zone B-cell Lymphomas (MALT lymphoma)		
Follicular, grade I	Follicular	B. Follicular, predominately small cleaved cell
Follicular, grade II	Follicular	C. Follicular, mixed small cell cleaved and large cell
Diffuse	Diffuse	E. Diffuse and small leaved cell
		F. Diffuse mixed small and large cell
High-grade non-Hodgkin's lymphomas		
Follicular, grade III	Follicular	D. Follicular large cell
Diffuse large B-cell lymphoma	Diffuse	G. Diffuse, large cell
Diffuse large B-cell lymphoma	Immunoblastic	H. Large cell immunoblastic
Primary mediastinal B-cell lymphoma		
Mantle cell lymphoma, blastoid variant	Centocytoid	
Burkitt's lymphoma	Burkitt's lymphoma	J. Small noncleaved Burkitt's and non-Burkitt's
Precursor B-cell lymphoma/leukemia	Lymphoblastic	L. Lymphoblastic
T-cell neoplasms		
Low-grade non-Hodgkin's lymphomas		
Chronic lymphocytic	Chronic lymphocytic	A. Small lymphocytic consistent with chronic lymphocytic lymphoma
Large granular lymphocytic leukemia		
Prolymphocytic leukemia	Prolymphocytic leukemia	
Mycosis fungoides/Sézary syndrome	Small cell cerebriform	
PTCL, lymphoepithelial type	Lymphoepithelioid (Lennert's) lymphoma	
Angioimmunoblastic T-cell lymphoma	Angioimmunoblastic	
PTCL, unspecified	T-zone lymphoma	
PTCL, medium-size cell	Pleomorphic, small cell	A. Small lymphocytic consistent with chronic lymphocytic lymphoma
Intestinal T-cell lymphoma		
Adult T-cell lymphoma/ leukemia		
High-grade non-Hodgkin's lymphomas		
PTCL, mixed medium and large cell	Pleomorphic, medium-sized and large cell	
PTCL, large cell	T-cell immunoblastic	
Anaplastic large cell lymphoma, T and null cell type	T-cell large cell anaplastic (Ki-1+)	
Precursor T-cell lymphoma, T-cell lymphoblastic lymphoma/leukemia	T-cell lymphoblastic	L. Lymphoblastic

MALT, Mucosa-associated lymphoid tissue; *PTCL,* peripheral T-cell lymphoma.

Helper cells are CD4-positive and express a full complement of other T-cell antigens. Suppressor T-cells are characterized by the presence of CD8 and also express a full complement of other T-cell antigens. These other antigens include CD2, CD3, CD5, and CD7. Normal T-cells do not coexpress CD4 and CD8. In a normal node, the number of CD4-positive cells is usually twice the number of CD8-positive cells. T-cell lymphomas are typically subset-restricted and express either CD4 or CD8. In reactive processes one may observe a predominance of either suppressor or helper T-cells, but as a general rule the CD4/CD8 ratios are higher in lymph nodes than in peripheral blood. Immature thymic phenotypes characterized by CD1, and CD4 and CD8 coexpression are rarely seen.

The ratio of T-cells to B-cells in a normal node is highly variable, but it should be close to one. B-cells are typically characterized by the presence of CD19, CD20, CD79a, and kappa or lambda SIg. B-cell differentiation may be classified by their relation to the germinal center. The prefollicular cells are characterized by either the lack of SIg or the presence of immunoglobulins M or D (IgM or IgD) on the cell surface. The follicular zone contains cells characterized by the presence of CD10 and SIg. The mantle zone contains memory B lymphocytes that manifest coexpression of CD5. The marginal zone contains lymphocytes that express CD11c. In a normal node, there are many diverse populations of B-cells, and no one clone is expressed more than any other clone. As a result of this diversity, the percentage of kappa-bearing B-cells is roughly 1.5 times the number of lambda-bearing B-cells but varies between 0.8 and 2.3. This ratio is an important one because it is the primary marker for monoclonality of B-cells.

Neoplastic Immunophenotypes

Low-grade B-cell lymphomas have B-cell antigens (CD19, CD20, CD79a), light chain restriction, and SIg expression.[68,69] Follicular center cell lymphomas often demonstrate CD10 and prominent SIg, but lack CD5.[70] Small lymphocytic lymphomas (SLLs) characteristically possess CD5 and weak SIg and are CD10-negative.[68,69,71] Marginal zone B-cell lymphomas are usually CD11C-positive and negative for CD5 and CD10.[72] Mantle cell lymphomas (MCLs) express CD5 and Leu 8 with restricted SIg.[73] They are also negative for CD23, which is usually positive in SLL.

High-grade lymphomas such as large cell or immunoblastic types have a mature B-cell phenotype (CD79a) but may not express SIg, CD19, or CD20.[69] Burkitt's lymphomas have a similar mature B-cell typing and often show cytoplasmic immunoglobulin (CIg) or SIg, usually IgM. Multiple myeloma and plasmacytomas have strong CIg but lack CD45 and B-cell surface antigens other than CD79a.

Peripheral T-cell lymphomas (PTCLs) are a heterogeneous group but express one or more pan–T-cell markers (CD2 and CD3) and most often have abnormal predominances of CD4 helper cells.[66,74,75] In others, CD8 cells may be overexpressed, CD4 and CD8 may be coexpressed, an immature T-cell antigen (e.g., CD1) may be expressed, and CD25 or CD38 activation antigens may be demonstrated.

Lymphoblastic lymphomas usually have an immature (thymic) T-cell phenotype with CD1 and terminal deoxynucleotidyl transferase, as well as CD4 and CD8 coexpression.[76,77] To distinguish these lymphomas in the mediastinum from thymomas, which may have similar lymphoid markers, correlation with cytomorphologic, demographic, and/or molecular diagnostic features is required.

Specific Entities

Nonspecific Reactive Lymphoid Hyperplasia

In many instances, the underlying cause of reactive lymphoid hyperplasia is never determined. Many antigens, including a number of viruses, may induce benign proliferative responses among various components of the lymphoid tissue within lymph nodes. Clinically, the most common picture is that of a solitary lymph node up to 3 to 4 cm in the head and neck region. The most common histologic pattern is that of follicular hyperplasia, in which well-delineated germinal centers, composed of a heterogeneous population of lymphocytes and tingible-body macrophages, are prominent. Less often, interfollicular expansion by plasmacytoid cells, immunoblasts, and histiocytes is the cause of the nodal enlargement. FNA biopsy in general does not affect the histologic interpretation of subsequently excised nodes.[78]

The crucial cytomorphologic feature of reactive hyperplasia is the recognition of a heterogeneous population of lymphoid cells.[40] A mixture of small lymphocytes and large lymphoid cells including immunoblasts is present with a complete spectrum of intermediate morphologic (stages of maturation) forms (Figure 24-6; see Figures 24-1 and 24-5). However, the small mature-appearing lymphocyte predominates numerically. Tingible-body macrophages with intracytoplasmic apoptotic debris, although characteristic, are not pathognomonic of a hyperplastic process; they may be seen in high-grade lymphomas such as Burkitt's lymphoma and other malignancies with a brisk proliferation rate (Figure 24-7). However, large numbers of tingible-body macrophages in the presence of a full spectrum of lymphoid cells with small lymphocytes predominating leads to a benign diagnosis.[6,11,52] Lymphohistiocytic aggregates of dendritic reticulum cells and large and small cleaved and noncleaved cells have their origin in germinal centers (Figures 24-8 and 24-9; see Figure 24-2). Capillaries may be prominent in smears (Figure 24-10).

In air-dried Romanowsky-stained smears, artifacts resulting from crush and slow air-drying may make it difficult to distinguish small mature lymphocytes from lymphoblasts and small cleaved cells. Thus, the smears should be examined for better-preserved and better-stained areas. Romanowsky-stained samples do yield excellent cytomorphology of lymphoid cells. Alcohol-fixed Pap-stained smears clearly show the lymphocyte cell membrane and highlight membrane or chromatin irregularities (Box 24-1).

Specific causes of lymphadenopathy should be carefully excluded by searching for markers such as caseous material, suggesting tuberculosis. The differential diagnosis of the polymorphic cellular smear includes Hodgkin's disease, SLL, and lymph nodes only partially involved by other neoplasms, including the non-Hodgkin's lymphomas. Reed-Sternberg (R-S) cells and eosinophils should be looked for specifically, especially along the edges of the smear.

Reactive hyperplasias yield variable flow cytometric results. A monoclonal population is absent, but subclones that greatly skew the kappa to lambda ratio may be present. A mixture of T- and B-cells is present, with roughly 50% of

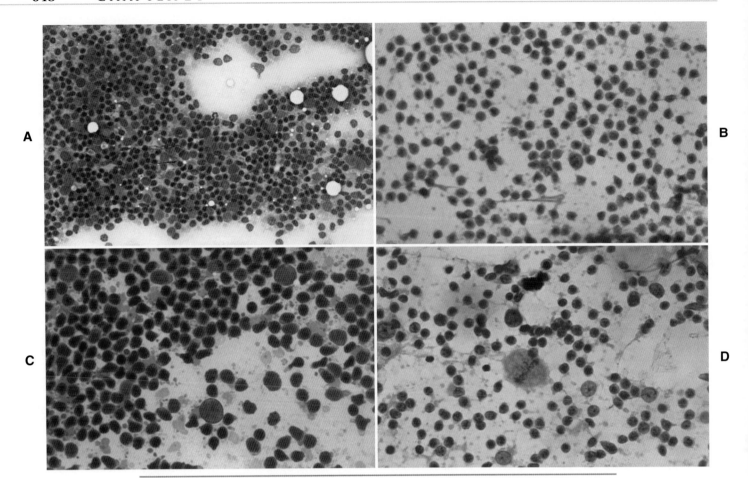

Figure 24-6 **Follicular hyperplasia. A,** In addition to high cellularity and a dissociative pattern of individual lymphocytes, a marked spectrum of lymphoid cell sizes and appearances is present. The predominant cell is the small mature lymphocyte that is characterized by a single round nucleus with dark, dense chromatin, inconspicuous nucleoli, and extremely high N:C ratios. The largest lymphoid cells have much more finely reticulated chromatin, small but distinct nucleoli, and at times, visible and faintly to darkly basophilic cytoplasm. Importantly, note the presence of intermediate or transitional lymphoid forms between the smallest and the largest cells. (DQ) **B,** With alcohol fixation, the marked polymorphism present in air-dried smears is somewhat more subtle. Still, a range in cellular sizes including large lymphoid cells with immature chromatin is recognizable. In addition, it is apparent that small, mature lymphocytes predominate numerically. Note the absence of intercellular cohesion and the presence of scattered lymphoglandular bodies. (Pap) **C,** The largest lymphoid cells have finely reticulated, uniformly dispersed chromatin granules and one or more small but obvious nucleoli. In addition, a visible rim of basophilic cytoplasm is evident. Some of the cells possess a few small vacuoles in their cytoplasm. The chromatin is much more condensed and smooth in appearance in the small lymphocytes. Intermediate forms are also evident. (DQ) **D,** With the Pap stain, the chromatin in the largest lymphoid cells is finely granular and often fairly pale stained. Minute nucleoli are evident, as is a thin rim of cyanophilic cytoplasm. The dark staining quality of the chromatin in the small lymphocytes is much more readily apparent. Note the dissociative pattern and the presence of a mitotic figure. Such mitotic figures may be seen in aspirates of benign lymphoid hyperplasia. (Pap)

each type of cell. Within the T-cell compartment, the number of helper CD4 cells is increased. A mixture of small and large cells can be seen by light scatter properties. All cells have a normal mature immunophenotype, and no antigen aberrancy is present, except in florid follicular hyperplasias, where the larger cells have increased CD20 expression and CD10 may not be present (Box 24-2).

Suppurative Lymphadenitis

Pyogenic infection of lymph nodes with secondary enlargement is seen more often in children than adults. Commonly, lymph nodes in the head and neck region are involved, presumably draining a regional bacterial infec-tion. The nodes may be painful, tender, and associated with fever; the overlying skin may also appear inflamed (see Table 24-1).

Aspiration smears are usually highly cellular and dominated by large numbers of intact and degenerated neutrophils (Figure 24-11).[11] Lymphocytes may also show well developed degenerative changes. Bacteria may be visualized, especially with the Romanowsky stains. Lupus lymphadenitis may yield a suppurative picture in smears requiring careful examination for systemic lupus erythematosus (SLE) cells, which are more easily seen with Romanowsky stains.[79] Rarely, Hodgkin's disease may present in aspirates as an acute inflammatory process[80] (Box 24-3).

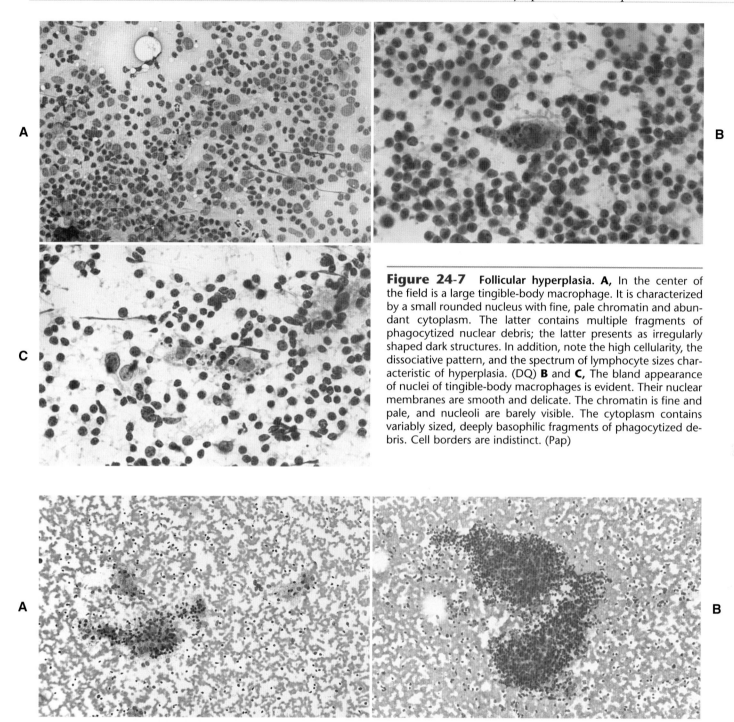

Figure 24-7 Follicular hyperplasia. **A,** In the center of the field is a large tingible-body macrophage. It is characterized by a small rounded nucleus with fine, pale chromatin and abundant cytoplasm. The latter contains multiple fragments of phagocytized nuclear debris; the latter presents as irregularly shaped dark structures. In addition, note the high cellularity, the dissociative pattern, and the spectrum of lymphocyte sizes characteristic of hyperplasia. (DQ) **B** and **C,** The bland appearance of nuclei of tingible-body macrophages is evident. Their nuclear membranes are smooth and delicate. The chromatin is fine and pale, and nucleoli are barely visible. The cytoplasm contains variably sized, deeply basophilic fragments of phagocytized debris. Cell borders are indistinct. (Pap)

Figure 24-8 Follicular hyperplasia. **A** and **B,** Lymphohistiocytic aggregates are comprised of irregularly shaped and sized clusters of lymphocytes and histiocytes. The relative proportion of the two cell types varies from aggregate to aggregate. As seen in **A,** when lymphocytes are relatively sparse, the abundant pale histiocytic cytoplasm stands out. By contrast, as witnessed in **B,** the aggregates appear relatively dark when lymphocytes are numerous. (DQ)

Flow cytometric evaluation is not needed; if performed, the findings are nonspecific. When using T- and B-cell antigens alone, many of the cells fail to stain. However, these cells are CD45-positive, indicating they are hematopoietic in origin. Myeloid antigens such as CD13 can demonstrate the presence of neutrophils. Staining with 7-actinomycin D often reveals numerous dead cells.[61] Necrosis also produces a substantial degree of nonspecific binding by the monoclonal antibodies.

Granulomatous Lymphadenitis

Granulomatous lymphadenitis is a form of chronic inflammation with numerous etiologic factors, which include sarcoidosis, foreign body reactions, and infections. Classically, infectious agents include mycobacteria and fungi. Sarcoid is a diagnosis of exclusion, whereas FNA biopsy may reveal the etiologic agent in many other diseases.[27]

In developed countries, mycobacterial infections had become an uncommon clinical event. Today, however, the ac-

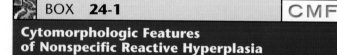

Figure 24-9   Follicular hyperplasia. A, A syncytial appearance is evident in the lympho-histiocytic aggregates as the cytoplasm of neighboring histiocytes and lymphocytes blends with each other. The lymphoid cells have relatively small and variably shaped nuclei with more condensed chromatin. Much more finely reticulated and even chromatin is evident in the nuclei of the histiocytic elements. (DQ) **B,** The dark chromatin in the lymphocytes contrasts sharply with the more abundant pale chromatin of the histiocytic nuclei. The two cell types appear to be randomly scattered within these aggregates. (Pap)

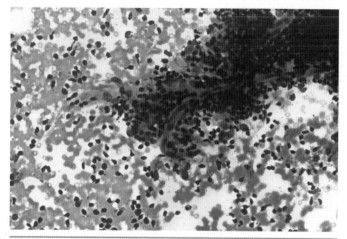

Figure 24-10   Follicular hyperplasia. Delicate branched capillaries are encased by lymphocytes. Although vascular fragments may be seen in aspirates of malignant lymphomas, especially those of the T-cell type, they are often more common in benign nodal aspirates. (DQ)

quired immune deficiency syndrome (AIDS) epidemic has led to a resurgence. Furthermore, tuberculosis remains a problem in developing nations.[81,168] Before AIDS, clinical infections by atypical mycobacteria were uncommon. Atypical mycobacteria have become a major cause of infections in immunosuppressed people, especially those with AIDS. The classic histopathologic change in tuberculosis consists of granulomatous inflammation associated with caseous necrosis, but in markedly immunocompromised patients, a well-developed granulomatous response may not occur. Rather, a proportion of patients with AIDS with tuberculosis may have nodal aspiration smears composed largely of neutrophils.

The typical feature of tuberculous lymphadenitis is epithelioid cell granulomas associated with necrosis (Figure 24-12). Epithelioid cells are modified histiocytes with a moderate amount of pale cytoplasm[11,12,14] and a solitary nu-

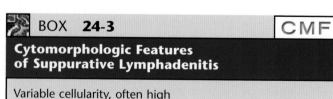

BOX   **24-1**   CMF

Cytomorphologic Features of Nonspecific Reactive Hyperplasia

Generally high cellularity
Mixture of dispersed lymphoid cells with a full spectrum of sizes and differentiation, in which small lymphocytes predominate
Plasma cells, plasmacytoid cells, and immunoblasts may be evident
Lymphohistiocytic aggregates
Tingible-body macrophages

BOX   **24-2**

Immunophenotype of Reactive Hyperplasia

Variable findings due to mixture of B- and T-cells
CD10 may be positive
Both kappa- and lambda-positive cells
Reactive T-cells (CD3 and CD4 predominate)

BOX   **24-3**   CMF

Cytomorphologic Features of Suppurative Lymphadenitis

Variable cellularity, often high
Predominant cell is neutrophil, both intact and degenerated
Neutrophils are both dispersed and loosely aggregated
Lymphocytes and macrophages, often degenerated
Bacteria may be seen, both within phagocytes and extracellularly

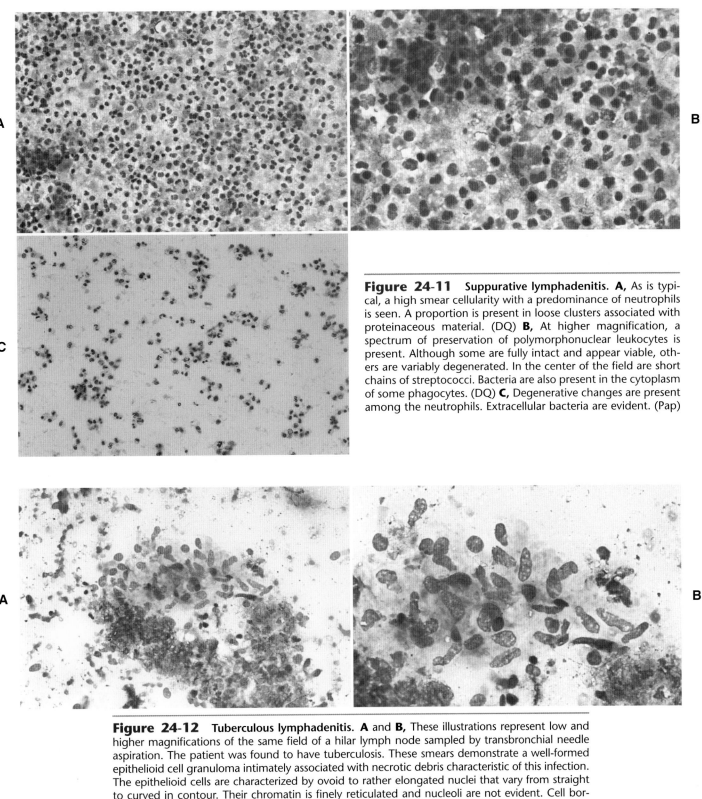

Figure 24-11 **Suppurative lymphadenitis. A,** As is typical, a high smear cellularity with a predominance of neutrophils is seen. A proportion is present in loose clusters associated with proteinaceous material. (DQ) **B,** At higher magnification, a spectrum of preservation of polymorphonuclear leukocytes is present. Although some are fully intact and appear viable, others are variably degenerated. In the center of the field are short chains of streptococci. Bacteria are also present in the cytoplasm of some phagocytes. (DQ) **C,** Degenerative changes are present among the neutrophils. Extracellular bacteria are evident. (Pap)

Figure 24-12 **Tuberculous lymphadenitis. A** and **B,** These illustrations represent low and higher magnifications of the same field of a hilar lymph node sampled by transbronchial needle aspiration. The patient was found to have tuberculosis. These smears demonstrate a well-formed epithelioid cell granuloma intimately associated with necrotic debris characteristic of this infection. The epithelioid cells are characterized by ovoid to rather elongated nuclei that vary from straight to curved in contour. Their chromatin is finely reticulated and nucleoli are not evident. Cell borders are indistinct because the cytoplasm in these cells blends with each other, creating a classic syncytial appearance. Note the relatively scant cellularity and clean smear background. (DQ)

cleus with a characteristic elongated, bent, or centrally indented shape (Figure 24-13). Nuclear membranes are delicate. Chromatin is very finely granular and pale stained; nucleoli are small and generally inconspicuous (Figure 24-14). Syncytial arrangement of these cells results in gran-

ulomas, which may be present in a background of necrotic, relatively agranular, (fluffy) debris. Multinucleated giant cells are present in variable numbers. Their nuclei are often arranged peripherally in a horseshoe rimming of the cytoplasm. Pandit and colleagues have described the *eosinophilic structure* as a characteristic component of smears from nodes involved by tuberculous lymphadenitis.[12] With the hematoxylin and eosin stain, these consist of sharply delineated masses of eosinophilic material containing no recognizable cells and surrounded by a clear zone or halo (Figure 24-15). They proposed that these represented further degeneration within granulomas.[12] However, they are not specific for tuberculosis.[13] Ellison and colleagues examined the sensitivity of FNA to diagnose mycobacterial lymphadenitis in the United States.[82] Using the presence of acid-fast bacilli or a positive culture as diagnostic, sensitivity was 46%. The most sensitive procedure appears to be the application of the polymerase chain reaction (PCR) to aspirated cellular material.[81,83] However, false-positive results may occur. PCR may also be used to detect drug resistance in tuberculous aspirates.[81]

Although sarcoidosis is a diagnosis of exclusion, FNA biopsies demonstrating prominent granulomatous inflammation without necrosis in the proper clinical setting assists in confirming the presence of sarcoidal inflammation in enlarged lymph nodes.[27] For example, transbronchial needle aspirates can diagnose sarcoidosis in hilar nodes. Reflecting the diffuse nature of the granulomatous process within the sampled node, the overall smear cellularity tends to be low because relatively few lymphocytes are present. The smears may be dominated by cohesive aggregates of epithelioid histiocytes, which may also occur as dispersed cells (Figure 24-16). Multinucleated inflammatory giant cells and mostly small lymphocytes may also be present. Necrotic debris should not be evident in the smear background. Negative acid-fast and methenamine silver-stained direct smears and cell blocks are considered mandatory by some in making the diagnosis. Aspirated material should be culture-negative (Box 24-4).

Such changes are often not present in patients who are immunosuppressed. Rather, smears may be dominated by dispersed macrophages with abundant pale cytoplasm, which in the Romanowsky stains may have a reticulated

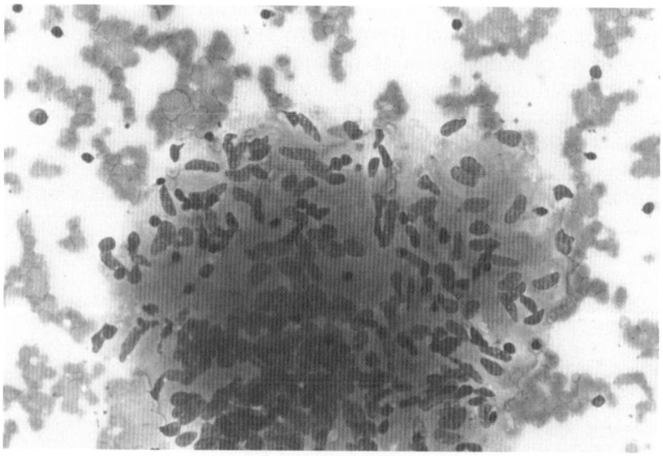

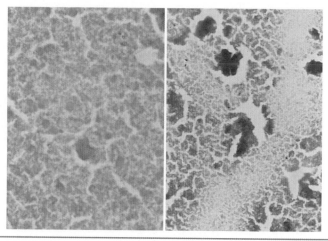

Figure 24-15 **Tuberculous lymphadenitis.** Eosinophilic structures probably represent largely degenerated granulomas in which distinct cellular detail is lost. They stand out from the surrounding amorphous necrotic debris on account of the peripheral clear zone. (Pap [left] and DQ [right])

Figure 24-13 **Granulomatous lymphadenitis.** This patient was thought to have sarcoid. The curved or bent appearance of the nuclei in many of the epithelioid cells is easily recognized, as is the lack of distinct cell borders. The frayed edges of the granuloma are also characteristic. (DQ)

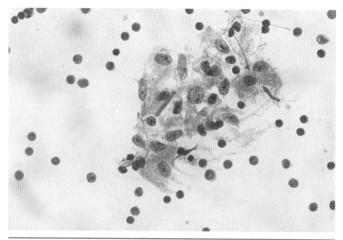

Figure 24-14 **Tuberculous lymphadenitis.** The nuclei of the epithelioid cells have extremely delicate smooth membranes, finely granular and pale chromatin with minute or inconspicuous nucleoli. Even within this loosely cohesive granuloma, the cell borders of the epithelioid cells remain indistinct. (Pap)

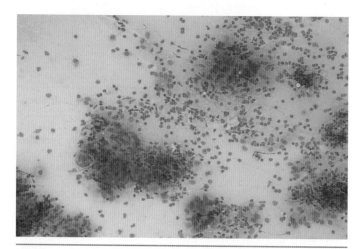

Figure 24-16 **Sarcoid lymphadenitis.** Tightly cohesive granulomas are composed of mononucleated epithelioid cells and rare multinucleated inflammatory giant cells. They are situated within a background of sparse lymphocytes. (DQ)

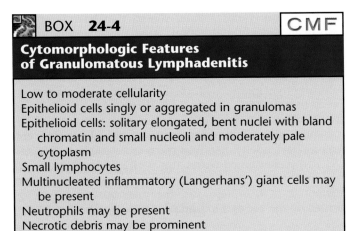

BOX 24-4 | CMF

Cytomorphologic Features of Granulomatous Lymphadenitis

Low to moderate cellularity
Epithelioid cells singly or aggregated in granulomas
Epithelioid cells: solitary elongated, bent nuclei with bland chromatin and small nucleoli and moderately pale cytoplasm
Small lymphocytes
Multinucleated inflammatory (Langerhans') giant cells may be present
Neutrophils may be present
Necrotic debris may be prominent

cross-hatched appearance due to numerous rodlike, nonstaining phagocytized bacilli (Figure 24-17).[11,15,16] These negative images of unstained bacilli may also be recognized extracellularly (Figure 24-18).[11,15,16] An acid-fast stain directly on the aspirated material can confirm their presence (Figure 24-19). Usually, these are atypical mycobacteria, but one study did not find reduced granulomatous inflammation in people with human immunodeficiency virus (HIV) with tuberculosis.[84] Aspirated material should be submitted for culture and sensitivity studies.

Vaccination with bacillus Calmette-Guérin (BCG) often results in lymphadenopathy, especially of regional draining lymph nodes. Although the cytomorphology overlaps with tuberculosis, neutrophils and necrotic debris occur much more often with BCG disease, whereas well-formed granulomas are seen less often (Figure 24-20).[85]

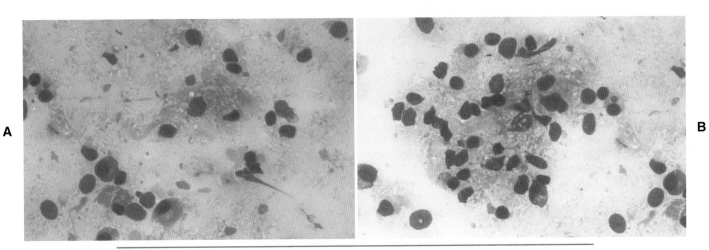

Figure 24-17 Acquired immune deficiency syndrome (AIDS)–associated mycobacterial lymphadenitis. **A,** A solitary large histiocyte is characterized by abundant pale gray cytoplasm punctuated by phagocytized bacilli. The latter present as nonstained or clear, minute, rod-shaped structures. Only a few lymphocytes and plasmacytoid elements are also present. (DQ) **B,** A loose cluster of similar modified histiocytes show numerous "negative images" of phagocytized mycobacteria in their cytoplasm. (DQ)

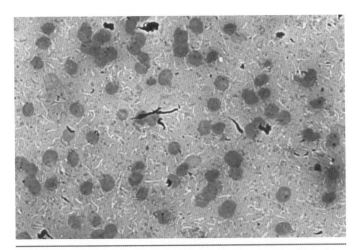

Figure 24-18 AIDS-associated mycobacterial lymphadenitis. Extracellular organisms occur in the background serum as clear rod-shaped structures. Note the complete absence of any inflammatory or immune-effector cells. (DQ)

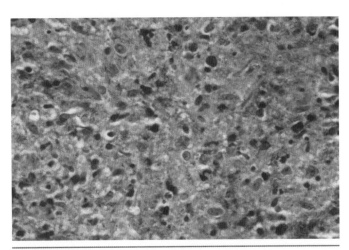

Figure 24-19 AIDS-associated mycobacterial lymphadenitis. Numerous extracellular organisms are highlighted by this acid-fast stain.

Toxoplasmosis

Toxoplasmosis, caused by infection with the protozoan *Toxoplasma gondii,* is often an asymptomatic process, but it may produce a wide spectrum of disease depending on several factors, most importantly, the route of transmission and the patient's immune status. The most common clinical manifestation in immunocompetent people with acute infection is lymphadenopathy. The cervical nodes, especially those posteriorly, are most often affected.

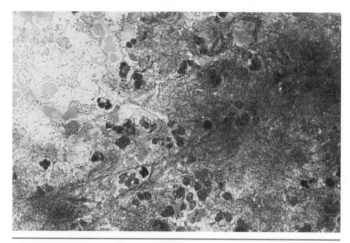

Figure 24-20 Bacillus Calmette-Guérin (BCG)–associated lymphadenitis. Numerous negative images (extracellular mycobacteria) are evident within the mixture of serum and fibrin. The predominate inflammatory cell is the neutrophil. (DQ)

FNA biopsy yields cellular smears that have lymphoid cells in all stages of maturation, tingible-body macrophages, lymphohistiocytic aggregates, single histiocytes, and the characteristic small clusters of histiocytic cells (Figure 24-21). The cytology reflects the typical histopathology of follicular hyperplasia, with small epithelioid cell clusters apposed to the germinal centers.[20-24] However, the monocytoid B-cell, which prominently expand sinuses in tissue sections, are more difficult to recognize in smears. Orell and colleagues have briefly described them as having large oval nuclei with pale-stained chromatin.[86] The presence of the actual organism is rare.[11,24] Whenever the cytomorphology is suggestive of toxoplasmosis, the diagnosis must be confirmed by the use of appropriate serologic tests (Box 24-5).

Cat-Scratch Disease

Cat-scratch disease is a self-limited benign inflammatory process of lymph nodes, typically cervical, that is often associated with exposure to cats. *Bartonella henselae* is the

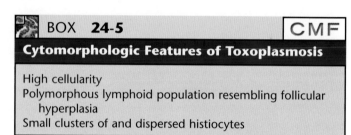

BOX 24-5 CMF

Cytomorphologic Features of Toxoplasmosis

High cellularity
Polymorphous lymphoid population resembling follicular hyperplasia
Small clusters of and dispersed histiocytes

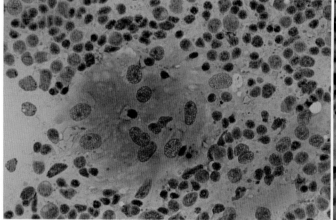

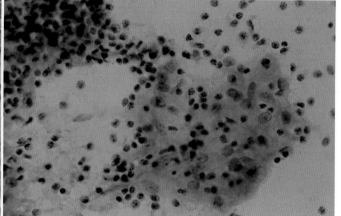

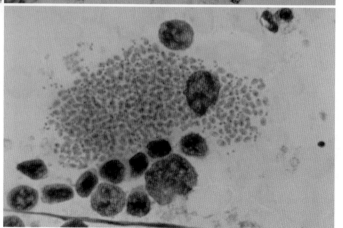

Figure 24-21 Toxoplasmic lymphadenitis. **A** and **B,** Clusters of macrophages with abundant pale cytoplasm, indistinct cellular borders with a syncytial appearance; round or slightly ovoid nuclei with delicate membranes; fine, pale chromatin; and small nucleoli are present and typical of aspirates of this entity. In contrast with well-formed granulomas, the nuclei are not the long, thin, and often bowed structures typical of epithelioid cells. Only rare lymphocytes appear to be intimately associated with these histiocytes, in contrast with the usual lymphohistiocytic aggregate. A polymorphic appearance of the adjacent lymphocytes is apparent. **C,** The cytoplasm in this histiocyte is distended because of numerous minute toxoplasmic trophozoites. (**A** and **C,** DQ; **B,** Pap) (From Geisinger KR, et al. Lymph nodes. In Geisinger KR, Silverman JF, editors. Fine needle aspiration cytology of superficial organs and body sites. New York: Churchill-Livingstone; 1999.)

usual etiologic agent. Many patients also have a rash and fever. Although it may occur at any age, most patients are children and young adults. The characteristic histologic picture includes a mixture of stellate microabscesses and associated granulomatous inflammation.

Aspiration smears show a polymorphous cell population of variably sized lymphocytes, lymphohistiocytic aggregates, tingible-body macrophages, neutrophils, and granulomas.[11,18,19] Suppurative granulomas, the most distinctive feature, consist of aggregates of epithelioid cells surrounding and infiltrated by neutrophils (Figure 24-22). Dispersed histiocytes with ingested neutrophils may be prominent. Granular cellular debris is present in the background. If granulomas are not evident, a combination of neutrophils and individually dispersed macrophages in a background of reactive lymphoid cells may suggest the diagnosis. Donnelly and colleagues demonstrated the causative pleomorphic microbes in the smears using a modified Steiner stain in most of their specimens.[18] A classic Warthin-Starry stain may also be used. In the absence of demonstrable organisms, a combination of clinical history, serology, and cytomorphology establishes the diagnosis of cat-scratch disease. The differential diagnosis of the neutrophilic infiltrate includes the causes of suppurative lymphadenitis (Box 24-6).

Infectious Mononucleosis

Infectious mononucleosis is usually a self-limited infection caused by the Epstein-Barr virus (EBV). Most often, adolescents and young adults are affected with fever, pharyngitis, splenomegaly, and a peripheral atypical lymphocytosis. The lymphadenopathy is usually cervical in distribution but may be generalized. In patients with a typical clinical picture, FNA biopsy is unlikely. However, an unusual presentation or prolonged lymphadenopathy may lead to FNA biopsy.

FNA biopsy smears are markedly cellular, with a heterogeneous lymphoid response resembling follicular hyperplasia but with increased numbers of plasmacytoid cells and immunoblasts (Figure 24-23).[25,26] The latter are large cells with solitary nuclei with smooth nuclear membranes, fine chromatin, and a large, often central nucleolus. The cytoplasm is eccentric, usually basophilic, and abundant (see Figure 24-23). FNA biopsy cannot make a specific diagnosis of infectious mononucleosis but rather can suggest this diagnosis that needs to be confirmed by serology. The differential diagnosis includes other florid nonspecific reactive changes, follicular center cell and large cell lymphomas, and Hodgkin's disease. The predominant cell remains the small lymphocyte. R-S cells lack the deep-blue eccentric cytoplasm of the occasional binucleated immunoblast of infectious mononucleosis. Although EBV uses the CD21 receptor to infect B-cells, many of the symptoms and the hypercellularity encountered with infectious mononucleosis are consequences of proliferating suppressor T-cells. These cells proliferate to destroy the immortalized B-cell clone, producing a characteristic predominance of CD8-positive cells with a normal complement of other T-cell antigens.[87] These cells do not coexpress CD4. Monotypic B-cells are not identified, and B-cells may be rare (Boxes 24-7 and 24-8).

Rosai-Dorfman Disease (Sinus Histiocytosis with Massive Lymphadenopathy)

This idiopathic disease characteristically involves the cervical neck nodes of children and young adults, particularly African-Americans. Characteristically, the lymphadenopathy is bilateral, painless, and often quite impressive in size.

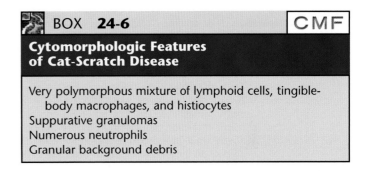

BOX 24-6 CMF

Cytomorphologic Features of Cat-Scratch Disease

Very polymorphous mixture of lymphoid cells, tingible-body macrophages, and histiocytes
Suppurative granulomas
Numerous neutrophils
Granular background debris

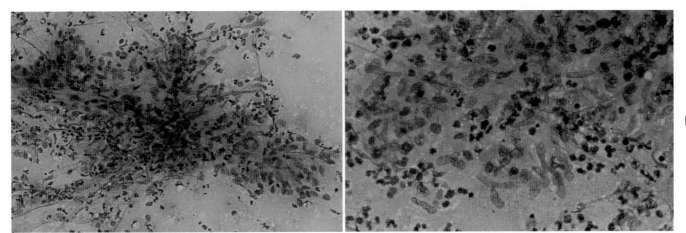

A   B

Figure 24-22 **Cat-scratch disease. A** and **B,** Neutrophils in varying stages of degeneration are intimately mixed with the epithelioid cells forming these granulomas. This suppurative granulomatous inflammation is characteristic but not diagnostic of cat-scratch disease. (DQ) (From Geisinger KR, et al. Lymph nodes. In Geisinger KR, Silverman JF, editors. Fine needle aspiration cytology of superficial organs and body sites. New York: Churchill-Livingstone; 1999.)

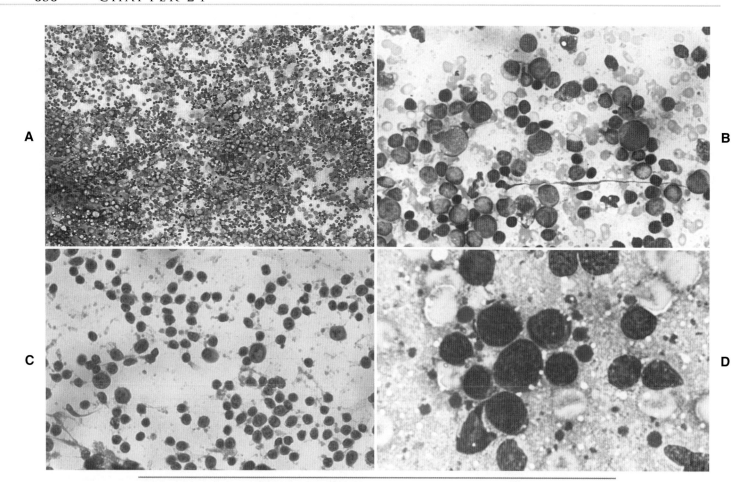

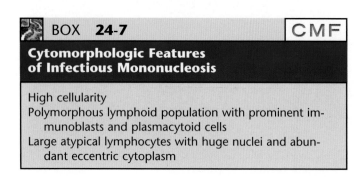

Figure 24-23   Infectious mononucleosis. A, An extremely cellular smear with numerous "activated" lymphoid cells are characteristic of this infection. Although small lymphocytes are certainly present, they appear outnumbered by moderately size and huge lymphoid elements. Thus, the polymorphism differs qualitatively from that of the usual follicular hyperplasia. (DQ) **B,** An admixture of lymphoid cell size is apparent but includes a large proportion of immunoblast-like cells. The latter are characterized by finely reticulated, evenly dispersed chromatin and distinct nucleoli. Also note the presence of an occasional plasmacytoid cell and a relatively small proportion of mature lymphoid elements. (DQ) **C,** With alcohol fixation, the diameters of all the cellular elements are somewhat more uniform. Still, a large proportion of cells are immunoblasts with finely granular, even chromatin and prominent nucleoli. A delicate rim of cytoplasm surrounds these huge nuclei. Rare plasmacytoid cells are also evident. (Pap) **D,** These immunoblasts have primitive or immature chromatin and basophilic cytoplasm. The latter contain an occasional vacuole. This picture demonstrates why a diagnosis should never be based on a single microscopic field. (DQ)

BOX   24-7   CMF

**Cytomorphologic Features
of Infectious Mononucleosis**

High cellularity
Polymorphous lymphoid population with prominent immunoblasts and plasmacytoid cells
Large atypical lymphocytes with huge nuclei and abundant eccentric cytoplasm

---

BOX   24-8

**Immunophenotype of Infectious
Mononucleosis**

Abundance of CD8-positive lymphocytes
Normal complement of other T-cell antigens
Rare B-cells

Histologically, lymph nodes are altered by prominent distention of the sinuses by benign histiocytes that have phagocytized erythrocytes and/or lymphocytes. Follicles are reduced in extent.

FNA biopsy smears may be moderately to highly cellular and include both small and large lymphocytes. The diag-

nostic feature is the large number of phagocytic histiocytes that contain viable-appearing lymphocytes and red blood cells (RBCs) in their pale cytoplasm (Figure 24-24).[11,28-30] To diagnose or suggest Rosai-Dorfman disease in an FNA biopsy, these cells need to be seen in large numbers. Although these cells are immunocytochemically positive

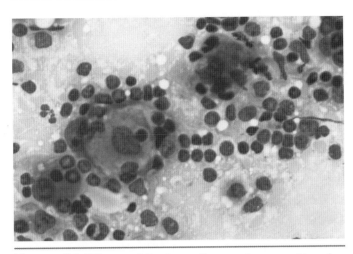

Figure 24-24 Rosai-Dorfman disease. A corona of lymphocytes surrounds several of the huge histiocytic elements characteristic of this disorder. In addition, the cytoplasm contains a few phagocytized lymphocytes (emperipolesis). (DQ)

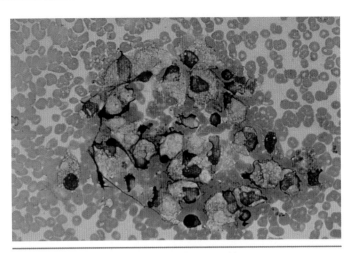

Figure 24-25 Kikuchi's lymphadenitis. A poorly cohesive aggregate of histiocytes with voluminous foamy cytoplasm dominates this field. Some of the benign nuclei have sickled shape and are closely opposed with the cell membrane. Note the absence of nuclear debris in their cytoplasm—that is, it does not represent tingible body macrophages. Lymphocytes are sparse. (DQ) (From Geisinger KR, et al. Lymph nodes. In Geisinger KR, Silverman JF, editors. Fine needle aspiration cytology of superficial organs and body sites. New York: Churchill-Livingstone; 1999.)

for S-100 protein, they lack the nuclear grooves and complex indented nuclei of the proliferating cells of Langerhans' histiocytosis. This entity cannot be diagnosed by flow cytometry. A huge population of CD45-negative cells suggests a nonlymphoid malignancy, but secondary markers demonstrate bright staining with CD38, indicating the presence of macrophages.

Kikuchi's Lymphadenitis

Histiocytic necrotizing (or Kikuchi's) lymphadenitis is an uncommon lymph node disorder that most often affects the cervical lymph nodes of young adult women, particularly those of Japanese or other Asian descent.[31,88,89] It is a benign self-limited process of unknown origin. Histopathologically, lymph nodes show karyorrhectic areas in the paracortex composed of phagocytic and nonphagocytic histiocytes, immunoblasts, plasmacytoid monocytes, karyorrhectic debris, and an almost complete absence of neutrophils.

Tsang and Chan described in detail a series of FNA biopsy of Kikuchi's lymphadenitis.[31] According to these authors, two characteristic cell types are seen in the smears. The phagocytic histiocyte, the most distinctive form, is a large cell with round contours and a crescent-shaped nucleus, the convex side of which appears to fuse with the cell membrane (Figure 24-25). These nuclei manifest irregular, twisted contours and inconspicuous nucleoli. Their abundant cytoplasm is pale and contains phagocytized eosinophilic and basophilic debris. Similar-appearing debris is also present extracellularly and at times extensive. The other typical cell type is the plasmacytoid monocyte, characterized by an eccentrically positioned round nucleus and basophilic cytoplasm without a perinuclear hof. Immunoblasts are always in the smears, at times in large numbers, whereas neutrophils are minimal or totally absent. However, these cell types are not specific for this disorder.[88]

Necrosis can also be seen in infarcted nodes and nodes involved by metastatic carcinoma (usually squamous) and high-grade lymphomas. However, in these cases neutrophils are usually present. SLE yields a polymorphic lymphoid infiltrate in which plasmacytoid cells are prominent with karyorrhectic debris, tingible-body macrophages, neutrophils, and the pathognomonic but rare hematoxylin bodies, which represent mauve cytoplasmic inclusions in inflammatory cells.[90]

Immunosuppressed Patients

During the last two decades an increase in the number of immunocompromised patients has occurred, including people undergoing treatment for solid and lymphoreticular malignancies, transplant recipients, and individuals with HIV. The diagnostic usefulness of FNA in these patients with lymphadenopathy is well established.[82,84,91-95] The general aim of the FNA in immunocompromised patients is to exclude an infectious agent, Kaposi's sarcoma, and lymphoma. Culture of FNA material is an essential component of the procedure in a group of patients whose inflammatory reactions to common agents may be both deficient and atypical, and in whom unusual agents may occur. A suppurative lymphadenitis, with its hallmarks of a necrotic background, large numbers of degenerated and viable neutrophils, and a minor component of macrophages and mixed lymphoid population should suggest either a conventional bacterial infection or a fungal infection.

Granulomatous lymphadenitis, with its characteristic epithelioid cells, multinucleated giant cells, small lymphocytes, and granulomatous tissue fragments should raise the traditional differential diagnosis of *Mycobacterium tuberculosis* or sarcoidosis.[84,93] In patients with HIV, however, the only finding may be large numbers of plump histiocytes with cross-hatched cytoplasm representing "negative image" bacilli, which are also found in the Romanowsky-stained background (see Figures 24-17 and 24-18).[15,16] Alternatively, segmented leukocytes may comprise the major inflammatory cell present. *Mycobacterium avium intracellulare* can be seen in the macrophages and smear background with acid

A **B**

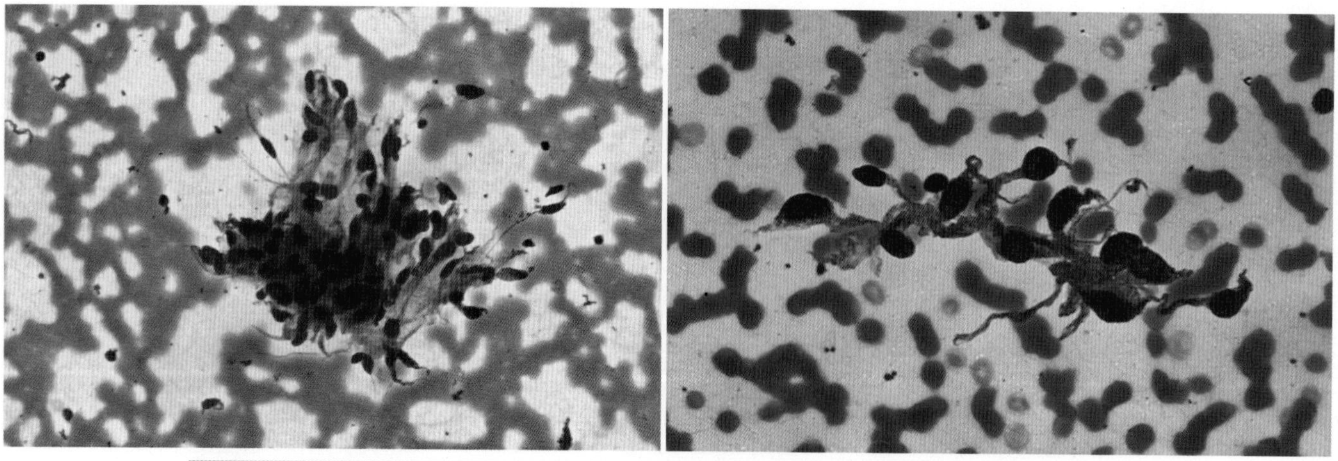

Figure 24-26 Kaposi's sarcoma. **A,** A small tissue fragment of tumor is present in an otherwise sparsely populated smear with a clean background. Neoplastic cells have solitary ovoid to elongated nuclei with smooth contours and inapparent nucleoli. In addition, they have long tapering tails of cytoplasm that blend with that of the adjacent neighboring cells. (DQ) **B,** The neoplastic cells are relatively small and homogeneous with solitary ovoid to elongated nuclei with finely reticulated chromatin and inconspicuous nucleoli. Cytoplasm is delicate and typically forms tapering tails. (DQ)

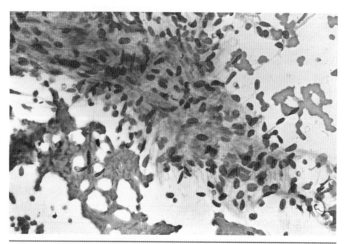

Figure 24-27 Kaposi's sarcoma. Clusters of cells from this neoplasm may simulate aspirated granulomas. The nuclei typically are plumper and do not show the indentations characteristic of benign epithelioid histiocytes. (DQ)

fast stains. If neutrophils are prominent and the patient does not have HIV, cat-scratch fever (neck and axillary nodes) and lymphogranuloma venereum (inguinal nodes) should be considered. Toxoplasmosis should also be considered when the smears have a polymorphic lymphoid population in which small lymphocytes predominate. Tingible-body macrophages, occasional small histiocytic clusters, and even rare toxoplasmal cysts assist in the diagnosis.

The histologic stages of HIV lymphadenopathy recognized in surgical pathology are not readily diagnosable on FNA.[96] However, some lymph node FNA biopsies in patients with HIV produce hypocellular smears with predominant plasmacytoid lymphocytes, consistent with HIV infection–related involution of the lymph node.

The cellular yield from lymph nodes containing Kaposi's sarcoma is often low, with the aspirate often yielding mostly blood with only scattered tissue fragments of spindle cells (Figure 24-26). These cells may be irregularly

arranged in these fragments, which may resemble granulomas with metachromatic stroma between the cells in the Romanowsky stain (Figure 24-27). The nuclei, which lack the "footprint" indentations of epithelioid histiocytes, are large, normochromatic, and only slightly variable. Nuclear crush artifact may be prominent.[97] If neutrophils are admixed with the spindle cells and histiocytes, then bacillary angiomatosis should be considered and a Warthin-Starry stain should be evaluated.

Most lymphomas seen in patients with HIV are intermediate to high-grade B-cell neoplasms, often presenting in soft tissues, central nervous system, gastrointestinal tract, and lymph nodes.[98] Burkitt's-like small noncleaved lymphoma accounts for one third of the lymphomas; it often has plasmacytoid features and cytologically overlaps with immunoblastic lymphoma. The other two thirds of lymphomas in patients with HIV are large cell, immunoblastic, and anaplastic large cell neoplasms with a common association with EBV. Often, classification on morphology alone is difficult because of the overlapping cell types. Flow cytometry is valuable in both categorization and distinction from benign proliferations.

The diagnosis of Hodgkin's disease can be suggested by FNA biopsy in patients with HIV, but distinction from viral lymphadenitis generally relies on excisional biopsy.[99]

Similarly, FNA biopsy of lymph nodes in transplant patients can provide a rapid diagnosis of the monoclonal proliferations identical to immunoblastic lymphoma, multiple myeloma, large cell lymphoma, or Burkitt's-like lymphoma.[100] However, distinguishing plasmacytic hyperplasias and polymorphic lymphoproliferations, with their mixed populations of small and large lymphocytes, in the spectrum of posttransplant lymphoproliferative disorders requires flow cytometry and probably histopathologic assessment (Figure 24-28).[100-105] Many of these proliferations regress when immunosuppression is decreased, whereas others progress with a high mortality rate, even with chemotherapy. Thus, a full diagnostic evaluation is required. T-cell lymphomas are uncommon in patients with HIV and posttransplant patients.

Overview of Malignant Lymphomas

The use of FNA biopsy to diagnose lymphomas has been controversial. A proportion of clinical oncologists and histopathologists regarded this application with a high level of suspicion and even disdain. However, the weight of the evidence in the literature and in practice shows that most malignant lymphomas can be diagnosed primarily and treated on the basis of FNA biopsy cytomorphology, at times supplemented with ancillary diagnostic procedures.* The judicious use of ancillary tests and recognizing certain limitations (most lymphomas including both Hodgkin's and non-Hodgkin's tumors) can be diagnosed and subclassified. The major differential diagnosis in most cases is nonspecific reactive hyperplasia.

The most important ancillary diagnostic tests involve the detection of specific lymphoid cell surface markers. Flow cytometry determines these antigens in aspirated cellular material, although immunocytochemical studies can also provide useful information and offer the advantage of direct correlation of cytomorphology and antigen expression.[53] The number of antigens evaluated depends on the number of aspirated cells available and the specific cytologic picture. Most important is the detection of kappa and lambda light chain restriction in monoclonal B-cell lymphoid populations. Other desirable markers include CD19, CD20, CD79a, CD5, CD10, CD3, and CD7. The first three are good markers of B-cell lymphomas. Normally a T-cell antigen, CD5 is aberrantly coexpressed in some small cell types of B-cell lymphomas. In many T-cell lymphomas, the neoplastic elements are positive for CD7 and negative for CD3, demonstrating an aberrant expression of T-cell antigens. A myeloid cell marker may be useful for the diagnosis of granulocytic sarcoma. Some institutions determine the proliferative activity of the lymphoma cells either by immunocytochemistry or flow cytometry to facilitate grading of the malignant lymphoma.[110] The authors have very little personal experience with this specific application. The use of molecular techniques to determine rearrangements of the genes for T-cell receptors or immunoglobulin chains has a role in this setting, but cell surface marker analysis usually provides sufficient information.[55,56]

Classification of Lymphomas

Of all malignant neoplasms, the lymphomas have probably been the group of tumors that have undergone the greatest and most substantial changes in their nomenclature and classification in the last few decades. In the last 20 years, tremendous progress has been made in both the clinical and scientific understanding of lymphoproliferative disorders related to contributions from the fields of immunology, molecular biology, and cytogenetics. This information has been incorporated into what is probably currently the most widely used classification system worldwide; this is the revised European-American classification of lymphoid neoplasms (REAL).[44] The REAL system was proposed by the International Lymphoma Study Group (Box 24-9; see Table 24-2).

Earlier heavily used classification schemes were based in large part on alterations in the lymph node architecture and/or immunologic functions of the normal counterparts of the neoplastic cells. In the REAL system, greater empha-

*References 45-48, 53, and 106-109.

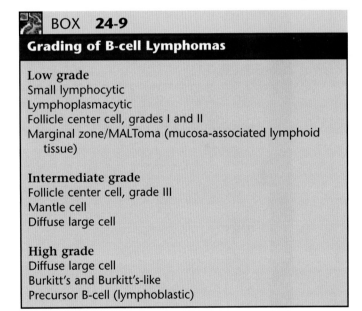

Figure 24-28 **Posttransplant lymphoproliferative disorder.** This cellular aspirate is characterized by individually dispersed lymphoid cells with a preponderance of atypical and immature forms. Many of the latter are relatively large with solitary round, smooth to irregularly contoured nuclei; finely reticulated chromatin; and nucleoli. Plasma cells and plasmacytoid lymphocytes are also present, as are small mature lymphoid elements. It is this highly variable appearance among the cells that should lead one to suspect that this is benign. (DQ)

BOX 24-9
Grading of B-cell Lymphomas

Low grade
Small lymphocytic
Lymphoplasmacytic
Follicle center cell, grades I and II
Marginal zone/MALToma (mucosa-associated lymphoid tissue)

Intermediate grade
Follicle center cell, grade III
Mantle cell
Diffuse large cell

High grade
Diffuse large cell
Burkitt's and Burkitt's-like
Precursor B-cell (lymphoblastic)

---

sis is placed on combining the cytomorphology of the neoplastic cells with their immunophenotypic profile, karyotype, and molecular analysis. With the REAL classification, the demonstration of monoclonality and defining the immunophenotypic features of neoplastic lymphoid elements are an integral part of the exact diagnosis (Table 24-3) The World Health Organization (WHO) has also created a new classification scheme that encompasses the REAL system with only minor modifications.[111] These two systems are thus more applicable to the FNA diagnosis of lymphomas.

The REAL and thus the WHO systems are relatively simplistic in that they define neoplasms that can be recognized consistently using currently available morphologic, immunologic, and genetic techniques. Thus, they conform to a list of well-defined neoplastic disease entities, many of which

TABLE 24-3
Lymphoma Reference Sheet

B-cell Lymphomas		L26	MB1	CD10	CD3	CD5	CD23	CD43	IgD	TdT	Cyclin	BCL-2	BCL-6	K vs L	p53	Other Facts
Follicular	Hyperplasia	F+	F+	F+	Neg	Neg	Neg	Neg	Neg	Neg	Neg	Neg	+	Poly	Neg	Mantles IgD+
	Progressive transformation (PTGC)	F+	F+	F+	Neg	Neg	Neg	Neg	Neg	Neg	Neg	Neg	+	Poly	Neg	t(14;18) bclu-2 ±
	Follicular lymphoma	F+	F+	F+	Neg	Neg	Neg	Neg	Neg	Neg	Neg	+	+	K>L	-/+	
Diffuse	Small lymphocytic lymphoma (SLL/CU)	+	+	Neg	Neg	+	+	+	+/-	Neg	Neg	+	Neg	Faint		Trisomy 12, 13q del
	Lymphoplasmacytic lymphoma (LPL)	+	+	Neg	Neg	Neg	Neg	+/-	+/-	Neg	Neg	+	Neg			t(9;14)
	Mantle call lymphoma (MCL)	+	+	-/+	Neg	+	Neg	+	+	Neg	+	+	Neg	L>K		t(11;14)
Starry-sky	Large cell lymphoma (LBCL)	+	+	-/+	Neg	-/+	Neg	Neg	Neg	Neg	Neg	-/+	-/+	+/-	-/+	t(14;18)
	Burkitt's lymphoma (BL)	-/+	+/-	+	Neg	Neg	Neg	Neg	Neg	Neg	Neg	Neg	+	Neg	-/+	t(8;14) > (2;8) > t(8;22); EBV
	Lymphoblastic lymphoma (B-LBL)	-/+	+/-	+/-	Neg	Neg	Neg	+/-	Neg	+	Neg	Neg	Neg	Neg	-/+	t(1;19), t(9;22), IgH +/-, TCI
Marginal/ Mantle	Nodal marginal zone lymphoma	+	+	Neg	Neg	Neg	Neg	+	Neg	Neg	Neg	+	Neg	+	Neg	Trisomy 3 -/+
	Malt-type marginal zone lymphoma	+	+	Neg	Neg	Neg	Neg	-/+	Neg	Neg	Neg	+	Neg	+	Neg	t(11;18)
	Splenic marginal zone lymphoma	+	+	Neg	Neg	Neg	Neg	Neg	+	Neg	Neg	+	Neg	+	Neg	
	Mantle cell lymphoma (MCL)	+	+	-/+	Neg	+	Neg	+	+	Neg	+	Neg	Neg	L>K	-/+	t(11;14)
Others	Lymphomatoid granulomatosis	+	-/+	Neg	Neg	Neg	Neg	Neg	Neg	Neg	Neg	-/+	Neg	-/+	-/+	EBV+
	Hairy cell leukemia	+	+	Neg	Neg	Neg	Neg	Neg	+/-	Neg	Neg	Neg	Neg	+	Neg	CD11c+, CD103+
	Plasma cell myeloma	-/+	+/-	Neg	Neg	Neg	Neg	+/1	Neg	Neg	Neg	Neg	Neg	+	Neg	CD30+, EMA+

Lymphomas with Reed-Sternberg Cells and Variants

	LCA	L26	MB-1	CD3	CD15	CD30	EMA	EBV	Other facts
Nodular sclerosis (NS)	Neg	Neg	Neg	Neg	+/-	+	Neg	-/+	Ig gene rearrangements
Mixed cellularity (MC)	Neg	Neg	Neg	Neg	+/-	+	Neg	+/-	
Lymphocyte depleted (LP)	Neg	Neg	Neg	Neg	+/1	+	Neg	+/-	
Lymphocyte predominant	+	+	-/+	Neg	-/+	-/+	Neg	Neg	
T-cell rich B-cell lymphoma	+	+	+/-	Neg	Neg	Neg	+/-	+/-	BCL-6+
Anaplastic large cell lymphoma	+	Neg	+/-	+/-	Neg	+	+	Neg	T(2;5), ALK

T-cell Lymphomas

	L26	CD3	CD4	CD8	TIA-1	Perforin	Tdt	CD30	EBV	Other Facts
Lymphoblastic lymphoma	Neg	+	+/-	-/+	Neg	Neg	+	Neg	Neg	TCR +/-; IgH -/+
Large granular lymphocytic leukemia	Neg	+	Neg	+	+	+/-	Neg	Neg	Neg	CD56-/+; TCR+; Hepatosplenomegaly
Angioimmunoblastic T-cell lymphoma	Neg	+	+	Neg	Neg	Neg	Neg	Neg	Neg	CD21+meshworks, TCR+, EBV+B-cells, trisomies 3 & 5
Extranodal NK/T-cell lymphoma	Neg	-/+	+/-	-/+	+	+	Neg	Neg	+	TCR usually
Adult T-cell leukemia/lymphoma (ATL)	Neg	+	+	Neg	Neg	Neg	Neg	Neg	Neg	HTLV-1 associated, CD25+
Anaplastic large cell lymphoma (ALCL)	Neg	+/-	+/-	Neg	+/-	Neg	Neg	+	Neg	t(2;5); ALK+; EMA +/-
Primary Cutaneous ALCL	Neg	+	Neg	Neg	+	Neg	Neg	+	Neg	ALK-; EMA-

Modified by Clark B, National Institutes of Health from Harris NL, et al. A revised European American classification of lymphoid neoplasms: a proposal from the International Lymphoma Study Group [see comments]. Review. Blood 1994; 84(5):1361-1392.

possess distinctive clinical presentations and natural histories. The REAL classification is divided into three major categories of lymphomas: B-cell neoplasms, T-cell neoplasms, and Hodgkin's disease.[44] Each of these major groups is divided into three subcategories: definite, provisional, and unclassifiable. Lymphoproliferative disorders were considered provisional if the experts creating the REAL classification felt that insufficient experience was obtained to be certain that it represented a distinct disease entity. Unclassifiable tumors were those that did not really fit into either the definite or provisional categories. Within both B-cell and T-cell lymphomas, the two major categories are precursor and peripheral neoplasms. Within each, the precursor neoplasms represent lymphoblastic leukemias and lymphomas. The PTCLs are more extensive and are classified according to their cytomorphologic attributes, their location within the lymphoid system, and possibly on the presumed function of the neoplastic cells. Within the B-cell and T-cell groups, the neoplasms are divided into three grades that tend to correlate with their degree of clinical aggressiveness. This grading is based on morphologic features including cellular and nuclear sizes, chromatin patterns, and proliferative activity.

Hodgkin's Disease

Accounting for approximately 40% of lymphoid neoplasms, Hodgkin's disease principally affects older adolescents or young adults, with a second smaller incidence peak in middle-age people. Supraclavicular, cervical, and mediastinal lymph nodes are those most often involved.

Hodgkin's disease is actually a heterogeneous condition that consists of several distinct clinical and pathologic entities. The REAL classification splits the lymphocyte-predominant type from classic Hodgkin's disease; this division is based on immunophenotypic and genotypic differences. In addition the REAL classification has a provisional type referred to as *lymphocyte-rich classic Hodgkin's disease*.[44] Morphologically, this resembles the lymphocyte-predominant type but possesses the phenotype of the classic forms of Hodgkin's disease. No more than 5% of all patients with Hodgkin's disease have the lymphocyte-predominant form. Although rarely this variant has a diffuse histologic architecture, the pattern usually is nodular. Classic binucleated R-S cells would be extremely unusual or absent. The diagnostic cells are mononucleated with highly lobulated nuclei, small nucleoli, and finely reticulated chromatin, creating the characteristic popcorn nuclei. In contrast with classic Hodgkin's disease, in the lymphocyte-predominant form the abnormal cells are B-cells. By immunocytochemistry, they are positive for leukocyte common antigen and are nonreactive with CD15. A FNA biopsy diagnosis of lymphocyte-predominant Hodgkin's disease is therefore difficult.[106] This is supported by the rarity in which it has been reported in the literature.

In both tissue sections and smears, benign inflammatory cells are often present. Eosinophilic leukocytes are especially noticeable and if seen to any extent in a lymph node aspirate, this is a clue that one should perform a diligent search for diagnostic R-S cells. Eosinophils may also be seen in nodal aspirates in association with parasitic infestations and allergic reactions, including those related to drugs. Granulomatous inflammation may also accompany Hodgkin's disease, and recently it has been suggested that the presence of individual epithelioid cells in smears is also a tip-off to the presence of this lymphoma.[112]

Smear cellularity tends to be relatively low, reflecting the prominent fibrosis of nodular sclerosing Hodgkin's disease, the most common form of this disease.[11,106,107,113-118] The smears demonstrate a polymorphous lymphoid population in which small mature lymphocytes predominate numerically and are mixed with eosinophils, plasma cells, and histiocytes (Figures 24-29 and 24-30). The diagnosis requires the presence of R-S cells and their mononuclear variants. R-S cells may possess abundant pale cytoplasm with two or more large complex or lobulated nuclei that are often eccentrically positioned (Figure 24-31). The nuclei have variably thickened membranes with irregular, often coarse

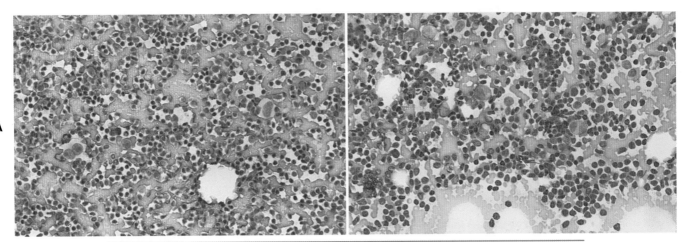

Figure 24-29 Hodgkin's disease. **A,** This is a relatively cellular aspirate that is composed mostly of small mature-appearing lymphocytes. Two neoplastic cells are present, one of which is a classic Reed-Sternberg (R-S) cell. The latter is characterized by two huge mirror image nuclei, each of which contains a solitary large macronucleolus. The surrounding cytoplasm is pale and basophilic. More cytoplasm is seen in the solitary mononucleated malignant cell. (DQ) **B,** Scattered large R-S cells and their variants are scattered among the much more numerous small lymphocytes. As in this particular field, it is important to search the edge of smears as large cells show a propensity to be concentrated in this portion of the smear. (DQ)

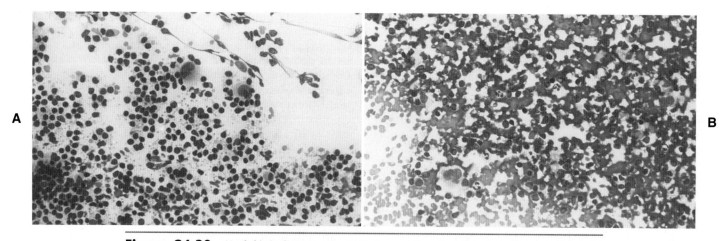

Figure 24-30 Hodgkin's disease. **A** and **B**, Rare scattered malignant cells are greatly outnumbered by small mature-appearing lymphocytes. Even at this low magnification, the large nuclei with their huge nucleoli stand out. (DQ)

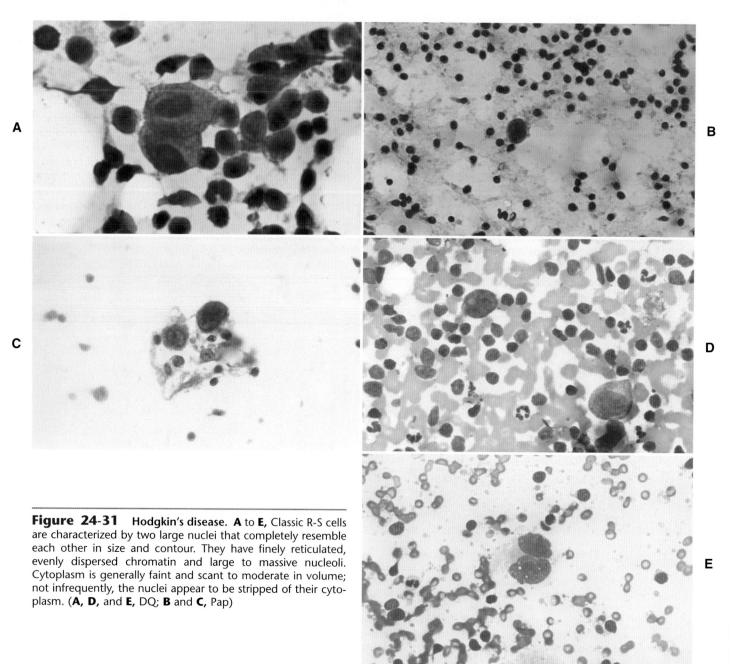

Figure 24-31 Hodgkin's disease. **A** to **E**, Classic R-S cells are characterized by two large nuclei that completely resemble each other in size and contour. They have finely reticulated, evenly dispersed chromatin and large to massive nucleoli. Cytoplasm is generally faint and scant to moderate in volume; not infrequently, the nuclei appear to be stripped of their cytoplasm. (**A, D,** and **E,** DQ; **B** and **C,** Pap)

chromatin and large variably shaped nucleoli. In alcohol-fixed Pap-stained smears, the malignant nature of the nuclei is readily apparent. Mononuclear variants have similar nuclear features. Although the R-S cells may be relatively sparse in the smears, they usually stand out because of their large size and are often located at the edge of the smear. One possible pitfall is the mistaken identification of benign immunoblasts as mononuclear variants. Immunoblasts usually are smaller, have smooth round nuclear and nucleolar contours, and have cytoplasm that appears more basophilic. In any smear in which small lymphocytes predominate, one must search for R-S cells to exclude Hodgkin's disease. The application of CD15 (Leu-M₁) staining is useful in confirming the diagnosis (Figure 24-32). Immunocytochemistry may be especially valuable in distinguishing Hodgkin's disease from T-cell rich B-cell lymphomas.[119] A host of malignancies may mimic Hodgkin's disease in aspirates. Several examples of metastatic nasopharyngeal carcinomas masquerading as Hodgkin's disease have been reported.[120]

An unusual form of Hodgkin's disease has recently been described in FNA biopsies.[80] These specimens were dominated by intact or degenerated neutrophils simulating suppurative lymphadenitis. However, small numbers of lymphoid cells and R-S cells were present. Only a high level of suspicion recognizes such malignant Hodgkin's cells.

A few aspirates of another unusual variant, namely interfollicular Hodgkin's disease are known. It is considered a form of mixed cellularity Hodgkin's disease. The smear is overall quite suggestive of follicular hyperplasia; scattered classic and variant R-S cells are present (Box 24-10).

For the following several reasons, no reliable method for detecting these neoplasms by flow cytometry exists[64]:
1. R-S cells are large and fragile, and thus many are lost in sample processing.
2. Hodgkin's disease has a cellular background of mixed benign cells. Attempts to enrich samples for R-S cells have not resulted in a useful product.
3. R-S cells may be coated by helper T-cells making them inaccessible to staining by monoclonal antibodies and increasing the percentage of CD4-positive cells. Accordingly, a greatly increased CD4 to CD8 ratio suggests but is not diagnostic of Hodgkin's disease.

Non-Hodgkin's Lymphoma

In the United States the Working Formulation has been the gold standard used to classify lymphoid neoplasms.[121] This scheme uses the morphologic appearance to classify lymphomas into low, intermediate, or high grades but does not take into account the biology or the pathogenesis of the neoplasm. A more recent classification scheme, REAL, uses morphologic, immunologic, and genetic features or combinations of such attributes.[44] Recently, Wakely has discussed the usefulness of FNA biopsy with the REAL system.[46] For instance, many mantle cell lymphomas (MCLs) express the *bcl-1* oncogene.[122] This protein is expressed as a novel fusion protein resulting from a translocation involving chromosomes 11 and 14. This is an entity with a specific marker and is so recognized by the REAL scheme.[44] Flow cytometry can assess the immunologic phenotype of a neoplasm for classification under the REAL system.[53,54] Symmans and colleagues have used the number of apoptotic bodies in smears to assess grade.[123]

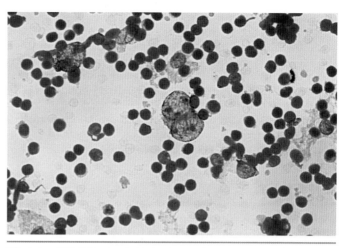

Figure 24-32 **Hodgkin's disease.** Binucleated and mononucleated R-S cells show intense cytoplasmic staining for CD15. Note that the small mature lymphocytes are nonreactive.

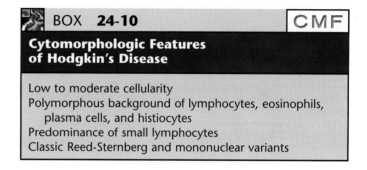

![] BOX **24-10**	CMF
Cytomorphologic Features of Hodgkin's Disease	

Low to moderate cellularity
Polymorphous background of lymphocytes, eosinophils, plasma cells, and histiocytes
Predominance of small lymphocytes
Classic Reed-Sternberg and mononuclear variants

The basic approach to lymphoma diagnosis in FNA biopsy relies on the morphologic assessment of cellularity, cell type, and special features, followed by ancillary studies, including flow cytometry and immunocytochemistry. Flow cytometry is generally recommended in almost all cases of primary diagnosis because cytomorphology alone cannot diagnose all the subcategories of non-Hodgkin's lymphomas. For example, follicular center cell lymphomas with a mixed cell population are challenging to differentiate from reactive lymph nodes.

The presence or absence of monoclonality is crucial in diagnosing lymphoid malignancies. Although it has been shown that some monoclonal proliferations behave as dysplastic processes, it is generally believed that monoclonal proliferations of lymphoid tissue represent a malignancy. For B-cells, monoclonality is documented by the presence or absence of kappa or lambda SIg restriction. Normal cells are admixed with neoplastic cells, so the percentage of kappa-positive or lambda-positive B-cells may sometimes be less than 100% in a B-cell non-Hodgkin's lymphoma. Although T-cell malignancies are also monoclonal, the T-cell receptor is far more complex, and the presence or absence of a range of antigens must be assessed.

The ability to diagnosis non-Hodgkin's lymphomas accurately has been appropriately questioned. This is difficult to assess by review of the literature for several reasons. First, some series include a diverse spectrum of lymphoma types including Hodgkin's disease, whereas others deal specifically with one type such as lymphoblastic lymphoma. Second, the proportion of primary vs. recurrent lymphoma diagnoses by FNA biopsy varies greatly from one study to another. Some authors do not provide sufficient data to calculate the levels of diagnostic sensitivity and specificity; some investigators include suspicious diagnoses as positive for malignancy in their calculation, whereas others do not. We are fortunate that Wakely has painstakingly reviewed the recent literature for levels of sensitivity and specificity in 30 published FNA biopsy series (Table 24-4). With the combination of cytomorphology and immunophenotyping, the diagnosis of non-Hodgkin's lymphomas in aspiration smears can successfully be achieved.

TABLE 24-4

Diagnostic Sensitivity and Specificity of FNA Biopsy of Non-Hodgkin's Lymphomas

Authors	Number of Non-Hodgkin's Lymphoma	Sensitivity (%)	Specificity (%)
30 series*	1997	89	99
Meda	179	85†	100

Modified from Wakely PE, Jr. Fine-needle aspiration cytopathology in diagnosis and classification of malignant lymphoma: accurate and reliable? Diagn Cytopathol 2000; 22:120-125.
*Only 27 provided sufficient data to calculate sensitivity and specificity.
†False-negative fine-needle aspiration diagnoses included 24 suspicious and four benign interpretations.

Large Cell Lymphoma

The most common lymphoma diagnosed by FNA biopsy is non-Hodgkin's large cell lymphoma. This neoplasm affects both adults and children and is relatively common in patients with AIDS and transplant recipients.

Aspiration smears are highly cellular and characterized by a monomorphic population of atypical noncohesive large lymphoid cells (Figure 24-33).[1,11,35,57,68] Specifically, it is this monomorphism of large atypical lymphoid cells that readily permits the diagnosis of this malignancy. Nuclei are large and irregular in shape, with membranes with thick and thin regions, variably clumped and cleared chromatin, and one to several prominent nucleoli (Figures 24-34 to 24-36). Cytoplasmic basophilia may be intense and vacuolization may be prominent, usually in the form of minute vacuoles. The cells may resemble large centrocytes (cleaved) or centroblasts (noncleaved immunoblasts) with single nucleoli in large nuclei with eccentric cytoplasm. Alternatively, they may have large, polylobated hyperchromatic nuclei. The nuclear features, although appreciable in Romanowsky-stained smears, are more clearly seen in Pap-stained smears; air-dried smears allow better assessment of cytoplasmic features. Tingible-body macrophages may be seen, and necrotic debris is occasionally present.

The differential diagnosis includes anaplastic carcinomas and malignant melanomas, both of which typically have a prominent dissociated cell population in smears (Figure 24-37). The presence of true cohesion and tissue fragments in carcinomas, the presence of pigment granules and the prominent nuclear pseudoinclusions in melanoma, and the

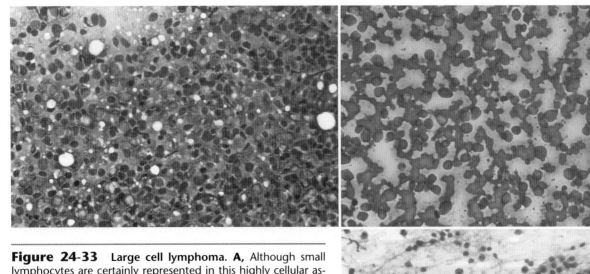

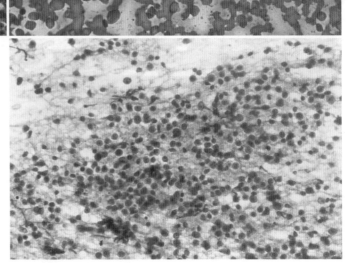

Figure 24-33   Large cell lymphoma. A, Although small lymphocytes are certainly represented in this highly cellular aspirate, the predominant components of this smear are the tumor cells derived from a large cell lymphoma. The latter are characterized by solitary round nuclei, finely reticulated chromatin, small but distinct nucleoli, and high N:C ratios. Note the characteristically high level of smear cellularity and total lack of intercellular cohesion. (DQ) **B,** The dispersed lymphomatous elements are quite uniform in appearance. They have finely reticulated chromatin, minute inconspicuous nucleoli, and almost no visible cytoplasm. Lymphoglandular bodies are present in the background. (DQ) **C,** With alcohol fixation, the neoplastic lymphocytes appear even more homogeneous. Note the dissociative pattern and the high cellularity. (Pap)

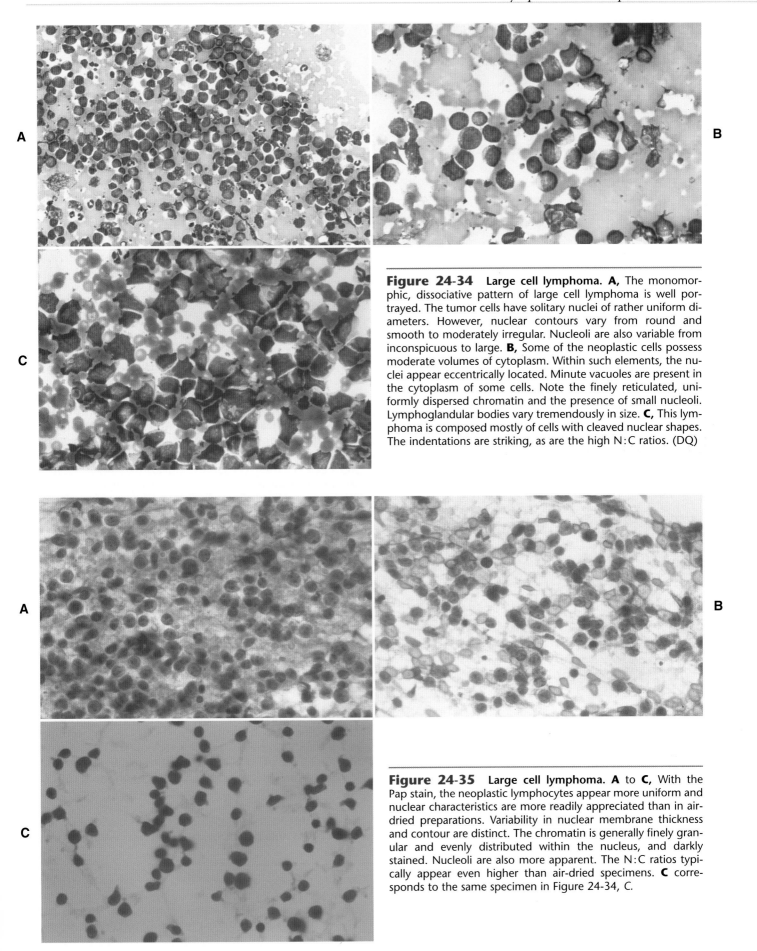

Figure 24-34 Large cell lymphoma. **A,** The monomorphic, dissociative pattern of large cell lymphoma is well portrayed. The tumor cells have solitary nuclei of rather uniform diameters. However, nuclear contours vary from round and smooth to moderately irregular. Nucleoli are also variable from inconspicuous to large. **B,** Some of the neoplastic cells possess moderate volumes of cytoplasm. Within such elements, the nuclei appear eccentrically located. Minute vacuoles are present in the cytoplasm of some cells. Note the finely reticulated, uniformly dispersed chromatin and the presence of small nucleoli. Lymphoglandular bodies vary tremendously in size. **C,** This lymphoma is composed mostly of cells with cleaved nuclear shapes. The indentations are striking, as are the high N:C ratios. (DQ)

Figure 24-35 Large cell lymphoma. **A** to **C,** With the Pap stain, the neoplastic lymphocytes appear more uniform and nuclear characteristics are more readily appreciated than in air-dried preparations. Variability in nuclear membrane thickness and contour are distinct. The chromatin is generally finely granular and evenly distributed within the nucleus, and darkly stained. Nucleoli are also more apparent. The N:C ratios typically appear even higher than air-dried specimens. **C** corresponds to the same specimen in Figure 24-34, **C.**

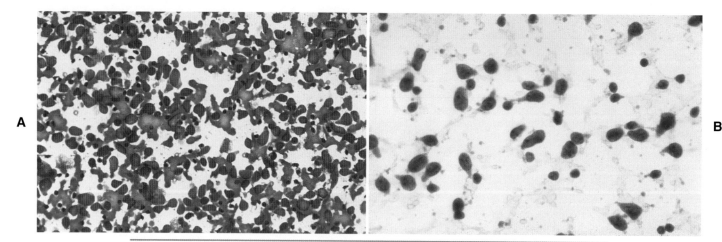

Figure 24-36 **Large cell lymphoma.** This lymphoma is characterized by neoplastic cells with blunt cytoplasmic tails, a most unusual finding in our experience. The neoplastic cells somewhat resemble those from the so-called hand mirror variant of acute lymphoblastic leukemia. Note the dissociative pattern of the neoplastic elements. (**A,** DQ; **B,** Pap)

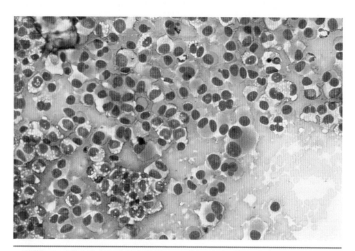

Figure 24-37 **Metastatic melanoma.** This aspirate is characterized by high cellularity and a dissociative pattern, superficially resembling malignant lymphoma. However, the cells possess much greater volumes of cytoplasm than are typically seen in large cell lymphomas. In addition, occasional cells manifest more than one nucleus, a feature most unusual in the usual lymphoma. (DQ)

nuclear and cytoplasmic features of lymphomas assist in the diagnosis (Figure 24-38). The use of flow cytometry and immunocytochemistry almost always confirms the diagnosis (Box 24-11).

Small Cleaved Cell Lymphoma

This malignancy is essentially restricted to the adult population. Histologically, the lymph node architecture is effaced by either a nodular or diffuse proliferation of small atypical lymphoid cells. In the Working Formulation, nodular and diffuse patterns are classified as low and intermediate grades, respectively, with prognostic differences. This distinction requires histologic examination.[121]

Smears are generally highly cellular and show a homogeneous population of dispersed small mononucleated lymphoid cells (Figure 24-39).[11,69] However, cellularity may be lowered if the node is sclerotic. The tumor cells have diameters up to double that of small mature lymphocytes, high nuclear to cytoplasmic (N:C) ratios, and thick, irregularly contoured nuclear membranes with clefts, deeper indentations, and linear creases (Figure 24-40). Areas of parachromatin clearing and small nucleoli may be evident. Aggregates of these cells in the smears may suggest a nodular architecture of the lymphoma (see Figure 24-39).[11,39] However, as stated above, histology is required for this distinction (Box 24-12).

Mixed Small Cleaved and Large Cell Lymphoma

As with small cleaved cell lymphoma, this follicular center cell neoplasm occurs almost exclusively in adults (Figure 24-41). In the Working Formulation, this is an intermediate-grade lymphoma and consists of an admixture of small and large atypical lymphoid cells, with a predominance of the former.[68,121] According to Sneige and colleagues, when large tumor cells represent 5% to 15% of the neoplastic elements, the specimen should be classified as a mixed lymphoma.[69] In their study, Young and colleagues used an upper threshold of 20% but in real-life practice used a cutoff of 25%.[124]

The major problem in the diagnosis is distinguishing this heterogeneous mixture of malignant lymphocytes from a benign reactive hyperplastic node, and immunophenotyping is often essential.[11] FNA biopsy of nodes with follicular hyperplasia can show various regions on the slides in which small cleaved cells and larger lymphoid cells can be quite prominent, to the exclusion of small lymphocytes. These areas, which represent smeared germinal centers, often have tingible-body macrophages, and by examining the entire smear, foci in which small lymphocytes predominate are seen.

Follicular center cell lymphomas account for the majority of non-Hodgkin's lymphomas. Many are associated with a chromosomal translocation that produces the *bcl-2* oncogene.[59] Immunologically, these lymphomas express pan–B-cell antigens with SIg expression. Most also coexpress CD10 and demonstrate increased CD20 expression com-

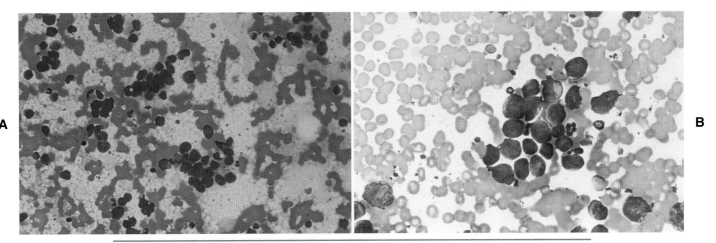

Figure 24-38 **Large cell lymphoma. A,** Small aggregates of lymphoma cells suggest the possibility of intercellular cohesion. This could lead to the misidentification of this primary lymphoproliferative disorder as a metastatic malignancy. **B,** At higher magnification, the cellular attributes of lymphomatous elements are evident. In addition, although closely clustered, true cohesion is lacking. Lymphoglandular bodies are present in the background. (DQ)

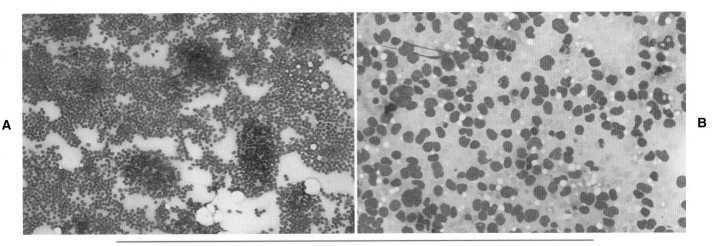

Figure 24-39 **Small cleaved cell lymphoma. A,** This highly cellular aspirate shows numerous individually dispersed small homogeneous tumor cells. In addition, three-dimensional clusters of the tumor cells are also present. This is an aspirate of a node that subsequently showed a mixed follicular and diffuse pattern. **B,** The high cellularity and dissociative pattern characteristic of malignant lymphomas are evident in this aspirate. The neoplastic cells are strikingly uniform with relatively small nuclei, moderately clumped chromatin, inconspicuous nucleoli, and extremely high N:C ratios. The prominent cleaved nature of the nuclear outline is readily evident. (DQ)

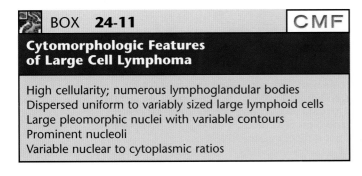

BOX **24-11**   CMF

**Cytomorphologic Features
of Large Cell Lymphoma**

High cellularity; numerous lymphoglandular bodies
Dispersed uniform to variably sized large lymphoid cells
Large pleomorphic nuclei with variable contours
Prominent nucleoli
Variable nuclear to cytoplasmic ratios

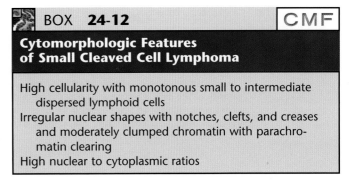

BOX **24-12**   CMF

**Cytomorphologic Features
of Small Cleaved Cell Lymphoma**

High cellularity with monotonous small to intermediate
  dispersed lymphoid cells
Irregular nuclear shapes with notches, clefts, and creases
  and moderately clumped chromatin with parachromatin clearing
High nuclear to cytoplasmic ratios

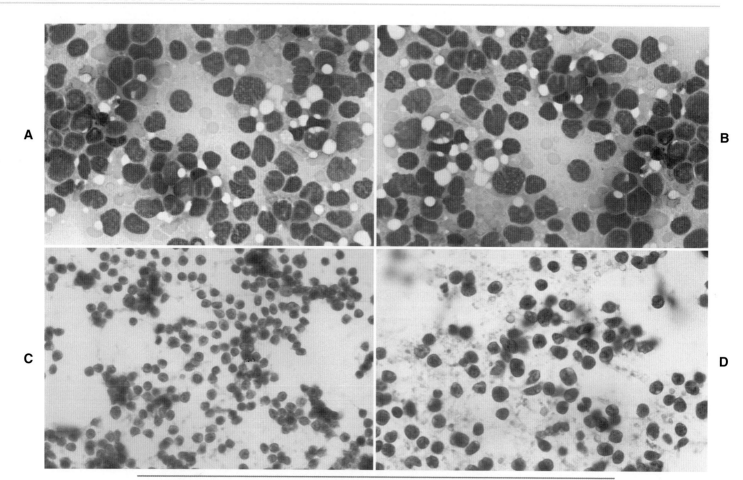

Figure 24-40 Small cleaved cell lymphoma. **A** to **D,** The highly irregular nuclear contours are even more evident at higher magnification. In some cells, the deep nuclear indentations are readily apparent. In other cells a linear nuclear groove marks the site of such cleavage. (**A** and **B,** DQ; **C** and **D,** Pap)

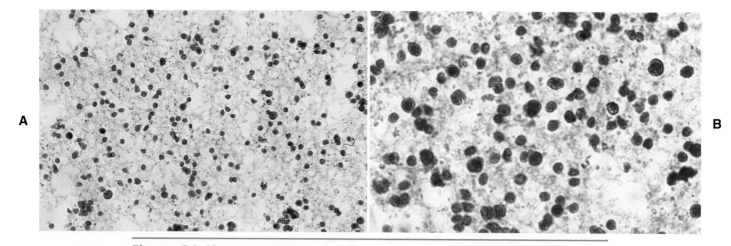

Figure 24-41 Mixed small cleaved-large cell lymphoma. **A,** This single cell pattern demonstrates the predominance of small cleaved cells with dark condensed chromatin. A minority of the cells is larger with more rounded nuclei and distinct nucleoli. **B,** These small cleaved cells resemble those seen in pure small cleaved cell lymphoma with thick irregular nuclear contours, condensed chromatin, inapparent nucleoli, and high N:C ratios. The large cell component has more finely granular chromatin and small but distinct nucleoli. (Pap)

pared with normal B-cells.[41,42] These cells lack other antigens such as CD5. These neoplasms may represent a progression from follicular, predominantly small cleaved cell lymphoma to diffuse, predominantly large cell lymphomas.[166] CD10 is less apt to be coexpressed and CD20 less likely to be abnormal as these lymphomas migrate toward the more aggressive end of the spectrum.

Follicular center cell lymphomas are generally easily detected by flow cytometry. Monotypic SIg can usually be found, but the type of heavy chain is variable. Furthermore, a small percentage of these lymphomas express pan–B-cell antigens but lack detectable SIg. Additional complications may occur as some florid follicular hyperplasias may also lack detectable SIg. In this situation, the flow cytometric findings are not diagnostic for a lymphoma but rather are suspicious (Box 24-13).

Small Lymphocytic Lymphoma

These neoplasms affect middle-age and older populations, progress slowly, and typically involve multiple lymphoid sites. They roughly correspond to chronic lymphocytic leukemia and are mainly B-cell neoplasms. This category of low-grade lymphomas is relatively common, but is seen relatively infrequently in FNA biopsy. The ability to separate them from benign conditions on morphologic grounds alone is difficult. Aspiration smears are highly cellular and composed of numerous dispersed small lymphocytes with high N:C ratios, clumped chromatin, and inconspicuous nucleoli (Figure 24-42). Leong and Stevens[6] have warned about the similarity with benign inactive lymph nodes, which yield a similar predominant small lymphocyte pattern. The demonstration of light chain restriction is essential for the FNA biopsy diagnosis of this lymphoma.

Chronic lymphocytic leukemia and its nodal counterpart, SLL characteristically coexpress pan–B-cell antigens, CD19 and CD20 as well as CD5 and can be detected by the presence of monotypic kappa or lambda SIg. However, immunologic findings are highly heterogeneous with respect to the density of antigen expression on the cell surface.[68] One constant feature is that the expression of CD5 is always weaker than in the normal T-cells present in the sample. The CD20 is also often weakly expressed and cannot be detected in some tumors. The CD19 is usually intensely expressed and is almost always brighter than the CD20.

SLL may undergo several transformations, notably Richter's and prolymphocytic. Richter's transformation is an aggressive change to a high-grade lymphoma with large and almost blastlike cells. No definitive means of detecting this process by flow cytometry exists because these cells have the same immunophenotype as the parent SLL.[71]

Prolymphocytic transformation has no specific immunologic features to distinguish it from SLL, but it may coexpress CD11c and have increased expression of CD20 and SIg expression compared with SLL.

A rare entity is the T-cell variant of SLL. It is a peripheral T-cell neoplasm, not a B-cell tumor. Immunologically, it is characterized by expression of either CD4 or CD8, and the cells have an aberrant immunophenotype. For flow cytometry, it is best to use a combination of CD5 or CD7 in conjunction with CD3.

Mantle Cell and Marginal Zone Lymphomas

Although SLL and its variants have in common the coexpression of CD5 and pan–B-markers, this finding is not specific because MCLs also have this pattern.[72,73,125,126] These lymphomas have a more aggressive course and are difficult to maintain in remission. MCL is composed of small lymphocytes with variably irregular nuclear outlines, some resembling small cleaved cells and others prolymphocytes.[72] The authors have demonstrated that MCL and SLL have overlapping morphologic features in aspiration smears (Figure 24-43).[127] However, most cases of MCL can be separated from SLL by flow cytometric data. Generally, MCL has much brighter expression of CD20 and SIg. SLL is a neoplasm of prefollicular center cells and thus tends to have IgM or IgD on its surface; MCL, a lymphoma of postfollicular center cells, tends to have surface IgG. Another discriminator is the use of CD23. This protein is expressed on SLL cells but not on MCL cells. Mantle cell lymphoma may present as or transform into more aggressive blastic or large cell variants (Figure 24-44).[125,126]

Overlapping cytomorphologic attributes can also be shown between MCL and marginal zone lymphoma (MZL).[127] In general, MZL cells manifest more prominent nuclear membrane contour irregularities compared with MCL cells (Figure 24-45). MZL also tends to present in smears with a greater degree of cytologic monotony compared with MCL. However, the two lymphomas cannot be distinguished reliably in a given case based solely on cytomorphology.[127]

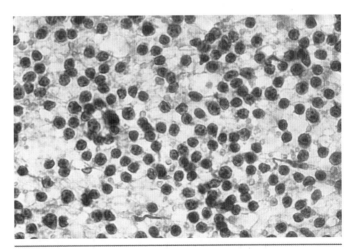

Figure 24-42 Small lymphocytic lymphoma. Strikingly uniform lymphocytes are characterized by perfectly round nuclei with distinct membranes, clumped dark chromatin, a lack of nucleoli, and high N:C ratios. (Pap)

> ### BOX 24-13
>
> ### Immunophenotyping of Follicular Center Cell Lymphomas
>
> Pan–B-cell markers (CD19, CD20, CD79a) expressed
> CD10 may be expressed
> Variably increased CD20 expression
> Monoclonal surface immunoglobulin

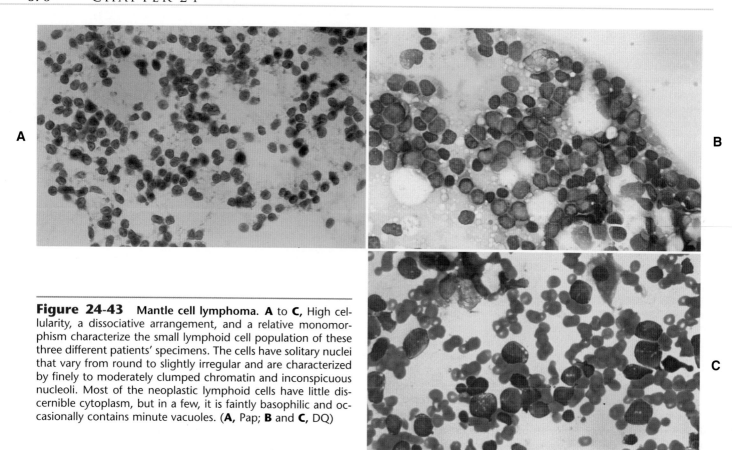

Figure 24-43 **Mantle cell lymphoma. A** to **C,** High cellularity, a dissociative arrangement, and a relative monomorphism characterize the small lymphoid cell population of these three different patients' specimens. The cells have solitary nuclei that vary from round to slightly irregular and are characterized by finely to moderately clumped chromatin and inconspicuous nucleoli. Most of the neoplastic lymphoid cells have little discernible cytoplasm, but in a few, it is faintly basophilic and occasionally contains minute vacuoles. (**A,** Pap; **B** and **C,** DQ)

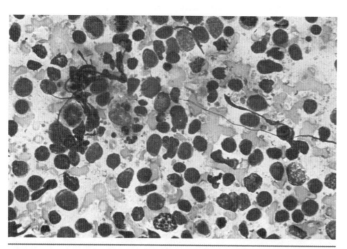

Figure 24-44 **Mantle cell lymphoma, blastic form.** Much more primitive chromatin, more irregular nuclear contours, and distinct nucleoli characterize this neoplasm. Also present are mitotic figures and a tingible-body macrophage; both of these are markers of the high proliferative rate of this variant. (DQ)

Small Noncleaved Cell Lymphoma

This neoplasm, categorized as a high-grade lymphoma in the Working Formulation, characteristically occurs in its nonendemic form as an intraabdominal tumor involving lymph nodes with infiltration of visceral organs. This lymphoma represents a large proportion of all lymphomas arising in patients with AIDS and is also fairly common in transplant recipients.[92] Aspiration smears are extremely cellular, with intermediate-size lymphoid cells with round nuclei, high to moderate N:C ratios, moderately to coarsely clumped chromatin, and one or more prominent small nucleoli (Figure 24-46).[11,128,129] Although nuclei often appear perfectly round, some may be polylobated or irregular. Multiple small nucleoli are typical of the Burkitt's variant, whereas solitary and larger nucleoli are expected in the non-Burkitt's type. The deeply basophilic cytoplasm is eccentric, varies from scanty to moderate in volume in air-dried Romanowsky smears, and contains small but prominent lipid vacuoles in some neoplastic cells. With alcohol fixation, the vacuoles are lost. Tingible-body macrophages are often a prominent attribute. Numerous mitotic figures and apoptotic bodies are evident (Box 24-14)

Burkitt's lymphoma has a characteristic phenotype, co-expressing pan–B-cell antigens and SIg. Often IgM lambda is detectable. As in follicular center cells, CD10 is present. When assessing these neoplasms, a proliferative fraction may be helpful because almost all the cells should be cycling and thus be positive for Ki-67; this is one of the most rapidly dividing human neoplasms (Box 24-15).

Lymphoblastic Lymphoma

This malignancy typically involves children, particularly teenage boys. In many cases, peripheral lymphadenopathy is associated with a mediastinal mass, which may actually call clinical attention to the disease. Lymphoblastic lymphoma is a high-grade neoplasm. Most are T-cell neoplasms.

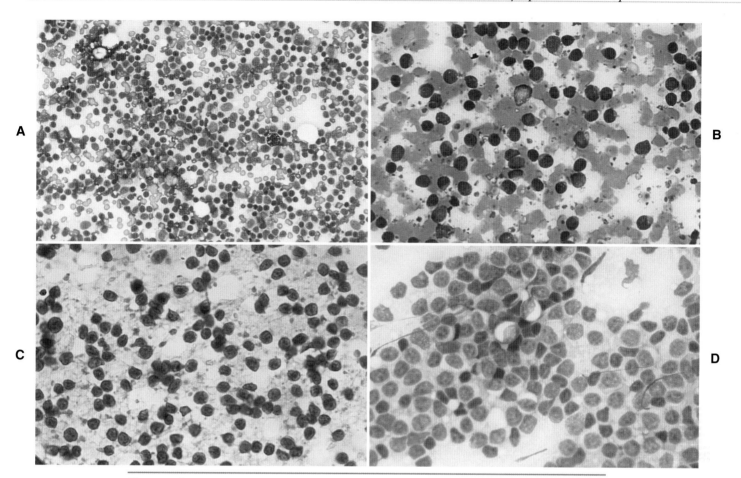

Figure 24-45 Marginal zone lymphoma. **A,** High cellularity and a single cell pattern typical of lymphoma are present in this aspirate. Although most of the neoplastic lymphocytes are rather small and homogeneous in appearance, a definite spectrum of nuclear size is apparent. Some of the larger nuclei have small but distinct nucleoli. **B,** Nuclear contours vary from round and smooth to quite irregular. The chromatin varies from finely to moderately reticulated and is uniformly dispersed. For the most part, nucleoli are not evident. Although variable from cell to cell, cytoplasm is generally quite scanty. Lymphoglandular bodies are numerous. **C,** With alcohol fixation, the nuclear membranes are more distinct, the chromatin is witnessed as finely granular and darkly stained, and nucleoli are remarkably variable. Although cytoplasm can be seen surrounding many of the nuclei, it is quite scant in volume. **D,** The neoplastic cells in this example are rather monotonous in appearance. They have small nuclei with generally smooth outlines; moderately clumped, even chromatin; inconspicuous nucleoli; and high N:C ratios. A few cells manifest greater cytoplasmic volumes. (**A, B,** and **D,** DQ; **C,** Pap)

Aspiration smears are usually extremely cellular, with a disassociated pattern of small uniform blastic cells.[11,76,77] The cells are 1.5 to two times the diameter of small mature lymphocytes, have extremely high N:C ratios, and manifest variable nuclear contours (Figure 24-47). Although the nuclei may appear round and smooth, most are quite irregular with convolutions and indentations. The chromatin is finely granular, almost powdery in consistency, and nucleoli are generally inconspicuous (Box 24-16).

The tumor cells demonstrate a thymic immunophenotype expressing CD1, TdT, CD7, and CD5, and may or may not coexpress CD3, which is a late T-cell antigen. Additionally, these cells may coexpress CD4 and CD8 on the same cell, or alternatively may lack both antigens. Lymphoblastic lymphomas rarely demonstrate B-cell differentiation and then are identical to acute lymphoblastic leukemias immunologically. These cells express CD19 and CD10 but lack SIg and CD20. Recall that acute lymphoblastic lymphomas that show SIg and CD20 are typically classified as having a Burkitt's immunophenotype (Box 24-17).

Peripheral T-Cell Lymphomas

In the REAL classification, the peripheral T-cell lymphomas (PTCLs) are those with a mature or postthymic phenotype.[44] They are subdivided into various forms. Probably the most common type to involve lymph nodes are those that are considered unspecified. They may be divided into those composed predominantly of medium-size cells, predominantly of large-size cells, and those with mixed medium and large neoplastic cells. This subclassification of the unspecified tumors has no known clinical significance.

Most of the literature that deals specifically with FNA biopsies of PTCL are case reports; in addition, a small mi-

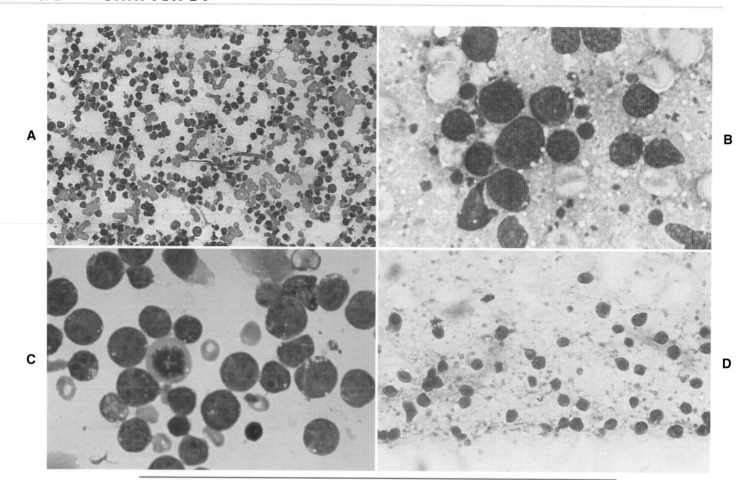

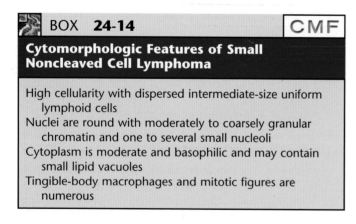

Figure 24-46   Small noncleaved cell lymphoma. A, Numerous dispersed medium-size lymphoid tumor cells with round nuclei are present in this abdominal aspirate. Degenerative changes are evident in a minority of the cells. A tingible-body macrophage is present in the center of the field. (DQ) **B** and **C,** Homogeneous-appearing lymphoblasts are characterized by moderately clumped chromatin, small but distinct nucleoli, and rounded nuclei. Cytoplasm is scant to moderate in volume and basophilic and at times contains sharply delineated vacuoles. (DQ) **D,** With alcohol fixation, the malignant cells appear even more uniform. Nuclear membranes are distinct and slightly irregular, the chromatin is clumped and dark, and small nucleoli are evident. (Pap)

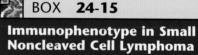

BOX 24-14	CMF

Cytomorphologic Features of Small Noncleaved Cell Lymphoma

High cellularity with dispersed intermediate-size uniform lymphoid cells
Nuclei are round with moderately to coarsely granular chromatin and one to several small nucleoli
Cytoplasm is moderate and basophilic and may contain small lipid vacuoles
Tingible-body macrophages and mitotic figures are numerous

BOX   24-15

Immunophenotype in Small Noncleaved Cell Lymphoma

Expression of surface immunoglobulin
Expression of a full complement of B-cell antigens
Expression of CD10
May coexpress CD34

nority of all lymphomas reported in large aspiration series are T-cell neoplasms. A large study was published by Katz and colleagues with 13 patients.[75] More recently, the series of Park and Kim included six PTCLs.[130] The majority of the cases from both studies had a mixed tumor cell size. Although Katz and colleagues reported hypercellular smears

in these patients, a proportion of those by Park and Kim were poorly cellular.[75,130] The smears demonstrate an intimate admixture of relatively small, medium-size, and large atypical lymphoid cells (Figures 24-48 and 24-49). The smallest tumor cells may be marginally larger than small mature-appearing lymphocytes, but they show pronounced irregularity of the nuclear contour with folds, deep indentations and protrusions, which are often better recognized with the Pap stain. The chromatin varies from finely granular to coarsely clumped with areas of parachromatin clear-

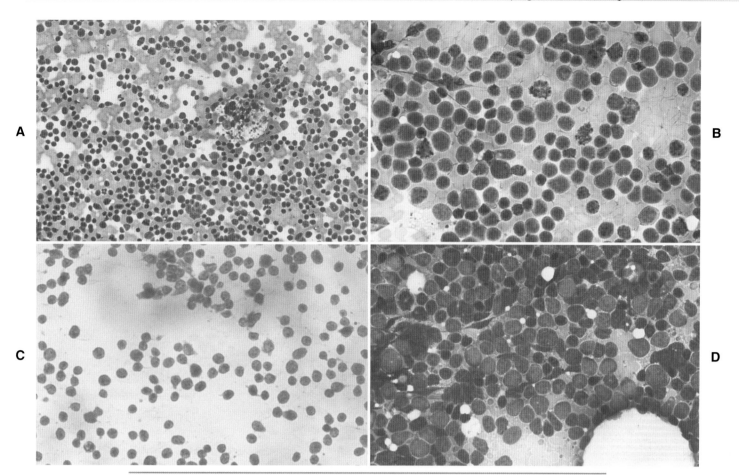

Figure 24-47   Lymphoblastic lymphoma. A, The vast majority of the sampled cells are small with solitary nuclei and extremely high N:C ratios. Their nuclei are smaller than that of the benign tingible-body macrophage. **B** and **C,** Individually dispersed small lymphoblasts are characterized by delicate nuclear membranes, very finely granular and evenly dispersed chromatin, and inapparent nucleoli. Mitotic figures are evident. Cytoplasm is difficult to discern. **D,** The velvety appearance of the chromatin is easily demonstrated in these small lymphoblasts. Again, nucleoli are not well developed and the N:C ratios are extremely high. (**A, B,** and **D,** DQ; **C,** Pap)

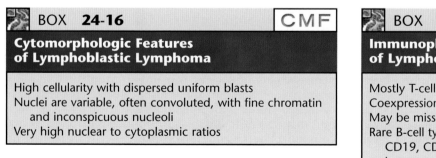

BOX **24-16**	CMF

**Cytomorphologic Features
of Lymphoblastic Lymphoma**

High cellularity with dispersed uniform blasts
Nuclei are variable, often convoluted, with fine chromatin and inconspicuous nucleoli
Very high nuclear to cytoplasmic ratios

BOX   **24-17**

**Immunophenotype
of Lymphoblastic Lymphoma**

Mostly T-cell
Coexpression of CD4 and CD8
May be missing some T-cell antigens, especially CD3
Rare B-cell type shows pre–B-cell immunophenotype with CD19, CD10, and CD34 but no CD20 or surface immunoglobulina

ing. Generally, nucleoli are poorly developed. On the other hand, the largest cells may have one or more massive nucleoli, creating a resemblance to R-S cells and their variants. These largest cells have huge nuclei that vary from smooth and round to quite irregular. Cytoplasm is variable but often more abundant than one appreciates in many of the B-cell neoplasms. In some cases, the cytoplasm is intensely basophilic. The intermediate-size lymphoma cells show fea-

tures resembling both the smaller and larger cells. Due to the admixture of cell sizes, the low magnification picture is one of heterogeneity that could superficially suggest reactive hyperplasia. However, on closer inspection, the cells are seen as highly atypical (very bizarre nuclei) and "left shifted" with small mature lymphocytes distinctly lacking.

By flow cytometry, almost all the sampled cells from unspecified PTCL show a T-cell immunophenotype. In some

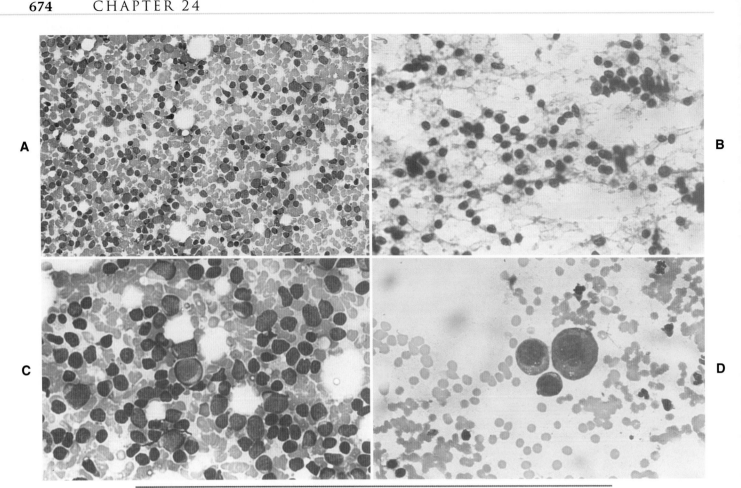

Figure 24-48 **Peripheral T-cell lymphoma, unspecified type, mixed medium and large cell variant. A** and **B,** A dissociative pattern of malignant lymphocytes is evident. They manifest a spectrum of nuclear and cellular sizes. This polymorphic appearance needs to be distinguished from that of benign lymphoid hyperplasia. **C,** This smear demonstrates a mixture of small, medium, and large malignant T-cells. The largest have finely reticulated chromatin, distinct nucleoli, and visible rims of cytoplasm. Often, the nuclei in these cells are peripherally located. The smallest neoplastic elements have condensed chromatin, inconspicuous nucleoli, and extremely scanty cytoplasm. The medium-size cells, which appear to dominate in this field, are sort of a hybrid between the two extremes; many have highly irregular nuclear outlines. **D,** In this field, only a few cells are evident, but they demonstrate striking pleomorphism. (**A, C,** and **D,** DQ; **B,** Pap)

but not all PTCLs, aberrant T-cell antigen expression may be found. Most commonly, the CD3 antigen is lacking. In other instances, a deletion of the CD7 antigen or a coexpression of CD4 and CD8 is found.

Rarely is a small cell lymphoma (or chronic lymphocytic leukemia) found, which is a T-cell type. Morphologically, it is indistinguishable from the much more common B-cell form of this neoplasm.

Mycosis fungoides and Sézary syndrome are PTCLs, which typically arise in the skin.[131] However, in many cases, the lymph nodes, especially axillary and inguinal, are involved and enlarged. In aspiration samples of lymph nodes involved by this lymphoma, the smears contain variable numbers of atypical lymphoid cells (Figure 24-50). The latter are characterized by highly irregular, convoluted (cerebriform) nuclei. The chromatin is moderately clumped and nucleoli are inconspicuous. The N:C ratios are high. However, nodes in patients with mycosis fungoides may be enlarged as a result of dermatopathic lymphadenitis and not lymphomatous in-

volvement. In dermatopathic lymphadenitis, the smears show a polymorphic picture characteristic of follicular hyperplasia plus histiocytes containing cytoplasmic melanin pigment.[132,133] Some of these histiocyte-like elements have elongated nuclei with longitudinal nuclear grooves. Such cells may also be found in smears of nodes involved by mycosis fungoides. Usually, the neoplastic T-cells are positive for CD3 and CD4 and negative for CD7 and CD8. The majority of cases in the series of Katz and colleagues expressed a similar helper phenotype.[75]

Another PTCL is a group known as the *anaplastic large cell lymphomas.* Although many of these present clinically as lymphadenopathy, others manifest first as cutaneous lesions or involvement of deep viscera. The definition of the anaplastic large cell lymphomas is still evolving.[134] The malignant cells manifest remarkable pleomorphism. Many resemble those of a large cell lymphoma, whereas others are smaller, resembling small cleaved cells and blasts. Still others are monstrous and often multinucleated; some may sim-

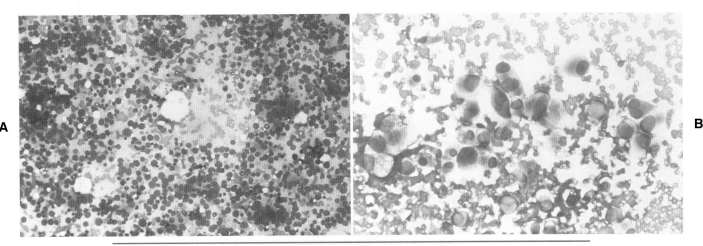

Figure 24-49 **Peripheral T-cell lymphoma, unspecified type, large cell variant.** **A,** Although a spectrum of cellular sizes is apparent in this highly cellular aspirate, a predominance of large tumor cells is evident. Although most of the neoplastic elements are individually dispersed, small pseudoaggregates of tumor cells are also evident. **B,** At higher magnification, the nuclei demonstrate irregular contours, finely reticulated chromatin, and variably distinct nucleoli. A few cells are binucleated. Most have moderate to abundant, almost clear-appearing cytoplasm. (DQ)

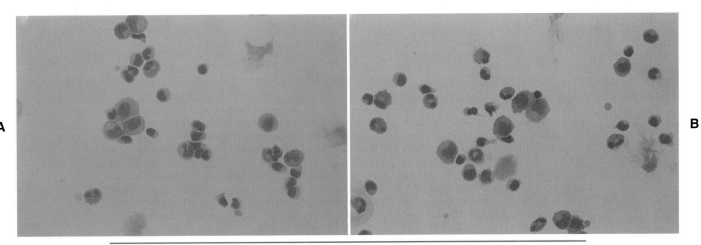

Figure 24-50 **Mycosis fungoides. A** and **B,** The small malignant lymphocytes have nuclei, which, although relatively uniform in maximal dimension, are highly variable in shape. Some appear to be round and smooth, whereas others have marked indentations, folds, and convolutions. The chromatin is clumped and nucleoli are not evident. (DQ)

ulate R-S cells. Nucleoli may or may not be prominent. Histologically, the tumor cells may resemble metastatic carcinoma in their pattern of lymph node involvement. However, in aspiration smears, a dissociated pattern is apparent, and pleomorphism is usually well developed.[135-140] The neoplastic cells are consistently positive for CD30 (and negative for CD15). Most instances of nodal anaplastic large cell lymphoma are associated with a specific reciprocal translocation between chromosomes 2 and 5. The majority of anaplastic large cell lymphomas are T-cell in type, but approximately 10% to 15% have a null cell phenotype. It is now thought that they are never of B-cell derivation. It is important to recognize that these neoplastic cells may be positive for epithelial membrane antigen.

Aspiration smears are usually highly cellular and show striking pleomorphism (Figures 24-51 and 24-52). Many neoplastic cells are huge with highly irregular nuclear contours and/or multinucleation. Prominent nucleoli are another morphologic hallmark. Somewhat incongruously, a small cell variant exists.[141] Although in histologic sections the neoplastic cells may appear cohesive, in FNA biopsies they are usually individually dispersed. Rarely, large numbers of neutrophils dominate the smears (see Figure 24-52).[140] A proteinaceous watery background is evident. Lymphoglandular bodies are often conspicuously absent.

Another variant of PTCL is referred to as *adult T-cell leukemia/lymphoma*. Although it is rare in the United States, it is more commonly seen in Asian countries. It is thought to be related to infection of T-cells by the human T-lymphotrophic virus-1. Smears contain a dispersed polymorphic mixture of small bland to large atypical forms with bizarre multilobated nuclei resembling clover leafs with coarse chromatin and prominent nucleoli (Figure 24-53).[142,143] Cytoplasm is typi-

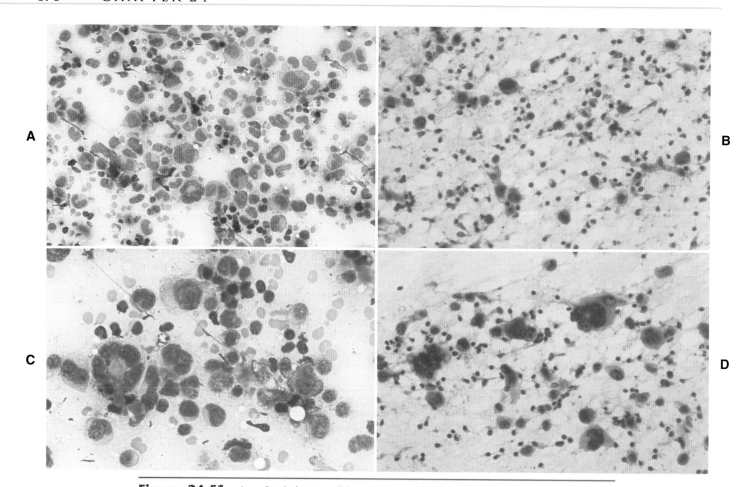

Figure 24-51 Anaplastic large cell lymphoma. **A** and **B,** Marked pleomorphism characterizes the low-power magnifications of aspirates of two different examples of this T-cell lymphoma. Neoplastic elements range from small cells with solitary round nuclei and high N:C ratios to huge multinucleated tumor giant cells. The latter has moderate to voluminous cytoplasm, which contains one or more hyperchromatic nuclei. In the largest nuclei, the chromatin is relatively finely reticulated and nucleoli are often prominent. A minority of the neoplastic cells shows the characteristic "wreath-arrangement" of the nuclei. **C,** A multinucleated tumor giant cell with a peripheral ring or wreath arrangement of the nuclei is present. Striking variability in tumor cell size is readily apparent. **D,** These same features are seen as in **C.** In addition, nuclear hyperchromasia is obvious. (**A** and **C,** DQ; **B** and **D,** Pap)

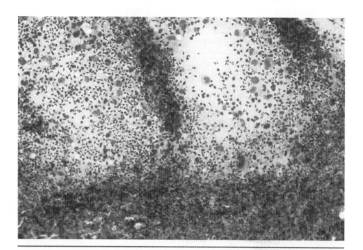

Figure 24-52 Neutrophil-rich anaplastic large cell lymphoma. Although obviously malignant tumor cells are present, the predominant cell in this specimen is the benign neutrophil. In other portions of this sample, the neoplastic elements were obscured by the inflammatory cell infiltrate. (DQ)

cally deeply basophilic and vacuolated. Plasmacytoid cells are also present.

Metastatic Neoplasms

The use of FNA biopsy of both superficial and deeply situated enlarged lymph nodes to diagnose metastatic tumors is widely practiced. Several authors have published their experiences in this setting.* Metastatic carcinoma is the most common diagnosis rendered on aspirated nodes in most institutions. This procedure provides rapid results, is minimally invasive in patients who are often quite sick or even terminal, and is inexpensive.

For example, Steel and colleagues reported their results in lymph node FNA biopsies in more than 1100 patients.[5] More than 80% of the malignant cytologic diagnoses were metastatic carcinoma or melanoma. The site most likely to contain cancer (85%) was the supraclavicular region. Their

---

*References 2, 3, 5, 11, 32, and 33.

diagnostic accuracy was 96% in carcinomas and 100% in melanomas; their rare false-negative specimens were thought to be the result of sampling errors. Of the 215 benign enlarged nodes, three false-positive and seven suspicious diagnoses were rendered. The suspicious diagnoses represented examples of granulomatous inflammation and an epidermal inclusion cyst. All three false-positive specimens were benign lymphoid hyperplasia mistaken for non-Hodgkin's lymphomas.

Cervin and colleagues retrospectively analyzed 152 FNA biopsies of supraclavicular lymph nodes (Virchow's node).[33] Two thirds of the patients had a malignant diagnosis. The left-sided nodes were involved more often by tumor than were the right nodes. Malignant neoplasms arising in the breast, lungs, and head and neck regions showed no difference in laterality of spread. However, 84% of all metastatic pelvic cancers and 100% primary abdominal neoplasms metastasized to the left supraclavicular nodes. Of the cancers, 10% represented lymphoreticular malignancies. More recently, Nasuti and colleagues and Jaffer and Zakowski examined supraclavicular and axillary aspirates, respectively.[144,145]

One important consideration is the presence of a small cell malignancy in FNA biopsy of lymph nodes. Careful scrutiny of the clinical data is essential. It is important to know the patient's age, the history of a previously diagnosed cancer, the site of the aspirated node, and a history of tobacco usage. In all age groups, non-Hodgkin's lymphomas need to be considered. In children, the most common nonlymphoreticular malignancy to metastasize to lymph nodes is neuroblastoma. The small tumor cells manifest varying degrees of intercellular cohesion, with the formation of small spherical aggregates, broad sheets, and pseudorosettes.[146] In addition, larger neoplastic cells representing maturing neuroblasts and ganglion cells may be present. Characteristically, the smear background contains a filamentous material that corresponds to neuropil.

The most common nonlymphoreticular small cell malignancy in adults is metastatic small cell undifferentiated (oat cell) carcinoma of bronchogenic origin. Many of these specimens are transbronchial FNA biopsy of hilar nodes. Nodal aspirates contain obviously malignant cells, both singly and clustered. The latter usually manifest nuclear molding, in which adjacent nuclei are compressed against one another. The carcinoma cells have angulated nuclear contours, darkly stained coarse chromatin, very high N:C ratios, and possibly minute nucleoli. Crushed nuclear debris and strands of smeared chromatin are usually prominent. Characteristically, small cell carcinomas are positive for synaptophysin and cytokeratin and negative for CD45.

In FNA biopsy of metastatic squamous cell carcinomas that contain tumor cells with obviously malignant nuclei, the diagnosis is almost always straightforward. However, metastases of squamous cell carcinoma in nodes may undergo extensive necrosis and keratinization and may be associated with neutrophils or a granulomatous reaction (see Table 24-1). This is especially common in nodes in the head and neck region. Thus, viable neoplastic cells may form only a thin rim near the periphery of the node. Aspiration smears may consist predominantly of anucleate squamous cells presenting as polygonal masses of cytoplasm; with the Pap stain, they often have an orangeophilic appearance, whereas they have a sky blue color with the Romanowsky stains. Centrally, empty holes may mark the grave site of

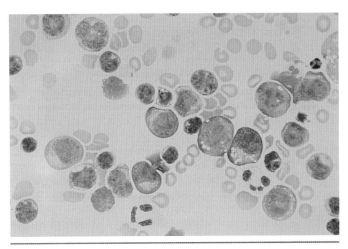

Figure 24-53 **Adult T-cell leukemia/lymphoma.** This aspirate is characterized largely by huge malignant lymphoid cells with solitary nuclei. The contours of the latter vary from rather smooth to markedly irregular. The chromatin varies from moderately to coarsely clumped and nucleoli are prominent. Some of the latter are large with irregular contours, whereas multiple nucleoli characterize other cells. Cytoplasm is moderate to voluminous, basophilic, and distinctly vacuolated. Note how large the cells are in comparison with the neutrophils. (DQ)

the malignant nuclei. In this setting, the differential diagnosis includes benign congenital and acquired squamous-lined cysts, including branchial cleft cysts.[147]

Melanomas often enter the differential diagnosis of dispersed cell patterns in FNA biopsy of nodes. Melanomas may feature bizarre nuclear pleomorphism, numerous nuclear pseudoinclusions, and cytoplasmic pigment. However, hemorrhage may produce pigment in tumor cells of other types of malignancy. Generally, the diagnosis can be rendered by demonstrating S-100 protein and HMB-45 in tumor cells immunocytochemically.

In women with carcinoma of the breast, the single most crucial predictor of clinical outcome is the status of their ipsilateral axillary lymph nodes—that is, are the nodes positive or negative for metastatic carcinoma.[147] The traditional manner in which the axillary nodes have been evaluated is through a routine axillary nodal dissection that accompanies other surgery, most commonly lumpectomy or mastectomy. Perhaps the most discussed topic with regard to treatment of breast cancer within the last several years had been the evaluation of sentinel lymph nodes.[148] In theory and usually in practice, the sentinel lymph node is the axillary lymph node that is the first one to receive the lymphatic drainage from the region of the breast tumor and thus the most likely one to harbor a metastasis. In practice, this lymph node is identified by injecting the region of the tumor with either a dye or radiolabeled particles, usually technetium 99m (^{99m}Tc). This permits the surgeon to identify and excise one or more sentinel nodes from patients for extensive histologic evaluation for the presence or absence of metastatic carcinoma. It is thought that the sentinel node generally reflects the status of the axillary lymph node contents overall. Thus, in a patient with a positive sentinel lymph node, the patient returns to the operating room for a second procedure, namely a complete axillary nodal dissection. Conversely, if the sentinel lymph node is negative for metastases, then the axillary dissection is not performed. Thus, in a significant proportion of women (approximately 40% of all women have a positive sentinel lymph node), the morbidity associated with axillary dissection is eliminated. It is important to recognize, however, that sentinel lymph nodes are not 100% accurate in predicting the status of all axillary nodes; skip metastases may occur in between less than 1% and 5% of all patients.

The intraoperative evaluation of sentinel lymph nodes in women with carcinoma of the breast may be considered a major step forward in their care.[149,150] This is predicated on the assumption that the assessment method is highly accurate. If the sentinel node is found to contain metastatic carcinoma intraoperatively, then the surgeon can proceed with the axillary dissection immediately during a single procedure instead of waiting for the results of a permanent histologic evaluation. Thus, the patient is spared a second visit to the operating room. Extremely high levels of diagnostic specificity are required in that a false-positive intraoperative diagnosis would lead potentially to an unnecessary dissection with its associated negative side effects. Recently, the College of America of Pathologists has recommended that if intraoperative evaluation of sentinel lymph nodes are to be performed, then touch preparation cytology is preferred over frozen sections.[151] The reported levels of diagnostic sensitivity for touch preparations of sentinel lymph nodes in patients with carcinoma of the breast has shown a tremendous range from about 30% to 96%. On the other hand, with rare exceptions, the reported levels of diagnostic specificity hover around 99% to 100%.

Sentinel lymph nodes are also widely used in patients with known malignant melanomas to determine whether a complete regional lymph node dissection will be performed. Again, if the sentinel lymph node contains metastatic melanoma, then additional surgery is performed, whereas if the sentinel lymph node is negative for metastasis, the patient is spared a lymphadenectomy.[167]

Sentinel lymph node mapping has also been used for patients with gastrointestinal carcinomas. However, the rationale behind sentinel lymph node mapping is different from that of either breast carcinoma or melanoma. The greatest use of sentinel lymph node mapping in patients with gastrointestinal malignancies is not to predict the status of the draining lymph nodes or to limit a lymphadenectomy but rather to identify those lymph nodes that are most apt to contain metastases.[152] Once identified, this lymph node(s) can be more intensively evaluated by numerous histologic sections and immunohistochemistry than is practical for all excised lymph nodes.[152] In this setting, although intraoperative cytology or frozen sections can be used, it is less clinically imperative than with melanoma or carcinoma of the breast.

 SPLEEN

Normally, the spleen lies in the left upper abdominal quadrant and generally is not palpable. However, splenomegaly, or enlargement of the spleen, may result from numerous conditions that systemically involve the lymphoreticular system. In many instances, the splenomegaly can be readily explained on the basis of known clinical data such as in patients who have hereditary spherocytosis, idiopathic

thrombocytopenic purpura, and infectious mononucleosis. In this country, the spleen is often involved because of changes in normal blood flow; this occurs most commonly in patients with cirrhosis and portal hypertension. In such patients, FNA biopsy would not be used for diagnosis. However, some authors have advocated splenic FNA biopsy to render primary diagnoses or to confirm the clinical impression of splenomegaly resulting from a number of conditions including amyloidosis and leishmaniasis.[153-158]

A less frequent indication for splenic FNA biopsy is the evaluation of a radiographically detected mass lesion or lesions within the spleen. This would be especially likely in this country in centers treating large numbers of patients with malignancies.[159-161]

In many parts of the world, splenic FNA biopsy enjoys relatively widespread usage. However, in the United States, this procedure appears to be underused. One possible explanation for this is that clinicians simply do not know in a given patient that the spleen is involved by a mass lesion. In other individuals with obvious clinical splenomegaly, the clinical picture has explained the cause of splenic enlargement and thus an FNA biopsy certainly would not be needed. However, we believe that a major reason is a fear of precipitating a serious hemorrhagic event subsequent to puncture of the spleen. As discussed later in this chapter, a review of the literature demonstrates that this is unfounded.

Normal Cytology

The smear cellularity is variable from specimen to specimen; one may also note a predominance of either red pulp elements or white pulp components. The red pulp is characterized in smears by numerous erythrocytes, occasional small lymphoid cells, plasma cells, platelet clumps, endothelial cells, and histiocytes (Figure 24-54).[153,155] The cytoplasm of the latter cells should not contain obvious phagocytized material.

The white pulp is represented by lymphoid elements with two patterns of presentation.[153,155] A proportion of the lymphocytes is dispersed as individual cells in flat monolayers. This population is polymorphic, similar to that of benign lymph nodes, although a greater proportion of immature-appearing lymphocytes is present. The second manifestation represents sampling of the periarteriolar lymphoid sheath. In smears, this occurs as three-dimensional cellular aggregates of lymphocytes that are associated with capillaries or other small vessels. These endothelial-lined structures may appear to penetrate and travel through the lymphoid clusters or abut tangentially along one outer edge. In the condition known as *white pulp hyperplasia*, which may be either a focal or diffuse process, the smears would be expected to be dominated by lymphocytes derived from the white pulp. However, it is our opinion that this would be difficult indeed to distinguish from normal.

If a smear consists solely of normal-appearing blood, then the aspirate should be considered inadequate or nonrepresentative of the spleen.

Infections

Malaria is the result of infection by one of the four species of the intraerythrocytic parasite Plasmodium. Infection by any four species may result in a long-standing moderate

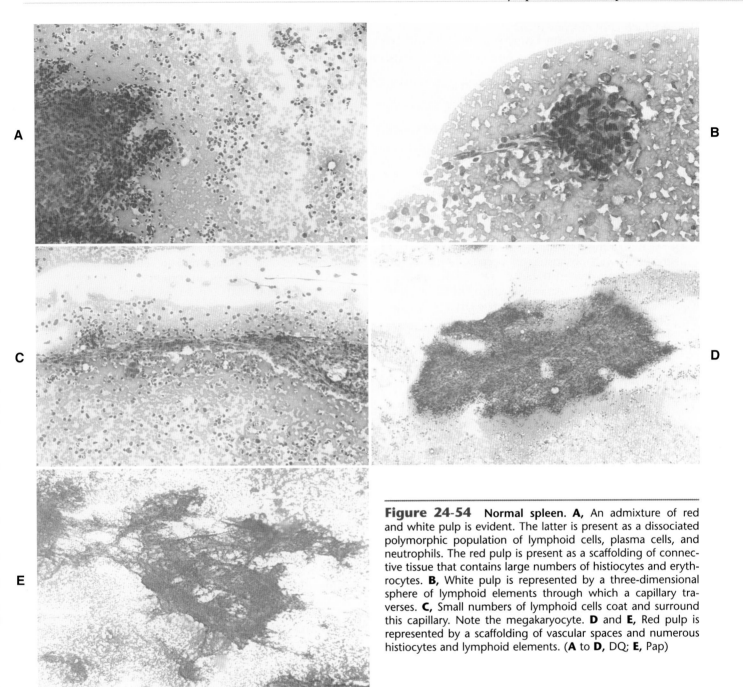

Figure 24-54 Normal spleen. A, An admixture of red and white pulp is evident. The latter is present as a dissociated polymorphic population of lymphoid cells, plasma cells, and neutrophils. The red pulp is present as a scaffolding of connective tissue that contains large numbers of histiocytes and erythrocytes. **B,** White pulp is represented by a three-dimensional sphere of lymphoid elements through which a capillary traverses. **C,** Small numbers of lymphoid cells coat and surround this capillary. Note the megakaryocyte. **D** and **E,** Red pulp is represented by a scaffolding of vascular spaces and numerous histiocytes and lymphoid elements. (**A** to **D,** DQ; **E,** Pap)

splenomegaly. In addition, infection by *Plasmodium falciparum* may result in an acute splenomegaly associated with a sequestration crisis. The authors have never personally seen a splenic FNA biopsy to diagnose malaria. Histologically, the spleen is enlarged mostly from an expansion of the histiocytic component of the red pulp as these cells attempt to phagocytize infected RBCs. The smears reflect this process by being dominated by enlarged histiocytes, the cytoplasm of which may contain the parasitized erythrocytes and/or a dark brown to black pigment, which represents a breakdown product of hemoglobin. The morphology of the intracytoplasmic parasite would depend on both the specific species and the various stages in the life cycle of this organism.

Although other species are occasionally implicated, *Leishmania donovani* is the major cause of visceral leishma-

niasis (Kala-azar). This disease is endemic in specific portions of the world and in particular eastern India, Pakistan, the Mediterranean basin, the Middle East, and parts of Africa, notably Kenya, Ethiopia, and Sudan. Occasional cases occur in various parts of Latin America. Kala-azar is seen only very rarely in the United States when an immigrant or a traveler from one of the endemic areas presents with clinical disease. On physical examination, the clinical hallmarks are enlargement of the spleen and liver. In endemic areas, FNA biopsy of the spleen is considered by many to be the diagnostic test of choice. In this setting, FNA biopsy of the spleen may result in a diagnosis in more than 95% of all patients.

The cytomorphologic features of visceral leishmaniasis has been well described by Haque and colleagues.[157] Splenic smears contain variable numbers of histiocytes, the cytoplasm of which contains one or more phagocytized organisms. In humans the parasite consists of the intracellular amastigote. These are ovoid structures that measure between 2 and 3 microns in maximal dimension. They contain a solitary nucleus that occupies approximately one half of the area of the organism. These parasites are best seen with Romanowsky-stained material. The cytoplasm of the amastigote contains a distinct rodlike structure, the kinetoplast, which corresponds to mitochondria. This latter structure is important to recognize in that it helps distinguish *L. donovani* from *Histoplasma,* which are otherwise quite similar in appearance.

Haque and colleagues reported a series of 210 splenic aspirates from children clinically suspected of having Kala-azar.[157] Of these, 147 were diagnostic for visceral leishmaniasis. Of the remaining 63 samples, 41 were negative for the organism and 22 were unsatisfactory because of scant cellularity. These authors demonstrated a direct relationship between the density of the parasites within the smears and the number of histiocytes aspirated.[157] The latter were larger than normal and often demonstrated irregular cell contours. These histiocytes often contained more than 10 amastigotes within their cytoplasm. In specimens with numerous parasites, the smears showed almost no evidence of white pulp lymphocytes; this is not surprising because Kala-azar is a red pulp disorder.

As discussed previously in this chapter, infectious mononucleosis usually is the result of an infection of B lymphocytes by EBV. More than half of all patients with infectious mononucleosis have clinically apparent splenomegaly. A major complication of this infection is splenic rupture, which may be associated with trauma or may occur spontaneously. Histologically, the white pulp is usually markedly expanded with marked polymorphism of the cells, similar to the histomorphology in lymph nodes. In an occasional patient, however, the white pulp is markedly atrophic in extent. The aspiration cytomorphology of infectious mononucleosis has been previously described in this chapter and would be expected to show the same picture in splenic aspirates. Recall that the lymphoid infiltrate may include benign cells that resemble R-S cells. In contrast with infectious mononucleosis, which produces a diffuse, uniform splenomegaly, however, distinct tumor nodules are typically in Hodgkin's disease. These may be palpable or detected by abdominal radiographic procedures. The authors have not yet personally experienced a splenic aspirate for the diagnosis of infectious mononucleosis.

Bacterial abscesses are clinically uncommon entities that may be solitary or multiple. In the authors' experience, FNA biopsy is used only rarely in an attempt to diagnose a splenic abscess. An example of aspergillosis-associated abscess has been seen in a patient with an underlying known T-cell lymphoma.[159] In addition to causative organisms, the smears contain numerous neutrophils that are not expected in aspirates of other splenic conditions.

Infection-associated hemophagocytosis syndromes result in clinical splenomegaly with some frequency. Although such infections may be the result of various types of organisms, viruses are most often the guilty culprit. Histologically, the red pulp is greatly expanded by histiocytes with prominent intracytoplasmic erythrocytes. These cells dominate aspiration smears. A similar aspiration picture could be seen if the spleen were sampled in certain he-

molytic anemias such as hereditary spherocytosis. Depending on whether the viral infection has stimulated or depleted the body's lymphoid cells, the smears may or may not contain evidence of white pulp. These smears may also contain normoblasts related to myeloid metaplasia. In this particular setting, these smears may also contain immature leukocytes and megakaryocytes. The latter especially could be confused with malignant cells.

Accumulation of Abnormal Materials

Primary or generalized amyloidosis is an idiopathic condition in which deposition amyloid protein is found in various organs. Most patients are middle-age or older adults who often present with nonspecific symptoms such as fatigue or weakness. Although the spleen often histologically demonstrates deposits of amyloid, clinical splenomegaly occurs in less than 10% of all patients.

In smears, amyloid appears as rather well-delineated masses of dense homogeneous material.[156] With the Romanowsky stains, it appears reddish-purple, whereas it is variably pale green to pink to orange with the Pap preparation. Although the edges of these clumps may appear fuzzy, usually they have sharply defined outlines. With the Congo red stain, the material is distinctly red or dark pink in color. With such slides, the directly aspirated material may be examined with polarized light and show its classic apple green color. In some instances, the fragments of amyloid protein are surrounded by lymphoid cells but often are totally acellular.

In 1974, Pasternack published a series of patients evaluated by splenic FNA biopsy for the diagnosis of amyloidosis.[156] In all 18 patients proven to have this disease, the smears were positive. In that author's hands, splenic aspiration had a high level of sensitivity for the diagnosis of amyloidosis compared with both rectal and renal biopsies. His study also included control patients (being evaluated for proteinuria), none of whom showed amyloid in their splenic aspirates.[156] Only rarely has amyloidosis of the spleen been described in other published series. Of the aspirates in the study from the M.D. Anderson Hospital, 2% were positive for amyloid.[161] Two other large series of aspirates for the investigation of splenomegaly with a combination of 205 FNA biopsies did not show a single example of amyloid in the smears.[154,155]

Infrequently, FNA biopsy has been used to document a storage disease resulting from an inborn error of metabolism.[153] In this setting, the Romanowsky stains would certainly be preferred over the Pap stain. This is because the engorged histiocytes in Gaucher's disease have a characteristic appearance that is appreciated in air-dried preparations. The cytoplasm has a reticulated or wrinkled tissue paper appearance. In many of the other storage diseases, the histiocytes possess a less specific foamy vacuolization.

Sarcoidosis

Sarcoidosis is a systemic disorder characterized by the presence of noncaseating granulomas in various organs. Although children may be affected, sarcoidosis is most commonly diagnosed in young adults. The majority of all patients are asymptomatic with the disease often first being suggested by an abnormal chest x-ray, which typically demonstrates bilateral hilar lymphadenopathy often associated with enlargement of the peritracheal lymph nodes. Clinical splenomegaly occurs in up to 10% of all involved individuals.

Depending on the extent of splenic involvement by sarcoid, the smears may be poorly cellular and contain predominantly epithelioid cell granulomas or may be quite cellular with components of both red and white pulp with only rare scattered granulomas. The granulomas are typically tightly aggregated clusters of characteristic epithelioid cells as described earlier in this chapter. They are characterized by solitary elongated nuclei with delicate membranes; very fine, pale chromatin; and minute nucleoli. They may show the characteristic indentation along their long axis. Multinucleated inflammatory giant cells and small lymphocytes may also be evident. The authors personally have not seen a splenic aspirate diagnostic of sarcoidosis. Taavitsainen and colleagues reported a series of splenic FNA biopsy in 101 patients who clinically were potentially thought to have sarcoid.[158] Of this initial group, 79 patients were subsequently shown to have sarcoid. In these, FNA biopsies demonstrated granulomous inflammation in 19 (24%). However, of the 19 individuals with splenic sarcoid demonstrated in the smears, most (84%) had a normal-size spleen as witnessed by ultrasound. These authors hypothesized that the diagnostic yield might be higher in patients with clinical splenomegaly.[158] It should be recalled that sarcoidosis occurs with a relatively high frequency in the Scandinavian nations. In a series by Lishner and colleagues, one patient had nonnecrotizing granulomas in the splenic aspirate and was subsequently shown to have sarcoid.[154] Small numbers of individuals in two other series demonstrated granulomatous inflammation, but the authors did not specifically ascribe this to sarcoidosis.[155,161]

Cysts

Cysts of the spleen are rare entities that clinically are most commonly found in children and young adults. Although many of these are completely asymptomatic, they may present clinically as a palpable mass in the left upper quadrant. Cysts may be divided into those related to parasitic infections and those unrelated to such infestations. The latter may be subdivided into true and false cysts. The former is lined by epithelium, whereas the latter consists of a dense fibrous wall that is often calcified but is not lined in any portion by epithelium. The pseudocysts account for at least 80% for the nonparasitic cystic lesions of the spleen. Histologically, the true cysts are lined by either a flat mesothelium-like cell layer or by stratified squamous epithelium that may be keratinized.

The authors have never seen an FNA biopsy of a primary splenic cyst. Furthermore, only rarely have such specimens been reported. Nerlich and Permanetter have described the FNA biopsies of two true (epidermoid) cysts.[162] In both patients, the smears were dominated by squamous epithelial cells, some showing pyknosis, without any evidence of dysplasia or malignancy (nuclear atypia). In addition, anucleated squames and scattered histiocytes were evident.

It is thought that the pseudocysts may result from traumatic damage to the spleen resulting in hematoma formation, which is walled off by fibrous connective tissue and in which the blood is variably resorbed. The authors are un-

aware of a report of an FNA biopsy of this entity. These smears would be expected to consist largely of lysed blood, hemosiderin, and histiocytes.

Vascular Neoplasms

The single most common primary neoplasm in the spleen is the hemangioma. Most patients are asymptomatic, but an occasional individual presents clinically as a result of either abdominal pain or a mass. Histologically, most splenic hemangiomas are cavernous in type. The authors have not yet seen and are unaware of any reported examples of splenic hemangiomas in FNA biopsies.

The littoral cell angioma is an endothelial proliferation that is specific for the spleen. In contrast with usual hemangiomas, patients present with splenomegaly. In histologic sections, vascular spaces are lined by endothelial cells with abundant cytoplasm and a cuboidal to columnar configuration. Although the nuclei may be larger than expected in usual hemangiomas, they are completely bland and benign in appearance. These plump endothelial cells may pile up on one another to form papillary structures, which project into vascular spaces. By immunohistochemistry, the neoplastic cells coexpress endothelial and histiocytic markers. We are unaware of a single example of a littoral cell angioma in a FNA biopsy.

The splenic hamartoma is an extremely uncommon and usually asymptomatic mass lesion of the spleen. These hamartomas occur as well-delineated but unencapsulated masses that typically bulge from the cut surface. Histologically, they consist of normal-appearing red pulp—that is, a proliferation of splenic cords and sinuses are found without any intervening white pulp. Kumar has reported four examples of splenic hamartomas occurring in three individuals in FNA biopsies.[163] The smears contained both individual cells and aggregates that varied from flat clusters to papillary-like structures. The individual cells had solitary round or ovoid nuclei that were darkly stained and scant cytoplasm, resulting in high N:C ratios. Large nucleoli were evident in a few of the aspirated cells. From the illustrations of Kumar, it is believed that these cells probably are largely endothelial in nature but may also include histiocytes.[163] A word of warning may be prudent here in that Kumar reported that all four aspirates were misinterpreted as metastatic neoplasms.[163] The smears contained a bloody background. Superficially, these smears may resemble those derived from a hemangioma, although the overall smear cellularity appears to be higher with the hamartoma.

Excluding lymphomas, the most common malignancy to arise in the spleen is angiosarcoma. Patients with primary splenic angiosarcoma often present with abdominal pain and splenomegaly; prognosis is dismal. FNA biopsies of angiosarcoma of the spleen would be suspected to resemble angiosarcomas aspirated in other body sites, as described in Chapter 28.

Malignant Lymphomas

Far and away, malignant lymphoreticular neoplasms are the most common primary cancers of the spleen. In addition, essentially any type of lymphoma may secondarily involve the spleen and often do; most splenic lymphomas are not primary in this organ. In general, most low-grade lymphomas composed of small lymphocytes have a diffuse involvement of the spleen, whereas the large cell non-Hodgkin's lymphomas and Hodgkin's disease typically occur as one or more tumoral masses.

The aspiration cytomorphology of these lymphomas will resemble those as described earlier in this chapter. In patients with known, previously characterized malignant lymphomas, immunocytochemistry is generally not necessary. On the other hand, when attempting to render an initial diagnosis of lymphoma with a splenic aspirate, immunophenotyping along with cytomorphology is often imperative.

Two specific forms of primary splenic lymphoma appear to be unique to this organ.[164,165] The first of these is the splenic marginal zone lymphoma, which is composed of small to moderately size lymphoid elements characterized by minimal nuclear pleomorphism and rather voluminous cytoplasm.[164] These are B-cell neoplasms that are typically negative for CD5. The second, hepatosplenic T-cell lymphoma, is even rarer.[165] This neoplasm typically occurs in young individuals with a marked male predominance as hepatosplenomegaly. Histologically, the spleen is diffusely infiltrated, especially the red pulp, by moderately sized to rather large malignant lymphocytes. The latter are characterized by solitary round to irregular nuclei with vesicular chromatin and abundant pale cytoplasm. By immunophenotyping, these cells are typically negative for both CD4 and CD8.[165] This is because this neoplasm consists of gamma/delta T-cells. The authors are unaware of any descriptions of FNA biopsies of these two primary splenic lymphomas.

Leukemias

Although many leukemias may infiltrate splenic parenchyma, a complete review of leukemic processes is beyond the scope of this text.[155] However, hairy cell leukemia is briefly described because splenomegaly is an intregal component of its clinical picture and may be the dominant attribute. However, lymphadenopathy is not a major component of this disease in which most patients are middle-age or older adults with a male predominance. Pancytopenia is characteristic, but the peripheral blood often does not have a leukemic picture. Histologically, the tumor cells concentrate in the red pulp.

FNA biopsies yield cellular specimens with rather monomorphic, medium-size lymphoid cells. The cells have moderate to abundant, variably basophilic cytoplasm. Very characteristically, the cell borders are frayed and may show long fingerlike projections. Nuclear contours are round to ovoid, often with small focal indentations. Their chromatin is finely granulated and evenly dispersed; nucleoli may be present but are inconspicuous.

A helpful diagnostic feature of the malignant cells is that their cytoplasm is tartrate-resistant, acid phosphatase (TRAP) positive. As demonstrated by Moriarty and colleagues, TRAP positivity may be demonstrated directly in splenic aspiration smears, confirming the diagnosis.[160] Hairy cell leukemias are B-cell proliferations that are positive for SIg, CD25, and CD11c; they are CD5 negative.

The somewhat related chronic myeloproliferative diseases are a group of related disorders that have in common the proliferation of a neoplastic pluripotential stem cell that is capable of producing granulocytic, erythroid, and megakaryocytic cell lines. Clinically, the spleen is invariably involved and in some patients, splenomegaly is marked. In most patients, the diagnosis is formed by a combination of clinical, peripheral blood, and bone marrow findings, and therefore the spleen is only rarely aspirated. The smear picture includes varying proportions of erythrocytic, segmented leukocytic, and megakaryocytic precursors and also more mature forms. The major diagnostic pitfalls include misinterpreting large, bizarre-appearing megakaryocytes as malignant cells derived from nonhematopoietic neoplasms and Hodgkin's disease. The megakaryocytes are characterized by multiple and/or very highly lobulated nuclei with moderately reticulated, dark chromatin and abundant cytoplasm. With the Pap stain, the chromatin may appear homogeneous and extremely hyperchromatic. As might be expected, the cells are more accurately evaluated with the Romanowsky preparations. The periphery of megakaryocytes and some of their earlier forms may possess ruffled cell borders associated with platelet formation. Another potential problem consists of misinterpreting blasts as neoplastic cells derived from malignant lymphomas. This can be overcome by recognizing that the most primitive cells form part of a spectrum of leukocytic differentiation that include eosinophils, which are easily recognized by their cytoplasmic granules.[153]

Metastases

In clinical practice, splenic metastases of nonlymporeticular neoplasms may go unrecognized. In part, this may result from the fact that the metastases do not cause splenomegaly. In other situations, metastases to other sites have already been recognized and documented, so the spleen is "ignored." Relatively small metastases may not be recognized unless the spleen is specifically studied by radiographic methods.

Metastases from various types of carcinomas have been reported infrequently in the literature in splenic FNA biopsies.[154,155,159,161] From the literature, which may not be a true reflection of real life, an overrepresentation in splenic FNA biopsy of ovarian carcinomas and testicular germ cell neoplasms is noted. Metastatic melanomas and sarcomas have also been reported in these samples.

Accuracy

To say the least, it is difficult to state with certainty the overall accuracy of FNA biopsy of the spleen. In large part, this is because of relatively few substantial published series. Second, some series do not include patients with malignant neoplasms. In a study by Caraway and Fanning, 50 patients underwent splenic FNA biopsy in a large cancer center.[161] No false-positive diagnoses were found for a diagnostic specificity of 100%. Excluding the six specimens that were considered nondiagnostic because of scant cellularity, the diagnostic sensitivity was approximately 96%. This series included four aspirates that were suspicious for malignant lymphoma. Two of the four individuals underwent splenectomy that showed lymphoma; the other two, who had histories of a prior diagnosis of lymphoma, were maintained on their therapy.[161]

An even larger series was published by Zeppa and colleagues with rather good results.[155] In cases of splenic aspirates that were followed by histologic confirmation, the levels of diagnostic sensitivity and specificity for neoplasia were 86% and 98%, respectively. The latter figure incorporates a false suspicious diagnosis as a statistical abnormality.

Complications

As stated at the beginning of this section on the spleen, it was the authors' belief that a major reason that some practitioners do not use splenic FNA biopsy is because of the fear of precipitating a serious bleeding problem. In most published series, investigators shy away from aspirating the spleen in patients with abnormal coagulation parameters. In the series by Zeppa and colleagues, two patients had serious splenic bleeding after FNA biopsy out of the total 140 patients; one of these led to a splenectomy.[155] In the smaller series by Silverman (11 patients), one patient had a significant hemorrhage necessitating a splenectomy.[159] By incorporating the data from 10 published series, a total of 614 patients who underwent splenic FNA biopsy can be evaluated.[154-163] This yields a rate of significant hemorrhage requiring splenectomy of 0.3%. Caraway and Fanning reported a single instance of pneumothorax which cleared spontaneously.[161] Thus, the authors believe that in patients with no obvious clotting abnormalities, splenic FNA biopsy should be considered a safe procedure that may be used when it is necessary to document disease within the spleen.

References

1. Frable WJ, Kardos TF. Fine needle aspiration biopsy. Applications in the diagnosis of lymphoproliferative diseases. Am J Surg Pathol 1989; 12(Suppl 1):62-72.
2. Cardillo MR. Fine-needle aspiration cytology of superficial lymph nodes. Diagn Cytopathol 1989; 5:166.
3. Gupta A, et al. Reliability and limitations of fine needle aspiration cytology of lymphadenopathies: an analysis of 1,261 cases. Acta Cytol 1991; 35:777.
4. Perkins SL, Segal GH, Kjoldsberg CR. Work-up of lymphadenopathy in children. Sem Diagn Pathology 1995; 12:284.
5. Steel BL, Schwartz MR, Ramzy I. Fine needle aspiration biopsy in the diagnosis of lymphadenopathy in 1,103 patients: role, limitations and analysis of diagnostic pitfalls. Acta Cytol 1995; 39:76.
6. Leong A SY, Stevens M. Fine-needle aspiration biopsy for the diagnosis of lymphoma: a perspective. Diagn Cytopathol 1996; 15:352-357.
7. Carter T, Feldman P, Innes D, et al. The role of FNA cytology in the diagnosis of lymphoma. Acta Cytol 1988; 32:848-853.
8. Pilotti S, DiPalma S, Alasio L, et al. Diagnostic assessment of enlarged superficial lymph nodes by fine needle aspiration. Acta Cytol 1993; 37:853-866.
9. Daskalopoulou D, Harhalakis N, Maouni N, et al. Institution fine needle aspiration cytology of non-Hodgkin's lymphomas: a morphologic and immunophenotypic study. Acta Cytol 1994; 39:180-186.
10. Prasad RRA, Narasimhau R, Sankaran V, et al. Fine-needle aspiration cytology in the diagnosis of superficial lymphadenopathy: an analysis of 2,418 cases. Diagn Cytopathol 1996; 15:382-386.
11. Geisinger KR, Rainer RO, Field AS. Lymph nodes. In: Geisinger KR, Silverman JF, editors. Fine needle aspiration cytology of superficial organs and body sites. New York: Churchill-Livingstone; 1999. pp.1-49.
12. Pandit AA, Khilneni PH, Prayag AS. Tuberculous lymphadenitis: extended cytomorphologic features. Diagn Cytopathol 1995; 12:23.
13. Arora VK, Singh N, Bhatia A. Are eosinophilic structures really a diagnostic criterion for tuberculosis? Diagn Cytopathol 1996; 15:360.
14. Gupta AK, et al. Critical appraisal of FNAB in tuberculous lymphadenitis. Acta Cytol 1992; 36:391.
15. Jannotta FS, Sidawy MK. The recognition of mycobacterial infections by intraoperative cytology in patients with acquired immunodeficiency syndrome. Arch Pathol Lab Med 1989; 113:120.
16. Stanley MW, Horwitz CA, Burton LG, et al. Negative images of bacilli and mycobacterial infection: a study of FNA smears from lymph nodes in patients with AIDS. Diagn Cytopathol 1990;6:118-121.
17. Alfonso F, Gallo L, Winkler B, et al. FNA cytology of peripheral lymph node cryptococcosis: a report of three cases. Acta Cytol 1994; 38:459-462.
18. Donnelly A, Hendricks G, Martens S, et al. Cytologic diagnosis of cat scratch disease (CSD) by fine-needle aspiration. Diagn Cytopathol 1995; 13:103.
19. Stastny FJ, Wakely PE Jr, Frable WJ. Cytologic features of necrotizing granulomatous inflammation consistent with cat-scratch disease. Diagn Cytopathol 1996; 15:108-115.
20. Christ ML, Feltes-Kennedy M. Fine-needle aspiration of toxoplasmic lymphadenitis. Acta Cytol 1982; 26:425-428.
21. Argyle JC, Schumann GB, Kjeldsberg CR, et al. Identification of *Toxoplasma* cyst by FNA. Am J Clin Pathol 1983; 80:256-258.
22. Jayaram N, Ramaprasad AV, Chethan M, et al. *Toxoplasma* lymphadenitis: analysis of cytologic and histologic criteria and correlation with serologic tests. Acta Cytol 1997; 41:653-758.
23. Gupta RK. Fine needle aspiration cytodiagnosis of toxoplasmic lymphadenitis. Acta Cytol 1997; 41:1031-1034.
24. Zaharpoulos P. Demonstration of parasites in toxoplasma lymphadenitis by fine-needle aspiration cytology: report of two patients. Diagn Cytopathol 2000; 22:11-15.
25. Kardos TF, Kornstein MJ, Frable WJ. Cytopathology and immunopathology of infectious mononucleosis. Acta Cytol 1988; 32:722.
26. Stanley MW, et al. Fine needle aspiration of lymph nodes in patients with acute infectious mononucleosis. Diagn Cytopathol 1990; 6:323.
27. Tambouret R, Geisinger KR, Powers CN, et al. The clinical application of fine needle aspiration biopsy in the diagnosis and management of sarcoidosis. Chest 2000; 117: 1004-1011.
28. Layfield LJ. Fine needle aspiration cytologic findings in a case of sinus histiocytosis with massive lymphadenopathy (Rosai-Dorfman syndrome). Acta Cytol 1990; 34:767.
29. Trautman BC, Stanley MW, Goding GS, et al. Sinus histiocytosis with massive lymphadenopathy (Rosai-Dorfman disease): diagnosis by fine needle aspiration. Diagn Cytopathol 1991; 7:513.
30. Stastny JF, Wilkerson ML, Hamati HF, et al. Cytologic features of sinus histiocytosis with massive lymphadenopathy: a report of three cases. Acta Cytol 1997; 41:871-876.
31. Tsang WYW, Chan JKC. Fine-needle aspiration cytologic diagnosis of Kikuchi's lymphadenitis: a report of 27 cases. Am J Clin Pathol 1994; 102:454.
32. Cochand-Priollet B, et al. Retroperitoneal lymph node aspiration biopsy in staging of pelvic cancer: a cytological study of 220 consecutive cases. Diagn Cytopathol 1987; 3:102.
33. Cervin JR, Silverman JF, Loggie B, et al. Virchow's node revisited: analysis with clinicopathologic correlation of 152 fine-needle aspiration biopsies of supraclavicular lymph nodes. Arch Pathol Lab Med 1995; 119:727.

34. Cafferty LL, et al. Fine needle aspiration diagnosis of intraabdominal and retroperitoneal lymphomas by a morphologic and immunocytochemical approach. Cancer 1990; 65:72.

35. Pontifex AH, Haley L. Fine-needle aspiration cytology in lymphomas and related disorders. Diagn Cytopathol 1989; 5:432.

36. Katz RL, Caraway NP. FNA lymphoproliferative disease: myths and legends. Diagn Cytopathol 1995; 12:99.

37. Tani EM, Christensson B, Porwit A, et al. Immunocytochemical analysis and cytomorphologic diagnosis on fine needle aspirates of lymphoproliferative diseases. Acta Cytol 1988;32:209.

38. Chorny J, Katz RL. Overlooking malignant lymphoma on FNA: a diagnostic pitfall. Pathologic Case Rev 1996; 1:92-95.

39. Kornstein MJ, Wakely PG Jr, Kardos TF, et al. Dendritic reticulum cells and immunophenotype in aspiration biopsies of lymph nodes: value in subclassification of non-Hodgkin's lymphomas. Am J Clin Pathologic 1990; 94:164-169.

40. Stani J. Cytologic diagnosis of reactive lymphadenopathy in fine needle aspiration biopsy specimens. Acta Cytol 1987; 31:8.

41. Braylan RC, Benson NA. Flow cytometric analysis of lymphomas. [Review]. Arch Pathol Lab Med 1989; 113: 627-633.

42. Borowitz MJ, et al. Monoclonal antibody phenotyping of B-cell non-Hodgkin's lymphomas: the Southeastern Cancer Study Group experience. Am J Pathol 1985; 121(3):514-521.

43. Borowitz MJ, et al. The phenotypic diversity of peripheral T-cell lymphomas: the Southeastern Cancer Study Group experience. Hum Pathol 1986; 17(6):567-574.

44. Harris NL, et al. A revised European-American classification of lymphoid neoplasms: a proposal from the International Lymphoma Study Group [see comments] review. Blood 1994; 84(5):1361-1392.

45. Young NA, Al-Saleem TI, Ehya H, et al. Utilization of fine-needle asiration cytology and flow cytometry in the diagnosis and subclassification of primary and recurrent lymphoma. Cancer Cytopathol 1998; 84:252-261.

46. Wakely PE Jr. Fine-needle aspiration cytopathology in diagnosis and classification of malignant lymphoma: accurate and reliable? Diagn Cytopathol 2000; 22:120-125.

47. Dunphy CH, Ramas R. Combining fine-needle aspiration and flow cytometric immunophenotyping in evaluation of nodal and extranodal sites for possible lymphoma: a retrospective review. Diagn Cytopathol 1997; 16:200-206.

48. Ravinsky E, Morales C, Kutryk E, et al. Cytodiagnosis of lymphoid proliferations by fine needle aspiration biopsy: adjunctive value of flow cytometry. Acta Cytol 1999; 43:1070-1078.

49. Simsir A, Fetsch P, Stetler-Stevenson M, et al. Immunophenotypic analysis of non-Hodgkin's lymphomas in cytologic specimens: a correlative study of imunocytochemical and flow cytometric techniques. Diagn Cytopathol 1999; 20:278-284.

50. Park IA, Kim C-W. FNAC of malignant lymphoma in an area with a high incidence of T-cell lymphoma: correlation of accuracy of cytologic diagnosis with histologic subtype and immunophenotype. Acta Cytol 1999; 43: 1059-1069.

51. Saikia UN, Dey P, Vohra H, et al. DNA flow cytometry of non-Hodgkins's lymphoma: correlation with cytologic grade and clinical relapse. Diagn Cytopathol 2000; 22: 152-156.

52. Stewart CJR, Duncan JA, Farquharson J, Richmond J. Fine needle aspiration cytology diagnosis of malignant lymphoma and reactive lymphoid hyperplasia. J Clin Pathol 1998; 51:197-203.

53. Meda BA, Buss DH, Woodruff RD, et al. Diagnosis and subclassification of primary and recurrent lymphoma: the usefulness and limitations of combined fine-needle aspiration cytomorphology and flow cytometry. Am J Clin Pathol 2000; 113:688-699.

54. Nicol TL, Silberman M, Rosenthal DL, et al. The accuracy of combined cytopathologic and flow cytometric analysis of fine-needle aspirates of lymph nodes. Am J Clin Pathol 2000; 114:18-29.

55. Lubnski J, et al. Molecular genetic analysis in the diagnosis of lymphoma in fine needle aspiration biopsies. I. Lymphomas versus benign lymphoproliferative disorders. Anal Quant Cytol Histol 1988; 10:391-398.

56. Katz RL, et al. The role of gene rearrangements for antigen receptors in the diagnosis of lymphoma obtained by fine-needle aspiration. Am J Clin Pathol 1991; 96:479-490.

57. Sneige N, et al. Cytomorphologic, immunocytochemical, and nucleic acid flow cytometry of 50 lymph nodes by fine-needle aspiration: comparison with results obtained by subsequent excisional biopsy. Cancer 1991; 67:1003-1010.

58. Molot RJ, et al. Antigen expression and polymerase chain reaction amplification in mantle cell lymphomas. Blood 1994; 83:1626-1631.

59. Capaccioli S, et al. A bcl-2/IgH antisense transcript deregulates *bcl-2* gene expression in human follicular lymphoma t(14;18) cell lines. Oncogene 1996; 13:105-115.

60. Nowell PC, Croce CM. Chromosome translocations and onocogenes in human lymphoid tissues. Am J Clin Pathol 1990; 94:229.

61. Schmid I, et al. Dead cell discrimination with 7-amino-actinomycin D in combination with dual color immuno-fluorescence in single laser flow cytometry. Cytometry 1992; 13(2):204-208.

62. Stelzer GT, et al. Detection of occult lymphoma cells in bone marrow aspirates by multi-dimensional flow cytometry. Prog Clin Biol Res 1992; 377:629-635.

63. Rainer RO, Hodges L, Seltzer GT. CD 45 gating correlates with bone marrow differential. Cytometry 1995; 22: 139-145.

64. Morgan KG, et al. Hodgkin's disease: a flow cytometric study. J Clin Pathol 1988; 41:365-369.

65. Ault KA. Detection of small numbers of monoclonal B lymphocytes in the blood of patients with lymphoma. N Eng J Med 1979; 300:1401-1405.

66. Horning SJ, et al. Clinical and phenotypic diversity of T cell lymphomas. Blood 1986; 67:1578-1582.

67. Kelsoe G. The germinal center: a crucible for lymphocyte selection. Sem Immunol 1996; 8:179-184.

68. Cossman J, et al. Low-grade lymphomas: expression of developmentally regulated B-cell antigens. Am J Pathol 1984; 115:117-124.

69. Sneige N, et al. Morphologic and immunocytochemical evaluation of 220 fine needle aspirates of malignant lymphoma and lymphoid hyperplasia. Acta Cytol 1990; 34:311.

70. Scott CS, et al. Membrane phenotypic studies in B cell lymphoproliferative disorders. J Clin Pathol 1985; 38(9):995-1001.

71. Cherepakhin V, et al. Common clonal origin of chronic lymphocytic leukemia and high-grade lymphoma or Richter's syndrome. Blood 1993; 82(10):3141-3147.

72. Sheibani K, et al. Monocytoid B cell lymphoma, clinico-pathologic study of 21 cases of a unique type of low-grade lymphoma. Cancer 1998; 62:1531.

73. Banks PM, et al. Mantle cell lymphoma: a proposal for unification of morphologic, immunologic and molecular data. Am J Surg Pathol 1992; 16:1637.

74. Winberg CD. Peripheral T cell lymphoma: morphologic and immunologic observations. Am J Clin Pathol 1993; 99:426.

75. Katz RL, Gritsman A, Cabanillas F. Fine needle aspiration cytology of peripheral T-cell lymphoma. Am J Clin Pathol 1989; 91:120.

76. Kardos TF, et al. Fine needle aspiration biopsy of lymphoblastic lymphoma and leukemia: a clinical, cytologic, and immunologic study. Cancer 1987; 60:2448.

77. Jacobs J, et al. Fine needle aspiration of lymphoblastic lymphoma: a multiparameter diagnostic approach. Acta Cytol 1992; 36:887.

78. Behm FG, O'Dowd GJ, Frable WF. Fine needle aspiration effects on benign lymph node histology. Am J Clin Pathol 1985; 82:195-198.

79. Pai MR, Adhikari P, Coimbatore RVR, et al. Fine needle aspiration cytology in systemic lupus erythematosus lymphadenopathy: a case report. Acta Cytol 2000; 44:67-69.

80. Vicandi B, Jimenez-Herrernan JA, Lopez-Ferrar P, et al. Hodgkin's disease mimicking suppurative lymphodenitis: a fine-needle aspiration report of five cases. Diagn Cytopathol 1999; 20:302-306.

81. Gong G, Lee H, Kang GH, et al. Nested PCR for diagnosis of tuberculous lymphadenitis and PCR-SSCP for identification of rifampicin resistance in fine-needle aspirates. Diagn Cytopathol 2002; 26:228-231.

82. Ellison E, Lapuerta P, Martin SE. Fine needle aspiration diagnosis of mycobacterial lymphadenitis: sensitivity and predictive value in the United States. Acta Cytol 1999; 43:153-157.

83. Singh KK, Muralidhar M, Kumar A, et al. Comparison of in house polymerase chain reaction with conventional techniques for the detection of *Mycobacterium tuberculosis* DNA in granulomatous lymphadenopathy. J Clin Pathol 2000; 53:355-361.

84. Lapeurta P, Martin S, Ellison E. Fine-needle aspiration of peripheral lymph nodes in patients with tuberculosis and HIV. Am J Clin Pathol 1997; 107:317-320.

85. Gupta K, Singh N, Bhatia A, et al. Cytomorphologic patterns in Calmed-Gorin bacillus lymphadenitis. Acta Cytol 1997; 41:348-350.

86. Orell SR, Sterrett GF, Walterns M N-I, et al. Manual and atlas of fine needle aspiration cytology. 2nd ed. Edinburgh: Churchill Livingstone; 1992. p.72.

87. Anagnostopoulus I, et al. Morphology, immunophenotype, and distribution of latently and/or productively Epstein-Barr virus-infected cells in acute infectious mononucleosis: implication for the interindividual infection route of Epstein-Barr virus. Blood 1995; 85:744-750.

88. Tong TRS, Chan OW, Lee K. Diagnosing Kikuchi disease in fine needle aspiration biopsy: a retrospective study of 44 cases diagnosed by cytology and 8 by histopathology. Acta Cytol 2001; 45:953-957.

89. Viguer JM, Jiménez-Herrerman JA, Perez P, et al. Fine-needle asiration cytology of Kikuchi's lymphadenitis: a report of ten casaes. Diagn Cytopathol 2001; 25:220-224.

90. Pai MR, Adhikari P, Coimbatore RVR, et al. Fine needle aspiration cytology in systemic lupus erythematosus lymphodenopathy: a case report. Act Cytol 2000; 44:67-69.

91. Strigle SM, Rarck MU, Cosgrove MM, et al. A review of FNA cytological findings in HIV infection. Diagn Cytopathol 1992; 8:41-52.

92. Strigle SM, Martin SE, Levine AM, et al. The use of FNA cytology in the management of HIV-related non-Hodgkin's lymphoma and Hodgkin's disease. J Acquir Immune Defic Syndr 1993; 6:1329-1334.

93. Margin-Bates E, Tanner A, Suvarna SK, et al. Use of FNA cytology for investigating lymphadenopathy in HIV-positive patients. J Clin Pathol 1993; 46:564-566.

94. Shabb N et al: Fine-needle aspiration evaluation of lymphoproliferative lesions in human immunodeficiency virus-positive patients. Cancer 1991; 67:1008.

95. Llatjos M, Roneu J, Clotet B, et al. A distinctive cytologic pattern for diagnosing tuberculosis lymphadenitis in AIDS. J Acquir Immune Defic Syndr 1993; 6:1335-1338.

96. Burns BF, Wood GS, Dorfman RF. The varied histopathology in the homosexual male. Am J Surg Pathol 1985; 9:287.

97. Hales M, Bottles K, Miller T, et al. Diagnosis of Kaposi's sarcoma by fine-needle aspiration biopsy. Am J Clin Pathol 1987; 88:20.

98. Knowles DM, et al. Lymphoid neoplasia associated with the acquired immunodeficiency syndrome. Ann Intern Med 1998; 108:744.

99. Tirelli U, et al. Hodgkin's disease and HIV infection: clinicopathologic and virologic features of 114 patients from the Italian Cooperative Group on AIDS and tumors. J Clin Oncol 1995; 13:1758.

100. Gattus P, Castelli MJ, Peng Y, et al. Post transplant lymphoproliferative disorders: a fine needle aspiration biopsy study. Diagn Cytopathol 1997; 16:392-395.

101. Siddiqui MT, Reddy VB, Castelli MJ, et al. Role of fine-needle aspiration in clinical management of transplant patients. Diagn Cytopathol 1997; 17:429-435.

102. Davey DD, Gulley ML, Walker WP, et al. Cytologic findings in posttransplant lymphoproliferative disease. Acta Cytol 1990; 34:304-310.

103. Collins BT, Ramos RR, Grosso LE. Combined fine needle aspiration biopsy and immunophenotypic and genotypic approach to posttransplantation lymphoproliferative disorders. Acta Cytol 1998; 42:869-874.

104. Dusenbery D, Nalesnik MA, Locker J, et al. Cytologic features of post-transplant lymphoproliferative disorder. Diagn Cytopathol 1997; 16:489-496.

105. Ponder TB, Collins BT, Bee CS, et al. Fine needle aspiration biopsy of a posttransplant lymphoproliferative disorder with pronounced plasmacytic differentiation presenting in the face; a case report. Acta Cytol 2002; 46:39-394.

106. Moreland WS, Geisinger KR. The utility and outcomes of fine needle aspiration biopsy in Hodgkin's disease. Diagn Cytopathol 2002; 26:278-282.

107. Jiménez-Hefferman JA, Vicandi B, López-Ferrer P, et al. Value of fine needle aspiration cytology in the initial diagnosis of Hodgkin's disease: analysis of 188 cases with an emphasis on diagnostic pitfalls. Acta Cytol 2001; 45:300-306.

108. Liu K, Stern RC, Rogers RT, et al. Diagnosis of hematopoietic processes by fine-needle aspiaration in conjunction with flow cytometry: a review of 127 cases. Diagn Cytopathol 2001; 24:1-10.

109. Chhieng DC, Cohen J-M, Cangiarella JF. Cytology and immunophenotyping of low- and intermediate-grade B-cell non-Hodgkin's lymphomas with a predominant small-cell component: a study of 56 cases. Diagn Cytopathol 2001; 24:90-97.

110. Stook L, et al. Growth fraction in non-Hodgkin's lymphomas and reactive lymphadenitis determined by Ki-67 monoclonal antibody in fine-needle aspirates. Diagn Cytopathol 1995; 12:234.

111. Harris NL, Jaffe ES, Diebold J, et al. The World Health Organization classification of hematologic malignancies report of the Clinical Advisory Committee Meeting, Arlie House, Virginia, November 1997. Modern Pathol 2000; 13:193-197.

112. Igengar KR, Mutha S. Discrete epithelioid cells: useful clue to Hodgkin's disease cytodiagnosis. Diagn Cytopathol 2002; 26:142-144.

113. Friedman M et al. Appraisal of aspiration cytology in management of Hodgkin's disease. Cancer 1980; 45:1653.

114. Kardos TF, et al. Hodgkin's disease: diagnosis by fine needle aspiration biopsy: analysis of cytologic criteria from a selected series. Am J Clin Pathol 1986; 86:286.

115. Moriarty A, et al. Cytologic criteria for subclassification of Hodgkin's disease using fine needle aspiration. Diagn Cytopathol 1989; 5:122.

116. Das DK, et al. Fine needle aspiration cytodiagnosis of Hodgkin's disease and its subtypes. I. Scope and limitations. Acta Cytol 1990; 34:329.

117. Fulciniti F, Vetrani A, Aeppa P, et al. Hodgkin's disease: diagnostic accuracy of fine needle aspiration, a report of 62 consecutive cases. Cytopathology 1994; 5:226-233.

118. Chhieng DC, Cangiarella JF, Symmans WF, et al. Fine-needle aspiration cytology of Hodgkin's disease: a study of 89 cases with emphasis on the false-negative cases. Cancer Cytopathol 2001; 93:52-59.

119. Tani E, Johansson B, Skoog L. T-cell-rich B-cell-rich lymphoma: fine needle aspiration cytology and immunocytochemistry. Diagn Cytopathol 1998; 18:1-7.

120. Chan MKM, McGuire LJ, Lee JCK. Fine needle aspiration diagnosis of nasopharyngeal carcinoma in cervical lymph nodes: a study of 40 cases. Acta Cytol 1989; 33:344-350.

121. Robb-Smith AH. U.S. National Cancer Institute working formulation of non-Hodgkin's lymphomas for clinical use. Lancet 1982; 2(8295):432-434.

122. Wojcik EM, et al. Diagnosis of mantle cell lymphoma on tissue acquired by fine needle aspiration in conjunction with immunocytochemistry and cytokinetic studies. Acta Cytol 1995; 39:909.

123. Symmans WF, Cangiarella JF, Symmans PJ, et al. Apoptotic index from fine needle aspiration as a criterion to predict histologic grade of non-Hodgkin's lymphoma. Acta Ctyol 2000; 44:194-204.

124. Young NA, Al-Saleem TI, Al-Saleem Z, et al. The value of transformed lymphocyte count in subclassification of non-Hodgkin's lymphoma by a fine-needle aspiration. Am J Clin Pathol 1997; 108:143-151.

125. Hughes JH, Caraway NP, Katz RL. Blastic variant of mantle-cell lymphoma: cytomorphologic, immunocytochemical, and molecular genetic features of tissue obtained by fine-needle aspiration biopsy. Diagn Cytopathol 1998; 19:59-62.

126. Lai R, Medeiros LJ. Pathologic diagnosis of mantle cell lymphoma. Clin Lymph 2000; 1:197-206.

127. Murphy BA, Meda BA, Buss DH, et al. Marginal zone cell and mantle cell lymphomas: assessment of cytomorphology in subtyping small B-cell lymphomas. Diagn Cytopathol 2003; 28:126-130.

128. Labrecque LG, Lampert I, Kazembe P, et al. Correlation between cytopathological results and an *in situ* hybridization on needle aspiration biopsies of suspected African Burkitt's lymphomas. Int J Cancer 1994; 59:591-596.

129. Stastny JF et al. Fine-needle aspiration biopsy and imprint cytology of small non-cleaved cell (Burkitt's) lymphoma. Diagn Cytopathol 1995; 12:201.

130. Park IA, Kim C-W. FNAC of malignant lymphoma in an area with a high incidence of T-cell lymphoma. Correlation of accuracy of cytologic diagnosis with histologic subtype and immunophenotype. Acta Cytol 1999; 43: 1059-1069.

131. Galindo LM, Garcia F, Hanan CA, et al. Fine-needle spiration biopsy in the evaluation of lymphadenopathy associated with cutaneous T-cell lymphoma (mycosis fungoides/Sézary syndrome). Am J Clin Pathol 2000; 113: 865-871.

132. Sudilousky D, Cha I. Fine needle aspiration cytology of dermatopathic lymphadenitis. Acta Cytol 1998; 1341-1346.

133. Iyer VK, Kapila K, Verma K. Fine needle aspiration cytology of dermatopathic lymphadenitis. Acta Cytol 1998; 42:1347-1351.

134. Jaffe ES. Anaplastic large cell lymphoma: the shifting sands of diagnostic hematopathology. Modern Pathol 2001; 14:219-228.

135. Akhtar M, Ali MA, Haider A, et al. Fine-needle aspiration biopsy of Ki-1 positive anaplastic large cell lymphoma. Diagn Cytopathol 1992; 8:242-247.

136. Zakowski MF, Feiner H, Finfer M, et al. Cytology of extranodal Ki-1 anaplastic large cell lymphoma. Diagn Cytopathol 1996; 14:155-160.

137. McCluggage WG, Anderson N, Herron B, et al. Fine needle aspiration cytology, histology and immunohistochemistry of anaplastic large cell Ki-1-positive lymphoma. Acta Cytol 1996; 40:779-785.

138. Sgrignoli A, Abati A. Cytologic diagnosis of anaplastic large cell lymphoma. Acta Cytol 1997; 41:1048,1052.

139. Bizjak-Schwarzbartl M. Large cell anaplastic Ki-1 positive non-Hodgkin's lymphoma vs. Hodgkin's disease in fine needle aspiration biopsy samples. Acta Cytol 1997; 41:351-356.

140. Creager AJ, Geisinger KR, Bergman S, Neutrophil-rich Ki-1 positive anaplastic large cell lymphoma: a report of 2 cases diagnosed by fine needle aspiration biopsy. Am J Clin Pathol 2002; 117:709-715.

141. Gatter KM, Rader A, Braziel RM. Fine-needle aspiration biopsy of anaplastic large cell lymphoma, small cell variant with prominent plasmacytoid features: case report. Diagn Cytopathol 2002; 26:113-116.

142. Oshima K, Tani E, Masuda Y, et al. Fine needle aspiration cytology of high grade T-cell lymphomas in human T-lymphotrophic virus type 1 carriers. Cytopathology 1992; 3:365-373.

143. Dahmoush L, Hijazi Y, Barnes E, et al. Adult T-cell leukemia/lymphoma (ATLL): a cytopathologic, immunocytochemical and flow cytometric study. Cancer Cytopathol 2002; 96:110-116.

144. Nasuti JF, Mahrota R, Gupta PK. Diagnostic value of fine needle aspiration of supraclavicular lymphadenopathy: a study of 106 patients and review of literature. Diagn Cytopathol 2001; 25:351-355.

145. Jaffer S, Zakowski M. Fine-needle aspiration biopsy of axillary lymph nodes. Diagn Cytopathol 2002; 26:69-74.

146. Geisinger KR, Silverman JF, Wakely PG Jr. Pediatric cytopathology. Chicago: ASCP Press; 1994. pp.307-313.

147. Engzell U, Zajicek J. Aspiration biopsy of tumors of the neck. I. Aspiration biopsy and cytologic findings in 100 cases of congenital cysts. Acta Cytol 1970; 14:51-57.

148. Krag D, et al. The sentinel lymph node biopsy in breast cancer: a multicenter validation study. N Eng J Med 1998; 339:941-946.

149. Kane JM III, Edge Sb, Winston JS, et al. Intraoperative evaluation of a breast cancer sentinel lymph node biopsy as a determinant for synchronous axillary lymph node dissection. Am Surg Oncol 2001; 8:361-367.

150. Creager AJ, Geisinger KR. Intraoperative evaluation of sentinel lymph nodes for breast carcinoma: current methodologies. Ann Anat Pathol 2002; 9:233-243.

151. Fitzgibbons PL, et al. Prognostic factors in breast cancer: College of American Pathologists Consensus Statement 1999. Arch Pathol Lab Med 2000; 124:966-978.

152. Waters GS, Geisinger KR, Garske DD, et al. Sentinel lymph node mapping for carcinoma of the colon: a pilot study. Am Surgeon 2000; 66:943-946.

153. Söderström N. How to use cytodiagnostic splenic puncture. Acta Med Scand 1976; 199:1-5.

154. Lishner M, Lang R, Halph E, et al. Fine needle aspiration biopsy in patients with diffusely enlarged spleens. Acta Cytol 1996; 40:196-198.

155. Zeppa P, Vetrani A, Luciano L, et al. Fine needle aspiration biopsy of the spleen: a useful procedure in the diagnosis of splenomegaly. Acta Cytol 1994; 38:299-309.

156. Pasternack A. Fine-needle aspiration biopsy of speen in diagnosis of genralized amyloidosis. Br Med J 1974; 2:20-22.

157. Haque I, Haque MZ, Krishnani N, et al. Fine needle aspiration cytology of the spleen in visceral leishmaniasis. Acta Cytol 1993; 37:73-76.

158. Taavitsainen M, Koivuniemi A, Helminen J, et al. Apsiration biopsy of the spleen in patients with sarcoidosis. Acta Radiol 1987; 28:723-725.

159. Silverman JF, Geisinger KR, Raab SS, et al. Fine needle aspiration biopsy of the spleen in the evaluation of neoplastic disorders. Acta Cytol 1993; 37:158-162.

160. Moriarty AT, Schwenk GR Jr, Chua C. Splenic fine needle aspiration biopsy in the diagnosis of lymphoreticular diseases: a report of four cases. Acta Cytol 1993; 37:191-196.

161. Caraway NP, Fanning CV. Use of fine-needle aspiration biopsy in the evaluation of splenic lesions in a cancer center. Diagn Cytopathol 1997; 16:312-316.

162. Nerlich A, Permanetter W. Fine needle aspiration cytodiagnosis of epidermoid cysts of the spleen: report of two cases. Acta Cytol 1991; 25:567-569.

163. Kumar PV. Splenic hamartoma: a diagnostic problem on fine needle aspiration cytology. Acta Cytol 1995; 39:391-395.

164. Wu CD, Jackson CL, Meideiros LJ. Splenic marginal zone lymphoma: an immunophenotypic and molecular study of six cases. Am J Clin Pathol 1996; 105:277-285.

165. Wong KF, Chan JKC, Matutes E, et al. Hepatosplenic T-cell lymphoma: a distinct aggressive lymphoma type. Am J Surg Pathol 1995; 19:718-726.

166. Symmans WF et al: Transformation of follicular lymphoma. Acta Cytol 1995; 39:673.

167. Creager AJ, Shiver SA, Shen P, et al. Intraoperative evaluation of sentinel lymph nodes for metastatic melanoma by imprint cytology. Cancer 2002; 94:3016-3022.

168. Sridhar CB, Kini U, Subhash K. Comparative cytologic study of lymph node tuberculosis in HIV-infected individuals and in patients with diabetes in a developing country. Diagn Cytopathol 2002; 26:75-80.

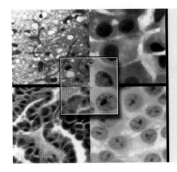

CHAPTER
25

The Pelvis and Scrotal Contents

The true pelvis is that portion of the body's trunk below and behind the abdomen. The pelvic cavity, which differs somewhat in contour in males and females, is separated superiorly from the abdominal cavity by an imaginary plane passing through the arcuate lines on the sacrum, ilium, and pubis. In the female, the cavity contains the ovaries, uterus, and the connecting fallopian tubes. In addition, this is the home of the urinary bladder, prostate, and lower portion of the gastrointestinal tract. The pelvis possesses an extremely rich lymphatic drainage system with predictable patterns of flow. The scrotum contains the testes, the epididimi, and the proximal segments of the vas deferens, in addition to the spermatic cords' neurovascular bundles and associated nonspecific soft tissues.

This chapter deals with fine-needle aspiration (FNA) biopsies of primary neoplasms arising in the pelvis and scrotum and other metastases; the latter are actually much more commonly biopsied. Overlap does exist between some of the neoplasms arising in the male and female gonads, especially the germ cell neoplasms; their aspiration cytomorphology is the same. In addition, this chapter discusses the use of aspiration biopsies in two additional settings, namely, the evaluation of clinically benign nonneoplastic cysts of the ovary and the investigation of infertility in males.

GYNECOLOGIC ORGANS

General Overview of Fine-Needle Aspiration Biopsy

In all likelihood, the most common indication for FNA biopsy of the pelvis is the investigation of women with suspected or known gynecologic cancers. In some portions of the world, aspiration biopsies are used for the primary diagnoses of such malignancies, and in particular, ovarian carcinomas.[1,2] On the other hand, in the United States, FNA biopsies are used only rarely in an attempt to render a primary diagnosis of a gynecologic neoplasm. Most applications have revolved about the use of FNA biopsy to identify recurrent or metastatic neoplasms in patients who have been previously treated for a gynecologic malignancy.[3-26] In this setting, reported levels of diagnostic sensitivity have

ranged from approximately 65% to 95%, whereas diagnostic specificities have had a much tighter spectrum from approximately 92% to 100%.[8-10]

In fact, false-positive diagnoses by FNA biopsy are only rarely reported. Perhaps in the largest single series that involved 405 aspirates in 287 women, largely to identify recurrent or metastatic neoplasm, only two false-positive interpretations were found.[20] Both of these were aspirates in women with prior diagnoses of ovarian carcinoma in which the smears contained macrophages misinterpreted as neoplastic cells. Similarly, benign histiocytes in an aspirate of a lymph node were misinterpreted as metastatic adenocarcinoma in a patient with a previous diagnosis of extramammary Paget's disease in a series reported by Belinson and colleagues; it was their solitary false-positive diagnosis.[5] The huge series (217 aspirates) by Moriarty and colleagues included three false-positive interpretations.[8] One of these was an aspirate of the cul-de-sac in a woman with a previous diagnosis of endometrial adenocarcinoma. The needle sampled a rectovaginal fistula that yielded benign glandular cells misinterpreted as recurrent adenocarcinoma. The second consisted of a biopsy of a vaginal nodule in a woman clinically thought to have carcinoma of the cervix. Although the aspirate was interpreted as malignant, the nodule was subsequently shown to be adenosis. Interestingly, at a later point in time, squamous cell carcinoma of the cervix was identified. Their third false-positive result was an aspirate of a soft tissue mass from the lower extremity in a woman with a prior diagnosis of carcinosarcoma of the endometrium. Although the mass was a lipoma, it was interpreted as malignant.

The reported levels of diagnostic sensitivity have not been as good as specificity. Several valid reasons can be offered for false-negative interpretations. Radiation and/or chemotherapy can stimulate a marked fibrotic reaction in surrounding tissues.[10,20] As elsewhere in the body, the presence of collagen-rich tissue may preclude sampling of sufficient numbers of neoplastic cells to render a frankly positive interpretation. Neoplasms may also undergo necrosis, either spontaneously or to the secondary effects of therapy. If the needle is present in a necrotic focus, then again sufficient numbers of viable tumor cells are not aspirated to permit making a malignant diagnosis. In this situation, it is prudent to recommend that a different portion of the lesion be aspirated and, in particular, the peripheral rim of the mass. This demonstrates the value of onsite evaluation of the aspirated material by laboratory personnel. Many of these aspirates are performed under radiologic guidance, and it is certainly true that instances occur in which the needle does not puncture the mass in question. Again, immediate interpretation of the sample would prompt an additional pass to obtain diagnostic material. Finally, certain low-grade malignancies may be interpreted as benign. This is most likely in borderline tumors of the ovary and possibly with well-differentiated squamous cell carcinoma.

Several authors have evaluated potential causes for false-negative interpretations of gynecologic neoplasms. For example, the series by Nash and colleagues had a sensitivity of 68%.[9] The authors concluded that false-negative diagnoses were not related to the site of the aspiration biopsy, the cell type of the underlying neoplasm, or a history of previous radiation therapy or chemotherapy. Similarly, Wojcik and colleagues did not find the type of primary neoplasm, the mode of radiologic guidance, prior treatment, or the period between diagnosis and recurrence to be statistically significant in this regard.[22] These authors did identify two factors that were significant for results: the size of the mass lesion (those greater than 3 cm in diameter were much likely to be positive) and the site of the mass. They stated, furthermore, that a history of prior radiation did lead to an increase in insufficient samples (in contrast to false negative interpretations).[22] On the other hand, both Layfield and colleagues and Imachi and colleagues stated that a history of previous radiation did indeed lead to false-negative diagnoses.[10,20] Essentially, when the clinical suspicion is strong enough that a mass represents recurrent or metastatic tumor but the aspiration biopsy is negative, additional evaluation is indicated. Generally, this implies either a repeat of the aspiration biopsy or an attempt to obtain material for histologic examination.

Moriarty and colleagues defined cytomorphologic criteria for considering an aspirate in this setting to be adequate.[8] Specifically, the specimen needed to include at least two slides, each of which contained a minimum of two groups of cells appropriate for the target site. Using these criteria, one fourth of the aspirates in their series were considered to be invalid (insufficient) for evaluation. Application of this criterion led to an increase in sensitivity from 73% to 92% in their series. Concurrent with this was an improvement in the predictive value of a negative test result from 70% to 84%.

Malstrom specifically compared the diagnostic results of FNA biopsy with tissue core biopsies in 85 women with clinically suspected recurrent gynecologic cancers.[21] The levels of diagnostic sensitivity were significantly higher for the aspiration biopsies compared to the cores (92% versus 73%). Relatively equal numbers of samples were considered insufficient by the two biopsy techniques. Malström concluded that both biopsy procedures were safe and diagnostically complementary.[21]

Ovarian Neoplasms

Overall, malignant neoplasms of the ovary account for approximately 5% to 10% of all malignancies in women. Excluding skin cancers, it is the fifth most common form of malignancy in women in the United States. However, be-

cause of the relatively vague and nonspecific symptoms of ovarian carcinoma, a large percentage of them are first detected when they have reached an advanced stage. Accordingly, they account for a disproportionate number of deaths from cancer. In fact, they are responsible for approximately 50% of all deaths related to malignant neoplasms of the female genital tract.

Three major categories of ovarian neoplasms have been cited.[27] By far the most common and important of these are tumors derived from the surface epithelium. They account for approximately 65% of all neoplasms of the ovary and 85% or more of all ovarian malignancies. Germ cell tumors are the second major category, accounting for 15% of all ovarian tumors and no more than 5% of the cancers. Sex cord–stromal neoplasms are slightly less common than the germ cell tumors but probably comprise a slightly greater proportion of all ovarian malignancies.

Three major types of ovarian neoplasms are of surface epithelial origin: benign, borderline (low malignant potential), and malignant.[27] Additionally, all three of these can be subdivided on the basis of the appearance of the predominant tumor cell type. The five major epithelial types include serous, endometrioid, mucinous, clear cell, and transitional. Although the clinical presentation and course differ on the basis of the biological category, cell type differences, in general, do not produce distinct manifestations. From Sweden, Kjellgren and colleagues published a classic article dealing with FNA biopsy of ovarian neoplasms.[1] The publication included both a prospective and a retrospective study. The prospective investigation included 80 women who presented with ovarian masses that were aspirated. The major goal of this study was to determine how accurately they could distinguish benign from malignant on the basis of aspiration cytomorphology. This included 39 benign and 41 malignant aspiration diagnoses. Three false-negative and two false-positive interpretations resulted in an overall accuracy of 93%.[1]

In their retrospective study, 60 women with a previous histologic diagnosis of ovarian cancer were evaluated in an attempt to see how well the pathologist could specifically state the cell type of the neoplasm.[1] Eight of the patients were excluded because of insufficient aspirated cellular material. The investigators did an excellent job in predicting a serous cell type of carcinoma on the basis of the aspiration cytomorphology; they were correct in 97% of the cases. They were also correct in identifying a mucinous adenocarcinoma in 90%. On the other hand, they did terribly in predicting an endometrioid histopathology from the cytologic features. In most of these cases, they considered the carcinomas to be of a serous type. As might be expected, the series did not include rare forms of primary malignancies.

Andersen and colleagues studied a series of 74 women with an aspiration biopsy of an ovarian mass in which histologic material was also available.[2] It is important to note that all of these represented newly diagnosed mass lesions and not recurrent or metastatic ovarian carcinomas. The benign lesions included both serous and mucinous cystadenomas, as well as nonneoplastic cysts. This series included five false-negative interpretations, all of which occurred in postmenopausal women. This is an age group in which epithelial ovarian neoplasms are more likely to be malignant and thus should raise a suspicion of an incorrect diagnosis. This study also involved four aspirates that were considered to be false positives.[2] However, in reality the actual cytologic diagnosis was either *atypical* or *equivocal*. Three of these were serous cystadenomas and one was a luteoma of pregnancy.

The most common cell type of ovarian neoplasms are serous.[27] Although serous cystadenomas are clinically relatively common, aspiration biopsies are uncommon. Smears of serous cystadenomas are characterized by extremely low cellularity.[11,28-32] Almost all the cells are present in cohesive aggregates, which are usually small flat sheets; rarely, papillary structures may be seen (Figure 25-1). The neoplastic cells typically have a columnar configuration with small, obviously benign round nuclei.

As with other epithelial ovarian neoplasms, serous borderline tumors are those that show a much greater degree of proliferation than benign cystadenomas but in which destructive stromal invasion by tumor cells is not present.[33] Obviously, such invasion is essentially impossible to demonstrate in aspiration smears. In general, aspiration biopsies of borderline serous neoplasms yield lower smear cellularity than specimens obtained from frankly malignant serous adenocarcinomas (Figure 25-2). Perhaps this is because of the fact that, in contrast with invasive tumors, large solid nests of neoplastic cells are not present. Furthermore, intercellular cohesion is well preserved so that in most examples, the neoplastic cells are present in either well-formed papillary structures or flat sheets. The papillae may be either simple or complex with prominent branching. Usually, the neoplastic cells are quite homogeneous within a given neoplasm. They are characterized by finely granular, evenly distributed chromatin and small nucleoli. The nuclear to cytoplasmic (N:C) ratios are uniformly high; in contrast, in aspirates of serous carcinomas, a greater variability may be seen within a given smear. Psammoma bodies may be numerous (Box 25-1).

Aspiration biopsies of serous adenocarcinomas are typically characterized by high levels of smear cellularity with both numerous individual neoplastic cells and cohesive aggregates (Figures 25-3 to 25-6).[1,11] The latter vary from spheres to branched papillary structures that are generally small. The individual neoplastic cells are characterized by solitary huge nuclei with hyperchromatic chromatin that may show an irregular distribution and distinct nucleoli. As stated above, the N:C ratios are variable. Pleomorphism can be minimal or extreme with multinucleated tumor giant cells. Psammoma bodies may be well formed and numerous (see Figure 25-5). In smears, they may be encased by neoplastic cells or "naked." These structures are round or slightly oval with smooth external contours. Within them, one or more concentric laminations are evident. These calcifications appear eosinophilic with a Pap stain and basophilic with the DQ stain. Although the neoplastic cells do not produce mucin to any extent, cytoplasmic vacuoles may be present; they tend to be solitary and sharply delineated from the adjacent cytoplasm (Box 25-2).

Despite extensive investigations by a number of authors, complete agreement on the classification of mucinous neoplasms of the ovary does not exist.[34,136] Most, but not all, authors believe that stromal invasion is necessary to diagnose a frank mucinous adenocarcinoma. Furthermore, within the last decade, it has become apparent that many neoplasms considered to be mucinous borderline tumors actually represent metastases from adenomas or well-differentiated adenocarcinomas of the appendix or large intestine.

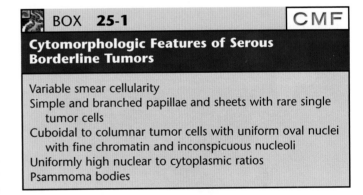

BOX 25-1   CMF

Cytomorphologic Features of Serous Borderline Tumors

Variable smear cellularity
Simple and branched papillae and sheets with rare single tumor cells
Cuboidal to columnar tumor cells with uniform oval nuclei with fine chromatin and inconspicuous nucleoli
Uniformly high nuclear to cytoplasmic ratios
Psammoma bodies

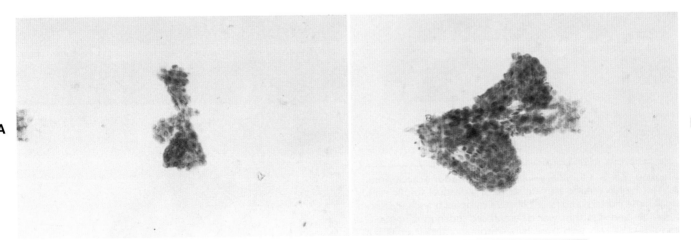

A   **B**

Figure 25-1 Ovarian serous cystadenoma. **A,** This scanning lens view demonstrates many of the tumor cells present in the aspirate of this benign neoplasm. Intercellular cohesion is well maintained because all of the neoplastic cells are present within three-dimensional papillary structures. Note their sharply defined, smooth edges. **B,** Small uniform ovoid nuclei with delicate membranes, extremely pale chromatin, and minutes nucleoli characterize the neoplastic cells which have nuclear to cytoplasmic (N:C) ratios. (Papanicolaou [Pap])

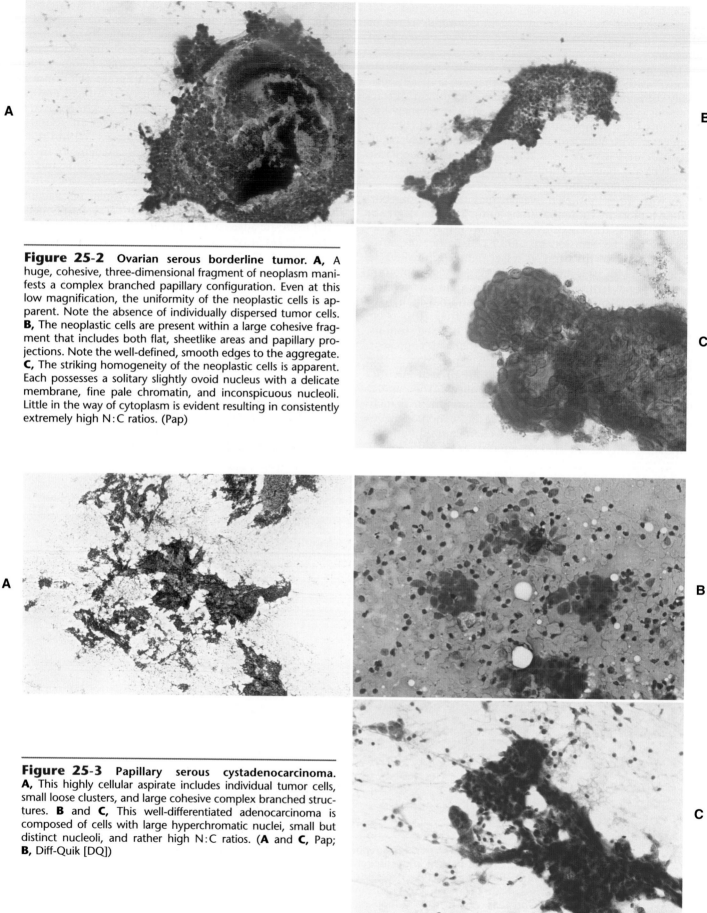

Figure 25-2 Ovarian serous borderline tumor. **A,** A huge, cohesive, three-dimensional fragment of neoplasm manifests a complex branched papillary configuration. Even at this low magnification, the uniformity of the neoplastic cells is apparent. Note the absence of individually dispersed tumor cells. **B,** The neoplastic cells are present within a large cohesive fragment that includes both flat, sheetlike areas and papillary projections. Note the well-defined, smooth edges to the aggregate. **C,** The striking homogeneity of the neoplastic cells is apparent. Each possesses a solitary slightly ovoid nucleus with a delicate membrane, fine pale chromatin, and inconspicuous nucleoli. Little in the way of cytoplasm is evident resulting in consistently extremely high N:C ratios. (Pap)

Figure 25-3 Papillary serous cystadenocarcinoma. **A,** This highly cellular aspirate includes individual tumor cells, small loose clusters, and large cohesive complex branched structures. **B** and **C,** This well-differentiated adenocarcinoma is composed of cells with large hyperchromatic nuclei, small but distinct nucleoli, and rather high N:C ratios. (**A** and **C,** Pap; **B,** Diff-Quik [DQ])

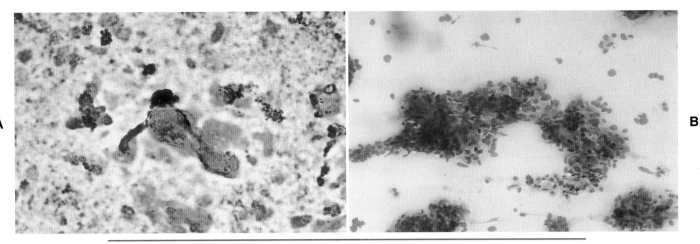

A   B

Figure 25-4 **Papillary serous cystadenocarcinoma. A** and **B,** The branched papillae have relatively smooth, well-defined edges. Such well-formed papillary structures would be unexpected in aspirates of other primary gynecologic carcinomas. Hyperchromasia is apparent. (**A,** Pap; **B,** DQ)

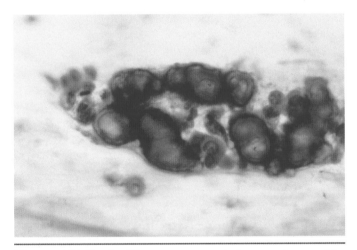

Figure 25-5 **Papillary serous cystadenocarcinoma.** The uniform neoplastic cells are associated with prominent psammoma bodies. The latter are characterized by basophilic coloration and concentric laminations. (Pap)

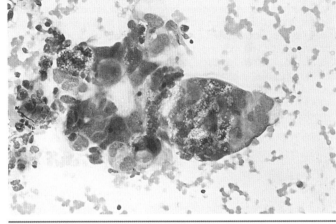

Figure 25-6 **Poorly differentiated serous cystadenocarcinoma.** Moderate to marked nuclear pleomorphism is apparent as is striking variability in nucleolar prominence and cytoplasmic volumes. (DQ)

Similar to serous cystadenomas, aspiration biopsies of mucinous cystadenomas yield scant smear cellularity. One striking feature is the presence of abundant mucinous material in the smear background. With the DQ stain, this mucin appears dense and pink, whereas it is much less apparent with the Pap stain. With the latter, it appears as a thin, watery pale pink to green substance. The neoplastic cells may be individually dispersed and present in small flat sheets with a distinct honeycomb arrangement of the cells. The latter have a columnar configuration with small basally oriented nuclei and abundant cytoplasmic mucin. This results in low N:C ratios.

With mucinous borderline neoplasms, smear cellularity of aspirates is also usually quite low. Although individually dispersed neoplastic cells may be evident, intercellular cohesion is usually well preserved with a majority of the tumor cells present in cohesive aggregates. The latter include both strips and sheets. As their nuclei are well polarized, palisading and honeycomb effects can be seen, respectively, within these aggregates. For the most part, the neo-

---

BOX 25-2   **CMF**

Cytomorphologic Features of Serous Adenocarcinoma

High smear cellularity with single tumor cells and aggregates

Aggregates vary from small spheres to large branched papillae

Columnar tumor cells with solitary large hyperchromatic nuclei with prominent nucleoli

High nuclear to cytoplasmic ratios

Psammoma bodies

---

plastic nuclei are small, round and homogeneous with evenly dispersed chromatin and inconspicuous nucleoli. However, in some borderline tumors, at least a proportion of the nuclei show distinct malignant features with larger sizes; thick, irregular nuclear membranes; hyperchromatic

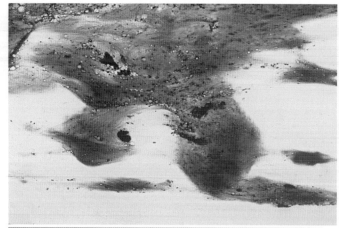

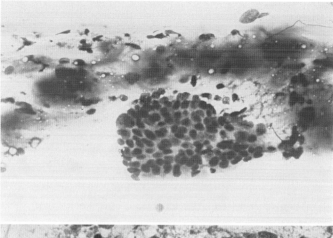

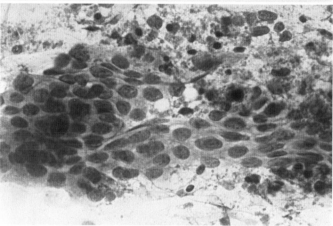

Figure 25-7 Ovarian mucinous adenocarcinoma. **A,** Abundant metachromatic, extracellular mucinous material dominates the smears of this well-differentiated adenocarcinoma. Embedded within the mucin are individual tumor cells and small cohesive aggregates. Most of the latter appear to be flat sheets. **B,** Mild variability in nuclear size and configuration is evident within the sheet of neoplastic epithelial cells. The nucleolar prominence is also variable. Note the rather sharply defined smooth edge to the sheet, the relatively even distribution of the nuclei, and the extracellular mucinous material, which has somewhat of a stringy appearance. **C,** The malignant nuclei are hyperchromatic with finely granular, uniformly dispersed chromatin and small nucleoli. Although polarity is not perfectly maintained, the nuclei are fairly evenly distributed within this cohesive sheet; such a well-formed honeycomb-like arrangement is unusual in the other ovarian carcinomas. (**A** and **B,** DQ; **C,** Pap)

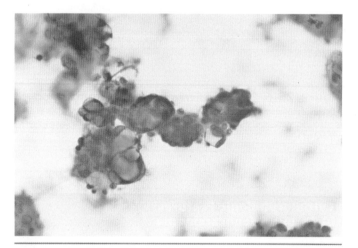

Figure 25-8 Metastatic endocervical adenocarcinoma. The cytoplasm of the malignant cells is distended by mucin vacuoles. In some cases, the nuclei are pushed to the very periphery of the cell. Hyperchromasia is not all that well developed. (Pap)

chromatin; and distinct nucleoli. The N:C ratios are quite variable.

With mucinous adenocarcinomas of the ovary, aspiration biopsies yield smears of variable cellularity that is generally lower than in serous carcinomas. This may be related to the relative abundance of extracellular mucin "pushing" the tumor cells apart on the slides. Typically, the smears contain individually dispersed malignant cells and cohesive aggregates (Figure 25-7). The latter vary from small spheres

> **BOX 25-3** CMF
>
> **Cytomorphologic Features of Mucinous Adenocarcinomas**
>
> Variable smear cellularity with single tumor cells and relatively small sheets and spheres
> Spectrum of nuclear appearances
> Cytoplasmic mucin; low nuclear to cytoplasmic ratios
> Extracellular mucin

to large flat sheets, but distinct papillary structures are not evident. Nuclear appearances are variable both within the same neoplasm and among different patients' specimens. Reports distinguishing the intestinal and endocervical histologic variants in aspiration smears are not known (Figure 25-8). Extracellular mucinous material may be prominent. With the Diff-Quik (DQ) stain, it appears metachromatic and somewhat stringy or striated. With alcohol fixation, the mucin has an even greater stringy look to it; it appears as a pale, watery green or pink substance. The presence of necrotic material has not been detailed in smears of these tumors (Box 25-3).

The second most frequent type of surface epithelial carcinoma is endometrioid adenocarcinoma, accounting for nearly one fourth of all ovarian epithelial malignancies. They are termed endometrioid as their histologic appearance recapitulates that of the more common primary adenocarcinoma of the endometrium. As with most other

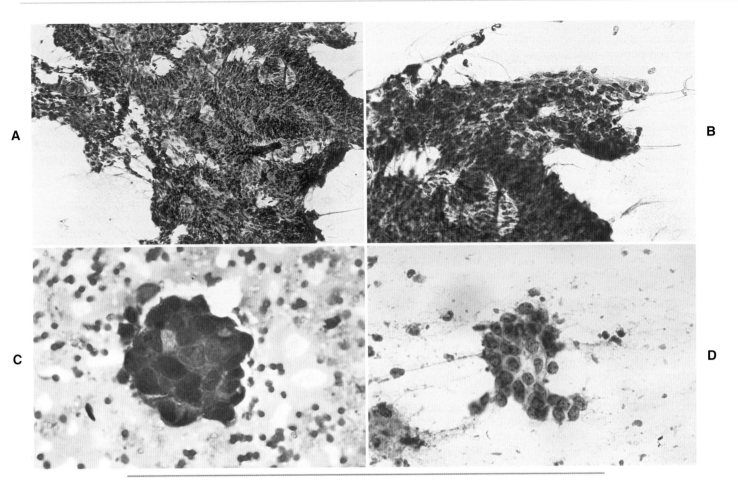

Figure 25-9 **Ovarian well-differentiated endometrioid adenocarcinomas. A,** This highly cellular aspirate is composed of a large cohesive fragment of obviously malignant epithelial cells. At low magnification, it is suggested that at least some of the neoplastic cells have a columnar contour associated with palisading at the edges of the aggregates. **B,** At higher magnification, the malignant cells are characterized by round hyperchromatic nuclei, small but distinct nucleoli, and scanty cytoplasmic volumes. Intercellular cohesion is well maintained. **C,** This spherical aggregate is composed of obviously malignant cells with variable and irregular nuclear contours and primitive chromatin. No specific differentiation is recognizable other than a nonspecific adenocarcinoma. **D,** The hyperchromatic chromatin in these tumor cells is finely granulated and uniformly distributed. Although small, nucleoli are evident. (**A, B,** and **D,** Pap; **C,** DQ)

frankly malignant ovarian carcinomas, patients most commonly present in the fifth and sixth decades of life. In contrast with the other surface epithelial malignancies, endometrioid adenocarcinomas of the ovary are often associated with pelvic (or even ipsilateral ovarian) endometriosis. At least one in five of these ovarian neoplasms are associated with, often synchronously, with a histologically similar neoplasm in the endometrium. These are often considered to be independent primary neoplasms rather than metastases from one site to the other. Borderline endometrial tumors are distinctly rare entities.

As is true of metastatic adenocarcinoma of the endometrium, aspiration biopsies of endometrioid ovarian carcinomas often yield high levels of smear cellularity (Figures 25-9 to 25-11). The vast majority of the neoplastic cells are present within cohesive aggregates that vary from dense spheres to large sheets. Classically, the neoplastic cells possess a columnar configuration, but this is quite variable and cells may appear to be more cuboidal. Their nuclei are usually easily recognized as malignant because of their darkly stained and coarsely granular chromatin and small but distinct nucleoli.

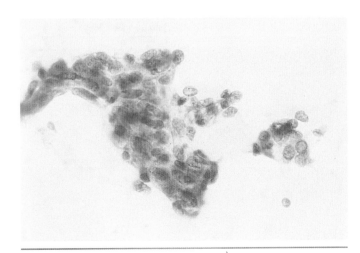

Figure 25-10 **Ovarian poorly differentiated endometrioid adenocarcinoma.** The malignant nuclei have thick irregular membranes, darkly stained chromatin, and distinct nucleoli. Despite the high histologic grade of this carcinoma, intercellular cohesion is well preserved. (Pap)

A significant minority of the endometrioid adenocarcinomas include neoplastic cells with squamous differentiation; this latter component usually possess bland, rather benign-appearing nuclei. The degree of gland formation by the neoplastic cells varies with the histologic grade of the underlying neoplasm; the majority of endometrioid adenocarcinomas are rather well-differentiated and thus, gland formation can be expected in aspirates from many of these neoplasms. Aspirates of endometrioid carcinomas may contain complex pseudopapillary structures (no true fibrovascular connective tissue core) that simulate serous carcinomas. This is one of the reasons the Kjellgren and colleagues had difficulty in classifying the endometrioid carcinomas correctly.[1] Potential helpful clues include relatively small nucleoli, the presence of squamous differentiation, and the rarity or absence of psammoma bodies (Box 25-4).

Analogous to the endometrioid type of ovarian surface epithelial neoplasms, most clear cell tumors are frankly malignant carcinomas—that is, benign and borderline neoplasms are uncommon. Overall, clear cell carcinomas account for no more than 10% of the epithelial malignancies of the ovary. A relatively high proportion of patients with pure clear cell carcinomas of the ovary are nulliparous. Although the clinical presentation is generally indistinguishable from other surface epithelial carcinomas, the clear cell carcinomas are much more commonly associated with the paraneoplastic syndrome of hypercalcemia. Histologically, it is not uncommon to find clear cell carcinomas mixed with either endometrioid or serous carcinoma. Clear cell carcinomas may also arise in the endometrium, cervix, and vagina. The latter are associated with vaginal adenosis.

Aspiration biopsies of clear cell carcinomas may present a distinctive picture (Figures 25-12 and 25-13).[35,36] Aspiration biopsy typically yields high smear cellularity in which there is an intimate admixture of neoplastic cells and dense homogeneous matrix material.[35-38] Malignant cells are characterized by abundant cytoplasm that varies from optically clear to cyanophilic. Cell borders are often well defined. Most neoplastic cells possess a single huge nucleus with a thick irregular membrane, finely granular vesicular chromatin, and one or more huge nucleoli. Fragments of the ex-tracellular material in the smears vary in contour from spheres to sheets to irregularly branched ribbon-like aggregates. With the DQ stain, the matrix appears metachromatic. With the Pap stain, it has a dense glassy green appearance. Some of these matrix fragments are acellular, whereas others are coated by neoplastic cells. With the latter, a hobnail pattern may be seen in which the neoplastic nuclei protrude away from the cellular base (Box 25-5).

Transitional cell or urothelial-like tumors include benign, borderline, and malignant entities such as Brenner tumors and papillary transitional cell carcinoma. They are not discussed in the cytologic literature.

Most germ cell tumors of the ovary are benign, representing cystic teratomas.[27] Of the germ cell neoplasms, 5% are malignant. In contrast with the surface epithelial carcinomas, the malignant germ cell tumors occur primarily in children, adolescents, and young women. Although many of them present as large pelvic masses, they may be associated with endocrine manifestations secondary to the production of human chorionic gonadotropin (HCG). In young girls, this would include isosexual precocious puberty and in adults, abnormal bleeding.

Relative to their frequency, benign cystic teratomas (dermoid cysts) of the ovary are only infrequently aspirated. The series by Allias and colleagues included 10 dermoids.[39] These were all correctly identified cytologically as benign and nonfunctional cystic lesions.

Aspiration biopsies show remarkably variable cellularity from case to case. Some are very poorly cellular, whereas others contain numerous cellular elements. By far, the most common cell type present is the anucleated squamous cell (Figure 25-14). These present in smears singly, in stacks, and in three-dimensional aggregates. With the Pap stain, their cytoplasm varies from transparent to dense and orangeophilic consistent with keratinization. With the DQ stain, the cytoplasm appears pale to dark blue. A minority

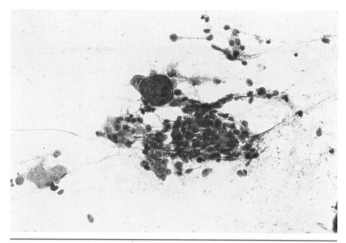

Figure 25-11 Endometrial adenosquamous carcinoma. This aspirate is characterized by malignant cells, some of which are glandular in type, whereas others manifest squamous differentiation. The latter have more abundant cyanophilic cytoplasm and centrally positioned nuclei. There is a suggestion of squamous "pearl" formation. (Pap)

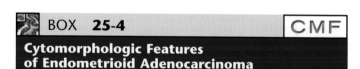

BOX 25-4   CMF

Cytomorphologic Features of Endometrioid Adenocarcinoma

High smear cellularity with mostly spheres and sheets
Columnar tumor cells with variable nuclear to cytoplasmic ratios and pseudostratified hyperchromatic nuclei, often with small but distinct nucleoli
Squamous differentiation possible

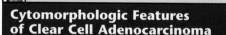

BOX 25-5   CMF

Cytomorphologic Features of Clear Cell Adenocarcinoma

High smear cellularity
Intimate mixture of tumor cells and dense matrix material
Large columnar tumor cells with abundant clear to cyanophilic cytoplasm and huge nuclei with fine chromatin and macronucleoli
Matrix fragments vary from sheets to spheres to complex branched structures
Matrix is metachromatic

of the squamous elements may contain a benign appearing nucleus, often with pyknotic chromatin. In addition, the smears may contain columnar respiratory epithelial cells with cilia, goblet cells, or intact sebaceous glandular cells. In the proper clinical setting, this diagnosis should be straightforward. Rarely, malignancies arise in these benign tumors. The most common type is squamous cell carcinoma. Aspiration biopsies have not been reported to show such an occurrence.

The authors' personal experience with aspiration biopsies of primary ovarian malignant germ cell tumors is quite limited.[40] It is more extensive with FNA biopsy of such neoplasms that represent metastases and primary extragonadal germ cell tumors.[41] The most common of the malignant germ cell tumors of the ovary is dysgerminoma. Aspiration biopsies yield moderately to highly cellular smears that contain a distinct biphasic pattern (Figure 25-15). In other words, an admixture of homogeneous large neoplastic cells

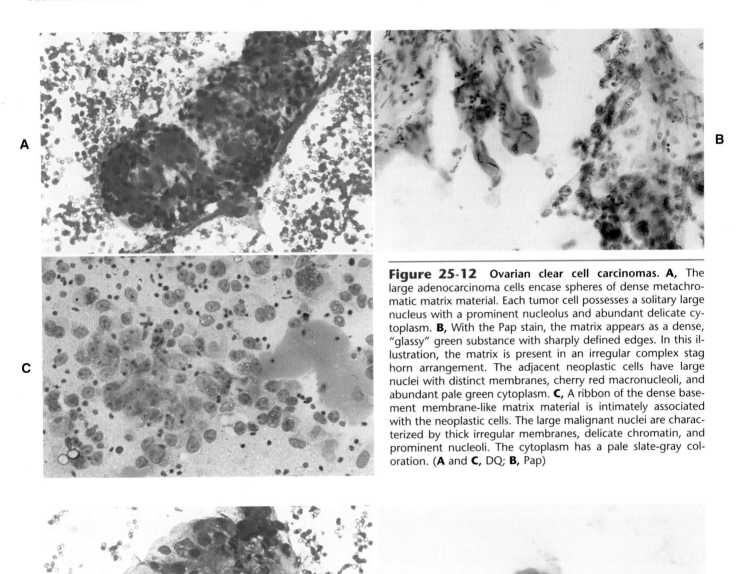

Figure 25-12 **Ovarian clear cell carcinomas. A,** The large adenocarcinoma cells encase spheres of dense metachromatic matrix material. Each tumor cell possesses a solitary large nucleus with a prominent nucleolus and abundant delicate cytoplasm. **B,** With the Pap stain, the matrix appears as a dense, "glassy" green substance with sharply defined edges. In this illustration, the matrix is present in an irregular complex stag horn arrangement. The adjacent neoplastic cells have large nuclei with distinct membranes, cherry red macronucleoli, and abundant pale green cytoplasm. **C,** A ribbon of the dense basement membrane-like matrix material is intimately associated with the neoplastic cells. The large malignant nuclei are characterized by thick irregular membranes, delicate chromatin, and prominent nucleoli. The cytoplasm has a pale slate-gray coloration. (**A** and **C,** DQ; **B,** Pap)

Figure 25-13 **Endometrial clear cell carcinoma. A,** Voluminous delicate pale cytoplasm dominates these huge malignant cells. Despite the presence of big nuclei, the cells possess relatively low nuclear-to-cytoplasmic ratios. **B,** With the Pap stain, the chromatin appears more darkly stained and cytoplasmic vacuolization is suggested. Nucleoli are prominent. (**A,** DQ; **B,** Pap)

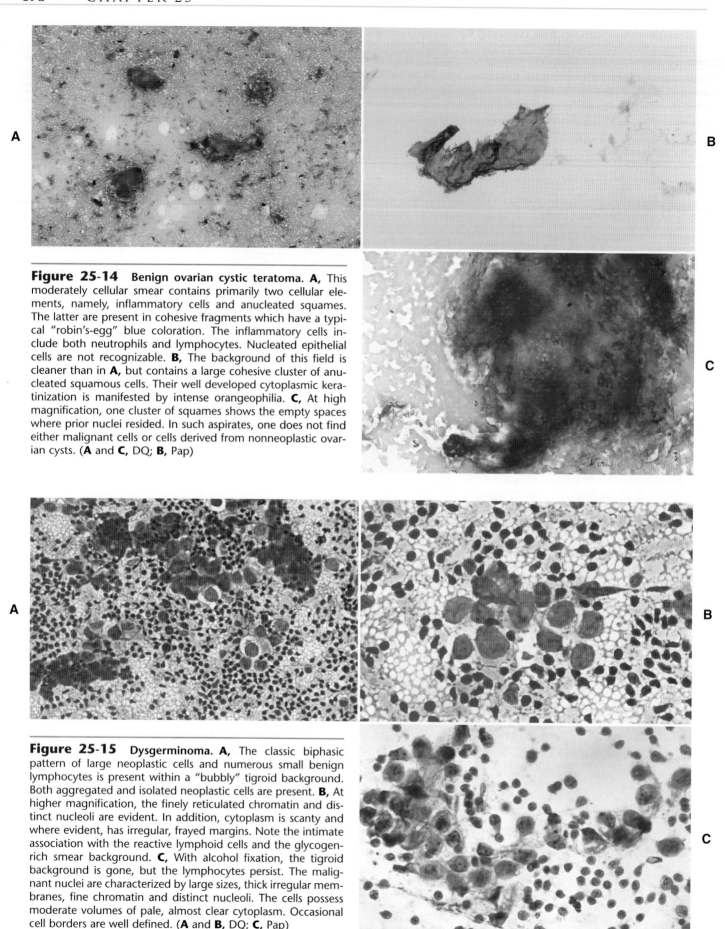

Figure 25-14 Benign ovarian cystic teratoma. **A,** This moderately cellular smear contains primarily two cellular elements, namely, inflammatory cells and anucleated squames. The latter are present in cohesive fragments which have a typical "robin's-egg" blue coloration. The inflammatory cells include both neutrophils and lymphocytes. Nucleated epithelial cells are not recognizable. **B,** The background of this field is cleaner than in **A,** but contains a large cohesive cluster of anucleated squamous cells. Their well developed cytoplasmic keratinization is manifested by intense orangeophilia. **C,** At high magnification, one cluster of squames shows the empty spaces where prior nuclei resided. In such aspirates, one does not find either malignant cells or cells derived from nonneoplastic ovarian cysts. (**A** and **C,** DQ; **B,** Pap)

Figure 25-15 Dysgerminoma. **A,** The classic biphasic pattern of large neoplastic cells and numerous small benign lymphocytes is present within a "bubbly" tigroid background. Both aggregated and isolated neoplastic cells are present. **B,** At higher magnification, the finely reticulated chromatin and distinct nucleoli are evident. In addition, cytoplasm is scanty and where evident, has irregular, frayed margins. Note the intimate association with the reactive lymphoid cells and the glycogen-rich smear background. **C,** With alcohol fixation, the tigroid background is gone, but the lymphocytes persist. The malignant nuclei are characterized by large sizes, thick irregular membranes, fine chromatin and distinct nucleoli. The cells possess moderate volumes of pale, almost clear cytoplasm. Occasional cell borders are well defined. (**A** and **B,** DQ; **C,** Pap)

that are obviously malignant and numerous small mature-appearing lymphoid cells are present. For the most part, the neoplastic cells show little in the way of intercellular cohesion and thus are largely dispersed as solitary elements. Each cell possesses a single huge nucleus with a thick irregular membrane, rather finely granular and evenly dispersed chromatin, and prominent nucleoli; usually the latter is centrally placed and solitary, but multiple nucleoli may also be recognized. Their cytoplasm is quite delicate and thus is often stripped away from the cells, resulting in numerous naked nuclei within the smears. In intact cells, the cytoplasm often appears as a thin, frayed rim about the nucleus. With the DQ stain, the cytoplasm has a slight gray color, whereas with the Pap, it varies from optically clear to green. The smear background is highly characteristic. In addition to the numerous lymphocytes, it typically appears frothy or bubbly; at times, this foamy material is present in a layered bandlike arrangement. It is referred to as having a *tigroid* appearance. Presumably, this results from the fragile glycogen-rich cytoplasm. This background appearance has recently been reported in an aspirate of clear cell carcinoma of the cervix.[42] Rarely, a granulomatous reaction can be intimately associated with the neoplastic cells. Where intercellular cohesion is preserved, the cell borders are often sharply defined. Mitotic figures are usually easily recognized. In contrast with other malignant germ cell tumors, the neoplastic cells are usually nonreactive for cytokeratin.

The second most common malignant ovarian germ cell neoplasm is the yolk sac tumor. In addition to arising in the ovary, yolk sac tumors are often primary neoplasms in the retroperitoneum of children and rarely in the mediastinum. Pure yolk sac tumors are not associated with endocrine manifestations, although serum levels of alpha fetoprotein (AFP) are often increased. Numerous histologic pictures can be seen in yolk sac neoplasms. Although not always present, the most distinctive is the endodermal sinus pattern that includes the presence of Schiller-Duval bodies. Similarly, in tissue sections, a spectrum of appearances can be seen among the neoplastic cells within a given tumor. They range from flat and endothelial or mesothelial-like cells to embryonal columnar epithelial elements to huge polygonal neoplastic cells with well defined cell borders. For the most part, the tumor cells possess a solitary, obviously malignant nucleus. The latter have round or ovoid contours, hyperchromatic finely granular chromatin, and often distinct nucleoli.

It is this myriad of tissue patterns and cytologic appearances that may create variability in the aspiration smears.[41,43] The smear background may contain necrotic debris and/or a watery myxoidlike material. Smears are moderately to highly cellular and include both individually dispersed cells and cohesive aggregates. The latter are characteristically spherical clusters, but sheets and papillae may also be evident. Another major component of the smears is a dense basement membrane–like matrix material. With the DQ stain, it appears metachromatic, whereas it is green and homogeneous with the Pap stain. Individual tumor cells may appear embedded within the matrix material and forming linear arrays at the edges of these matrix fragments. In the authors' experience with aspiration biopsies of yolk sac tumors, the neoplastic cells are more homogeneous in appearance than they are in histologic preparations. In aspirates, the neoplastic cells tend to have polygonal contours, relatively scanty cytoplasm, and solitary hyperchromatic nuclei, often with distinct nucleoli. The tumor cells appear clearly epithelial in nature, which corresponds to their positive immunocytochemical reaction for cytokeratin. One final component that may be seen in FNA biopsy smears are round dense globules of matrix material that have tinctorial qualities similar to the basement membrane–like material. These globules may be present both within the cytoplasm of neoplastic cells and also free and extracellular.

Yang has recently described the aspiration appearance of a yolk sac tumor (of testicular origin) in which there were numerous Schiller-Duval bodies histologically.[44] The aspiration smears contained an anastomosing network of branched rigid vascular channels were lined by neoplastic cells. These channels, which varied remarkably in diameter, formed highly complex structures. Her beautifully illustrated publication demonstrates many of these Schiller-Duval bodies in smears that, at low magnification, have a distinct papillary-like appearance. This could certainly lead to diagnostic confusion with epithelial neoplasms with a prominent papillary configuration, and in particular, serous carcinomas. However, as adroitly pointed out by Yang, these complex anastomosing channels differ from papillae.[44] The latter term is used to describe an epithelial lined fibrovascular stalk that terminates at its tip.

Embryonal carcinoma is a relatively uncommon primary pure ovarian germ cell tumor that theoretically is thought to demonstrate somatic differentiation of primordial neoplastic germ cells. These neoplasms may be associated with the production of both AFP and/or HCG. Thus, it may be associated with endocrine syndromes that vary depending on the age of the patient. Histologically, this neoplasm is composed of large polygonal neoplastic cells with moderate volumes of cytoplasm and solitary centrally positioned nuclei with a distinct membrane and often multiple nucleoli. The neoplastic cells may be arranged in glandular structures, papillae, and solid sheets. Especially in the latter, a syncytial arrangement may be evident as cell borders appear indistinct.

Aspiration biopsies of embryonal carcinoma typically yield highly cellular smears that may contain necrotic debris in the background. Basically, the carcinoma presents as a high-grade adenocarcinoma.[41] The authors are unaware of any distinguishing cytomorphologic features. The neoplastic cells are typically present in variably contoured, three-dimensional cohesive aggregates, including papillae that may have a syncytial appearance. As in the histologic preparations, the neoplastic cells are characterized by solitary huge nuclei with prominent and often multiple deeply basophilic nucleoli. For the most part, the N:C ratios are quite high. In contrast with many other forms of adenocarcinoma, one does not find evidence of mucin production by the tumor cells.

Based purely on cytomorphology, the differential diagnosis of embryonal carcinoma needs to include dysgerminoma, a high-grade surface epithelial carcinoma, and metastatic carcinoma. The distinction from the former is based on larger tumor cell size, greater degrees of pleomorphism, the presence of multiple nucleoli, a much greater retention of intercellular cohesion, and the lack of a tigroid background. In addition, the neoplastic cells are positive by immunocytochemistry for both cytokeratin and AFP; both of these markers are generally negative in dysgerminoma.

Pure nongestational choriocarcinomas primary in the ovary are extremely rare neoplasms of children and young adults.[45] These neoplasms secrete HCG and thus, in the pediatric population, may be associated with isosexual precocious puberty. Histologically, these consist of an admixture of two types of malignant cells: cytotrophoblast and syncytiotrophoblast.

The former cell type is characterized by an epithelial appearance with well-defined cell borders, scanty clear to eosinophilic cytoplasm, and a single, obviously malignant nucleus that may or may not contain nucleoli. The syncytiotrophoblasts are comprised of huge multinucleated neoplastic cells. They have abundant cytoplasm that is basophilic and often finely vacuolated; the cytoplasm contains multiple, clearly malignant, hyperchromatic and irregularly contoured nuclei; chromatin may appear structureless (pyknotic-like).

Aspiration biopsies of pure choriocarcinomas are quite limited. Even at low magnification, striking pleomorphism of cellular size and appearance is evident.[41] The mononucleated tumor cells are characterized by solitary darkly stained nuclei, distinct nucleoli, and high N:C ratios. They may occur singly but more often within flat mosaic sheets. The huge multinucleated malignant cells have abundant dense cytoplasm that may appear finely vacuolated and numerous malignant nuclei. The latter have large sizes, irregular contours, and very darkly stained chromatin. In fact, they are so hyperchromatic that nucleoli may not be evident.

As stated earlier, the vast majority of teratomas of the ovary are benign and cystic in type. Less than 1% of all ovarian teratomas are immature teratomas representing an uncommon form of malignant ovarian germ cell tumor. By definition, the tumor is composed of elements derived from ectoderm, endoderm, and mesoderm. Although some of these tissues may show complete histologic maturation, others are primitive or embryonal in appearance. Histologically, these elements appear to be haphazardly scattered throughout the neoplasm. Most often, the ectodermal component is neural tissue that includes neuroblastic cells, ganglion cells, neuroepithelium, glia, and ocular components. Endodermal components are usually represented by glandular or tubular structures lined by columnar epithelial cells that typically do not manifest distinctive differentiation; however, well-formed bronchial and/or gastrointestinal mucosal components may be present. Overall, these neoplasms are clinically quite aggressive. Their degree of aggressiveness, and therefore, potential therapy, may in part be based on their histologic grade. In general, the greater the proportion of immature or primitive tissue components and the higher the mitotic activity, then the higher the grade and hence, the worse the prognosis.

Aspiration smears may be extremely cellular and often are dominated by the neural component. As in neuroblastoma, the primitive neuroblasts have small round hyperchromatic nuclei and extremely high N:C ratios. The cells are arranged individually, in spheres, and in sheets; within the latter, pseudorosettes may be evident. One may also recognize in the smears more mature-appearing ganglion cells, cartilage, bone, and glandular or squamous epithelial cells.

It is the presence of both immature, but not anaplastic cells, and elements from two or three germ layers that allow one to make a specific diagnosis.

It is important to recognize that in many cases, primary ovarian germ cell tumors are mixed in type—that is, two or more of the previously described germ cell neoplasms are admixed with one another in the same mass. Furthermore, metastases from ovarian germ cell tumors may show components that are different from those recognized histologically in the primary neoplasm. All of this may contribute to confusion in constructing the correct diagnosis in aspiration smears.

The third major group of ovarian neoplasms are the sex cord–stromal tumors. These account for less than 10% of all ovarian neoplasms. Many of these are benign, representing simple fibromas of ovarian stroma. Although these may be incidental findings, fibromas may also present as either a mass lesion or rarely with effusions.

By far, the most common and clinically important neoplasm in this category is the adult granulosa cell tumor. These neoplasms, which represent no more than 2% of all ovarian tumors, occur most often in perimenopausal and postmenopausal women. Their most striking clinical manifestation is related to the fact that they are usually estrogenic. The most common manifestation in the older patient is abnormal vaginal bleeding. In younger women, menorrhagia is common. These clinical manifestations are associated with a relatively high frequency of hyperplasia and to a lesser extent, adenocarcinoma of the endometrium. It should be pointed out that rare adult granulosa cell tumors produce androgens, rather than estrogens, in excess and may be associated with virilization. Histologically, the neoplastic granulosa cells are homogeneous in appearance with solitary ovoid or slightly angulated nuclei and very high N:C ratios. The chromatin is pale stained, the nuclear membranes are often highly irregular resulting in nuclear grooves, and nucleoli are inconspicuous. In contrast with the uniformity of the tumor cells, the architectural patterns present within a given neoplasm and among different granulosa cell tumors is striking. Patterns include microfollicular, macrofollicular, trabecular, and solid. The most characteristic is the microfollicular pattern, which includes small central spaces that contain eosinophilic fluid and are surrounded by somewhat palisaded neoplastic cells. These are referred to as Call-Exner bodies. Although surgical excision of the neoplasm is often completely curative, all granulosa cell tumors need to be considered at least potentially malignant. Recurrences and metastases within the pelvis are the typical manifestation of malignancy. These may appear more than two decades after the diagnosis of the original neoplasm. Overall, the 10-year survival rate is nearly 90%.

Aspiration biopsies of granulosa cell tumors may produce a distinctive cytomorphologic picture.[11,46] The smears are usually quite cellular and include both individually dispersed and aggregated neoplastic cells (Figure 25-16). The cohesive clusters typically have sharply defined outlines. As one would expect from histology, the neoplastic cells are strikingly uniform in appearance: they have solitary ovoid nuclei with delicate membranes, fine pale chromatin, inconspicuous nucleoli, and grooves. Only scanty rims of nondescript cytoplasm surround each nucleus resulting in

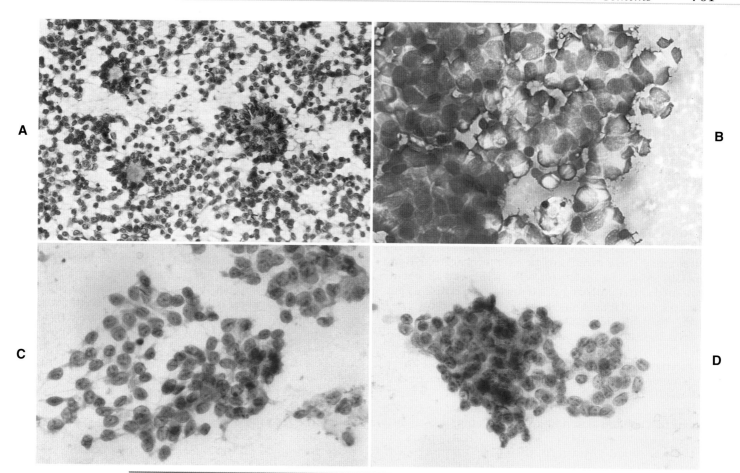

Figure 25-16 Granulosa cell tumors. **A,** This highly cellular aspirate is composed largely of individually dispersed tumor cells and small loosely cohesive clusters. In addition, well-developed Call-Exner bodies are present. The latter are composed of one or more peripheral rims of neoplastic cells surrounding amorphous matrix material. This material stains pale green with the Pap technique. At this magnification, it is obvious that the tumor cells are strikingly homogeneous in appearance. They have solitary ovoid nuclei with pale chromatin and inconspicuous nucleoli and only scanty rims of cytoplasm. **B,** The uniformity of the cells is striking with ovoid nuclei with smooth outlines, extremely finely reticulated and uniformly dispersed chromatin, and a lack of prominent nucleoli. In fact, nucleoli are not perceptible in the vast majority of these cells. Note that most of the cells possess extremely high N:C ratios. Still, nuclear molding is not evident, despite the crowding. **C,** Longitudinal nuclear grooves are evident in several of these homogeneous neoplastic cells. Note the absence of mitotic figures, nucleoli, and necrotic debris. **D,** The uniformity of the neoplastic cells is striking; along with the bland nuclear chromatin, these features point directly to the diagnosis of a granulosa cell tumor. Note the rudimentary Call-Exner body formed by a single row of neoplastic cells surrounding homogeneous cyanophilic material. The smear background is clean. (**A, C,** and **D,** Pap; **B,** DQ)

very high N:C ratios. Within cohesive aggregates, structures consistent with Call-Exner bodies may be evident. By immunocytochemistry, the tumor cells are positive for vimentin, inhibin, and the sex steroid hormone receptors (Box 25-6).

The differential diagnosis includes small cell carcinoma, endometrial stromal sarcoma (both discussed later), and carcinoid tumors.[47,48] The latter may arise as a monodermal derivative of a teratoma or represent a metastasis to the ovary, generally, from the gastrointestinal tract. The neoplastic cells of a carcinoid may have more distinctly granular chromatin,

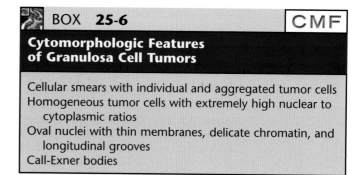

BOX **25-6**　　　　　　　　　　　CMF

Cytomorphologic Features of Granulosa Cell Tumors

Cellular smears with individual and aggregated tumor cells
Homogeneous tumor cells with extremely high nuclear to cytoplasmic ratios
Oval nuclei with thin membranes, delicate chromatin, and longitudinal grooves
Call-Exner bodies

more abundant cytoplasm, and lack nuclear grooves. The center of rosettes in carcinoids is composed of cytoplasm, not the matrix material of Call-Exner bodies. Immunocytochemistry would be very useful in this distinction. Granulosa cell tumors are immunocytochemically reactive for vimentin and inhibin, whereas carcinoids are positive for keratin and neuroendocrine markers (e.g., synaptosin).

Sertoli-Leydig cell tumors account for much less than 1% of all ovarian neoplasms. Experience with aspiration biopsies of these neoplasms, which are often androgenic, is remarkably scant.[12]

Although not definitely classifiable among the sex cord–stromal neoplasms, one tumor often considered in this setting is the fortunately uncommon primary small cell carcinoma.[49] This neoplasm typically presents in women under age 40 years. Its most characteristic association is hypercalcemia. These neoplasms are extremely aggressive and generally fatal. The malignant cells have small irregularly contoured and sharply angulated nuclei with coarsely granular and very darkly stained chromatin and scanty cytoplasm. Nucleoli are small, and they may or may not be evident. In histologic sections, the neoplastic cells are characteristically arrayed in a diffuse sheetlike pattern with little intervening stroma. Punctuated throughout the sheets are structures resembling thyroid follicles; the lumens contain watery eosinophilic fluid.

Aspiration biopsies yield moderately to highly cellular smears that contain a monotonous population of obviously malignant small cells (Figure 25-17).[47,50] Their solitary nuclei appear round to irregular; they have a distinct membrane and finely to coarsely granular and hyperchromatic chromatin. Minute nucleoli may be evident. The cells are scattered individually and in cohesive aggregates. Similar to the much more common bronchogenic small cell carcinoma, nuclear molding may be evident within cohesive aggregates. Necrotic debris is common in the background. A major item in the differential diagnosis includes granulosa cell tumors; several cases have been seen in consultation in which the initial diagnosis was thought to be a granulosa cell tumor. However, the neoplastic cells from these two tumors are distinctly different in appearance. Whereas the chromatin is very darkly stained in small cell carcinoma, it is very pale and finely granular in granulosa cells. Although the neoplastic cells in granulosa cell tumors may be densely packed within aggregates, molding is not evident. Neither necrotic debris nor mitotic figures are expected in aspirates of adult granulosa cell tumors; they are common with small cell carcinoma. Finally, Call-Exner bodies are not found in the latter aggressive neoplasm.

Nonneoplastic Functional Ovarian Cysts

Worldwide, aspiration cytology is increasing in use to evaluate ovarian cysts that are clinically thought to be benign.[28-30,39,51-57] These aspirates may be performed during laparotomy or laparoscopy or through a transvaginal, transrectal, or transabdominal approach. Many of these women are being evaluated for either pelvic pain or infertility. The most common of these nonneoplastic lesions are follicular and corpus luteum cysts. Both of these may be defined as *cystic masses* that exceed 3 cm in diameter. At times, they may be related to an abnormal release of gonadotropins. Follicular cysts occur throughout a rather broad age range, being present even in newborns and rarely in postmenopausal women; however, they do present most often during the reproductive years. Corpus luteum cysts have a much more restricted age spectrum occurring almost exclusively in women during their reproductive period. Clinically, both of these cystic lesions may present either as an adnexal mass or through clinical evidence of an elevated estradiol level, most commonly, irregularities of the menstrual cycle. Fortunately, many of these cystic masses regress spontaneously within a few months. Histologically, these cysts are comprised of an inner layer of granulosa cells and an outer layer of theca interna cells. Both cell types may or may not be luteinized to varying degrees. When an-

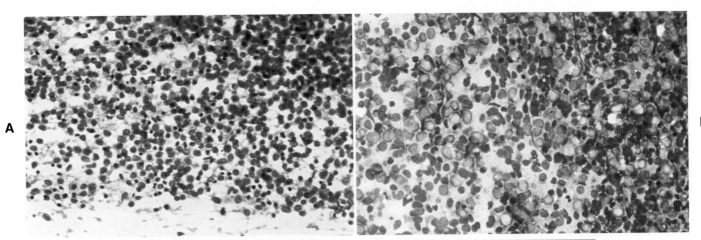

Figure 25-17 Ovarian small cell carcinoma. **A** and **B,** These obviously malignant cells show no evidence of specific differentiation. They have solitary small to moderately sized nuclei that vary from round to ovoid to sharply irregular with angulations. Their chromatin is markedly hyperchromatic and nucleoli are not apparent. In addition, cytoplasm is scanty resulting in high N:C ratios. Numerous apoptotic tumor cells are evident. Nuclear molding is strongly suggested in both illustrations. (**A,** Pap; **B,** DQ)

alyzed biochemically, the cyst fluid typically manifests a high level of estradiol; this is in sharp contrast with the low or absent levels of this estrogenic hormone in neoplastic cysts such as serous and mucinous cystadenomas and benign teratomas.

It is difficult to compare directly the results of different published series of aspiration biopsies of these functional, nonneoplastic cystic ovarian lesions. Differences include the actual type of aspiration performed, the clinical indication for the aspiration biopsy, the use of different types of radiologic guidance, differences in biochemical techniques and quantitative thresholds for measuring estradiol, and cytomorphologic criteria for considering an aspirate to be inadequate. In 1995, Kreuzer and colleagues published a series of histologically examined cysts from 203 women.[28] Each patient underwent a clinical examination that included abdominal ultrasound and laparoscopy with aspiration of the cyst contents. An aliquot of the aspirated fluid was submitted for convention cytology, whereas another portion was submitted for the biochemical determination of estradiol. For these authors, a measurement of less than 800 picograms per mm was considered diagnostic of neoplasm.[28] This series included 60 functional cysts, nine endometriotic cysts, and 101 neoplastic cysts, 15% of which proved to be malignant. Kreuzer and colleagues compared the ability of the clinical examination, including ultrasound, aspiration cytomorphology, and estradiol measurements, to predict the histology of the associated cyst.[28] Both the clinical examination and the cytomorphology correctly identified all 15 malignancies. A single false-negative interpretation was made by the estradiol determination. On the other hand, estradiol measurements were superior to both cytology and the clinical examination for identification of true neoplasms. Relatively equivalent results were achieved for all three test modalities for the nonneoplastic functional cysts. The authors stated that the results of the three test modalities often provided contradictory data.

One year later, Mulvany and colleagues reported a series of 235 ovarian cyst aspirates.[29] In contrast with the preceding study, Mulvany's investigation used transvaginal ultrasound and aspiration biopsies. Again, cyst fluid contents were divided for cytology and estradiol determinations. For Mulvany and colleagues, estradiol level greater than 20 millimoles per liter was considered diagnostic of a functional cyst.[29] The reason for this is readily apparent. Of the 52 follicular cysts in their series, 92% had an estradiol level exceeding 20 and over 75% had a level greater than 132 millimoles per liter. Of the 140 nonfunctional cysts in the series, none of them had an estradiol level exceeding 20. These authors considered the aspiration cytomorphology of more than half the aspirates to be nondiagnostic, largely because of poor cellularity. By combining the results of cytomorphology and estradiol measurements, Mulvany determined the levels of diagnostic sensitivity and specificity for the different histologic types of cysts.[29] Follicular cysts had extremely high levels of both sensitivity and specificity. However, for the other cyst types, the levels of sensitivity were quite low; specificity hovered around 100%.

More recently, Allias and colleagues evaluated 122 ultrasound diagnosed adnexal cysts that were aspirated and then surgically excised.[39] In addition to cytomorphology, the fluids in 90 of these cysts were also assayed for estradiol content. The authors compared the ability of ultrasound, cyto-

morphology, and estradiol measurement to predict whether the cyst was functional or nonfunctional. They made the correct prediction in 51%, 55%, and 94%, respectively.[39] By combining the results of all three tests, this discrimination was improved to 98% of the cysts (Figures 25-18 to 25-21 and Box 25-7).

Carcinoma of the Uterine Cervix

Worldwide, carcinoma of the cervix is the second most common type of cancer in women. In some relatively underdeveloped nations in Southeast Asia and South America, this neoplasm is a major cause of death in female patients. On the other hand, the United States and other more modernized nations have witnessed a remarkable decline in the incidence and death rate from invasive cervical carcinoma; in large part, this is because of the widespread usage of good cytologic cervicovaginal screening as discussed elsewhere in this text.[58] Today, approximately 80% of all cervical cancers are squamous cell carcinomas, with most of the remainder representing adenocarcinomas.

In women who fail their initial therapy for invasive carcinoma of the cervix or in those who present in an advanced stage, local pelvic recurrence is very common and often associated with significant morbidity and mortality. In large part, this may be related to local obstruction of the urinary tract. Thus, pelvic FNA biopsy can play a very important clinical role in the diagnosis of metastatic or recurrent cervical carcinoma. In the United States, nearly 14,000 women are diagnosed each year with invasive carcinoma; the 5-year survival rate is about 35%.

Squamous cell carcinoma of the cervix is the second most common malignancy seen in FNA biopsy of recurrent gynecologic malignancies, after ovarian carcinoma. Less often, squamous cell carcinomas originate in the vulva or vagina. To an extent, the aspiration pictures of squamous cell carcinoma varies with the histologic degree of differentiation. In the better-differentiated neoplasms, intercellular

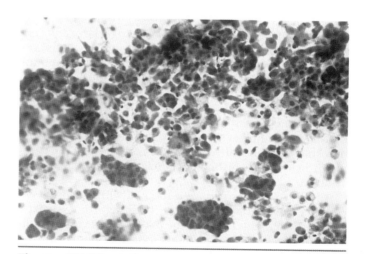

Figure 25-18 Follicular cysts. This highly cellular aspirate is characterized by relatively uniform benign granulosa cells which are present both individually and in cohesive aggregates. Some of the latter appear to include three-dimensional spheres. These cells have solitary oval nuclei and scant to moderate volumes of cyanophilic cytoplasm. Although highly cellular, there is no evidence of pleomorphism, and nuclear features are distinctly benign. (Pap)

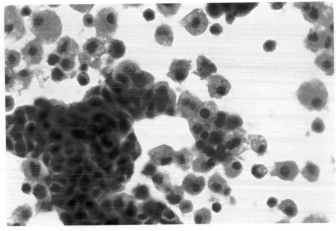

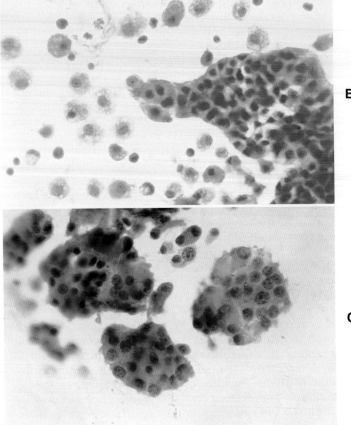

Figure 25-19   Partially luteinized follicular cysts. **A** and **B,** The cohesive cluster of nonluteinized granulosa cells is composed of elements with solitary darkly stained ovoid nuclei which are devoid of nucleoli and only scanty rims of cytoplasm resulting in high N:C ratios. Longitudinal nuclear grooves are not evident. Additionally, loosely clustered and individual luteinized cells are present. They are characterized by much more voluminous cytoplasm and by more rounded nuclei. The latter frequently contain small but distinct nucleoli. Their cytoplasm varies from finely granular to foamy to distinctly vacuolated. **C,** Features of luteinization are present in these aggregated clusters of benign cells. The nuclei are round with delicate membranes, fine pale chromatin, and micronucleoli. Cytoplasm is scant to moderate and cyanophilic; some of the latter shows distinct granularity or foaminess. (Pap)

cohesion is relatively well preserved in the smears. Thus, the aspirates contain large fragments of tumor and individually dispersed malignant cells. The neoplastic cells are often large with voluminous opaque cytoplasm. One of the beauties of the Pap stain is that it specifically stains keratin a bright orange or yellow; thus, many of the neoplastic cells have orangeophilic cytoplasm. With the DQ stain, the cytoplasm has a characteristic "robin's-egg" blue appearance. Typically, the neoplastic cells possess a single large and centrally positioned nucleus with sharply angulated or squared-off contours. Classically, the chromatin appears dense and dark simulating pyknosis. Intercellular cohesion is less well preserved in the less differentiated neoplasms. Thus, a greater proportion of the tumor cells in the smears are individually dispersed. Lower volumes of cytoplasm translate into higher N:C ratios. In addition, the nuclei may manifest qualitative differences. Specifically, the chromatin may appear distinctly granular, and in general, nucleoli are more prominent.

These carcinomas may be associated with extensive necrosis, either spontaneously or resulting from therapy (Figure 25-22). This is one of the potential difficulties in diagnosing metastatic squamous cell carcinoma in the pelvis—that is, relatively few neoplastic cells are mixed with the neutrophils and the granular necrotic material. One may have to conduct a diligent search to identify the malignant squamous cells. This is especially difficult in the radiologic suite with on-site evaluation and the DQ stain. This is further complicated by the fact that many patients with cervical carcinoma have been irradiated. As stated ear-

BOX   25-7   CMF

Cytomorphologic Features of Functional Ovarian Cysts

Extremely variably cellular smears with both single and clustered granulosa cells
Solitary round to oval nuclei with smooth membranes, often dark chromatin, and inconspicuous nucleoli
No nuclear grooves
With luteinization, nuclei are rounder and have more vesicular chromatin and distinct nucleoli
In nonluteinized, cells, scanty indistinct cytoplasm
With luteinization, abundant foamy to granular cytoplasm

lier, the intense fibrotic reaction incited by radiation may preclude the aspiration of sufficient numbers of neoplastic cells to feel comfortable in rendering a frank diagnosis of recurrence. In addition, as pointed out by Bottles and colleagues, such therapy may produce cytologic atypia in benign cellular elements which may simulate malignancy.[24]

Over the last four to five decades, both the absolute and relative incidences of adenocarcinoma of the cervix have increased dramatically.[58] In part, this appears to be because of the reduction in the incidence of invasive squamous cell carcinoma resulting from cytologic screening programs. Today, adenocarcinoma accounts for approximately 20% to 25% of all invasive neoplasms of the cervix. A variety of

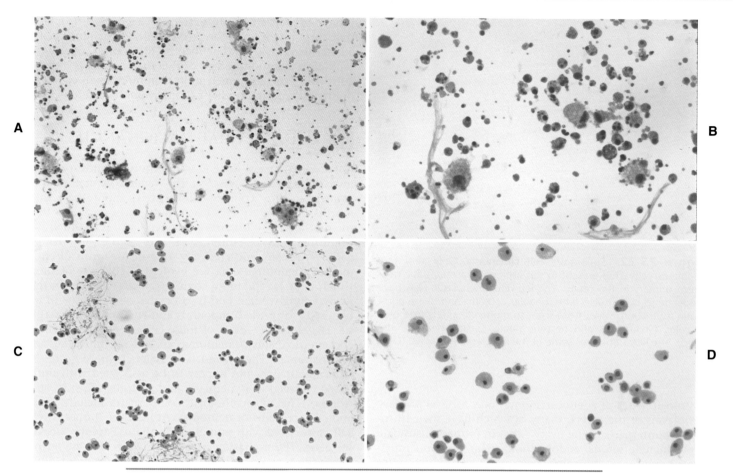

Figure 25-20 **Corpus luteum cysts. A** and **B,** Many of the luteinized cells of this speci-men show degenerative changes with pyknotic nuclei and detached fragments of cytoplasm. In the more intact cells, the nuclei remain round with delicate chromatin and small nucleoli. **C** and **D,** This specimen contains less cellular degeneration. Individually dispersed luteinized cells dom-inate the smear. Each cell has voluminous cytoplasm and rounded contours with solitary small round nuclei. The positions of the latter vary from central to very peripheral. However, the nu-clei otherwise are uniform in appearance. Blood is present focally in the background. (Pap)

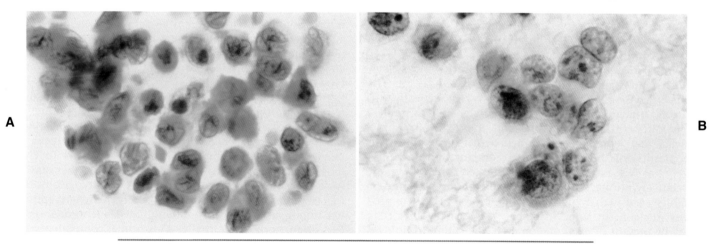

Figure 25-21 **Atypical follicular cysts. A,** This specimen is characterized by cells with markedly irregularly contoured nuclei. This is witnessed by irregularly shaped and thickened nu-clear membranes. In addition, hyperchromasia is evident, as are an occasional well-developed nucleolus. The N:C ratios are obviously extremely high. The irregularities in the nuclear outline include grooves. Also in this sample, mitotic figures were moderate in number. **B,** The variably shaped nuclei in this cellular sample show fine to moderately granulated chromatin and distinct nucleoli. Only scanty rims of cytoplasm surround each nucleus. This specimen was markedly cel-lular. (Pap)

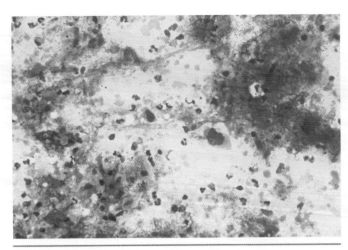

Figure 25-22 Squamous cell carcinoma. Only very rare neoplastic cells were present in this aspirate of a metastatic neoplasm primary in the cervix. The individual neoplastic cells have moderate to huge nuclei with irregular contours and dense chromatin. Cytoplasm varies from scant to moderate and is pale blue in color. Neutrophils and necrotic debris occupy much of the smear. The latter obscures some of the neoplastic elements. (DQ)

histologic types of adenocarcinomas may arise as primary neoplasms of the cervix, many of which have their histologic counterparts in the ovary—that is, primary histologic types include serous, endometrioid, clear cell, and mucinous carcinomas (this same spectrum of adenocarcinomas also occurs as primary neoplasms of the endometrium and fallopian tube). However, in the cervix, the relative incidences of these various histologic forms differ greatly from that of primary ovarian carcinomas. By far, the most common type arising in the endocervix is mucinous adenocarcinomas. Many of the latter histologically resemble, to a degree, normal endocervical mucinous cells. On the other hand, serous adenocarcinomas are rare as primary neoplasms in the uterine cervix. The second most common type arising in the cervix is endometrioid adenocarcinomas. Less than 5% of all primary adenocarcinomas of this site are of the clear cell type.

Similar to squamous cell carcinomas of the cervix, adenocarcinomas may recur as pelvic mass lesions that of course may be the target of FNA biopsy. Histologically, the primary mucinous carcinomas are usually well or moderately differentiated neoplasms and thus, the aspiration smears may contain well-formed acinar structures. The neoplastic cells have a columnar configuration and relatively low N:C ratios. The malignant nuclei often maintain a relatively normal basal polarity; they tend to be round or slightly oval with hyperchromatic chromatin and prominent nucleoli. In some instances, neoplastic goblet cells may be present or even predominate the cytomorphologic picture. Rarely is distinct signet-ring differentiation encountered (see Figure 25-8). As might be expected, the aspiration cytomorphology of serous, endometrioid, and clear cell adenocarcinomas closely mimic and are morphologically indistinguishable from those described in the ovarian section.

Small cell neuroendocrine carcinomas account for less than 5% of all primary cervical malignancies.[59] This is for-

tunate in that these are extremely aggressive neoplasms that carry a worse prognosis than either squamous cell or adenocarcinomas. As described by Shin and Caraway, the aspiration cytomorphology of these neoplasms is indistinguishable from the much more common small cell carcinoma of the lung or other extrapulmonary locations.[47]

 ENDOMETRIAL MALIGNANCIES

Adenocarcinoma of the endometrium is the most common invasive cancer to arise in the female genital tract in women in this country. Fortunately, more than three fourths of these are diagnosed in an early stage and thus, the mortality resulting from this neoplasm is less than that resulting from carcinomas of the cervix and ovaries. Pathogenetically and clinically, two major forms of endometrial adenocarcinoma are evident.[60] The first of these, which is by far the more common, tends to occur in relatively young women and is associated with the use of unopposed estrogenic compounds and endometrial hyperplasia. Histologically, most of these correspond to the classic endometrioid adenocarcinomas and the rare mucinous adenocarcinomas. The second type is much more aggressive clinically. It does not appear to be associated with unopposed estrogen or hyperplasia and typically arises in older women. The histopathologic counterparts include serous and clear cell adenocarcinomas. At least the former is typically associated with mutations in the *p53* tumor suppressor gene. The aspiration cytomorphology of these adenocarcinomas again cannot be distinguished from those arising in the ovary (see Figure 15-11).

The most common *sarcomatous* malignancy of the uterus is the carcinosarcoma or malignant mixed müllerian tumor.[61] This neoplasm accounts for no more than 2% of all uterine cancers but is an extremely aggressive neoplasm with a poor prognosis. Most patients are postmenopausal. Histologically, these are biphasic neoplasms in that they include both malignant epithelial and stromal components. Most commonly, the epithelial element is a high-grade adenocarcinoma that may resemble serous or endometrioid adenocarcinoma. The malignant stromal component most often consists of nonspecific malignant spindled cells that are arranged in fascicles and sheets. When this is the only type of sarcomatous element present, the neoplasm is referred to as a *homologous carcinosarcoma*. When the malignant stroma includes elements such as cartilage, bone, or skeletal muscle, then the neoplasm is referred to as a *heterologous carcinosarcoma*. These neoplasms often recur as pelvic mass lesions and thus may be subjected to FNA biopsy. Furthermore, these neoplasms may metastasize widely, again forming a target for biopsy. Histologically, the metastases most often consist of a purely malignant epithelial tumor, usually poorly differentiated adenocarcinoma. Less often, both the epithelial and stromal components are present or only the sarcomatous elements are found (Figure 25-23).

The largest study dedicated to the FNA biopsy of carcinosarcomas was published Mourad and colleagues.[14] These authors studied the aspirates of six recurrent and ten metastatic carcinosarcomas. In all sixteen instances, the specimens demonstrated carcinoma, but in only three were definite glandular differentiation evident. In other words,

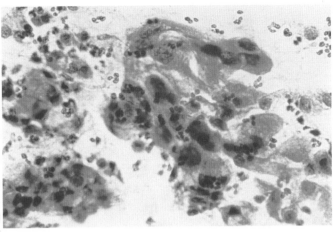

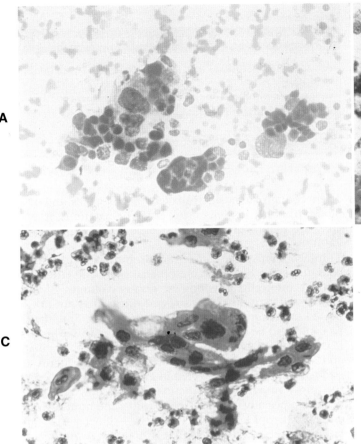

Figure 25-23 **Endometrial carcinosarcoma. A,** This aspirate is from a pelvic lymph node in a woman with a prior diagnosis of uterine carcinosarcoma. Only a high-grade adenocarcinomatous component was present in this sample. The cells have obviously malignant nuclei with marked pleomorphism and prominent nucleoli. This specimen did not show evidence of specific endometrial differentiation or sarcomatous elements. **B** and **C,** Obviously malignant sarcomatous elements are present in this aspirate of a pelvic recurrence of a previously diagnosed endometrial carcinosarcoma. The neoplastic cells have one or more huge nuclei with obviously hyperchromatic chromatin and moderate volumes of dense cyanophilic cytoplasm. In a proportion of the cells, the cytoplasm forms tapering tails that appear to blend imperceptibly into the smear background. (**A,** DQ; **B** and **C,** Pap)

these were poorly differentiated neoplasms in the smears. In addition, in five of the aspirates, homologous sarcomatous cells were present along with the carcinoma. As stated by these authors, in the majority of cases, the cytologic diagnosis of a carcinosarcoma may be impossible without knowing the previous history of such a neoplasm in a given patient.[14] They did find that the biphasic nature of the neoplasm was more easily recognizable in accompanying cell block preparations.

Endometrial stromal sarcomas are uncommon malignancies, many of which occur in premenopausal patients (in contrast with most other malignancies of the uterine corpus).[62] Histologically, these can be divided into low-grade and high-grade forms. The former is composed of neoplastic cells that, to a degree, resemble the normal stromal elements of a proliferative phase endometrium. Thus, the neoplastic cells possess solitary round nuclei with evenly dispersed and somewhat darkly stained chromatin and minute or inconspicuous nucleoli. The cells have scant to moderate volumes of cytoplasm with poorly visualized cell borders. These neoplasms are highly vascular and characteristically possess arterioles that resemble the normal spiral arterioles of the endometrium. The histologic picture acceptable for a diagnosis of high-grade stromal sarcoma varies among different pathologists. In any case, the neoplastic cells have larger nuclei than in the low-grade forms, more coarsely granular chromatin, and more prominent nucleoli. Mitotic activity is usually much greater than that seen in the low-grade neoplasms.

Low-grade stromal sarcomas pursue a relative indolent course. Many patients are cured by their primary surgery. However, it is not rare for these low-grade neoplasms to recur, generally within the pelvis. These recurrences may occur more than two decades after the original diagnosis. The neoplastic cells in the low-grade neoplasms are often positive for both estrogen and progesterone receptors, and hormonal therapy may be quite beneficial in patients with recurrent tumor. On the other hand, high-grade stromal sarcomas are more aggressive neoplasms. These may present as recurrent pelvic masses but also may be seen in more widely disseminated metastatic sites.

Only uncommonly has the aspiration cytomorphology of endometrial stromal sarcomas been described.[15,18,48] The low-grade stromal sarcomas present in smears as small homogeneous cells with solitary round dark nuclei and high N:C ratios. Although they may occur as individually dispersed cells, they are often present within cohesive tissue fragments. With the DQ stain, metachromatic fibrillar matrix material appears to "cement" the neoplastic cells. According to Yang, this material corresponds to the fine reticulum fiber network that envelops individual neoplastic cells and small groups of such cells.[48] On the other hand, this matrix material is not evident in the Pap-stained smears. The latter stain, however, is beneficial in that the relatively bland appearance of the neoplastic nuclei is demonstrated and arterioles passing through the cohesive tumor fragments are present. Aspirates of high-grade stromal sarcomas show cells that are clearly

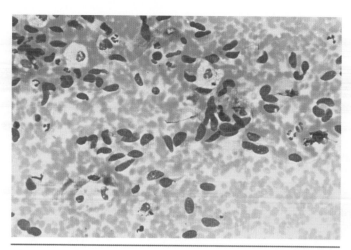

Figure 25-24 **Endometrial stromal sarcoma.** Individual tumor cells dominate this aspiration smear. They are characterized by rather uniform large elongated nuclei. The latter vary from having sharply pointed tips to blunt rounded contours. However, the chromatin is uniform from cell to cell with an even condensed appearance and a lack of nucleoli. Also poorly developed is cytoplasm; in a minority of cells, delicate tails are evident. (DQ)

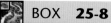

BOX   25-8   **CMF**

Cytomorphologic Features of Endometriosis

Admixture of glandular and stromal cells with small benign nuclei
Columnar epithelial cells in flat honeycomb sheets
Round to elongated stromal cells, both individually and in loose syncytia
Hemosiderin containing histiocytes

malignant (Figure 25-24). The nuclei vary from round to irregular in contour, have more irregularly distributed chromatin granules, and nucleoli. Although the N:C ratios are usually high, some of the neoplastic cells may possess greater volumes of cytoplasm. One may not find the metachromatic extracellular matrix material or arterioles in these specimens.[18,48]

 ## DISEASES OF THE PERITONEUM

Endometriosis

Endometriosis is the presence of endometrial tissue outside of the endometrium and myometrium proper. In most cases, both endometrial stroma and epithelium are evident histologically, often with evidence of prior bleeding (hemosiderin). Endometriosis often involves the pelvic peritoneum, the rectovaginal septum, ligaments of the uterus, and ovaries. Less frequently, these ectopic tissues may be found in the upper abdomen and even in the lungs and pleura. The vast majority of patients are women in the reproductive years. Clinical manifestations vary from completely asymptomatic to the production of one or more mass lesions to incapacitating pain.

In FNA biopsy, both the epithelial and stromal components must be identified to render a diagnosis of endometriosis with certainty (Figures 25-25 and 25-26).[29,30,63-65] The glandular cells have a low columnar configuration and are typically present in smears in cohesive aggregates that vary from spheres to acinar structures to large flat sheets. On the other hand, the stromal cells have a round to elongated appearance with very high N:C ratios. They may be individually dispersed or present within very loose syncytial clusters. Furthermore, decidualization of stroma may result in cells with much lower N:C ratios.[65] Both cell types possess benign-appearing nuclei with fine, pale chromatin and generally inconspicuous nucleoli. In addition, the smears will

often contain hemosiderin-laden macrophages and lysed blood. In our experiences, cell block preparations, if available, are helpful in the correct aspiration diagnosis (Box 25-8).

In FNA biopsy, the differential diagnosis includes simple contamination by pelvic mesothelial cells. The latter have distinct intercellular windows, greater volumes of cytoplasm, and centrally placed round nuclei that are not expected in benign endometrial glandular cells. Endometriosis could also be confused with endosalpingiosis. The latter is composed of bland epithelial cells that may be ciliated and associated with psammoma bodies. Hemosiderin and stromal cells are not expected in endosalpingiosis. Perhaps the most important distinction is with low-grade neoplasms, especially ovarian serous borderline tumors. In the latter, the neoplastic cells occur in three-dimensional papillae and sheets, and have higher N:C ratios. Again, distinct stromal elements and hemosiderin are not be present.

Papillary Serous Neoplasms

Primary neoplasms arising in the pelvic peritoneum may histologically be indistinguishable from their serous neoplastic counterparts in the ovary. This includes serous borderline neoplasms that typically do not appear to invade the underlying tissues.[33] These patients, who are often quite young, have a relatively indolent clinical course. At the other end of the spectrum are primary high-grade serous adenocarcinomas. These tumors invade deeply and may metastasize; they are almost uniformly fatal. Somewhat intermediate between these two extremes are tumors known as *psammoma carcinomas*.[66] Histologically, these tumors have low-grade malignant nuclear features, extremely numerous psammoma bodies, and invasion of tissues underlying the peritoneum. Fortunately, they usually have a rather good prognosis, similar to the serous borderline tumors of the peritoneum.

The cytomorphology of these serous neoplasms resemble completely that of their ovarian counterparts.[1,11,67] In the rare examples of psammoma carcinoma that we have seen, the smears may be "jam-packed" with psammoma bodies.[68] Neoplastic cells comprise a small proportion of these specimens and are typically attached to the external surfaces of the psammoma bodies.

Mesotheliomas

Two major forms of mesotheliomas may arise in the peritoneum. One of these is the diffuse tubulopapillary (epithelial) malignant mesothelioma that morphologically resem-

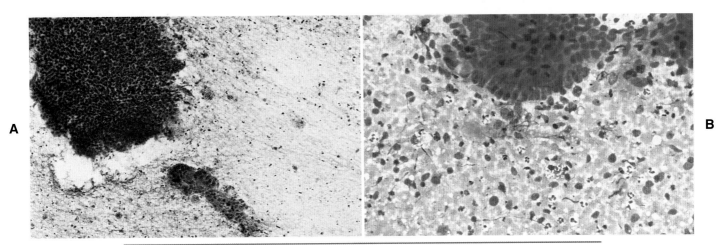

Figure 25-25   Pelvic endometriosis. **A,** In this scanning lens view, it can be recognized that the benign endometrial epithelial cells are present in cohesive and generally flat aggregates. Even at this low magnification, the maintenance of normal cohesion and polarity is apparent. The latter is manifested by the uniform distribution of the nuclei within the sheets. The benign quality of these cells is also apparent in this classic honeycomb arrangement with small uniform bland nuclei. Individually dispersed cells are also present. Presumably, many of these represent stromal elements with ovoid nuclei and very scanty cytoplasm. Finally, hemosiderin-laden histiocytic elements are also present. **B,** At higher magnification, a peripheral palisading of the benign nuclei is apparent within the sheet of glandular elements. Again, note the strikingly bland and uniform appearance of these cells and their nuclei. Individual stromal cells with ovoid to elongated contours, solitary dark nuclei, and very high N:C ratios are present, as are hemosiderin-laden macrophages. (**A,** Pap; **B,** DQ)

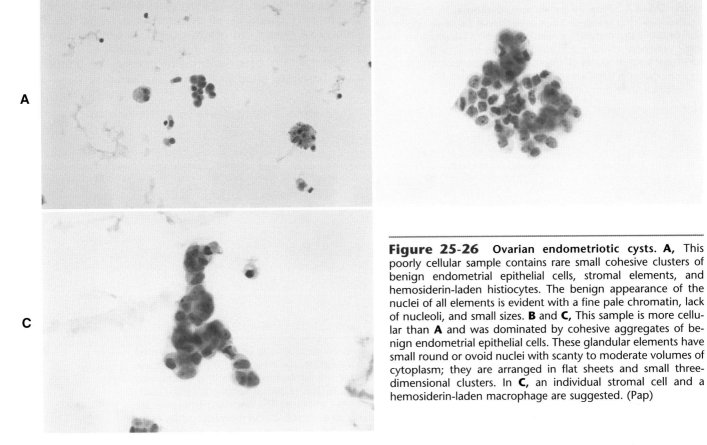

Figure 25-26   Ovarian endometriotic cysts. **A,** This poorly cellular sample contains rare small cohesive clusters of benign endometrial epithelial cells, stromal elements, and hemosiderin-laden histiocytes. The benign appearance of the nuclei of all elements is evident with a fine pale chromatin, lack of nucleoli, and small sizes. **B** and **C,** This sample is more cellular than **A** and was dominated by cohesive aggregates of benign endometrial epithelial cells. These glandular elements have small round or ovoid nuclei with scanty to moderate volumes of cytoplasm; they are arranged in flat sheets and small three-dimensional clusters. In **C,** an individual stromal cell and a hemosiderin-laden macrophage are suggested. (Pap)

bles its more common brethren primary in the pleura. Both aspiration and exfoliative cytomorphology of this malignant mesothelioma are indistinguishable from those arising in the thorax (Figure 25-27). The other form is the multicystic mesothelioma. This extremely rare benign neoplasm occurs almost exclusively in young adults with the majority of patients being females. Grossly, multiple small to large cystic masses can be seen involving the peritoneum, including that within the pelvis. They have been described as having the appearance of raindrops. In tissue sections, the masses consist largely of cystic spaces that are lined by benign-appearing homogenous mesothelial cells. Bland connective tissue may separate the different locules with

scattered fibroblasts. In addition, in these more solid areas, the neoplasm may resemble adenomatoid tumors.

Only rarely has the multicystic mesothelioma been described in aspiration biopsies.[69,70] The aspirates are moderately cellular and dominated by uniform benign mesothelial cells present within cohesive aggregates. The latter typically are large flat sheets in which a honeycomb arrangement can be seen at low magnification. Within these monolayers, intercellular spaces (windows) may be evident. The cells have dense cyanophilic cytoplasm with peripheral pallor, the picture that all cytologists would recognize as characteristic of mesothelial cells in effusions. Further, the nuclei are quite bland in appearance; they are perfectly round with finely granular evenly dispersed chromatin that is often pale and stained, with minute but distinct nucleoli. These mesothelial cells may appear entrapped within dense connective tissue. Some of the mesothelial cells may have prominent cytoplasmic vacuoles; when these cells are numerous focally, it may resemble an adenomatoid tumor (Figure 25-28).[71,72]

URINARY BLADDER

Urothelial (Transitional Cell) Carcinoma

Although urothelial carcinoma of the bladder may arise in young individuals, most patients are older adults, most commonly between the ages of 60 and 70 years. Men are affected more often than women. Painless hematuria is by far the most common initial symptom in patients with urothelial carcinoma. Irritative manifestations occur less often. In contradistinction to exfoliative urinary tract cytology, in the United States, FNA biopsy plays no significant role in the primary diagnosis of urothelial carcinoma. On the hand, FNA biopsy can be quite useful in confirming local recurrences and metastases of these neoplasms.

Histologically, the noninvasive portions of urothelial carcinomas are often papillary in appearance. These are

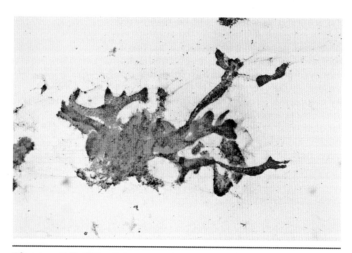

Figure 25-27 **Primary pelvic mesothelioma.** In this scanning lens view, the complex three-dimensional papillary configuration of the malignant cells is readily apparent. Obviously, intercellular cohesion is well maintained. On the basis of this single microscopic field, it would be impossible to distinguish this specimen from that of a papillary serous adenocarcinoma. (Pap)

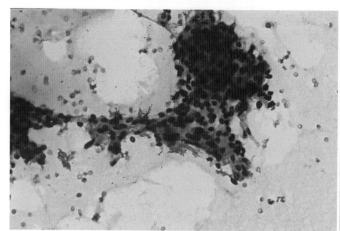

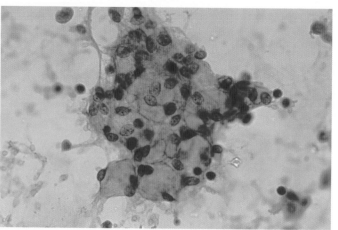

Figure 25-28 **Multicystic mesothelioma. A,** Uniform neoplastic cells appear embedded within metachromatic matrix material. At this magnification, the neoplastic elements appear very homogeneous with solitary round dark nuclei that are surrounded by scant to voluminous cytoplasm. No true distinguishing features are evident. **B,** This cluster of neoplastic cells is characterized by small, bland, uniform nuclei and abundant cytoplasm. The nuclear membranes are delicate, the chromatin is fine, and the nucleoli are barely perceptible. The morphologically helpful feature is the highly vacuolated cytoplasm with peripherally oriented nuclei, as are seen in aspiration biopsies of adenomatoid tumors. (**A,** DQ; **B,** Pap)

comprised of relatively delicate fibrovascular connective tissue cores coated by multiple layers of neoplastic urothelial cells. Both the number of cellular layers and the appearance of the neoplastic cells is variable, not only among neoplasms, but also at times, within the same tumor. In well-differentiated neoplasms, the tumor cells are morphologically indistinguishable from normal urothelial elements. Maturation may be seen within the layers of epithelium. As the neoplasm becomes less differentiated, progressive loss of this maturation, often increased layers of tumor cells, and progressively anaplastic and pleomorphic neoplastic cells occur. The tumor cells characteristically have oval to angulated solitary nuclei that are very hyperchromatic. The chromatin varies from finely to coarsely granular or structureless. Nucleoli are also quite variable from case to case. The cytoplasm is moderate in volume and amphophilic. This papillary architecture is characteristically lost as the tumor invades underlying stroma. The typical invasive picture is that of variably sized and sharply demarcated nests

of malignant cells that may show peripheral palisading and small clusters and individual tumor cells.

Chagnon and colleagues reported the results of aspiration biopsies of pelvic lymph nodes in 101 patients with carcinoma of the bladder.[74] Aspirates were performed after lymphangiography. The overall accuracy of aspiration biopsy in these patients was 93% with a specificity of 100%. Very similar results were also reported by Piscioli and colleagues.[75] More recently, both computed tomography (CT) and magnetic resonance imaging (MRI) scanning has been used to delineate possible targets for FNA biopsy including pelvic masses and enlarged lymph nodes.[76] The results may alter subsequent surgery.

Aspirates of urothelial carcinoma reflect the underlying level of histologic differentiation, which is usually high grade.[77-80] Smears are often quite cellular and include individually dispersed neoplastic cells; small, flat, loose monolayers; and three-dimensional cohesive aggregates (Figures 25-29 to 29-31). However, true papillary structures are often

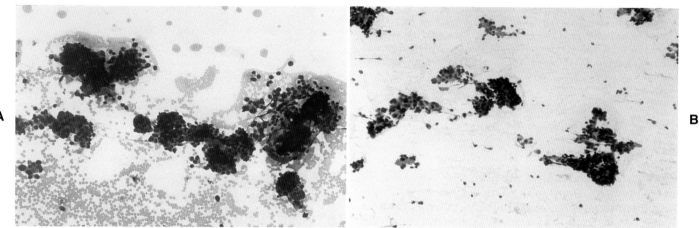

Figure 25-29　**Well-differentiated urothelial carcinoma. A** and **B,** Cohesive clusters of relatively uniform-appearing neoplastic cells dominate these aspiration smears. The aggregates are clearly three-dimensional but distinct papillary differentiation is not readily apparent—that is, fibrovascular cores cannot be seen running through the center of these clusters. Hyperchromasia is obvious. (**A,** DQ; **B,** Pap)

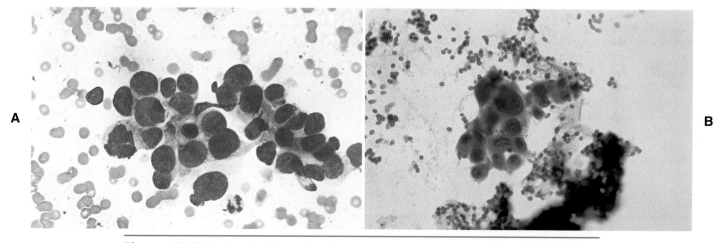

Figure 25-30　**Poorly differentiated urothelial carcinoma. A** and **B,** Cohesive clusters of obviously malignant and poorly differentiated carcinoma cells are present. No specific lineage differentiation is evident. The cells have large nuclei with primitive chromatin, which is darkly stained and distinct nucleoli. In **A,** a mitotic figure is apparent. (**A,** DQ; **B,** Pap)

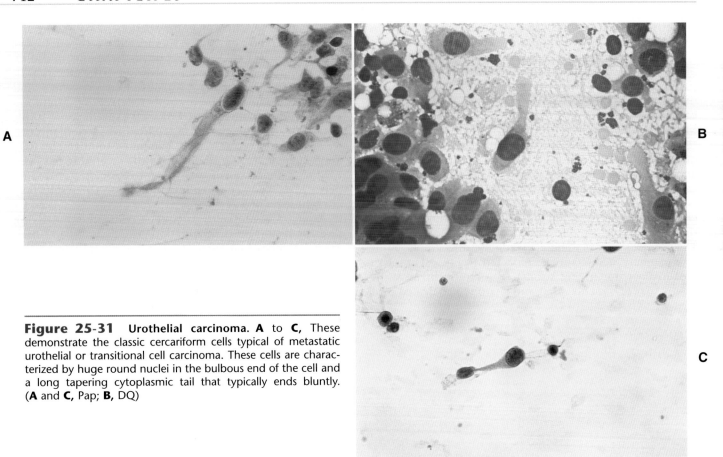

Figure 25-31   Urothelial carcinoma. A to **C,** These demonstrate the classic cercariform cells typical of metastatic urothelial or transitional cell carcinoma. These cells are characterized by huge round nuclei in the bulbous end of the cell and a long tapering cytoplasmic tail that typically ends bluntly. (**A** and **C,** Pap; **B,** DQ)

not evident. The contours of the neoplastic cells are quite variable, ranging from oval to polygonal to spindled. Recent attention has been paid to the so-called cercariform cells.[78-80] Several groups have stated that such cellular elements are characteristic of urothelial carcinoma in aspiration smears. As defined by Hida and Gupta, these elements are characterized as malignant cells with a rounded or globular cytoplasmic body that contains the nucleus and a solitary (unipolar) nontapering cytoplasmic process (see Figure 25-31).[80] The distal end of this cytoplasmic process may appear flat, notched, or bulbous. For the most part, the cytoplasm is dense and homogeneous, although vacuoles may be present especially in the tip of the cytoplasmic tail. These cercariform cells are not specific for urothelial carcinoma in aspiration smears, but when present in large numbers, this does strongly favor the interpretation of a metastatic urothelial carcinoma. Most of the neoplastic cells are uninucleated. The nuclei vary from round or oval and smooth to highly irregular and angulated. The nuclear membranes may be quite thickened. The chromatin, which is always hyperchromatic, varies from finely to coarsely granular or pyknotic-like (Box 25-9).

One morphologic variant that necessitates specific mention is sarcomatoid urothelial carcinoma. These neoplasms often have a distinct gross appearance presenting as a polyp that grows into the bladder lumen. The neoplasm is defined histologically, however, by its admixture of malignant epithelial and malignant spindle-shaped neoplastic cells. The carcinomatous component most often resembles the usual type of urothelial carcinoma, but squamous cell carcinoma is also seen with some frequency. Ill-defined bundles of spindle-

---

BOX   25-9   CMF

Cytomorphologic Features of Urothelial Carcinoma

Variably cellular smears with many individual tumor cells, sheets, spheres, papillae
Pleomorphic tumor cell size and shapes: round, polygonal, spindled, or cercariform with dense cyanophilic cytoplasm
Pleomorphic nuclei with hyperchromatic chromatin
Highly variable nucleoli

---

shaped neoplastic cells without any evidence of specific differentiation is the typical appearance of the sarcomatoid component. This neoplasm is associated with an aggressive clinical course. Sarcomatous appearing cells may dominate aspirates of this tumor. If the histology of the patient's primary carcinoma is known, then the diagnosis should be straightforward. Furthermore, at least a small proportion of the malignant cells should be positive for cytokeratin.

Adenocarcinoma

No more than 1% to 2% of all primary malignancies of the urinary bladder are adenocarcinomas.[137] The two major types of bladder adenocarcinomas are those arising from the urothelium and the less common form arising from urachal remnants. The distinction between these two is important in that the latter typically arise within the wall of the dome of the bladder (rather than from the urothelial surface). Histologic types include an intestinal variant that morphologically may be indistinguishable from primary colonic adenocarcinomas, mucinous adenocarcinomas, and clear cell adenocarcinomas; the latter resemble those arising in the female genital tract. The authors are unaware of any publications dealing specifically with the aspiration cytomorphology of primary adenocarcinomas of the urinary bladder.

Small Cell Carcinoma

Small cell carcinoma is a rare and extremely aggressive form of malignancy that may arise in the urinary bladder. Not uncommonly, metastases are present at the time of initial diagnosis. Histologically, the neoplasm resembles small cell carcinoma arising in other body sites such as the lung or cervix. The aspiration cytomorphology also resembles small cell carcinomas arising in other body sites.[47] No specific clues suggest origin in the bladder. Recent data suggest the importance of including multiagent chemotherapy in the initial treatment of patients with this neoplasm.

Rhabdomyosarcoma

A number of different histologic types of sarcoma may arise in the urinary bladder. Perhaps the most distinctive is rhabdomyosarcoma, as it occurs primarily in young children, in contrast to most other cancers of this organ. Boys are affected more often than girls. The most common histologic type is embryonal rhabdomyosarcoma. Accordingly, small primitive malignant cells infiltrate the bladder wall. Most of the tumor cells possess a single round hyperchromatic nucleus with a small but distinct nucleolus and a high N:C ratio. Most neoplastic cells do not show any evidence of specific differentiation at the light microscopic level. One morphologic variant is sarcoma botryoides in which grossly the neoplasm occurs as multiple aggregated polyploid masses. In this setting, the malignant rhabdomyoblasts are concentrated in a layer just beneath the urothelium.

As described in detail in Chapter 28, aspiration biopsies of embryonal rhabdomyosarcoma present a cellular picture with both dispersed and loosely cohesive clusters of tumor cells.[81] With the DQ stain, the chromatin is seen as finely reticulated, one or more small nucleoli may be apparent, and cytoplasm appears basophilic. Sharply punched-out glycogen vacuoles may be present within the cytoplasm. As a result, rhabdomyosarcoma is one of the neoplasms that may have a tigroid smear background, in addition to seminoma. In a child with a prior diagnosis of rhabdomyosarcoma of the bladder, the aspiration cytomorphology of recurrence or metastasis would be certainly sufficiently characteristic to render a specific diagnosis. However, in a patient without a prior histologic diagnosis, immunocytochemistry (or electron microscopy) is required to render a specific diagnosis of rhabdomyosarcoma.

 ## PROSTATE

The prostate gland, which is a hormonally responsive secondary sex organ, is a common site of disease in adult men. Three major areas of abnormalities are discussed in this section: inflammation, nodular hyperplasia, and malignancies. The prostate gland can be sampled by FNA biopsy, usually by a transrectal approach. This employs a special aspiration device that fits on one hand so that the index finger can palpate suspicious nodules and direct the aspiration needle into these targeted sites. The opposite hand is used to provide a vacuum on the syringe for the aspiration procedure. In the United States, FNA biopsy of the prostate gland enjoyed only a limited and terse period of success. Before it could gain popularity as a diagnostic procedure (over transurethral resection sampling), multiple quadrant sextant tissue core biopsies prevailed. This histologic sampling procedure is used widely throughout this country and has essentially supplanted aspiration biopsy of the prostate. However, in other countries, FNA biopsy of the prostate remains a mainstay in the evaluation of prostatic nodules and the diagnosis of prostatic carcinoma.

Inflammation

Inflammation of the prostate may be acute or chronic in nature and may be related to an identifiable microbial agent or noninfectious in origin. Acute inflammation of the prostate is often related to infection by gram-negative bacteria especially *Escherichia coli*. Although it may affect individuals at almost any age, it tends to be seen more often in relatively young adult males. Characteristic symptomatology includes frequency and urgency of urination, often associated with discomfort of varying degrees. Perineal pain may also be present as may fever and chills. On palpation, the gland is enlarged, boggy, and tender. It is unusual for the prostate to be sampled for pathologic exam in this setting. Generally, the patient is treated with antibiotics and discharged. Neutrophils dominate smears (Figure 25-32).

Chronic inflammation involving the prostate takes several different forms. The most common consists of infiltrates of lymphocytes closely associated with epithelial structures and is often associated with urinary tract infections. Thus, symptoms include urgency, frequency, and possibly a dull discomfort in the perineal region. A wide spectrum of findings can be detected by rectal palpation. As with the acute form of inflammation, the prostate is generally not examined pathologically in this setting. However, Matsumoto and colleagues studied a series of patients with chronic prostatitis by FNA biopsy.[82] The smears demonstrated mostly neutrophilic leukocytes and histiocytes; lymphocytes and plasma cells were relatively sparse. An attempt was made to culture pathogenic organisms in aspirated cellular material. This was successful in only one (4%) patient. The authors hypothesized that this failure to identify a specific bacterial agent was related to focal colonization of the gland and thus sampling error.

A specific form of chronic inflammation needs to be discussed, namely, granulomatous prostatitis.[83] Although some examples may be related directly to infection with mycobacteria or fungal organisms, most instances appear to be unrelated to infections. The two most common types are termed *nonspecific granulomatous prostatitis* and *granulomatous inflammation related to prior biopsies*.[83] On palpation, the prostate may feel nodular and hard, simulating carcinoma. Both of these forms of prostatitis may be related to damage to epithelial structures with release of "foreign" material into the stroma inciting a granulomatous response. Aspira-

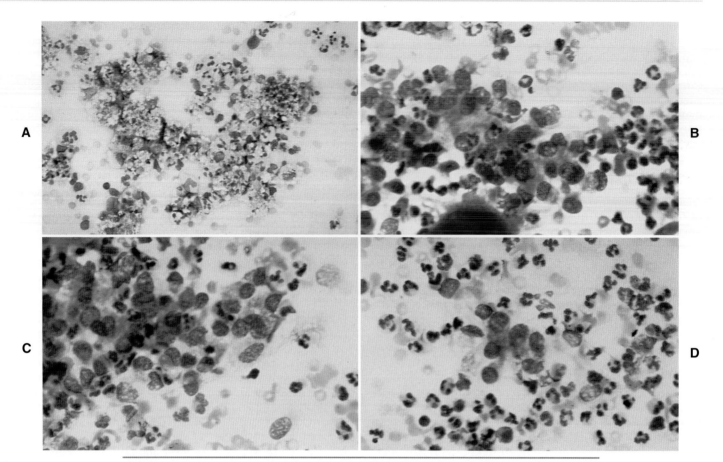

Figure 25-32 Acute prostatitis. **A** to **D,** Small loose clusters of benign epithelial cells are mixed with much more numerous segmented leukocytes. The epithelial nuclei are small and uniform, although they occasionally contain a nucleolus. Although cohesion is generally well maintained, with this degree of acute inflammation, rare individual epithelial cells are present, but they maintain benign attributes. In the presence of such a degree of acute inflammation, one should never make a diagnosis of adenocarcinoma. (DQ)

tion biopsies show a mixed inflammatory picture including epithelioid cells, multinucleated inflammatory giant cells, lymphocytes, plasma cells, and segmented leukocytes (Figure 25-33).[84,85] Epithelial elements represent only a small proportion of all the cellular elements present within the smears; they may demonstrate reactive atypical features.

Nodular Hyperplasia

Benign nodular hyperplasia of the prostate is the most common disease to involve this organ. It is so common that it may almost be considered a normal occurrence. The major reason that nodular hyperplasia is clinically important is that it causes urinary tract obstruction. This results in varying degrees of difficulty in urination. The prostate gland progressively increases in size after puberty, and hyperplasia is found in at least half of all men age 60 years and in almost all men over age 80 years. Although the cause(s) of nodular hyperplasia is unknown, it is believed that steroid hormones play significant roles in the proliferation of both the epithelium and the stroma. Nodular hyperplasia is not a premalignant condition.

Histologically, the glandular component of the hyperplasia consists of an admixture of small to large acinar structures, many of which have a stellate contour. This lat-

ter feature is related to papillary projections of the epithelium with fibrovascular cores into the lumen. The glands are lined by tall columnar epithelial cells with small nuclei and low N:C ratios and by small and at times difficult-to-recognize basal epithelial cells. The latter have high N:C ratios and scanty clear cytoplasm (by immunohistochemistry, they are positive for high molecular weight cytokeratins). The spindle-shaped stromal cells, which include smooth muscle, may form concentric coronas about the glandular structures.

Aspiration smears obtained from nodular hyperplasia may or may not be highly cellular (Figure 25-34). This probably is related to the proportions of epithelial and stromal components involved in this proliferative process. Almost all of the benign glandular cells are present in small to large honey-combed sheets with sharply defined, smooth edges.[84,86,87] The glandular cells are strikingly homogeneous in appearance with distinct cell borders creating polygonal contours, relatively scant clear to pale granular cytoplasm, and solitary nuclei. The latter appear perfectly round, are small, have evenly dispersed chromatin, and inconspicuous nucleoli. The staining intensity of the chromatin and the distinctness of its granularity is variable. Only infrequently are definite acinar structures present within the smear. The smear background is clean. If the prostate contains a con-

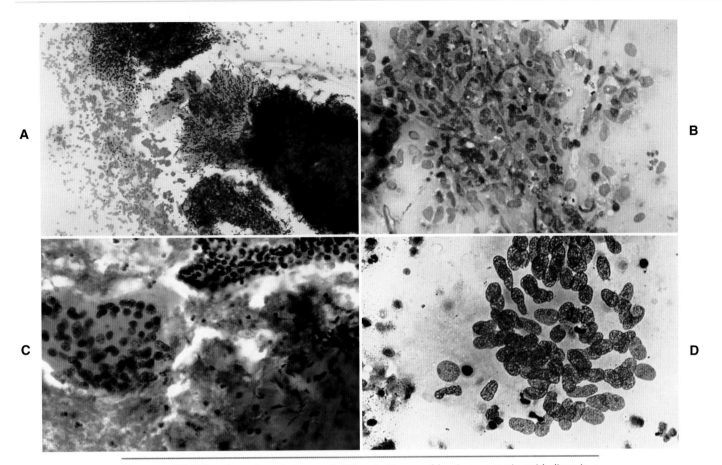

Figure 25-33 Granulomatous prostatitis. A, Sheets of benign prostatic epithelium in a honeycomb arrangement are attached to elements of granulomatous inflammation including multinucleated giant cells. **B,** The granulomas are composed of epithelioid cells with elongated nuclei and moderate volumes of cytoplasm with indistinct cell borders, leading to a syncytial arrangement. The nuclei of the epithelioid cells have such delicate membranes that they are indistinct from the chromatin that is very evenly dispersed. Nucleoli are not evident. Some of the nuclei have central folds or indentations. **C,** A huge multinucleated inflammatory giant cell with numerous round nuclei is adjacent to a flat sheet of benign of prostatic epithelium. The nuclei of the latter are smaller, somewhat more darkly stained, and more crowded than those of the giant cells. **D,** An admixture of individual epithelioid cells and multinucleated inflammatory giant cells characteristic of granulomatous inflammation is present in this aspirate. Although the presence of granulomatous inflammation does not exclude the concurrent possibility of adenocarcinoma, one should always hesitate to diagnose malignancy in the presence of intense inflammation. (**A** and **C,** Pap; **B** and **D,** DQ)

current acute inflammatory reaction, reactive atypia may be present within the epithelium resulting in well formed, obvious nucleoli. The nucleoli, along with rare acinar structures, may create a confusion with well-differentiated adenocarcinoma. However, most of the specimens consist of flat monolayers with evenly distributed small nuclei lacking nucleoli. In addition, the presence of inflammatory cells, especially neutrophils, should increase one's threshold for rendering the diagnosis of adenocarcinoma. Such inflammatory elements are generally not seen in aspirates of carcinoma.

Adenocarcinoma

In the United States, malignant neoplasms of the prostate are the most common form of cancer in adult men. For the most part, this refers to adenocarcinoma of the prostate gland, although other forms of malignant neoplasms also do occur. Many of these appear to be clinically insignificant cancers. Still, only carcinoma of the lung kills more American men than prostatic adenocarcinoma. It is believed that the pathogenesis of prostatic adenocarcinoma, at least in part, is related to hormonal influences. It is generally thought that a morphologic precursor to adenocarcinoma is prostatic intraepithelial neoplasia (PIN), which is discussed later in this chapter.[88,89]

Clinically, adenocarcinoma of the prostate does not produce any distinguishing symptomatology. Most often, it is inapparent to the patient and is detected either through rectal palpation with the observation of a hard irregular nodule in the region of the prostate or through an elevation of the serum level of prostatic specific antigen. Unfortunately, a small but significant proportion of patients presents with metastatic disease. As stated earlier, in the United States, the prostate is examined pathologically with sextant needle core biopsies that are generally 18-gauge. On the

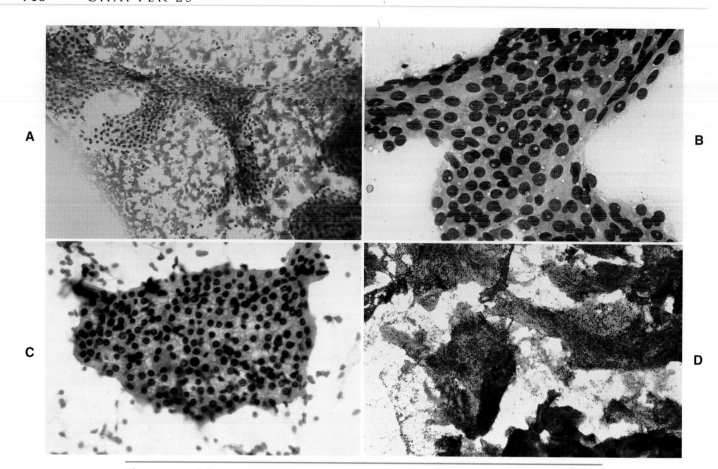

Figure 25-34   Prostatic nodular hyperplasia. A, Large flat cohesive sheets of benign prostatic epithelium are present. Even at this low magnification, the bland appearance of the uniform small round nuclei and the maintenance of normal polarity (honeycomb pattern) are readily apparent. One does not see acinar formation, individual tumor cells, or any evidence of pleomorphism. The smear background is clean. **B,** At higher magnification, the uniformity of the benign epithelial nuclei is apparent. They are round or slightly oval with smooth outlines, finely reticulated evenly dispersed chromatin, and lack nucleoli. They are evenly spaced within the sheet. At the periphery of the sheet are cells that have flatter elongated nuclei, which presumably represent basal epithelial cells. **C,** The clearly benign nature of this sheet of epithelium is apparent at low magnification with the maintenance of cohesion; polarity; and small, uniform, benign nuclei. **D,** Some aspirates of nodular hyperplasia may be dominated, as in this case, by fragments of prostatic stroma. The latter is characterized by eosinophilic matrix and small rather uniformly spaced mesenchymal nuclei. The latter vary from round to oval to elongated. (**A** and **B,** DQ; **C** and **D,** Pap)

other hand, FNA biopsy persists as the procedure of choice for diagnosing prostatic nodules, especially in northern Europe.

Histologically, adenocarcinoma of the prostate generally forms acinar structures. These represent generally small round glandular structures with central lumens and neoplastic cells with relatively high N:C ratios, round nuclei, distinct and often prominent nucleoli, and scanty amphophilic cytoplasm. Histologic grading of prostatic adenocarcinoma of the acinar type correlates with clinical stage and prognosis. Worldwide, the most widely used histologic grading system was devised by Gleason.[90] Importantly, the Gleason classification scheme is based solely on architectural arrangement of the malignant cells and not on their individual cytomorphologic attributes.

As in histologic sections, in aspiration smears, the cytomorphologic picture of prostatic adenocarcinoma is related in large part to the degree of differentiation of the neoplasm

(Figures 25-35 to 25-37).[84,87] In general, epithelial cellularity in smears is greater in samples from adenocarcinomas than from nodular hyperplasia. In well-differentiated adenocarcinomas, the most common characteristic feature is the presence of large numbers of acinar groupings (see Figure 25-35). These consist of central cytoplasm around which is a circumferential ring of glandular nuclei. The acinar structures may be present singly within the smears or may comprise a proportion of monolayered sheets. In the latter situation, the edges of the sheets may be frayed and irregular resulting from a loss of cohesion, in contrast with the well-defined edges of benign prostatic epithelium. Furthermore, rather than the evenly distributed nuclei of the honeycomb pattern of benign cells, acinar structures punctuate and may dominate the cellular sheets. The nuclei may be larger than in benign epithelial cells with a greater degree of anisonucleosis. In general, hyperchromasia may not be evident and nucleoli are often not well developed. At the expense of rep-

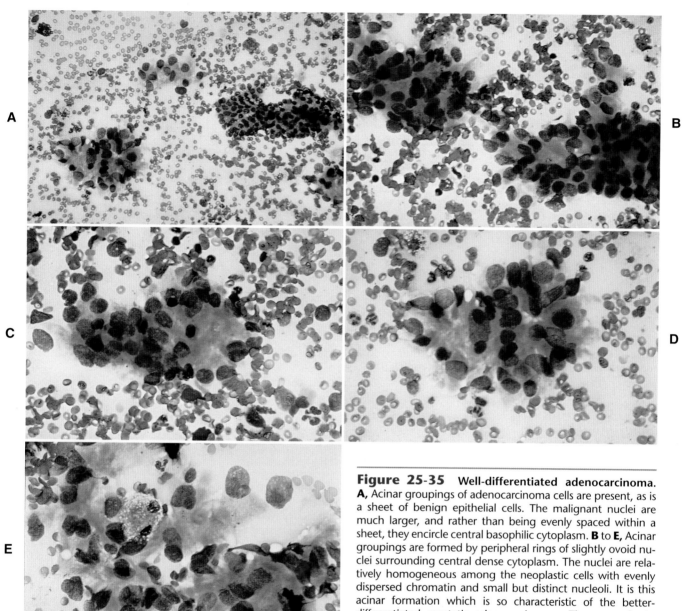

Figure 25-35 Well-differentiated adenocarcinoma. **A,** Acinar groupings of adenocarcinoma cells are present, as is a sheet of benign epithelial cells. The malignant nuclei are much larger, and rather than being evenly spaced within a sheet, they encircle central basophilic cytoplasm. **B** to **E,** Acinar groupings are formed by peripheral rings of slightly ovoid nuclei surrounding central dense cytoplasm. The nuclei are relatively homogeneous among the neoplastic cells with evenly dispersed chromatin and small but distinct nucleoli. It is this acinar formation which is so characteristic of the better-differentiated prostatic adenocarcinomas. The smear backgrounds are clean. (DQ)

etition, it is the finding of large numbers of glandular or acinar structures that allows the rendering of a diagnosis of well-differentiated prostatic adenocarcinoma.

In moderately differentiated adenocarcinoma, the number of individually dispersed neoplastic cells is greatly increased compared with well-differentiated neoplasms (see Figure 25-36).[84,87] Importantly, nuclear atypia is much more prominent including larger sizes, greater irregularity in contour, and hyperchromasia; in addition, nucleoli are generally enlarged and prominent.

Poorly differentiated adenocarcinomas generally yield highly cellular smears with large numbers of individually dispersed malignant elements.[84,87] Accompanying this dissociative pattern are nuclear alterations that include marked pleomorphism and markedly enlarged nucleoli (see Figure 25-37). A morphologic variant is sarcomatoid carcinoma. In aspiration smears, this resembles largely a spindle

cell sarcoma with areas mimicking a pleomorphic soft tissue sarcoma. However, the aspirates may show areas of "residual" adenocarcinoma.[91] It is well recognized by histopathologists that inadvertent sampling of skeletal muscle, the seminal vesicles, or other adjacent structures may result in a diagnostic problem (Figures 25-38 to 25-41). Some of the normal epithelium of the seminal vesical has huge, irregularly contoured and very darkly stained nuclei that simulate malignancy. If encountered in an aspiration biopsy, this could lead to a false-positive interpretation.[92]

Aspirated cellular material from the prostate has been studies by a variety of ancillary tests. Although the results of some of these studies may be helpful in diagnosis, they are largely an attempt to acquire prognostic information. Perhaps the most widely studied is the DNA ploidy of prostatic carcinoma cells by either image analysis or flow cytometry.[93-96] For example, Forsslund and colleagues evaluated

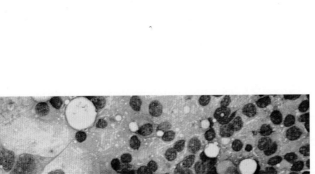

Figure 25-36 **Moderately differentiated adenocarcinoma. A** to **C,** Although acinar groupings are still typical of these neoplasms, other features include a greater degree of reduced intercellular cohesion with individual tumor cells and more marked variability in nuclear diameters. (DQ)

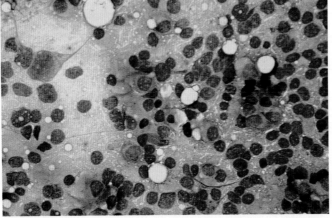

Figure 25-37 **Poorly differentiated adenocarcinoma.** Isolated or individually distributed tumor cells characterize this neoplasm. The latter have moderate variability in size and prominent nucleoli. (DQ)

Feulgen-stained aspiration smears of prostatic adenocarcinoma from a series of 145 men.[93] The neoplasms were divided into three major categories (diploid, tetraploid, and aneuploid). With a follow-up of up to 23 years, patients with aneuploid neoplasms had a much more rapidly progressive course and worse prognosis than those in the other two categories. The results were statistically significant. More recently, Buhmeida and colleagues have demonstrated that the ploidy determined by image analysis of prostatic aspirates

depends in part on which cells are analyzed.[95] Specifically, when individually dispersed tumor cells were analyzed, aneuploidy was more likely than when clusters of cells were examined. Using flow cytometric analysis of prostatic aspirates, Paz-Bouza and colleagues found that 39% of their carcinomas were aneuploid and all examples of hyperplasia were diploid.[94] Furthermore, the incidence of aneuploidy increased progressively as the degree of differentiation of the neoplasms decreased. These authors also analyzed cell cycle kinetics in this series of neoplasms.[94] Adenocarcinomas showed a greater proliferative activity than did hyperplasias; among the carcinomas, aneuploid neoplasms also showed a greater degree of proliferation than diploid tumors.

It is thought that an inverse correlation exists between the grade of the carcinoma and the amount of intracellular prostatic markers, namely, prostate-specific antigen (PSA) and prostatic acid phosphatase. In a recent series of 67 patients treated hormonally for prostatic carcinoma, Stege and colleagues measured the PSA levels and ploidy of aspirated carcinomas.[96] In addition to cytologic grade, these results were correlated with clinical neoplastic progression. In a multivariate analysis, both the cytomorphologic differentiation and the tissue content of PSA were statistically significant in predicting which neoplasms would progress; statistically, ploidy was less important. As determined by image analysis, nuclear diameters and contours were larger and more irregular, respectively, in carcinoma cells compared to benign prostatic epithelial elements.[97] This examination will probably never find clinical usefulness.

Recently, Hautmann and colleagues evaluated the ability of sextant needle core biopsies and FNA biopsies to detect

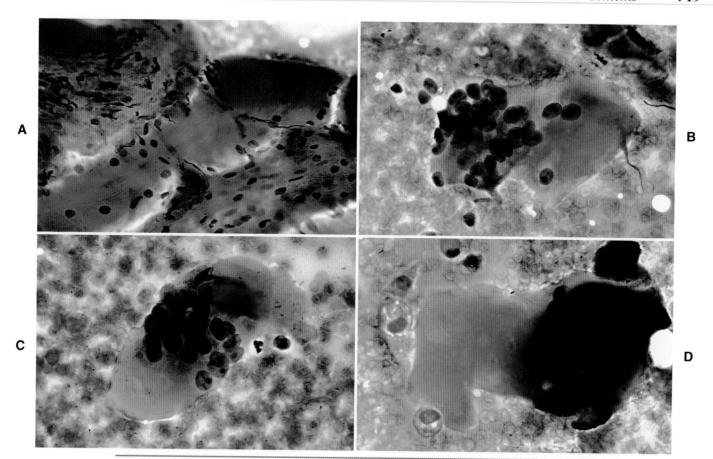

Figure 25-38 **Normal skeletal muscle. A,** When skeletal muscle is unaltered in appearance, it can be easily recognized even by the novice cytologist. It consists of sarcolemmal bands of tissue with uniform, peripherally oriented nuclei and basophilic cytoplasm within which one may occasionally appreciate striations. **B** to **D,** With degenerative changes in skeletal muscle, the nuclei may agregate or even appear to fuse. Thus, they could be confused with acinar arrangements of well-differentiated adenocarcinoma or the tumor cells derived from high-grade or sarcomatoid carcinoma. (DQ)

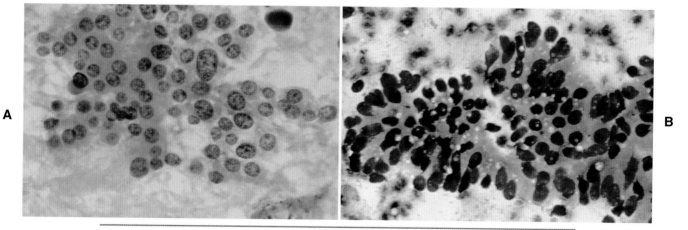

Figure 25-39 **Normal seminal vesicle. A,** Benign epithelial cells are present in a flat sheet. The nuclei manifest moderate variability in size. However, otherwise they are completely benign in appearance with perfectly round delicate membranes; fine, pale chromatin; and inconspicuous to absent nucleoli. A similar appearance is recognized in **B.** However, focally, acinar formation is suggested, which could be easily confused with well-differentiated adenocarcinoma. One helpful clue is that many of these cells have a columnar configuration when seen on end. They have abundant cytoplasm which is focally vacuolated (often not seen with prostatic carcinoma) and very elongated nuclei. Nucleoli are not evident. (DQ)

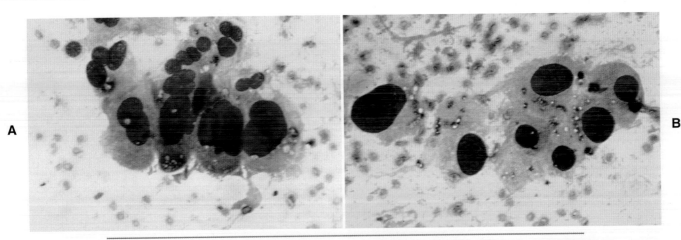

Figure 25-40   **Normal seminal vesicle. A,** Marked variation in nuclear size is evident within this field. As in specimen **B,** it is the uniform homogeneity or smudginess of the chromatin, which may be helpful in recognizing that these cells are derived from the seminal vesicles. In addition, as witnessed in **B,** lipofuscin pigment granules are evident in the cytoplasm. The latter is an important tip-off that one is probably dealing with elements derived from the seminal vesicles. (DQ)

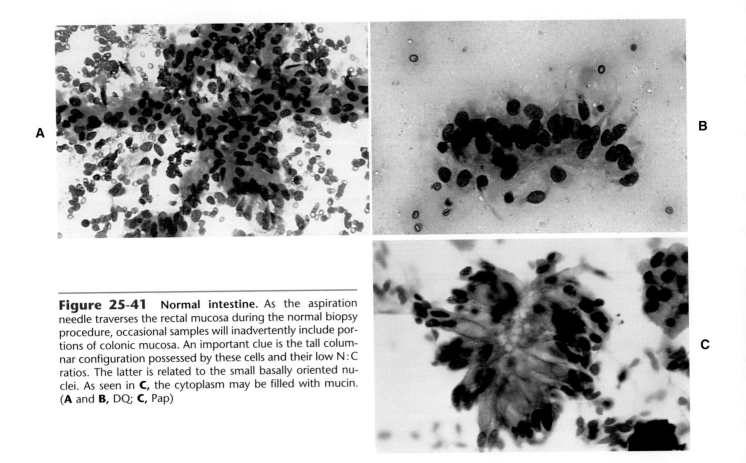

Figure 25-41   **Normal intestine.** As the aspiration needle traverses the rectal mucosa during the normal biopsy procedure, occasional samples will inadvertently include portions of colonic mucosa. An important clue is the tall columnar configuration possessed by these cells and their low N:C ratios. The latter is related to the small basally oriented nuclei. As seen in **C,** the cytoplasm may be filled with mucin. (**A** and **B,** DQ; **C,** Pap)

clinically insignificant adenocarcinoma (defined by these authors as a tumor volume of no more than 0.5 cubic centimeters).[98] The two techniques were equivalent in so doing. Furthermore, aspiration biopsies detected a higher proportion of larger prostatic neoplasms than did the sextant biopsies. However, caution is necessary in applying this data to the clinical situation. First, both biopsies were performed on radical prostatectomy specimens and not directly in patients. Second, 20-gauge needles were used for the aspiration biopsies, a larger caliber than would be used clinically. On the other hand, several groups have provided data in patients that do support the ex vivo work of Hautmann and colleagues.[98-102] A few investigations have also studied the potential for transrectal prostatic aspiration biopsy as a screening procedure for the detection of early (low-stage) adenocarcinoma.[103,104] Diagnostic sensitivity in this setting is low and thus, aspiration biopsy is not useful in screening, rather than as a diagnostic, modality.

As mentioned earlier, PIN is considered by many to be an immediate precursor to invasive adenocarcinoma. PIN is generally divided into low- and high-grade proliferations. Basically, PIN consists of cytologically abnormal epithelial cells within the confines of preexisting acini and ducts. In high-grade PIN, the nuclei and nucleoli resemble those present in many adenocarcinomas.[89] Markham has used FNA biopsy to follow patients with a prior diagnosis of PIN.[88]

A morphologic variant of the common acinar type of prostatic adenocarcinoma is ductal or endometrioid adeno-carcinoma. These rare neoplasms grow in the prostatic utri-cle or large periurethral ducts. A specific diagnosis requires the demonstration of involvement of these structures. Histologically, the neoplasm grows as glandular or papillary structures lined by malignant columnar epithelial cells with pseudostratification of their ovoid nuclei. Although serum levels of PSA are generally lower than in the conventional acinar carcinoma, the clinical behavior and prognosis are essentially the same as those for the much more common carcinoma. In fact, a large percentage of patients with duc-tal carcinoma have a coexistent acinar adenocarcinoma elsewhere in the prostate gland.

Only infrequently has the aspiration biopsy cytomor-phology of the endometrioid variant been described.[105,106] In the case reported by Masood and colleagues, much of the neoplasm had a papillary configuration in the smears.[106] Furthermore, approximately 10% of the neoplastic cells had nuclear grooves, similar to papillary thyroid carcinoma.

Small Cell Carcinoma

As in many other body sites, small cell neuroendocrine car-cinoma may arise in the prostate gland. In a proportion of cases, an associated typical acinar adenocarcinoma also oc-curs. It may be that some neuroendocrine carcinomas arise through dedifferentiation of a preexisting adenocarcinoma. The clinical presentation of small cell carcinoma is not sig-nificantly different from the acinar adenocarcinomas. Histologically, they resemble the classic small cell carci-noma of the lung.

The largest published cytologic series of prostatic small cell carcinoma involved the documentation of metastases in a dozen men.[107] Cytomorphologically, these specimens resembled aspirates of bronchogenic small cell carcinoma. Caraway and colleagues suggested the following features to distinguish small cell carcinoma from high grade adenocar-cinoma of the prostate: uniformly small cell sizes, poorly developed nucleoli, finely granular chromatin, and high proportions of individually dispersed malignant cells.[107]

Sarcomas

Primary sarcomas of the prostate are fortunately extremely rare neoplasms. The two major forms are rhabdomyosarco-ma and leiomyosarcoma. The former occurs primarily in boys under the age of 10 years. Histologically, most of these are embryonal rhabdomyosarcomas. Treatment with surgery, radiation, and chemotherapy has improved prog-nosis tremendously and the majority of patients today may be survivors. In adults, the most common sarcoma of the prostate is leiomyosarcoma. Unfortunately, prognosis is dis-

mal. Neither sarcoma is associated with elevated levels of serum prostatic markers. The histopathology and aspiration cytomorphology of these sarcomas resembles that as de-scribed in Chapter 28.[108,109]

Hessel and colleagues have described the aspiration cyto-morphology of a very rare cystic neoplasm, namely, a malig-nant mixed epithelial-stromal neoplasm of the prostate.[110] The tumor was massive, filling much of the patient's pelvis. The aspiration smears contained epithelial (glandular and urothelial) cells as well as a spindled stromal component, both of which were morphologically malignant.

Metastases

Most American cytologists do not examine FNA biopsies of the prostate itself. However, FNA biopsy can be used to de-tect metastatic carcinoma and most pathologists have had exposure to this arena. This is especially true in the follow-up of individuals with a prior diagnosis of prostatic malig-nancy. Pelvic lymph nodes and soft tissues are common tar-gets for such aspirates, but essentially, any part of the body may be sampled. Several groups have also reported the use of aspiration biopsies in a preoperative setting, namely, to look for pelvic nodal metastases of adenocarcinoma before a radical prostatectomy. These aspirates are performed un-der radiographic (ultrasound, computerized tomography, lymphangiography) guidance. In this setting, acceptable levels of diagnostic sensitivity and high levels of specificity have been reported.[111-113]

 ## SCROTAL CONTENTS

The major organs within the scrotum are the paired testes and epididymides. These organs are encased by the tunica vaginalis, which is an extension of the peritoneum into the scrotum that normally loses its connection with the peri-toneal cavity at or about the time of birth. Mass lesions may affect any of these structures and be a target for FNA biopsy.[114]

As described by Perez-Guillermo and Sola Perez, the most common masses represent cyst-like lesions, namely, hydro-cele and spermatocele.[114] On physical examination, the hy-drocele typically presents as a relatively diffuse enlargement in that the tunica vaginalis surrounds the entire testis. It represents an abnormal accumulation of fluid within the tunica. Hydrocele may either congenital or acquired and accumulation of fluid may be result from either excess production or reduced resorption. Variable amounts of clear yellow fluid are obtained through aspiration biopsy. Cellularity is extremely low and the specimen requires a concentration technique in order to detect the cells, most of which are benign mesothelial elements.[114] If the hydro-cele has been associated with trauma, the fluid may contain blood (hematocele).

Similar to hydroceles, spermatoceles transmit light on physical examination. However, the spermatocele is a local-ized cystlike lesion of the epididymis and therefore is more localized and lateral within the scrotum. Spermatoceles consist of variable distension of portions of the epididymis with its secretions that normally contain large numbers of spermatozoa; these usually arise as a result of an obstruc-tion to outflow from the epididymis. Aspiration biopsy yields a cloudy, white fluid. In smears, spermatozoa are the predominant cell type present.[114]

Epididymitis

In addition to spermatocele, true neoplasms and inflammatory lesions may present as a palpable mass. Far and away, epididymitis is much more common than are tumors. Most instances of acute and chronic epididymitis are thought to be infectious in origin, often related to retrograde spread from the prostate. Although variable in relation to the severity and duration of the inflammatory process, epididymitis is usually associated with pain and tenderness. The patient may also suffer from symptoms of urinary tract infection and systemic manifestations such as fever. In acute epididymitis, aspiration biopsies yield large numbers of intact, degenerated neutrophils and sheets of reparative epithelium.[114] However, this diagnostic procedure is very uncommon in that this is generally a clinical diagnosis that is treated with antibiotics and rest. Similarly, chronic epididymitis usually does not prompt aspiration biopsies. Smear cellularity is generally lower than with an acute process and demonstrates a mixed inflammatory picture.[114] Although most cases of acute epididymitis are bacterial in origin, Secil and colleagues reported the diagnosis of bilateral epididymal abscesses secondary to *Candida albicans* by aspiration biopsy.[118]

A painless, long-standing enlargement of the epididymis is more likely associated with a true neoplasm. Most of these are benign with the most common being an adenomatoid tumor. Aspiration biopsies may be quite cellular and are dominated by cohesive arrangements of uniform-appearing epithelial-like cells. The cells present in flat monolayers, three-dimensional cords, and glandlike structures. The cells actually represent benign mesothelial elements. However, in contrast with a typical mesothelial cell, nuclei are characteristically eccentrically positioned within the abundant cytoplasm. The nuclei are benign with delicate membranes; fine, pale chromatin; and small but distinct nucleoli. Cytoplasm is moderate to voluminous in amount and distinctly vacuolated. This creates a benign signet ring cell appearance.[71]

Another similar mass lesion that may involve the epididymis is spermatic granuloma. These are typically preceded by trauma to the area and represent an inflammatory reaction to exuded spermatozoa. Aspiration smears have two major elements.[116] The first is a granulomatous inflammatory reaction with epithelioid and multinucleated inflammatory giant cells, in addition to lymphocytes, eosinophils, and plasma cells. The second major component consists of spermatozoa; many of these lie free within the smear background but others have been phagocytized by the epithelioid cells.[116]

 # TESTIS

Mass lesions of the testis generally represent either an inflammatory process or a neoplasm, most of which are malignant. In the United States, aspiration biopsies to diagnose testicular masses are quite uncommon. However, in other nations, FNA biopsy is used with some frequency as the first step in the pathologic evaluation of these lesions.[114-117] In addition, a number of centers worldwide are using testicular FNA biopsy to evaluate infertility; again, this is most unusual in the United States.[120]

Orchitis

Testicular inflammation may be acute or chronic in nature and is often infectious in origin. Neutrophils predominate the smears in aspirates from patients with acute orchitis, whereas a less cellular aspirate consists largely of chronic inflammatory cells in chronic orchitis.[114,121] The latter may include a prominent granulomatous inflammatory reaction. Outlines of necrotic seminiferous tubules may be seen.

Germ Cell Tumors

At least 95% of true neoplasms of the testis represent germ cell tumors, the most common of which is the seminoma. With some exceptions, most of these neoplasms present in young adult men with a peak age of about 30 years. Pure seminomas tend to occur in older males, whereas pure yolk sac tumors predominate in young boys less than age 3 years. Histologically, the malignant germ cell tumors of the testis completely resemble those that arise in the ovary. The one exception is the rare benign spermatocytic seminoma. In contrast with the ovarian germ cell neoplasms, in the testis a precursor lesion has been identified histologically. This is known as *intratubular germ cell neoplasia* and occurs as an *in situ* proliferation within the seminiferous tubules.[122] The spermatocytic seminoma is not associated with this precursor. Most often, the malignant germ cell tumors present as a painless mass involving one of the testes. This may be discovered by the patient or on a routine physical examination. In some patients, dull pain accompanies the mass. The aspiration cytomorphology of primary germ cell tumors of the testis completely resemble those of the ovary. Thus, they are not discussed in this portion of the chapter.[114,115,121]

Sex Cord-Stromal Tumors

Less than 5% of all testicular neoplasms are sex cord-stromal tumors. By far, the most common of these is the Leydig cell tumor; others include Sertoli cell tumor and granulosa cell tumor.[114,115]

The Leydig cell tumor has a bimodal age presentation. One in five patients are in the pediatric age range, but the majority are adults. Clinical presentation in boys almost always represents virilization resulting from excessive androgen production, whereas in adults the most common presentation is a painless testicular mass. In both age groups, gynecomastia may also be present. Approximately 90% of Leydig cell tumors are benign. Based on the histopathology, it is impossible to determine precisely which neoplasms will pursue a malignant course.

Histologically, a sheet-like growth of large uniform neoplastic cells is most characteristic of the Leydig cell tumor. The neoplastic cells are characterized by polygonal contours with distinct membranes, voluminous cytoplasm that is characteristically foamy and eosinophilic, and solitary round dark nuclei with a single large nucleolus. The cytoplasm may also contain lipofuscin pigment granules and rod-shaped crystals of Reinke.

Only rarely has the aspiration cytomorphology of the Leydig cell tumor been described.[114,115,121,123] The smears are dominated by cohesive aggregates of uniform epithelial-like cells. The latter have abundant granulated cytoplasm and solitary nuclei. The latter appear perfectly round with distinct delicate membranes; fine, even pale chromatin; and a single prominent central nucleolus. The most diagnostic feature is the identification of the crystals of Reinke in the cytoplasm of the neoplastic cells. With the DQ stain, these crystals appear as rod-shaped negative images, whereas with the Pap stain, they are eosinophilic.[118,120]

Testicular Evaluation of Male Infertility

In a large proportion of infertile couples, pathology in the male genitourinary tract appears to be the underlying pathogenic problem. The "gold standard" in this evaluation has been the surgical biopsy of a testis with subsequent histologic evaluation. Histologically, the infertile testis has been divided into several categories on the basis of the presence or absence of normal spermatogenesis, spermatogenic maturation arrested at various stages, a complete absence of seminiferous cells within the tubules (Sertoli cell only), and thickening and hyalization of the tubular basement membranes. For a number of decades, FNA biopsy of the testis has been advocated by a few workers as an alternative approach to evaluate testicular morphology in infertile males. However, only within the last decade or so has this been used to any extent, as reflected by appropriate publications.[120,121,124-130]

In 1988, Schenck and Schill detailed the normal and abnormal cytomorphology of the human testis in aspiration biopsies.[124] These authors used a Romanowsky stain (although some authors prefer hematoxylin and eosin or Pap stains). Aspiration biopsies of the nonneoplastic testes typically include two major cell types: the spectrum of germ cell components and Sertoli cells (Figure 25-42). The latter cell type is somewhat bigger than the largest of the normal germ cell elements. Sertoli cells are characterized by solitary round nuclei with distinct smooth membranes, vesicular chromatin, and a prominent centrally positioned nucleolus. In addition, the cells possess moderate to voluminous amounts of cytoplasm, which is characterized as eosinophilic to faintly basophilic, is often vacuolated, possibly contains spermatozoa, and has frayed edges. The latter reflects the fragility of the cells' cytoplasm; this is also recognized in smears by numerous stripped nuclei from these cellular elements. Regardless of the underlying conditions within the testis, Sertoli cells are almost always found within the smears.

The series of germ cells are characterized by progressive reduction in overall cellular diameters and increased chromatin condensation.[124] The early primary spermatocytes are characterized by relatively large sizes and high N:C ratios as the germ cells possess relatively scanty volumes of deeply basophilic cytoplasm (less apparent with the Pap stain). They possess one, or less often two, perfectly round nuclei with variably distributed chromatin. They may have a distinct concentration of the chromatin on the inner surface of the nuclear membrane. As the germ cells mature, a concurrent reduction in size and increase in chromatin density occurs. Spermatids are characterized by more ovoid to elongated nuclei with dark dense chromatin and scanty vacuolated cytoplasm. These cells are quite small but are still larger than

the final product, namely, the spermatozoa. The latter have a small ovoid nucleus with biphasic chromatin staining, a dense paranuclear acrosome, and a long tapering tail.

From the authors' study of the literature, those who routinely evaluate testicular aspirates in the work-up of infertility are divided roughly into two camps. One group of investigators are quantitative in that they actually perform cellular counts to create various types of ratios or indices, which they then relate to the associated testicular histopathology. For example, Batra and colleagues enumerated between 200 and 500 consecutive cells in aspiration smears to produce three different indices.[128] These are the spermatic index that was defined as the ratio of spermatozoa to all germ cells, the sperm-Sertoli cell index that was the ratio of spermatozoa to Sertoli cells, and the Sertoli cell index that is the ratio of Sertoli to all spermatogenic elements. Arora and colleagues performed a differential count on 500 germ cells and also determined the ratio of the number of Sertoli cells for every 500 spermatogenic cells.[129] This created their spermatic and Sertoli cell indices, respectively. In their study, correlation with the histologic diagnosis occurred in 82% of the patients.

Other authors have been only semiquantitative in their analysis and have used pattern recognition in their assessment of testicular aspirates in infertile men (Figures 25-43 through 25-45).[120,125-127] In one of the earlier papers, Ali and colleagues evaluated a huge series (272 infertile men with azoospermia) and divided the aspiration smears into five patterns.[125] Fifty-two males also had testicular biopsies for histology. They noted an excellent correlation between the cytologic and histologic assessment of the underlying testicular problem. The only large investigation from the

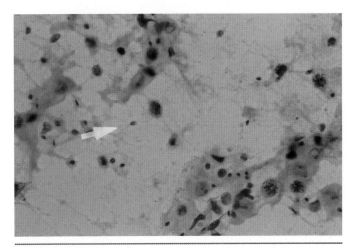

Figure 25-42 **Normal spermatogenesis.** This testicular aspirate was highly cellular and included all levels of maturation of germ cells. Primary spermatogonia are characterized by large round smooth nuclei with delicate membranes, distinctly granulated pale chromatin, and prominent centrally positioned nucleoli. These cells also possess a moderate volume of pale cyanophilic cytoplasm and relatively distinct cell borders. Spermatids are characterized by round to ovoid darkly stained nuclei and scanty cytoplasm, resulting in high N:C ratios. Spermatozoa have a slightly smaller ovoid nucleus and a long delicate tapering tail. With the Pap stain, the chromatin shows an irregular distribution within the nucleus with most of the staining intensity polarized towards the end from which the tail emanates. The *arrow* points to a spermatid. (Pap)

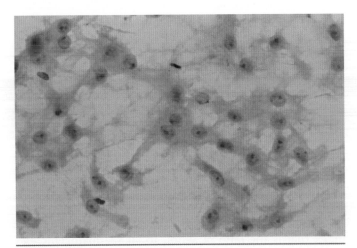

Figure 25-43 **Sertoli cell only syndrome.** This contains Sertoli cells without any of the germ cell line represented. Sertoli cells have solitary round to ovoid nuclei with pale chromatin and small but distinct nucleoli. The cells typically possess abundant cyanophilic cytoplasm, which may appear vacuolated or foamy. Cell borders are indistinct and the cells characteristically have a columnar or pyramidal contour. Smears are generally poorly cellular. (Pap)

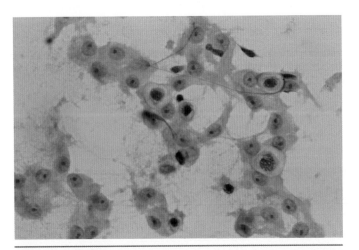

Figure 25-44 **Early maturation arrest.** These aspirates are highly cellular and as seen in this particular field are dominated by the presence of only primary spermatocytes. An absence of spermatids and spermatozoa is evident. (Pap)

United States was recently published by Meng and colleagues.[120] These authors required the finding of between 10 and 20 spermatozoa per high microscopic field in normal spermatogenesis. These smears were generally highly cellular and included numerous primary spermatocytes and spermatids. In hypospermatogenesis, a broad decline in all three types of germ cells and an overall poor smear cellularity occurred (Sertoli cells were always present). The authors divided maturation arrest into two categories, early and late. In the former situation, large numbers of primary spermatocytes were evident in the smears, but no spermatids or spermatozoa were present (see Figure 25-44). However, with late maturation arrest, only spermatozoa were absent (see Figure 25-45). All three germ cell types were deficient with only Sertoli cells in the smears in pa-

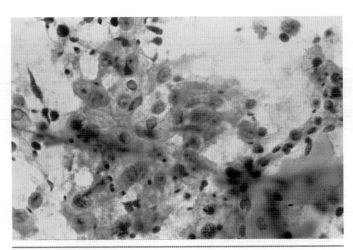

Figure 25-45 **Late maturation arrest.** These cellular aspirates contain both primary spermatocytes and spermatids but lack spermatozoa. (Pap)

tients in whom the histology showed seminiferous tubules lined solely by Sertoli cells (see Figure 25-43). In this study, the authors claimed that a major limitation to aspiration evaluation of the testis in infertility was the inability to evaluate the tubular basement membrane.

Leukemia

Leukemia is a form of malignancy that most often spreads to involve the testes. This is especially true in children who have acute lymphoblastic leukemia (ALL); with improvement in therapy for ALL, including central nervous system prophylaxis, involvement of the testes has been increasing in incidence. Most often, it presents as either unilateral or bilateral firm enlargement of these structures, typically long after clinical remission appears sustained. It has been proposed that these organs represent a "safe sanctuary" for the leukemic elements from systemic chemotherapy. Examination of open testicular biopsy is the traditional method to evaluate for potential relapse. Rarely, acute myeloblastic leukemia (AML) may also involve the testis. A number of studies have indicated that testicular FNA biopsy is a reliable, safe method to diagnose involvement by ALL and AML with high levels of sensitivity and specificity.[137-142]

 ## MISCELLANEOUS ENTITIES

Pelvic Malacoplakia

Malacoplakia is an extremely uncommon granulomatous process that most commonly involves the urinary bladder. Only rarely does it present as a soft tissue mass extrinsic to viscera. Histologically, the hallmark is an accumulation of histiocytic cells with abundant granular cytoplasm, some of which contain inclusions often referred to as *Michaelis-Gutmann bodies*. The latter are round concentric laminations that usually are basophilic and stain positively for iron and calcium. It is believed that malacoplakia results from an impairment in the ability of the histiocytes to destroy completely phagocytized bacteria that are usually co-liforms and in particular *Escherichia coli.*

Only rare examples of malakoplakia have been described in aspiration biopsies.[131,132] Pérez-Barrios reported an example of soft tissue pelvic malakoplakia.[131] The highly cellular smears included numerous neutrophils, plasma cells, and lymphocytes. In addition, large numbers of macrophages were characterized by abundant foamy cytoplasm and obviously benign nuclei. The cytoplasm of some of these histiocytes contained round basophilic inclusions that often demonstrated concentric laminations. With special stains and electron microscopy, they were confirmed to be Michaelis-Gutmann bodies. This example probably arose as primary involvement of the urinary bladder with extension into the extravesical soft tissues.

Retrocystic Hamartoma

An extremely uncommon congenital abnormality consists of the retrocystic hamartoma or tailgut cyst. The authors are aware of only a single report of an aspiration biopsy of this entity.[133] The aspiration smears contained mixed inflammatory cells and numerous benign squamous epithelial cells.

Aggressive Angiomyxoma

Aggressive angiomyxoma is an uncommon soft tissue proliferation which occurs primarily in the pelvis and peritoneum, almost exclusively in women. Although this neoplasm does not appear to metastasize, the clinical course is often characterized by recurrences. Histologic sections demonstrate a poorly cellular neoplasm in which small benign-appearing spindled and stellate mesenchymal cells are situated within an abundant myxoid matrix material. Characteristically, the vasculature includes thick-walled blood vessels that do not manifest the branching patterns of angiosarcoma.

The authors are aware of a single case report of the aspiration cytomorphology of aggressive angiomyxoma.[134] The aspiration cytomorphology reflected the underlying histopathology. The smears were hypocellular and dominated by a myxoid smear background. In addition to the large numbers of erythrocytes, spindled or stellate cells with long thin cytoplasmic tails and small benign nuclei were present. For the most part, these cells were individually dispersed. A specific cytologic diagnosis was not rendered. In fact, Layfield and Dodd stated that such is probably not possible and that the cytologic report should recommend a surgical biopsy for definitive diagnosis.[134]

Penile Neoplasms

The vast majority of malignant neoplasms of the penis represent squamous cell carcinomas, many of which are related to human papillomavirus infection. Usually, but not always, these occur in uncircumcised men. Little attention has been paid by the cytologic literature to the aspiration biopsy diagnosis of tumors of the penis. Skoog and colleagues reported a series of 11 patients who presented to the Karolinska Hospital for an evaluation of a mass lesion on the penis.[135] Five of these represented squamous cell carcinomas

of which three were for primary diagnosis. Interestingly, one represented a metastasis from a primary bronchogenic carcinoma. Three other neoplasms were a metastasis from the large intestine, urinary bladder, and prostate. Although unusual, it appears as if aspiration biopsy can be used quite successfully to render accurate cytologic diagnoses in such patients.

References

1. Kjellgren O, Angstrom T, Bergman F, et al. Fine needle aspiration biopsy in diagnosis, and classification of ovarian carcinomas. Cancer 1979; 28:967.
2. Andersen WA, Nichols GE, Avery SR, et al. Cytologic diagnosis of ovarian tumors: factors influencing accuracy in previously undiagnosed cases. Am J Obstet Gynecol 1995; 173:457-463.
3. Sevin B-U, Greening SE, Nadju M, et al. Fine needle aspiration cytology in gynecologic oncology. 1. Clinical aspects. Acta Cytol 1979; 23:277.
4. Bonfiglio TA, Macintosh PK, Patten SF, et al. Fine needle aspiration cytopathology in retroperitoneal lymph nodes in the evaluation of metastatic disease. Acta Cytol 1979; 23:126.
5. Belinson JL, Lynn JM, Papillo JL, et al. Fine-needle aspiration cytology in the management of gynecologic cancer. Am J Obstet Gynecol 1981; 139:148.
6. Flint A, Terhart K, Murad TM, et al. Confirmation of metastases by fine needle aspiration biopsy in patients with gynecologic malignancies. Gynecol Oncol 1982; 14:382.
7. Fortier KJ, Clarke-Pearson DL, Creasman WT, et al. Fine-needle aspiration in gynecology: evaluation of extrapelvic lesions in patients with gynecologic malignancy. Obstet Gynecol 1985; 65:67.
8. Moriarty AT, Glant MD, Stehman FB. The role of fine needle aspiration cytology in the management of gynecologic malignancies. Acta Cytol 1986; 30:59.
9. Nash JD, Burke TW, Woodward JE, et al. Diagnosis of recurrent gynecologic malignancy with fine needle aspiration cytology. Obstet Gynecol 1988; 71:333.
10. Layfield LJ, Heaps JM, Berek JS. Fine-needle aspiration cytology accuracy with palpable gynecologic neoplasms. Gynecol Oncol 1991; 40:70.
11. Ramzy I, Delaney M. Fine needle aspiration of ovarian masses. I. Correlative cytologic and histologic study of celomic epithelial neoplasms. Acta Cytol 1979; 23:97.
12. Ramzy I, Delaney M, Rose P. Fine needle aspiration of ovarian masses. II. Correlative cytologic and histologic study of non-neoplastic cysts and noncelomic epithelial neoplasms. Acta Cytol 1979; 34:185.
13. Nguyen GK, Berendt RC. Aspiration biopsy cytology of metastatic endometrial stromal sarcoma and extragenital mixed mesodermal tumor. Diagn Cytopathol 1986; 2:256.
14. Mourad WA, Sneige N, Katz RL, et al. Fine-needle aspiration cytology of recurrent and metastatic mixed mesodermal tumors. Diagn Cytopathol 1944; 11:328.
15. Finley JL, Silverman JF, Cappellari JO, Geisinger KR. Fine needle aspiration cytology of gynecologic sarcomas and mixed tumors. Cytopathol Ann 1996; 1:267-287.
16. Nadji M, et al. Fine-needle aspiration cytology of palpable lesions of the lower female genital tract. Intern J Gynecol Pathol 1996; 13:54-61.
17. Dey P, et al. Fine needle aspiration biopsy in gynecologic malignancies: recurrent and metastatic lesions. Acta Cytol 1994; 38:698-701.

18. Liu K, et al. Hyaline matrix material in high-grade endometrial stromal sarcoma diagnosed by fine-needle aspiration: a case report. Diagn Cytopathol 1997; 16:151-155.

19. Cappellari JO, et al. Utility of transvaginal fine-needle aspiration biopsy in the management of patients with gynecologic malignancies. Am J Clin Pathol 1996; 105:501.

20. Imachi M, Tsukamoto N, Shigematsu T, et al. Fine-needle aspiration cytology in patients with gynecologic malignancies. Gynecol Oncol 1992; 46:309-312.

21. Malström H. Fine needle aspiration cytology versus core biopsies in the evaluation of recurrent gynecologic malignancies. Gynecol Oncol 1997; 65:69-73.

22. Wojcik EM, Salvaggi SM, Johnson SC, et al. Factors influencing fine-needle aspiration cytology in the management of recurrent gynecologic malignancies. Gynecol Oncol 1992; 46:281-286.

23. Silverman JF, Geisinger KR. Fine needle aspiration cytology of the thorax and abdomen. Churchill Livingstone, New York, 1996; pp.243-254.

24. Bottles K, Winkler B, Lacey CG, et al. Fine-needle aspiration biopsy in the management of cervical carcinoma following primary therapy. Gynecol Oncol 1987; 28:68-73.

25. Miller B, Morris M, Rutledge F, et al. Aborted exenterative procedures in recurrent cervical cancer. Gynecol Oncol 1993; 50:90-99.

26. Picharadi, LR, Attal H. Fine needle aspiration cytology of vaginal cuff lesions. Acta Cytol 2000; 44:147-150.

27. Katsube Y, Berg JW, Silverberg SG. Epidemiologic pathology of ovarian tumors. Int J Gynecol Pathol 1982; 1:3-16.

28. Kreuzer GF, et al. Neoplastic or nonneoplastic ovarian cyst? The role of cytology. Acta Cytol 1995; 39:882-886.

29. Mulvany NJ. Aspiration cytology of ovarian cysts and cystic neoplasms. A study of 235 aspirates. Acta Cytol 1996; 40:911-920.

30. Greenbaum E, et al. Fine needle aspiration of cystic ovarian lesions: detection, cytologic analysis, ancillary techniques. Cytopathol Ann 1996; 1:175-195.

31. Wojcik EM, Selvaggi SM. Fine-needle aspiration cytology of cystic ovarian lesions. Diagn Cytopathol 1994; 11:9.

32. Ganjei P, et al. Aspiration cytology of neoplastic and nonneoplastic ovarian cysts: is it accurate? Int J Gynecol Pathol 1995;15:94-101.

33. Hart WR. Ovarian epithelial tumors of borderline malignancy (carcinomas of low malignant potential). Hum Pathol 1977;8:541-549.

34. Lee KR, Scully RE. Mucinous tumors of the ovary: a clinicopathologic study of 196 borderline tumors (of intestinal type) and carcinoma, including an evaluation of 11 cases with *Pseudomyxoma peritonei*. Am J Surg Pathol 2000; 24:1447-1464.

35. Matthews LJ, Geisinger KR. The cytopathology of Mullerian clear cell carcinoma. Mod Pathol 1996; 9:35.

36. Hughes JH, Jensen CS, Donnelly AD, et al. The role of fine-needle aspiration cytology in the evaluation of metastatic clear cell tumors. Cancer Cytopathol 1999; 87:380-389.

37. Ito H, et al. Excessive formation of basement membrane substance in clear-cell carcinoma of the ovary: diagnostic value of the "raspberry body" in ascites cytology. Diagn Cytopathol 1997;16:500-504.

38. Atahan S, Ekinci C, Icli F, et al. Cytology of clear cell carcinoma of the female genital tract in fine needle aspirates and ascites. Acta Cytol 2000; 44:1005-1009.

39. Allias F, Chanoz J, Blache G, et al. Value of ultrasound-guided fine-needle aspiration in the management of ovarian and parovarian cysts. Diagn Cytopathol 2000; 22:70-80.

40. Akhtar M, Ali MA, Hug M, et al. Fine-needle aspiration biopsy of seminoma and dysgerminoma: cytologic, histologic, and electron microscopic correlations. Diagn Cytopathol 1990;6:99.

41. Collins KA, Geisinger KR, Wakely PE Jr, et al. Extragonadal germ cell tumors: a fine-needle biopsy study. Diagn Cytopathol 1995;12:223.

42. Hirokawa M, Shimizu M, Nakamura E, et al. Basement membrane material and tigroid background in a fine needle aspirate of clear cell adenocarcinoma of the cervix. A case report. Acta Cytol 2000; 44:251-254.

43. Dominguez-Franjo P, Vargas J, Rodriguez-Peratto JL, Martinez-Gonzalez MA et al. Fine needle aspiration biopsy findings in endodermal sinus tumors: a report of four cases with cytologic, immunocytochemical and ultrastructural findings. Acta Cytol 1993; 37:209-215.

44. Yang GCH. Fine-needle aspiration cytology of Schiller-Duval bodies of yolk-sac tumor. Diagn Cytopathol 2000; 23:228-232.

45. Vance RP, Geisinger KR. Pure nongestational choriocarcinoma of the ovary: report of a case. Cancer 1985; 56: 2321-2325.

46. Ehya H, Lang WR. Cytology of granulosa cell tumor of the ovary. Am J Clin Pathol 1986; 85:402.

47. Shin HJC, Caraway NP. Fine-needle aspiration biopsy of metastatic small cell carcinoma from extrapulmonary sites. Diagn Cytopathol 1998; 19:177-181.

48. Yang GCH. Fine needle aspiration cytology of low grade endometrial stromal carcinoma. Acta Cytol 1995; 39: 701-705.

49. Young RH, et al. A clinicopathologic analysis of primary small cell carcinoma of the ovary. Acta Cytol 1995; 39: 1023.

50. Matthews LJ, et al. A clinicopathologic analysis of primary small cell carcinoma of the ovary. Acta Cytol 1995; 39:1023.

51. Selvaggi SM. Cytology of nonneoplastic cysts of the ovary. Diagn Cytopathol 1990; 6:77.

52. Stanley MW, Horowitz CA, Frable WJ. Cellular follicular cyst of the ovary: fluid cytology mimicking malignancy. Diagn Cytopathol 1991; 7:48.

53. Selvaggi SM. Fine-needle aspiration cytology of ovarian follicle cysts with cellular atypia from reproductive-age patients. Diagn Cytopathol 1991; 7:189.

54. Nunez C, Diaz JI. Ovarian follicular cysts: a potential source of false positive diagnoses in ovarian cytology. Diagn Cytopathol 1991; 7:48.

55. Greenebaum E, Mayer JR, Stangel JJ, et al. Aspiration cytology of ovarian cysts in in vitro fertilization patients. Acta Cytol 1992; 36:11.

56. Mulvany N, et al. Evaluation of estradiol in aspirated ovarian cystic lesions. Acta Cytol 1995; 39:663-668.

57. Rubenchik I, et al. Fine-needle aspiration cytology of ovarian cysts in in vitro fertilization patients. A study of 125 cases. Diagn Cytopathol 1996; 15:341-344.

58. Nieminen P, Kallio M, Hakama M. The effect of mass screening on the incidence and mortality of squamous and adenocarcinoma of cervix uteri. Obstet Gynecol 1995; 85:1017-1021.

59. Abeler VM, et al. Small cell carcinoma of the cervix. A clinicopathologic study of 26 patients. Cancer 1994; 73:627-677.

60. Sherman ME. Theories of endometrial carcinogenesis: a multidisciplinary approach. Mod Pathol 2000; 13:295-308.

61. Silverberg SG, Major FJ, Blessing JA, et al. Carcinosarcoma (malignant mixed mesodermal tumor) of the uterus: a Gynecologic Oncology Group pathologic study of 203 cases. Int J Gynecol Pathol 1990; 9:1-19.

62. Chang KL, Crabtree GS, Lim-Tan SK, et al. Primary uterine stromal neoplasms: a clinicopathologic study of 117 cases. Am J Surg Pathol 1990; 14:415-438.

63. Leiman G, Markowitz S, Veiga-Ferreria MM, et al. Endometriosis of the rectovaginal septum: diagnosis by fine needle aspiration cytology. Acta Cytol 1986; 30:313-316.

64. Tabbara SO, Covell JL, Abbitt PL. Diagnosis of endometriosis by fine needle aspiration cytology. Diagn Cytopathol 1991; 6:606-610.

65. Berardo MD, Valente PT, Powers CN. Cytodiagnosis and comparison of nondecidualized and decidualized endometriosis: a report of two cases. Acta Cytol 1991; 36: 957-962.

66. Gilks CB, Bell DA, Scully RE. Serous psammomacarcinoma of the ovary and peritoneum. Int J Gynecol Pathol 1990; 9:110-121.

67. Tauchi PS, et al. Serous surface carcinoma of the peritoneum: useful role of cytology in differential diagnosis and follow-up. Acta Cytol 1996; 40:429-436.

68. Chen KTK. Psammomacarcinoma of the peritoneum. Diagn Cytopathol 1994; 10:224.

69. Baddoura FK, Varma VA. Cytologic findings in multicystic peritoneal mesothelioma. Acta Cytol 1990; 34:524-528.

70. Devaney K, Kragel PJ, Devaney EJ. Fine-needle aspiration cytology of multicystic mesothelioma. Diagn Cytopathol 1992; 8:68-72.

71. Perez-Guillermo M, Thor A, Löwenhagen T. Peritesticular adenomatoid tumors: the cytologic presentation in fine-needle biopsies. Acta Cytol 1989; 33:6-10.

72. Rege JD, Amarapur Kar AD, Phatak AM. Fine needle aspiration cytology of adenomatoid tumor: a case report. Acta Cytol 1999; 43:495-497.

73. Epstein JF, Amin MB, Reuter VR, Mostofi FK. The World Health Organization/International Society of Urological Pathology consensus classification of urothelial (transitional cell) neoplasms of the urinary bladder. Am J Surg Pathol 1998; 22:1435-1448.

74. Chagnon S, Cochand-Priollet B, Gzaeil M, et al. Pelvic cancers: staging of 139 cases with lymphography and fine-needle aspiration biopsy. Radiology 1989; 173:103-106.

75. Piscioli F, Scappini P, Luciani L. Aspiration cytology in the staging of urologic cancer. Cancer 1985; 56:1173-1180.

76. Jager GJ, Barentsz JO, Oosterhof GO, et al. Pelvic adenopathy in prostatic and urinary bladder carcinoma: MR imaging with a three-dimensional T1-weighted magnetization-prepared-rapid gradient echo sequence. AJR 1996; 167:1503-1507.

77. Johnson TL, Kini SR. Cytologic features of metastatic transitional cell carcinoma. Diagn Cytopathol 1993; 9:270-278.

78. Powers CN, Elbadwi A. "Cercariform" cells: a clue to the cytodiagnosis of transitional cell origin of metastatic neoplasms? Diagn Cytopathol 1995; 13:15-21.

79. Renshaw AA, Madge R. Cercariform cells for helping distinguish transitional cell carcinoma from non-small cell carcinoma in the fine needle aspirates. Acta Cytol 1997; 41:999-1007.

80. Hida CA, Gupta PK. Cercariform cells: are they specific for transitional cell carcinoma? Cancer Cytopathol 1999; 87:69-74.

81. Akhtar M, Ali MA, Bakry M, et al. Fine needle aspiration biopsy of childhood rhabdomyosarcoma: cytologic, histologic, and ultrastructural correlations. Diagn Cytopathol 1992; 8:465-474.

82. Matsumato T, Soejima T, Tanaka M, et al. Cytologic findings of fine needle aspirates in chronic prostatitis. Int Urol Nephrol 1992; 24:43-47.

83. Epstein JI, Hutchins GM. Granulomatous prostatitis: distinction among allergic, non-specific, and post-transurethral lesions. Hum Pathol 1984; 15:818-825.

84. Zajicek J. Aspiration biopsy cytology: cytology of infradiaphregmatic organs. pt. 2. Basel: S. Karger; 1979. pp.129-166.

85. Mendal A. Mukherjee B, Ghosh E. Transrectal fine needle aspiration cytology of granulomatous prostatitis. Indian J Pathol Microbiol 1994; 37:275-279.

86. Esposti PL, Cytologic malignancy grading of prostatic carcinoma by transrectal aspiration biopsy: a five-year follow-up study of 469 hormone-treated patients. Scand J Urol Nephrol 1971; 5:199-209.

87. Casey JH, Silenieks AI. Fine-needle aspiration cytology of prostate: experience in a nonacademic practice. Sem Diagn Pathol 1988; 5:294-300.

88. Markham CW. Prostatic intraepithelial neoplasia: detection and correlation with invasive cancer in fine-needle biopsy. Urology 1989; 34:57-61.

89. Berner A, Skjorten FJ. Fossa SD. Follow-up of prostatic intraepithelial neoplasia. Eur Urol 1996; 30:256-260.

90. Gleason DF. Classification of prostatic carcinomas. Cancer Chemotherapy Rep 1966; 50:125-128.

91. Renshaw AA, Granter SR. Metastatic sarcomatoid and PSA- and Pap-negative prostatic carcinoma: diagnosis by fine-needle aspiration. Diagn Cytopathol 2000; 23:199-201.

92. Ibarrala de Andres C, Castellano Megias VM, Perez Barrias A, et al. Seminal vesical epithelium as a potential pitfall in the diagnosis of preserved masses: a report of two cases. Acta Cytol 2000; 44:399-402.

93. Forsslund G, Esposti PL, Nilsson B, et al. The prognostic significance of nuclear DNA content in prostatic carcinoma. Cancer 1992; 15:1432-1439.

94. Paz-Bouza JI, Orfao A, Abad M, et al. Transrectal fine needle aspiration biopsy of the prostate combining cytomorphologic, DNA ploidy status and cell cycle distribution. Pathol Res Pract 1994; 190:682-689.

95. Buhmeida A, Kuopio T, Collan Y. Influence of sampling practices on the appearance of DNA image histograms of prostate cells in FNAB samples. Anal Cell Pathol 1999; 18: 95-102.

96. Stege R, Tribukait B, Lundh B, et al. Quantitative estimation of tissue prostate specific antigen, deoxyribonucleic acid ploidy and cytologic grade in fine needle aspiration biopsies for prognosis of hormonally treated prostatic carcinoma. J Urol 1992; 148:833-837.

97. Buhmedia A, Kuopio T, Collan Y. Nuclear size and shape in fine needle aspiration biopsy samples of the prostate. Anal Quant Cytol Histol 2000; 22:291-298.

98. Hautmann SHE, Conrad S, Henko RP, et al. Detection rate of histologically insignificant prostate cancer with systematic sextant biopsies and fine needle aspiration cytology. J Urol 2000; 163:1734-1738.

99. Adolfssen J, Skoog L, Lowenhagen T, et al. Franzen transrectal fine-needle biopsy versus ultrasound-guided transrectal core biopsy of the prostate gland. Acta Oncol 1991; 30:152-160.

100. Engelstein D, Mukamel E, Cytron S, et al. A comparison between digitally-guided fine needle aspiration and ultrasound-guided transperineal core needle biopsy of the prostate for the detection of prostate cancer. Br J Urol 1994; 74:210-213.

101. Deliveliotis C, Stavropoulos NJ, Macrychoritis C, et al. Int Urol Nephrol 1995; 27:173-177.

102. Al-Abadi H. Fine needle aspiration biopsy vs. ultrasound-guided transrectal random core biopsy of the prostate. Comparative investigations in 246 cases. Acta Cytol 1997; 41:981-986.

103. Suhrland MJ, Deitch D, Schreiber K, et al. Assessment of fine needle aspiration as a screening test for occult prostatic carcinoma. Acta Cytol 1988; 32:495-498.

104. Palmer LS, Laor E, Skinner WK, et al. Prostatic cancer screening using fine-needle aspiration cytology prior to open prostatectomy. Eur Urol 1995; 27:96-98.

105. Howell LP, Treplitz RL. Papillary carcinoma of prostate ductal origin: a cytologic case report with immunochemical and quantitative DNA correlation. Diagn Cytopathol 1989; 5:211-216.

106. Masood S, Swartz DA, Meneses M, et al. Fine needle aspiration cytology of papillary endometrioid carcinoma of the prostate: the grooved nucleus as a cytologic marker. Acta Cytol 1991; 35:451-455.

107. Caraway NP, Fanning CV, Shin HJ, et al. Metastatic small-cell carcinoma of the prostate diagnosed by fine-needle aspiration biopsy. Diagn Cytopathol 1998; 19:12-16.

108. Cookingham CL, Kumar NB. Diagnosis of prostatic leiomyosarcoma with fine needle aspiration cytology. Acta Cytol 1985; 29:170-172.

109. Moroz K, Crespo P, de las Morenas A. Fine needle aspiration of prostatic rhabdomyosarcoma: a case report demonstrating the value of DNA ploidy. Act Cytol 1995; 39:785-790.

110. Hessel RG, Royes CV, Jensen J, et al. Malignant cystic epithelial-stromal tumor of the prostate. Diagn Cytopathol 1993; 9:314-317.

111. Oyen RH, Van Pappel HP, Ameye FF, et al. Lymph node staging of localized prostatic carcinoma with CT and CT-guided fine-needle aspiration biopsy: prospective study of 285 patients. Radiology 1994; 190:315-322.

112. Wolf JS Jr, Cher M, Dall'era M, et al. The use and accuracy of cross-sectional imaging and fine needle aspiration cytology for detection of pelvic lymph node metastases before radical prostatectomy. J Urol 1995; 153:993-999.

113. Rorvik J. Halvorsen OJ, Albertsen G, Hankaas S. Lymphangiography combined with biopsy and computer tomography to detect lymph node metastases in localized prostate cancer. Scand J Urol Nephrol 1998; 32:116-119.

114. Perez-Guillermo M, Sola Perez J. Aspiration cytology of palpable lesions of the scrotal contents. Diagn Cytopathol 1990; 6:169-177.

115. Assi A, Patetta R, Fava C, et al. Fine-needle aspiration of testicular lesions: report of 17 cases. Diagn Cytopathol 2000; 23:388-392.

116. Pettinato G, Insabato L, DeChiara A, et al. Fine needle aspiration cytology of a large cell calcifying Sertoli cell tumor of the testis. Acta Cytol 1987; 31:578-582.

117. Berner A, Franzen S, Heilo A. Fine needle aspiration cytology in the diagnosis of epidermoid cyst in testis. Cytopathology 1998; 9:126-129.

118. Secil M, Goktay AY, Dicle O. Yorukoglu K. Bilateral epididymal Candida abscesses: sonographic findings and sonographically guided fine-needle aspiration. J Clin Ultrasound 1998; 26:413-415.

119. Perez-Guillermo M, Thor A, Lowhagen T. Spermatic granuloma: diagnosis by fine needle asiration cytology. Acta Cytol 1989; 33:1-5.

120. Meng MV, Cha I, Ljung B-M, et al. Testicular fine-needle aspiration in infertile men. Correlation of cytologic pattern with histology. Am J Surg Pathol 2001; 25:71-79.

121. Zakicek J. Aspiration biopsy cytology: cytology of infradiaphragmatic organs. pt 2. Basel: S. Karger; 1979; 104-128.

122. Hittmair A, Rogatsch H, Feichtinger H, et al. Carcinoma in situ of the testis detected by DNA flow cytometry of testicular fine-needle aspirates. Cytometry 1994; 17:327-331.

123. Assi A, Sironi M, Bacchioni AM, Pasquinelli G, et al. Leydig cell tumor of the testis: a cytohistological, immunohistochemical, and ultrastructural case study. Diagn Cytopathol 1997; 16:262-266.

124. Schenck U, Schill W-B. Cytology of the human seminiferous epithelium. Acta Cytol 1988; 32:689-696.

125. Ali MA, Akhtar M, Woodhouse N, et al. Role of testicular fine-needle aspiration biopsy in the evaluation of male infertility: cytologic and histologic correlation. Diagn Cytopathol 1991; 7:128-131.

126. Gottschalk-Sabag S, Glick T, Weiss DB. Fine needle aspiration of the testis and correlation with testicular open biopsy. Acta Cytol 1993; 37:67-72.

127. Rammou-Kinia R, Anagnostopoulou, Tassiopoulas F, et al. Fine needle of the testis. Correlation between cytology and histology. Acta Cytol 1999; 43:991-998.

128. Batra VV, Khadgawat R, Agarwal A, et al. Correlation of cell counts and indices in testicular FNAB with histology in male infertility. Acta Cytol 1999; 43:617-623.

129. Arora VK, Singh N, Bhatia A, et al. Testicular fine needle aspiration cytology for the diagnosis of azoospermia and oligospermia. Acta Cytol 2000; 44:349-356.

130. Dey P, Mondal AK, Singh SK, et al. Quantitation of spermatogenesis by DNA flow cytometry from fine-needle aspiration cytology material. Diagn Cytopathol 2000; 23: 386-387.

131. Pérez-Barrios A, Rodriguez-Peralto JL, Martinez-Gonzalez MA, et al. Malacoplakia of the pelvis: report of a case with cytologic and ultrastructural findings obtained by fine needle aspiration. Acta Cytol 1992; 36:377-380.

132. Saad AJ, Donovan TM, Truong LD. Malakoplakia of the vagina diagnosed by fine needle aspiration cytology. Diagn Cytopathol 1993; 9:559-561.

133. Young NA, Neeson T, Bernal D, et al. Retrorectal cystic hamartoma diagnosed by fine-needle aspiration biopsy. Diagn Cytopathol 1990; 6:359-363.

134. Layfield LJ, Dodd LG. Fine-needle aspiration cytology findings in a case of aggressive angiomyxoma: a case report and review of the literature. Diagn Cytopathol 1997; 16:425-429.

135. Skoog L, Collins BT, Tani E, et al. Fine needle aspiration cytology of penile tumors. Acta Cytol 1998; 42:1336-1340.

136. Rodriguez IM, Prat J. Mucinous tumors of the ovary: a clinicopathologic analysis of 75 borderline tumors (of intestinal type) and carcinomas. Am J Surg Pathol 2002; 26:138-152.

137. El-Mekresh MM, el-Baz MA, Abol-Enein H, et al. Primary adenocarcinoma of the urinary bladder: a report of 185 cases. Br J Urol 1998; 82:206-212.

138. Jahnukainen K, Salmi TT, Kristinsson J, et al. The clinical indications for identical pathogenesis of isolated and non-isolated testicular relapses in acute lymphoblastic leukemia. Acta Paediatr 1998; 87:638-643.

139. Layfield LJ, Hilborne LH, Ljung BM, et al. Use of a fine needle aspiration cytology for the diagnosis of testicular relapse in patients with acute lymphoblastic leukemia. J Urol 1988; 139:1020-1022.

140. Akhtar M, Ali MA, Burgess A, et al. Fine-needle aspiration biopsy (FNAB) diagnosis of testicular involvement in acute lymphoblastic leukemia in children. Diagn Cytopathol 1991; 7:504-507.

141. de Almeida MM, Chagas M, de Sousa JV, Mendonca ME. Fine-needle aspiration cytology as a tool for the early detection of testicular relapse of acute lymphoblastic leukemia in children. Diagn Cytopathol 1994; 10:44-46.

142. Kumar PV. Testicular leukemia relapse. Fine needle aspiration findings. Acta Cytol 1998; 42:312-316.

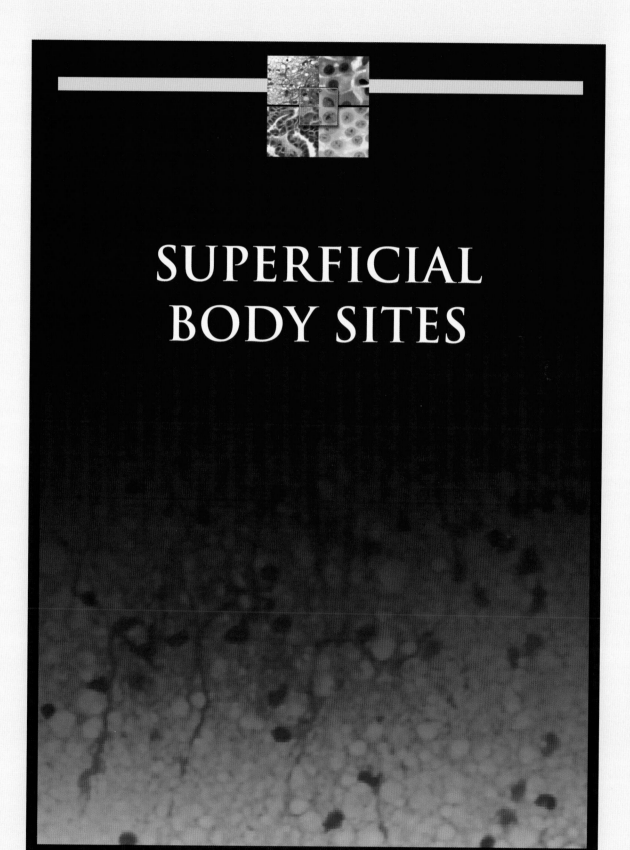

SUPERFICIAL BODY SITES

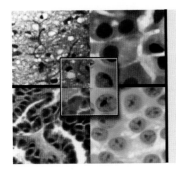

Thyroid Gland Fine Needle Aspiration

CHAPTER

26

Thyroid nodules are one of the most commonly detected physical examination abnormalities, having a prevalence in the general population of 4% to 7%.[1] In the year 2001, approximately 275,000 thyroid nodules were detected in the United States.[2] The vast majority of these nodules are benign. However, each year in the United States, about 17,000 new cases of thyroid cancer are diagnosed and about 1200 deaths occur as a result of thyroid malignancy.[3] Thyroid cancer constitutes from 1% to 2% of all malignant neoplasms in North America.[3] Clinicians dealing with patients who have a thyroid nodule want to determine which thyroid nodules are benign and which are malignant. Although history, signs, symptoms, and clinical laboratory findings may suggest that malignancy is present, they are not definitively diagnostic.

Thyroid gland fine-needle aspiration (FNA) biopsy generally is viewed as the diagnostic panacea.[4-40] Before the widespread acceptance of FNA in North America, surgical excision was the definitive diagnostic procedure to determine if a thyroid gland nodule was neoplastic or nonneoplastic. Before FNA, up to 90% of all excised thyroid gland nodules were benign. The introduction of thyroid gland FNA markedly reduced the number of operative procedures. Currently, every major medicine and endocrine textbook advocates thyroid gland FNA as the first line screening *and* diagnostic test.[41-43] Thyroid gland FNA is used to determine which subset of patients with nodules needs an operative procedure. Thyroid gland FNA is reportedly cost effective[44-56] because it is less expensive than surgery and produces information far faster than thyroid gland suppression. By using FNA, the cost of care may be reduced by as much as $1000 per patient.[46] Thyroid gland FNA also is safer than surgery, which has a higher morbidity rate.

 THE CLINICIAN'S KNOWLEDGE

The following section outlines the thyroid gland's function and structure and the diagnostic tests available to the clinician. This information serves as a scaffold for the FNA diagnosis. By knowing the context of how an FNA diagnosis is used by the clinician, we are better able to fulfill our role as diagnostic consultants.

The thyroid gland produces thyroid hormone and calcitonin. Thyroid hormone (thyroxine [T_4] and thriiodothyronine [T_3]) is essential for normal cellular growth, development, and function, and either thyroid hormone excess or deficiency may result in serious consequences. Thyroid hormone is manufactured in the follicle, the functional unit of the thyroid gland. Follicles are composed of a single layer of epithelium, known as *follicular cells,* which surround a viscous fluid called colloid. The shape and size of the follicle become more heterogeneous with age (i.e., cuboidal cells with little colloid in the fetus and flattened cells with lots of colloid and more heterogeneity in the adult). The thyroid gland contains a second cellular population known as *C cells,* which secrete calcitonin. Calcitonin counters the action of parathormone (produced by the parathyroid) and thus is involved in calcium regulation. The C cells comprise only a small percentage of the parenchyma because more than 99.9% of thyroid gland FNAs concern the cells making thyroid hormone. For the cytologist, the only significant disease involving the C cells is medullary carcinoma.

Thyroid gland endocrinology is predicated on an understanding of the hypothalamic-pituitary-thyroidal axis and of the control of thyroid hormone production.[57] Thyrotropin-releasing hormone (TRH), produced in the hypothalamus, stimulates pituitary production of thyrotropin (TSH), which stimulates production of thyroid hormone by the thyroid gland follicular cells. The major secretory products of the follicular cells are the hormones T_4 and T_3. Intrapituitary and central nervous system conversion of T_4 to T_3 results in inhibition of TRH and TSH and subsequent reduction in production of thyroid hormone by the thyroid gland. T_3 is the biologically active form of the hormone. The majority of T_4 and T_3 are bound to proteins in the circulation, and only 0.02% of the T_4 produced and 0.3% of the T_3 produced are free.[57]

In evaluating a patient with a thyroid nodule and/or possible thyroidal dysfunction, laboratory evaluation may include the following[58,59]:
1. Tests assessing overall thyroid function (e.g., radioactive iodine uptake)
2. Tests assessing the hypothalamic-pituitary-thyroidal axis (e.g., sensitive TSH)

3. Tests assessing peripheral thyroid hormone binding (e.g., total T_4 and T_3, free T_4 and T_3)
4. Imaging tests (e.g., ultrasound, iodine 131 [^{131}I], technetium 99m [^{99m}Tc]scans)
5. Miscellaneous tests (e.g., antithyroid antibodies, thyroglobulin, calcitonin, basal metabolic rate)

Depending on the patient's history and the clinician, one or more of these tests may have been obtained before an FNA. TSH measurement has been recommended in all patients who have a nodular thyroid.[60] Subnormal or suppressed TSH levels suggest an autonomously functioning adenoma or Graves' disease. Because a hyperfunctioning nodule rarely contains a cancer, confirmation of hyperthyroidism by thyroid scintigraphy may preclude the need for further testing. A high TSH level indicates hypothyroidism and suggests one of the more common causes, such as Hashimoto's thyroiditis. In summary, abnormal TSH testing does not exclude cancer but makes it less likely. Most patients who undergo an FNA have either normal or high TSH titers.

Hypothyroidism is a clinical disease state characterized by decreased T_4.[61] It may be a primary thyroid disorder or a pituitary disorder. Primary causes include Hashimoto's thyroiditis, granulomatous thyroiditis, subacute lymphocytic (painless) thyroiditis, and drugs (e.g., propylthiouracil), which may lead to nodular hyperplasia. Hyperthyroidism is increased thyroid hormone synthesis.[61] *Thyrotoxicosis*, on the other hand, is defined as an elevated serum/plasma concentration of T_4 and/or T_3. Thyrotoxicosis may or may not be the result of hyperthyroidism. Causes of thyrotoxicosis *and* hyperthyroidism include Graves' disease, nodular hyperplasia, and Plummer's disease (solitary functioning nodule). In these diseases, the thyroid gland shows increased radioactive iodine uptake. Causes of thyrotoxicosis *not resulting from* hyperthyroidism include granulomatous thyroiditis, subacute lymphocytic (painless) thyroiditis, and metastatic thyroid cancer. In these diseases, the thyroid gland does not show increased radioactive iodine uptake. Thus, patients who undergo FNA may be hyperthyroid, hypothyroid, or euthyroid (normal thyroid gland functioning). It is also important to remember that some diseases are associated with either hyperthyroidism or hypothyroidism.

Radioisotope (tracer) scanning provides data on the iodine-trapping function of a nodule compared with the surrounding tissue.[57] The normal uptake of a tracer is uniform throughout both lobes. Depending on how much tracer is taken up, nodules may be classified as *hot* (increased uptake in the nodule with decreased uptake in the surrounding thyroid), *warm* (uptake identical to that of the surrounding tissue), and *cold* (decreased uptake).[2] Of all nodules, 85% are cold, 10% warm, and 5% hot.[2] A hot nodule is seldom malignant, precluding the need for FNA in most cases.[47,62] An FNA may be performed on a hot nodule if suppressive therapy is unsuccessful. From 5% to 15% of cold nodules are malignant and are the target of most aspirates.[47,63]

Ultrasonography is unsurpassed in its detection of thyroid nodules and provides an accurate assessment of nodule size and characteristics.[51,64-71] It is excellent at identifying a cystic component and the majority of cystic nodules are benign.[64] Ultrasonography has a low specificity in separating benign from malignant.[72,73] Small, nonpalpable nodules may be aspirated under ultrasound guidance.

Technique

Palpable thyroid gland lesions are aspirated by cytologists or clinicians. For noncystic lesions, most cytologists perform three to five passes.[74] For cystic lesions that produce a lot of fluid, cytologists, on average, perform two to four passes. If the lesion is cystic and a residual nodule is still palpated after aspiration, additional passes should be performed. Aspirates are performed using 22- to 27-gauge needles. The authors use 25- to 27-gauge needles, with their experience being that the lower-gauge (i.e., less than 25-gauge) needles produce a bloody aspirate that is difficult to interpret. Some aspirators use a disposable syringe, and some perform the aspirate without using suction.[75-78] If a pass is particularly bloody, additional passes without suction may be preferred. After performing two aspirates, some cytologists check for adequacy by using a Diff-Quik (DQ) stain, before additional aspirates are performed. After all the passes are performed, most cytologists examine from six to 20 slides, half of which are air-dried, and half of which are alcohol-fixed and stained with the Papanicolaou (Pap) stain. If the aspirates are bloody, a cell block may be prepared. Some laboratories use monolayer preparations exclusively. Fluid from cysts often is spun down. Deep-seated, nonpalpable thyroid gland lesions are aspirated using ultrasound guidance by the radiologist. Because these FNAs are often bloody, cell blocks are prepared more commonly.

Diagnostic Categories

The diagnostic categories of thyroid gland FNA reflect the screening and diagnostic nature of the test. In a screening sense the clinician needs to know whether the thyroid nodule should be excised. Thus, thyroid gland diagnoses may be divided into neoplastic, possibly neoplastic (suspicious), nonneoplastic, and unsatisfactory (Table 26-1). Unsatisfactory aspirates generally should be reaspirated. In a diagnostic sense, the neoplastic, possibly neoplastic, and nonneoplastic categories all may be further subdivided; the clinician may or may not derive benefit from this subdivision. Of course, the proper use of these categories depends on the manner in which treatment is rendered at specific institutions.

Diagnostic Accuracy

Calculating the accuracy of thyroid gland FNA is difficult and depends on how the diagnostic categories are determined. Although most authors use the measures of sensitivity, specificity, positive predictive value, and negative predictive value, these measures are not the most appropriate because they do not account for the suspicious category and the category of follicular neoplasm, which may be benign or malignant.[14,79] Measures such as sensitivity and specificity are only appropriate for tests with binary diagnoses.[14,79] The use of these measures has led to a wide range of reported sensitivity and specificity because authors count the diagnostic categories differently. Few researchers have used more appropriate measures of accuracy, such as likelihood ratios or receiver operating characteristic curves.[14,79]

Depending on the study, 2% to 15% of thyroid gland FNAs are diagnosed as unsatisfactory, 50% to 75% as benign, 15% to 30% as atypical or suspicious, and 5% to 10% as malignant.[24,51,53,60,80-88] Variation in these numbers de-

TABLE 26-1	
Thyroid Diagnostic Categories	
Diagnoses	**Examples**
Unsatisfactory	
Benign lesions	Acute thyroiditis
	Hashimoto's thyroiditis
	Granulomatous thyroiditis
	Subacute lymphocytic (painless) thyroiditis
	Nodular hyperplasia
	Graves' disease
	Hyperfunctioning nodule (Plummer's disease)
	Riedel's thyroiditis
Neoplastic lesions	Papillary carcinoma
	Follicular neoplasm, including Hürthle cell tumors
	Medullary carcinoma
	Insular carcinoma
	Malignant lymphoma
	Salivary gland-type neoplasms
	Metastasis
Suspicious lesions	Atypical, but not diagnostic of follicular neoplasm
	Atypical cyst
	Rare atypical groups
	Suspicious for papillary carcinoma

pends mainly on the patient population but also on the individuals performing and interpreting the FNA. Accuracy correlates with the experience of the aspirator and the interpreter.[24,45,64,80,89] After excluding the unsatisfactory aspirates the reported sensitivity ranges from 57% to 99%, and the specificity ranges from 90% to 99%.* Some have estimated that the diagnostic accuracy of thin-layer preparations is lower than that of smears.[90] Others have reported no decrease in accuracy using thin-layer preparations, although some classic cytologic features are lost.[91,92] A positive diagnosis of malignancy raises the individual patient probability of malignancy by up to 90%, and a negative diagnosis lowers the probability of malignancy to as low as 1%.[60,80-87,89,93,94] If diagnoses of unsatisfactory, follicular, and suspicious neoplasms are excluded, the overall false-positive rate ranges from 0.5% to slightly over 1%.[64,86,87] The majority of false-positive diagnoses result from overinterpretation of papillary carcinoma. Causes of error include misinterpretation of reparative changes as neoplastic, papillary-like structures as evidence of papillary carcinoma, and nuclear changes (e.g., nuclear grooves) as diagnostic of papillary carcinoma. If the same categories of diagnosis are excluded, the false-negative rate ranges from 5% to 10%.[44,87,95-98] The main reason for a false-negative diagnosis is inadequate sampling.[29,84]

Approximately 20% to 60% of suspicious diagnoses have malignant histologic follow-up.[51,80,97] This wide range is mainly a reflection of interpreter skill and adequacy of spec-

imen. Benign follow-up is obtained in approximately 20% to 40% of follicular neoplasm diagnoses.* In the majority of cases, these benign lesions are nodular hyperplasia. Most clinicians recommend removal of lesions classified as follicular neoplasm and are not too concerned with these "false-positive" results.[72,103,113,114] Interestingly, clinicians accept the fact that a follicular neoplasm diagnosis is probabilistic and that follow-up shows benign entities. This acceptance is hardly the rule in other areas of diagnostic cytology.

 ## THE UNSATISFACTORY DIAGNOSES

The percentage of cases diagnosed as unsatisfactory depends on the skill of the aspirator (experienced FNA cytologists are better than most clinicians), diagnostic criteria, the number of passes, and the skill of the interpreter. In some studies, up to 20% of aspirates are unsatisfactory, and anecdotally, some clinicians have unsatisfactory rates of more than 50%. Those who perform the aspiration with immediate interpretation have far fewer unsatisfactory aspirates than those who do not. As the number of aspirations increase, the unsatisfactory rate decreases. Although many aspirators perform from two to six passes, some experts, such as Hamburger, performed more than 10 per patient.[103,115]

Experts use different criteria to determine if a thyroid gland FNA is satisfactory.[24,27,51,72,115-121] If tumor is present, the diagnosis may be made on a scantily cellular specimen. If tumor is not present, most criteria for adequacy are based on cell counting. Some authors report that more than six cell clusters (with 10 cells per cluster) are necessary on at least two slides for the specimen to be considered adequate.[72,115] Others report that at least six smears containing 10 to 15 groups of follicular cells are needed for the FNA to be satisfactory.[24,51] In the practices of the authors, the number of cells are not counted. Other features, such as the amount of obscuring blood, are taken into consideration before rendering a satisfactory diagnosis. With less stringent criteria for cell numbers, more satisfactory FNAs result, but diagnostic accuracy is reduced because more false-negative diagnoses occur. If a specimen is adequate and the specimen contains few cells, the Bethesda Committee recommends using the term *limited*.[122]

Experts disagree on the criteria of adequacy for a cystic specimen.[24,122,123] FNAs of benign cysts may contain only a few follicular groups and are dominated by abundant colloid and break down products. If no epithelium is present, Aktinson recommends that this type of specimen be classified as *unsatisfactory*.[122] Others are less stringent and sign out these cases as "cyst" with a comment that no epithelium was obtained. The overwhelming majority of cysts without epithelial representation are benign, although an occasional papillary carcinoma may present as a cystic mass and the neoplastic epithelium may not be sampled. The majority of these have a worrisome clinical presentation (e.g., recurrence of the mass) that should evoke a clinical response.[23,60,110,124-128] The authors are personally unaware of a cystic papillary carcinoma that was aspirated and showed no epithelium and an excessive amount of colloid. The

---

*References 24, 51, 53, 60, 81-87, and 89.

*References 5, 44, 51, 53, 60, 64, 80, 81, 84, 89, and 99-112.

clinician has not been done a favor if every cyst with scant epithelium is diagnosed as nondiagnostic.

THE NONNEOPLASTIC LESIONS

The lesions that are most often aspirated and generally do not need to be excised include the hyperplasias and the thyroiditises (Box 26-1). Remember a benign diagnosis only lowers the probability that a lesion is neoplastic and never completely excludes it. If the clinical suspicion (based on physical signs and symptoms) is low, patients with benign FNA diagnoses may be followed or repeat FNAs may be obtained. If the clinical suspicion is high, such as with a rapidly growing nodule, signs of invasive disease, or lymphadenopathy, even lesions with benign FNA diagnosis should be excised. Consider the role of thyroid gland FNA similar to the role of breast FNA as part of the "triple test." The FNA diagnoses serve as only a *piece* of the clinical puzzle.

Hyperplasias

Nodular Hyperplasia (Benign Thyroid Nodule)

Depending on the population, 60% to 85% of thyroid gland FNAs are from patients with a dominant nodule in nodular hyperplasia or nontoxic goiter.[44,51,60,100] The term *benign thyroid nodule* describes these aspirates. Nodular hyperplasia is the most common cause of a goiter or thyroid gland enlargement.[129] (Goiter is a French word derived from the Latin *guttur,* meaning throat.) It is estimated that at least 4% of the population in iodine-sufficient areas have a nontoxic goiter, which is six times more common in women than in men.[129] Nontoxic goiter may be classified as *endemic,* meaning it is prevalent in certain geographic regions (more than 10% of the population), or *sporadic,* meaning it affects only a small percentage of the population. Endemic goiter tends to predominate in developing nations, where public health measures may not be widely practiced and food supplies are limited.[44] Most patients are euthyroid and a small number of patients are hyperthyroid. In some patients, the gland becomes quite large and may cause tracheal obstruction. Occasionally, nodules may hemorrhage, resulting in pain (Box 26-2) and sudden enlargement. In developed nations, most goiters are sporadic and the most probable cause is an inherited biosynthetic defect in the formation or secretion of thyroid hormone.[130,131] Other causes include diet (e.g., vegetables such as turnips and cabbage), drugs (e.g., lithium and thiocarbamide), and chemicals (calcium fluoride).

Grossly, the thyroid gland appears enlarged and nodular with variation in size and appearance of nodules. Histologically, a wide spectrum of appearances are seen, although the underlying change is regions of hyperplasia adjacent to regions of normal or less hyperplastic thyroid.[132,133] The hyperplastic regions may be palpated as nodules, and a dominant or single nodule may raise clinical concern.[64,129] Areas of fibrosis, hemorrhage, and calcification are common. For the practicing cytologist, the main problem is separating a nodular hyperplasia from a follicular neoplasm. The only time a cytologist may encounter a "normal" thyroid gland FNA is if a thyroid lesion is missed.

The cytology of a benign thyroid nodule is varied with variable proportions of different cellular and tissue components. Smears may contain follicular cells, Hürthle cells, foam cells, crystals, and colloid (Box 26-3).[60,81,134,135] The cytologic hallmark of nodular hyperplasia is the presence of colloid. If colloid is not present, the diagnosis of nodular hyperplasia should not be made.

In an FNA from a benign thyroid nodule, follicular cells may form large, flat, honeycombed sheets or small groups (Figure 26-1).[136,137] Fewer large groups and more small or dissociated groups are found in liquid-based preparations.[136-138] The predominance of microfollicles (e.g., small rosettes) should raise the suspicion of a follicular neoplasm.[106,138,139] True papillae (i.e., follicular cells surrounding a fibrovascular core) are exceedingly rare, although pseudopapillary structures are not uncommon (Figure 26-2).[54,140-142] Pseudopapillae consist of elongated groups of follicular cells without the fibrovascular core. Depending on the needle gauge, microtissue fragments may be seen.[27] Atkinson reported that intact single follicular cells are rarely seen in benign thyroid nodules.[122]

The follicular cells have different appearances, depending on the physiologic activity of the cell.[143] The more active is the cell in producing thyroxine, the more abundant the cytoplasm. In such cells the cytoplasm is fragile, and on aspiration, extensive stripping of the nuclei may occur (Figure 26-3). Stripped follicular cell nuclei resemble lymphocytes, although on close inspection, lymphocytes should contain a rim of cytoplasm.[136] The follicular cell cytoplasm has a

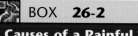

BOX 26-2

Causes of a Painful Thyroid

Granulomatous thyroiditis
Bleeding in a nodule of nodular hyperplasia
Acute thyroiditis
Malignant lymphoma
Anaplastic carcinoma
Hashimoto's thyroiditis

BOX 26-1

The Benign Thyroid Diagnoses

Nodular hyperplasia (benign thyroid nodule)
Graves' disease
Diffuse hyperplasia
Acute thyroiditis
Granulomatous thyroiditis
Riedel's thyroiditis
Hashimoto's thyroiditis
Nonspecific lymphocytic thyroiditis
Subacute lymphocytic (painless) thyroidits

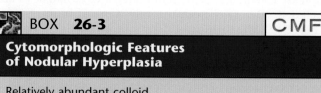

BOX 26-3   CMF

Cytomorphologic Features of Nodular Hyperplasia

Relatively abundant colloid
Varying size groups of cells
Mixed population of follicular and Hürthle cells
Relatively low cellularity

wispy texture, and cell borders are poorly defined, looking like a one-dollar haircut.[136,144] On the DQ stain the cytoplasm is light blue to purple, and with the Pap stain the cytoplasm is light green to brown. Degenerating follicular cells are characterized by foamy, vacuolated cytoplasm.

Follicular cell nuclei are generally nonoverlapping, small and round, or slightly oval.[136,144] The more overlapping the nuclei, the more worrisome for a neoplasm.[145] In nonfunctioning cells, the nuclear to cytoplasmic (N:C) ratio may be high, although the nuclei are not increased in size. The nuclei generally have smooth nuclear membranes, although the presence of nuclear irregularity, characterized by the nuclear groove is not unusual (Figure 26-4).[146-148] In fact, if examined close enough, one may find occasional nuclear grooves in most benign thyroid nodules. However, if the nuclei are grooved like a shar-pei (i.e., several are found), papillary carcinoma is considered.[146-150] Benign follicular

cell nucleoli are single and small, unless the cells are active. The chromatin has a finely granular texture and is relatively hyperchromatic.[136]

As the activity of the follicular cells increases, fewer honeycomb sheets are seen.[151-153] The cytoplasm of a hyperfunctioning follicular cell is bubbly and vacuolated, and the vacuoles may be as large as the nucleus.[153] With the DQ stain, the vacuoles stain pink to red; because the vacuoles are located predominantly at the cell periphery, the cell may have a flamelike appearance (Figure 26-5).[154] Flames are not seen with the Pap stain. Flame cells are more often associated with Graves' disease, mainly because the vacuoles are increased in number.[154] Flame cells also are present in other benign and neoplastic entities.[155]

Hürthle cells, also known as *oncocytes* or *oxyphil cells*, are nonfunctional or poorly functioning follicular cells.[156-158] Hürthle cells are filled with mitochondria so the cytoplasm

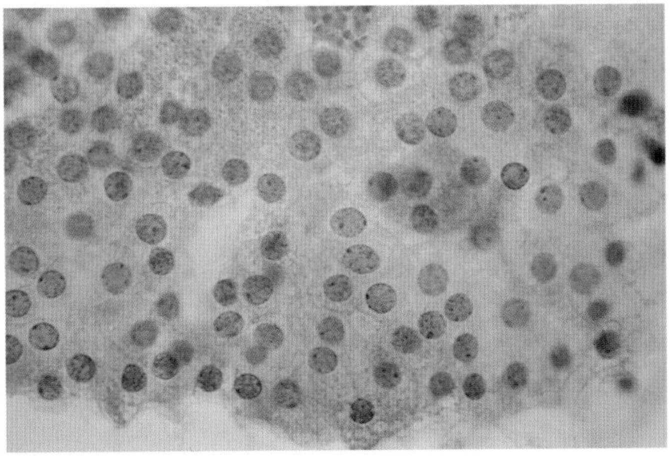

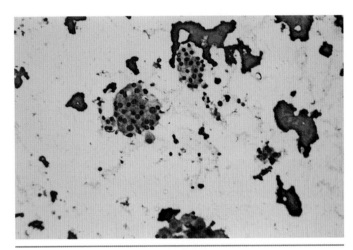

Figure 26-1 **Nodular hyperplasia.** The aspirate smear shows a honeycomb sheet of follicular cells having abundant granular cytoplasm. At the edges of the groups, the cytoplasm is wispy and the cell borders are for the most part indistinct. The nuclei are round and although the nuclei are crowded in some areas, there is an absence of nuclear overlap. The chromatin pattern is finely granular and a small nucleus is present in some of the cells. (Papanicolaou [Pap])

Figure 26-3 **Nodular hyperplasia.** Clusters of active benign follicular cells are present in a background of watery colloid and blood. The follicular cells are arranged in small honeycomb sheets without nuclear overlapping. Scattered, stripped follicular cell nuclei are present. (Diff-Quick [DQ])

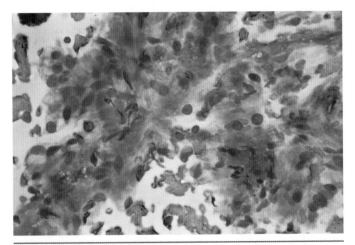

Figure 26-2 **Nodular hyperplasia.** A pseudopapillary structure composed of a fibrovascular core with spindled endothelial cells is present. Fibrin is attached to the fragment and scattered follicular cells are present. Even though a fibrovascular core is present, the follicular cells lack the features of a papillary carcinoma. (DQ)

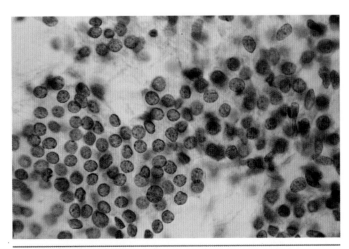

Figure 26-4 **Nodular hyperplasia.** In this case of nodular hyperplasia, slight nuclear crowding and even occasional nuclear overlap is seen. Some of the cells contain intranuclear grooves. An absence of intranuclear pseudoinclusions is evident, and the cells contain granular rather than metaplastic cytoplasm. (Pap)

is granular and dense. It is purple to blue with the DQ stain and orange with the Pap stain (Figure 26-6). Hürthle cells have a polygonal appearance with well-defined cell borders. Hürthle cell nuclei are eccentric and often enlarged. Prominent nucleoli may be seen, and multiple nucleoli are not unusual. A pure population of Hürthle cells is worrisome, although a mixed population of Hürthle cells and follicular cells is expected in nodular hyperplasia.[159]

Because benign thyroid nodules often bleed, degenerative and reparative features may be seen in the follicular and supporting stromal cells (Figure 26-7).[159,160] Thyroidal repair looks similar to cervical or soft tissue repair that has been previously discussed. Simply put, the cells may look atypical. Epithelial cell repair may be quite frightening because the epithelial cells are enlarged and have high N:C ratios (similar to follicular carcinomas).[159,160] The tip-off that

one is dealing with repair in a nodular hypoplasia, rather than a neoplasm, is that the benign groups are admixed with the reparative groups.[102] With neoplasms, more uniformity of the cells occurs. Neoplasms are not characterized by a little bit of atypia mixed with lots of bland material. However, if in doubt, some cytologists prefer to classify lesions with possible repair in the suspicious category.[110]

Colloid, the sine qua non of the benign thyroid nodule, is variably described as watery or dense.[161] The more active the gland, the more watery the colloid; the less active the gland, the denser the colloid. In nodular hyperplasia, parts of the gland are active and parts of the gland are relatively inactive; consequently both watery and dense colloid are often seen in combination. Colloid tends to fall off the slide during processing and is better preserved on air-dried preparations. For better adherence of colloid, allow alcohol smears to fix for at least 30 minutes before staining.

Watery colloid is difficult to recognize and is easily confused with serum (Figure 26-8). Watery colloid may disappear completely on liquid-based preparations.[91] Watery colloid is light blue with the DQ stain and light green with the Pap stain.[161] A hint that one may be dealing with watery colloid comes if one assists with the aspiration. If watery colloid is abundant, the slides have a tendency not to stick, which is not the case if only blood is present. Grossly, smears with watery colloidal have a slightly brown tinge. Microscopically, watery colloid has a tendency to crack and is described as having a cellophane or rumpled tissue paper appearance. Watery colloid also has a tendency to surround follicular cells, whereas serum accumulates at the edges of the slide and around platelets, fibrin, blood clots, or foreign material. During processing, watery colloid may fall off the slide leaving behind the erythrocytes lined up in rows.

Dense colloid is relatively easy to spot with both the Pap (colored pink to dark blue) and the DQ (colored purple) stains (Figure 26-9). Muscle cells may mimic dense colloid fragments, although in contrast with colloid, muscle fragments are lined by nuclei and have cross striations. The differential diagnosis of thick colloid includes amyloid,

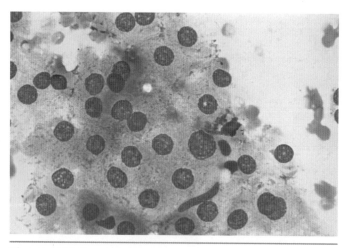

Figure 26-5   **Nodular hyperplasia.** A small cluster of benign follicular cells is present. These cells contain nuclei of variable size, and the cytoplasm has a blue, granular appearance. The cells are hyperfunctioning, and the cytoplasm at the periphery of the cell contains small red granules. These cells have a flamelike appearance. (DQ)

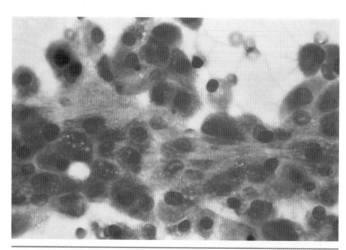

Figure 26-6   **Nodular hyperplasia.** The Hürthle cells in this case of nodular hyperplasia have cytoplasm with a granular or dense appearance. The cytoplasmic borders are well-defined. Watery colloid is present in the background. Despite the cytoplasmic appearance, the cells lack the nuclear features of a papillary carcinoma. (DQ)

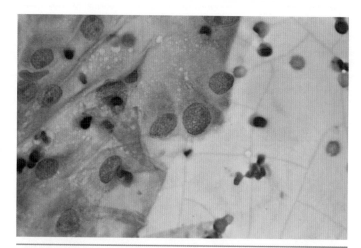

Figure 26-7   **Nodular hyperplasia.** These benign follicular cells show reparative change. The cells contain abundant cytoplasm and are variable in size. The nuclei are round to oval and eccentrically placed. A prominent nucleolus is seen in some of the cells. The background shows a watery colloid with a cracked appearance. In reparative change, the benign cells often have a more metaplastic appearing cytoplasm. (DQ)

mucin, and fibrous tissue.[162-164] Similar to watery colloid, lesser quantities of dense colloid may be seen on a monolayer preparation compared with a conventional smear.[91]

In addition to colloid and follicular cell variants, other findings in an FNA of nodular hyperplasia include lymphocytes, histiocytes, crystals, calcifications, and pigments (Figure 26-10).[136,165] An abundance of lymphocytes should raise the possibility of a thyroiditis, and thyroiditis may occur in combination with nodular hyperplasia. More than a few groups of lymphocytes are required before making a thyroiditis diagnosis. Histiocytes and cholesterol crystals are seen in cystic degeneration of a benign thyroid nodule. Reid described oxalate crystals occurring in all types of thyroid disease, including benign thyroid nodules.[165] Hemosiderin pigment is seen intracellularly in macrophages or extracellularly and is a sign of prior bleeding. Dystrophic calcification may occur in areas of fibrosis and repair, providing a gritty sensation to the aspiration. Before ascribing calcification to a benign thyroid nodule, be certain that they are not, in reality, psammoma bodies, which are seen

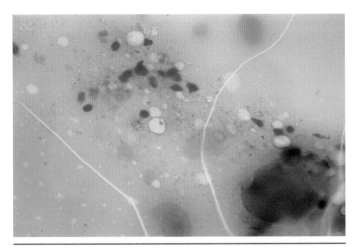

Figure 26-8 **Nodular hyperplasia.** Abundant watery colloid is present in the background of the smear. The colloid has a cracked appearance, and the follicular cells appear degenerated. Stripped nuclei are present. (DQ)

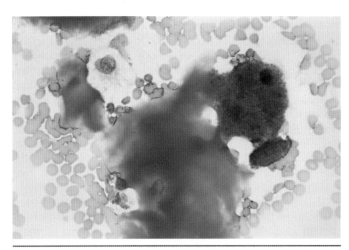

Figure 26-9 **Nodular hyperplasia.** Dense colloid is present and has a purple to blue color on the DQ stain. The borders of the colloid are well-defined. A macrophage is present. (DQ)

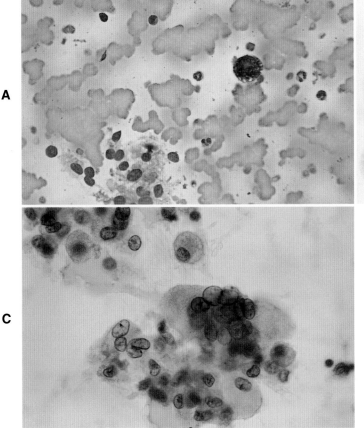

A

B

C

Figure 26-10 **Nodular hyperplasia. A,** In this case of nodular hyperplasia, cystic degeneration with occasional histiocytes and abundant watery colloid are present. The follicular cells have a degenerated appearance and the follicular cell nuclei may be dissociated from the fragmented cytoplasm. **B,** Hemosiderin-laden histiocytes are admixed with a cluster of follicular cells. **C,** Clusters of histiocytes including multinucleated giant cells are seen in this smear showing cystic degeneration. The histiocytes may have a hard metaplastic cytoplasm, although their nuclear chromatin is open and a small nucleolus is seen. (**A,** DQ; **B** and **C,** Pap)

in papillary carcinoma.[140,166] Melanin pigment is associated with tetracycline or minocycline therapy.[167,168]

Although several neoplastic processes may be confused with a nodular hyperplasia, the most common one is the follicular neoplasm.* The authors use the term *follicular neoplasm* to mean follicular adenoma and carcinoma (and sometimes other neoplasms such as the follicular variant of papillary carcinoma). The authors use the term *follicular lesion* to mean nodular hyperplasia and follicular neoplasm. The separation of follicular lesions into follicular neoplasms and nodular hyperplasia is the bread and butter of thyroid gland cytology.

The two major cytologic criteria useful in this separation are cellularity and colloid content. Other criteria are also important, but the majority of lesions may be separated by these two criteria alone. Figure 26-11 is divided into three regions. Region 1 corresponds to nodular hyperplasia (Benign Lesions), Region 2 to uncertain neoplastic potential lesions (Suspicious Lesions), and Region 3 to the follicular neoplasms (Neoplastic Lesions). Some argue to further subdivide Region 2 lesions.[172] For the clinician, Region 1 generally corresponds to those lesions that may be followed medically, and Region 3 generally corresponds to those lesions that should be excised. Region 2 lesions are more problematic.

Based on surgical pathology follow-up (i.e., the gold standard), more than 95% of Region 1 lesions are dominant nodules in nodular hyperplasia, indicating that most of these dominant nodules contain abundant colloid and relatively few cells.[44,60,134] Some follicular neoplasms and other benign entities (e.g., thyroiditises) also may show similar features.[44,60,173] Less than 5% of Region 1 lesions actually are neoplastic (i.e., a false negative) and the majority of these false negatives are follicular adenomas rather than follicular carcinomas.[173] The literature indicates that 1% of lesions called *nodular hyperplasia* on cytology prove to be a follicular carcinoma.[44,60,134] However, approximately 25% to 30% of Region 3 lesions have benign follow-up, indicating that FNAs of nodular hyperplasia may be highly cellular and contain little colloid.[139,159] Some refer to these lesions as cellular nodules. In a sense, these are false-positive results, although this somewhat low specificity does not unduly rankle most clinicians. Remember that without thyroid FNA, most of these nodules would be surgically removed, so explaining which lesions should *not* be excised is of the utmost importance.

Follow-up of Region 2 lesions show both nodular hyperplasia and neoplasms, and as expected, the proportion of each falls in between the proportions in Regions 1 and 3. The nodular hyperplasias that fall in Region 2 contain more cells and less colloid than usual. Although colloid and cellularity are the kingpins for prognostication, other important clues are cell types, architecture, nuclear overlapping, and degeneration. Utilizing these criteria may help categorize a lesion into Region 1 or 3, rather than Region 2. Features supporting the benign thyroid nodule include more than one follicular cell type (i.e., "normal" follicular cells *and* Hürthle cells), cell groups of different sizes, a lack of microfollicles, a lack of nuclear overlapping, and degenerative features (Figure 26-12).* For a neoplastic process, look for the opposite.

Classifying cystic nodular hyperplasia also may be problematic. In this instance the difficulty lies in separating a cystic nodule in nodular hyperplasia from a cystic papillary carcinoma. Both lesions degenerate, leading to the formation of a cyst. By definition, a thyroid lesion is cystic if more than 1 ml of fluid is removed.[51] Biochemical analysis is not helpful in the differential diagnosis.[110,174,175] For cystic nodular hyperplasia, the FNA may be curative in up to 60% of cases, because the cyst contents are completely removed.[60,110,125,176] The FNA of a benign cyst may contain abundant material and few epithelial cells (Figure 26-13). Smears or cytospins show blood, macrophages, occasional giant cells, colloid, and cholesterol crystals. Fragments of fibrous tissue and reparative mesenchymal or follicular cells may be present. If few epithelial cells are present, cytologists may use the diagnostic terminology of "cyst, favor degenerated benign thyroid nodule."

---

*References 82, 106, 108, 110, 135, 138, 139, 159, and 169-171.

*References 95, 106, 108, 110, 138, 139, 145, 159, and 160.

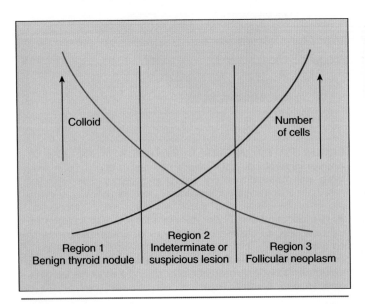

Figure 26-11 Separation of follicular neoplasms and benign thyroid nodules.

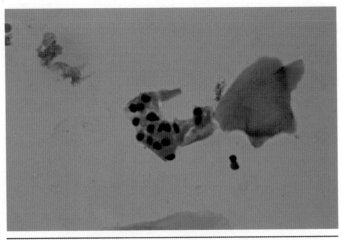

Figure 26-12 **Nodular hyperplasia.** Degenerated follicular cells are admixed with metachromatic hard colloid. The follicular cell nuclei are hyperchromatic and small. A background of watery colloid is present. (Pap)

Although the vast majority of nodules in nodular hyperplasia are cold, rarely they are hot. FNAs of hot nodules may show similar findings to those from cold nodules.[151] Sometimes the FNA smears show signs of hyperactivity and appear identical to the smears from patients with Graves' disease.[152,154] The differential diagnosis then includes a follicular neoplasm and papillary carcinoma. The cytologic features of Graves' disease and its distinction from neoplasms are discussed in the next section. Follicular adenomas, follicular carcinomas, and papillary carcinomas rarely are hot nodules.[151,177]

Graves' Disease (Diffuse Hyperplasia)

Graves' disease (diffuse toxic hyperplasia or thyrotoxicosis) typically is manifested in a young woman (age 20 to 50) by diffuse thyroid gland enlargement and hyperthyroidism. Other clinical manifestations may include exophthalmus, irritability, weight loss, increased appetite, tachycardia, and muscle weakness. Late manifestations include myxedema and clubbing of the fingers and toes. Graves' disease is the most common cause of hyperfunction and is a result of circulating thyroid receptor immunoglobulins that are directed against the thyrotropin receptor.[178-180] For patients with diffuse disease, FNA usually is not necessary for diagnosis. Some even believe that FNA is contraindicted because of the risk of precipitating a thyroid storm. However, nodules may form in Graves' disease resulting from more exuberant areas of hyperplasia or fibrosis. The incidence of malignancy in hyperthyroidism varies from 1% to 9%, and nearly all are small papillary carcinomas.[181] The risk of cancer in cold nodules in Graves' disease is much higher (approaching 50%).[182,183] Consequently, well-formed nodules (particularly if cold) in patients with known Graves' disease may be aspirated.[183]

The treatment of Graves' disease consists of antithyroid drugs such as propylthiouracil and carbimazole, destruction of the gland with radioactive iodine, or partial excision. Medical treatment may mask some of the more typical histologic or cytologic findings.[184] Graves' disease is closely related to Hashimoto's thyroiditis (both are autoimmune diseases) and, on occasion, both diseases may show similar cytologic features.[153,155,185]

The histology of Graves' disease is characterized by follicles that show marked activity with papillary infolding. FNAs are usually cellular with numerous follicular cells and watery colloid[186] (Box 26-4). Hürthle cells and lymphocytes may be seen but usually are not a major feature.[139,153,187] The follicular cell cytoplasm appears foamy (containing glycogen or lipid) and characteristic flame cells are seen in DQ preparations (Figure 26-14).[154] Flame cells have marginal cy-

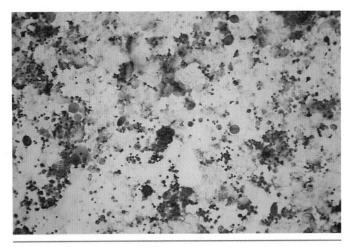

Figure 26-13　Nodular hyperplasia. At this low power, extensive degeneration within a cyst is present. Macrophages, benign follicular cells, and watery colloid are present. The epithelial cells are few in number. (DQ)

BOX　**26-4**	**CMF**
Cytomorphologic Features of Graves' Disease	

Cellular smear
Small and large groups of cells
Flame cells
Scant colloid

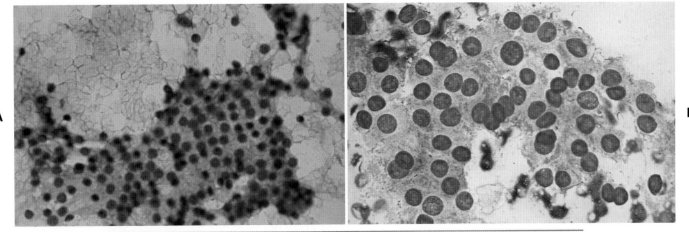

A　　　　　　　　　　　　　　　　　　　　　　　　　　　　　　　**B**

Figure 26-14　Graves' disease. A, Aspirates of Graves' disease may show extensive hypercellularity with both large and small clusters of follicular cells. The cells generally are present in honeycomb sheets, although occasional single cells are present. Nuclear overlap and crowding are common. Watery colloid admixed with blood is present in the background. **B,** A higher power of Graves' disease shows the variability in nuclear size and the crowding of the nuclei. Numerous flame cells with eosinophilic nuclear borders are seen. In this case, abundant colloid is not present within the background. (**A,** Pap; **B,** DQ)

toplasmic vacuoles containing red to pink granular material, which corresponds ultrastructurally to phagolysosomes. Marginal cytoplasmic vacuoles also may be seen in diseases with focal hyperplasia, such as Hashimoto's thyroiditis, benign nodular goiter, follicular neoplasm, and follicular variant of papillary carcinoma.[155,188-190] The cytologic features of Graves' disease are not specific. Thus, before a cytologic diagnosis of Graves' disease is made, the appropriate clinical history should be obtained.

In Graves' disease, microfollicles may be abundant, and considerable nuclear atypia may occur, including nuclear enlargement and overlapping and enlarged nucleoli.[152,154,191] Psammoma bodies and giant cells also have been reported.[139,153,192] The high cellularity and presence of microfollicles raises the possibility of a follicular neoplasm.[152,154] The identification of watery colloid (an argument to use the DQ stain) and the cellular signs of hyperactivity (e.g., flame cells) should suggest Graves' disease. The overwhelming majority of follicular adenomas and carcinomas do not show such marked signs of hyperactivity. The cellular atypia and presence of pseudopapillary groups raise the possibility of a papillary carcinoma. However, the nuclear and cytoplasmic features of papillary carcinoma are absent in Graves' disease.[193]

Thyroiditises

Acute Thyroiditis

Acute thyroiditis is seen most commonly in women 20 to 40 years old, although it may also occur in the extremes of age. Although very rare, it is one of the causes of a painful thyroid (see Box 26-1). More than 50% of patients have pre-existing thyroid disease and 70% have concurrent upper respiratory tract symptoms.[194] The cause is bacterial (either staphylococci or streptococci) in 68%, fungal in 15%, and parasitic in less than 1% of patients.[194-197] The onset is sudden, and the symptoms in more than 90% of patients include anterior neck pain, fever, and dysphagia. Patients are initially hyperthyroid, then euthyroid, then hypothyroid, then euthyroid (full recovery). In most instances, the entire thyroid gland is enlarged and the diagnosis is made without aspiration. However, some medical textbooks advocate FNA for diagnosis even in nonnodular disease if acute thyroiditis is suspected. In rare instances, a solitary mass, or abscess, may be observed. Clinically, the differential diagnosis includes hemorrhage into a cyst and neoplasm. Antithyroid antibodies are absent.

The FNA smears of acute thyroiditis show numerous neutrophils, degenerated debris, and occasional reactive follicular cells with prominent nucleoli (Box 26-5). Infectious organisms may be seen in the background (Figure 26-15).[194-201] Often the only finding is pus, and using

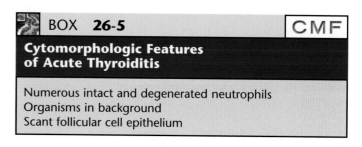

BOX 26-5   CMF

Cytomorphologic Features of Acute Thyroiditis

Numerous intact and degenerated neutrophils
Organisms in background
Scant follicular cell epithelium

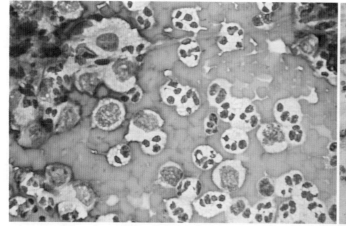

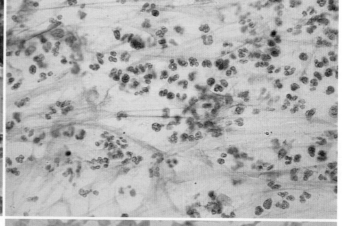

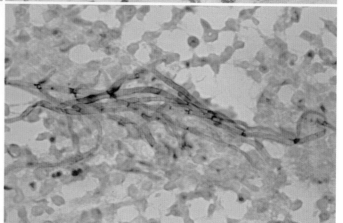

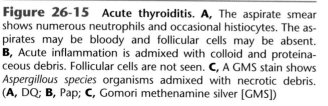

Figure 26-15 **Acute thyroiditis. A,** The aspirate smear shows numerous neutrophils and occasional histiocytes. The aspirates may be bloody and follicular cells may be absent. **B,** Acute inflammation is admixed with colloid and proteinaceous debris. Follicular cells are not seen. **C,** A GMS stain shows *Aspergillous species* organisms admixed with necrotic debris. (**A,** DQ; **B,** Pap; **C,** Gomori methenamine silver [GMS])

a sufficiently large bore needle may completely drain an abscess. The differential diagnosis includes an anaplastic carcinoma, papillary carcinoma, infected thyroglossal cyst, and palpation thyroiditis. The cells of an anaplastic carcinoma are sufficiently pleomorphic that they should not be confused with reactive follicular cells.[202] Cystic papillary carcinomas also may contain neutrophils, although the epithelial elements of the papillary carcinoma usually preclude making a false-negative diagnosis.[116] As the name implies, palpation thyroiditis occurs after the thyroid gland has been handled previously or perhaps too roughly.[203] Palpation thyroiditis may be seen on smears of repeat aspirates performed up to several weeks after the initial aspirate. In contrast with acute thyroiditis, neutrophils are not as abundant and more follicular cells and colloid are present. For an acute thyroiditis, culture may be key to establishing the correct diagnosis.

Granulomatous Thyroiditis (Subacute Thyroiditis)

Granulomatous thyroiditis (subacute or de Quervain's thyroiditis) may represent a postviral syndrome.[204,205] Of patients, 80% are women 20 to 50 years old, and the disease is rare in the geriatric and pediatric age groups. Granulomatous thyroiditis is seasonal, occurring more often in the summer and fall. A genetic predisposition is suggested, because two thirds of patients have HLA-Bw35. A patient with granulomatous thyroiditis has a tender thyroid gland and viral-like symptoms such as malaise, fatigue, and chills. Neck pain is usually unilateral. Some patients are slightly hyperthyroid because of colloid leak resulting from inflammation with follicular damage. Patients with granulomatous thyroiditis classically have a high erythrocyte sedimentation rate and may have a slight elevation in antithyroid antibodies. The disease usually is self-limited (treated with nonsteroidals) and resolves in 2 to 3 months. In most patients the thyroid gland is diffusely enlarged, although a minority of patients show unilateral enlargement. In more severe forms of the disease, the gland becomes anchored to surrounding structures, because of inflammation and fibrosis.[205,206] In later stages the gland may be nodular and occasionally, a single large nodule is palpated. These are the patients who may undergo aspiration, particularly if the signs and symptoms are not classic (e.g., male, nontender thyroid, no viral-like prodrome).

Aspirating a patient with granulomatous thyroiditis is not pleasant for the patient or the aspirator. The procedure is often intensely painful, thought secondary to stretching of the gland's capsule. Other diseases associated with capsular stretching and pain are shown in Table 26-1. A frustrating aspect of performing the FNA in a patient with granulomatous thyroiditis is that the specimen usually is paucicellular, because of underlying fibrosis.[207] Thus, a tendency exists to want to perform more aspirates, which, unfortunately, does not facilitate the physician-patient relationship!

Histologically, granulomatous thyroiditis begins with necrosis of the follicular epithelium and ends with fibrosis and follicular regeneration.[205,206,208] The damage to the follicles results in colloid leak, macrophage scavenging, and granuloma formation. The cytologic findings depend on the stage of the disease, although most aspirations are performed in the later stages when the granulomas are well formed (Box 26-6). In the earliest stages of disease, smears contain neutrophils and reactive follicular epithelial cells; granulomas

are scarce.[209] In the later stages, smears contain granulomas, giant cells, a few neutrophils, eosinophils, plasma cells, lymphocytes and fibrous tissue fragments (Figure 26-16).[207,210] The granulomas are well formed and should have the appearance of foreign body granulomas. Some of the epithelioid histiocytes encircle specks of colloid.[207,210] Necrotic debris associated with the granulomas should be absent. The giant cells may be monstrous in size. Follicular epithelium is scant, and Hürthle cells are rare. The epithelium may appear reactive, and even slightly atypical, because of the inflammation.[211] The diagnostic features of follicular neoplasms or papillary carcinoma are lacking. Abundant colloid should not be seen in all stages of disease.[209]

The differential diagnosis includes other causes of granulomatous disease (Box 26-7). Some, such as sarcoid and drug reaction, require clinical history to exclude. Polarization may help rule out foreign body granulomas, caused by agents such as Teflon.[212] The infectious causes of granulomatous thyroiditis are often associated with caseation necrosis, and organisms may be seen on special stains or cultured.[194,213] Although tertiary syphilis is rare, it may involve the thyroid gland and is characterized by granulomas and abundant plasma cells.[194] In Hashimoto's thyroiditis, granulomas also may form, resulting from follicular destruction and colloid leak.[210] However, in Hashimoto's thyroiditis, the granulomas are few and smears are dominated by Hürthle cells and lymphocytes. In nodular hyperplasia the granulomas are few, and colloid is abundant. Palpation thyroiditis may appear cytologically identical to granulomatous thyroiditis.[203] Papillary carcinoma may be associated with granulomas and giant cells, particularly in the cystic forms,[140,202,214] but granulomatous thyroiditis is not associated with cyst formation.

Chronic Thyroiditis

Chronic thyroiditis includes Riedel's thyroiditis, Hashimoto's thyroiditis, nonspecific thyroiditis, and subacute lymphocytic (painless) thyroiditis. These diseases affect the entire thyroid gland, although large, dominant nodules may form. The FNA smears of all the chronic thyroiditises are characterized by the presence of lymphocytes, which are present in varying amounts. Other disease processes that are also characterized by lymphocytes are papillary carcinoma, malignant lymphoma, drug reaction, Graves' disease, and anaplastic carcinoma. Except for malignant lymphoma, the lymphocytes in these other conditions are fewer in number.

Riedel's thyroiditis (Riedel's struma). Riedel's thyroiditis is a chronic, fibrosing thyroiditis that develops as a painless mass. Riedel's thyroiditis is extremely rare (1 : 100,000).[215-217] Some argue that it is not a *true* thyroiditis because it is an

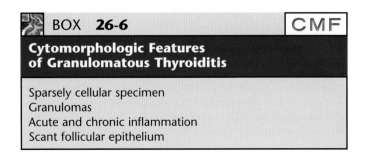

BOX 26-6 CMF

Cytomorphologic Features of Granulomatous Thyroiditis

Sparsely cellular specimen
Granulomas
Acute and chronic inflammation
Scant follicular epithelium

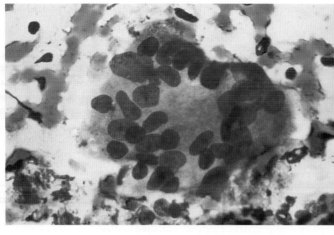

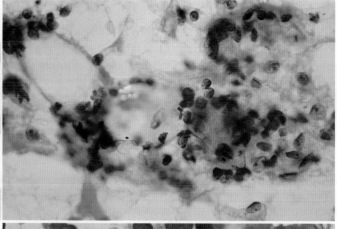

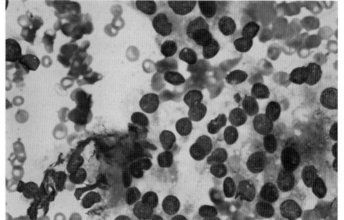

Figure 26-16   Granulomatous thyroiditis. A, In the later stage of granulomatous thyroiditis, giant cells and granulomas are seen. The epithelioid histiocytic nuclei may be markedly enlarged and elongated and may contain a prominent nucleolus. **B,** At this lower power, giant cells and granulomas are admixed with other chronic inflammatory cells such as lymphocytes. Colloid usually is absent, and follicular cells may be hard to identify. **C,** Reactive epithelial cells show nuclear enlargement and nuclear overlap. Cellular dissociation is common. Small microfollicles may be present; the cellularity and microfollicles may be suggestive of a follicular neoplasm. (**A** and **C,** DQ; **B,** Pap)

BOX 26-7

Causes of Granulomas

Granulomatous thyroiditis
Sarcoid
Infection (mycobacterial, fungal, ricketsial, parasitic)
Foreign body giant cell reaction
Drugs
Palpation thyroiditis
Nodular hyperplasia
Papillary carcinoma

BOX 26-8   CMF

Cytomorphologic Features of Riedel's Thyroiditis

Fibrous tissue fragments
Scantly cellular aspirate
Degenerated follicular cells
Scant colloid

---

inflammatory process that involves more than just the thyroid gland (i.e., other neck structures).[186] The classic patient who develops Riedel's thyroiditis is a middle-age woman (it is four times more common in women than men) who has had a history of nodular hyperplasia.[215-218] Patients with Riedel's thyroiditis may have elevated levels of antithyroid antibodies, although not as high as the levels in patients with Hashimoto's thyroiditis. The thyroid gland is nontender, and the majority of patients are euthyroid; in later stages of the disease, the patients may become hypothyroid. On palpation the thyroid gland feels rock hard, and clinically, tumor is suspected. The gland feels attached to the trachea, soft tissues, and other neck structures (some patients even progress to dysphagia). The process is asymmetric and only involves portions of the thyroid gland. Riedel's thyroiditis is related to other inflammatory fibroscleroses such as mediastinal or retroperitoneal fibrosis.[186]

The FNA smears are almost always paucicellular and mainly show fibrous tissue fragments, spindled stromal cells, and chronic inflammatory cells, including lymphocytes and histiocytes (Box 26-8).[27,122,219] Few, if any, follicular cells are seen, and one may be tempted to make an unsatisfactory diagnosis. The rare follicular cells present have a degenerated and even atypical appearance (Figure 26-17).[27,220] Granulomas are not seen. The differential diagnosis includes Hashimoto's thyroiditis (atrophic phase) and sclerotic malignant processes such as anaplastic carcinoma and metastases.[221,222] Hashimoto's thyroiditis may be excluded on clinical grounds (e.g., the gland in Hashimoto's thyroiditis is diffusely involved and firm, not rock hard; the gland in Riedel's thyroiditis is fixed and only focally involved) and on cytologic grounds (e.g., more Hürthle cells in Hashimoto's thyroiditis). Although the cells may look atypical in Riedel's thyroiditis, they lack the anaplasia of the cells in the more sclerotic malignancies that may involve the thyroid.

Hashimoto's thyroiditis (lymphocytic thyroiditis). Hashimoto's thyroiditis is an autoimmune disease that usually

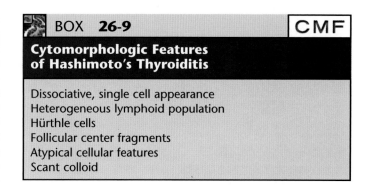

Figure 26-17 Riedel's thyroiditis. **A,** The aspirate smears typically are paucicellular and contain only fibrous tissue fragments and rare follicular cells. Abundant blood may be present. In this smear, spindled mesenchymal cells consistent with fibrous tissue are observed. Follicular cells are not seen. **B,** At this low power, clusters of follicular cells are admixed with blood clot. Colloid is absent in the background. (**A,** Pap; **B,** DQ)

presents with diffuse thyroid gland enlargement in middle-age women, with a female to male ratio of 9:1.[223] A strong genetic predisposition is related to the inheritance of HLA-B8 and DR5 antigens.[224] Hashimoto's thyroiditis is the most common cause of hypothyroidism in areas with sufficient dietary iodine.[225] Hashimoto's thyroiditis is also the most common cause of thyroid enlargement in the pediatric age group. The gland may have a firm, multinodular quality, and up to 10% of patients have a dominant nodule.[226] Although the exact risk is controversial, patients who have Hashimoto's thyroiditis may develop malignant lymphoma, papillary carcinoma, or Hürthle cell neoplasms.[207,227-230] Thus, neoplasia must be excluded even in patients who have known Hashimoto's thyroiditis and a nodule.[231] Treatment of Hashimoto's thyroiditis depends on disease severity. In mild forms, no treatment may be rendered. As the disease intensifies, replacement thyroid hormone is given. Occasionally, surgical excision is performed if the gland is large or if pressure symptoms are present.

Clinically, Hashimoto's thyroiditis is manifested by hypothyroidism, an enlarged gland, and high serum levels of antithyroid antibodies.[223,224] The underlying disease process is characterized by progressive destruction of thyroid follicles mediated through several autoimmune mechanisms.[223,224,231-233] In many patients a deficiency of suppressor T-cells is noted. As the follicular cells express HLA-DR antigen, cytotoxic T cells attack and eradicate these follicular cells. A number of antibodies may be produced, including antimicrosomal (present in more than 90% of cases; titers of greater than 1:2500 are virtually diagnostic), antithyroglobulin, and anti-TSH receptor antibodies. In most patients, the diagnosis of Hashimoto's thyroiditis is based on physical examination and bloodwork. Antibody titers may be low, and the clinical diagnosis may be uncertain; in this scenario, a cytologic diagnosis of Hashimoto's thyroiditis may be especially rewarding.[227] However, in most patients, the clinician generally is trying to rule out a neoplasm and not establish a Hashimoto's diagnosis. If the aspiration findings are not diagnostic per se, and you are contemplating a Hashimoto's thyroiditis diagnosis, a call to the clinician generally will help.

BOX 26-9 CMF

Cytomorphologic Features of Hashimoto's Thyroiditis

Dissociative, single cell appearance
Heterogeneous lymphoid population
Hürthle cells
Follicular center fragments
Atypical cellular features
Scant colloid

As Hashimoto's thyroiditis progresses, the histologic appearance changes.[186,221] Early, the thyroid gland is full of lymphocytes that infiltrate the follicles and may even form germinal centers. This stage is known as the *lymphoid* or *early phase.* As the gland becomes more involuted, the lymphocytes decrease in number and the gland becomes more fibrotic.[221] Not surprisingly, this stage is known as the *atrophic* or *fibrotic phase.* As many of the follicles are being destroyed, the majority of follicular cells are inactive and have an oncocytic appearance.[234,235] Foci of non-Hürthle cell epithelium also may be present. Nodules may consist of epithelial hyperplasia (follicles trying to maintain proper hormone production in a background of destruction) surrounded by regions of fibrosis.

The lymphoid phase is more commonly aspirated than the atrophic phase (Box 26-9). The definitive diagnosis of Hashimoto's thyroiditis rests on identifying lymphoid cells and Hürthle cells (Figure 26-18). Both criteria must exist to make this diagnosis. At low power, the smear may resemble a smear from a lymph node. The lymphoid population is heterogeneous, and lymphoid tangles, follicular center fragments, tingible body macrophases and lymphoglandular bodies are abundant.[19,207,226] Be careful to separate true lymphoid cells from stripped follicular cell nuclei. A complete absence of epithelial cells should raise the possibility that the needle was placed in a perithyroidal or intrathyroidal lymph node. Although background blood is the staple of most thyroid aspirates, Hashimoto's thyroiditis smears tend to be less bloody than those from most other thyroid lesions.

The epithelium is readily apparent on medium to high power and consists of a mixture of non-Hürthle and Hürthle cells.[207,226,230] The non-Hürthle cell epithelium appears only in small clusters, and the big flat sheets seen in nodular hyperplasia are not present. The Hürthle cells generally lack prominent nucleoli and do not form large three-dimensional clusters. Some have reported that epithelial cells may be lacking in the lymphoid phase of Hashimoto's thyroiditis, although with adequate sampling, the authors have not seen this.[236] The non-Hürthle cell epithelium may appear degenerated and the cells contain small amounts of cytoplasm.[122] Often, the lymphocytes are present in and intimately admixed with the epithelial aggregates.[207] It is not

unexpected to see considerable Hürthle cell atypia with increased N:C ratios, prominent nucleoli, and nuclear irregularity.[122] Atypia is more pronounced in aspirates from Hashimoto's thyroiditis than in aspirates from Hürthle cell neoplasms (Figure 26-19). Colloid is scant, and other features of inflammation may be present.[237] These features include foam cells, giant cells, fibrous tissue fragments, and granulomas. The granulomas form as a result of follicular destruction and leak of colloid.

In the atrophic phase of Hashimoto's thyroiditis, the smears are less cellular. Lymphocytes still predominate and the epithelial cells are even less numerous. In end-stage Hashimoto's thyroiditis, more fibrous tissue fragments are seen, although Hürthle cells and lymphocytes still should be present. Diagnosing the specific stage of Hashimoto's thyroiditis usually is not important.

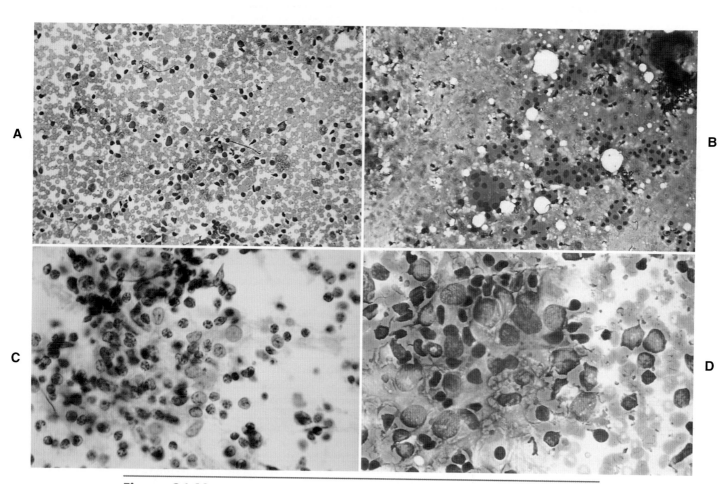

Figure 26-18   **Hashimoto's thyroiditis. A,** At a low power, the aspirate smears may resemble lymph node aspirate smears. Lymphocytes of varying size are admixed with blood and occasional crushed cellular groups. At a low power, the differential diagnosis includes an intrathyroidal lymph node and a malignant lymphoma. **B,** At a higher power, a mixture of Hürthle cells and lymphocytes are observed. The Hürthle cells are usually seen in small clusters and form occasional microfollicles. The lymphocytes may be seen within the clusters and are present outside the epithelial cell groups. The background of the smear consists predominantly of serum rather than watery colloid. Note the presence of the vacuoles within the serum; watery colloid of this amount usually would show cracking and red cell rouleaux. **C,** A follicular center cell fragment consisting of numerous lymphocytes and macrophages having larger, round to oval nuclei with prominent nucleoli is seen. The lymphocytes may exhibit crushing and show abundant cellular overlap. The lymphocytes are variable in size and include reactive lymphoid cells and small mature lymphocytes. **D,** A heterogeneous lymphoid population is present. The lymphocytes consist of large cells with prominent nucleoli admixed with small lymphoid cells. Lymphoglandular bodies are present in the background. (**A, B,** and **D,** DQ; **C,** Pap)

The differential diagnosis of a Hashimoto's thyroiditis FNA includes nodular hyperplasia, other thyroiditises, malignant lymphoma, follicular neoplasm (particularly the Hürthle cell variant), and papillary carcinoma.[238] Aspirates of nodular hyperplasia are less cellular, contain more colloid, and lack the predominance of Hürthle cells. Nonspecific thyroiditis, Riedel's thyroiditis, and granulomatous thyroiditis also may be confused with Hashimoto's thyroiditis. Because these disease processes may exhibit similar features, cytologists sometimes use the generic diagnosis of *thyroiditis* with a comment favoring one of the processes. Clinical data generally allows this distinction to be made.

The large cell type of malignant lymphoma is the most common malignant lymphoma associated with Hashimoto's thyroiditis.[186,227,239,240] FNAs of large cell malignant lymphoma show a monotonous appearance of large neoplastic cells, whereas the lymphocytes in Hashimoto's thyroiditis show a spectrum of sizes with a predominance of small lymphoid cells.[207,241] Epithelium is more often absent in FNAs of malignant lymphoma. Clinically, malignant lymphoma occurs in an older population and often presents as an abrupt enlargement.

Hürthle cell neoplasms lack the predominance of lymphocytes and show a greater epithelial cellularity.[207,226,242] The more monomorphic the Hürthle cell population, the more likely a Hürthle cell neoplasm.[243-245] Hürthle cell proliferations that lack encapsulation have been described in Hashimoto's thyroiditis, and the cytologic distinction of this process from a Hürthle cell neoplasm is virtually impossible.[122] Aspirates from both lesions show Hürthle cells and an absence of lymphocytes. Fortunately, the occurrence of a nonneoplastic dominant Hürthle cell nodule in Hashimoto's thyroiditis is rare.

Papillary carcinomas may be distinguished from Hashimoto's thyroiditis by their specific nuclear features,

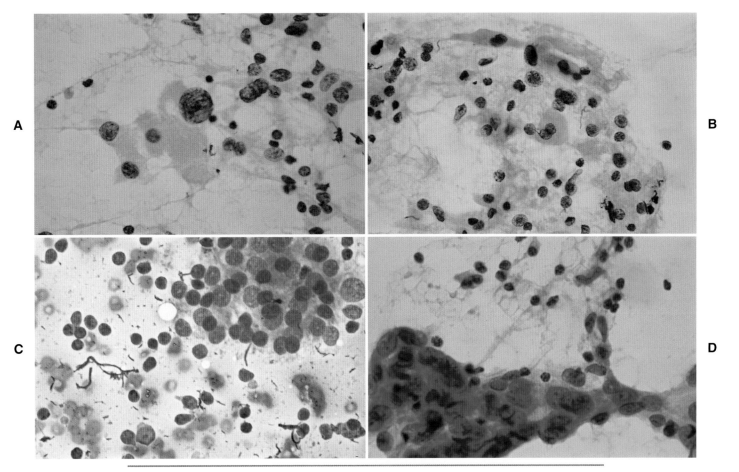

Figure 26-19 **Hashimoto's thyroiditis.** **A,** Hürthle cell atypia is common in Hashimoto's thyroiditis. In this case a cluster of Hürthle cells including a large Hürthle cell with abundant cytoplasm and an enlarged round nucleus is present. The numerous lymphocytes and the absence of microfollicles are indicative that this is a lymphocytic thyroiditis rather than a Hürthle cell neoplasm. **B,** Reactive Hürthle cell atypia is seen. The Hürthle cells may exhibit multinucleation, spindling, and nuclear enlargement. Stripped Hürthle cell nuclei are admixed with lymphocytic nuclei. **C,** A monolayer of Hürthle cells are infiltrated by numerous lymphocytes. Lymphoglandular bodies are present in the background. The Hürthle cell nuclei vary in size and shape, and in this case, it appears that several microfollicles are adjoined. **D,** A cluster of atypical Hürthle cells is admixed with lymphocytes. The follicular cells exhibit nuclear overlapping gland granular chromatin. The nuclei are enlarged and are slightly hyperchromatic. The cells lack features of either papillary carcinoma or follicular carcinoma. (**A, B,** and **D,** Pap; **C,** DQ)

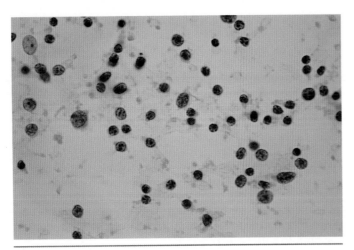

Figure 26-20 **Nonspecific lymphocytic thyroiditis.** A mixed population of lymphoid cells is present. Lymphoglandular bodies are seen in the background. (Pap)

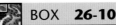

BOX 26-10

The Neoplastic Lesions

Papillary carcinoma
Follicular neoplasms
Hürthle cell neoplasms
Medullary carcinoma
Insular carcinoma
Malignant lymphoma
Salivary gland type tumors
Metastases

fewer lymphocytes, and lack of Hürthle cells.[139-141] In most cases, the diagnosis of Hashimoto's thyroiditis is relatively straightforward, and one does not have to comb every cell group for a lurking papillary carcinoma. Occasionally, smears of Hashimoto's thyroiditis may show epithelial cells with prominent nuclear grooving and even rare nuclear pseudoinclusions and these findings may lead to a false-positive diagnosis.

Nonspecific lymphocytic thyroiditis. The classic histologic description of Hashimoto's thyroiditis was very specific regarding the percentage of epithelial cells that had to show Hürthle cell change. Today, many pathologists are not that rigid and will make a diagnosis of Hashimoto's thyroiditis when lymphocytic infiltrates are present (regardless of the Hürthle cell count). Others are more demanding and would prefer to classify Hashimoto's thyroiditis as a subtype of lymphocytic thyroiditis and classify the non-Hashimoto's thyroiditises as *nonspecific* or simply lymphocytic thyroiditis. Mizukami established a classification system that separates Hashimoto's thyroiditis from other lymphocytic thyroidites.[225] Some of the nonspecific thyroiditises also are immune related and may be clinically identical to Hashimoto's thyroiditis. However, a subset of lymphocytic thyroiditises, apart from immune thyroiditises, also exist.[225,233,246,247] Many of these patients have an underlying nodular hyperplasia.[248]

The only clinical manifestation of a nonspecific thyroiditis is a nodular thyroid (antithyroid antibody titers may be absent or low). Smears from nonspecific thyroiditis look like a cross between smears from a nodular hyperplasia and smears from a Hashimoto's thyroiditis. Aspirates show follicular cells and hard colloid, similar to the smears of a benign thyroid nodule. The smears also show a heterogeneous lymphoid population similar to the smears of Hashimoto's thyroiditis (Figure 26-20). However, Hürthle cells are rare.[246-248] Consequently, if the lymphoid cells are in sufficient numbers to suggest Hashimoto's thyroiditis but the Hürthle cells are lacking, a diagnosis of nonspecific thyroiditis is appropriate.

Subacute lymphocytic (painless) thyroiditis. Subacute lymphocytic thyroiditis typically occurs sporadically (90%) or postpartum (10%).[249-251] The postpartum form has an autoimmune basis, and these patients have elevated antithyroid antibody titers (antimicrosomal antibodies are found in 10% of postpartum patients).[249,250] The sporadic form may have a viral etiology.[249] The disease follows a temporal course similar to granulomatous thyroiditis (e.g., abrupt onset) and most patients completely recover. One third of patients become hyperthyroid, one third hypothyroid, and one third hyperthyroid and then hypothyroid.[252] In most patients the thyroid gland is diffusely enlarged, although not to the extent to cause pain. Occasionally, a nodule arises. Clinically, the differential diagnosis includes Graves' disease.[249] Aspiration smears show a heterogeneous population of lymphocytes admixed with follicular epithelial cells that are present in large and/or small groups. Reactive epithelial changes usually are not pronounced. Colloid is sparse and Hürthle cells are absent or few in number.[249] Thus, the smears look similar to the smears of a Hashimoto's thyroiditis without Hürthle cells.

THE NEOPLASTIC LESIONS

This category contains lesions that may be surgically removed (follicular neoplasm, Hürthle cell neoplasm, hyalinizing trabecular adenoma, papillary carcinoma, medullary carcinoma, anaplastic carcinoma, insular carcinoma, and salivary gland-type neoplasms) and/or portend a bad prognosis (malignant lymphoma and metastasis) (Box 26-10). The 10-year relative survival rates for United States patients with papillary, follicular, Hürthle cell, medullary, and anaplastic carcinoma are 93%, 85%, 76%, 75%, and 14% respectively.[253]

Follicular Neoplasms

Follicular neoplasms include follicular adenomas and follicular carcinomas.[74] The follicular variant of papillary carcinoma, discussed here and in the section on papillary carcinoma, sometimes may cytologically mimic a follicular neoplasm. The closely related Hürthle cell neoplasms are discussed in the next section.

Follicular adenomas are benign neoplasms (usually cold nodules), which are completely encapsulated and lack invasion.[186] The presence or absence of a capsule is critical in determining if a lesion is an adenoma (no capsule: nodular hyperplasia; capsule: adenoma). Histologically, adenomas should be solitary, and if multiple nodules are present, the more appropriate diagnosis is nodular hyperplasia.[254] Adenomas may be subtyped according to their histologic

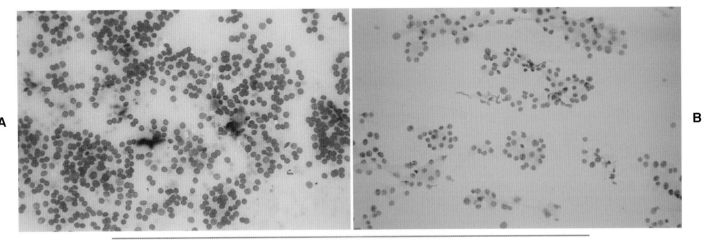

Figure 26-21 Follicular neoplasm. **A,** At a low power a hypercellular lesion is present. Numerous microfollicles, large clusters of cells and stripped nuclei are seen. Colloid is absent in the background. **B,** Small clusters of follicular cells are observed. Many of these cells are arranged in microfollicles, containing from five to 12 nuclei arranged around a central area of cytoplasm. Occasional stripped follicular cell nuclei are present. Even at a low power the variability in nuclear size can be appreciated. Colloid is absent in the background. (**A,** DQ; **B,** Pap)

appearance (i.e., simple, microfollicular, macrofollicular, trabecular, embryonal, and fetal), although subclassification has no clinical importance.[186] Joensuu and colleagues have hypothesized that a subset of adenomas are carcinoma in situ (aneupoid population in 27%), and the biologic potential is uncertain.[255] However, for practical purposes, if the adenoma is excised and adequately studied, it will not recur or metastasize.[186] A small subset of adenomas have markedly atypical histologic features (mitoses, pleomorphism, necrosis, increased cellularity), and these adenomas are known as *atypical adenomas*.[256,257] Despite the atypia, these lesions are not viewed as having malignant potential.

Follicular carcinoma comprises about 5% of all thyroid carcinomas.[258,259] This percentage increases (up to 40%) in iodine-deficient areas, because the number of papillary carcinomas decreases.[258,259] LiVolsi and colleagues report that approximately 2% to 3% of all follicular neoplasms show invasive characteristics.[186] In actuality the true incidence of follicular carcinoma is difficult to determine because the follicular variant of papillary carcinoma may be placed, often incorrectly, in this group. Backdahl reported that only 60% of follicular carcinomas are aneuploid, which indicates that a follicular carcinoma cannot be excluded on the basis of diploid analysis on FNA material.[260] In contrast with papillary carcinoma, follicular carcinoma typically metastasizes through the bloodstream into bone, lungs, brain, and liver and not the lymphatics.[261,262] Patients who have a follicular carcinoma confined to the thyroid gland do well (survival greater than 80% at 10 years).[263,264] Patients who have widely disseminated disease do poorly (overall survival of 50%).[263-266]

Follicular carcinomas are separated from follicular adenomas by the presence of capsular and/or vascular space invasion.[267] This *requires* histologic examination. The definition of capsular invasion is controversial and need not concern the cytologist.[268,269] Histologically, both follicular adenomas and carcinomas are composed of follicles, and in many cases, the neoplastic cells of a follicular carcinoma appear identical to the cells of a follicular adenoma. Not all

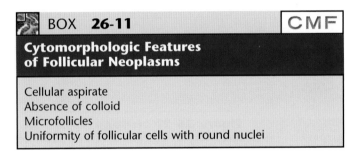

BOX 26-11   CMF

Cytomorphologic Features of Follicular Neoplasms

Cellular aspirate
Absence of colloid
Microfollicles
Uniformity of follicular cells with round nuclei

follicular carcinomas are well differentiated, and anaplastic follicular carcinomas may be widely invasive.[263,264,268]

Cytologically, follicular adenomas and carcinomas are classified *together* under the rubric follicular neoplasm because the cells from both neoplasms appear the same and the cytologist cannot evaluate the features definitive for separation (i.e., vascular or capsular invasion).[74] The main task for the cytologist is separating a follicular neoplasm from a dominant nodule of nodular hyperplasia, which is not always easy.

Follicular neoplasms occupy Region 3. Remember that the two criteria important in the separation are epithelial cellularity and amount of colloid (Box 26-11). Smears from follicular neoplasms are cellular and contain little colloid (Figure 26-21).[106,138,139,270] Surgical pathology follow-up of Region 3 lesions show that 85% to 95% are follicular adenomas or carcinomas.* Approximately 20% of Region 3 lesions are follicular carcinomas (range: 15% to 50%).† Only a small percentage (approximately 1%) of Region 1 lesions are follicular carcinomas on follow-up (meaning that a small subset of follicular carcinomas contain significant amounts of colloid).[44,60,134]

---

*References 31, 44, 53, 84, 100, 102, 103, 106, 109, 110, 271, and 272.
†References 31, 44, 53, 84, 100, 102, 103, 106, 109-112, 134, 269, and 271.

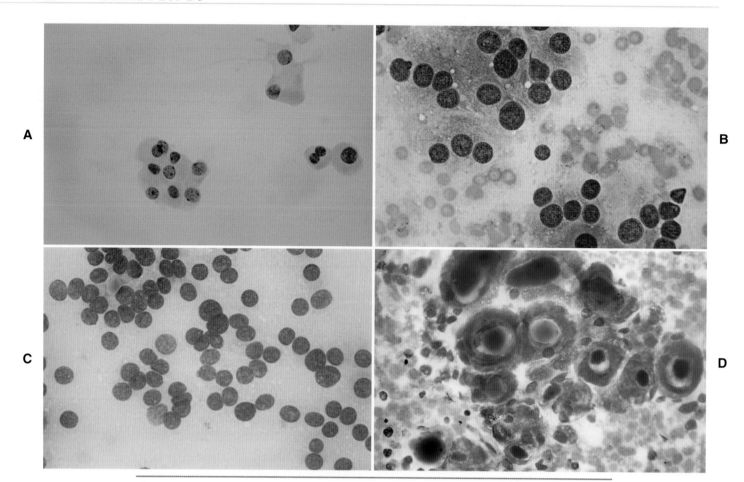

Figure 26-22   Follicular neoplasm. A, A microfollicle is present in the center of the smear and several single follicular cells are seen. The microfollicle contains nine follicular cell nuclei that are all round to regular and contain a granular chromatin pattern. An occasional small nucleus is seen. Note that the intact single cells also contain cytoplasm. This is an unusual feature for non-neoplastic conditions. **B,** A Diff-Quik (DQ) stain shows several microfollicles. Several of these microfollicles are aligned back to back and the nuclei are slightly crowded and enlarged. The chromatin pattern is finely granular. Occasional stripped follicular cell nuclei are seen. **C,** Numerous stripped follicular cell nuclei are seen. A relative absence of cytoplasm is seen, although the nuclei still are present in small clusters and small microfollicles. Nuclear overlap is present. **D,** In this lesion, the small microfollicles contain central areas of colloid. The colloid is often hard, and watery colloid is relatively absent. Several hard colloid fragments may be seen outside of microfollicles. The follicular cell nuclei appear small and round. (**A,** Pap; **B-D,** DQ)

Other cytologic features also are useful in the separation of a dominant nodule of nodular hyperplasia from a follicular neoplasm. Architecturally, microfollicles are often present in follicular neoplasms (Figure 26-22).[106,138,139,273] Microfollicles are cellular rosettes with a ring of five to 15 follicular cells, sometimes surrounding a little ball of colloid.[24] Large, flat honeycomb sheets of cells tend to be absent. Cell clusters, including the microfollicles, show nuclear overlapping and crowding. Stripped single cells with intact cytoplasm are present in aspirations from follicular neoplasms.[24,108,110,137,274]

The follicular cells tend to be more monotonous and uniform in a follicular neoplasm than in nodular hyperplasia.[110,159,160,170] The presence of the two epithelial cell types (follicular cells *and* Hürthle cells) and cellular degeneration support the diagnosis of nodular hyperplasia.[102,170] Reparative features and focal cellular atypia are

uncommon in follicular neoplasms.[122,275] In follicular adenomas and carcinomas, the nuclei are usually slightly increased in size (larger than a lymphocyte) but do not show significant irregularities or changes in chromatin appearance (Figure 26-23).[108,145,274,276,277] Mai and colleagues report that some follicular neoplasms may have fine chromatin.[278] Nucleoli are often small and inconspicuous. Follicular neoplasms may show a slight increase in the nuclear to cytoplasmic (N:C) ratio, although this finding is subtle.[137,274,277] The cytoplasm of the neoplastic cells is similar in appearance and texture to the cytoplasm of non-neoplastic follicular cells.

The more poorly differentiated follicular carcinomas have more recognizable cytologic atypia (Figure 26-24).[107,108,277,279] Aspirates show three-dimensional groups (in addition to disorganized microfollicles), increased numbers of single cells with intact cytoplasm, nuclear pleomorphism and mem-

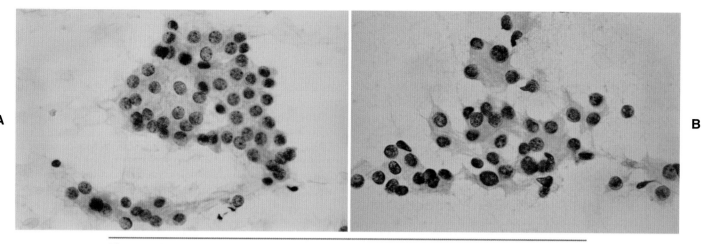

Figure 26-23 **Follicular neoplasm.** **A,** The chromatin pattern in this follicular neoplasm is evenly dispersed and finely granular. Thus, in this case the chromatin pattern of the neoplastic follicular cells appears similar to the chromatin pattern in benign follicular lesions. In this case, the follicular cell nuclei are slightly increased in size. The architectural features of high cellularity and microfollicles are indicative of a follicular neoplasm. Colloid is absent. **B,** In this follicular neoplasm the follicular cells contain round, regular, slightly enlarged nuclei. Nuclear membrane irregularities are absent. Nuclear overlap also is present. (**A-B,** Pap)

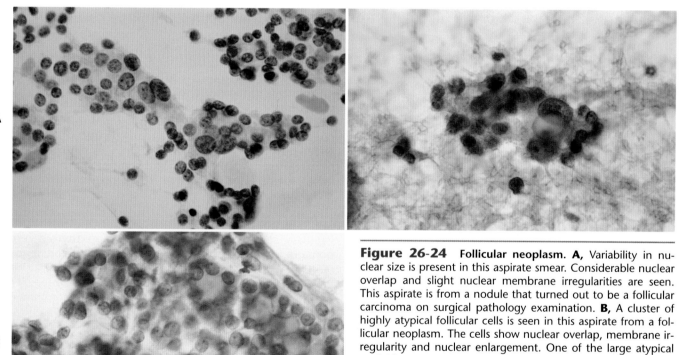

Figure 26-24 **Follicular neoplasm.** **A,** Variability in nuclear size is present in this aspirate smear. Considerable nuclear overlap and slight nuclear membrane irregularities are seen. This aspirate is from a nodule that turned out to be a follicular carcinoma on surgical pathology examination. **B,** A cluster of highly atypical follicular cells is seen in this aspirate from a follicular neoplasm. The cells show nuclear overlap, membrane irregularity and nuclear enlargement. One of the large atypical nuclei has a prominent nucleolus. On histologic follow-up, this patient was found to have a follicular carcinoma. **C,** Extensive nuclear overlapping is seen in this large cluster of follicular cells. Several microfollicles are observed in the upper right and the nuclei of these follicles show overlap. Nucleoli and nuclear grooves are present in many of the nuclei. On histologic follow-up this patient had a follicular carcinoma. (**A-C,** Pap)

brane irregularities, prominent nucleoli, frequent mitoses, greater nuclear overlapping, higher N:C ratios, necrosis, and denser cytoplasm (Box 26-12).* Miller and colleagues and Kini report that by using specific criteria, 70% to 82% of follicular carcinomas may be diagnosed correctly.[73,277] Based on the experience of other authors, such a high percentage of follicular carcinomas cannot be diagnosed with certainty. In fact, using statistical analysis, Rout and Shariff report that cytologic criteria were not effective in separating follicular adenomas from carcinomas.[281] In many laboratories the term *follicular carcinoma* is not used on FNA. This is because, provided the *definition* of follicular carcinoma, examination of surgical tissue is necessary for the diagnosis.[143] Because atypical features may be seen in benign conditions and adenomas (atypical adenoma), most laboratories use the diagnosis of follicular carcinoma very infrequently.[188,282] Thus, these laboratories usually only suggest a diagnosis of follicular carcinoma (follicular neoplasm, favor follicular carcinoma) in cases with marked cytologic atypia and a high clinical indication of malignancy (e.g., large mass).

If the nuclear and cytoplasmic features of papillary carcinoma are seen in smears that otherwise look like a follicular neoplasm, the diagnosis of a follicular variant of papillary carcinoma should be considered.[108,214,283-288] Yan and colleagues report that, in some cases, the diagnosis of follicular variant of papillary carcinoma may be suggested by the presence of branched monolayer sheets, instead of the presence of microfollicles.[72,108,214,283,285-288]

Hürthle Cell Neoplasms

Hürthle cell neoplasms are a variant of follicular neoplasms. Hürthle cell neoplasms compose approximately 10% of all thyroid neoplasms and include Hürthle cell adenoma and Hürthle cell carcinoma.[289] Not all collections of Hürthle cells are neoplastic; as with their follicular counterpart, Hürthle cell neoplasms are a subset of Hürthle cell lesions. Benign aggregates of Hürthle cells may be seen in nodular hyperplasia and Hashimoto's thyroiditis.[156,290,291] The separation of a Hürthle cell neoplasm from a Hürthle cell nodule may be accomplished with the criteria in Figure 26-11. Few Hürthle cells and abundant colloid are found in a Hürthle cell nodule.[207,292] Criteria supportive of nodular hyperplasia include flat, large sheets of Hürthle cells; cellular degeneration; focal

---

*References 106, 108, 116, 188, 277, 279, and 280.

cellular atypia; few single cells; and a mixed population of Hürthle cells and follicular cells.[207,292-294] Few studies have examined the follow-up of Region 2 Hürthle cell lesions. To separate a dominant Hürthle cell nodule in Hashimoto's thyroiditis from a Hürthle cell neoplasm, larger numbers of lymphocytes and more cellular atypia favor Hashimoto's thyroiditis.[207,237,292-294]

Hürthle cell adenomas are benign tumors that are encapsulated and lack invasion.[272,289,295] Previously, some authors considered all Hürthle cell neoplasms, whereas other authors consider Hürthle cell neoplasms larger than 2 cm in diameter as malignant.[294] These considerations are no longer valid. Hürthle cell carcinomas are defined by the presence of capsular or vascular space invasion.[272,289,295] Size, cellular pleomorphism, mitoses, nuclear atypia, and histologic subtype are not predictive of behavior.[296,297] Between 30% and 40% of Hürthle cell neoplasms are carcinomas.[272,295] Similar to their follicular counterparts, the separation of Hürthle cell adenoma from Hürthle cell carcinoma depends on histologic features. Cytologically, the term *Hürthle cell neoplasm* is used in reporting the authors' findings.

FNA smears of Hürthle cell neoplasms are cellular and show scant colloid and few lymphocytes (Figure 26-25 and Box 26-13).[237,243] The neoplastic Hürthle cells are arranged in large and small clusters, papillary structures, and singly.[237,243,292,298,299] Occasional microfollicles with small, centrally placed colloid balls are present. The nuclei are round to oval with distinctly granular chromatin,[237] and multinucleation is common.[243] The cells may show considerable atypia, including increased N:C ratios, nuclear pleomorphism, macronucleoli, atypical mitoses, and large groups.[243,289,298] Features favoring a Hürthle cell carcinoma include macronucleoli, crowded groups, ill-defined cytoplasm, and marked pleomorphism.[237,243,289,298,300] Intranuclear pseudoinclusions have been reported in Hürthle cell neoplasms.[243,299,301] Of course, if many pseudoinclusions are seen, a Hürthle cell variant of papillary carcinoma should be considered. Calcification and psammoma bodies also have been reported in Hürthle cell neoplasms.

Papillary Carcinoma

Papillary carcinoma is the most common thyroid carcinoma in all age groups with a mean age at initial diagnosis of 40 years.[259,302,303] In a small percentage of cases, a prior history of radiation exposure may be obtained.[304,305] Papillary carcinoma is up to four times more common in

---

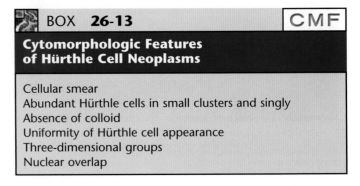

BOX 26-12 CMF

Cytomorphologic Features of Follicular Carcinoma

Cellular smears
Microfollicles
Follicular cell atypia
Nuclear overlap
Cellular dissociation
Nuclear enlargement
Prominence of nucleoli
Absence of colloid

BOX 26-13 CMF

Cytomorphologic Features of Hürthle Cell Neoplasms

Cellular smear
Abundant Hürthle cells in small clusters and singly
Absence of colloid
Uniformity of Hürthle cell appearance
Three-dimensional groups
Nuclear overlap

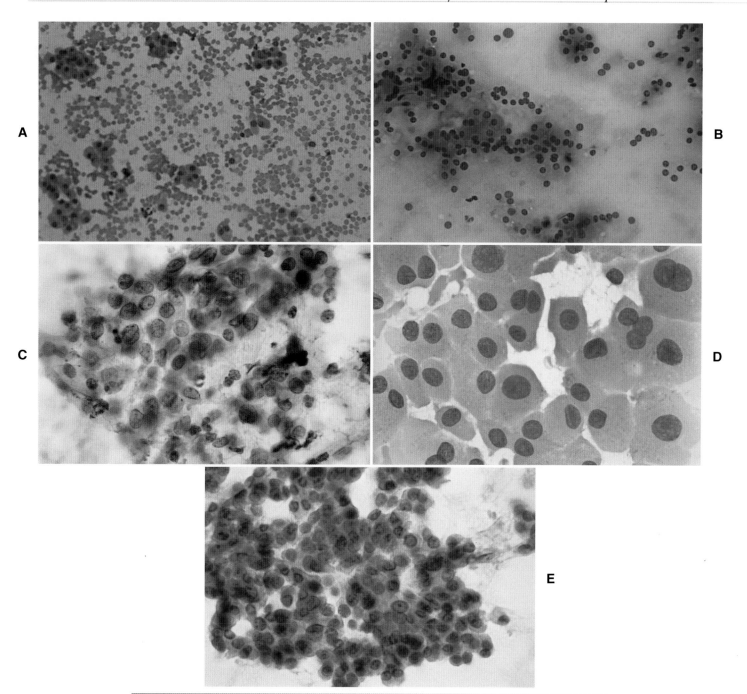

Figure 26-25 **Hürthle cell neoplasm.** **A,** On this low power, small clusters of Hürthle cells are admixed with blood. The clusters contain from five to 10 cells arranged in small microfollicles. Colloid is absent in the background. At this power, the cells appear very monomorphic. **B,** At this medium power, clusters of Hürthle cells and stripped Hürthle cell nuclei are present. A microfollicle is seen in the upper center. The nuclei exhibit slight variation in size, although the variation is nothing more than would be seen in benign Hürthle cell processes. The cytoplasm is slightly frayed and ill-defined in the larger groups. **C,** A three-dimensional group of atypical Hürthle cells is present. The cells are variable in size and the nuclei are round to oval. The nuclei contain a prominent nucleolus. On histologic follow-up, this patient had a Hürthle cell carcinoma. **D,** On this high power, numerous Hürthle cells are present. Occasional cells exhibit binucleation and the cells have abundant cytoplasm. The nuclei are round to oval and many contain a prominent nucleolus. The cytoplasm has a hard to granular appearance. In some areas, distinct cell borders are not identified. **E,** This smear is cellular and shows three-dimensional clusters of Hürthle cells. The cells exhibit considerable nuclear overlap. The cells have higher nuclear to cytoplasmic (N:C) ratios compared with the Hürthle cells seen in Figure 26-24, *D,* and the nucleoli are more prominent. Colloid is absent in the background. On histologic follow-up this patient was found to have a Hürthle cell carcinoma. (**A, B,** and **D,** DQ; **C** and **E,** Pap)

women.[266,306] Almost all patients present with evidence of disease in the neck, and papillary carcinoma usually presents as a cold nodule.[267] Tumor is confined to the thyroid in 67% of cases, to the thyroid gland and lymph nodes in 13%, and to lymph nodes alone in 20%. Interestingly, the presence of lymph node metastases does not correlate with poorer prognosis, although it does portend an increased probability of recurrence.[307] Papillary carcinoma usually metastasizes through the lymph system (hence the high percentage of lymph node metastases).[267,308] Papillary carcinoma also may metastasize through the blood, and the most common sites of metastasis are the lungs, followed by bones and the central nervous system.[266,306] Patients who have a worse prognosis are older; are men; or have larger tumors, extrathyroidal extension, distant metastases, anaplastic histologic foci, or multicentric tumor foci.[309-311] Although recurrence occurs in approximately 10% of patients, papillary carcinoma is one of those tumors that may recur many years after the initial presentation.[312] Most patients, however, have an excellent prognosis with a 20-year survival of more than 90%.[137,267]

When papillary carcinoma is first detected in a lymph node, without obvious gross thyroid involvement, the carcinoma most likely is occult.[313] Careful sectioning of the thyroid gland usually shows a small focus of tumor.[314] Depending on the definition, occult carcinomas measure less than 1 or 1.5 cm in diameter.[266,267] Not all occult carcinomas are papillary (follicular carcinomas, Hürthle cell carcinomas, and medullary carcinomas also may be occult), although the majority are.[313] In most cases, occult papillary carcinomas are detected incidentally (i.e., thyroid removed for some other disease) and do not present with extrathyroidal disease.[313,315,316] Harach reported occult carcinomas in 35.6% of all thyroid glands.[314] Based on autopsy studies, however, most authors report an incidence of occult carcinoma ranging from 4% to 7%.[313,315] Patients who have an occult papillary carcinoma have an excellent prognosis (5-year survival of approximately 99%).[287]

Grossly, the typical papillary carcinoma appears as a solid, nonencapsulated nodule, although up to 15% are encapsulated.[317,318] Papillary carcinomas often are partially cystic and up to 10% of papillary carcinomas are entirely cystic. The proportion of multicentric tumors varies greatly between 20% and 80%.[287,319] Multicentricity is the reason why endocrine surgeons despise the less than definitive papillary carcinoma diagnoses (e.g., *atypical grooved cells, possibly suspicious for a papillary neoplasm*). The diagnosis of a papillary carcinoma results in a total thyroidectomy (to remove all possible tumor foci), whereas suspicious lesions and follicular neoplasm diagnoses yield a lobectomy (with possible frozen section).

Papillary carcinoma has a classic form and several variants. The classic form is what is seen with most FNA specimens. Histologically, the classic papillary carcinoma shows papillary regions mixed with follicular regions.[320] Less than half of the cases show a pure papillary architecture.[321] In addition to true papillae with connective tissue stalks, other histologic features supportive of a papillary carcinoma diagnosis are nuclear crowding, ground glass nuclei, intranuclear pseudoinclusions, nuclear grooves, and psammoma bodies.[267,287,320,322] The ground glass nuclei, also known as *Orphan Annie eye nuclei,* are seen on formalin-fixed sections and are not seen in cytologic preparations.[323,324]

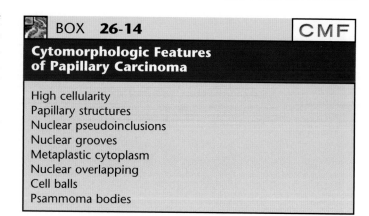

Accounting for up to 15% of papillary carcinomas, the follicular variants are composed almost exclusively of neoplastic follicles and lack true papillary structures.[286,287,321,325] Histologically and cytologically, this variant maintains the characteristic nuclear features.[286,321,326-329] The authors are unaware of a good study measuring interobserver diagnostic variability (i.e., Do experts agree on the classification of papillary carcinoma versus follicular neoplasm?), although, based on anecdotal evidence, considerable disagreement is evident. The follicular variant behaves similarly to a classic papillary carcinoma (less aggressively) compared with a true follicular carcinoma.[321] Although some authors report a higher rate of distant metastases with the follicular variant of papillary carcinoma compared with the classic papillary carcinoma, the prognosis of patients with the follicular variant of papillary carcinoma is excellent.[267,321] The follicular variant of papillary carcinoma may not be outright diagnosable on FNA. Nair and colleagues reported that less than a third of the follicular variant subtype was correctly identified on aspiration.[330] However, the possibility of a follicular variant of papillary carcinoma may be raised so that a frozen section could be obtained at the time of surgical intervention.[331]

On cytologic preparations, classic papillary carcinoma has a number of distinctive features so that the diagnosis is relatively straightforward (Box 26-14). The smears usually are cellular, and papillary structures are present (Figure 26-26).[89,136,141,166] A true papillary structure contains a fibrovascular core and does not consist of just an elongated folded group of follicular cells (i.e., pseudopapilla). True papillae are present in up to 60% of cases.[140,141] The neoplastic cells are arranged in a three-dimensional, hobnail fashion along the core, although cellular dissociation is common. In some cases of cystic papillary carcinoma, papillary groups may be present only on the cell block. Although highly suggestive of papillary carcinoma, true papillae also may be seen in other thyroid diseases, such as Graves's disease, nodular hyperplasia, the thyroiditises, and other neoplasias.[53,141,166]

The neoplastic cells also may be arranged in large or small groups, balls, microfollicles, and singly.[140,166,283] The presence of three-dimensional cell balls is highly suggestive of papillary carcinoma (Figure 26-27).[140] The literature reports that the presence of follicular structures may occur in up to 85% of cases.[140,141,166] This raises a cautionary note about microfollicles: before signing out a case as a follicular neoplasm, remember to look for the nuclear features of a

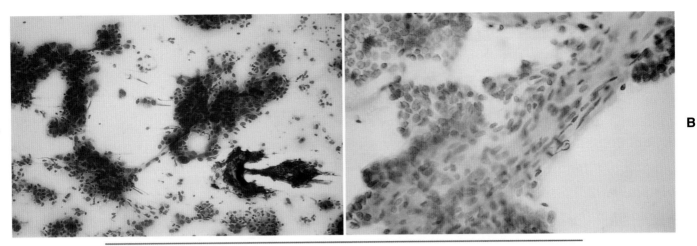

A

B

Figure 26-26 **Papillary carcinoma. A,** On this low-power view, large groups of epithelial cells are seen. Several of the groups contain endothelial cell fragments suggestive of a fibrovascular core. A large fragment of bubble-gum colloid is seen in the lower right. **B,** A true papillary structure is depicted. A fibrovascular core is seen in the center. Surrounding this core are numerous neoplastic cells. The cells exhibit three-dimensional piling and overlap. The N:C ratio is high. Although true fibrovascular cores may be seen in benign conditions, their presence is worrisome for a papillary carcinoma. (**A,** DQ; **B,** Pap)

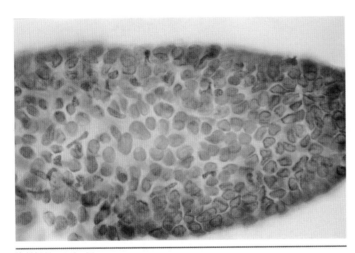

Figure 26-27 **Papillary carcinoma.** At this medium power, a three-dimensional cell ball is depicted. Note that artifactually less piling up occurs in the center of the cluster than at the edges. Thus, the nuclear details are better observed in the center fragments of these large neoplastic cell balls. At the edge the nuclei show molding. The chromatin pattern is finely dusty and a nuclear groove is identified in many of the nuclei. The neoplastic cell borders are indistinct. Note the lack of individual cell dissociation and the crisp border to the cellular ball. (Pap)

papillary carcinoma (one may be dealing with the follicular variant).[331] In many of the cell groups the nuclei appear crowded and may exhibit obvious overlapping. Nuclear crowding persists in microfollicles, which may be a subtle sign that one is dealing with a follicular variant of papillary carcinoma rather than a true follicular neoplasm. Although nuclear stripping may occur in papillary carcinoma, the majority of single cells retain their cytoplasm, an unusual feature in benign thyroid entities.

The cytoplasm of the neoplastic cells is variable (Figure 26-28). In many tumors, the cytoplasm is homogeneous and *metaplastic,* meaning it has a hard or squamoid ap-

pearance (more than 70% of cases) with well-defined cytoplasmic borders.[140,141] In up to 40% of papillary carcinomas, actual squamous differentiation with well-defined cytoplasmic borders is present.[332] On the DQ stain the cytoplasm stains blue, and on the Pap stain the cytoplasm stains dark orange to green. In other cases the cytoplasm remains hard but has a more granular quality so that the neoplastic cells resemble Hürthle cells, particularly on the DQ stain. In the follicular variant of papillary carcinoma, the cytoplasm may be finely granular. This dense cytoplasmic appearance is unexpected in follicular neoplasms. Metaplastic cytoplasm also may be seen in benign thyroid conditions such as the hyperplasias, particularly the degenerated cystic nodular hyperplasia, and the thyroiditises.[139,186,333] In these cases the metaplastic appearance of the benign follicular cells results from inflammation, repair, or degeneration.

Vacuolated cytoplasm is another feature commonly seen in papillary carcinoma, particularly the cystic variant.[140] These vacuoles may be large, and they may actually indent the nucleus. Some vacuolated papillary carcinoma cells resemble macrophages, although in contrast with macrophages, the tumor cell cytoplasm surrounding the vacuoles maintains a hard, waxy appearance.[140]

The neoplastic nuclei are oval, uniform, and larger than normal follicular cell nuclei (Figure 26-29). The nuclear membrane is irregular in contour and often folded.* Nuclear grooves, which result from nuclear folding, are a distinctive feature and are best seen on the Pap stain.[334] Other lesions that have grooved nuclei are the thyroiditises, nodular hyperplasia, follicular adenoma, and follicular carcinoma.[146-150] Beware of overinterpreting the occasional nuclear groove as diagnostic for papillary carcinoma; this mistake has led to more than one false-positive diagnosis. The grooves seen in papillary carcinomas are observed in many cells and in many microscopic fields. Chhieng and col-

---

*References 147, 149, 150, 267, 334, and 335.

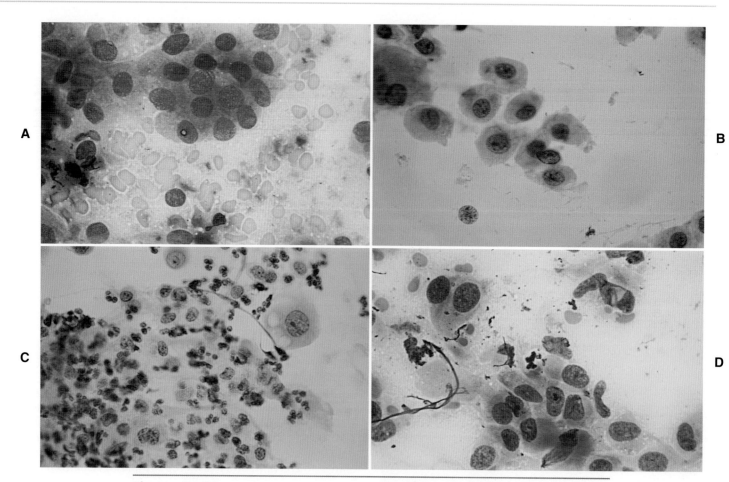

Figure 26-28   Papillary carcinoma. A, The neoplastic cells of this papillary carcinoma show metaplastic cytoplasm. The nuclei are enlarged, although the N:C ratio is not markedly high. Occasional stripped neoplastic cell nuclei are present. A grungy background is observed. **B,** On the Pap stain the metaplastic cytoplasm is cyanophilic to slightly eosinophilic. The nuclei tend to be eccentrically placed and a nuclear groove is observed in several of the nuclei. Note the presence of a multinucleated neoplastic cell in the upper left. **C,** In some instances of papillary carcinoma, the cytoplasm may have a slightly vacuolated appearance as is seen in the neoplastic cell in the upper right. This smear is from a patient who had a cystic papillary carcinoma and the cyst exhibited rupture and acute inflammation. The vacuolization within the cytoplasm may be a reparative feature. In some instances, these atypical cells may be mistaken for reactive histiocytes. **D,** In this papillary carcinoma, considerable cell dissociation occurs, although the majority of neoplastic cells contain cytoplasm. The nuclei are eccentrically placed and variably shaped. Even in the DQ stain, nuclear grooves are appreciated. The cytoplasm has a hard metaplastic squamoid appearance. (**A** and **D,** DQ; **B** and **C,** Pap)

leagues reported that CD44 is useful in separating papillary carcinomas from other thyroid lesions with nuclear grooves; CD44 reportedly is positive only in papillary carcinoma.[336] Nasser and colleagues reported that cytokeratin 19 differentially stained thyroid papillary carcinomas (in contrast with other thyroid lesions).[337]

Intranuclear pseudoinclusions are the most pathognomonic cytologic feature of papillary carcinoma (Figure 26-30).[140,141,149,214,338] True inclusions are large and occupy from one third to one half of the nuclear area. Nuclear pseudoinclusions have a sharp margin, and nuclear material should not be present within them. Pseudoinclusions represent invaginations of the nuclear membrane.[322] Pseudoinclusions are present in more than 90% of cases.[149,322,324,338] Overcalling pseudoinclusions is another cause of misdiagnosing papillary carcinoma. The most common mistake is misinterpreting nuclear degeneration,

which may have a clear appearance, as a pseudoinclusion. True pseudoinclusions may be seen in benign diseases, but they are the exception. Benign diseases that reportedly show nuclear pseudoinclusions include nodular hyperplasia and Hashimoto's thyroiditis.[29,84,140,292] One caution is that if a pseudoinclusion is present and a benign process is suspected, one must be absolutely certain that an adequate specimen has been obtained. The needle may have passed through the lesion and only obtained rare neoplastic cell groups. Pseudoinclusions also are reported in other neoplasms such as follicular neoplasms (possibly misdiagnosed follicular variants of papillary carcinoma), Hürthle cell neoplasms, medullary carcinoma, anaplastic carcinoma, insular carcinoma, hyalinizing trabecular adenoma, and metastases.[140,147,301,339,340] Again, the point cannot be stressed enough that if a pseudoinclusion is present, papillary carcinoma must be considered.

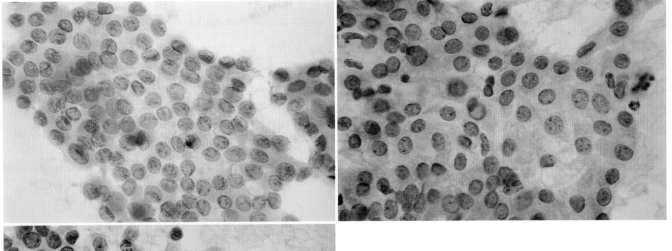

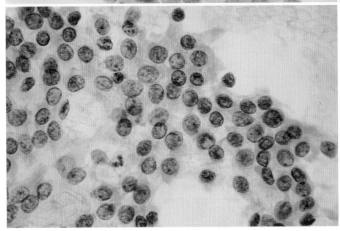

Figure 26-29 Papillary carcinoma. A, A sheet of neoplastic cells is present. The neoplastic nuclei tend to have pale chromatin with thick nuclear membranes. Nuclear grooves are easily identified in many of the neoplastic cells. **B,** A large flat cluster of neoplastic cells is seen. The nuclear shape varies from round to oval to slightly elongated. An occasional nucleolus is present. Many of the cells exhibit a nuclear groove. **C,** A relatively flat sheet of neoplastic cells is seen in this example. The cytoplasm has a degenerated appearance, although the nuclei are well-preserved. Slight nuclear overlap and occasional nucleoli are seen. Nuclear grooves are evident. (**A-C,** Pap)

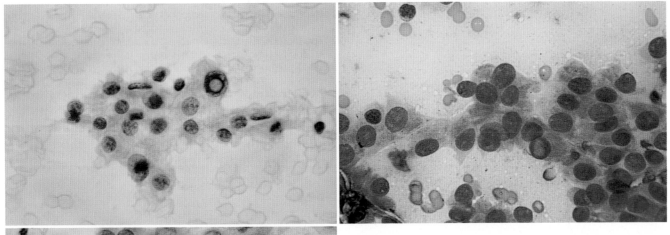

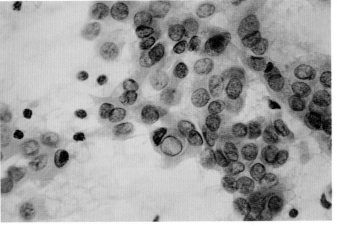

Figure 26-30 Papillary carcinoma. A, A small cluster of neoplastic cells from a papillary carcinoma is admixed with blood. Note the presence of a large intranuclear pseudoinclusion. This pseudoinclusion occupies greater than half the nuclear volume and has a thick nuclear border. **B,** Intranuclear pseudoinclusions are easily identified on the DQ stain. In this case, a cell with an intranuclear pseudoinclusion is seen in the center of the field. **C,** A large intranuclear pseudoinclusion is seen in the lower center field. This inclusion occupies almost the entire nucleus, giving the nucleus a "cleared" appearance with a thickened nuclear rim. The surrounding nuclei have irregular nuclear membranes and are variable in size and shape. (**A** and **C,** Pap; **B,** DQ)

The chromatin pattern of papillary carcinoma generally is pale and finely granular so that the papillary carcinoma nuclei are less hyperchromatic than benign follicular cell nuclei (Figure 26-31).[320] On the Pap stain the nuclei may appear washed out. Nucleoli are small, multiple (up to four per nucleus), and peripherally located, although some papillary carcinomas have large central nucleoli.[320,341] Most papillary carcinomas lack significant anaplasia, mitoses, and necrosis.

If colloid is present, it often has a thick, hard (bubble-gum) appearance and appears pink to purple on the DQ stain and green to blue on the Pap stain (Figure 26-32).[214] It has a stretched, irregular stranded appearance.[139,140] Bubble-gum colloid may be abundant, mimicking hard colloid, leading to the consideration of nodular hyperplasia![140] Bubble-gum colloid is present in up to 25% of cases but also may be seen in benign diseases such as Graves' disease.[139] In the follicular areas of a papillary carcinoma, thick, tight

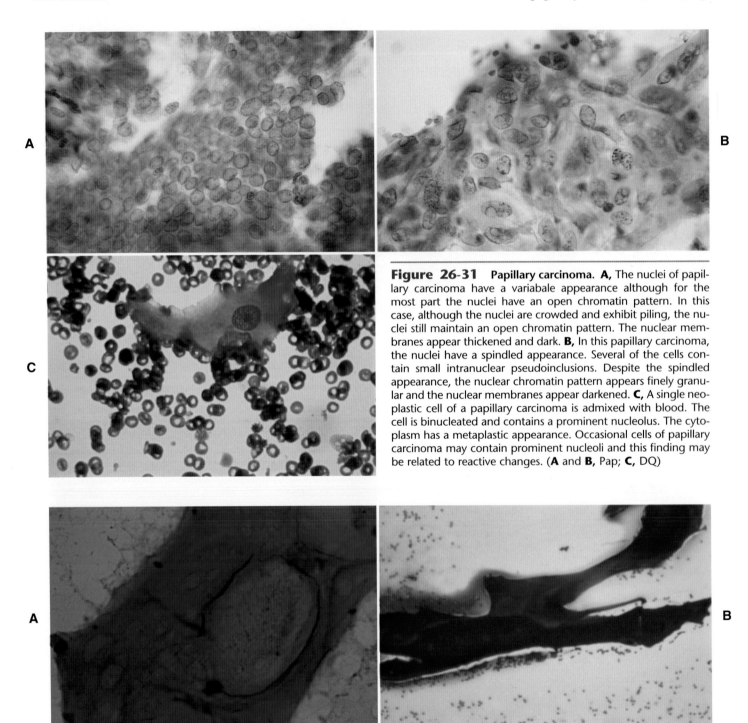

Figure 26-31 **Papillary carcinoma. A,** The nuclei of papillary carcinoma have a variabale appearance although for the most part the nuclei have an open chromatin pattern. In this case, although the nuclei are crowded and exhibit piling, the nuclei still maintain an open chromatin pattern. The nuclear membranes appear thickened and dark. **B,** In this papillary carcinoma, the nuclei have a spindled appearance. Several of the cells contain small intranuclear pseudoinclusions. Despite the spindled appearance, the nuclear chromatin pattern appears finely granular and the nuclear membranes appear darkened. **C,** A single neoplastic cell of a papillary carcinoma is admixed with blood. The cell is binucleated and contains a prominent nucleolus. The cytoplasm has a metaplastic appearance. Occasional cells of papillary carcinoma may contain prominent nucleoli and this finding may be related to reactive changes. (**A** and **B,** Pap; **C,** DQ)

Figure 26-32 **Papillary carcinoma. A,** A large fragment of bubble-gum colloid is depicted on the Pap stain. The colloid has a well-defined boundary and exhibits variable internal thickness. **B,** A fragment of bubble-gum colloid is depicted on the DQ stain. The colloid has a pulled appearance. Fragments of bubble-gum colloid are often massive. (**A,** Pap; **B,** DQ)

balls of colloid are present within small microfollicles or are free floating. The presence of watery colloid in papillary carcinoma is highly unusual.

Kini and colleagues have stressed the importance of giant cells as a key diagnostic feature of papillary carcinoma (Figure 26-33).[166] Giant cells are present in up to 50% of cases.[140,202] Giant cells may have a macrophage or epithelioid appearance.[166,342] The macrophage type cells contain foamy cytoplasm and may be multinucleated.[140] The epithelioid type cells have hard cytoplasm without vacuoles. These cells may be monstrous in size. The nuclei of both cell types are elongated, hypochromatic, and not particularly suggestive of tumor although nuclear grooves may be present.[342] Giant cells may be present in other thyroid neoplasms, Hashimoto's thyroiditis, and nodular hyperplasia. Other inflammatory cell types seen in papillary carcinoma include lymphocytes and occasional neutrophils.[202]

The presence of psammoma bodies in smears should immediately raise the suspicion of papillary carcinoma, although they have been described in other neoplasms (e.g., medullary carcinoma, mucoepidermoid carcinoma) and benign conditions (nodular hyperplasia, Graves' disease, and Hashimoto's thyroiditis) (Figure 26-34).[64,140,166,343-346] Psammoma bodies should be distinguished from fragments of calcification, which are seen in many benign diseases such as nodular hyperplasia.[344] Psammoma bodies are concentric and laminated, and stain clear to dark blue on the DQ stain and red to purple on the Pap stain. Tumor cells are often seen outlining the psammoma body. Psammoma bodies are present in up to 40% of papillary carcinoma cases.[140,166,214]

With all these good criteria to chose from, which are the most important for the diagnosis of papillary carcinoma? Experts disagree and several studies have been performed to identify key diagnostic criteria.[139-141] The most sensitive cri-

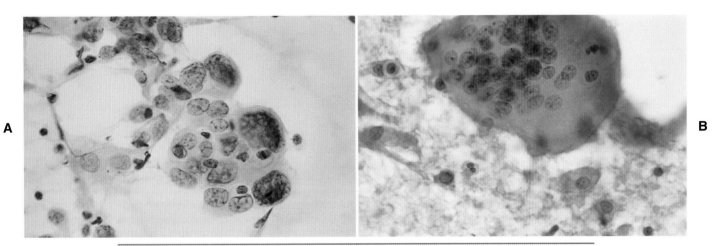

Figure 26-33 **Papillary carcinoma. A,** Multinucleated giant cells are commonly seen in some examples of papillary carcinoma. These giant cells contain five to eight overlapping nuclei. The cytoplasm of the giant cells has a metaplastic appearance. In this case the giant cells are adjacent to neoplastic mononuclear cells. The nuclei of the giant cells have a similar appearance to the nuclei of the mononuclear cells. **B,** A multinucleated giant cell is present. This cell has the appearance of multinucleated histiocyte. These cells are commonly seen in papillary carcinoma and often are seen in the cystic variant. (**A-B,** Pap)

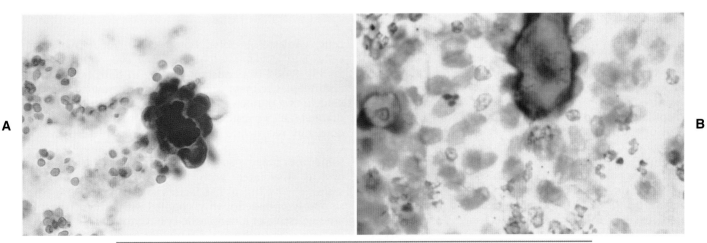

Figure 26-34 **Papillary carcinoma. A,** A psammoma body is present in the center field and is surrounded by neoplastic cell nuclei. **B,** A psammoma body is present in the upper center. In this case, many of the neoplastic cell nuclei are out of the plane of focus or have an air-dried appearance. Psammoma bodies are three-dimensional and the large ones often show a thick border. (**A-B,** Pap)

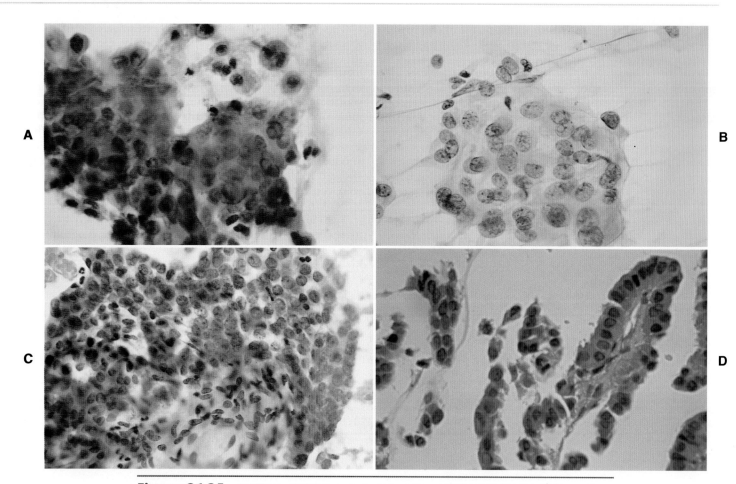

Figure 26-35 Papillary carcinoma. A, In the cystic variant of papillary carcinoma, large clusters of neoplastic cells may be observed. These large clusters exhibit nuclear crowding and overlap. In the upper portion of the photomicrograph, hemosiderin-laden macrophages and other inflammatory cells are observed. **B,** A relatively flat sheet of neoplastic cells is seen in this cystic variant of papillary carcinoma. Scattered inflammatory cells are overlying. In this case, the neoplastic cells exhibit a reactive appearance with variable cytoplasmic tincture and cytoplasmic "pulling" that may be seen on the cells to the left. The nuclei exhibit a greater degree in variability in size and shape. Nuclear grooves still are evident, although many of the cells also display a small nucleolus. **C,** In this case of a cystic papillary carcinoma, a true papillary fragment capped by neoplastic cells is seen. In the lower center, a fibrovascular core is observed. **D,** In this cell block preparation of a cystic papillary carcinoma, a true papillary fragment containing a fibrovascular core lined by a single layer of neoplastic cells is observed. (**A-C,** Pap; **D,** Hematoxylin and eosin [H&E])

teria (when used in combination) are nuclear pseudoinclusions, nuclear grooves, papillary structures or cell balls, and metaplastic cytoplasm.[139-141,166] If all these criteria are simultaneously present, a papillary carcinoma diagnosis is almost guaranteed.

Papillary carcinoma is the most common cystic neoplasm of the thyroid gland.[64,267,347] Other neoplasms that may be cystic include follicular adenoma and Hürthle cell adenoma. Underdiagnosing cystic lesions as benign is one of the more common causes of a false-negative diagnosis. The risk of malignancy in a surgically excised cyst ranges from 3% to 25%.[348,349] It is estimated that up to 50% of purely cystic papillary carcinomas may be missed on FNA.[125,350-352] In actual practice, this figure is most likely much lower. Grossly, the color of the cyst fluid is not a good predictor of malignancy.[125,330,352]

The difficulty in diagnosing cysts on aspirates is that the epithelium may be scant, and foamy macrophages, giant cells, cholesterol clefts, hemosiderin, reparative stromal cells, and degenerated debris may predominate (Figure 26-35). Blood is a constant finding in both nonneoplastic and neoplastic cysts. Signs that a cyst is not neoplastic include a cyst diameter less than 3 cm; the cyst is completely drained (i.e., no residual mass is present after FNA); the cyst does not recur; and no atypical cells are seen cytologically.[23,64,126,353] If atypical cells are seen, many experts will sometimes make a suspicious diagnosis. Recurrence of the cyst is associated with neoplasm in up to 10% of cases.[60,123,125] Clinical risk factors such as vocal cord paralysis and lymphadenopathy, coupled with a "cyst" diagnosis, are suggestive of a neoplastic cyst. Cytologic features that a cyst may be harboring a papillary carcinoma include increased cellularity, epithelial cytologic atypia, and psammoma bodies.[141,169] The macrofollicular variant of papillary carcinoma has similar cytologic findings as the cystic variant.[348,349] In summary, always cytologically examine the

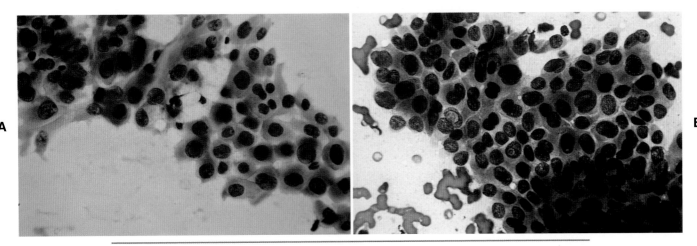

Figure 26-36 **Papillary carcinoma: tall cell variant. A,** The aspirate smear shows a honeycombed group of neoplastic cells. By definition, the cells are twice as tall as they are wide. **B,** The cells have a large amount of cytoplasm and eccentrically placed nuclei. Like the conventional variant, the cytoplasm of the neoplastic cells has a metaplastic appearance. (**A,** Pap; **B,** DQ)

contents of cysts. It should go without saying that patients with thyroid cysts should have close clinical follow-up.

Papillary carcinoma has several variants that generally have a poorer prognosis than the classic type.[267,354] These variants include tall cell, Hürthle cell, sclerosing, and columnar cell papillary carcinoma. The tall cell variant, which is the most common of the variants (up to 10% of all papillary carcinomas), has by definition, cells that are twice as tall as they are wide (Figure 26-36).[267,355] The cells have a granular cytoplasm (like Hürthle cell cytoplasm) and smears show numerous papillae and mitoses.[193,197,267,355-358] The elongated nature of the cells may aid in the diagnosis.[197] The Hürthle cell variant looks like a Hürthle cell neoplasm (Figure 26-37).[27,320,359-361] FNAs of the sclerosing variant may show numerous fibrotic fragments and psammoma bodies with little epithelium (Figure 26-38).[182,362-364] The columnar cell variant consists of elongated cells with elongated nuclei and cytoplasm that may have a clear appearance.[365-367] Importantly, to confirm the diagnosis of papillary carcinoma, look for the classic nuclear features in all these variants.[365,366] The follicular cell variant of papillary carcinoma may be difficult to separate from follicular neoplasms (Figure 26-39).

Hyalinizing Trabecular Adenoma

Hyalinizing trabecular adenoma, also known as *paraganglioma-like adenoma (PLAT),* is considered a benign tumor.[368,369] This neoplasm is much more common in women.[370] Histologically, the hyalinizing trabecular adenoma is composed of nests of cells surrounded by dense hyaline matrix.[368,369] The tumor resembles a paraganglioma, although the neoplastic cells stain for thyroglobulin and do not stain for calcitonin (however, they may stain for other neuroendocrine markers).[369,371] On FNA the hyalinizing trabecular adenoma may be confused with papillary carcinoma and medullary carcinoma.[368-371] Similar to papillary carcinoma, smears of hyalinizing trabecular adenoma may show psammoma bodies and cells with fine chromatin, nuclear grooves, and nuclear pseudoinclusions (Figure 26-40).[372-375] In contrast with papillary carcinoma, papillary structures and bubble

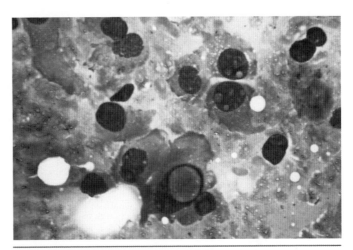

Figure 26-37 **Papillary carcinoma: Hürthle cell variant.** The neoplastic cells have abundant squamoid to granular cytoplasm. The nuclei are eccentrically placed and a nucleolus is visible in some of the nuclei. One cell has a prominent intranuclear pseudoinclusion, and small pseudoinclusions are seen in several other of the neoplastic cell nuclei. (DQ)

gum colloid are absent.[372-374] FNA smears of hyalinizing trabecular adenoma characteristically show cells separated by a metachromatic stromal substance.[376] This material resembles amyloid (thus the confusion with medullary carcinoma).[376] In addition, as in medullary carcinoma, the cells are very dissociative or are present in small follicular groups. Spindle cells may be present.[374] Cytoplasmic granules are absent in hyalinizing trabecular adenoma.

Medullary Carcinoma

Medullary carcinoma arises from the C cell or the parafollicular cell and is a neuroendocrine carcinoma. Medullary carcinoma comprises 5% to 17% of all thyroid carcinomas.[377] Approximately 80% of cases are sporadic.[377] Most sporadic cases present as a solitary nodule in the upper pole, although up to 40% of cases may be multifocal. The

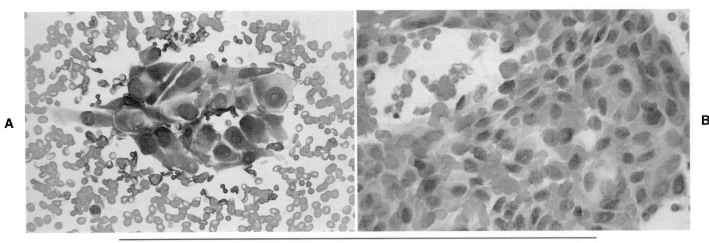

Figure 26-38   Papillary carcinoma: sclerosing variant. A, The aspirate smears show neoplastic cells with a spindled appearance. These cells have elongated nuclei and relatively high N:C ratios. **B,** A cluster of neoplastic cells having elongated nuclei is seen. (**A,** DQ; **B,** Pap)

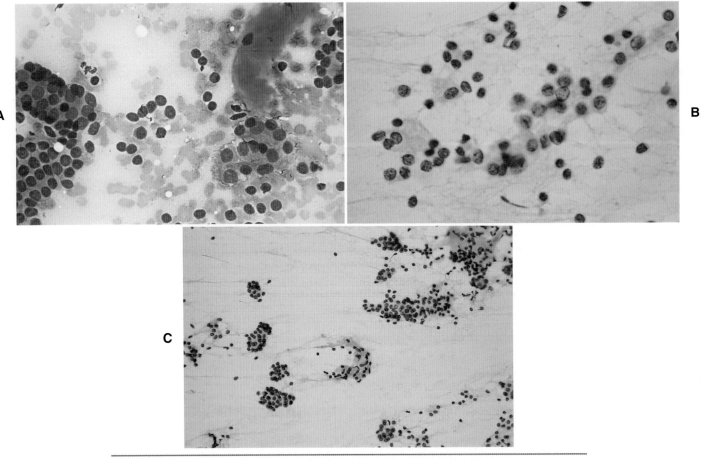

Figure 26-39   Papillary carcinoma: follicular variant. A, The specimen is hypercellular and shows scattered microfollicles. Similar to the findings seen in follicular adenomas and carcinomas, the aspirate smears of the follicular variant of papillary carcinoma show microfollicles with nuclear overlapping and crowding. The features of papillary carcinoma may be difficult to observe and in many cases, a definitive diagnosis of papillary carcinoma cannot be rendered. The cytologic nuclear features of papillary carcinoma may be seen focally. In this case, nuclear pseudoinclusions and grooves are not observable. **B,** In this high power, microfollicles and stripped neoplastic cell nuclei are observed. The chromatin pattern is finely granular although a rare nuclear groove may be observed. **C,** At this low power, the specimen is hypercellular and small clusters of neoplastic cells are observed. At this power, a follicular adenoma or carcinoma cannot be distinguished from a follicular variant of papillary carcinoma. (**A,** DQ; **B** and **C,** Pap)

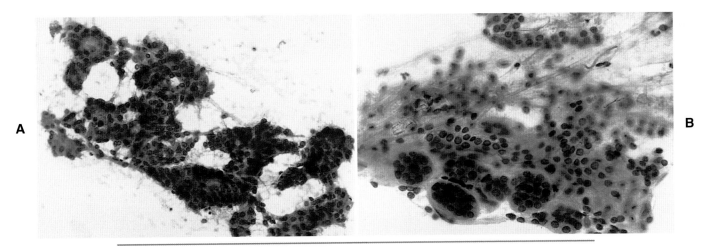

Figure 26-40 Hyalinazing trabecular adenoma. **A,** At a low power, the cells show pseudopapillary clusters adjoined to small microfollicles. **B,** At a higher power, small follicles are admixed with an amorphous ground substance. **(A-B,** Pap)

sporadic form is more common in women (female to male ratio of 3:2), and most patients are between the ages 30 to 50. The familial form of medullary carcinoma (20% of patients) presents in a younger age group (patients are in their twenties) and the tumors are usually multifocal. In the familial form, medullary carcinoma is most likely found in conjunction with the multiple endocrine neoplasm syndrome (MEN) II.[378,379] MEN IIA (Sipple's syndrome) consists of medullary carcinoma, pheochromocytoma, and parathyroid hyperplasia or adenoma.[378,379] MEN IIB or III (mucosal neuroma syndrome) consists of medullary carcinoma, pheochromocytoma, and mucocutaneous ganglioneuromas (and inconstantly parathyroid hyperplasia and a Marfanoid habitus).[380,381] The childhood form of medullary carcinoma is invariably familial. Medullary carcinomas run a more aggressive course than papillary and follicular carcinomas and metastasize in up to 50% of cases.[186,382-384] Metastatic disease to neck lymph nodes may be the first sign of disease.[382-384] In up to one third of patients, medullary carcinoma metastasizes to the lungs, bones, and liver. Prognosis is related to stage and clinical presentation.[186,377,385] Five-year survival in patients with medullary carcinoma is only about 50%.[377,385]

The two distinguishing FNA features of medullary carcinoma are neuroendocrine cells and amyloid (Box 26-15).[386] The smears are often bloody because of the highly vascular nature of the tumor. The cellularity is inversely proportional to the amount of amyloid (Figure 26-41)[387] Medullary carcinomas manifest a wide spectrum of appearance.[387-389] On low power, smears of some have a dissociated appearance with mostly single cells and may even resemble smears from a lymph node or Hashimoto's thyroiditis.[389,390] The neoplastic cells also may form microfollicles, large sheets, small clusters, or papillae.[213,390,391] Medullary carcinoma is the "syphilis" of thyroid tumors, because medullary carcinoma has the ability to mimic any of the other tumor types (i.e., papillary carcinoma, follicular carcinoma, Hürthle cell carcinoma, malignant lymphoma, and metastasis).[213,387,388,390-393]

Amyloid is seen in up to 80% of FNAs of medullary carcinoma.[387,388,390] Amyloid appears very similar to hard colloid and stains blue to purple with the DQ stain and green

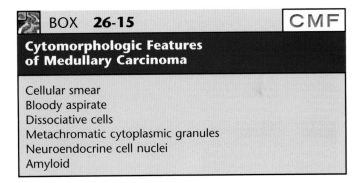

BOX **26-15** | CMF

Cytomorphologic Features of Medullary Carcinoma

Cellular smear
Bloody aspirate
Dissociative cells
Metachromatic cytoplasmic granules
Neuroendocrine cell nuclei
Amyloid

to orange with the Pap stain.[394] Amyloid fragments are variable in size and shape but often have rounded edges (Figure 26-42). The neoplastic cells may be interspersed in the amyloid fragments, a tip that one is not dealing with colloid. In some cases, the neoplastic cells completely surround little amyloid balls, mimicking a follicular neoplasm. A Congo red stain produces the characteristic apple green birefringence on polarization in medullary carcinoma. The presence of amyloid is not 100% diagnostic of medullary carcinoma, and other lesions that contain amyloid include amyloidosis and plasmacytoma.[162,163,395] Other background smear findings in medullary carcinoma include fibrous tissue fragments, acute and chronic inflammatory cells, and calcified particles.[387,388] Large chunks of calcification may be seen (Figure 26-43), similar to the findings in nodular hyperplasia. The calcification even may be detected radiographically. Psammoma bodies are seen in 10% of cases of medullary carcinoma.[396]

The diagnostic northern star of medullary carcinoma is the neuroendocrine nuclear appearance (Figure 26-44). Medullary carcinoma nuclei are round to oval and have a granular (salt and pepper) texture with relatively thick, regular nuclear membranes.[387,388] Binucleated cells are commonly seen.[387,389] Nuclear eccentricity is the rule, and true nuclear pseudoinclusions are evident (another pitfall for papillary carcinoma) in up to 50% of cases.[213,387] Mitoses are present in 15% of cases.[387] Nucleoli generally are not prominent.

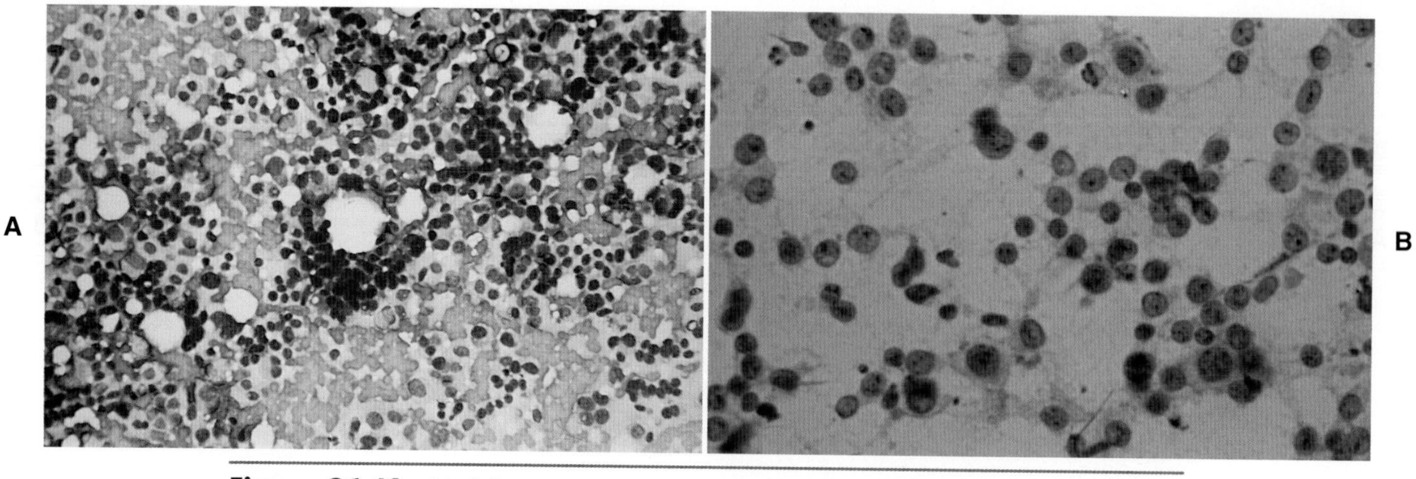

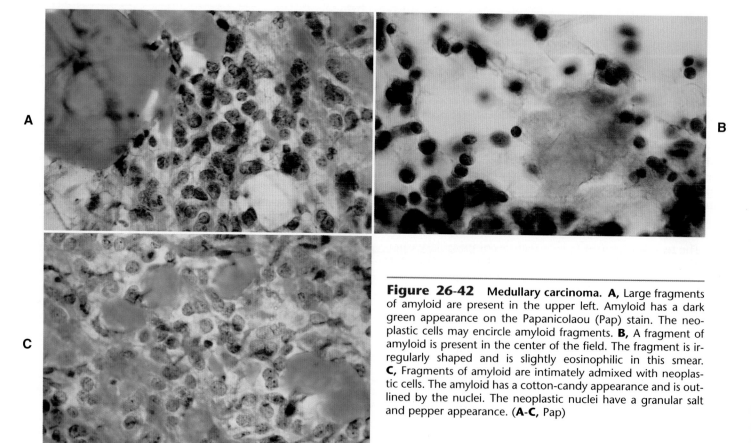

Figure 26-41   Medullary carcinoma. A, At a low power, aspirate smears of medullary carcinoma may show extensive cellular dissociation and the differential diagnosis includes thyroidal lymphoid lesions. In this case, clusters of cells alternate with single cells. The cells are variable in size and shape and in the amount of cytoplasm. **B,** Although medullary carcinomas have many appearances, this smear shows marked cellular dissociation with numerous stripped neoplastic cell nuclei. Small clusters of cells with indistinct cytoplasmic boundaries are observed. The nuclei are variable in size and shape, and prominent nucleoli are seen in many of the cells. The chromatin pattern appears finely granular and the cells have high nuclear to cytoplasmic ratios. Colloid is absent in the background. (**A,** DQ; **B,** Pap)

Figure 26-42   Medullary carcinoma. A, Large fragments of amyloid are present in the upper left. Amyloid has a dark green appearance on the Papanicolaou (Pap) stain. The neoplastic cells may encircle amyloid fragments. **B,** A fragment of amyloid is present in the center of the field. The fragment is irregularly shaped and is slightly eosinophilic in this smear. **C,** Fragments of amyloid are intimately admixed with neoplastic cells. The amyloid has a cotton-candy appearance and is outlined by the nuclei. The neoplastic nuclei have a granular salt and pepper appearance. (**A-C,** Pap)

The cytoplasmic features are the most variable and give rise to the naming of several of the medullary carcinoma variants (Table 26-2). Pleomorphism of cell size and contour is the rule.[397] The neoplastic cells may be plasmacytoid, spindled, granular, clear, giant, or combinations thereof.[397] In all these types, the cytoplasmic borders are well-defined.[387,389] In the plasmacytoid cell the cytoplasm has a hard, squamoid to granular quality (Figure 26-45).[388] These cells may appear identical to the neoplastic elements of a carcinoid tumor. The cytoplasm stains blue with the DQ stain and green to blue on the Pap stain. With the DQ stain, red granules, corresponding to neurosecretory granules, may be seen in most cases.[387,391] However, only a minority of cells (less than 20%) stain in each case.[387,388]

The granularity of the cytoplasm may be so pronounced that the neoplastic cells have a Hürthle cell appearance, and the FNA may mimic a Hürthle cell neoplasm. These cases are known as the *oncocytic variant* of medullary carcinoma.[398] In other cases the cytoplasm has a vacuolated appearance. The vacuoles are large and indent the nucleus, producing a signet ring cell appearance.[396] Some of these cells are mucin positive, which is not characteristic of most other thyroid neoplasms.[396,399] The clear cell variant of medullary carcinoma appears similar (again, the nuclei are diagnostic) to clear cell neoplasms from other sites (e.g., kidney, breast, etc.).[400] The clear cell variant stains negatively for mucin and glycogen. The spindle cells of medullary carcinoma have elongated processes and are irregular in shape.[389] The spindle cell variant may resemble a sarcoma (Figure 26-46).[389] Metastatic melanoma must be separated from the melanotic variant.

The more poorly differentiated variants of medullary carcinoma are the small cell and the anaplastic variants. The small cell medullary carcinoma variant appears identical to a metastasis from a small cell lung carcinoma; therefore, a lung primary should always be excluded before making this diagnosis.[142] The anaplastic variant contains numerous giant cells and may resemble an anaplastic carcinoma (see the section on Anaplastic Carcinoma).[401]

TABLE 26-2	
Medullary Carcinoma Variants	
Variant	**Other lesions to rule out**
Papillary	Papillary carcinoma
Anaplastic	Anaplastic carcinoma metastases
Plasmacytoid	Hematolymphoid lesions
Granular	Hürthle cell lesions
Spindle cell	Spindle cell papillary carcinoma, sarcoma
Clear cell	Papillary carcinoma, follicular
Giant cell	Anaplastic carcinoma
Melanaocytic	Metastatic melanoma

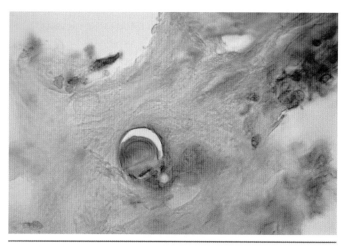

Figure 26-43 **Medullary carcinoma.** On the cell block section, a focus of calcification is in the center of this large fragment. (H&E)

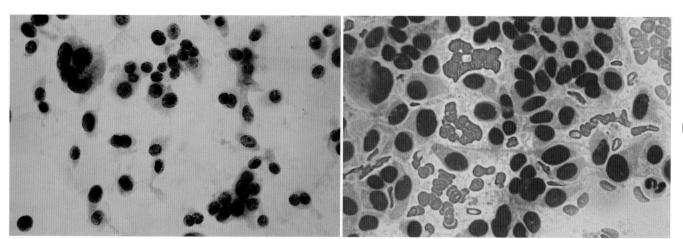

A

B

Figure 26-44 **Medullary carcinoma. A,** In this high-power view of a medullary carcinoma, multinucleated neoplastic cells are admixed with single cells. The single cells have a slightly spindled appearance with eccentrically placed nuclei that are round to oval in shape. The nuclear membranes are relatively regular in contour, although the size of the nuclei vary considerably. **B,** The cells in this example of medullary carcinoma have a plasmacytoid appearance with nuclear eccentricity and cytoplasmic tails. (**A,** Pap; **B,** DQ)

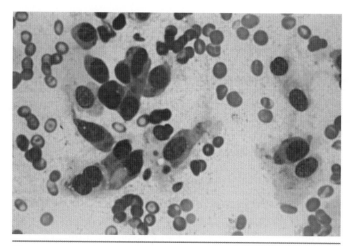

Figure 26-45   Medullary carcinoma. In this DQ preparation, the cells have a plasmacytoid appearance with nuclear eccentricity. Note the cell in the upper left that has a round regularly shaped nucleus and a small amount of cytoplasm that mimicks a plasma cell. Several of the cells contain cytoplasmic vacuoles. Note the absence of lymphoglandular bodies. (DQ)

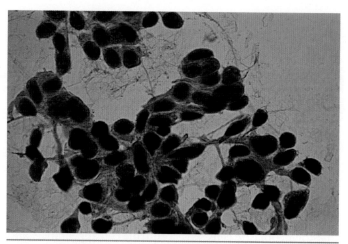

Figure 26-46   Medullary carcinoma: spindle cell variant. In this case of medullary carcinoma, the cells have a spindled appearance with elongated nuclei and cytoplasmic tails. Wispy fragments of cytoplasm connect several of the cell groups. In this case, the cytoplasm has a hard metaplastic appearance. (DQ)

For the special stain buffs, medullary carcinoma is a gold mine. In addition to amyloid and mucin stains, silver stains (e.g., Grimelius) and a calcitonin immunostain may be helpful. Most tumors stain positively for Grimelius and up to 95% of cases are positive for calcitonin.[387,396,402] Interestingly, more than 30% positive of cases stain positively for thyroglobulin, and therefore a calcitonin stain will not exclude a medullary carcinoma.[396]

Anaplastic Carcinoma

Anaplastic carcinoma is the deadliest of thyroid malignancies, with 85% of patients dying within a year of diagnosis. Anaplastic carcinoma represents 10% of all thyroid carcinomas.[403-405] This tumor more commonly is found in women (female to male ratio of 3:1) and in older adults (age 65 and older).[403-405] Anaplastic carcinomas often are infiltrating, although the differential diagnosis of a rapidly growing nodule also includes hemorrhage into a cyst and lymphoma. Patients with anaplastic carcinoma may present emergently with symptoms of airway obstruction. In some of these cases, a correct FNA diagnosis leads to immediate radiation therapy. Unfortunately, anaplastic carcinomas do not respond well to either radiation or surgery.[406]

The cell of origin of anaplastic carcinomas is uncertain. Presumably, these tumors arise from either follicular cells or C cells, since the majority of these tumors are keratin positive.[407] Some cases of papillary, follicular, or medullary carcinoma contain anaplastic elements, and if the more well-differentiated elements are present, then the tumor should be classified as one of these other carcinomas.[406,408] A neoplasm may be called anaplastic if these well-differentiated elements are not seen. On an FNA, because sampling may be a problem, many cytologists classify a tumor as anaplastic but comment that the tumor could represent a poorly differentiated papillary, follicular, or medullary carcinoma.

The FNA smears of anaplastic carcinoma usually are highly cellular, although fibrotic tumors may yield little material (Box 26-16).[222,408] Cellular dissociation is the rule,

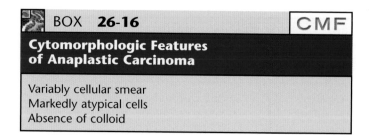

BOX   **26-16**   CMF

**Cytomorphologic Features
of Anaplastic Carcinoma**

Variably cellular smear
Markedly atypical cells
Absence of colloid

and the smears resemble those from high grade sarcomas (Figure 26-47).[408,409] Characteristically, neutrophils and necrotic debris are seen in the background.[24] The neoplastic cells are large, even gigantic, often with high N:C ratios.[389,408-410] The cytoplasm is variable and may be vacuolated or squamoid.[389,410] Cell contours vary from round to polygonal to spindled to highly irregular. Cell borders are usually distinct. Mesenchymal components such as cartilage or bone may be seen.[408,409] The nuclei are hyperchromatic, irregular in shape, and have thick nuclear membranes. Mitotic figures are readily identified, and nuclear pseudoinclusions may be present. The atypia and pleomorphism of anaplastic carcinomas far outstrips the changes seen in repair.

The differential diagnosis includes a soft tissue sarcoma (e.g., malignant fibrous histiocytoma, angiosarcoma, fibrosarcoma), metastasis (particularly lung), and high-grade malignant lymphoma, in addition to a poorly differentiated component in the more common thyroid carcinomas. Immunohistochemical stains may be of use in sorting out these tumors. Thyroglobulin staining in anaplastic carcinoma is negative or only weakly positive.[411]

Malignant Lymphoma

The majority of thyroid gland malignant lymphomas are secondary because 15% of patients with systemic lymphoma have thyroidal involvement.[240,407,412-415] However,

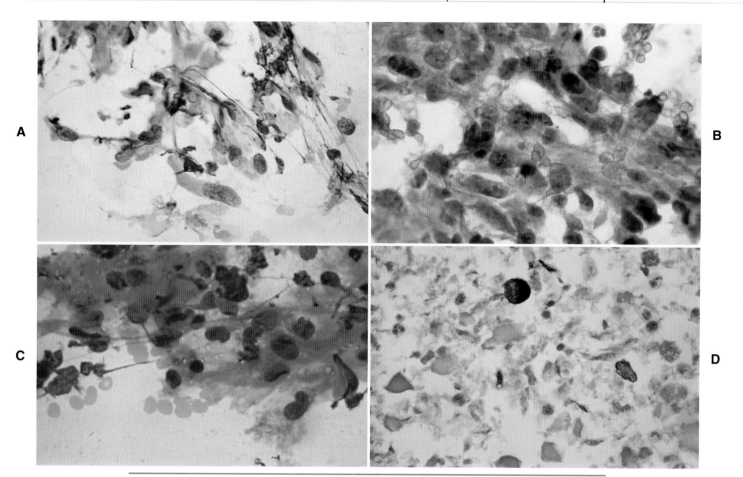

Figure 26-47 Anaplastic carcinoma. **A,** Anaplastic carcinomas often appear poorly differentiated and in this case, several neoplastic cells are admixed with necrotic and crushed debris. The cell in the lower center has the appearance of a spindle cell with an enlarged elongated nucleus and a cytoplasmic tail. In this case, the neoplastic cells have a sarcomatous appearance. **B,** The neoplastic cells have a pleomorphic appearance exhibiting spindled shapes with marked nuclear membrane irregularity. The chromatin distribution is irregular and several of the cells contain a prominent nucleolus. **C,** Necrotic cells and stripped neoplastic nuclei are admixed with malignant cells. Distinct cytoplasmic borders are not present and nuclear streak artifact is observed. **D,** A cytokeratin CAM 5.2 immunostain shows reactivity of the neoplastic cells. This smear is from the same case as depicted in **C.** (**A** and **B,** Pap; **C,** DQ; **D,** Chromogranin immunoperoxidase [Chromo])

malignant lymphomas comprise up to 2% of all primary thyroid gland malignancies.[240,407,412] The typical patient is older (most patients are older than 60 years) and female (female to male ratio of 4:1).[412,416,417] Patients may have a history of Hashimoto's thyroiditis, and 15% have a long history of nodular hyperplasia.[417,418] The classic clinical presentation is a rapidly growing thyroid gland mass. Primary thyroid gland malignant lymphomas often behave aggressively, although the disease is curable (75% cure rate) if confined to the thyroid gland.[418] It has been proposed that at least some thyroid gland malignant lymphomas are a tumor of mucosal associated lymphoid tissue (MALT).[267,419]

Although, most primary malignant lymphomas are non-Hodgkin's, large B-cell type,[239,407,420] other B-cell types including small lymphocytic and small cleaved occur. T-cell lymphomas have been reported.[421] Primary Hodgkin's disease of the thyroid gland is exceedingly rare.[422] Other lymphoreticular malignancies involving the thyroid gland include plasma cell dyscrasia, leukemia, and Langerhans' cell histiocytosis.[416,423,424]

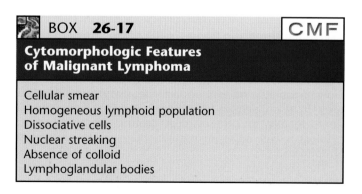

BOX **26-17**   CMF

Cytomorphologic Features of Malignant Lymphoma

Cellular smear
Homogeneous lymphoid population
Dissociative cells
Nuclear streaking
Absence of colloid
Lymphoglandular bodies

FNA smears of malignant lymphoma of the thyroid gland are similar to smears of malignant lymphoma of other body sites. Recognizable thyroid elements may not be apparent. The FNA smears of large cell malignant lymphoma are composed of a monotonous population of dissociated cells (Box 26-17).[240,241,425,426] These cells have high N:C ratios and fine

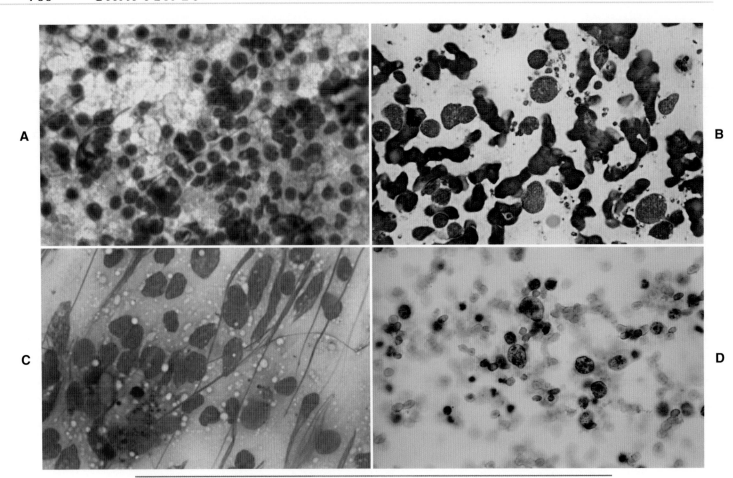

Figure 26-48   Malignant lymphoma. **A,** At a low power, the smear is hypercellular showing numerous single neoplastic cells. The background appears frothy, consistent with cytoplasmic debris. The nuclei are fragile and nuclear streaking is observed. At this power, clusters of neoplastic cells are observed and a carcinoma cannot be completely excluded. **B,** A relatively monomorphic population of large neoplastic cells is observed. The cells contain scant cytoplasm that has a cyanophilic appearance. Lymphoglandular bodies are prominent. This smear is from a patient who has a primary large cell B-cell lymphoma of the thyroid gland. **C,** Numerous single large malignant lymphoid cells are present. Extensive nuclear streaking is observed. Note the presence of a crushed tingible body macrophage in the left center field. This patient has a malignant large cell B-cell lymphoma. **D,** In this patient with a large cell B-cell malignant lymphoma, large neoplastic cells are mixed with necrotic single nuclei. (**A** and **D,** Pap; **B** and **C,** DQ)

to granular chromatin (Figure 26-48).[240,241] Prominent nucleoli are classically present. Lymphoglandular bodies should be appreciated in the background. Necrosis often is apparent in smears of the high-grade malignant lymphoma types. Flow cytometry or immunocytochemistry are important tools in the diagnosis.[425] If flow cytometry demonstrates monoclonality and the cytologic features are classic, most cytologists will make an outright diagnosis of malignant lymphoma.

The differential diagnosis includes metastatic disease (particularly pulmonary small cell carcinoma), medullary carcinoma, anaplastic carcinoma, and Hashimoto's thyroiditis. Metastatic small cell carcinoma, in contrast with large cell malignant lymphoma, shows more cellular clumping, larger cells, more necrosis, and an absence of nucleoli and lymphoglandular bodies. Medullary carcinomas with abundant plasmacytoid cells lack the nuclear characteristics and lymphoglandular bodies of large cell malignant lymphoma. The small cell variant of medullary carci-

noma also may be confused with malignant lymphoma, although this variant more closely resembles a small cell carcinoma metastasis.[368] Large atypical lymphocytes may be present in Hashimoto's thyroiditis, although most Hashimoto's aspirates should contain more Hürthle cells and lack a monotonous lymphoid population. Again, flow cytometry is helpful to demonstrate monoclonality in malignant lymphoma.

Salivary Gland–Type Tumors (Mucoepidermoid Carcinoma and Adenoid Cystic Carcinoma)

Primary salivary gland type tumors are exceedingly rare. A proportion of primary thyroid mucoepidermoid carcinomas are associated with intense tissue eosinophilia and an underlying Hashimoto's thyroiditis. On FNA, these tumors appear like their salivary gland counterparts.[271,427-429] Mucoepidermoid carcinomas may be confused with papillary carcinoma, because the neoplastic cells in papillary carci-

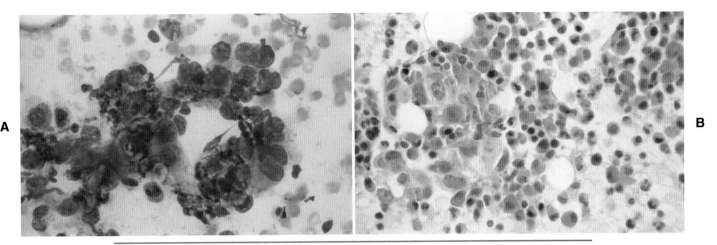

A   B

Figure 26-49   Mucoepidermoid carcinoma. **A,** Clusters of neoplastic cells are present and eosinophils are seen in the lower center field. The cells have high N:C ratios and squamoid cytoplasm. **B,** In this Pap stain, abundant eosinophils are admixed with a neoplastic cell fragment. The cells have prominent nucleoli and granular chromatin. (**A,** DQ; **B,** Pap)

noma have a squamoid appearance (Figure 26-49).[271,427-430] The neoplastic cells in papillary carcinoma also may have vacuolated cytoplasm (suggestive of mucinous differentiation), which is seen in mucoepidermoid carcinoma. In contrast with mucoepidermoid carcinoma, papillary carcinoma should not be mucin positive. Adenoid cystic carcinoma may be confused with follicular neoplasms.

Insular Carcinoma (Poorly Differentiated Carcinoma)

Similar to medullary carcinoma, insular carcinomas are more aggressive than follicular carcinoma and papillary carcinoma and less virulent than anaplastic carcinomas.[403,431,432] FNA smears are cellular and morphologically resemble a cross between smears of follicular carcinoma and papillary carcinoma (Figure 26-50).[433,434] Similar to papillary carcinoma, the neoplastic cells appear relatively monomorphic; contain cytoplasmic vacuoles; and possess slightly irregular nuclei with nuclear grooves, occasional nuclear pseudoinclusions, and possibly psammoma bodies.[433-435] In contrast with papillary carcinoma, papillae are absent, nuclear grooves are infrequent, and metaplastic cytoplasm is absent. Similar to follicular neoplasms, the smears contain numerous small groups and microfollicles with almost no colloid.[433,434] Abundant single cells may be present.[436] The fine, dusty chromatin of insular carcinoma is unlike the darker chromatin in follicular neoplasms.[433] In contrast with follicular and papillary carcinoma, necrosis is a frequent finding in insular carcinoma.[431-434,437] Some insular carcinomas show greater pleomorphism with variation in cell size, giant cells, Hürthle cell change, greater hyperchromasia, and mitotic figures; these cases may be inseparable on FNA from anaplastic follicular or papillary carcinoma.[431]

 ## METASTASES

Metastases reach the thyroid by direct extension, lymphatic spread, or hematogeneously.[413,438,439] The majority correspond to direct spread of primary neoplasms of the pharynx,

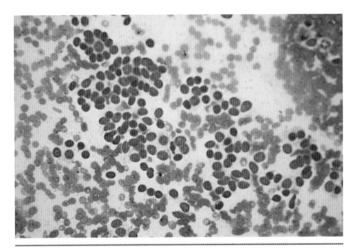

Figure 26-50   Insular carcinoma. This low power of an insular carcinoma has a similar appearance to that of a follicular adenoma or carcinoma. The specimen is cellular, showing clusters of cells and single neoplastic cells. In an insular carcinoma, the nuclei appear slightly enlarged and there is considerable nuclear overlap. On cytologic specimens, these aspirates are often included within the follicular neoplasm diagnosis. (DQ)

larynx, and esophagus (Figure 26-51).[438] Most metastases are recognized clinically, and very rarely does a patient present with a thyroid lesion that represents a metastasis from an unknown primary. Metastases represent less than 0.5% of thyroid tumors in most FNA series.[440] Of patients who have known extrathyroidal malignancies and a thyroid nodule, FNA shows 71% benign lesions, 17% metastases, and 6% primary tumors.[441] Cytologically, metastases do not resemble primary thyroid malignancies, and if a poorly differentiated or "unusual" tumor is seen, a metastasis should be suspected.[136,343,439,440,442-444] Some metastases, from such sites as breast, kidney, or lung, may mimic a primary thyroid neoplasm (Table 26-3).[439,440,442,443,445,446] Immunostains may be helpful in the separation.[447] Primary thyroid tumors generally are reactive for cytokeratin 7, thyroglobulin, and thyroid transcription factor 1, and negative for cytokeratin 20.[448]

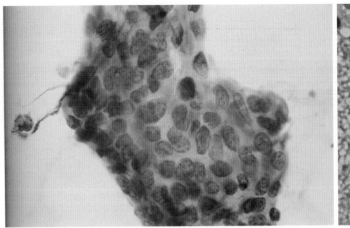

A

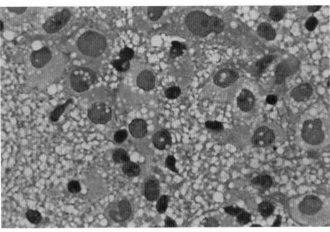

B

Figure 26-51 Metastasis. **A,** A large cluster of neoplastic cells is present. Note the absence of colloid and the marked anaplasia within this cellular group. This smear represents a metastatic pulmonary adenocarcinoma to the thyroid gland. **B,** In this aspirate smear the neoplastic cells are dissociated and the background has a bubbly appearance. The cytoplasm of the neoplastic cells is vacuolated, and the neoplastic cell nuclei are variable in size and shape. Many of the cells contain a prominent nucleolus. This aspirate smear represents a metastatic renal cell adenocarcinoma. (**A,** Pap; **B,** DQ)

TABLE 26-3

Metastases to the Thyroid Gland That Mimic Primary Neoplasms

Primary Thyroid Lesion	Site of Origin of Metastasis
Follicular neoplasm	Breast, kidney
Papillary carcinoma	Breast, kidney, ovary
Hürthle cell neoplasms	Kidney (granular cell variant)
Clear cell carcinoma (papillary, follicular, Hürthle, or medullary)	Kidney, breast
Mucoepidermoid or squamous cell carcinoma	Head and neck, esophagus, lung
Anaplastic carcinoma	Lung, pancreas, or soft tissue (sarcoma)
Malignant lymphoma	Small cell carcinoma
Sarcomas (very rare)	Soft tissue (sarcoma)

Two very rare primary tumors must be distinguished from metastases (in fact, the metastasis is more common than the primary). The first is primary squamous cell carcinoma, which purportedly arises in patients with a history of nodular hyperplasia.[449-451] Metastases from the head and neck are much more likely.[449] The second tumor is a clear cell tumor. Clear cell change may occur in follicular cells and C cells and in all the primary thyroid gland tumor subtypes.[141,452-454] The most common clear cell tumor of the thyroid, however, is a metastasis from the kidney.[455-458]

 ## THE SUSPICIOUS LESIONS

In practice, not all thyroid gland FNAs can be neatly placed in the previously discussed diagnostic categories. The main problems arise when FNAs are categorized in Region 2 (see

BOX 26-18

The Suspicious Lesions

Region 2 lesions
Atypical cells
Atypical cysts
Neoplasm, not otherwise specified

Figure 26-11) as atypical cells (cannot rule out follicular neoplasm or papillary carcinoma) or as atypical cysts (Box 26-18). These diagnoses are problematic because clinicians may not understand the import of these diagnoses. The significance of these categories depends on their frequency of use and the follow-up. Although the reporting of suspicious lesion diagnoses varies, in many institutions it ranges from 5% to 30%.[51,60,100] The main cause of a suspicious diagnosis is a marginally adequate specimen which contains few representative elements or is heavily admixed with blood. If one assists in immediate FNA interpretation and suspects that the final diagnosis could be a suspicious lesion, more tissue should be obtained. If one issues a suspicious diagnosis, a repeat FNA may be in order. Suspicious diagnoses carry a risk for neoplasia (a higher risk than a benign diagnosis) and the clinician should treat every diagnosis probabilistically.

Region 2 Lesions

Follicular lesions and Hürthle cell lesions may be classified in Region 2 if the colloid content and cellularity are either high or low. It is more likely that both are low. These lesions are diagnosed using a wide range of terminology. The majority of these lesions are benign.

If both the colloid content and cellularity are high, the lesion probably is a cellular nodule in nodular hyperplasia or a macrofollicular follicular neoplasm.[139,159] Additional passes usually do not help in the differentiation. If the gland is multinodular (an ultrasound study may help here), follow-up probably will show a nodular hyperplasia. In such a lesion, favoring one process or the other may be helpful to the clinician. Look for the secondary criteria to aid in diagnosis. Focal atypia, relative absence of microfollicles, mixture of groups of different sizes, degeneration, mixed cellular pattern (Hürthle cells and follicular cells), absence of nuclear overlapping, and no noticeable increase in nuclear size all support a nodular hyperplasia diagnosis. The opposite findings support the diagnosis of a follicular or Hürthle cell neoplasm.

If both the colloid content and cellularity are low, the specimen is probably marginal and repeat aspirations are helpful. The majority of these lesions turn out to be benign.[47] Again, the diagnosis should depend on the observation of secondary criteria. Look for nuclear overlapping, microfollicles, and uniform atypia across all the cells to support a follicular or Hürthle cell neoplasm diagnosis.

Atypical Cells (Rule out Papillary Carcinoma or Follicular Neoplasm)

One of the more difficult diagnostic conundrums is when focal cellular atypia is present and a temptation exists to classify the lesion as *atypical*. If the lesion otherwise looks like a nodular hyperplasia, one *should* expect to see focal atypia (e.g., cellular enlargement, hyperchromasia, slight nuclear overlap).[159,433] Commenting on the atypia may be appropriate, but most likely the lesion is benign. Thus, many cytologists do not use the diagnosis *rare atypical cells suspicious for follicular neoplasm* because in a follicular neoplasm the cells generally are all atypical or are all bland.

A more difficult problem occurs when signs suggestive for papillary carcinoma are present. These cytologic features include nuclear pseudoinclusions, nuclear grooves, metaplastic cytoplasm, papillary structures, and psammoma bodies.[139,140,166] If the specimen is scantily cellular, consider reaspirating, because most papillary carcinomas produce cellular aspirates (or are fibrotic, in which case calcification and psammoma bodies may be present).[139,140] Pseudoinclusions have been reported in Hashimoto's thyroiditis and other benign lesions with Hürthle cells. Expect to see a few nuclear grooves (but not a lot!) in almost all benign processes. Metaplastic, or even squamous cytoplasm may be seen in nodular hyperplasia, reparative thyroid lesions, remnant thymic tissue, and thyroglossal duct cysts. For most of the benign lesions, only a few metaplastic cells should be present. Papillary structures have been described in nodular hyperplasia and Graves' disease, although in both of these processes, the nuclear features of papillary carcinoma are lacking. Psammoma bodies have been reported in Hashimoto's thyroiditis and reparative processes.[345]

Atypical Cysts

Cysts may pose a diagnostic problem either when they are acellular or when focal atypia is present. As mentioned previously, if the cyst is acellular, many cytologists simply comment on the lack of epithelium. Some cytologists use the terms *atypical cyst, hypercellular cyst,* or *cyst with atypical epithelial cells*. The majority of these cysts are benign.[64] Expect to see focal epithelial atypia (e.g., nuclear enlargement, mild nuclear hyperchromasia, slight nuclear membrane irregularities, etc.), although the majority of the epithelium should appear benign. Reparative features commonly are seen. High cellularity in cysts should be concerning.[348] Also, be certain to examine the specimen for the nuclear features of a papillary carcinoma, remembering that some papillary carcinomas are completely cystic.[287]

Suspicious or Indeterminate Lesions

In a subset of *thyroid gland FNAs,* the smears are certain to be neoplastic, but one is not certain of the neoplastic cell type (papillary carcinoma, follicular neoplasm, Hürthle cell neoplasm, medullary carcinoma, and so on). As thyroid gland FNA is partly a screening test, we do not need to always specifically classify neoplastic entities; neoplastic diagnoses generally result in a*n operative procedure*. The neoplasms that should be excluded include metastasis and malignant lymphoma because most of these are secondary and surgery is *usually* not done for systemic malignant lymphoma. Cytologists may use the term *thyroid gland neoplasm, or neoplasm, not otherwise specified type* if they are uncertain of tumor type.

Core biopsy has been shown to be useful in patients who have suspicious or unsatisfactory FNA diagnoses. Compared with FNA, core biopsy alone has more complications, more inadequate specimens, and a higher cost.[54,64,111,459] However, in some cases, core biopsy produces information in which FNA fails.[87,459-462] Core biopsy is not widely practiced in North America.

Intraoperative consultation with frozen section also may provide benefit following suspicious or unsatisfactory FNA diagnoses.[463-468] FNA and frozen section are complementary.[18,103,173,465,469-471] Scrape preparations of surgical material are a useful adjunct to frozen section.[472] Some surgeons perform a complete thyroidectomy for patients with a papillary carcinoma and a lobectomy for patients with a follicular neoplasm (a follicular carcinoma may be followed by a completion thyroidectomy). Thus, for *neoplasm, not otherwise specified type* diagnoses, a frozen section may be beneficial because it allows for appropriate patient triage.

References

1. Risgway E. Clinical evaluation of solitary thyroid nodules. In: Ingbar SH, Braverman LE, editors. Werner's the thyroid: a fundamental and clinical text, 5th ed. Philadelphia: JB Lippincott; 1986. pp.1377-1383.
2. Castro M, Gharib H. Thyroid nodules and cancer. Postgrad Mod 2000; 107:113-124.
3. Landis S, Murray T, Boden S, et al. Cancer statistics, 1999. CA Cancer J Clin 1999; 49:8-31.
4. Cristallini E, Bolis G. Fine-needle aspiration biopsy in the preoperative diagnosis of solitary thyroid nodules. Appl Pathol 1989; 7:149-153.
5. Clark K, Moffat F, Ketcham A. Nonoperative techniques for tissue diagnosis in the management of thyroid nodules and goiters. Semin Surg Oncol 1991; 7:76-80.
6. Frable W. The treatment of thyroid cancer: the role of fine-needle aspiration cytology. Arch Otolaryngol Head Surg 1986; 112:1200-1203.
7. Morayati S, Freitas J. Guiding thyroid nodule management by fine-needle aspiration. Fam Pract Res J 1962; 11:379-386.
8. Cohen J, Cho H. The role of needle aspiration biopsy in the selection of patients for thyroidectomy. Laryngoscope 1988; 98:35-39.

9. VanVliet G, Glinoer D, Verelst J. Cold thyroid nodules in childhood: is surgery always necessary? Eur J Pediatr 1987; 146:378-382.

10. Piromalli D, Martelli G, delPrato I. The role of fine needle aspiration in the diagnosis of thyroid nodules: analysis of 795 consecutive cases. J Surg Oncol 1992; 50:247-250.

11. Garcia-Mayor R, Mendez L, Paramo C. Fine-needle aspiration of thyroid nodules: impact on clinical practice. J Endocrinol Invest 1997; 20:482-487.

12. Baskin H, Guarda L. Influence of needle biopsy on management of thyroid nodules: reasons to expand its use. South Med J 1987; 80:702-705.

13. Lin J, Hsueh C, Chao T, et al. Thyroid follicular neoplasms diagnosed by high-resolution ultrasonography with fine-needle aspiration cytology. Acta Cytol 1997; 41:687-691.

14. Raab S, Silverman J, Elsheikh T, et al. Pediatric thyroid nodules: disease demographics and clinical management as determined by fine-needle aspiration biopsy. Pediatrics 1995; 95:46-49.

15. Scanlan P, Dowling M, Dervan P. Fine needle aspiration cytology of thyroid nodules: review of 36 months experience. Irish J Med 1993; 162:177-179.

16. Anderson J, Webb A. Fine needle aspiration biopsy and the diagnosis of thyroid cancer. Br J Surg 1987; 74:292-296.

17. Godinho-Matos L, Kocjan G, et al. Contribution of fine needle aspiration cytology to diagnosis and management of thyroid disease. J Clin Pathol 1992; 45:391-395.

18. Aguilar-Diosdado M, Contreras A, Gavilan I, et al. Thyroid nodules: role of fine needle aspiration and intraoperative frozen section examination. Acta Cytol 1997; 41:677-682.

19. Tani E, Skoog L, Lowhagen T. Clinical utility of fine-needle aspiration cytology of the thyroid. Ann Rev Med 1988; 39:255-260.

20. Sidawy M, DelVecchio D, Knoll S. Fine-needle aspiration of thyroid nodules: correlation between cytology and histology and evaluation of discrepant cases. Cancer 1997; 25:253-259.

21. Bodo M, Dobrossy L, Sinkovics I. Fine-needle biopsy of thyroid gland. J Surg Oncol 1979; 12:289-297.

22. Tsung J. Fine needle aspiration biopsy of thyroid nodules. Ind Med 1988; 81:701-705.

23. Crile G, Hawk W. Aspiration biopsy of thyroid nodules. Surg Gynecol Obstet 1973; 136:241-245.

24. Gharib H, Goellner J, Johnson D. Fine-needle aspiration cytology of the thyroid: a 12-year experience with 11,000 biopsies. Clin Lab Med 1993; 13:699-709.

25. Einhorn J, Franzen G. Thin-needle biopsy in the diagnosis of thyroid disease. Acta Radiol 1962; 58:321-336.

26. Colacchio T, LoGerfo P, Feind C. Fine-needle cytologic diagnosis of thyroid nodules: review and report of 300 cases. Am J Surg 1980; 140:568-571.

27. Nguyen G-K, Ginsberg J, Crockford P. Fine-needle aspiration biopsy cytology of the thyroid: its value and limitations in the diagnosis and management of solitary thyroid nodules. Pathol Ann 1991; 26:63-91.

28. Shapiro M, Batang E. Needle aspiration biopsy of the thyroid and parathyroid. Otolaryngol Clin North Am 1990; 23:217-229.

29. Hall T, Layfield L, Philippe A. Sources of diagnostic error in fine needle aspiration of the thyroid. Cancer 1989; 63:718-725.

30. Grant C, Hay I, Gough I. Long-term follow-up of patients with benign thyroid fine-needle aspiration cytologic diagnoses. Surgery 1989; 106:980-986.

31. Leonard N, Melcher D. To operate or not to operate? The value of fine-needle aspiration cytology in the assessment of thyroid swellings. J Clin Pathol 1997; 50:941-943.

32. Carmeci C, Jeffrey R, McDougall I, et al. Ultrasound-guided fine-needle aspiration biopsy of thyroid masses. Thyroid 1998; 8:283-289.

33. Lioe T, Elliott H, Allen D, et al. A 3-year audit of thyroid fine-needle aspirates. Cytopathology 1998; 9:188-192.

34. Boyd L, Earnhardt R, Dunn J, et al. Preoperative evaluation and predictive value of fine-needle aspiration and frozen section of thyroid nodules. J Am Coll Surg 1998; 187:494-502.

35. Khurana K, Labrador E, Izquierdo R, et al. The role of fine-needle aspiration biopsy in the management of thyroid nodules in children, adolescents, and young adults: a multi-institutional study. Thyroid 1999; 9:383-386.

36. Raab S, Veronezi-Gurwell A. Thyroid nodules in the elderly: clinical management and incidence of malignancy as determined by fine-needle aspiration biopsy. Oncol Rep 1995; 2:1151-1156.

37. Bennedback F, Perrild H, Hegedus L. Diagnosis and treatment of the solitary thyroid nodule: results of a European survey. Clin Endocrinol (Oxf) 1999; 50:357-363.

38. Cap J, Ryska A, Rehorkova P, Hovorkova E, et al. Sensitivity and specificity of the fine-needle aspiration biopsy of the thyroid: clinical point of view. Clin Endocrinol (Oxf) 1999; 51:509-515.

39. Mandreker S, Nadkarni N, Pinto R, et al. Role of fine-needle aspiration cytology as the initial modality in the investigation of thyroid lesions. Acta Cytol 1995; 39:898-904.

40. Oertel Y, Oertel J. Diagnosis of malignant epithelial thyroid lesions: fine-needle aspiration and histopathologic correlation. Ann Diagn Pathol 1998; 2:377-400.

41. Wartofsky L. Diseases of the thyroid. In: Fauci A, Braunwald E, Isselbacher K, editors. Harrison's principles of internal medicine. 14th ed. New York: McGraw-Hill.

42. Dolan J. Thyroid nodules. In: Panzar RJ, Black ER, Griner PF, editors. Diagnostic strategies for common medical problems. American College of Physicians, Philadelphia; 1991. pp.385-393.

43. American Association of Clinical Endocrinologists and American College of Endocrinology. Endocrinology: AACE clinical practice guidelines for the management of thyroid carcinoma. Endocrinology. Vol 3; 1997.

44. Gharib H, Goellner J. Fine-needle aspiration biopsy of the thyroid: an appraisal. Ann Intern Med 1993; 118:282-289.

45. Gharib H. Fine-needle aspiration biopsy of thyroid nodules: advantages, limitations, and effect. Mayo Clin Proc 1994; 69:44-49.

46. Caplan R, Kisken W, Strut P. Fine-needle aspiration biopsy of thyroid nodules: a cost-effective diagnostic plan. Postgrad Med 1991; 90:183-199.

47. Ashcraft M, VanHerle A. Management of thyroid nodules. I. History and physical exaimination, blood tests, x-ray tests, and ultrasonography. Head Neck Surg 1981; 3:216-230.

48. Wool M. Thyroid nodules: the place of fine-needle aspiration biopsy in management. Postgrad Med 1993; 94:111-122.

49. Hanni C, Bratt H, Dean R. Fine-needle aspiration biopsy: a reliable diagnostic tool in the management of thyroid nodules. Am Surg 1984; 50:485-487.

50. Khafagi F, Wright G, Castles H. Screening for thyroid malignancy: the role of fine-needle biopsy. Med J Aust 1988; 149:302-307.

51. Caruso D, Mazzaferri E. Fine needle aspiration biopsy in the management of thyroid nodules. Endocrinologist 1991; 1:194-202.

52. Caplan R, Wester S, Kisken W. Fine-needle aspiration biopsy of solitary thyroid nodules: effect on cost of management, frequency of thyroid surgery, and operative yield of thyroid malignancy. Minn Med 1986; 69:189-192.

53. Silverman J, West R, Larkin E. The role of fine-needle aspiration biopsy in the rapid diagnosis and management of thyroid neoplasm. Cancer 1986; 57:1164-1170.

54. Silverman J, West R, Finley J. Fine-needle aspiration versus large-needle biopsy or cutting biopsy in evaluation of thyroid nodules. Diagn Cytopathol 1986; 2:25-30.

55. Rimm D, Stastny J, Rimm E, et al. Comparison of the costs of fine-needle aspiration and open surgical biopsy as methods for obtaining a pathologic diagnosis. Cancer 1997; 81:51-56.

56. Thomas J, Amanguno A, Adeyi O, et al. Fine needle aspiration (FNA) in the managment of palpable masses in Ibadan: impact on the cost of care. Cytopathology 1999; 10:206-210.

57. Arqueta R, Whitaker M. When a thyroid abnormality is palpable. Postgrad Med 2000; 107:100-110.

58. Gurza E. Thyroiditis. In: Rakel RE, editor. Saunder's manual of medical practice. Philadelphia: WB Saunders; 1996. pp.646-650.

59. Helfand M, Redfern C, Sox H. Screening for thyroid disease. Ann Intern Med 1996; 129:141-143.

60. Rojeski M, Gharib H. Nodular thyroid disease: evaluation and management. N Engl J Med 1985; 313:428-436.

61. Watts R. Hyperthyroidism. In: Rakel R, editor. Saunders' manual of medical practice. Philadelphia: WB Saunders; 1996.

62. Giuffrida D, Gharib H. Controversies in the management of cold, hot, and occult thyroid nodules. Am J Med 1995; 99:642-650.

63. Gharib H, Goellner J. Evaluation of nodular thyroid disease. Endocrinol Metab Clin North Am 1988; 17:511-526.

64. Ashcraft M, VanHerle A. Management of thyroid nodules. II. Scanning techniques, thyroid suppressive therapy and fine needle aspiration. Head Neck Surg 1981; 3:297-322.

65. Shulkin B, Shapiro B. The role of imaging tests in the diagnosis of thyroid carcinoma. Endocrinol Metal Clin North Am 1990; 19:523-543.

66. Boland G, Lee M, Mayo-Smith W. Efficacy of sonographically guided biopsy of thyroid masses and cervical lymph nodes. AJR 1993; 161:1053-1056.

67. Watters D, Ahuja A, Evans R. Role of ultrasound in the management of throid nodules. Am J Surg 1992; 164:654-657.

68. Rosen I, Azadian A, Walfish P. Ultrasound-guided fine-needle aspiration biopsy in the management of thyroid disease. Am J Surg 1993; 166:346-349.

69. Goldfinger M, Rothberg R, Stoll S. Sonographic guidance of thyroid needle biopsy. J Can Assoc Radiol 1986; 37:186-188.

70. Tambouret R, Szyfelbein W, Pitman M. Ultrasound-guided fine-needle aspiration biopsy of the thyroid. Cancer 1999; 87:299-305.

71. Danese D, Sciacchitano S, Farsetti A, et al. Diagnostic accuracy of conventional versus sonography-guided fine-needle aspiration biopsy of thyroid nodules. Thyroid 1998; 8:15-21.

72. Hamburger J. Needle aspiration for thyroid nodules: skip ultrasound—do initial assessment in the office. Postgrad Med 1988; 8:61-66.

73. Miller J, Kini S, Hamburger J. The diagnosis of malignant follicular neoplasms of the thyroid by needle biopsy. Cancer 1985; 55:2812-2817.

74. Lowhagen T. Thyroid. In: Zajizek J, editor. Aspiration biopsy cytology. I. Cytology of supradiaphragmatic organs; 1974.

75. Jayaram G, Gupta B. Nonaspiration fine needle cytology in diffuse and nodular thyroid lesions. Acta Cytol 1991; 35:789-790.

76. Santos J, Leiman G. Nonaspiration fine needle cytology: application of a new technique to nodular thyroid disease. Acta Cytol 1988; 32:353-356.

77. Mair S, Dumbar F, Becker P, et al. Fine needle cytology: is aspiration suction necessary? Acta Cytol 1989; 33:809-813.

78. Kumarasinghe M, Sheriffdeen A. Fine needle sampling without aspiration. Pathology 1995; 27:330-332.

79. Raab S. Probabilities in the cytologic diagnosis of thyroid gland lesions. Am J Clin Pathol 2000; 113:765-768.

80. Frable M, Frable W. Thin needle aspiration biopsy of the thyroid galnd. Laryngoscope 1980; 90:1619-1625.

81. LaRosa G, Belfiore A, Giuffrida D. Evaluation of the fine needle aspiration biopsy in the preoperative selection of cold thyroid nodules. Cancer 1991; 67:2137-2141.

82. Akerman M, Tennval J, Bioklund A. Sensitivity and specificity of fine needle aspiration cytology in the diagnosis of tumors of the thryoid gland. Acta Cytol 1985; 29:850-855.

83. Bugis S, Young J, Archibald S. Diagnostic accuracy of fine-needle aspiration biopsy versus frozen section in solitary thyroid ndules. Am J Surg 1986; 152:411-416.

84. Caraway N, Sneige N, Samaan N. Diagnostic pitfalls in thyroid fine-needle aspiration: a review of 394 cases. Diagn Cytopathol 1993; 9:345-350.

85. Varhaug J, Segadal E, Heimann P. The utility of fine needle aspiration biopsy cytology in the management of thyroid tumors. World J Surg 1981; 5:573-577.

86. Layfield L, Mohrmann R, Kopald K. Use of aspiration cytology and frozen section examination for management of benign and malignant thyroid nodules. Cancer 1991; 68:130-134.

87. Boey J, Hsu C, Collins R. A prospective controlled study of fine-needle aspiration and tru-cut needle biopsy of dominant thyroid nodules. World J Surg 1984; 8:458-465.

88. Charles M, Heller K. Cytologic determinants of well-differentiated thyroid cancer. Am J Surg 1997; 174:545-547.

89. Goellner J, Gharib H, Grant C. Fine needle aspiration cytology of the thyroid, 1980 to 1986. Acta Cytol 1987; 31:587-590.

90. Frost A, Sidawy M, Ferfelli M. Utility of thin-layer preparations in thyroid fine-needle aspiration: diagnostic accuracy, cytomorphology, and optimal sample preparation. Cancer 1998; 84:17-25.

91. Biscotti C, Hollow J, Toddy S. ThinPrep versus conventional smear cytologic preparations in the analysis of thyroid fine-needle aspiration specimens. Am J Clin Pathol 1995; 104:150-153.

92. Leung C, Chiu B, Bell V. Comparison of ThinPrep and conventional preparations: nongynecologic cytology evaluation. Diagn Cytopathol 1997; 16:368-371.

93. Molitch M, Beck J, Dreisman M. The cold thyroid nodule: an analysis of diagnostic and therapeutic options. Endocrinol Rev 1984; 5:185-199.

94. Erdogan M, Kamel N, Aras D, et al. Value of re-aspirations in benign nodular thyroid disease. Thyroid 1998; 8:1087-1090.

95. Stavric G, Karanfilski B, Kalamaras A. Early diagnosis and detection of clinically non-suspected thyroid neoplasia by the cytologic method: a critical review of 1536 aspiration biopsies. Cancer 1980; 45:340-344.

96. Hsu C, Boey J. Diagnostic pitfalls in the fine needle aspiration of thyroid nodules: a study of 555 cases in Chinese patients. Acta Cytol 1987; 31:699-704.

97. Nathan A, Rainesf K, Lee Y-T. Fine-needle aspiration biopsy of cold thyroid nodules. Cancer 1988; 62:1337-1342.

98. Lowhagen T, Granberg P-O, Lundell G. Aspiration biopsy cytology (ABC) in nodules of the thyroid gland suspected to be malignant. Surg Clin North Am 1979; 59:3-18.

99. Smeds S, Lennquist S. The role of aspiration cytology in the management of thyroid nodules. Eur J Cancer Clin Oncol 1988; 24:293-297.

100. Gharib H, Goellner J, Zinsmeister A. Fine-needle aspiratioin biopsy of the thyroid: the problem of suspicious cytologic findings. Ann Intern Med 1984; 101:25-28.

101. Schlinkert R, vanHeerden J, Goellner J. Factors that predict malignant thyroid lesions when fine-needle aspiration is "suspicious for follicular neoplasm." Mayo Clinic Proc 1997; 72:913-916.

102. Atkinson B, Ernst C, LiVolsi V. Cytologic diagnoses of follicular tumors of the thyroid. Diagn Cytopathol 1986; 2:1-3.

103. Hamburger J, Hamburger S. Fine needle biopsy of thyroid nodules: avoiding the pitfalls. NY State J Med 1986; 86:241-249.

104. Layfield L, Reichman A, Bottles K. Clinical determinants for the management of thyroid nodules by fine-needle aspiration cytology. Arch Otolaryngol Head Neck Surg 1992; 118:717-721.

105. LoGerfo P, Starker P, Weber C. Incidence of cancer in surgically treated thyroid nodules based on method of selection. Surgery 1985; 98:1197-1201.

106. Aggarwal S, Jayaram G, Kakar A. Fine needle aspiration cytologic diagnosis of the solitary coled thyroid noeule: comparison with ultrasonography, radionuclide perfusion study and xeroradiography. Acta Cytol 1989; 33:41-47.

107. Gagneten C, Roccatagliata G, Lowenstein A. The role of fine needle aspiration biopsy cytology in the evaluation of the clinically solitary thyroid nodule. Acta Cytol 1987; 31:595-598.

108. Kini S, MIller J, Hamburger J. Cytopathology of follicular lesions of the thyroid gland. Diagn Cytopathol 1985; 1:123-132.

109. Silver C, Loiodice J, Johnson J. Needle aspiration biopsy of thyroid nodules. Surg Gynecol Obstet 1981; 152: 469-472.

110. Block M, Failey G, Block M. Thyroid nodules indeterminate by needle biopsy. Am J Surg 1983; 145:72-78.

111. Brauer R, Silver C. Needle aspiration biopsy of thyroid nodules. Laryngoscope 1984; 94:38-42.

112. Altavilla G, Pascale M, Nenci I. Fine needle aspiration cytology of thyroid gland diseases. Acta Cytol 1990; 34: 251-256.

113. Kapoor V, Sikora S. Solitary thyroid nodule: what to do? 1989; 65:642-644.

114. Reeve T, Delbridge L, Sloan D. The impact of fine-needle aspiration biopsy on surgery for single thyroid nodules. Med J Aust 1986; 145:308-311.

115. Hamburger J. Fine needle biopsy diagnosis of thyroid nodules: perspective. Thyroidology 1988; 1:21-34.

116. Kini S. The thyroid. Guides to clinical aspiration biopsy. Kline TS, editor. New York: Igaku Shoin; 1987.

117. Schmidt T, Riggs M. Significance of nondiagnostic fine-needle aspiration of the thyroid. South Med J 1997; 90:1183-1186.

118. Musgrave Y, Davey D, Weeks J, et al. Assessment of fine-needle aspiration sampling technique in thyroid nodules. Diagn Cytopathol 1998; 18:76-80.

119. Burch H, Burman K, Reed H, et al. Fine needle aspiration of thyroid nodules: determinants of insufficiency rate and malignancy yield at thyroidectomy. Acta Cytol 1996; 40:1176-1183.

120. MacDonald L, Yazdi H. Nondiagnostic fine needle aspiration biopsy of the thyroid gland: a diagnostic dilemma. Acta Cytol 1996; 40:423-428.

121. Kulkarni H, Kamal M, Arjune D. Improvement of the Mair scoring system using structural equations modeling for classifying the diagnostic adequacy of cytology material from thyroid lesions. Diagn Cytopathol 1999; 21:387-393.

122. Atkinson B. Fine needle aspiration of the thyroid. Monogr Pathol 1993; 35:166-199.

123. McHenry C, Slusarczyk S, Khiyami A. Recommendations for management of cystic thyroid disease. Surgery 1999; 126:1167-1172.

124. Crile G. Treatment of thyroid cysts by aspiration. Surgery 1966; 59:210-212.

125. Cusick E, McIntosh C, Krukowski Z. Cystic change and neoplasia in isolated thyroid swellings. Br J Surg 1988; 75:982-983.

126. Walfish P, Hazani E, Strawbridge H. Combined ultrasound and needle aspiration cytology in the assessment and management of hypofunctioning thyroid nodule. Ann Intern Med 1977; 87:270-274.

127. O'Leary T, Walker T. Thyroid cysts: does cancer at pathology mean clinical cancer? Arch Intern Med 1991; 151:1228.

128. Grant C, Hay I, Ryan J. Diagnostic and prognostic utility of flow cytometric DNA measurements in follicular thyroid tumors. World J Surg 1990; 14:283-290.

129. LiVolsi V, Montone K, Sack M. Pathology of thyroid disease. In: Diagnostic surgical pathology. 3rd ed. Philadelphia: Lippincott Williams and Wilkins.

130. Kennedy J. The pathology of dyshormonogentetic goiter. J Pathol 1969; 99:251-264.

131. Lever E, Medeiros-Neto G, DeGroot L. Inherited disorders of thyroid metabolism. Endocr Rev 1983; 4:213-239.

132. Peter H, Studer H, Smeds S. Pathogenesis of heterogeneity in human multinodular goiter. J Clin Invest 1985; 76: 1992-2002.

133. Ramelli R, Studer H, Bruggiesser D. Pathogenesis of thyroid nodules in multinodular goiter. Am J Pathol 1982; 109:215-223.

134. Harach H. Usefulness of fine needle aspiration of the thyroid in an endemic goiter region. Acta Cytol 1989; 33:31-35.

135. Jayaram G. Fine needle aspiration cytologic study of the solitary thyroid nodule: profile of 308 cases with histologic correlation. Acta Cytol 1985; 29:967-973.

136. Kini S, Miller J, Hamburger J. Cytopathology of thyroid nodules. Henry Ford Hosp Med J 1982; 30:17-24.

137. Suen K. How does one separate cellular follicular lesions of the thyroid by fine-needle aspiration biopsy? Diagn Cytopathol 1988; 4:78-81.

138. Busseniers A, Oertel Y. Cellular adenomatoid nodules of the thyroid: review of 219 fine-needle aspirates. Diagn Cytopathol 1993; 9:581-589.

139. Basu D, Jayaram G. A logistic model for thyroid lesions. Diagn Cytopathol 1992; 8:23-27.

140. Miller T, Bottles K, Holly E. A step-wise logistic regression analysis of papillary carcinoma of the thyroid. Acta Cytol 1986; 30:285-293.

141. Kaur A, Jayaram G. Thyroid tumors: cytomorphology of papillary carcinoma. Diagn Cytopathol 1991; 7:462-468.

142. Rosai J, Carcangiu M, DeLellis R. Tumors of the thyroid gland. In: Rosaij, editor. Atlas of tumor pathology, Series 3, Fascicle 5. Washington, DC: Armed Forces Institute of Pathology; 1993.

143. Soderstrom N. Puncture of goiters for aspiration biopsy: a preliminary report. Acta Med Scand 1952; 144:237-244.

144. Wright R, Castles H. Variability of thyroid cell nuclear size with Romanowsky stains. Acta Cytol 1987; 31:526-527.

145. DeJong S, Demeter J, Castelli M. Follicular cell predominance in the cytologic examination of dominant thyroid nodules indicates a sixty percent incidence of neoplasia. Surgery 1990; 108:794-800.

146. Gould E, Watzak L, Chamizo W. Nuclear grooves in cytologic preparations: a study of the utility of this feature in the diagnosis of papillary carcinoma. Acta Cytol 1989; 33:16-20.

147. Scopa C, Melachrinous M, Saradopoulou C. The significance of the grooved nucleus in thyroid lesions. Mod Pathol 1993; 6:691-694.

148. Deligeorgi-Politi H. Nuclear crease as a cytodiagnostic feature of papillary thyroid carcinoma in fine-needle aspiration biopsies. Diagn Cytopathol 1987; 3:307-310.

149. Rupp M, Ehya H. Nuclear grooves in the aspiration cytology of papillary carcinoma of the thyroid. Acta Cytol 1989; 33:21-26.

150. Chan J, Saw D. The grooved nucleus: a useful diagnostic criterion of papillary carcinoma of the thyroid. Am J Surg Pathol 1986; 10:672-679.

151. Liel Y, Zirking H, Sobel R. Fine needle aspiration of the hot thyroid nodule. Acta Cytol 1988; 32:866-867.

152. Walfish P, Strawbridge H, Rosen I. Management implications from routine needle biopsy of hyperfunctioning thyroid nodules. Surgery 1986; 98:1179-1187.

153. Jayaram G, Singh G, Marwaha R. Grave's disease: appearance in cytologic smears from fine needle aspirates of the thyroid gland. Acta Cytol 1989; 33:36-40.

154. Soderstrom N, Nilsson G. Cytologic diagnosis of thyrotoxicosis. Acta Med Scand 1979; 205:263-265.

155. Nilsson G. Marginal vacuoles in fine needle aspiration biopsy smears of toxic goiters. Acta Pathol Microbiol Scand Sec 1972; 80:289-293.

156. Friedman N. Cellular involution in thyroid gland: significance of Hürthle cells in myxedema, exhaustion atrophy, Hashimoto's disease and reaction to irradiation, thiouracil therapy and subtotal resection. J Clin Endocrinol Metal 1949; 9:874-882.

157. Harcourt-Webster J, Stott N. HIstochemical study of oxidative and hydrolytic enzymes in the human thyroid. J Pathol Bacteriol 1960; 30:353-361.

158. Tremblay G. Histochemical study of cytochrome oxidase and adenosine triphosphatase in Askanazy cells (Hürthle cells) of the human thyroid. Lab Invest 1962; 11:514-517.

159. Harach H, Zusman S, Day E. Nodular goiter: a histocytological study with some emphasis on pitfalls of fine-needle aspiration cytology. Diagn Cytopathol 1992; 8:409-419.

160. Anderson R, Pragasam P, Nazeer T. Atypical, retrogressive and metaplastic changes in nodular goiters: potential pitfalls in aspiration cytology of the thyroid. Acta Cytol 1990; 34:715-716.

161. Soderstrom N. Identification of normal tissue and tumors by cytologic aspiration biopsy. Acta Soc Med 1958; 65: 53-87.

162. Gharib H, Goellner J. Diagnosis of amyloidosis by fine-needle aspiration biopsy of the thyroid. N Engl J Med 1981; 305:586.

163. Kapila K, Verma K. Amyloid goiter in fine needle aspirates. Acta Cytol 1993; 37:257-258.

164. Rigaud C, Bogomoletz W. "Mucin secreting" and "mucinous" primary thyroid carcinomas: pitfalls in mucin histochemistry applied to thyroid tumors. J Clin Pathol 1987; 40:890-895.

165. Reid J, Choi C-H, Oldroyd N. Calcium oxalate crystals in the thyroid: their identification, prevalence, origin and possible significance. Am J Clin Pathol 1987; 87:443-454.

166. Kini S, Miller J, Hamburger J. Cytopathology of papillary carcinoma of the thyroid by fine needle aspiration. Acta Cytol 1980; 24:511-521.

167. Attwood H, Dennett X. A black thyroid and minocycline treatment. Br J Med 1976; 2:1109-1110.

168. Wajda K, Wislon M, Lucas J. Fine needle aspiration cytologic findings in the black thyroid syndrome. Acta Cytol 1988; 32:862-865.

169. Kung I, Yuen R. Fine needle aspiration of the thyroid: distinction between colloid nodules and follicular neoplasms using cell blocks and 21-gauge needles. Acta Cytol 1989; 33:53-60.

170. Ravinsky E, Safneck J. Fine needle aspirates of follicular lesions of the thyroid gland: the intermediate-type smear. Acta Cytol 1990; 34:813-820.

171. Deshpande V, Kapila K, Sai K, et al. Follicular neoplasms of the thyroid. Decision tree approach using morphologic and morphometric parameters. Acta Cytol 1997; 41:369-376.

172. Poller D, Ibrahim A, Cummings M, et al. Fine-needle aspiration of the thyroid: importance of an indeterminate diagnostic category. Cancer 2000; 90:239-244.

173. Mazzaferri E. Thyroid cancer in thyroid nodules: finding a needle in a haystack. Am J Med 1992; 93:359-362.

174. Wolf P. Biochemical biopsy of thyroid cysts vs cytologic diagnosis: which is preferable? Arch Pathol Lab Med 1993; 117:593-594.

175. Clark O, Okerlung M, Cavalieri R. Diagnosis and treatment of thyroid, parathyroid, and thyroglossal duct cysts. J Colin Endocrinol Metab 1979; 48:983-988.

176. Franklyn J, Sheppard M. Aspiration cytology of the thyroid. Br Med J 1987; 295:510-511.

177. Smith M, McHenry C, Jarosz H. Carcinoma of the thyroid in patients with autonomous nodules. Ann Surg 1988; 54:448-449.

178. DeGroot L, Quintans J. The causes of autoimmune thyroid disease. Endocrinol Rev 1989; 10:537-562.

179. Utiger R. The pathogenesis of autoimmune thyroid disease. N Engl J Med 1991; 325:278-279.

180. Furmaniak J, Nakajima Y, Hashim F. The TSH receptor: structure and interaction with autoantibodies in thyroid disease. Acta Endocrinol (Copenh) 1987; 28:157-165.

181. Shapiro S, Friedman N, Perzik S. Incidence of thyroid carcinoma in Graves' disease. Cancer 1970; 26:1261-1270.

182. Caruso G, Tabarri B, Lucchi I. Fine needle aspiration cytology in a case of diffuse sclerosing carcinoma of the thyroid. Acta Cytol 1990; 34:352-354.

183. Belfiore A, Garofalo M, Giuffrida D. Increased aggressiveness of thyroid cancer in patients with Graves' disease. J Clin Endocrinol Metabol 1990; 70:830-835.

184. Spjut H, Warren W, Ackerman L. Clinical-pathologic study of 76 cases of recurrent Graves' disease, toxic (nonexophthalmic) goiter, and nontoxic goiter. Am J Clin Pathol 1957; 27:367-392.

185. Bhalotra R, Jayaram G. Overlapping morphology in thyroiditis (Hashimoto's and subacute) and Graves' disease. Cytopathology 1990; 1:371-372.

186. LiVolsi V, Merino M. Squamous cells in the human thyroid gland. Am J Surg Pathol 1978; 2:133-140.

187. Nilsson G. Lymphoid infiltration in toxic goiters studies with fine needle aspiration biopsy. Acta Endocrinol 1972; 71:480-490.

188. Friedman M, Shimaoka K, Getaz P. Needle aspiration of 310 thyroid lesions. Acta Cytol 1979; 23:194-203.

189. Panke T, Croxson M, Parker J. Triiodothyronine-secreting (toxic) adenoma of the thyroid gland: light and electron microscopic characteristics. Cancer 1978; 41:528-537.

190. Das D, Jain S, Tripathi R. Marginal vacuoles in thyroid aspirates. Acta Cytol 1998; 42:1121-1128.

191. Smejkal V, Smejkalova, Rosa M. Cytologic changes simulating malignancy in thyrotoxic goiters treated with carbimazole. Acta Cytol 1985; 29:173-178.

192. Patchefsky A, Hoch W. Psammoma bodies in diffuse toxic goiter. Am J Clin Pathol 1972; 57:551-556.

193. Cameselle-Teijeiro J, Febles-Perez C, Cameselle-Teijeiro J, et al. Cytologic clues for distinguishing the tall cell variant of thyroid papillary carcinoma: a case report. Acta Cytol 1997; 41:1310-1316.

194. Berger S, Zonszein J, Villamena P. Infectious diseases of the thyroid gland. Rev Infect Dis 1983; 5:108-122.

195. Kirkland R, Kirkland J, Rosenberg H. Solitary thyroid nodules in 30 children and report of a child with a thyroid abscess. Pediatrics 1973; 51:85-90.

196. Singh S, Agrawal J, Kumar M. Fine needle aspiration cytology in the management of acute suppurative thyroiditis. Ear Nose Throat J 1994; 73:415-417.

197. Kaw Y. Fine needle aspiration cytology of the tall cell variant of papillary carcinoma of the thyroid. Acta Cytol 1994; 38:282-283.

198. Guttler R, Singer P. Pneumocystis carinni thyroiditis: report of three cases and review of the literature. Arch Intern Med 1993; 153:393-396.

199. Drucker D, Bailey D, Rotstein L. Thyroiditis as the presenting manifestation of disseminated extrapulmonary pneumocystis carinii infection. J Clin Endocrinol Metab 1990; 71:1663-1665.

200. Kline T. The thyroid. In: Kline T, editor. Handbook of fine needle aspiration biopsy cytology. 2nd ed. New York: Churchill Livingstone; 1988. pp.153-198.

201. Torres A, Agrawal S, Peters S, et al. Invasive aspergillosis diagnosed by fine-needle aspiration of the thyroid gland. Thyroid 1999; 9:1119-1122.

202. Lowhagen T, Sprenger E. Cytologic presentation of thyroid tumors in aspiration biopsy smear: a review of 60 cases. Acta Cytol 1974; 18:192-197.

203. Carney J, Moore S, Northcutt R. Palpation thyroiditis (multifocal granulomatous folliculitis). Am J Clin Pathol 1975; 64:639-647.

204. Greene J. Subacute thyroiditis. Am J Med 1971; 51:97-108.

205. Woolner L, McConahey W, Beahrs O. Granulomatous thyroiditis (de Quervain's thyroiditis). J Clin Endocrinol Metal 1957; 17:1202-1221.

206. Volpe R. The pathology of thyroiditis. Hum Pathol 1978; 9:429-438.

207. Guarda L, Baskin H. Inflammatory and lymphoid lesions of the thyroid gland: cytopathology by fine-needle aspiration. Am J Clin Pathol 1987; 87:14-22.

208. Meachim G, Young M. de Quervain's subacute granulomatous thyroiditis: histological identificaiton and incidence. J Clin Pathol 1963; 16:189-199.

209. Ofner C, HIttmair A, Kroll I. Fine needle aspiration cytodiagnosis of subacute (de Quervain's) thyroiditis in an endemic goiter area. Cytopathology 1994; 5:33-40.

210. Jayaram G, Marsaha R, Gupta R. Cytomorphologic aspects of thyroiditis: a study of 541 cases with functional, immunologic and ultrasonographic data. Acta Cytol 1987; 31:687-693.

211. Sidawy M, Costa M. The significance of paravacuolar granules of the thyroid: a histologic, cytologic and ultrastructural study. Acta Cytol 1989; 33:929-933.

212. Wilson R, Gartner W. Teflon granuloma mimicking a thyroid tumor. Diagn Cytopathol 1987; 3:156-158.

213. Das A, Gupta S, Banerjee A. Atypical cytologic features of medullary carcinoma of the thyroid: a review of 12 cases. Acta Cytol 1992; 36:137-141.

214. Leung C-S, Hartwick R, Bedard Y. Correlation of cytologic and histologic features in variants of papillary carcinoma of thyroid. Acta Cytol 1993; 37:645-650.

215. Hay I. Thyroiditis: a clinical update. Mayo Clin Proc 1985; 60:836-843.

216. Katsikas D, Shorthouse A, Taylor S. Riedel's thyroiditis. Br J Surg 1976; 63:929-931.

217. Hines R, Scheuermann H, Royster H, et al. Invasive fibrous (Riedel's) thyroiditis with bilateral fibrous parotitis. JAMA 1970; 213:869-871.

218. Schwaegerle SM, Bauer TW, Esselstyn CB. Riedel's thyroiditis. Am J Clin Pathol 1988; 90:715-722.

219. Al-Hilaly M, Koshi P, Nasr A, et al. Riedel's thyroiditis: case report. Acta Chir Scand 1990; 156:237-239.

220. Blumenfeld W. Correlation of cytologic and histologic findings in fibrosing thyroiditis: a case report. Acta Cytol 1997; 41:1337-1340.

221. Katz S, Vickery JA. The fibrous variant of Hashimoto's thyroiditis. Hum Pathol 1974; 5:161-170.

222. Guarda L, Peterson C, Hall W, et al. Anaplastic thyroid carcinoma: cytomorphology and clinical implications of fine-needle aspiration. Diagn Cytopathol 1991; 7:63-67.

223. Volpe R. Etiology, pathogenesis, and clinical aspects of thyroiditis. Pathol Annu 1978; 13:399-412.

224. Volpe R. The immunoregulatory disturbance in autoimmune thyroid disease. Autoimmunity 1988; 2:55-72.

225. Mizukami Y, Michigishi T, Kawato M, et al. Chronic thyroiditis; thyroid function and histologic correlations in 601 cases. Hum Pathol 1992; 23:980-988.

226. Friedman M, Shimaoka K, Rao U. Diagnosis of chronic lymphocytic thyroiditis (nodular presentation) by needle aspiration. Acta Cytol 1981; 25:513-522.

227. Holm L-E, Blomgren H, Lowhagen T. Cancer risks in patients with chronic lymphocytic thyroiditis. N Engl J Med 1985; 312:601-604.

228. Sclafani A, Valdes M, Cho H. Hashimoto's thyroiditis and carcinoma of the thyroid: optimal management. Laryngoscope 1993; 103:845-849.

229. Ott R, Calandra D, McCall A, et al. The incidence of thyroid carcinoma in patients with Hashimoto's thyroiditis and solitary cold nodules. Surgery 1985; 98:1202-1206.

230. Tseleni-Balafouta S, Kyroudi-Voulgari A, Paizi-Biza P, et al. Lymphocytic thyroiditis in fine-needle aspirates: differential diagnostic aspects. Diagn Cytopathol 1989; 5:362-365.

231. McKee R, Krukowski Z, Matheson N. Thyroid neoplasia coexistent with chronic lymphocytic thyroiditis. Br J Surg 1993; 80:1303-1304.

232. Volpe R. Immunoregulation in autoimmune thyroid disease. N Engl J Med 1987; 316:44-45.

233. Harris M. The cellular infiltrate in Hashimoto's disease and focal lymphocytic thyroiditis. J Clin Pathol 1969; 22:326-333.

234. Lindsay S, Dailey M, Friedlander J, et al. Chronic thyroiditis: a clinical and pathological study of 354 patients. J Clin Endocrinol Metab 1952; 12:1578-1600.

235. Marshall S, Meissner W, Smith D. Chronic thyroiditis. N Engl J Med 1948; 238:758-766.

236. Gutteridge D, Orell S. Non-toxic goiter: diagnostic role of aspiration cytology, antibodies and serum thyrotrophin. Clin Endocrinol 1978; 9:505-514.

237. Kini S, Miller J, Hamburger J. Cytopathology of Hürthle cell lesions of the thyroid gland by fine needle aspiration. Acta Cytol 1981; 25:647-652.

238. Nguyen G, Ginsberg J, Crockford P, et al. Hashimoto's thyroiditis: cytodiagnostic accuracy and pitfalls. Diagn Cytopathol 1997; 16:531-536.

239. Maurer R, Taylor C, Terry R, et al. Non-Hodgkin lymphomas of the thyroid: a clinico-pathological review of 29 cases applying the Lukes-Collins classifications and an immunoperoxidase method. Virchows Arch Path Anat Histol 1979; 383:293-317.

240. Matsuzuka F, Miyauchi A, Katayama S, et al. Clinical aspects of primary thyroid lymphoma: diagnosis and treatment based on our experience of 119 cases. Thyroid 1993; 3:93-99.

241. Detweiler R, Katz R, Alapat C, et al. Malignant lymphoma of the thyroid: a report of two cases diagnosed by fine-needle aspiration. Diagn Cytopathol 1991; 7:163-171.

242. Carson H, Castelli M, Gattuso P. Incidence of neoplasia in Hashimoto's thyroiditis: a fine-needle aspiration study. Diagn Cytopathol 1996; 14:38-42.

243. Vodanovic S, Crepinko I, Smoje J. Morphologic diagnosis of Hürthle cell tumors of the thyroid gland. Acta Cytol 1993; 37:317-322.

244. Bondeson L, Bondeson A-G, Lindholm K, et al. Morphometric studies on nuclei in smears of fine needle aspirates from oxyphilic tumors of the thyroid. Acta Cytol 1983; 27:437-440.

245. MacDonald L, Yazdi H. Fine needle aspiration biopsy of Hashimoto's thyroiditis: sources of diagnostic error. Acta Cytol 1999; 43:400-406.

246. Kurashima C, Hirokawa K. Focal lymphocytic infiltration of thyroids in elderly people. Survey Synth Pathol Res 1985; 4:457-466.

247. Williams E, Doniach I. The postmortem incidence of focal thyroiditis. J Pathol Bacteriol 1962; 83:255-264.

248. Weaver DK, Batsakis JG, Nishiyama RH. Relationship of iodine to "lymphocytic goiter." Arch Surg 1969; 98:183-186.

249. Dahlberg P, Jansson R. Different etiologies in post-partum thyroiditis? Acta Endocrinol (Copenh) 1983; 104:195-200.

250. Reith P, Kyner J. Postpartum thyroiditis: a common cause of thyrotoxicosis and/or hypothyroidism after pregnancy. Nebr Med J 1984; 69:356-359.

251. Woolf P, Daly R. Thyrotoxicosis with painless thyroiditis. Am J Med 1976; 60:73-79.

252. Mizukami Y, Michigishi T, Nonomura A, et al. Postpartum thyroiditis: a clinical, histologic, and immunopathologic study of 15 cases. Am J Clin Pathol 1993; 100:200-205.

253. Hundahl S, Gleming I, Fremgen A, et al. A national cancer data base report on 53,856 cases of thyroid carcinoma treated in the United States, 1985-1995. Cancer 1998; 83: 2638-2648.

254. Al-Moussa M, Berk J. Histometry of thyroids containing few and multiple modules. J Clin Pathol 1986; 39:483-488.

255. Joensuu H, Klemi P, Eerola E. DNA aneuploidy in follicular adenomas of the thyroid gland. Am J Pathol 1987; 124:373-376.

256. Harzard J, Kenyon R. Atypical adenoma of the thyroid. Arch Pathol Lab Med 1954; 58:554-563.

257. Lang W, Georgii G, Stauch G, Kienzie E, et al. The differentiation of atypical adenomas and encapsulated follicular carcinomas in the thyroid gland. Virchows Arch (A) 1980; 385:125-141.

258. Williams E. Pathology and natural history. In: Duncan W, editor. Thyroid cancer. Berlin: Springer-Verlag; 1980. pp.47-55.

259. Williams ED, Doniach I, Bjarnason O, Michie W. Thyroid cancer in an iodide rich area. Cancer 1977; 39:215-222.

260. Backdahl M. Nuclear DNA content and prognosis in papillary, follicular, and medullary carcinomas of the thyroid: doctoral thesis. Stockholm: Karolinska Medical Institute; 1985.

261. Ruegemer J, Hay I, Bergstrith E, et al. Distant metastases in differentiated thyroid carcinoma: a multivariate analysis of prognostic variables. J Clin Endocrinol Metab 1988; 67:501-508.

262. Evans H. Follicular neoplasms of the thyroid. Cancer 1984; 54:535-540.

263. Schroder S, Baisch H, Rehpenning W, et al. Morphologie und prognose des follicularen Schilddrusencarcinoms: eine klinicsh pathologische und DNS-cytometrische untersuchung an 95 tumoren. Langenbecks Arch Chir 1987; 370:3-24.

264. Lang W, Choritz H, Hundeshagen H. Risk factors in follicular thyroid carcinomas: a retrospective follow-up study covering a 14-year period with emphasis on morphological findings. Am J Surg Pathol 1986; 10:246-255.

265. Franssila K. Prognosis in thyroid carcinoma. Cancer 1975; 36:1138-1146.

266. Woolner O. Thyroid carcinoma: pathologic classification with data on prognosis. Semin Nucl Med 1971; 1:481-502.

267. LiVolsi V. Papillary neoplasms of the thyroid: pathologic and prognostic features. Anat Pathol 1992; 97:426-434.

268. Franssila K, Ackerman L, Brown C, et al. Follicular carcinoma. Semin Diagn Pathol 1985; 2:101-102.

269. Lang W, Georgii G. Minimal invasive cancer in the thyroid. Clin Oncol 1982; 1:527-537.

270. Klemi P, Joensuu H, Nylamo E. Fine needle aspiration biopsy in the diagnosis of thyroid nodules. Acta Cytol 1991; 35:434-438.

271. Larson R, Wick M. Primary mucoepidermoid carcinoma of the thyroid: diagnosis by fine-needle aspiration biopsy. Diagn Cytopathol 1993; 9:438-443.

272. Bronner M, LiVolsi V. Oxyphilic (Askanazy/Hürthle cell) tumors of the thyroid: microscopic features predict biologic behavior. Surg Pathol 1988; 1:137-150.

273. Kaur A, Jayaram G. Thyroid tumors: cytomorphology of follicular neoplasms. Diagn Cytopathol 1991; 7:469-472.

274. Boon M, Lowhagen T, Willems J-S. Planimetric studies on fine needle aspirates from follicular adenoma and follicular carcinoma of the thyroid. Acta Cytol 1980; 24:145-148.

275. Walts A, Pitchon H. Pneumocystis carinii in FNA of the thyroid. Diagn Cytopathol 1991; 7:615-617.

276. Fadda G, Rabitti C, Minimo C. Morphologic and planimetric diagnosis of follicular thyroid lesions on fine needle aspiration cytology. Anal Quant Cytol Histol 1995; 17:247-256.

277. Kini S. Needle aspiration biopsy of the thyroid: revisited. Diagn Cytopathol 1993; 9:249-251.

278. Mai K, Yazdi H, Commons A, Perkins D, et al. Neoplastic non-papillary thyroid carcinoma lesions with a fine chromatin pattern. Pathol Int 1999; 49:601-607.

279. Montironi R, Braccischi A, Scarpelli M, et al. Value of quantitative nucleolar features in the preoperative cytological diagnosis of follicular neoplasias of the thyroid. J Clin Pathol 1991; 44:509-514.

280. Faroux M, Pluot M, Delisle M, et al. Evaluation of morphological criteria in the cytological diagnosis of thyroid cold nodules: a preliminary study. Pathol Res Pract 1990; 186:330-335.

281. Rout P, Shariff S. Diagnostic value of qualitative and quantitative variables in thyroid lesions. Cytopathology 1999; 10:171-179.

282. Backdahl M, Wallin G, Lowhagen T, et al. Fine-needle biopsy cytology and DNA analysis: their place in the evaluation and treatment of patients with thyroid neoplasms. Surg Clin North Am 1987; 67:197-211.

283. Yan Z, Yang GC, Waisman J. A low-power "architectural" clue to the follicular variant of papillary thyroid adenocarcinoma in aspiration biopsy. Acta Cytol 2000; 44:211-217.

284. Hamburger J, Husain M. Semiquantitative criteria for fine-needle biopsy diagnosis: reduced false-negative diagnoses. Diagn Cytopathol 1988; 4:14-17.

285. Miller JM, Hamburger JI, Kini SR. The needle biopsy diagnosis of papillary thyroid carcinoma. Cancer 1981; 48:989-993.

286. Tielens E, Sherman S, Hruban R, et al. Follicular variant of papillary thyroid carcinoma: a clinicopathologic study. Cancer 1994; 73:424-431.

287. Carcangiu M, Zampi G, Pupi A, et al. Papillary carcinoma of the thyroid: a clinicopathologic study of 241 cases treated at the University of Florence, Italy. Cancer 1985; 55:805-828.

288. Hugh J, Duggan M, Chang-Poon V. The fine-needle aspiration appearance of the follicular variant of thyroid papillary carcinoma: a report of three cases. Diagn Cytopathol 1988; 4:196-201.

289. Gonzalez-Campora R, Herrero-Zapatero A, Lerma E, et al. Hürthle cell and mitochondrion-rich cell tumors: a clinicopathologic study. Cancer 1986; 57:1154-1163.

290. Bastenie P, Ermans A. Thyroiditis and thyroid function: clinical, morphological and physiopathological studies. Oxford: Pergamon Press; 1972.

291. Kendall CH, McCluskey E, Meagles IN. Oxyphil cells in thyroid disease: a uniform change? J Clin Pathol 1986; 39:908-912.

292. Ravinsky E, Safneck J. Differentiation of Hashimoto's thyroiditis from thyroid neoplasms in fine needle aspirates. Acta Cytol 1988; 32:854-861.

293. Jayaram G. Problems in the interpretation of Hürthle cell populations in fine needle aspirates from the thyroid. Acta Cytol 1983; 27:84-85.

294. Thompson N, Dunn E, Batsakis J, et al. Hürthle cell lesions of the thyroid gland. Surg Gynecol Obstet 1974; 139:555-560.

295. Watson R, Brennan M, Goellner J, et al. Invasive Hürthle cell carcinoma of the thyroid: natural history and management. Mayo Clin Proc 1984; 59:851-855.

296. Galera-Davidson F, Bibbo M, Bartels P, et al. Correlation between automated DNA ploidy measurements of Hürthle cell tumors and their histopathologic and clinical features. Anal Quant Cytol Histol 1986; 8:158-167.

297. Bondeson L, Azavedo E, Bondeson A, et al. Nuclear DNA content and behavior of oxyphil thyroid tumors. Cancer 1986; 58:672-675.

298. Gonzalez JL, Wang HH, Ducatman BS. Fine-needle aspiration of Hürthle cell lesions: a cytomorphologic approach to diagnosis. Am J Clin Pathol 1993; 100:231-235.

299. Blumenfeld W, Nair R, Mir R. Diagnostic significance of papillary structures and intranuclear inclusions in Hürthle-cell neoplasms of the thyroid. Diagn Cytopathol 1999; 20:185-189.

300. Nguyen GK, Husain M, Akin MR. Cytodiagnosis of benign and malignant Hürthle cell lesions of the thyroid by fine-needle aspiration biopsy. Diagn Cytopathol 1999; 20:261-265.

301. Thranov I, Francis D, Olsen J. Intranuclear cytoplasmic invaginations in a Hürthle-cell carcinoma of the thyroid. Acta Cytol 1983; 27:341-344.

302. Mills S, Allen M. Congenital occult papillary carcinoma of the thyroid gland. Hum Pathol 17:1179-1181.

303. Cady B. Papillary carcinoma of the thyroid. Semin Surg Oncol 1991; 7:81-86.

304. Favus M, Schneide A, Stachura M. Thyroid cancer occurring as a late consequence of head and neck irradiation: evaluation of 1056 patients. N Engl J Med 1976; 294:1019-1025.

305. Reteloff S, Harrison J, Karanfilski BT, et al. Continuing occurrence of thyroid carcinoma after irradiation to the neck in infancy and childhood. N Engl J Med 1975; 292:171-175.

306. Woolner L, Beahrs O, Black B, et al. Classification and prognosis of thyroid carcinoma: a study of 885 cases observed over a thirty-year period. Am Surg 1961; 102:354-387.

307. Cady B, Sedgwick CE, Meissner WA, et al. Changing clinical, pathologic, therapeutic, and survival patterns in differentiated thyroid carcinoma. Ann Surg 1976; 187:541-553.

308. McConahey WM, Hay IO, Woolner LB, et al. Papillary thyroid cancer treated at the Mayo Clinic, 1946 through 1970: initial manifestations, pathologic findings, therapy and outcome. Mayo Clin Prac 1986; 61:978-996.

309. Noguchi S, Noguchi A, Murakami N. Papillary carcinoma of the thyroid. I. Developing pattern of metastasis. Cancer 1970; 26:1053-1060.

310. Tollsfsen H, DeCosse J, Hutter R. Papillary carcinoma of the thyroid: a clinical and pathological study of 70 fatal cases. Cancer 1964; 17:1035-1044.

311. Tubiana M, Schlumberger M, Rougier P, et al. Long-term results and prognostic factors in patients with differentiated thyroid carcinoma. Cancer 1985; 55:794-804.

312. DeGroot LJ, Kaplan EL, McCormick M, et al. Natural history, treatment, and course of papillary thyroid carcinoma. J Clin Endocrinol Metab 1990; 71:414-424.

313. Lawson W, Biller H. The solitary thyroid nodule: diagnosis and management of malignant disease. Am J Otolaryngol 1983; 4:43-73.

314. Harach HR, Franssila KO, Wasenius VM. Occult papillary carcinoma of the thyroid: a "normal" finding in Finland. A systematic autopsy study. Cancer 1985; 556:531-538.

315. Franssila K, Harach H. Occult papillary carcinoma of the thyroid in children and young adults: a systemic autopsy study in Finland. Cancer 1986; 58:715-719.

316. Martinez-Tello FJ, Martinez-Cabruja R, Fernandez-Margin J, et al. Occult carcinoma of the thyroid: a systematic autopsy study from Spain of two series performed with two different methods. Cancer 1993; 71:4022-4029.

317. Evans H. Encapsulated papillary neoplasms of the thyroid: a study of 14 cases followed for a minimum of 10 years. Am J Surg Pathol 1987; 11:592.

318. Schroder S, Bocker W, Dralle H. The encapsulated papillary carcinoma of the thyroid: a morphologic subtype of the papillary thyroid carcinoma. Cancer 1984; 54:90.

319. Katoh R, Sasaki J, Kurihara H, et al. Multiple thyroid involvement (intraglandular metastasis) in papillary thyroid carcinoma: a clinicopathologic study of 105 consecutive patients. Cancer 1992; 40:1585-1590.

320. Rosai J. Papillary carcinoma. Monogr Pathol 1993; 35:138-165.

321. Rosai J, Zampi G, Carcangiu ML. Papillary carcinoma of the thyroid: a discussion of its several morphologic expressions, with particular emphasis on the follicular variant. Am J Surg Pathol 1983; 7:809-817.

322. Soderstrom N, Biorklund A. Intranuclear cytoplasmic inclusions in some types of thyroid cancer. Acta Cytol 1973; 17:191-197.

323. Dominguez-Malagon HR, Szymanski-Gomez JJ, Gaytan-Garcia SR. Optically clear and vacuolated nuclei: two useful signs for the transoperative diagnosis of papillary carcinoma of the thyroid. Cancer 1988; 62:105-108.

324. Akhtar M, Ali M, Huq M, et al. Fine needle aspiration biopsy of papillary thyroid carcinoma: cytologic, histologic and ultrastructural correlations. Diagn Cytopathol 1991; 7:373-379.

325. Albores-Saavedra J, Gould E, Vardaman C, et al. The macrofollicular variant of papillary thyroid carcinoma: a study of 17 cases. Hum Pathol 1991; 22:1195.

326. Zacks J, Morenas A, Beazley R, et al. Fine-needle aspiration cytology diagnosis of colloid nodule versus follicular variant of papillary carcinoma of the thyroid. Diagn Cytopathol 1998; 18:87-90.

327. Mesonero C, Jugle J, Wilbur D, et al. Fine-needle aspiration of the macrofollicular and microfollicular subtypes of the follicular variant of papillary carcinoma of the thyroid. Cancer 1998; 84:235-244.

328. Goodell WM, Saboorian MH, Ashfaq R. Fine-needle aspiration diagnosis of athe follicular variant of papillary carcinoma. Cancer 1998; 84:349-354.

329. Baloch Z, Gupta P, Yu G, et al. Follicular variant of papillary carcinoma: cytologic and histologic correlation. Am J Clin Pathol 1999; 111:216-222.

330. Nair M, Kapila K, Karak A, et al. Papillary carcinoma of the thyroid and its variants: a cytohistological correlation. Diagn Cytopathol 2001; 24:167-173.

331. Logani S, Gupta P, LiVolsi V, et al. Thyroid nodules with FNA cytology suspicious for follicular variant of papillary thyroid carcinoma: follow-up and management. Diagn Cytopathol 2000; 23:380-385.

332. Meissner W, Warren S. Tumors of the thyroid gland. Fascicle 4, Second Series. Washington, DC: Armed Forces Institute of Pathology; 1969.

333. Kobayashi T, Okamoto S, Maruyama H. Squamous metaplasia with Hashimoto's thyroiditis presenting as a thyroid nodule. J Surg Oncol 1989; 40:139-142.

334. Shurbaji MS, Gupta PK, Frost JK. Nuclear grooves: a useful criterion in the cytopathologic diagnosis of papillary thyroid carcinoma. Diagn Cytopathol 1988; 4:91-94.

335. Francis I, Das D, Sheikh Z. Role of nuclear grooves in the diagnosis of papillary thyroid carcinoma: a quantitative assessment of fine needle aspirate smears. Acta Cytol 1995; 39:409-415.

336. Chhieng DC, Ross JS, McKenna BJ. CD44 immunostaining of thyroid fine-needle aspirates differentiates thyroid papillary carcinoma from other lesions with nuclear grooves and inclusions. Cancer 1997; 81:157-162.

337. Nasser S, Pitman M, Pilch B, Faquin W. Fine-needle aspiration biopsy of papillary thyroid carcinoma: diagnostic utility of cytokeratin 19 immunostaining. Cancer 2000; 90:307-311.

338. Christ M, Haja J. Intranuclear cytoplasmic inclusions (Invaginations) in thyroid aspirations: frequency and specificity. Acta Cytol 1979; 23:327-331.

339. Glant M, Berger E, Davey D. Intranuclear cytoplasmic inclusions in aspirates of follicular neoplasms of the thyroid: a report of two cases. Acta Cytol 1984; 28:576-580.

340. Solares J, Lacruz C. Fine needle aspiration cytology diagnosis of an extracranial meningioma presenting as a cervical mass. Acta Cytol 1987; 31:502-504.

341. Chan J. Papillary carcinoma of thyroid: classical and variants. Histol Histopathol 1990; 5:241-257.

342. Shabb N, Tawil A, Gergeos F, et al. Multinucleated giant cells in fine-needle aspiration of thyroid nodules: their diagnostic significance. Diagn Cytopathol 1999; 21:307-312.

343. Satoh Y, Sakamoto A, Yamada K, et al. Psammoma bodies in metastatic carcinoma to the thyroid. Mod Pathol 1990; 3:267-270.

344. Riazmontazer N, Bedayat G. Psammoma bodies in fine needle aspirates from thyroids containing nontoxic hyperplastic nodular goiters. Acta Cytol 1991; 35:563-566.

345. Dugan J, Atkinson B, Avitabile A, et al. Psammoma bodies in fine needle aspirate of the thyroid in lymphocytic thyroiditis. Acta Cytol 1987; 31:330-334.

346. Ellison E, Lapuerta P, Margin S. Psammoma bodies in fine-needle aspirates of the thyroid: predictive value for papillary carcinoma. Cancer 1998; 84:169-175.

347. Goellner J, Johnson D. Cytology of cystic papillary carcinoma of the thyroid. Acta Cytol 1982; 26:797-799.

348. de las Santos E, Keyhani-Rofagha S, Cunningham J, et al. Cystic thyroid nodules: the dilemma of malignant lesions. Arch Intern Med 1990; 150:1422-1427.

349. Hammer M, Wortsman J, Folse R. Cancer in cystic lesions of the thyroid. Arch Surg 1982; 117:1020-1023.

350. Jayaram G, Kaur A. Cystic thyroid nodules harboring malignancy: a problem in fine needle aspiration cytodiagnosis. Acta Cytol 1989; 33:941-942.

351. Muller N, Cooperberg P, Suen K, et al. Needle aspiration biopsy in cystic papillary carcinoma of the thyroid. AJR 1985; 144:251-253.

352. Sarda A, Bal S, Gupta S, et al. Diagnosis and treatment of cystic disease of the thyroid by aspiration. Surgery 1988; 103:593-596.

353. Miller J, Zafar S, Karo J. The cystic thyroid nodule: recognition and management. Radiology 1974; 110:257-261.

354. Damiani S, Dina R, Eusebi V. Cytologic grading of aggressive and nonaggressive variants of papillary thyroid carcinoma. Am J Clin Pathol 1994; 101:651-655.

355. Hawk W, Hazard J. The many appearances of papillary carcinoma of the thyroid. Cleve Clin Q 1976; 43:207-216.

356. Johnson TL, Lloyd RV, Thompson NW, et al. Prognostic implications of the tall cell variant of papillary thyroid carcinoma. Am J Surg Pathol 1988; 12:22-27.

357. Pisani T, Giovagnoli M, Intrieri F, et al. Tall cell variant of papillary carcinoma coexisting with chronic lymphocytic thyroiditis: a case report. Acta Cytol 1999; 43:435-438.

358. Filie A, Chiesa A, Bryant B, et al. The tall cell variant of papillary carcinoma of the thyroid: cytologic features and loss of heterozygosity of metastatic and/or recurrent neoplasms and primary neoplasms. Cancer 1999; 87:238-242.

359. Beckner M, Heffess C, Oertel J. Oxyphil papillary thyroid carcinomas. Am J Clin Pathol 1995; 103:280-287.

360. Chen K. Fine-needle aspiration cytology of papillary Hürthle-cell tumors of thyroid: a report of three cases. Diagn Cytopathol 1991; 7:53-56.

361. Doria M, Attal H, Wang H, et al. Fine needle aspiration cytology of the oxyphil variant of papillary carcinoma of the thyroid: a report of three cases. Acta Cytol 1996; 40:1007-1011.

362. Vickery A, Carcangiu M, Johannessen J, et al. Papillary carcinoma. Semin Diagn Pathol 1985; 2:90-100.

363. Carcangiu M, Bianchi S. Diffuse sclerosing variant of papillary thyroid carcinoma. Clinicopathologic study of 15 cases. Am J Surg Pathol 1989; 13:1041-1049.

364. Kumarasinghe M. Cytomorphologic features of diffuse sclerosing variant of papillary carcinoma of the thyroid: a report of two cases in children. Acta Cytol 1998; 42:983-986.

365. Gaertner E, Davidson M, Wenig B. The columnar cell variant of thyroid papillary carcinoma: case report and discussion of an unusually aggressive thyroid papillary carcinoma. Am J Surg Pathol 1995; 19:940-947.

366. Hui PK, Chan JK, Cheung PS, et al. Columnar cell carcinoma of the thyroid: fine needle aspiration findings in a case. Acta Cytol 1990; 34:355-358.

367. Perez F, Llobet M, Garijo G, et al. Fine-needle aspiration cytology of columnar-cell carcinoma of the thyroid: report of two cases with cytohistologic correlation. Diagn Cytopathol 1998; 18:352-356.

368. Carney J, Ryan J, Goellner J. Hyalinizing trabecular adenoma of the thyroid gland. Am J Surg Pathol 1987; 11:583-591.

369. Bronner M, LiVolsi V, Jennigs T. PLAT: paraganglioma-like adenomas of the thyroid. Surg Pathol 1988; 1:383.

370. Hicks M, Batsakis J. Hyalinizing trabecular adenoma of the thyroid gland. Ann Otol Rhinol Laryngol 1993; 1993.

371. Katoh R, Jasani B, Williams E. Hyalinizing trabecular adenoma of the thyroid: a report of three cases with immunohistochemical and ultrastructural studies. Histopthology 1989; 15:211-224.

372. Cerasoli S, Tabarri B, Farabegoli P, et al. Hyalinizing trabecular adenoma of the thyroid: report of two cases, with cytologic, immunohistochemical and ultrastructural studies. Tumori 1992; 78:274-279.

373. Goellner J, Carney J. Cytologic features of fine-needle aspirates of hyalinizing trabecular adenoma of the thyroid. Am J Clin Pathol 1989; 91:115-119.

374. Strong C, Garcia B. Fine needle aspiration cytologic characteristics of hyalinizing trabecular adenoma of the thyroid. Acta Cytol 1990; 34:359-362.

375. Akin M, Nguyen G. Fine-needle aspiration biopsy cytology of hyalinizing trabecular adenomas of the thyroid. Diagn Cytopathol 1999; 20:90-94.

376. Bondeson L, Bondeson A-G. Clue helping to distinguish hyalinizing trabecular adenoma from carcinoma of the thyroid in fine-needle aspirates. Diagn Cytopathol 1994; 10:25-29.

377. Saad MF, Ordonez NG, Rashid RK, et al. Medullary carcinoma of the thyroid: a study of the clinical features and prognostic factors in 161 patients. Medicine 1984; 63:319-342.

378. Sipple J. The association of pheochromocytoma with carcinoma of the thyroid gland. Am J Med 1961; 31:163-166.

379. Manning P, Molnar G, Lack B, et al. Pheochromocytoma, hyperparathyroidism and thyroid carcinoma occurring coincidentally. N Engl J Med 1963; 268:249-265.

380. Schimke R. Multiple endocrine adenomatosis syndromes. Adv Intern Med 1976; 21:249-265.

381. Block M, Horn R, Miller J, Barrett J, Brush B. Familial medullary carcinoma of the thyroid. Ann Surg 1967; 166:403-412.

382. Freeman D. Medullary carcinoma of the thryoid gland: a clinicopathological study of 33 patients. Arch Pathol Lab Med 1965; 80:575-582.

383. Sizemore G. Medullary carcinoma of the thyroid gland. Semin Oncol 1987; 54:89-112.

384. Tashjian A, Melvin K. Medullary carcinoma of the thyroid gland. N Engl J Med 1968; 279:279-283.

385. Albores-Saavedra J, LiVolsi V, Williams E. Medullary carcinoma. Semin Diagn Pathol 1985; 2:137-146.

386. Halliday B, Silverman J, Finley J. Fine-needle aspiration cytology of amyloid associated with non-neoplastic and malignant lesions. Diagn Cytopathol 1998; 18:270-275.

387. Bose S, Kapila K, Verma K. Medullary carcinoma of the thyroid: a cytological, immunocytochemical, and ultrastructural study. Diagn Cytopathol 1992; 8:28-32.

388. Kini S, Miller J, Hamburger J. Cytopathologic features of medullary carcinoma of the thyroid. Arch Pathol Lab Med 1984; 108:156-159.

389. Kaur A, Jayaram G. Thyroid tumors: cytomorphology of medullary, clinically anaplastic, and miscellaneous thyroid neoplasms. Diagn Cytopathol 1990; 6:383-389.

390. Geddie S, Bedard Y, Strawbridge T. Medullary carcinoma of the thyroid in fine-needle aspiration biopsies. Am J Clin Pathol 1984; 82:552-558.

391. Mendonca M, Ramos S, Soares J. Medullary carcinoma of the thyroid: a re-evaluation of the ltytological criteria of diagnosis. Cytopathology 1991; 2:93-102.

392. Forrest C, Frost F, DeBoer W, et al. Medullary carcinoma of the thyroid: accuracy of diagnosis of fine-needle aspiration cytology. Cancer 1998; 84:295-302.

393. Green I, Ali S, Allen E, Zakowski M. A spectrum of cytomorphologic variations in medullary thyroid carcinoma: fine-needle aspiration findings in 19 cases. Cancer 1997; 81:40-44.

394. Boey J, Hsu C, Collins R. False-negative errors in fine-needle aspiration biopsy of dominant thyroid nodules: a prospective follow-up study. World J Surg 1986; 10:623-630.

395. Fukuzawa M, Maejima T, Sano K, et al. Immunohistochemical, electron microscopic, and immunoelectron microscopic features of plasmacytoma of the thyroid with amyloid deposition. Ultrastruct Pathol 1993; 17:681-686.

396. Uribe M, Fenoglio-Preiser CM, Grimes M, et al. Medullary carcinoma of the thyroid gland: clinical, pathological and immunohistochemical features with review of the literature. Am J Surg Pathol. 1985; 9:577-594.

397. Kumar P, Hodjati H, Monabati A, et al. Medullary thyroid carcinoma: rare cytologic findings. Acta Cytol 2000; 44:181-184.

398. Dominguez-Malagon H, Delgago-Chavez, Torres-Najera M, et al. Oxyphil and squamous variants of medullary thyroid carcinoma. Cancer 1989; 63:1183-1188.

399. Haleem A, Akhtar M, Ali M, et al. Fine-needle aspiration biopsy of mucus-producing medullary carcinoma of thyroid: report of a case with cytologic, histologic, and ultrastructural correlations. Diagn Cytopathol 1990; 6:112-117.

400. Landon G, Ordonez N. Clear cell variant of medullary carcinoma of the thyroid. Hum Pathol 1985; 16:844-847.

401. Mendelsohn G, Baylin SB, Bigner SH, Wells SA, et al. Anaplastic variants of medullary thyroid carcinoma: a light-microscopic and immunohistochemical study. Am J Surg Pathol 1980; 4:333-341.

402. Collins B, Cramer H, Tabatowski K, et al. Fine needle aspiration of medulary carcinoma of the thyroid: cytomorphology immunocytochemistry and electron microscopy. Acta Cytol 1995; 39:920-930.

403. Rosai J, Saxen E, Woolner L. Undifferentiated and poorly differentiated carcinoma. Semin Diagn Pathol 1985; 2: 123-136.

404. Lampertico P. Anaplastic (sarcomatoid) carcinoma of the thyroid gland. Semin Diagn Pathol 1993; 10:159.

405. Venkatesh Y, Ordonez N, Schultz P, et al. Anaplastic carcinoma of the thyroid: a clinicopathologic study of 121 cases. Cancer 1990; 66:321.

406. Nishiyama R, Dunn E, Thompson N. Anaplastic spindle-cell and giant cell tumors of the thyroid gland. Cancer 1972; 30:113-127.

407. Samaan N, Ordonez N. Uncommon types of thyroid cancer. Endocrinol Metab Clin North Am 1990; 19:637-648.

408. Brooke P, Hameed M, Zakowski M. Fine-needle aspiration of anaplastic thyroid carcinoma with varied cytologic and histologic patterns: a case report. Diagn Cytopathol 1994; 11:60-63.

409. Berry B, MacFarlane J, Chan N. Osteoclastoma-like anaplastic carcinoma of the thyroid: diagnosis by fine needle aspiration cytology. Acta Cytol 1990; 34:248-250.

410. Carcangiu M, Steeper T, Zampi G, et al. Anaplastic thyroid carcinoma: a study of 70 cases. Am J Clin Pathol 1985; 83:135-158.

411. Hurlimann J, Gardiol D, Scazziga B. Immunohistology of anaplastic thyroid carcinoma: a study of 43 cases. Histopathology 1987; 11:567-580.

412. Aozasa K, Inoue A, Tajima K, et al. Malignant lymphomas of the thyroid gland: analysis of 79 patients with emphasis on histologic prognostic factors. Cancer 1986; 58:100-104.

413. Shimaoka K, Sokal J, Pickren J. Metastatic noeplasms in the thyroid gland: pathological and clinical findings. Cancer 1962; 15:557-565.

414. Lam K, Lo C, Kwong D, Lee J, et al. Malignant lymphoma of the thyroid: a 30-year clinicopathologic experience and an evaluation of the presence of Epstein-Barr virus. Am J Clin Pathol 1999; 112:263-270.

415. Derringer G, Thompson L, Frommelt R, et al. Malignant lymphoma of the thyroid gland: a clinicopathologic study of 108 cases. Am J Surg Pathol 2000; 24:623-639.

416. Compagno J, Oertel J. Malignant lymphoma and other lymphoproliferative disorders of the thyroid gland: a clinicopthologic study of 245 cases. Am J Clin Pathol 1980; 74:1-11.

417. Burke J, Butler J, Fuller L. Malignant lymphomas of the thyiod: a clinical pathologic study of 35 patients including ultrastructural observations. Cancer 1977; 39:1587-1602.

418. Hamburger J, Miller J, Kini S. Lymphoma of the thyroid. Ann Intern Med 1983; 99:685-693.

419. Lovchik J, Lane M, Clark D. Polymerase chain reaction-based detection of B-cell clonality in the fine needle aspiration biopsy of a thyroid mucosa-associated lymphoid tissue (MALT) lymphoma. Hum Pathol 1997; 28:989-992.

420. Chak L, Hoppe R, Burke J, et al. Non-Hodgkin's lymphoma presenting as thyroid enlargement. Cancer 1981; 48:2712-2716.

421. Dunbar J, Lyall M, MacGillivray J, et al. T-cell lymphoma of the thyroid. Br Med J 1977; 2:679.

422. Vailati A, Marena C, Aristia L, et al. Primary Hodgkin's disease of the thyroid: report of a case and a review of the literature. Haematologica 1991; 76:69-71.

423. El-Halabi D, El-Sayed M, Eskaf W, et al. Langerhan's cell histiocytosis of the thyroid gland: a case report. Acta Cytol 2000; 44:805-808.

424. Kirchgraber P, Weaver M, Arafah B, et al. Fine needle aspiration cytology of Langerhan's cell histiocytosis involving the thyroid: a case review. Acta Cytol 1994; 38:101-106.

425. Jayaram G, Rani S, Raina V, et al. B cell lymphoma of the thyroid in Hashimoto's thyroiditis monitored by fine-needle aspiration cytology. Diagn Cytopathol 1990; 6:130-133.

426. Matsuda M, Sone H, Koyama H, et al. Fine-needle aspiration cytology of malignant lymphoma of the thyroid. Diagn Cytopathol 1987; 3:244-249.

427. Rhatigan R, Roque J, Bucher R. Mucoepidermoid carcinoma of the thyroid gland. Cancer 1977; 39:210-214.

428. Mizukami Y, Matsubara F, Hashimoto T, et al. Primary mucoepidermoid carcinoma in the thyroid gland. Cancer 1984; 53:1741-1745.

429. Nguyen G-K, Vogelsang P, Schumann G. Follicular carcinoma of the thyroid with an adenoid cystic pattern: report of a case with aspiration biopsy cytology, immunohistochemistry and electron microscopy. Acta Cytol 1993; 37:740-744.

430. Geisinger K, Steffe C, McGee R, et al. The cytomorphologic features of sclerosing mucoepidermoid carcinoma of the thyroid gland with eosinophilia. Am J Clin Pathol 1998; 109:294-301.

431. Carcangiu M, Zammpi G, Rosai J. Poorly differentiated (insular) thyroid carcinoma. Am J Surg Pathol 1984; 8:655-668.

432. Papotti M, Micca F, Favero A, et al. Poorly differentiated thyroid carcinomas with primordial cell component: a group of aggressive lesions sharing insular, trabecular and solid patterns. Am J Surg Pathol 1993; 17:291-301.

433. Pietribiasi F, Saino A, Papotti M, et al. Cytologic features of poorly differentiated "insular" carcinoma of the thyroid, as revealed by fine-needle aspiation biopsy. Am J Clin Pathol 1990; 94:687-692.

434. Flynn S, Forman B, Stewart A, et al. Poorly differentiated (insular) carcinoma of the thyroid gland: an aggressive subset of differentiated thyroid neoplasms. Surgery 1988; 104:963-970.

435. Kuhel W, Kutler D, Santos-Buch C. Poorly differentiated insular thyroid carcinoma: a case report with identification of intact insular with fine needle aspiration biopsy. Acta Cytol 1998; 42:991-997.

436. Guiter G, Auger M, Ali S, et al. Cytopathology of insular carcinoma of the thyroid. Cancer 1999; 87:196-202.

437. Layfield L, Gopez E. Insular carcinoma of the thyroid: report of a case with intact insular and microfollicular structures. Diagn Cytopathol 2000; 23:409-413.

438. Mortenson J, Woolner L, Bennett W. Secondary malignant tumors of the thyroid gland. Cancer 1965; 19:306-309.

439. Ivy H. Cancer metastatic to the thyroid gland: a diagnostic problem. Mayo Clin Proc 1984; 59:856-859.

440. Schmid K, Hittmair A, Ofner C, et al. Metastatic tumors in fine needle aspiration biopsy of the thyroid. Acta Cytol 1991; 35:722-724.

441. Fanning T, Katz R. Evaluation of thyroid nodules in cancer patients. Acta Cytol 1986; 30:572.

442. Watts N. Carcinoma metastatic to the thyroid: Prevalence and diagnosis by fine-needle aspiration cytology. Am J Med Sci 1987; 293:13-17.

443. Chacho M, Greenebaum E, Moussouris H, et al. Value of aspiration cytology of the thyroid in metastatic disease. Acta Cytol 1987; 31:705-712.

444. Lam K, Lo C. Metastatic tumors of the thyroid gland: a study of 79 cases in Chinese patients. Arch Pathol Lab Med 1998; 122:37-41.

445. Chen H, Nicol T, Udelsman R. Clinically significant, isolated metastatic disease to the thyroid gland. World J Surg 1999; 23:177-180.

446. Nakhjavani M, Gharib H, Goellner J, et al. Metastasis to the thyroid gland: a report of 43 cases. Cancer 1997; 79:574-578.

447. Judkins A, Roberts S, LiVolsi V. Utility of immunohistochemistry in the evaluation of necrotic thyroid tumors. Hum Pathol 1999; 30:1373-1376.

448. Bejarano P, Nikiforov Y, Swenson E, et al. Thyroid transcription factor-1, thyroglobulin, cytokeratin 7, and cytokeratin 20 in thyroid neoplasms. Appl Immunohistochem Molecul Morphol 2000; 8:189-194.

449. Huang T-Y, Assor D. Primary squamous cell carcinoma of the thyroid gland: a report of four cases. Am J Clin Pathol 1971; 55:93-98.

450. Simpson W, Carruthers J. Squamous cell carcinoma of the thyroid gland. Am J Surg 1988; 156:44-46.

451. Kumar P, Malekhusseini S, Talei A. Primary squamous cell carcinoma of the thyroid diagnosed by fine needle aspiration cytology: a report of two cases. Acta Cytol 1999; 43:659-662.

452. Carcangiu M, Sibley R, Rosai J. Clear cell change in primary thyroid tumors. Am J Surg Pathol 1985; 9:705-722.

453. Civantis F, Albores-Saavedra J, Nadji M, et al. Clear cell variant of thyroid carcinoma. Am J Surg Pathol 1984; 8:187-192.

454. Harach H, Virgilil E, Soler G, et al. Cytopathology of follicular tumors of the thyroid with clear cell change. Cytopathology 1991; 2:125-135.

455. Halbauer M, Kardum-Skelin I, Vranesic D, et al. Aspiration cytology of renal-cell carcinoma metastatic to the thyroid. Acta Cytol 1991; 35:443-446.

456. Gritsman A, Popok S, Ro J, et al. Renal-cell carcinoma with intranuclear inclusions metastatic to thyroid: a diagnostic problem in aspiration cytology. Diagn Cytopathol 1988; 4:125-129.

457. Linsk J, Franzen A. Aspiration cytology of metastatic hypernephroma. Acta Cytol 1984; 28:250-260.

458. Hughes J, Jensen C, Donnelly A, et al. The role of fine-needle aspiration cytology in the evaluation of metastatic clear cell tumors. Cancer 1999; 87:380-389.

459. Nishiyama R, Bigos S, Goldfarb W, et al. The efficacy of simultaneous fine-needle aspiration and large-needle biopsy of the thyroid gland. Surgery 1986; 100:1133-1137.

460. Miller J. Evaluation of thyroid nodules: accent on needle biopsy. Med Clin North Am 1985; 69:1063-1077.

461. Schwartz A, Nieburgs H, Davies T, et al. The place of fine needle biopsy in the diagnosis of nodules of the thyroid. Surg Gynecol Obstet 1982; 155:54-58.

462. Liu Q, Castelli M, Gattuso P, et al. Simultaneous fine-needle aspiration and core-needle biopsy of thyroid nodules. Am Surg 1995; 61:628-633.

463. Keller M, Crabbe M, Norwood S. Accuracy and significance of fine-needle aspiration and frozen section in determining the extent of thyroid resection. Surgery 1987; 101:632-635.

464. Shaha A, DiMario T, Webber C, et al. Intraoperative decision making during thyroid surgery based on the results of preoperative needle biopsy and frozen section. Surgery 1990; 108:964-971.

465. McHenry C, Rosen I, Walfish P. Influence of fine-needle aspiration biopsy and frozen section examination on the management of thyroid cancer. Am J Surg 1993; 166:353-356.

466. Rodriquez J, Parrilla P, Sola J. Comparison between preoperative cytology and intraoperative frozen-section biopsy in the diagnosis of thyroid nodules. Br J Surg 1994; 81:1151-1154.

467. Chang H, Lin J, Chen J, et al. Correlation of fine needle aspiration cytology and frozen section biopsies in the diagnosis of thyroid nodules. J Clin Pathol 1997; 50:1005-1009.

468. Paphavasit A, Thompson G, Hay I, et al. Follicular and Hürthle cell thyroid neoplasms: is frozen section evaluation worthwhile? Arch Surg 1997; 132:674-679.

469. Hamburger J, Hamburger S. Declining role of frozen section in surgical planning for thyroid nodules. Surgery 1985; 98:307-312.

470. Kopald K, Layfield L, Mohrmann R, et al. Clarifying the role of fine-needle aspiration cytologic evaluation and frozen section examination in the operative management of thyroid cancer. Arch Surg 1989; 124:1201-1205.

471. Chow T, Venu V, Kwok S. Use of fine-needle aspiration cytology and frozen section examination in diagnosis of thyroid nodules. Aust N Z J Surg 1999; 69:131-133.

472. Basolo F, Baloch Z, Baldanzi A, et al. Usefulness of Ultrafast Papanicolaou-stained scrape preparations in intraoperative management of thyroid lesions. Mod Pathol 1999; 12:653-657.

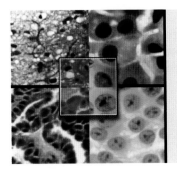

Salivary Gland Masses

CHAPTER
27

 GENERAL CONSIDERATIONS

Approaches to Salivary Gland Fine-Needle Aspiration

Considered in its entirety, the literature outlines three general approaches for using fine-needle aspiration (FNA) to address salivary gland masses[1,2] (Box 27-1). Some believe that FNA should be employed early and often, perhaps playing a role in most masses in this area. However, citing significant false-negative and false-positive rates for diagnosis of salivary gland neoplasms, others feel that this technique should be reserved almost exclusively for triage of new masses arising in patients with an established history of head and neck malignancy.

Other workers are even more restrictive in their application of FNA to the salivary glands. These physicians not only cite limited diagnostic accuracy but also mention the types of post-FNA infarction and repair that they feel might ultimately limit histologic interpretation of tissues excised after preoperative FNA. Thus, while agreeing that FNA has a place in evaluation of lymph node enlargements and thyroid disease, confirmation of suspected infectious or inflammatory masses, and in demonstration of recurrent malignancy, these investigators would argue that FNA does not merit inclusion in schemes for salivary gland mass evaluation. Unanimity of approach will not be achieved in the near future. The authors' experience indicates that when efficient, high-quality FNA services are available, many head and neck surgeons embrace the method, using it very early in the evaluation of most masses.

Accuracy of Salivary Gland Mass Diagnosis by Fine-Needle Aspiration

Reliable accuracy measures can be difficult to obtain because some series are small. Furthermore, some authors exclude unsatisfactory or nondiagnostic cases from summary calculations, whereas others do not. Several papers tabulate relatively numerous aspirations that contain only normal tissues. Without more detailed information than is often published, many reviewers would consider these unsatisfactory, or at least *nondiagnostic.* Definitions of false-negative FNA also vary. For example, some feel that a Warthin's tumor interpreted cytologically as chronic inflammation would represent a false-negative diagnosis; others would not. A sparsely cellular aspirate showing mostly mucus may suggest low-grade mucoepidermoid carcinoma and should direct further clinical investigations toward the appropriate interventions. However, the FNA report for such an aspirate rarely contains an unequivocal diagnosis of malignancy so that this aspiration may be considered as a false negative for the purpose of publishing statistical accuracy assessments. However, is this clinically useful report a false negative? Would the patient have benefited from having the FNA considered unsatisfactory?

True false-negative interpretations, however, remain a problem. Most involve malignancies that yield sparsely cellular smears or contain only cells of low cytologic grade. In other instances, rare diagnostic elements are overwhelmed by copious benign tissue or inflammatory cells. Low-grade mucoepidermoid carcinoma, small cell malignant lymphoma, acinic cell carcinoma, and Hodgkin's disease may result in samples with these problems. Others result from sampling error, particularly when small metastatic deposits are evaluated.

Thus, one should interpret published accuracy figures for salivary gland FNA cautiously. Using detection of malignancy as the diagnostic goal, sensitivity rates range from 64% to 100%, whereas those for specificity are usually much higher (94% to 100%). Given the low-grade mucoepidermoid carcinoma scenario cited in the preceding paragraph, published rates for unsatisfactory aspirations are also subject to interpretation. Such figures in part reflect procedural and interpretive skills, as well as the experience and orientation of the individuals involved. Overall nondiagnostic rates for salivary gland or general head and neck FNA are approximately 10% in most series, but some report up to 21%.

It is useful to compare FNA with the only other major means for rapid tissue diagnosis, the intraoperative frozen section applied to surgically excised tissues. Aspiration actually allows more time for reflection, consultation and special studies than does frozen section analyses that are performed during surgery. The rates for correct recognition of malignancy by these two procedures are similar in many studies and can be as low as 60%. Some series show FNA to be slightly more accurate, whereas others suggest that frozen sections lead to fewer diagnostic errors. Both meth-

BOX 27-1

Clinical Approaches to Salivary Gland Fine-Needle Aspiration

Use fine-needle aspiration (FNA) early and often for most salivary gland masses
Use FNA rarely, and only in special circumstances
Use FNA for thyroid and cervical lymph nodes but not for the salivary glands

BOX 27-2

Factors Complicating Salivary Gland Tumor Diagnosis by Fine-Needle Aspiration

Great tumor diversity
Many tumors are rare
Some malignancies are cytologically low grade
A variety of secondary alterations is shared by several tumors
The same types of neoplasms can occur in many sites, often outside the major glands
The same types of neoplasms can arise in aberrantly situated salivary gland tissue

ods can lead to false-positive and false-negative diagnoses; both have been blamed for unnecessarily radical surgery resulting from false-positive interpretations.

Higher-grade malignancies are more readily interpreted both in FNA and on frozen sections, and accuracy figures for both tests will depend in part on the case mix in the material available for review. Uncommon malignancies, low-grade (mucoepidermoid) carcinomas, cystic (or partially cystic) masses, and complex lesions with multiple components (some mixed tumors and most carcinomas ex pleomorphic adenoma) may be very difficult to interpret using either medium of rapid diagnosis. Inflammatory and fibrotic masses are also likely to be difficult.

One important consequence of these observations is that diagnostic problems remaining after FNA may not be addressed effectively by intraoperative frozen sections. Even though recommending cryostat "confirmation" for difficult cytologic diagnoses is a common practice, resolution of diagnostic problems may not be possible until well after completion of the surgery, when paraffin-embedded permanent sections become available. The parallels between FNA and surgical pathology are so extensive and so compelling that, if a case is difficult at FNA, it is likely to be just as difficult at the time of frozen section. Both methods have limitations, and these often converge on the same residuum of very difficult diagnoses.

Some have found that using combined FNA and frozen section improves the overall accuracy of salivary gland diagnosis prior to definitive resection. Some investigators suggest that both methods should be applied to the majority of patients in whom surgery for salivary gland tumors is performed. Because the complication rate of FNA is negligible, repeated aspiration of clinically worrisome masses can be safely employed as necessary. Furthermore, even if FNA fails to provide useful information, it will have cost relatively little and caused virtually no delay in application of other diagnostic approaches.

Many physicians feel that FNA is a useful test for preoperative evaluation of salivary gland masses. However, the foregoing brief overview indicates that this test has areas of considerable interpretational difficulty, as well as occasional false-positive and false-negative results. Reasons for these problems include the extraordinary diversity of morphology in salivary gland neoplasms and the fact that many are rare. The low-grade cytology of some malignancies and the frequent superimposition of inflammation or cystic change on many masses exacerbate this already difficult situation. The former is in contrast with the fact that the most common cause of false-positive diagnoses is "atypia" in benign

mixed tumors. Thus, the authors feel that salivary gland FNA is useful, only if performed and interpreted with skill and experience and if its limitations are kept in mind.

INTRODUCTION TO SALIVARY GLAND CYTOLOGY

The salivary glands host an extraordinary array of mass lesions. Many of these can be complicated by cystic alterations, inflammation, clear cell change, or metaplasias of various types. For these reasons, the cytologic range of any given type of mass can be very broad. Interpretation is made even more difficult by the fact that many tumors are so uncommon that most of us do not acquire adequate experience (Box 27-2).

The complexity of head and neck anatomy also makes it difficult to determine the site of origin for some lesions. Tumors can seem to be in the lower parotid, when they may actually represent the gland itself, a lymph node within the parotid, a cervical lymph node that is not within the parotid, a lateral neck cyst, a dermal-based mass, or a soft tissue swelling. In some instances, FNA may direct clinical thinking by providing confirmation of the mass's location, even if a specific diagnosis is not obtained.

The authors' approach to the cytology of these diverse masses is based on the differential diagnosis of certain key pictures that are usually apparent early in the evaluation of a case (Box 27-3). Most of these are common to a number of lesions so that a list of differential diagnostic possibilities flows from our recital of each key finding. The next step is identification of additional features that indicate a more specific diagnosis or that permit refinement of the list of possible diagnoses. If neither of these is possible, then it must be recognized that one of the limits inherent in salivary gland cytology has been reached.

This chapter is organized around these key findings that often form one's first impression of an aspirate. Lesions that are cytologically similar or even indistinguishable (e.g., mixed tumor, benign metastasizing mixed tumor, and most examples of carcinoma ex pleomorphic adenoma) are discussed together. This scheme is more useful in organizing differential diagnostic thinking than the traditional catalog of benign lesions followed by a list of malignancies.

The discussion that follows attempts to recapitulate and illustrate the thinking that goes into our cytologic interpre-

BOX **27-3**

Initial Classification of Salivary Gland Aspirates

Normal salivary gland tissues (acinar, ductal)
Normal tissues from adjacent sites
Inflammation (acute, chronic, granulomatous, with crystal formation)
Pleomorphic adenoma
Warthin's tumor
Cysts
Epithelial neoplasms of small cell type
Epithelial neoplasms of large cells with low nuclear grade
Epithelial neoplasms of large cells with high nuclear grade
Spindle cell processes with low nuclear grade
Spindle cell neoplasms with high nuclear grade
Hematopoietic lesions

BOX **27-5**

Salivary Gland Masses that May Have Lymphoid Stroma

Sialadenitis
Cystic lesions due to duct obstruction
Warthin's tumor
Sebaceous lymphadenoma
Lymphoepithelial cyst
Lymphoepithelial lesion
Oncocytic lesions
Acinic cell carcinoma
Mucoepidermoid carcinoma
Primary lymphoepithelioma-like carcinoma
Metastatic lymphoepithelioma
Other metastatic malignancies

BOX **27-4**

Cytologic Findings Shared by Many Salivary Gland Masses

Lymphoid stoma
Cystic change
Clear cell alterations
Oncocytic cells
Sebaceous differentiation

BOX **27-6**

Salivary Gland Masses that May Have Cystic Change

Congenital cysts
Human immunodeficiency virus (HIV)–associated cysts
Stones or other obstructive lesions
Pleomorphic adenoma
Monomorphic adenoma
Warthin's tumor
Mucoepidermoid carcinoma
Acinic cell carcinoma
Metastatic carcinoma
Malignant lymphoma

tation of these complex masses. These discussions include occasional lesions that are not salivary gland tumors but that must be considered in certain cytologic situations. Pleomorphic adenoma and Warthin's tumor are sufficiently common and (usually) distinctive to be listed as primary considerations around which thinking can be organized. The other categories result from the authors' initial impressions of an aspirate and may eventuate in a variety of final diagnoses. Some tumor types appear in more than one category, reflecting the complexity of certain differential diagnoses. Such lesions are discussed in the context of their most common or vexing mimics.

Clinical Expectations

Most clinically apparent salivary gland masses are located in the parotid. A smaller number can be found in the submaxillary glands, and occasional lesions occur in the sublingual gland or in submucosal minor salivary glands. Furthermore, approximately 20% of individuals harbor accessory parotid tissue along Stenson's duct. The parotid may have an anteriorly situated facial lobe. Heterotopic salivary gland tissue may occur in several head and neck sites.[1] Accordingly, a wide range of salivary gland masses, including malignancies, may occasionally be found in unusual locations. These tumors must be considered, despite clinical suggestions that the lesion may be based in other tissues. Up to 50% of aberrantly located salivary gland neoplasms are malignant, with mucoepidermoid carcinoma being the most common type.

The patients' age range and one's referral patterns influence the types of salivary gland masses likely to be encountered. Pathologists who often study material from patients with acquired immune deficiency syndrome (AIDS) are more likely to see masses from younger individuals with a correspondingly low rate of malignancy, especially carcinomas. It has been said that 80% or parotid tumors are benign and that 80% of these represent pleomorphic adenoma. In more detailed studies, it was noted that 71% to 96% of parotid tail masses unaccompanied by clinical signs of malignancy (pain, facial nerve damage, trismus, or fixation) represented mixed tumors (sensitivity of 88% to 91%, with specificities of 50% to 84%, respectively). Spontaneous pleomorphic adenoma infarction associated with pain is rare.

Cytologic Features Shared by Several Lesions

Several cytologic features overlap a number of diagnoses. Lymphoid stroma, sebaceous differentiation, cystic change, squamous metaplasia, clear cell change, and oncocytic features are all cytologic findings present in several types of masses (Boxes 27-4 to 27-9). Care must clearly be exercised in using these as important diagnostic criteria. Taken alone, each outlines only a differential diagnosis. This overlap contributes to the difficulty of salivary gland cytology and

BOX 27-7

Salivary Gland Masses that May Have Clear Cell Alterations

Mucoepidermoid carcinoma
Acinic cell carcinoma
Oncocytic lesions
Epithelial-myoepithelial carcinoma
Adenocarcinoma
Clear cell carcinoma
Some metastatic carcinomas

BOX 27-8

Salivary Gland Masses that May Have Oncocytic Cells

Warthin's tumor
Pleomorphic adenoma
Mucoepidermoid carcinoma (rarely)
Acinic cell carcinoma
Oncocytic lesions
Oncocytoid adenocarcinoma
Metastatic Hürthle cell carcinoma

BOX 27-9

Salivary Gland Masses that May Have Sebaceous Differentiation

Normal salivary tissue (all sites)
Sebaceous adenoma
Sebaceous lymphadenoma
Monomorphic adenoma
Pleomorphic adenoma
Warthin's tumor
Mucoepidermoid carcinoma

BOX 27-10

Cytomorphologic Features of Normal Salivary Gland Tissue

Rounded clusters of acinar cells
Flat sheets of uniform ductal cells
Tubular structures composed of ductal cells
Variable numbers of adipocytes
Naked nuclei of damaged acinar cells
Granulovacuolar background debris from damaged
    acinar cells

BOX 27-11

Sialosis

Nonneoplastic, noninflammatory, nonpainful enlargement
Usually bilateral
Parotids involved more often than submandibular glands
Idiopathic or associated with other conditions
Fine-needle aspiration yields normal-appearing salivary
    gland tissue
Enlargement of nuclei and cells detected by morphometry

serves to emphasize the need for excellent specimen collection and diagnostic limitations of the method. Although each of these may be cytologically impressive or may even be the predominant attribute, each is useful only in concert with other features. As evidence of this approach, the authors note that none of these findings figures into the first level of our rapid triage approach to salivary gland FNA.

ASPIRATION OF NORMAL SALIVARY GLAND TISSUE OR ADIPOSE TISSUE

The authors have previously commented on the fact that in some series, up to 20% of salivary gland aspirates yield only normal tissue. Cytologically, this shows acinar cells in characteristic round, basket-like arrangements. These oval to wedge-shaped cells have small, uniform, eccentrically placed round nuclei surrounded by abundant granular or vacuolated cytoplasm. Ductal tissue fragments manifest the honeycomb cell arrangement typical of many benign glandular tissues. Often, large branching duct fragments are present. These two types of tissue may be closely associated or

may be found separately. Variable numbers of adipocytes accompany these epithelial elements (Figure 27-1). Acinar cells are large and fragile, so that smears usually show some cell damage. As a result, naked acinar cell nuclei and granulovacuolar cytoplasmic debris may litter the smear background. These naked nuclei should not be interpreted as lymphocytes. Hematopoietic cells should be required to show a thin, intact rim of basophilic cytoplasm for positive identification. Both lymphocytes and the cytoplasmic residua of damaged acinar cells are more easily assessed in air-dried than in fixed material (Box 27-10).

Sialosis

This nonneoplastic salivary gland enlargement shows no evidence of inflammation and does not cause pain. The increase in size is slowly progressive, and the lesion has often been present for months or years before diagnosis. Physical examination shows a doughy swelling without distinct borders.[4,5] Most cases are bilateral, and the parotids are more commonly involved than the submandibular glands. Sialosis may be associated with nutritional deficiencies. Hence, the term *nutritional mumps*. Other patients experience diabetes mellitus, alcoholism, cirrhosis, or endocrine deficiencies. Still other examples have been associated with drugs such as phenylbutazone, iodine-containing compounds, some antibiotics, and adrenergic agents. Many cases are idiopathic (Box 27-11).

The affected glands show normal histologic architecture, but the acinar cells are said to be hypertrophic, with abundant cytoplasm. In one FNA study, aspiration of four bilateral parotid examples of sialosis were more cellular than most aspirates of normal tissue but did not include lymphocytes. (The authors' experience suggests that the latter observation would be very difficult to use as a diagnostic criterion in an individual case because most high-quality aspirates of normal tissue are very cellular.) The mean aci-

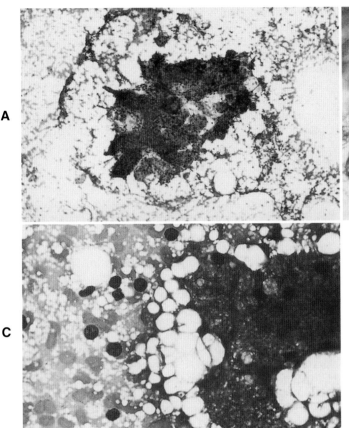

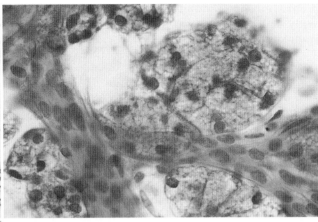

Figure 27-1 **Normal parotid tissue. A,** This low magnification image shows a large cohesive fragment of normal parotid tissue. An arborizing network of ducts is surrounded by acinar tissue. (Papanicolaou [Pap]) **B,** The ducts in this normal parotid tissue are composed of small uniform cells. The acinar cells are larger, with abundant granular cytoplasm and innocuous-appearing nuclei. (Pap) **C,** In air-dried smears the acinar cells' cytoplasm stains darkly. During the smearing process, some cells are damaged. Their cytoplasm forms a granular or bubbly background while their nuclei are stripped. The latter should not be mistaken for lymphocytes. (Diff-Quik [DQ]) (From Geisinger K, Silverman J. Fine needle aspiration cytology of superficial organs and body sites. New York: Churchill-Livingstone; 1999.)

nar cell diameter in sialosis (75 μm) was significantly greater than that of normal parotid tissue (56 μm). The utility of this diagnostic criterion remains to be more fully investigated. In contrast with the bilateral nature of sialosis, symptomatic stones are usually unilateral. Clinicopathologic comparisons of sialosis, lipoma, lipomatosis, and sampling error are discussed next.

Salivary Gland Lipomatosis and Lipomas

Aspiration of normal adipose tissue from salivary gland enlargements may suggest lipoma.[6] Clinically, these masses are soft and boggy, thus resembling Warthin's tumors, but are less often bilateral. The cytologic impression of a lipoma can be confirmed, when computed tomography (CT) or magnetic resonance imaging (MRI) images show a lesion with the density of fat that is located within the gland.

Bilateral fatty infiltration (lipomatosis) is similar to sialosis at physical examination and can share some of the same endocrine, metabolic, or drug-related associations. Acinar enlargement can also be noted. Radiographic studies show diffuse infiltration of the glands with tissue of fatty density rather than a mass. Sialosis and lipomatosis may give identical FNA findings, and it has been suggested that lipomatosis represents an end stage of sialosis.

Aspirates Showing Only Normal Salivary Gland Tissue

Sialosis, lipoma, and lipomatosis are uncommon conditions not often encountered in most FNA practices. Without strong clinical and radiographic support of the types previously described, recovery of such material from a mass le-

BOX 27-12

Differential Diagnosis of Aspirates Showing Normal Acinar, Ductal, or Adipose Tissue

The aspirator missed the target lesion
Sialosis
Lipoma
Lipomatosis
Except for the first, each of these is rare

sion is usually interpreted as nondiagnostic or unsatisfactory (Box 27-12). This stance is often reasonable, and it is motivated by a desire to minimize false-negative diagnoses that result from sampling error. However, given excellent aspiration technique and careful clinical correlation, selected examples of sialosis can be diagnosed or at least suggested by FNA. Furthermore, small masses that would previously have been followed without sampling often make very challenging FNA targets. Some of these will not be successfully aspirated, and this may explain the relatively frequent identification of normal tissue in some series.

When only normal or hypertrophic acinar tissue is recovered by FNA, one may consider a diagnosis of acinic cell carcinoma. If the aspirate material is reasonably cellular and adequately representative, the intimate admixture of ductal elements with acinar tissue will eliminate this consideration. Whether a small lesion has been missed altogether is more difficult to ascertain. In the authors' series reviewing normal tissue aspirated from 18 unilateral and two bilateral parotid or submandibular gland enlargements, the only missed neoplasm that subsequently came to light was a single pleomorphic adenoma measuring 0.5 cm in diameter; this lesion was correctly diagnosed by repeat FNA.[3] An example of false-negative findings in a metastatic squamous cell carcinoma has also been reported.

These data suggest that if physical examination, FNA, and follow-up are well performed and carefully coordinated, then the chance of missing a significant neoplasm is probably low. However, in situations that are less than ideal, aspiration of normal tissue from a salivary gland mass should still be considered evidence that the lesion has probably not been targeted accurately. FNA is easy to repeat and enjoys excellent patient acceptance. In many instances, repeat aspiration may be all that is needed to resolve problems related to sampling.[1]

Interestingly, the findings presented previously suggest that the clinical definition of sialosis might be expanded to include masses that are unilateral, submandibular, or unassociated with other clinical problems. Acinar diameter measurements deserve further evaluation in this regard.

 INFLAMMATORY SALIVARY GLAND MASSES

One of the immediate benefits of successful FNA is that it can quickly triage mass lesions into either inflammatory or neoplastic categories. Most of the former do not require surgery. In the salivary glands, relatively few masses referred for FNA are inflammatory. The most common clinical causes of sialadenitis include mumps and sialolithiasis. Mumps does not require cytologic diagnosis, and stone disease is rarely addressed by these means. Although inflammatory in their primary manifestations, duct obstructive lesions (including sialolithiasis) are discussed later with the cystic lesions because this is the category in which most of the relevant differential diagnostic considerations are to be found.

Acute Inflammation

Diagnosis of infectious salivary gland lesions by FNA is uncommon. Still, these may be seen in patients with AIDS or as lesions resulting from duct obstruction, such as those caused by stones. Most purulent aspirates are regarded as nonspecific, but material for cultures should be obtained. Aspirates of a purulent mass show a mixture of inflammatory cells dominated by neutrophils, fibrin, and debris. Necrotic neoplasms can give rise to acute inflammation so

that a careful search for malignant cells is also required. However, in the setting of marked acute inflammation, cells shed from the normal salivary glands may show striking cytologic atypia. Cautious interpretation is required, if one is to avoid false-positive diagnoses of malignancy. In most cases, a diagnosis of salivary gland carcinoma in the presence of acute inflammation is in error. A tumor, usually metastatic would need to manifest obvious high-grade malignant nuclear features for a diagnosis of cancer.

Chronic Inflammation and Its Differential Diagnosis

A wide variety of salivary gland mass lesions may be accompanied by chronic inflammatory cells (Table 27-1; see Box 27-5). When other diagnostic elements are not seen or are scanty, many of these aspirates are interpreted cytologically as nonspecific chronic inflammation. Some aspirates with chronic inflammatory cells represent hyperplastic intraparotid lymph nodes. Lymphoid proliferations that persist after FNA are suggestive of a neoplasm. The neoplasm that is most commonly mistaken for inflammation is the Warthin's tumor, from which oncocytes may be difficult to recover. This difficulty is the result of sampling error in a partially cystic lesion.

In addition to mixed acute and chronic inflammatory cells and foam cells, aspirates from chronic inflammatory lesions may show squamous metaplasia or stringy extracellular mucus and epithelial atypia as described in acute inflammation. Such features may lead to an erroneous diagnosis of mucoepidermoid carcinoma. This error can be very difficult to avoid, given the occasional occurrence of considerable chronic inflammation in aspirates from this malignancy. Fibrotic masses may yield sparely cellular nondiagnostic aspirates. Alternatively, fragments of metachromatic, fibrillary, collagenous stroma may be reminiscent of the matrix of pleomorphic adenomas. The previously described distinction between acinar cell nuclei and lymphocytes is useful in avoiding an erroneous diagnosis of acinic cell carcinoma in some cases of chronic sialadenitis.

Postirradiation sialadenitis is characterized by chronic inflammation, fibrosis, and acinar atrophy; the duct system is usually somewhat preserved. Clinically, this can cause very firm glands that are difficult to distinguish from carcinoma. Aspirates are often scanty and may show variable degrees of cytologic atypia. Cohesion within cell groups usually suggests a benign condition, but clusters of duct cells can mimic squamous cell carcinoma or low-grade mucoepidermoid carcinoma. Other salient features of these neoplasms should be

TABLE 27-1		
Errors in Diagnosis of Sialadenitis		
Type of Inflammation	**Cytologic Feature that may be Present**	**Erroneous Diagnosis**
Neutrophilic	Reactive epithelial cell atypia	Carcinoma
Lymphocytic	Lymphocytes mixed with various epithelial and stromal components	See Box 27-5
Mixed	Squamous metaplasia, mucous, cytologic atypia	Low-grade mucoepidermoid carcinoma
Fibrosis	Decreased cellularity, metachromatic collagen	Pleomorphic adenoma
Postradiation	Fibrosis and atypia	Carcinoma

sought, especially in difficult cases. Specimens with marked radiation-associated cytologic atypia have been mistaken for undifferentiated carcinoma. Diagnostic accuracy can be improved when the cytopathologist draws on experience gained from body sites in which this type of atypia is more commonly encountered. These include the lungs (Chapter 15) and the uterine cervix (Chapter 4).

The benign lymphoepithelial cyst in patients with AIDS and the benign lymphoepithelial lesion associated with Sjøgren's syndrome are discussed when cystic lesions are considered. Aspirates contain polymorphous lymphocytes, plasma cells, macrophages, and germinal center fragments. Lacking epimyoepithelial cell clusters or groups of spindled myoepithelial cells, this cytologic picture is nonspecific, and the diagnosis must be supported by clinicopathologic correlation. The most common alternative interpretation is Warthin's tumor. The lymphoid tissue of this neoplasm is more monomorphous and less likely to show germinal center fragments than the benign lymphoepithelial lesion. The finding of chronic inflammation and stone-like fragments requires distinction from sialolithiasis by clinical criteria. Another consideration, the malignant lymphoepithelial lesion, is discussed subsequently, when it is contrasted with other malignancies that show mostly small cells.

Hematopoietic neoplasms are discussed in other chapters, and only specific observations related to the salivary glands are summarized here. Ideally, one would like to identify these lesions in FNA samples so that the necessary studies can be instituted; in many cases, surgery can and should be avoided. Reactive lymphocytes may be confused with cells representing a low-grade malignant lymphoma. Usually, however, they are more polymorphous than their neoplastic counterparts. Nevertheless, aspiration of well-differentiated lymphoid neoplasms often leads to false-negative diagnoses because they are thought to represent lesions such as Warthin's tumor, congenital cyst, intragland lymph nodes, or benign inflammation. Mixtures of reactive and neoplastic lymphoid elements may further complicate the diagnosis, with polymorphism that belies the nature of the underlying process. In salivary gland lymphomas of the MALT type, residual entrapped epithelial cells can lead to an erroneous diagnosis of a benign lymphoepithelial lesion. High-grade hematopoietic neoplasms are more readily recognized as malignant but may be mistaken for small cell carcinoma. Difficulties are minimized, if high technical standards attend specimen preparation (Chapter 2). Consideration of the patient's previous history and application of marker studies resolve most difficult cases.

Hodgkin's disease is encountered only rarely in salivary gland aspirates. The possibility of false-negative diagnoses has been mentioned; these occur when Reed-Sternberg cells are rare or absent. Such cases are usually thought to represent nonspecific chronic inflammation. Other examples have been confused with pleomorphic adenoma, metastatic carcinoma, malignant melanoma, and undifferentiated carcinoma. Acute leukemia in salivary gland aspirates is rarely described (Table 27-2). Diagnosis and characterization of hematopoietic neoplasms with immunophenotyping and cytogenetic studies are considered more fully in Chapter 24.

Granulomatous Inflammation

Granulomatous sialadenitis may be either unilateral or bilateral but is an uncommon FNA diagnosis in salivary gland sites. A number of etiologic factors must be considered. Sarcoidosis may involve the salivary glands or intraglandular lymph nodes. Rupture of salivary gland ducts or cysts leads to extravasation of secretory material that can precipitate a giant cell reaction and mesenchymal repair. Furthermore, this reactive pattern may be superimposed on a variety of benign and malignant processes. In low-grade mucoepidermoid carcinomas, for example, atypia in benign stromal cells reacting to mucus extravasation can far outweigh that of the carcinoma cells, leading to a rather confusing FNA picture (Figure 27-2).

TABLE 27-2	
Diagnostic Errors in Hodgkin's Disease Cytology	
Cytologic Difficulty	**Erroneous Diagnosis**
RS cells absent or not identified	Benign lymphoid hyperplasia
	Warthin's tumors
	Other lymphocyte-rich process (see Box 27-5)
Mononuclear RS cells mistaken for myoepithelial cells	Pleomorphic adenoma
Mononuclear RS cells mistaken for epithelial cells	Primary or metastatic carcinoma
RS cells (typical or mononuclear) located but not identified correctly	Malignant melanoma

RS, Reed-Sternberg.

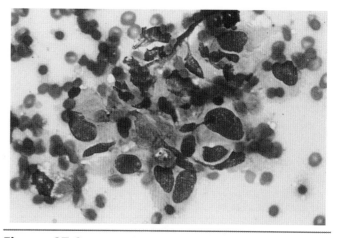

Figure 27-2 **Pseudomalignant reactive stromal cell atypia.** This group of atypical spindle cells was present in an otherwise sparsely cellular aspirate from a low-grade mucoepidermoid carcinoma. (DQ) (From Geisinger K, Silverman J. Fine needle aspiration cytology of superficial organs and body sites. New York: Churchill-Livingstone; 1999.)

Sialadenitis With Crystal Formation

This special type of sialadenitis is uncommon in FNA material.[7] Clinically, this is a lesion of adults, and most have been over age 70. Sialadenitis with crystal formation can involve either the parotid or the submandibular gland and causes physical findings that suggest carcinoma. The patients have usually been symptomatic for weeks or months. Crystals of various types can be seen as a nonspecific finding in normal salivary gland tissue, cysts, nonspecific chronic sialadenitis, pleomorphic adenoma, and Warthin's tumor. However, the crystals of this lesion consist of α-Amylase. They measure 20 μm to 300 μm in length and up to 100 μm in width (Figure 27-3). They are associated with various combinations of duct cells, acinar cells, and granulation tissue. Bacteria are not identified, and this process may recur after administration of antibiotics.

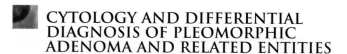

CYTOLOGY AND DIFFERENTIAL DIAGNOSIS OF PLEOMORPHIC ADENOMA AND RELATED ENTITIES

Pleomorphic Adenoma (Benign Mixed Tumor)

Many salivary gland aspirates represent pleomorphic adenomas. Physical examination shows a well-circumscribed mass that is usually very firm, often with a lobulated surface. This presents a different sensation to the fingertips than the softer surface of a Warthin's tumor.[1] The cytologic diagnosis is usually straightforward, and 80% or more are correctly interpreted at the time of aspiration.[8]

Smears show three components and differ largely in the relative proportions of these basic elements (Figure 27-4 and Box 27-13). Mixed tumors are given to a wide variety of

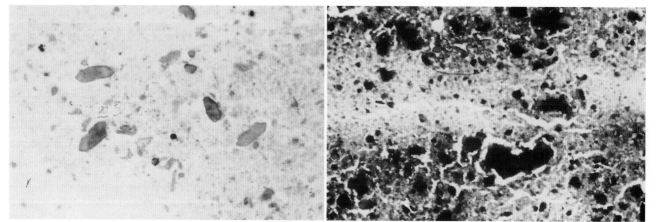

Figure 27-3   **Sialadenitis with crystal fomation. A,** When seen in fixed smears, sialadenitis with crystal formation is very distinctive. One may encounter duct cells or acinar cells, but much of the material will consist of debris and numerous crystals as illustrated here. (Pap) **B,** Air drying accentuates the background material, but renders the crystals very difficult to visualize. (DQ) (From Geisinger K, Silverman J. Fine needle aspiration cytology of superficial organs and body sites. New York: Churchill-Livingstone; 1999.)

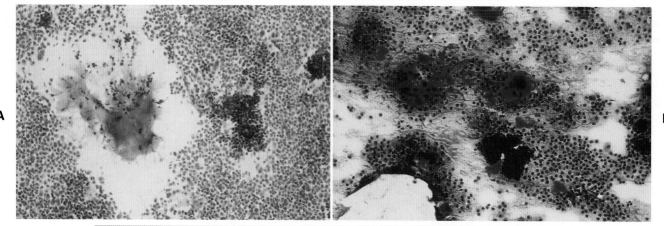

Figure 27-4   **Pleomorphic adenoma.** In both the fixed **(A)** and air-dried **(B)** smears, this mixed tumor shows all three types of tissue found in this neoplasm. Darkly staining cohesive clusters of ductal cells are three dimensional, whereas the myoepithelial cells lie singly. Fragments of stroma are pale on the fixed preparation and brightly metachromatic on the dried smear. The low-magnification images indicate that many examples can be immediately recognized by smear pattern. **(A,** Pap; **B,** DQ) (From Geisinger K, Silverman J. Fine needle aspiration cytology of superficial organs and body sites. New York: Churchill-Livingstone; 1999.)

alterations that can be seen singly or in combinations (Boxes 27-14 and 27-15). Ductal cells are usually small and cuboidal with very bland nuclear morphology, but moderate pleomorphism in a minority of cells is common. They may be arranged in flat sheets, glands, trabecula, or large branching tissue fragments. Squamous metaplasia, oncocytic change, cystic alteration, mucin production, or sebaceous differentiation may complicate the cytologic picture. Myoepithelial cells are usually present and may be either spindled or plasmacytoid. The latter show dissociation, and the single plasmacytoid cells are sometimes mistaken for hematopoietic elements. Myoepithelial cells can also be present in the chondroid matrix. In many aspirates this tripartite panorama allows immediate diagnosis by pattern recognition.

The epithelial and myoepithelial elements of pleomorphic adenomas are sufficiently complex and diverse to raise many diagnostic considerations. In general, however, the chondromyxoid matrix is the more specific and diagnostically helpful feature. This material may be mimicked by other types of collagenous stroma. This is most significant when the desmoplastic stroma of a carcinoma is mistaken for mixed tumor matrix. When associated with a low nuclear grade malignancy, this can result in severe diagnostic difficulties.

When fixed and prepared by the method of Pap, the matrix of pleomorphic adenomas is pale and gray to cyanophilic and closely resembles the chondroid material as it appears in histologic sections. When air-dried and stained by a Romanowsky method, this matrix is metachromatic and shows a distinctly fibrillary substructure. The latter can often be appreciated best at the edge of tissue particles, where it presents as frayed edges.

The Pap stain may show myoepithelial cells sequestered within the matrix to good advantage; they appear stellate or spindled and have small dense nuclei without prominent nucleoli. They may be widely dispersed through a large fragment of the matrix material, which imparts a distinctly chondro-osseous appearance. Air-dried preparations render these cells as pale smudgy blue outlines, that are largely obscured by the densely staining matrix in which they lie. However, the inability to see their nuclear details on air-dried smears does not result in diagnostic difficulties. The appearance of these tissue particles with their ghost-like myoepithelial inhabitants is characteristic and diagnostic (Figure 27-5; see Box 27-15).

When a mixed tumor aspirate contains relatively little matrix material, the risk of an incorrect diagnosis increases considerably. Small amounts of this material can be more easily detected by review of air-dried, Romanowsky-stained slides. In preparations of this type, its presence is trumpeted by bright metachromasia, rather than muted by its translucent quality in fixed material. Other findings occasionally embellish the cytology of mixed tumors. Intranuclear cytoplasmic inclusions may be seen. These distinctive structures are reminiscent of papillary thyroid carcinoma. However, they may also be seen in paragangliomas and meningiomas, so that their utility as a diagnostic criterion is not great, even in an aspirate from the neck. Tyrosine crystals may be found in sections of pleomorphic adenomas, reflecting the normal gland's ability to concentrate this amino acid. However, these needle-like or rosette-forming crystals are rarely found in FNA samples. Tyrosine crystals are not, as previously suggested, diagnostic of pleomorphic adenoma, as they have been identified in cysts, carcinomas ex pleomorphic adenoma, and at least one example of polymorphous low-grade adenocarcinoma.

FNA-associated infarction and squamous metaplasia in pleomorphic adenomas has been described. Furthermore, the potential parallels between these events and the pathogenesis of necrotizing sialometaplasia have been noted. Warthin's tumors are more often affected by post-FNA infarction than pleomorphic adenomas. The sudden onset of dental-like pain associated with enlargement that is not responsive to antibiotics may herald this type of infarction. These signs, however, may be mistaken clinically for a post-FNA infection, but in the authors' experience, this is a vanishingly rare event that is usually not the cause of unexpected patient difficulties (Chapter 2).

Spontaneous infarction of pleomorphic adenomas in the absence of antecedent FNA is an even rarer event. Aspirates

---

BOX 27-13 | CMF

Cytomorphologic Features of Pleomorphic Adenoma

Clusters of ductal cells
Spindled or plasmacytoid myoepithelial cells
Extracellular matrix material
Myoepithelial cells entrapped within matrix
These components vary widely in relative quantity

BOX 27-14

Epithelial Alterations in Pleomorphic Adenoma

Cystic change
Squamous metaplasia
Oncocytic change
Mucin production
Sebaceous differentiation

BOX 27-15

Matrix of Mixed Tumors

Fixed Pap-stained smears
- Pale gray or cyanophilic
- May resemble chondroid material
- Spindled or stellate myoepithelial cells well seen
- Small amounts of matrix difficult to see

Air-dried, Romanowsky-stained slides
- Metachromatic staining
- Dense and fibrillary
- Entrapped myoepithelial cells partially obscured
- Small amounts of matrix easily seen

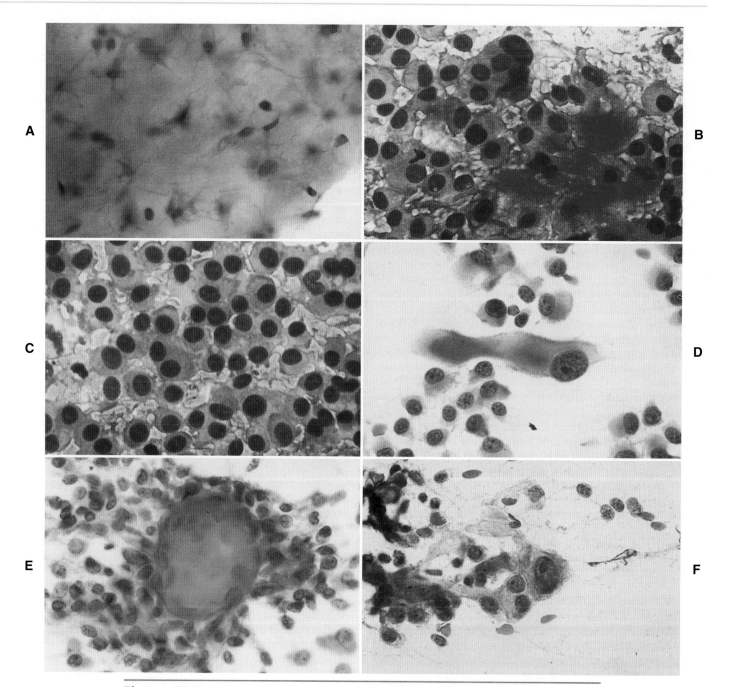

Figure 27-5 Pleomorphic adenoma—details and alterations. **A,** This fragment of matrix material from a pleomorphic adenoma has a distinctly chondro-osseous appearance that closely resembles its histologic counterpart. Scattered through this large three-dimensional matrix fragment are numerous stellate myoepithelial cells at various levels of focus. (Pap) **B,** In air-dried smears the same material is metachromatic and has a fibrillary quality. The latter is most apparent at the edge of large tissue fragments. Myoepithelial cells that are trapped in the matrix are pale and show little detail. Free-lying myoepithelial cells are plasmacytoid and more easily visualized. (DQ) **C,** Myoepithelial cells can be plasmacytoid (hyaline cells) and have been mistaken for a hematopoietic neoplasm. (DQ) **D,** When fixed, these plasmacytoid myoepithelial cells lack the chromatin structure usually associated with lymphoid malignancies. Occasional large forms should not be considered evidence of malignancy. (Pap) **E,** Morular squamous metaplasia can complicate the cytology of mixed tumors. In this example, the involved duct is surroiunded by numerous myoepithelial cells. (Pap) **F,** Oncocytic metaplasia and other types of atypia can occur in mixed tumors. The large nuclei and prominent nucleoli of atypical cells may be mistaken for carcinoma. However, cells with oncocytic cytoplasmic features are more likely to be metaplastic than neoplastic. (DQ)

Continued

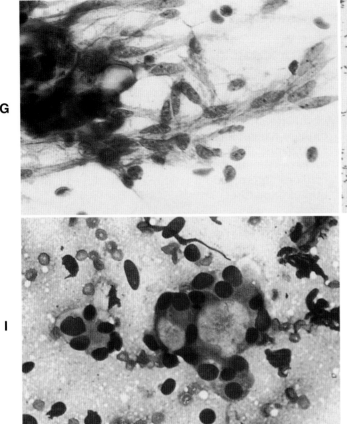

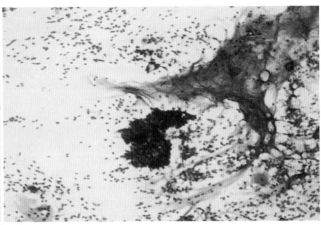

Figure 27-5, cont'd **G,** Myoepithelial cells can also be spindled. (Pap) **H,** This mixed tumor aspirate shows cystic change, with epithelial cell clusters scattered through mucinous appearing fluid. The resemblance to low-grade mucoepidermoid carcinoma can be quite misleading. (Pap) **I,** Cellular degeneration with vacuole formation furthers the similarity of this cystic mixed tumor to mucoepidermoid carcinoma. (DQ) (From Geisinger K, Silverman J. Fine needle aspiration cytology of superficial organs and body sites. New York: Churchill-Livingstone; 1999.)

show necrosis with atypia. Before excision, FNA diagnoses of squamous cell carcinoma or mucoepidermoid carcinoma may be considered.

Differential Diagnostic Considerations

Problems in the cytologic diagnosis of mixed tumors may originate in any of this tumor's three major components (Box 27-16). Distinction from low-grade mucoepidermoid carcinoma is a common issue because the matrix may be mistaken for mucus. This is compounded if squamous metaplasia is present. Cystic change with foam cells and a predominance of epithelium over matrix further heighten this difficulty. Still, careful attention to the extracellular material can help resolve this diagnostic dilemma; mucus lacks the fibrillary quality of true matrix material and usually stains much less densely.

The nonspecific collagenous stroma of many lesions may resemble mixed tumor matrix. It too is metachromatic and can show both dense staining and a fibrillary substructure. Less commonly, the necrosis of metastatic carcinoma has been mistaken for this matrix material. In this way, lesions as diverse as sialadenitis, sialolithiasis with fibrosis, metastases from cutaneous basal cell or squamous cell carcinomas, and a single example of malignant peripheral nerve sheath tumor have all been interpreted as mixed tumor at the time of FNA. Finally, a chordoma that invades the parotid may also be mistaken for mixed tumor.

One of the most common problems leading to false-positive diagnoses in salivary gland FNA is misinterpretation of atypical epithelial or myoepithelial cells aspirated

---

BOX 27-16

Problems in the Diagnosis of Pleomorphic Adenoma

Matrix mistaken for mucus resulting a diagnosis of mucoepidermoid carcinoma

Squamous metaplasia, foam cells, and cystic change may suggest mucoepidermoid carcinoma

Cylindromatous foci may mimic adenoid cystic carcinoma

Collagenous stoma of many other lesions can be mistaken for matrix

Atypical epithelial or myoepithelial cells may suggest malignancy

Pleomorphic adenoma is very difficult to distinguish from polymorphous low grade adenocarcinoma

Spindled myoepithelial cells may suggest a sarcoma

Plasmacytoid myoepithelial cells can mimic malignant lymphoma or plasmacytoma

More cellular or matrix-deficient examples resemble various small blue cell tumors

---

from pleomorphic adenomas. Cells suggestive of various malignancies, including carcinoma ex pleomorphic adenoma, feature enlarged nuclei with irregular contours, marconucleoli, and clumped chromatin. Such cells may originate in either the ductal or the myoepithelial areas.

The first step in avoiding diagnostic errors is recognizing the most characteristic feature of mixed tumor cytology, which is the matrix. When this component of the smear suggests the diagnosis of pleomorphic adenoma, this finding should override concern over focal atypia, even if it is severe. In the vast majority of instances, mixed tumor will be the correct interpretation. Mixed tumors with striking but clinically meaningless atypia are relatively common. On the other hand, carcinoma ex pleomorphic adenoma is rarely recognized in FNA.

Whether studied by frozen sections, or in FNA samples, pleomorphic adenomas can be mistaken for adenoid cystic carcinoma. This usually occurs when the matrix is scanty or absent so that the mixed tumor is hypercellular. Furthermore, duct lumina may mimic cylinder formation, or frankly cylindromatous foci may be identified. The cytology and the histology of these cellular mixed tumors approach the appearance of basal cell adenomas in that they show little of the diagnostic chondromyxoid matrix. The term *minimally pleomorphic adenoma* has been employed to illustratively describe this histologic circumstance. Distinction of these cases from adenoid cystic carcinoma, particularly its solid (anaplastic) variant, is very difficult at the time of FNA. Because these cases are cytologically similar to basal cell adenomas, they are discussed more fully with the other small cell epithelial neoplasms.

Polymorphous low-grade adenocarcinoma can closely resemble mixed tumor. A tumor's location may provide an important clue to the diagnosis because the carcinomas usually occur in the minor salivary glands, whereas mixed tumors are often located in the major glands. When polymorphous low-grade adenocarcinoma does arise in the parotid, it is commonly found within carcinoma ex pleomorphic adenoma. Histologically, the encapsulation of mixed tumors contrasts with the infiltrative nature of the carcinomas and with their proclivity for perineural growth. Unfortunately, these key histologic signs of malignancy cannot be assessed in cytologic samples. The epithelial-myoepithelial carcinoma is another rare low-grade malignancy that may show mixed tumor-like foci. Adequate sampling based on several FNA passes can resolve some diagnostic problems.

Plasmacytoid myoepithelial cells may be mistaken for plasmacytoma or plasmacytoid malignant lymphoma. Individual myoepithelial cells may be large, and multinucleated. The suspicion of malignancy can be very great, unless other evidence that the aspirate represents a mixed tumor is evaluated carefully. The authors have even seen this type of scattered large myoepithelial cell with multiple nuclei and a background of small uniform myoepithelial cells mistaken for Hodgkin's disease. The differential diagnosis of myoepithelial cells with a spindle shape, including myoepithelioma and malignant myoepithelioma is discussed subsequently with other spindle cell proliferations.

The cytologic diagnosis of mixed tumors is usually straightforward, but the foregoing descriptions emphasize the complexity and variability of this neoplasm. They also illustrate that the most secure cytologic diagnoses are those that are based on multiple criteria. Cells within the chondromyxoid matrix of mixed tumors are often positive with immunostains for glial fibrillary acid protein (GFAP). This may form the basis for resolution of some diagnostic difficulties related to myoepithelial cells. Furthermore, the epithelia of mixed tumors can often be decorated by immunoreagents that recognize the breast antigen GCDFP-15 (gross cystic disease fluid protein). This might be exploited to exclude diagnoses of polymorphous low-grade adenocarcinoma and adenoid cystic carcinoma, both of which are negative for this marker.

Benign Metastasizing Pleomorphic Adenoma

Histologically typical examples pleomorphic adenoma may rarely result in distant metastases. Pulmonary and osseous deposits have been approached by FNA. Myxoid matrix and bland-appearing epithelial cells may be confused with pulmonary hamartoma. Bone lesions may be destructive and radiographically mistaken for malignant fibrous histiocytoma or chondrosarcoma. All historical, radiographic, and cytologic information is required for the correct interpretation of these cases.

Malignant Mixed Tumor (True Carcinosarcoma) and Carcinoma ex Pleomorphic Adenoma

Mixed tumors that are large, or that show prognostically meaningless cytologic atypia are much more common than carcinoma ex pleomorphic adenoma.[9-11] The malignant areas in the rare carcinoma ex pleomorphic adenoma can be very focal. Thus, false-negative aspirations are common and smears show only the mixed tumor portion of the mass with no evidence of malignancy. A much less common sampling problem arises when only the carcinoma is aspirated, with no cytologic evidence of the associated mixed tumor.

The malignancy encountered in carcinoma ex pleomorphic adenoma is variable and may be poorly differentiated with little resemblance to the common carcinomas of this organ. Rare examples of low-grade mucoepidermoid carcinoma ex pleomorphic adenoma have been described in FNA samples. Because the neoplastic cells are of low nuclear grade, this diagnosis is problematic at the time of FNA.

True carcinosarcoma (malignant mixed tumor) occurs much less often than the carcinoma ex pleomorphic adenoma. Most are recognized as malignant when aspirated. Concurrent cytologic demonstration of both sarcomatous and carcinomatous components is unusual. One case studied by FNA showed both poorly differentiated squamous cell carcinoma and chondrosarcoma (Box 27-17).

BOX 27-17
Malignancy in Pleomorphic Adenoma

Benign metastasizing pleomorphic adenoma
No histologic evidence of aggressive behavior
No special cytologic features
Metastases to lung and bone
Least common type of malignant mixed tumor

Carcinoma ex pleomorphic adenoma
Carcinomas of various types
Residual benign pleomorphic adenoma
Significant sampling issues in FNA
Most common type of malignant mixed tumor

Carcinosarcoma (true malignant mixed tumor)
Malignant epithelial component
Malignant mesenchymal component
Ten percent of malignant mixed tumors

WARTHIN'S TUMOR: CYTOLOGY AND RELATED ENTITIES

Warthin's Tumor

Warthin's tumors are softer than mixed tumors at physical examination; they often feel like fluid-filled cysts.[1] Aspirates of Warthin's tumors may show three components in varying proportions: oncocytic epithelium, lymphocytes, and cyst fluid[12-14] (Box 27-18 and Figure 27-6). Any of these may be absent or scanty. Some examples show only nonspecific cyst fluid or lack the diagnostic oncocytes. Intact papillary tissue fragments with epithelium overlying lymphoid tissue are sometimes seen and recapitulate this tumor's histology.

Oncocytes typically occur in flat cohesive sheets. The nuclei of these cells are subject to the same enlargement, variability, and nucleolar prominence that attends oncocytic metaplasia in other tissues, such as in chronic lymphocytic thyroiditis. The abundant cytoplasm is usually sufficient to impart a low nuclear to cytoplasmic (N : C) ratio. In air-dried smears the cytoplasm is dense, whereas on fixed preparations, it often appears finely granular. Oncocytes are often cyanophilic in Pap-stained FNA samples, thus failing to recapitulate the eosinophilia typical of histologic preparations. The reason for this is that the H&E stain provides only eosin as a cytoplasmic stain. The Pap stain, in contrast, offers several cytoplasmic counterstains, allowing the cells several tinctorial options. For this reason, eosinophilia should not be a requirement for designation of cells as oncocytic. In addition to oncocytes, Warthin's tumors may show sebaceous, squamous, or mucinous differentiation as well as pleomorphic adenoma-like foci.

The lymphoid tissue may consist mostly of free-lying mature cells that feature thin rims of basophilic cytoplasm surrounding densely hyperchromatic nuclei. As previously discussed the lymphoid cells in Warthin's tumors tend to be more monotonous and to show fewer germinal center fragments (lymphohistiocytic aggregates) than usually seen in lymph node aspirates. In some instances, however, they are polymorphous and resemble reactive lymphoid tissue. *Lymphoid tangles* represent another manifestation of lymphoid tissue and appear as smeared strands of darkly staining chromatinic material. *Lymphoglandular bodies* are small detached cytoplasmic droplets that represent cells damaged in the smearing process. These general features of lymphoid cell cytology are discussed in more detail in Chapter 24.

Warthin's tumor aspirations vary widely from a few drops to one ml or more of brown turbid cyst fluid. These tumors are only partially cystic and cannot be drained completely by FNA. The fluid can be sparsely cellular so that concentration is essential, if occasional oncocytic clusters are to be identified. Furthermore, several smears from a centrifuge pellet may be required to find even a few diagnostic oncocyte clusters. In addition to lymphoid tissue and oncocytes, the fluid itself is represented by debris and precipitated protein that give the slide a "dirty" background. Cholesterol crystals may also be seen in air-dried preparations and have the same "window-pane" appearance noted in thyroid cyst fluids (Chapter 26).

Warthin's Tumors: Differential Diagnostic Considerations

When all of the elements discussed above are present, the diagnosis of Warthin's tumors is straightforward, and 60% to 88% are correctly diagnosed at the time of initial FNA. When the cytologic picture is less clear, several other entities may be considered (Box 27-19). Those cases that yield fluid lacking oncocytes and prominent lymphoid tissue must be distinguished from several other cystic salivary gland lesions that are discussed more fully later in this text. Unfortunately, the epithelial cells required for diagnosis of most other cystic masses are also absent. This means that one is left with a nondiagnostic cyst fluid specimen similar to those sometimes obtained by thyroid aspiration. Repeat aspiration may be useful because most Warthin's tumors are only partially cystic and the initial sampling will have left a palpable mass. On the other hand, such fluids should not be interpreted as unequivocally benign without other compelling evidence that leads to a specific diagnosis. Furthermore, the association of neutrophils with a cyst fluid does not automatically connote an infection or other primarily inflammatory process.

If the clusters and sheets of oncocytes are extremely prominent, an oncocytic neoplasm may be suggested, especially since these lesions may show abundant lymphoid stoma. Conversely, a cytologic diagnosis of Warthin's tumor may be suggested after study of a cyst fluid with debris and lymphocytes. Ultimately, however, it is impossible to make this diagnosis without positive identification of oncocytic epithelium.

The fluid aspirated from Warthin's tumors may also show foam cells and stringy precipitated material that can

---

BOX 27-18   `CMF`

Cytomorphologic Features of Warthin's Tumor

Cyst fluid with foam cells, macrophages, and debris
Oncocytes usually in flat sheet
Oncocytes show abundant cytoplasm and may have prominent nucleoli
Free lymphocytes that may appear monomorphous
Lymphoid tangles
Germinal center fragments
Lymphoglandular bodies are present if the lymphoid tissue is abundant

---

BOX 27-19

Differential Diagnosis of Warthin's Tumor

Nonspecific cyst fluid
Oncocytic neoplasms
Low-grade mucoepidermoid carcinoma
Chronic inflammation
Lymph node hyperplasia
Well-differentiated malignant lymphoma
Squamous cell carcinoma
Acinic cell carcinoma

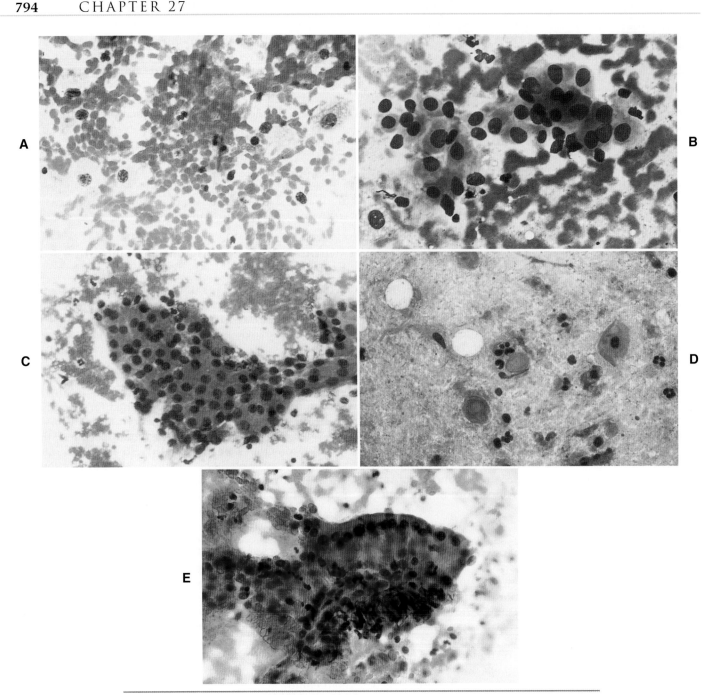

Figure 27-6 Warthin's tumor. **A,** Aspirates from Warthin's tumor often consist of cyst fluid. This must be concentrated and gives the smears a background of proteinaceous material, scattered inflammatory cells, and occasional foam cells. (Pap) **B,** Oncocytes usually form flat sheets and feature nuclei of varying size, abundant cytoplasm, and occasional nucleoli. (DQ) **C,** Oncocytes from a fixed smear of a Warthin's tumor are shown here. In Warthin's tumor aspirates it is important to scan the entire smear at intermediate magnification to identify what can be a very few clusters of these diagnostic cells. (Pap) **D,** Squamous metaplasia is common in Warthin's tumors. The keratinized cells shown here are evidence of this process. Significant degenerative atypia can be noted in such cells and may lead to a mistaken diagnosis of a cystic metastasis of squamous cell carcinoma. (Pap) **E,** This tissue fragment recapitulates the histology of Warthin's tumor, as oncocytes rest atop lymphoid tissue. (Pap) (From Geisinger K, Silverman J. Fine needle aspiration cytology of superficial organs and body sites. New York: Churchill-Livingstone; 1999.)

resemble extracellular mucus. Thus, in the setting of an oncocyte-deficient aspirate, a diagnosis of low-grade mucoepidermoid carcinoma may be considered. When lymphocytes are the most prominent element of the aspirate, one may suggest chronic inflammation, follicular hyperplasia, or a low-grade malignant lymphoma. Conversely, a salivary gland aspirate of a small cell malignant lymphoma may be interpreted as the much more common Warthin's tumor. Cell marker studies can resolve this diagnostic problem.

The papillary fronds in Warthin's tumor often undergo squamous metaplasia with marked individual cell keratosis. In some cases, this can be associated with considerable cytologic atypia or degenerative nuclear hyperchomasia that can mimic squamous cell carcinoma. The most important maneuvers in preventing an inappropriate diagnosis of carcinoma are repeating any questionable or sparsely cellular aspirates and adequately concentrating any fluid that is recovered. A diligent search usually shows oncocytes, and this should lead to the correct diagnosis.

Lymphocytes and cystic change may both be features of acinic cell carcinoma. Furthermore, the cells of this carcinoma closely resemble oncocytes and further its similarity to Warthin's tumor in aspirate smears. In the authors' experience, however, most aspirates of acinic cell carcinoma contain many more epithelial cells than usually recovered from Warthin's tumors and also show a much higher ratio of epithelial cells to lymphocytes. Furthermore, the zymogen granules of acinic cells are a useful differential diagnostic feature because they are coarser than the fine cytoplasmic granularity of oncocytes. Cell block sections are useful in demonstrating these granules.

Distinction between Warthin's tumor and acinic cell carcinoma is an uncommon but occasionally difficult problem, as is the distinction between other oncocytic lesions and acinic cell carcinoma. Oncocytic neoplasms, including rare malignant examples, and oncocytoid adenocarcinoma are discussed in the next section, where they are placed in the context of other large cell epithelial neoplasms of low nuclear grade.

CYSTIC SALIVARY GLAND MASSES

Cystic change in excised surgical specimens is often a secondary embellishment of diagnoses based primarily on other criteria. At the time of FNA, however, the presence of fluid is often the first apparent morphologic feature of a patient's mass not ascertained solely by physical examination or radiographic investigation. Thus, it often initiates and begins to organize the pathologist's differential diagnosis. The simple fact that a mass is cystic or partially cystic requires that a large array of diagnostic possibilities be considered. Furthermore, problems are compounded by the fact that any diagnostic cellular elements are probably diluted in a considerable specimen volume. This emphasizes the need for multiple careful aspirations. Special clinical considerations such as human immunodeficiency virus (HIV) infection may also alter the diagnostic approach to cystic lesions.[15]

Several lesions that may occasionally be cystic are more commonly solid (e.g., squamous cell carcinoma, other metastatic carcinomas, pleomorphic adenoma, monomorphic adenomas, or acinic cell carcinoma) and are usually recognized by the expected criteria. These are discussed in other sections in this chapter, where they present more frequent or urgent dilemmas. Partially cystic Warthin's tumors were considered earlier.

Lymphoepithelial Cysts and Lymphoepithelial Lesions

Benign lymphoepithelial cysts of the parotid gland were known before the AIDS epidemic but were uncommon. It has been suggested that these lesions originate in salivary gland inclusions within cervical lymph nodes or as branchial cleft developmental abnormalities. The cyst is surrounded by hyperplastic lymphoid tissue, and its lining can consist of squamous, mucinous, columnar, ciliated, or sebaceous cells in various patterns. Distinction must be made between benign lymphoepithelial lesions that are seen mostly in autoimmune disease and the relatively common AIDS-associated lymphoepithelial cysts. In the former, the gland parenchyma is replaced by a lymphohistiocytic infiltrate with residual epimyoepithelial islands and variable degrees of cystic alteration. The AIDS-related lesions are predominantly cystic with surrounding lymphoid tissue. Furthermore, the cysts are often situated within more normal-appearing salivary gland tissue than usually accompanies the diffuse pathology of benign lymphoepithelial lesions of Sjøgren's syndrome.

The benign lymphoepithelial cysts of AIDS are more common in the parotid, but they may also be found in submandibular glands. They may be unilateral or bilateral, and are often multicystic. Their apparent size and extent increase when physical examination is supplemented by CT scans. These cysts are often associated with extensive cervical lymphadenopathy. It has been suggested that progressive intraglandular lymphoid hyperplasia leads from entrapment to obstruction to cystic dilatation of the gland's ducts. They may recur whether simply drained by a needle or excised. For this reason, repeat aspiration rather than excision has been recommended for palliation.

Cytologically, benign lymphoepithelial cyst aspirates show various epithelial cells of the types mentioned previously and polymorphous lymphocytes. Lymphohistiocytic aggregates indicating germinal center formation, plasma cells, crystals, and parakeratotic squamous cells have also been described. In some cases, epithelial cells are not identified so that the impression is that of a benign lymph node. Alternatively, this picture can lead to consideration of several primary salivary gland masses including sialadenitis, Warthin's tumor, or the classic type of benign lymphoepithelial lesion. If squamous cells are prominent, one may consider pleomorphic adenoma with metaplasia, mucoepidermoid carcinoma, squamous cell carcinoma, or a congenital cyst. Clinical and radiographic factors contribute to a correct diagnosis.

When salivary gland masses in AIDS patients are considered, cysts and lymphoid hyperplasia are more common than malignancy. Furthermore, the probability of finding malignancy is much lower when a parotid mass is cystic than when it is solid. Most salivary gland malignancies associated with AIDS represent either Kaposi's sarcoma or malignant lymphoma.

Duct Obstruction as a Cause of Cystic Salivary Gland Enlargement

Long-standing duct obstruction has several causes, in addition to the previously described intraglandular lymphoid hyperplasia of lymphoepithelial cysts in patients with AIDS. Those usually operative in patients referred for FNA include sialolithiasis, compression by an adjacent mass, and radiation fibrosis. At physical examination, these glands are usually well-circumscribed and firm. These findings can mimic recurrent or metastatic malignancy and are excellent targets for FNA.

Obstruction leads to atrophy of the acinar parenchyma, extensive fibrosis, chronic periductal inflammation, and dilatation of the residual duct (Box 27-20). The epithelium of entrapped ducts may be flattened, or can show various combinations of squamous, mucinous and ciliated metaplasia. The lumina of these structures are often filled with mucoid or granular secretory material. If duct rupture supervenes, a foreign body reaction and cytologic atypia associated with mesenchymal repair can be part of an exuberant inflammatory mass (see Figure 27-2).

The combination of cyst-like spaces with complex lining epithelium, a background of fibrous tissue, inflammation, and abundant extracellular mucus is strongly suggestive of low-grade mucoepidermoid carcinoma with both cytology and frozen section. The distinction between these two conditions on cytologic grounds is often impossible (Figure 27-7).

Sialolithiasis

Sialolithiasis is a specific subtype of tumefactive duct obstruction. Varying degrees of the pathology described above can be seen in longstanding cases. Sialolithiasis is second only to mumps as a cause of sialadenitis. However, because very few stones occur in children, it is the most common cause in older individuals. Stones are more common in women than in men. The parotids are involved less often than the submandibular glands, with masses that are more likely to be unilateral than bilateral. Some are discovered incidentally on dental radiographs, whereas a significant minority (20%) are not radiographically visible (Box 27-21).

The presence of stones does not imply associated abnormalities of calcium metabolism. The classical symptoms include pain and swelling at mealtime. Some individuals may be symptomatic for many years. Alternatively, a stone may present as an otherwise asymptomatic hard mass that suggests malignancy. Others come to medical attention only after a secondary infection supervenes. In the latter instance, FNA for morphologic diagnosis and possibly for cultures may be requested. Only occasional applications of FNA to evaluation of sialolithiasis have been reported.[16-17] The diagnosis is straightforward, if stone fragments are identified in aspirate material. Also, if ciliated metaplastic

BOX   27-20

Morphology Salivary Gland Duct Obstruction

Parenchymal atrophy
Extensive fibrosis
Chronic periductal inflammation
Dilatation of the residual duct
Squamous, mucinous or ciliated metaplasia of the duct lining
Foreign body reaction after duct rupture
Mesenchymal repair atypia after duct rupture

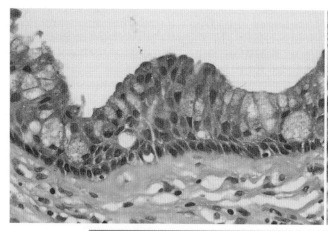
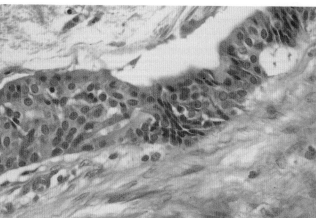

Figure 27-7   Epithelium in nonneoplastic duct obstruction compared with low-grade mucoepidermoid carcinoma. **A,** This histologic section from a dilated salivary gland duct was taken from a firm enlarged gland that showed diffuse radiation fibrosis. The surrounding fibrous tissue contains no acini and shows a few chronic inflammatory cells. The duct lining is thickened by a complex epithelium with squamous, mucinous, and immature metaplastic cells. The latter resemble the intermediate cells of low-grade mucoepidermoid carcinoma. The central mucinous contents and foam cells are not well seen in this illustration. (H&E) **B,** This cystic space represents a portion of a low-grade mucoepidermoid carcinoma. Its lining epithelium and mucinous contents are similar to those in nonneoplastic duct obstruction. Hence, the difficulty in distinguishing these two processes at the time of FNA. (H&E) (From Geisinger K, Silverman J. Fine needle aspiration cytology of superficial organs and body sites. New York: Churchill-Livingstone; 1999.)

cells are present, a benign condition is suggested, but in the absence of stone fragments, a specific diagnosis may not be possible. Examples of sialolithiasis interpreted as congenital cysts based on the finding of ciliated cells have been seen (Figure 27-8 and Box 27-22).

BOX 27-21

Sialolithiasis

More common in women than in men
Most common in the submandibular gland
Most are unilateral
Some incidentally discovered on dental radiographs
Some not radio-opaque
Presentations: pain and swelling at mealtime, mass, or secondary infection
Cytology: cystic aspirate with mucus and a few cells
Major fine-needle aspiration differential diagnosis: low-grade mucoepidermoid carcinoma

The greatest diagnostic danger with aspirates from sialolithiasis occurs when both stones and ciliated metaplasia are absent. In these cases, extracellular mucus with scattered foam cells and occasional epithelial cell groups strongly suggest low-grade mucoepidermoid carcinoma. The danger is greatest when the cell clusters show complex and variable mixtures of squamous and vacuolated cells. It is paradoxical that aspiration of sialolithiasis often yields more epithelial cells with a greater nuclear atypia than sampling of the typical low-grade mucoepidermoid carcinoma.

In addition, only one patient in a series of five sialolithiasis cases studied by FNA had the typical history.[16] This is an important clinical consideration and suggests that patients referred for FNA are not a typical sample of stone-bearing individuals. Rather, they are most likely to be those in whom a diagnosis of malignancy is under clinical consideration. Because inflammation can be a prominent component of low-grade mucoepidermoid carcinoma, this finding is not a helpful differential diagnostic consideration. Thus, the cytopathologist sees a patient with a firm mass and no history of pain or swelling at mealtime. The aspirate

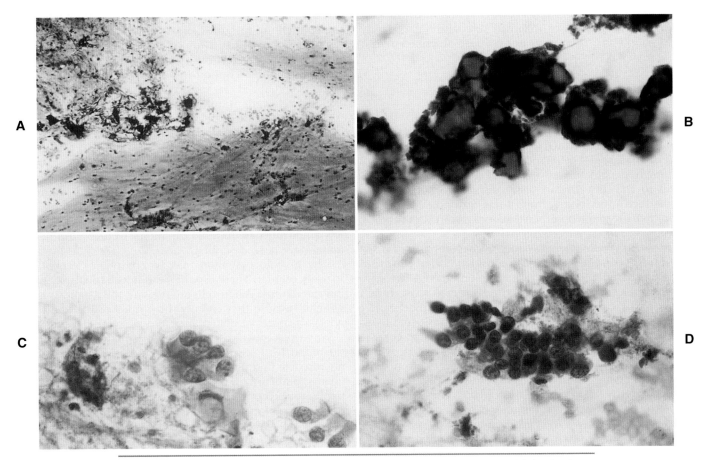

Figure 27-8 Sialolithiasis. **A,** At low magnification this aspirate of sialolithiasis shows abundant mucus through which are scattered several cell clusters. At this level and at the bedside where mucinous fluid will have been recovered, this process closely mimics low-grade mucoepidermoid carcinoma. (DQ) **B,** Some aspirates of sialolithiasis show stone fragments such as these. (Pap) **C,** In some cases the fluid of sialolithiasis contains ciliated cells. Although nonspecific, such elements indicate a benign metaplasia. (DQ) **D,** In fixed material, the cells of sialolithiasis may show more atypia than usually seen in low-grade mucoepidermoid carcinoma. These cells show crowding, nuclear hyperchromasia, and some degree of chromatin clearing. Nuclear smudging and cytoplasmic collapse indicate degeneration. (Pap) (From Geisinger K, Silverman J. Fine needle aspiration cytology of superficial organs and body sites. New York: Churchill-Livingstone; 1999.)

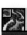

BOX 27-22

Sialolithiasis: Cytologic Findings

Cystic fluid
Mucus and foam cells
Variable numbers of squamous cells
Ciliated cells in some cases
Stone fragments in some cases
Differential diagnosis: low-grade mucoepidermoid
carcinoma

BOX 27-23

Low-Grade Mucoepidermoid Carcinoma

Fine-needle aspiration usually yields a small volume of
mucoid fluid
Very sparse cellularity
Foam cells resemble those in any cyst fluid
Lymphocytes may be prominent
Epithelial cells may be squamous, mucinous, or
intermediate
Intermediate cells resemble immature squamous metapla-
sia (Chapter 3)
No obvious malignant nuclear features

yields mucus and a few clusters of atypical epithelial cells. An incorrect diagnosis of low-grade mucoepidermoid carcinoma may be unavoidable. In this setting, the authors have made both possible errors.

As discussed more fully in the following section on Mucoepidermoid Carcinoma, many such aspirates lead to a diagnosis of "mucinous cyst," with a comment regarding the differential diagnostic possibilities.

Psammomatous calcifications can be found in histologic sections of the normal or inflamed submandibular gland and its neoplasms. These have not yet been described in cytologic material.

Low-Grade Mucoepidermoid Carcinoma

In the experience of many investigators, this is a difficult diagnosis in cytologic samples. One reason for this is its similarity to the duct-obstructive conditions discussed earlier. Cystic change, sparse cellularity, low-grade nuclear features, inflammation, and various epithelial metaplasias all contribute to the difficulty in distinguishing low-grade mucoepidermoid carcinoma from some examples of lymphoepithelial cyst, pleomorphic adenoma, Warthin's tumor, chronic sialadenitis, and sialolithiasis.[18-20]

Histologic grading schema for mucoepidermoid carcinoma must form the basis for the consideration of its cytologic manifestations. Several classifications have been advanced, and a complete review of this subject is beyond the scope of this chapter. In general, most mucoepidermoid carcinomas that are largely cystic would be considered low grade; those that are mostly solid are designated high grade.

This type of classification is readily adopted for use with FNA. The older cytology literature, however, is often unclear about grading, and various histologies are combined under the term *mucoepidermoid carcinoma*. These publications are thus difficult to interpret when addressing problems with the diagnosis and classification of this neoplasm. Furthermore, the term *high-grade mucoepidermoid carcinoma* has been rather loosely applied to a wide range of carcinomas that have little in common other than high nuclear grade.

Thus, the concept that low grade mucoepidermoid carcinoma is predominantly cystic is a reasonable starting point. This is the initial impression at the time of FNA because aspiration generally yields clear to turbid mucoid fluid. The smears are sparsely cellular and show a few foam cells and epithelial cell clusters in a background of abundant extracellular mucus. The histopathology of this neoplasm's epithelium prompts a search for combinations of mature squamous cells, the less mature intermediate cells, and mucinous cells. The latter are most often single foam cells that are cytologically indistinguishable from the macrophages that inhabit almost any cyst fluid. Vacuolated cells may also be situated within cohesive epithelial cell clusters. In this setting, one can be more confident that they truly represent the epithelium. Intermediate squamous cells are an important component of this tumor and form part of its definition in histologic sections. Cytologically, these cells have relatively high N:C ratios; in our experience, they can best be conceptualized as looking like immature squamous metaplastic cells familiar from gynecologic cytology (Chapter 3) (Figure 27-9 and Box 27-23).

The cytologic diagnosis of low-grade mucoepidermoid carcinoma is further confused by the presence of inflammation, which it shares with several of its mimics. Oncocytic variants are rare. However, they are important, because most other oncocytic masses are benign. Clear cell change and foci of sebaceous differentiation may be present, leading to diagnostic difficulties. Rare examples of low-grade mucoepidermoid carcinoma ex pleomorphic adenoma have been described.

The mucoid cyst fluid may be completely acellular or sparsely cellular. These aspirates often lead to false-negative interpretations. When cells are present, the diagnosis is still difficult because they usually show none of the traditional nuclear features of malignancy and are often degenerated.

Any thick mucoid salivary gland aspirate should be considered at least suspicious for carcinoma regardless of the microscopic findings. This includes specimens that are acellular or that contain only isolated foam cells. It should certainly not be concluded that the mass is benign, based on the absence of malignant-appearing cells; additional evaluation is indicated. It is our practice to give a diagnosis of "mucinous cyst aspirate," with a listing of differential diagnostic possibilities.

This discussion of low-grade mucoepidermoid carcinoma highlights the practical diagnostic utility of our approach to salivary gland masses (see Box 27-3). Low- and high-grade carcinomas of this type are often discussed together. However, one gives a sparsely cellular aspirate that must usually be distinguished from various benign lesions. The other is an obviously malignant epithelial neoplasm that must only be compared with other such carcinomas. Although the linking of these entities is interesting in our overall conceptualization of salivary

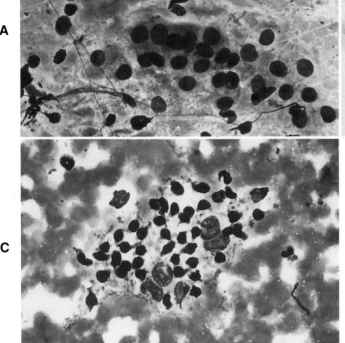

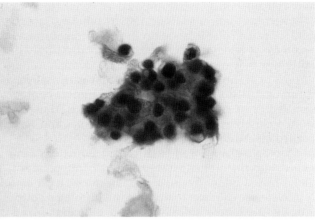

Figure 27-9 **Low-grade mucoepidermoid carcinoma.** **A,** Cell groups such as the one shown here are usually scattered widely through abundant cyst fluid. Free-lying foam cells are typical, but nonspecific. The remaining cells have a somewhat squamoid appearance and probably correspond to the intermediate cells in histologic preparations. (DQ) **B,** The background mucus is much less apparent in fixed material. These epithelial cells are much more bland than those depicted previously from a case of sialolithiasis (see Figure 27-8, *D*). In this example, the cells show degeneration, with collapsed nuclei that lack chromatin detail. (Pap) **C,** Chronic inflammation is commonly seen in aspirates of low-grade mucoepidermoid carcinoma. (DQ) (From Geisinger K, Silverman J. Fine needle aspiration cytology of superficial organs and body sites. New York: Churchill-Livingstone; 1999.)

gland tumors, their separation at the time of FNA has considerable practical utility.

SMALL CELL EPITHELIAL NEOPLASMS

Individually, most small cell epithelial neoplasms of the salivary glands are uncommon. However, the authors' experience indicates that as a group, they comprise a significant portion of the most difficult differential diagnostic dilemmas in salivary gland FNA. Hence, for the purpose of cytodiagnosis, these lesions are conceptualized as a group, despite great diversity in clinical presentation and outcome. This approach is highlighted in Box 27-3 and expanded in Box 27-24. An interesting and incompletely explored facet of this subject is that several of the primary salivary gland lesions in this category seem to share a common origin from the intercalated duct.

Cutaneous neoplasms, including pilomatrixoma and dermal eccrine cylindroma, should be considered with these lesions, particularly if adenoid cystic carcinoma is cytologically suspected. Clinical and radiographic findings usually suffice to exclude ameloblastoma from consideration. Metastatic carcinomas may also enter the differential diagnosis.[21]

Monomorphic Adenoma and Its Distinction from Adenoid Cystic Carcinoma

Historically, the term *monomorphic adenoma* has been applied a disparate group of salivary gland neoplasms. Their most important shared features were embodied by the con-

 BOX 27-24

Epithelial Neoplasms With Small Cells*

Monomorphic adenoma
Pleomorphic adenoma (with little chondromyxoid matrix)
Carcinoma ex monomorphic adenoma
Adenoid cystic carcinoma
Dermal eccrine cylindroma
Pilomatrixoma
Basal cell adenocarcinoma
Primary small cell carcinoma
Primary lymphoepithelioma-like carcinoma
Metastatic carcinomas
• Small cell carcinoma (includes Merkel cell carcinoma)
• Cutaneous basal cell carcinoma
• Nasopharyngeal carcinoma
Malignant lymphoma or leukemia

*Some of the entities are not of salivary gland origin but may enter the differential diagnosis of a parotid or submandibular mass at the time of FNA.

cept that they were benign neoplasms of a glandular organ (i.e., adenomas) that were not *pleomorphic*. Thus, the major import of this term seems to be in distinguishing these lesions from mixed tumors. More recently, however, oncocytomas, Warthin's tumors, and neoplasms with sebaceous differentiation have been classified separately. Currently, the term *monomorphic adenoma* is usually applied to basal cell adenomas.

Basal cell adenomas are composed of small uniform cells.[22-24] Architectural subclassification as tubular, trabecular, solid, or canalicular is based on the predominant histologic pattern. (The dermal *analogue* or *membranous type* is a special entity that more closely resembles dermal eccrine cylindroma or adenoid cystic carcinoma than other salivary gland tumors.) Histologically, some mixed tumors contain only small foci of chondromyxoid matrix; thus, these tumors often closely resemble basal cell adenomas and have been called *minimally pleomorphic adenomas*.[22]

The cytologic diagnosis of basal cell adenoma has been reconciled with the ultimate histopathologic interpretation as cellular mixed tumor by use of the illustrative term *minimally pleomorphic adenoma* to describe the histologic entity. Fortunately, the more clinically relevant differential diagnosis is not between adenomas that may or may not be pleomorphic. Rather, it involves distinctions between the monomorphic (or minimally pleomorphic) adenomas and certain carcinomas with which they share a common cytologic presentation as monotonous small cells.

FNA of a basal cell adenoma shows the numerous small blue cells that are associated with variable amounts of collagenous stroma (Box 27-25). The latter component is cyanophilic in alcohol-fixed preparations and metachromatic with Romanowsky stains. Tumors with a more solid growth pattern may show little or no stroma on aspirate smears. Single cells and naked nuclei may be numerous. Basosquamous whorls and sebaceous differentiation are seen rarely. Spontaneous infarction of basal cell adenomas may occur.

The collagenous stoma in aspirates of basal cell adenoma represents the interstitial connective tissue between nests and cords of epithelial cells. Thus, it contains scattered fibroblast-like spindle cells and capillaries. This feature has been found diagnostically useful in both cytologic and histologic samples. The interface between this stroma and the epithelial tumor cells is irregular. Wisps of frayed collagenous material interdigitate among the epithelial cells in a tissue particle (Figure 27-10).

These stromal components and the features of the cell-stoma interface are important in the consideration of the differential diagnosis of basal cell adenoma with adenoid cystic carcinoma. Aspiration of this carcinoma also yields uniform small blue cells associated with stroma. In both

neoplasms, the stroma is brightly metachromatic in air-dried preparations. This is probably the reason that basal cell adenomas often lead to false-positive diagnoses of adenoid cystic carcinoma in FNA material.

The extracellular material in adenoid cystic carcinoma is of two types. The first consists of whoring reduplicated basal lamina material elaborated by the tumor cells. Because it is not truly a connective tissue stroma, this material is always acellular and avascular. Furthermore, it has a sharp, linear interface with the surrounding small blue epithelial cells. However, these invasive lesions also feature tumor cells that are associated with desmoplastic tumor stroma that does not form spheres and cylinders. This second type of stroma interdigitates with small epithelial cells in the same manner noted for basal cell adenoma. This limits the diagnostic use of evaluating the stroma as a means of distinguishing these types of tumors. The problem is most severe, when we consider the solid (anaplastic) type of adenoid cystic carcinoma in which few, if any, spheres or cylinders exist.

Some investigators suggest that adenoid cystic carcinoma can be distinguished from adenomas, if sufficient attention is given to subtle nuclear features. These authors have not found this to be the case. Most examples of both entities show bland uniform nuclei. These are small and round to oval, with tiny or inapparent nucleoli and smooth chromatin.[24] We find no diagnostically useful differences in nucleus morphology between the adenomas and the carcinomas. The nuclei of adenoid cystic carcinoma do not show the traditional cytologic features of malignancy.

The most common small blue cell tumor encountered in salivary gland cytology is adenoid cystic carcinoma.[25-27] The celebrated spheres and cylinders of metachromatic extracellular matrix material surrounded by uniform small blue cells reflect the prominent cribriform pattern of this tumor's histology (Figure 27-11). Naked tumor cell nuclei litter the smear background. The extracellular spheres are sharply demarcated (Box 27-26).

Unfortunately, some cytology literature leaves the reader with the impression that the cylindromatous ap-

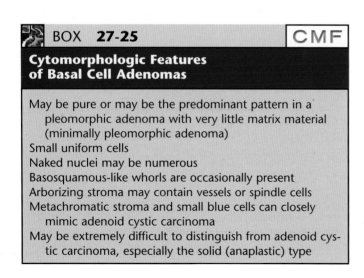

BOX 27-25   CMF

Cytomorphologic Features of Basal Cell Adenomas

May be pure or may be the predominant pattern in a pleomorphic adenoma with very little matrix material (minimally pleomorphic adenoma)
Small uniform cells
Naked nuclei may be numerous
Basosquamous-like whorls are occasionally present
Arborizing stroma may contain vessels or spindle cells
Metachromatic stroma and small blue cells can closely mimic adenoid cystic carcinoma
May be extremely difficult to distinguish from adenoid cystic carcinoma, especially the solid (anaplastic) type

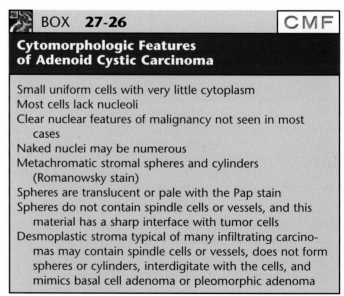

BOX 27-26   CMF

Cytomorphologic Features of Adenoid Cystic Carcinoma

Small uniform cells with very little cytoplasm
Most cells lack nucleoli
Clear nuclear features of malignancy not seen in most cases
Naked nuclei may be numerous
Metachromatic stromal spheres and cylinders (Romanowsky stain)
Spheres are translucent or pale with the Pap stain
Spheres do not contain spindle cells or vessels, and this material has a sharp interface with tumor cells
Desmoplastic stroma typical of many infiltrating carcinomas may contain spindle cells or vessels, does not form spheres or cylinders, interdigitate with the cells, and mimics basal cell adenoma or pleomorphic adenoma

pearance is pathognomonic for adenoid cystic carcinoma, and that this diagnosis is straightforward. However, when studied in FNA samples, several other neoplasms can mimic adenoid cystic carcinoma. Pleomorphic adenomas, basal cell adenomas, dermal analogue tumor, basal cell adenocarcinoma, epithelial-myoepithelial carcinoma, and polymorphous low-grade adenocarcinoma all show small uniform cells and may feature frankly cylindromatous areas (Box 27-27). This problem is not unique to FNA cytology because the same difficulties can arise at the time of frozen section. The small uniform cells of adenoid cystic carcinoma can result in false-negative diagnoses, especially

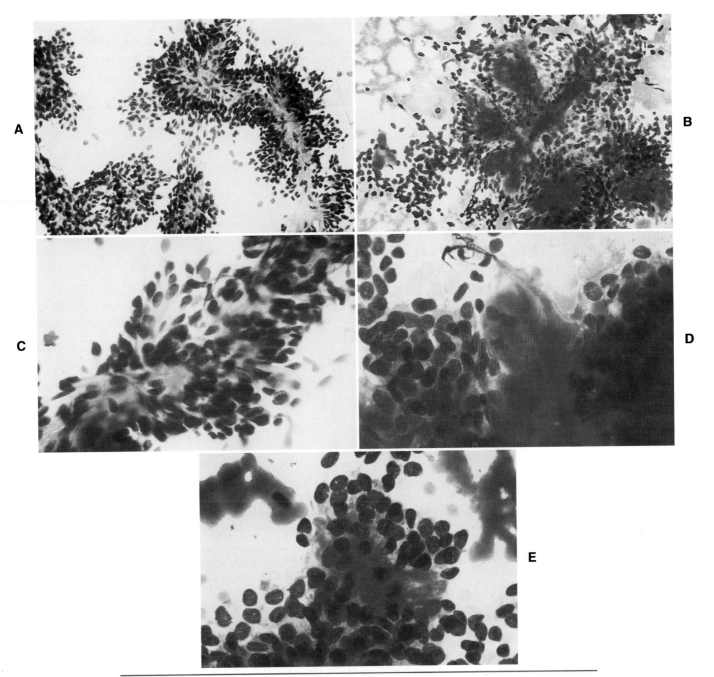

Figure 27-10   Basal cell adenomas. A, Basal cell adenomas usually give highly cellular aspirates. Narrow bands of collagenous stroma are decorated by uniform, small, darkly staining epithelial cells. Naked nuclei are numerous in the background. (Pap) **B,** In air-dried material, the stroma is rendered prominent by its metachromasia. This picture of metachromatic stroma and numerous small dark cells is often mistaken for adenoid cystic carcinoma. (DQ) **C,** The stroma interdigitates with the epithelial cells. (Pap) **D,** Details of the cell-stoma interface are clearly defined in air-dried smears. (DQ) **E,** Some examples of basal cell adenoma have very little stoma. Several small cell neoplasms must be considered in the differential diagnosis of such cases. (Pap) (From Geisinger K, Silverman J. Fine needle aspiration cytology of superficial organs and body sites. New York: Churchill-Livingstone; 1999.)

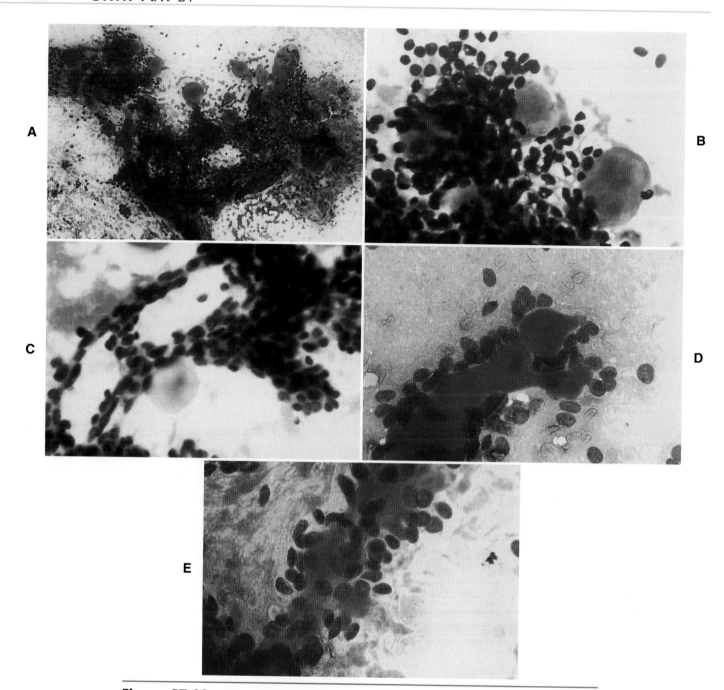

Figure 27-11 Adenoid cystic carcinoma. **A,** At low magnification, smears from the cribriform type of adenoid cystic carcinoma are highly cellular. This pattern of small blue cells and metachromatic stroma is mimicked by basal cell adenomas. (DQ) **B,** The celebrated appearance of blue cells and red balls typical of cribriform adenoid cystic carcinoma is shown here. (DQ) **C,** In fixed smears, the extracellular matrix is translucent. It is easily missed, if present in small quantities. (Pap) **D,** In adenoid cystic carcinoma, the interface between the cells and the stroma is extremely sharp. In some areas, a linear clearing occurs between the two. (DQ) **E,** This photomicrograph highlights the irregular cell-stroma interface that, although typical of basal cell adenomas, is seen in adenoid cystic carcinoma. This is because these tumors have desmoplastic stroma that is distinct from the more characteristic spheres and cylinders. (DQ) (From Geisinger K, Silverman J. Fine needle aspiration cytology of superficial organs and body sites. New York: Churchill-Livingstone; 1999.)

if the sample is sparsely cellular or if the matrix component is not well represented. This pattern of uniform small cells has also been mistaken for small cell anaplastic ("oat cell") carcinoma.

The cytologic similarity between basal cell adenomas and the uncommon solid type of adenoid cystic carcinoma has previously been noted[24] (Figure 27-12). Smears of the latter are usually cellular and show small uniform blue cells that may lie singly or in groups. Cylinders and spheres of extracellular matrix are absent or extremely rare. Fibrillary collagenous fragments of metachromatic desmoplastic stroma may be encountered. This material has been mis-

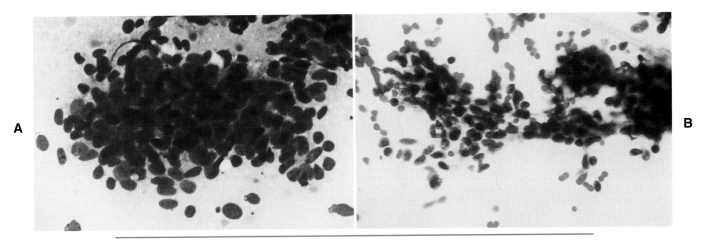

Figure 27-12 Solid adenoid cystic carcinoma. **A,** Aspirates from the solid (anaplastic) variant of adenoid cystic carcinoma show the same uniform small blue cells seen in the cribriform type. However, the metachromatic spheres and cylinders are either absent or extremely rare. (DQ) **B,** This solid adenoid cystic carcinoma cannot be indistinguishable from basal cell adenomas, unless tumor necrosis is unequivocally identified. The cell's nuclei lack the traditional cytomorphologic features of malignancy. (Pap) (From Geisinger K, Silverman J. Fine needle aspiration cytology of superficial organs and body sites. New York: Churchill-Livingstone; 1999.)

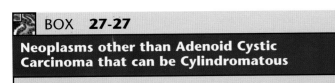

BOX 27-27

Neoplasms other than Adenoid Cystic Carcinoma that can be Cylindromatous

Pleomorphic adenoma
Basal cell adenoma
Dermal analogue tumor
Dermal eccrine cylindroma
Basal cell adenocarcinoma
Epithelial-myoepithelial carcinoma
Polymorphous low-grade adenocarcinoma

taken for the matrix component of pleomorphic adenoma and the extracellular connective tissue of basal cell adenoma. Some authors have suggested that these tumors can be distinguished by careful attention to subtle nuclear features that indicate malignancy. Other investigators have not found this to be the case and leave behind the important but disconcerting concept that these two prognostically very different entities are virtually identical in cytologic material. If one can unequivocally identify necrosis, adenoid cystic carcinoma should be the preferred diagnosis. In these authors' experience, only about half of anaplastic adenoid cystic carcinoma aspirates show necrosis in smear material.[24]

Reviewing these considerations and their own extensive experience, Drs. Löwhagen, Tani, and Skoog indicated considerable reluctance to render an unequivocal diagnosis of adenoid cystic carcinoma on cytologic evidence alone. They write that "in our institution, we refuse to take the full diagnostic responsibility for a radical surgical procedure in which sacrifice of the facial nerve may be necessary in cases where there may be classic cytologic findings of adenoid cystic carcinoma but the patient is symptom free."[27] We would add that, if this stance is justified for the cribriform pattern, it is even more appropriate for the solid variant. In most cases, we are able to offer the clinician only a differential diagnosis.

Uncommon Lesions With a Small Cell Cytologic Pattern

The membranous form of basal cell adenoma is also known as the *dermal analogue* type of monomorphic adenoma. Its histology closely resembles that of dermal cylindroma, and it can be associated with either benign or malignant cutaneous adnexal tumors in a synchronous or metachronous fashion. Cytologically, this tumor may mimic adenoid cystic carcinoma because it grows as large rounded cell nests that are outlined by basement membrane material. The tissue particles recovered by FNA consist of small blue cells surrounded by sheaths of this hyaline material. These are virtually impossible to distinguish from adenoid cystic carcinoma.

Ideally, aspirates of pilomatrixoma should be polymorphous, and should show material representing each of its several components (Figure 27-13). These include small hyperchromatic basal cells, anucleate shadow ("ghost") cells, and multinucleated giant cells. In some examples, bits of calcified material can be appreciated. Rarely, calcific material may dominate the cytologic picture. The shadow cells may lie singly and clearly manifest squamous features, or they may be compacted into clumps in which the squamous nature of individual cells is difficult to recognize. Mitotic figures may be identified among the small basaloid cells.

Shadow cells are essential for positive identification of this tumor in aspirate samples. Often, however, they are difficult to identify or are absent altogether. This is the major reason that other diagnoses are considered in up to 75% of pilomatrixomas described in the FNA literature. Often, important differential diagnostic considerations are suggested by the prominent small blue cell component. Basal cell carcinoma, metastatic small cell anaplastic carcinoma, various salivary gland tumors, the small blue cell tumors of childhood, and metastatic nasopharyngeal carcinoma are likely to be misdiagnoses. Nasopharyngeal carcinoma has been emphasized as a pitfall for those working with Chinese patients with pilomatrixoma in whom a relatively high incidence of the former neoplasm occurs. Because this malignancy can often present as a high cervical lymph node metastasis, it can clinically simulate a pilomatrixoma.

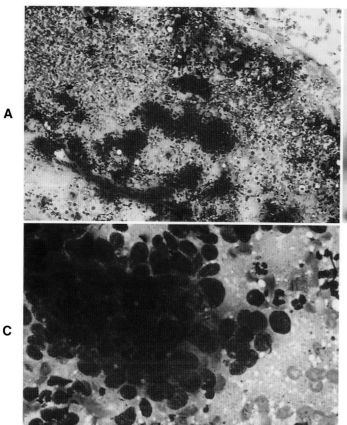

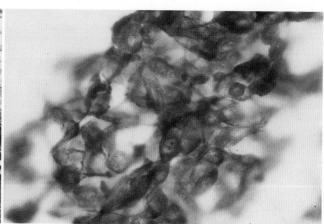

Figure 27-13 Pilomatrixoma. **A,** At low magnification, the pilomatrixoma shows large tissue particles composed of small darkly staining cells that often suggest a malignant neoplasm. (DQ) **B,** The ghost cells may be aggregated into large masses where their squamous nature may be difficult to recognize. (Pap) **C,** At high magnification, the basal cell component may further simulate a malignancy, if not placed in context by recognition of the ghost cells. (DQ) (From Geisinger K, Silverman J. Fine needle aspiration cytology of superficial organs and body sites. New York: Churchill-Livingstone; 1999.)

Pilomatrixomas are very firm to palpation, and this can further elevate clinical suspicion so that when a troublesome aspirate is encountered, the likelihood of an incorrect diagnosis of carcinoma may be very great indeed. Other problems may occur when this tumor is located in sites other than the head and neck. Finally, some pilomatrixomas can show striking atypia so that the expected small blue cell pattern is replaced by a proliferation of atypical cells that suggest large-cell types of carcinoma. If unfortunate circumstances combine several of these difficulties, correct diagnosis of pilomatrixoma may be extremely difficult. For example, one of the authors encountered striking large-cell type cytologic atypia and a paucity of shadow cells in a lesion on the forearm of a young man recently treated for testicular endodermal sinus tumor. It was incorrectly interpreted that the aspirate was probable evidence of metastatic malignancy, albeit before serum tumor marker studies were available. The cytologic atypia was also noted in the excised tumor. In this case, the prominent enlargement and atypia of the usually small blue cells may have been induced by chemotherapy. If so, aspiration of pilomatrixomas in cancer patients with suspected tumor recurrences might represent a special problem that remains incompletely explored at this time.

Carcinoma ex monomorphic adenoma arises in the parotid, where it usually appears approximately 10 years after diagnosis of the original adenoma. This neoplasm behaves in a locally aggressive fashion. It has been described histologically as a caricature of the adenoma that shows infiltrative growth, and variable combinations of necrosis, mitotic activity and nuclear pleomorphism. Some cases arise in a background of dermal analogue tumor. Examples of carcinoma ex monomorphic adenoma have not yet been described in the FNA literature.

Basal cell adenocarcinoma usually occurs in the parotid but can be seen in the submandibular and minor salivary glands.[28] Histologically, it closely resembles metastatic basal cell carcinoma of cutaneous origin. This carcinoma shares its immunocytochemical profile with basal cell adenoma but shows an infiltrative growth associated with local recurrence. Metastases can occur in up to 10% of cases.

Aspirates of basal cell adenocarcinoma have the same architectural pattern as basal cell adenoma and solid adenoid cystic carcinoma. Some three-dimensional cell clusters may be papillary or filiform, with palisading of peripheral nuclei. Individually, the cells show a high nucleocytoplasmsic ratio, fine chromatin and prominent nucleoli. Mitotic figures may be identified. The smear background can be myxoid or can show necrosis; the latter finding suggests a possible diagnosis of solid adenoid cystic carcinoma. A relationship between basal cell adenocarcinoma with carcinoma ex monomorphic adenoma has been postulated.

Small cell anaplastic carcinoma can arise as a primary salivary gland neoplasm, mostly in the parotid. Virtually all cases show immunocytochemical evidence of neuroendocrine differentiation. Cytologically, primary small cell carcinoma recapitulates the pattern that is familiar from similar neoplasms of the lung (Chapter 16) and other sites. Paranuclear blue cytoplasmic inclusions similar to those to be discussed in Merkel cell carcinoma have been noted.

Metastases from one of the other organs that more commonly host small cell carcinomas are much more common than primary small cell anaplastic carcinoma in a salivary gland site. Following this type of FNA diagnosis, a search for a primary tumor in the lung, or the head and neck (Merkel cell carcinoma) should be considered.

A single case of well-differentiated neuroendocrine carcinoma has been reported in FNA of a parotid mass.[29] Free-lying plasmacytoid tumor cells resulted in a smear pattern that was strongly reminiscent of medullary thyroid carcinoma. These cells gave a positive reaction when stained with anti-cytokeratin immunoreagents.

Primary lymphoepithelioma-like carcinoma of the parotid or submandibular gland is also known as malignant lymphoepithelial lesion, or Eskimo tumor. Poorly differentiated malignant cells with abundant lymphocyte-rich stroma cause this tumor to closely resemble nasopharyngeal carcinoma. FNA of metastatic nasopharyngeal carcinoma with an occult primary is more common than cytologic evaluation of a primary salivary gland tumor with this histology. The former often presents as an intraparotid or high cervical lymph node and may appear clinically to represent a primary parotid lesion.

Primary lymphoepithelioma-like carcinoma and metastatic lymphoepithelioma are morphologically identical and distinction should be based on clinical and radiographic findings. The cells are pleomorphic, and show high nucleocytoplasmic ratios, finely granular chromatin, and a single prominent nucleolus. Mitotic figures are often numerous. The associated lymphoid tissue varies in quantity, but should be polymorphous, in keeping with its benign nature. Acinic cell carcinoma consists of large cells and may have prominent lymphoid infiltrates, but it lacks the high-grade cytology of lymphoepithelioma.

Metastatic Carcinomas That Involve the Salivary Glands and Show a Small Cell Pattern

Metastatic basal cell carcinoma of cutaneous origin has an FNA smear pattern of small blue cells[21] (Figure 27-14). Variable amounts of necrosis and occasional squamous pearls can be superimposed on this picture. Individual cells show scanty cytoplasm, fine chromatin, and a single small nucleolus. Peripheral palisading of nuclei has been noted in some cases as a feature in favor of basal cell carcinoma, but it is not seen uniformly. These findings are very similar to those noted in aspirations of the primary cutaneous lesions.

In a salivary gland site, it may be clinically impossible to distinguish between metastases to the gland itself or to a lymph node. If a previous history of basal cell carcinoma is available, at the time of FNA, the material should be reviewed. However, metastases have been noted up to 30 years after excision of a primary skin lesion. Furthermore, cutaneous basal cell carcinomas are very common, but metastases are rare. Thus, patients, clinicians, and pathologists may not relate a new salivary gland area mass to the original diagnosis. One case was initially mistaken for pleomorphic adenoma. The history of basal cell carcinoma was not available, and desmoplastic tumor stroma was felt to incorrectly represent mixed tumor matrix.

FNA of Merkel cell carcinoma has been described. Metastatic deposits show the small cell anaplastic carcinoma cytology familiar from other sites. Perinuclear blue inclusions ("buttons") are a characteristic finding on air-dried smears but are not seen in fixed preparations. Ultrastructurally, they consist of intermediate filaments and are immunocytochemically positive for cytokeratin and

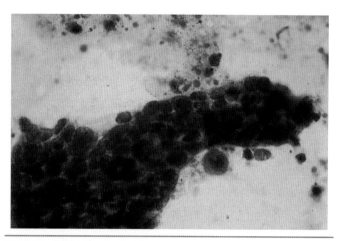

Figure 27-14 Metastatic cutaneous basal cell carcinoma. Without a good clinical history, nothing specific is noted about this small blue cell neoplasm to indicate its origin in a cutaneous basal cell carcinoma. The necrotic background helps prevent a false negative diagnosis. (Pap) (From Geisinger K, Silverman J. Fine needle aspiration cytology of superficial organs and body sites. New York: Churchill-Livingstone; 1999.)

neurofilaments. In smears, they can be seen as crescentic intracytoplasmic bodies, or as free-lying round structures in the background. These inclusions are apparently rare in non–small cell carcinoma and malignant lymphoma. Unfortunately, they are less specific than previously suggested because similar structures have been described in primary small cell carcinoma of the salivary glands and in small cell lung carcinoma as well as in rhabdomyosarcoma.

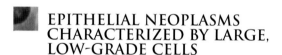

EPITHELIAL NEOPLASMS CHARACTERIZED BY LARGE, LOW-GRADE CELLS

Acinic Cell Carcinoma

Box 27-28 provides a list of these neoplasms.

Aspirates from acinic cell carcinomas are usually quite cellular, with numerous large cells that are present singly and in groups[30-33] (Figure 27-15). A few rounded acinar arrangements may be present. Larger tissue particles are often organized around a wide, thin-walled venule-sized central vessel that may branch and ramify through microbiopsy fragments of considerable size. These fragments have irregular borders, as tumor cells fall away to lie singly in the background[15] (Box 27-29). Well-differentiated acinic cell carcinoma differs in part from normal salivary gland tissue by the absence of duct cells and adipocytes. However, any admixture of neoplastic cells with tissue from the surrounding normal gland can considerably complicate interpretation.

Many of these large fragile tumor cell can be damaged in the smearing process so that numerous naked nuclei litter the smear background. These are occasionally mistaken for the lymphocytes of sialadenitis or Warthin's tumor. The background debris of Warthin's tumor is not present, unless one is dealing with a cyst variant of acinic cell carcinoma. The distinction between naked epithelial cell nuclei and lymphocytes was discussed previously in this chapter. These difficulties are compounded when true lymphocytic infiltrates accompany an acinic cell carcinoma. In other cases, the cells' granular cytoplasm has been thought to indicate the vacuoles of mucoepidermoid carcinoma.

The intact tumor cells have abundant finely granular cytoplasm and may be difficult to distinguish from oncocytes. Nucleoli range from inconspicuous to prominent but striking cytologic features of frank malignancy are not usually noted. For this reason, some cases are falsely interpreted as

negative. Pulmonary metastases of acinic cell carcinoma are occasionally diagnosed by FNA.

Several variants in the pattern of acinic cell carcinoma have been described in histopathology and in FNA material. Clear cell change may be very extensive and suggest metastatic renal cell carcinoma. Usually, however, cells more typical of acinic cell carcinoma are associated with the clear cell component. The papillary cystic variant is difficult to diagnose in aspirate samples. FNA yields cyst fluid contain-

---

BOX 27-28

Epithelial Neoplasms With Large Cells of Low Nuclear Grade

Acinic cell carcinoma
Oncocytic lesions
Polymorphous low-grade carcinoma
Epithelial-myoepithelial carcinoma
Predominantly sebaceous neoplasms
Squamous cell carcinoma (may alternatively show high nuclear grade)
Clear cell carcinoma
Metastases

BOX 27-29   CMF

Cytomorphologic Features of Acinic Cell Carcinoma

Most aspirates are highly cellular
Lacks association with ductal cells and adipose tissue
Large tumor cells are easily damaged by smearing
Numerous naked nuclei result from cell damage
Granular background material represents the cytoplasm of cells damaged during the smearing process
Large tissue particles show intact cells
Prominent blood vessels often traverse the larger particles
Cells show abundant cytoplasm and variably prominent nucleoli

---

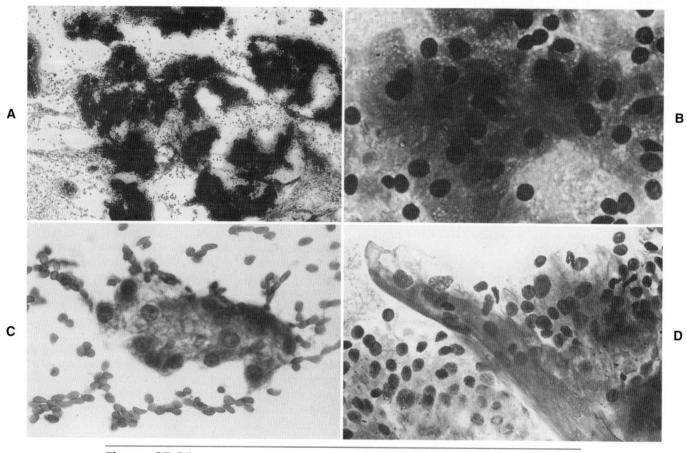

Figure 27-15   Acinic cell carcinoma. **A,** This acinic cell carcinoma aspirate is highly cellular. (DQ) **B,** The cells are large, with abundant finely granular cytoplasm, and resemble oncocytes. (DQ) **C,** In a fixed smear, the cytoplasm appears more clear than granular, and the nuclei are round. (Pap) **D,** A frequent feature of this tumor is the presence of large blood vessels around which tumor cells cluster. (DQ) (From Geisinger K, Silverman J. Fine needle aspiration cytology of superficial organs and body sites. New York: Churchill-Livingstone; 1999.)

ing flat sheets of large granular cells that suggest a Warthin's tumor; vacuolated cells may resemble low-grade mucoepidermoid carcinoma. Some aspirates contain psammoma bodies, but other features of papillary thyroid carcinoma are not present.

Most acinic cell carcinomas are slowly progressive and many do not recur or metastasize for 5 to 20 years. Thus, in considering their diagnosis, it is advisable to investigate the patient's history.

Oncocytic Neoplasms

Oncocytes occur in mature organs and are large cells with abundant granular cytoplasm with numerous mitochondria. Some cells without this ultrastructural finding can still appear oncocytoid at the light microscopic level. Cells of this type can be seen in normal salivary glands, and in a variety of neoplasms. Their cytologic features were described during the consideration of Warthin's tumor (Figure 27-16 and Box 27-30).

Most oncocytomas are benign, regardless of the pleomorphism that the smears or sections occasionally show.[34-38] Differential diagnostic problems relate to the similarity of oncocytes to acinic cells, and to other neoplasms that show oncocytic foci or features. Oncocytic neoplasms can be mistaken for Warthin's tumor, especially if lymphocytes are prominent. This is not a problem that is likely to alter pa-

tient care adversely. The dirty cyst fluid of Warthin's tumor is usually not seen in oncocytoma.

Distinction between oncocytoma and acinic cell carcinoma may require electron microscopy, and must often await surgical excision; FNA gives only a differential diagnosis in difficult cases. Clear cell change may be associated with more typical oncocytic features in other areas. Squamous metaplasia, mucinous change, and necrosis of cell nests may occur.

Oncocytomas often show nuclear pleomorphism but still behave in a benign fashion; malignant oncocytoma is a rare entity. Histologic or clinical evidence of aggressive behavior is required to override our usual tolerance for cytologic atypia in oncocytic neoplasms. Thus, it is not possible to diagnose malignant oncocytoma from FNA samples. Oncocytoid adenocarcinoma is probably more common than true malignant oncocytomas. Such tumors show lesser degrees of mitochondrial hyperplasia.

Polymorphous Low Grade Adenocarcinoma

Polymorphous low-grade adenocarcinoma is also known as *terminal duct carcinoma,* or lobular carcinoma. It is most common in minor salivary gland sites, but rare cases occur in the submandibular or parotid glands. In the latter instance, this tumor is most likely to represent a component of carcinoma ex pleomorphic adenoma.

Histologically, uniform cells with bland nuclear features grow in architecturally diverse combinations of tubular, solid, cribriform, and papillary pattern. These can be easily mistaken for adenoid cystic carcinoma. Follow-up shows local recurrences, but regional node metastases are rare. Tumors that show extensive areas of papillary growth tend to be more aggressive and are usually classified separately.[39-41]

Cytology of the few reported cases confirms that this tumor is very difficult to distinguish from adenoid cystic carcinoma or pleomorphic adenoma.[39-41] Uniform cells show fine chromatin, tiny nucleoli, and moderate amounts of cytoplasm. These are arranged in sheets, glands, and solid rounded groups. Tyrosine crystals may be identified.

BOX 27-30

Oncocytic Neoplasms

Most are benign
Oncocytes have abundant granular cytoplasm
Some cells may be atypical with enlarged nuclei and
   prominent nucleoli
May be very difficult to distinguish from acinic cell
   carcinoma

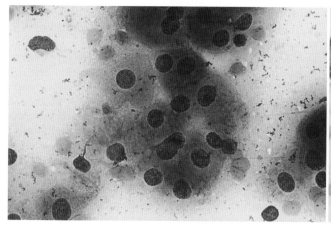
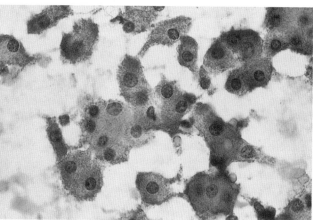

Figure 27-16 Oncocytoma. **A,** This oncocytoma shows a monotonous population of large cells with abundant dense cytoplasm. Cell borders are difficult to discern, and occasional nucleoli are evident. (DQ) **B,** In contrast with their appearance in histologic sections, oncocytes are not always eosinophilic in cytologic samples. (Pap) (From Geisinger K, Silverman J. Fine needle aspiration cytology of superficial organs and body sites. New York: Churchill-Livingstone; 1999.)

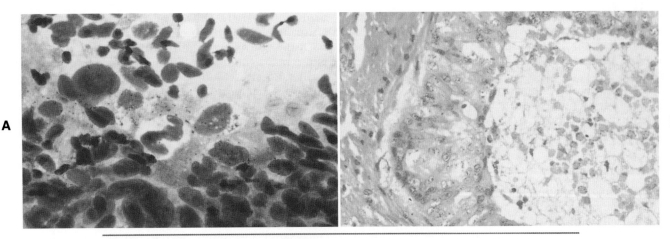

Figure 27-17 Salivary duct carcinoma. **A,** This aspirate from a parotid mass in an older adult male shows a non–small cell carcinoma with no distinguishing features. (DQ) **B,** Histologically, the resemblance of this neoplasm to breast carcinoma is striking and results in a diagnosis of ductal carcinoma of the parotid. (H&E) (From Geisinger K, Silverman J. Fine needle aspiration cytology of superficial organs and body sites. New York: Churchill-Livingstone; 1999.)

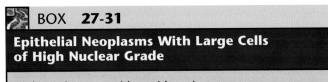

BOX **27-31**

Epithelial Neoplasms With Large Cells of High Nuclear Grade

High-grade mucoepidermoid carcinoma
High-grade carcinoma, NOS
Squamous cell carcinoma:
• Primary
• Metastatic
• Direct extension from adjacent sites
Ductal carcinoma
Metastatic nonsquamous carcinoma
Metastatic malignant melanoma

NOS, Not otherwise specific.

Epithelial-Myoepithelial Carcinoma

The histology of this neoplasm is reflected in aspirate smears, which show a combination of large myoepithelial cells and tubules formed by small, dark, uniform duct cells. Numerous naked nuclei are present. Cell clusters are associated with acellular hyaline material. In some cases, small cells and hyaline matrix predominate, and thus, one may consider a diagnosis of adenoid cystic carcinoma. Clear myoepithelial cells may suggest clear cell carcinoma, acinic cell carcinoma with clear cell change, or sebaceous carcinoma. None of these has a component of small duct cells. Furthermore, epithelial-myoepithelial carcinoma-like areas can occur in pleomorphic adenoma. Confident diagnosis should be based on thorough sampling.[42,43]

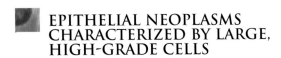

EPITHELIAL NEOPLASMS CHARACTERIZED BY LARGE, HIGH-GRADE CELLS

Box 27-31 provides a list of these neoplasms.

The salivary glands can be involved by direct extension of carcinomas derived from the head and neck mucosal surfaces or the skin. Metastatic lesions may involve an intraglandular lymph node or a major salivary gland. The parotid is more often involved than the submandibular gland. Malignant melanoma and squamous cell carcinoma are the most common tumors in this setting. FNA of malignant melanoma is discussed in other chapters. Additional metastases that are occasionally encountered include seminoma, sebaceous carcinoma, and astrocytoma.

Distinction between primary and metastatic carcinoma is of great clinical importance, and FNA may address this issue very well. Those who perform the aspiration and interpret the smears should always be provided any available history of previous malignancy. However, in the authors' series of nine metastatic high-grade carcinomas, only six patients had malignancies that were recognized in their primary sites prior to salivary gland FNA.[29] A metastasis should always be considered, especially if the sample does not appear typical of a well-characterized type of salivary gland tumor.

With high-grade mucoepidermoid carcinoma, the highly cellular aspirate of large carcinoma cells must be distinguished from metastatic carcinoma and from other primary high-grade carcinomas. Extensive clear cell change can suggest other diagnoses.

Salivary gland duct carcinoma is operatively defined by its histologic resemblance to breast carcinoma. The cells of this tumor can be arranged in solid, cribiform, or papillary patterns (Figure 27-17). Other features may include occasional psammoma bodies, keratinized cells, or comedo-like necrosis. Occasional cases yield low grade malignant cells and collagenous stroma in a pattern mistaken for a pleomorphic adenoma (Figure 27-18). Based on cytologic findings alone, this can be a formidable diagnostic dilemma.[44-47] Clinical findings can be helpful in this regard; ductal carcinoma usually occurs in older adult men, whereas mixed tumors are more common in women in the middle years.

SPINDLE CELL LESIONS

Primary spindle cell lesions of the salivary glands are not commonly studied by FNA. We divide these into groups with

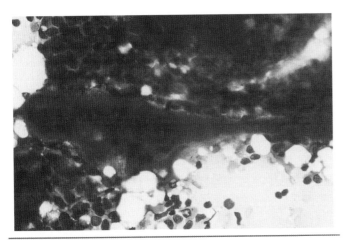

Figure 27-18   **Salivary duct carcinoma.** This example of salivary gland duct carcinoma shows low-grade nuclei and fragments of desmoplastic stroma. This aspirate was mistaken for pleomorphic adenoma at the time of FNA. (DQ) (From Geisinger K, Silverman J. Fine needle aspiration cytology of superficial organs and body sites. New York: Churchill-Livingstone; 1999.)

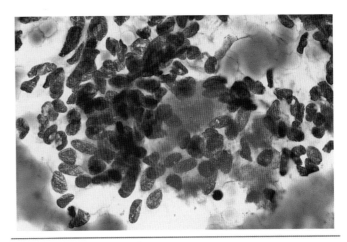

Figure 27-19   **Spindle cell myoepithelioma.** This example of benign myoepithelioma (myoepithelial adenoma) shows spindle cells that vary somewhat in size and fragments of collagenous stroma. (DQ)

BOX   27-32

Spindle Cell Lesions of Low Nuclear Grade

Nonspecific reactive proliferations
Nodular fasciitis
Hemangioma
Myoepithelioma
Kaposi's sarcoma

BOX   27-33

Spindle Cell Lesions of High Nuclear Grade

Primary sarcoma
Sarcoma from adjacent tissues
Malignant myoepithelioma
Squamous cell carcinoma
Metastatic carcinoma
Metastatic malignant melanoma

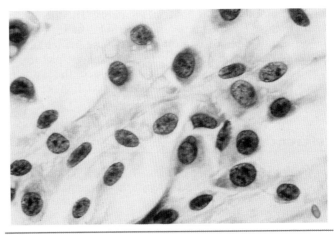

Figure 27-20   **Malignant myoepithelioma.** This malignant myoepithelioma shows loosely cohesive malignant spindle cells. (Pap) (From Geisinger K, Silverman J. Fine needle aspiration cytology of superficial organs and body sites. New York: Churchill-Livingstone; 1999.)

---

either high or low nuclear grade (Boxes 27-32 and 27-33). Most examples are reported in large series where they receive limited treatment and include hemangioma, lymphangioma, and hemangiopericytoma. A single case of nodular fasciitis was followed nonsurgically after FNA and resolved.[48]

The cells of myoepithelioma can be either spindled or plasmacytoid. However, plasmacytoid cells in pleomorphic adenomas lack ultrastructural and immunocytochemical features of myoepithelial differentiation.

Most myoepitheliomas are located in the parotid, but submandibular and rare extraglandular cases occur. Cytologically, these neoplasms usually show monotonous spindle cells that resemble those of a leiomyoma and are identical to the same cell type occasionally aspirated from mixed tumors[49] (Figure 27-19; see Figure 27-5, *G*). These cells are associated with variable amounts of collagenous stroma. When

this picture is encountered in smears, other low-grade spindle cell neoplasms must be considered because the cytologic findings are nonspecific. Electron microscopic or immunocytochemical confirmation can be sought for difficult cases. The plasmacytoid type of myoepithelioma can show striking nuclear enlargement and atypia in single cells similar to those derived from pleomorphic adenomas (see Figure 27-5, *D*).

Malignant myoepithelioma can arise *de novo,* or within a preexisting pleomorphic adenoma. Only a few examples have been described in the FNA literature.[49] These have shown a poorly cohesive proliferation of mitotically active spindle cells with high-grade nuclear features (Figure 27-20). Definitive diagnosis requires ultrastructural or immunocytochemical demonstration of myoepithelial differentiation. Hemangiopericytoma has been cytologically mistaken for malignant myoepithelioma.

Aspiration of a single salivary gland anlage tumor (congenital pleomorphic adenoma) was reported by Bondeson

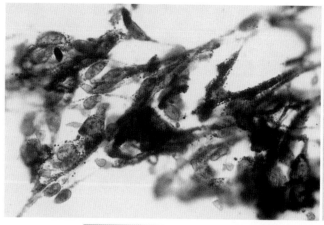
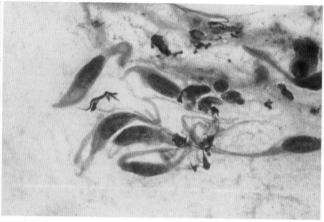

Figure 27-21   **Metastatic malignant melenoma. A,** Metastatic malignant melanoma can show a spindle cell pattern. In this case, heavy pigment makes the diagnosis simple. (DQ) **B,** Other metastatic melanomas may present a diagnostic problem, when pigment is not identified. (Pap) (From Geisinger K, Silverman J. Fine needle aspiration cytology of superficial organs and body sites. New York: Churchill-Livingstone; 1999.)

and colleagues.[50] Smears showed a combination of small uniform spindle cells and ductal elements. This neoplasm occurs exclusively in the neonatal period. The differential diagnosis must include teratoma; most of the small blue cell tumors of childhood do not share this cytologic picture.

Spindle cell malignancies can also reach the salivary glands by metastasis or direct extension. Malignant melanoma may present in this manner (Figure 27-21).

References

1. Stanley MW, Löwhagen T. Fine needle aspiration of palpable masses. Stoneham, Mass: Butterworth-Heinnemann; 1993.
2. Cohen MB. Editorial comments: FNAB of salivary gland. Diagn Cytopathol 1993; 9:224-225.
3. Henry-Stanley MJ, Beneke J, Bardales RH, et al. Fine needle aspiration of normal tissue from enlarged salivary glands: sialosis, or missed target? Diagn Cytopathol 1995; 13:300-303.
4. Waldron CA. Face, lips, teeth, oral soft tissue, jaws, salivary gland and neck: enlargements related to malnutrition, hormonal disturbances, and alcoholic cirrhosis (sialosis). In: Kissane JM, editor. Anderson's pathology, vol 2, 9th ed. St Louis: Mosby; 1990.p.1128.
5. Ascoli V, Albedi FM, De Blasiis R, et al. Sialadenosis of the parotid gland: report of four cases diagnosed by fine-needle aspiration cytology. Diagn Cytopathol 1993; 9:151-155.
6. Layfield LJ, Glasgow BJ, Goldstein N, et al. Lipomatous lesions of the parotid gland: potential pitfalls in fine needle aspiration biopsy diagnosis. Acta Cytol 1991; 35:553-556.
7. Johnson FB, Oertel YC, Ammann K. Sialadenitis with crystalloid formation: a report of six cases diagnosed by fine-needle aspiration. Diagn Cytopathol 1995; 12:76-80.
8. Viguer JM, Vicandi B, Jiménez-Heffernan JA, et al. Fine needle aspiration of pleomorphic adenoma: an analysis of 212 cases. Acta Cytol 1997; 41:786-794.
9. Luna MA, Batsakis JG, Tortoledo ME, et al. Carcinomas ex monomorphic adenoma of salivary glands. J Laryngol Otol 1989; 103:756-759.
10. Kim T, Yoon GS, Kim O, et al. Fine needle aspiration diagnosis of malignant mixed tumor (carcinosarcoma) arising in pleomorphic adenoma of the salivary gland: a case report. Acta Cytol 1998; 42:1027-1031.
11. Anand A, Brockie ES. Cytomorphological features of salivary duct carcinoma ex pleomorphic adenoma: diagnosis by fine-needle aspiration. Diagn Cytopathol 1999; 20:375-378.
12. Klijaniennko J, Vielh P. Fine-needle samping of salivary gland lesions. II. Cytology and histology correlation of 71 cases of Warthin's tumor (adenolymphoma). Diagn Cytopathol 1997; 16:221-225.
13. Chen KTK. Letter to the editor: aspiration cytology of metaplastic Warthin's tumor mimicking squamous-cell carcinoma. Diagn Cytopathol 1991; 7:330-331.
14. Ballo MS, Shin HJ, Sneige N. Sources of diagnostic error in the fine-needle aspiration diagnosis of Warthin's tumor and clues to correct diagnosis. Diagn Cytopathol 1997; 17:230-234.
15. Tao L-C, Gullane PJ. HIV infection-associated lymphoepithelial lesions of the parotid gland: aspiration biopsy cytology, histology, and pathogenesis. Diagn Cytopathol 1991; 7:159-162.
16. Stanley MW, Bardales RH, Beneke J, et al. Sialolithiasis: differential diagnostic problems in fine needle aspiration cytology. Am J Clin Pathol 1996; 106:229-233.
17. Frierson HF, Fechner RE. Chronic sialadenitis with psammoma bodies mimicking neoplasia in a fine-needle aspiration specimen from the submandibular gland. Am J Clin Pathol 1991; 95:884-888.
18. Cohen MB, Fisher PE, Holly EA, et al. Fine needle aspiration biopsy diagnosis of mucoepidermoid carcinoma: statistical analysis. Acta Cytol 1990; 34:43-49.
19. Hayes MMM, Cameron RD, Jones EA. Sebaceous variant of mucoepidermoid carcinoma of the salivary gland: a case report with cytohistologic correlation. Acta Cytol 1993; 37:237-241.
20. Kumar N, Kapila K, Verma K. Fine needle aspiration cytology of mucoepidermoid carcinoma: a diagnostic problem. Acta Cytol 1991; 35:357-359.
21. Stanley MW, Horwitz CA, Bardales RH, et al. Basal cell carcinoma metastatic to the salivary glands: differential diagnosis in fine needle aspiration cytology. Diagn Cytopathol 1997; 16:247-252.
22. Stanley MW, Horwitz CA, Rollins SD, et al. Basal cell (monomorphic) and minimally pleomorphic adenomas of the salivary glands: distinction from the solid (anaplastic) type of adenoid cystic carcinoma in fine needle aspiration. Am J Clin Pathol 1996; 106:35-41.

23. López JI, Ballestin C. Fine-needle aspiration cytology of a membranous basal cell adenoma arising in an intraparotid lymph node. Diagn Cytopathol 1993; 9:668-672.

24. Stanley MW, Horwitz CA, Henry MJ, et al. Basal-cell adenoma of the salivary gland: a benign adenoma that cytologically mimics adenoid cystic carcinoma. Diagn Cytopathol 1998; 4:342-346.

25. Kapidia SB, Dusenbery D, Dekker A. Fine needle aspiration of pleomorphic adenoma and adenoid cystic carcinoma of salivary gland origin. Acta Cytol 1997; 41:487-492.

26. Lee SS, Cho KJ, Ham EK. Differential diagnosis of adenoid cystic carcinoma of the salivary gland on fine needle aspiration cytology. Acta Cytol 1996; 40:1246-1252.

27. Löwhagen T, Tani EM, Skoog L. Salivary glands and rare head and neck lesions. In: Bibbo M, editor. Comprehensive cytopathology. Philadelphia: WB Saunders; 1991. pp.627-634.

28. Pisharodi LR. Basal cell adenocarcinoma of the salivary gland: diagnosis by fine-needle aspiration cytology. Am J Clin Pathol 1995; 103:603-608.

29. Stanley MW, Bardales RH, Farmer CE, et al. Primary and metastatic high grade carcinomas of the salivary glands: a cytologic-histologic correlation study of twenty cases. Diagn Cytopathol 1995; 13:37-43.

30. Nagel H, Laskawi R, Büter JJ, et al. Cytologic diagnosis of acinic-cell carcinoma of salivary glands. Diagn Cytopathol 1997; 16:402-412.

31. Sauer T, Jebsen PW, Olsholt R. Cytologic features of papillary-cystic variant of acinic-cell adenocarcinoma: a case report. Diagn Cytopathol 1994; 10:30-32.

32. Whitlatch SP. To the editor: psammoma bodies in fine-needle aspiration biopsies of acinic cell tumor. Diagn Cytopathol 1986; 2:268-269.

33. Klijanienko J, Vielh P. Fine-needle sample of salivary glands lesions. V. Cytology of 22 cases of acinic cell carcinoma with histologic correlation. Diagn Cytopathol 1997; 17:347-352.

34. Gray SR, Cornog JL, Seo IS. Oncocytic neoplasms of salivary glands: a report of fifteen cases including two malignant oncocytomas. Cancer 1976; 38:1306-1317.

35. Taxy JB. Necrotizing squamous/mucinous metaplasia in oncocytic salivary gland tumors: a potential diagnostic problem. Am J Clin Pathol 1992; 97:40-45.

36. Laforga JB, Aranda FI. Oncocytic carcinoma of parotid gland: fine-needle aspiration and histologic findings. Diagn Cytopathol 1994; 11:376-379.

37. Austin MB, Frierson HF, Feldman PS. Oncocytoid adenocarcinoma of the parotid gland: cytologic, histologic and ultrastructural findings. Acta Cytol 1987; 31:351-356.

38. Brandwein MS, Huvos AG. Oncocytic tumors of major salivary glands: a study of 68 cases with follow-up of 44 patients. Am J Surg Pathol 1991; 15:514-528.

39. Ritland F, Lubensky I, LiVolsi VA. Polymorphous low-grade adenocarcinoma of the parotid salivary gland. Arch Pathol Lab Med 1993; 117:1261-1263.

40. Simpson RH, Clarke TJ, Sarsfield PT, et al. Polymorphous low-grade adenocarcinoma of the salivary glands: a clinicopathological comparison with adenoid cystic carcinoma (see comments). Histopathology 1991; 19:121-129.

41. Haba R, Kobayashi S, Miki H, et al. Polymorphous low-grade adenocarcinoma of submandibular gland origin. Acta Pathol J 1993; 43:774-778.

42. Arora VK, Misra K, Bhatia A. Cytomorphologic features of the rare epithelial-myoepithelial carcinoma of the salivary gland. Acta Cytol 1990; 34:239-242.

43. Stewart CJ, Hamilton S, Brown IL, et al. Salivary epithelial-myoepithelial carcinoma: report of a case misinterpreted as pleomorphic adenoma on fine needle aspiration (FNA). Cytopathology 1997; 8:203-203.

44. Fyrat P, Cramer H, Feczko JD, et al. Fine-needle aspiration biopsy of salivary duct carcinoma: report of five cases. Diagn Cytopathol 1997; 16:526-530.

45. Khurana KK, Pitman MB, Powers CN, et al. Diagnostic pitfalls of aspiration cytology of salivary duct carcinoma. Cancer Cytopathol 1997; 81:373-378.

46. Garcia-Bonafe M, Catala I, Tarragona J, et al. Cytologic diagnosis of salivary duct carcinoma: a review of seven cases. Diagn Cytopathol 1998 19:120-123.

47. Gilcrease MZ, Guzman-Paz M, Froberg K, et al. Salivary duct carcinoma: Is a specific diagnosis possible by fine needle aspiration cytology? Acta Cytol 1998; 42:1389-1396.

48. Stanley MW, Skoog L, Tani EM, et al. Nodular fasciitis: spontaneous resolution following diagnosis by fine needle aspiration. Diagn Cytopathol 1993; 9:322-324.

49. Torlakovic E, Ames E, Manivel JC, et al. Benign and malignant neoplasms of myoepithelial cells: cytologic findings. Diagn Cytopathol 1993; 9:655-660.

50. Bondeson L, Andreasson L, Olsson M, et al. Salivary gland anlage tumor: cytologic features in a case examined by fine-needle aspiration. Diagn Cytopathol 1997; 16:518-521.

51. Layfield LJ, Glasgow BJ: Diagnosis of salivary gland tumors by fine-needle aspiration cytology: a review of clinical utility and pitfalls. Diagn Cytopathol 1991; 7:267-272.

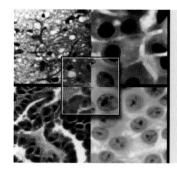

CHAPTER
28

Soft Tissue and Bone

Fine needle aspiration (FNA) biopsies have become an established tool in the diagnostic armamentarium of many clinical practices. The initial diagnosis of many mass lesions in both superficial (e.g., breast and thyroid) and deep (e.g., lung and pancreas) body sites can often be readily and safely assessed by FNA biopsy. One of the few remaining frontiers for FNA biopsy is the evaluation of primary tumors of soft tissue and bone.[1-21,143]

 ## GENERAL CONSIDERATIONS

Several important challenges exist that are inherent in the FNA biopsy evaluation of neoplasms of soft tissue and bone. First, many of these lesions, especially the sarcomas, are quite rare. In the United States, less than 6000 soft tissue sarcomas are diagnosed each year, yielding an incidence of 1.4 per 100,000 in the population. Bone sarcomas are even less common with only approximately 2000 annually, for an incidence of 0.5 new cases per 100,000 individuals. Accordingly, most practicing pathologists do not encounter these neoplasms on a routine basis and may not be intimately familiar with their morphologic, clinical, and radiographic features. Another reason that pathologists may be reluctant to evaluate these tumors is that they possess overlapping histopathologic and cytomorphologic attributes, which is further compounded by the morphologic heterogeneity that may be present within some of these mass lesions. The increasing recognition of borderline tumors or neoplasms of intermediate malignancy make the interpretation of FNA biopsy of orthopedic masses even more problematic. For these reasons, some pathologists and surgeons, in particular those from Scandinavia, have advocated that the diagnoses and treatment of many lesions, especially sarcomas, should occur within centralized medical facilities.[2,18]

FNA biopsy possess a number of distinct, well recognized advantages which require consideration for its application in evaluating mesenchymal neoplasms.[1,3,12] Aspiration biopsy, compared with other techniques, is a rapid outpatient procedure that may provide an immediate diagnosis. This permits the orthopedic surgeon to discuss potential additional diagnostic procedures and therapy with the patient during the initial visit. This also facilitates further processing or triaging of the patient by the surgeon. Patients suffer relatively little pain or discomfort from the aspiration procedure, and in most circumstances, local anesthesia is not necessary. A major advantage of FNA biopsy over core needle biopsies is the much greater sampling of a mass lesion. By altering the direction of the needle during a single puncture, multiple portions of the mass may be aspirated. If necessary, multiple separate needle punctures may be performed during a single patient visit. Cellular material may be obtained during the same biopsy setting for cell blocks. Cell blocks are preferable to direct smears for immunocytochemical studies that may assist in determining the histogenesis of a neoplasm. Material may also be obtained by FNA biopsy for electron microscopy, cytogenetics, and molecular biologic analysis.[144]

FNA biopsy also has a low incidence of significant clinical complications, and in the majority of patients, none are evident. Occasionally, some individuals may experience bleeding or develop edema at the biopsy site. Still, the procedure does not disrupt tissue planes or contaminate the subsequent surgical site. Thus, if not diagnostic, FNA biopsy can be followed by another biopsy procedure, which is not always the case with excisional biopsies. No documented instance of needle tracking of sarcomatous tumor cells by a fine needle has been noted.

Unfortunately, however, FNA biopsy possess several distinct disadvantages, some of which are relatively specific for bone and soft tissue lesions.[1,3,12,21,22] In general, FNA biopsy procures only relatively small samples of the tumor. Furthermore, dispersion of individual cells is inherent in the aspiration technique with at least partial loss of recognizable diagnostic tissue patterns. These limitations inevitably can result in less specific diagnoses with regard to histologic type and subtype of tumors. Thus, even if the neoplasm can be identified as sarcomatous, the cytopathologist may not be able to define more specifically the exact type of malignant mesenchymal tumor. It is difficult to distinguish among benign cellular lesions, borderline tumors, and low-grade sarcomas. Accurate grading of many sarcomas is impossible when using current histopathologic classification schemes. Finally, these aspirates inherently have relatively high rates of insufficiency. Insufficient specimens may result from structural features of the lesions themselves, such as in aspirates of osteoblastic and densely sclerotic tumors, highly vascular lesions, and cysts. All of these types of lesions may fail to yield sufficient numbers of diagnostic lesional cells to allow one to make a specific diagnosis. This is especially likely when the cortical bone is intact, as is often the case with benign bone lesions.

It is important to emphasize that the diagnosis of a bone or soft tissue tumor by FNA biopsy always requires the intimate cooperation and interaction of surgeons, radiologists, and pathologists. This is absolutely necessary to optimize the integration of all clinically relevant information to achieve the best cytologic diagnosis. Whenever possible, a rapid on-site evaluation of the aspirate by the pathologist is preferred. This provides the opportunity for the pathologist to review important imaging studies, discuss the mass lesion with the surgeon, and possibly examine the patient.[3,12]

 ## SOFT TISSUE TUMORS

General Sarcoma Classification

Soft tissue sarcomas can be classified into six general categories on the basis of the predominant appearance of the specimen in aspiration smears: myxoid, spindle cell, pleomorphic, polygonal cell, round cell, and miscellaneous.[12] The round cell and pleomorphic sarcomas can generally be considered high-grade sarcomas. Conversely, most myxoid sarcomas would often fall into the low-grade category. It is more difficult to grade with any degree of certainty the spindle cell and polygonal cell sarcomas. The miscellaneous category includes diverse entities that may occasionally be difficult to distinguish from benign mesenchymal proliferations. The best example is the well-differentiated liposarcomas. Because of the prominent overlap in certain features among various malignant and benign soft tissue tumors, their interpretations in FNA biopsy are approached by concentrating on the sarcomas.

Myxoid Sarcomas

This category includes myxoid liposarcoma, myxoid malignant fibrous histiocytoma (myxofibrosarcoma), extraskeletal myxoid chondrosarcoma, and fibromyxoid sarcoma.[12,23,24] At low magnification, the most apparent feature of the aspirate smears is voluminous extracellular matrix material (Figures 28-1 and 28-2). Often, this material presents as irregularly shaped, moderately sized fragments with or without embedded tumor cells. With the Romanowsky stains, the matrix appears as a reddish-purple substance and varies from fibrillar to structureless and homogeneous in appearance. The matrix may appear metachromatic, especially in the extraskeletal chondrosarcomas. With the Pap stain, the matrix is cyanophilic and typically appears as a relatively watery pale green substance. The edges of the fragments of matrix material may appear sharply defined or blend irregularly with the background as delicate spicules may extend from the body of the fragment. Within the smear, the tumor cells are present as individually dispersed elements and in small aggregates, both embedded within the matrix material and free in the smear background. The malignant cells are relatively small and have stellate, spindled, or rounded contours (Figure 28-3; see Figures 28-1 and

28-2). Their precise shapes are more apparent when they are unencumbered by the matrix. Most cells possess a solitary nucleus that is small to moderate in size and often densely hyperchromatic. Nucleoli are generally small and inconspicuous in the majority of the cells. Few to moderate numbers of multinucleated giant tumor cells may also be randomly distributed within the smears[23,24] (Box 28-1).

Gonzalez-Campora and colleagues reported an FNA biopsy series of 16 myxoid soft tissue tumors, five of which were benign and 11 of which were malignant.[23] Their opinion that the only cell type of diagnostic value in smears was lipoblasts in the lipomatous tumors. In the authors' experience, lipoblasts may be sparse, requiring a careful search for their identification. Lipoblasts are characterized by rounded contours and scant to moderate volumes of cytoplasm, which is occupied by one or more sharply defined lipid vacuoles (see Figure 28-3). These vacuoles may be uniform in size or vary in diameter, but they characteristically displace the solitary nucleus to an eccentric cellular position and indent its membrane with a resultant scalloped contour.[24] Their nuclei show mild to moderate variability in size and are generally hyperchromatic. Another highly distinctive feature that is evident at low magnification in smears of myxoid liposarcomas is the presence within the matrix material of branched delicate capillary arrays (Figures 28-4 and 28-5; see Figures 28-1 and 28-2).[3,23-26] The smears also contain unspecialized small mesenchymal cells with high nuclear to cytoplasmic (N:C) ratios and spindled or stellate contours that are indistinguishable from many tumor cells in myxoid malignant fibrous histiocytoma (MFH). Aspirates of poorly differentiated myxoid liposarcoma will contain larger round tumor cells with high N:C ratios and occasional lipid vacuoles (Figure 28-6). The finding of a low-grade component mixed with the obviously malignant round cells in the same aspirate is a helpful clue to the correct classification of the latter. Only very rarely has the aspiration appearance of lipoblastoma been described.[27] It may be indistinguishable from myxoid liposarcoma.

Aspirates from myxoid MFH have abundant matrix material within the smears and demonstrate three morphologic cell types: small spindle-shaped fibroblast-like cells, histiocytic cells and multinucleated tumor giant cells (Figures 28-7 to 28-9).[28] In the authors' practices, it is the last cell type that distinguishes this tumor from other myxoid sarcomas. Aspirate smears from intramuscular myxomas are poorly cellular and are characterized by voluminous matrix material with scattered spindled and stellate cells manifest-

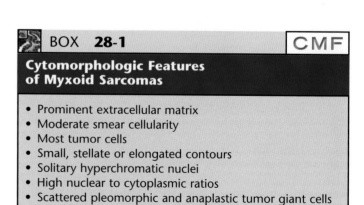

BOX 28-1   CMF

Cytomorphologic Features of Myxoid Sarcomas

- Prominent extracellular matrix
- Moderate smear cellularity
- Most tumor cells
- Small, stellate or elongated contours
- Solitary hyperchromatic nuclei
- High nuclear to cytoplasmic ratios
- Scattered pleomorphic and anaplastic tumor giant cells

ing no atypia and fragments of atrophic muscle fibers.[29] Gonzalez-Campora and colleagues warned about two potential diagnostic pitfalls in this setting: the misidentification of macrophages as lipoblasts and the misinterpretation of atrophic muscle fibers as multinucleated tumor giant cells.[23] In the former situation, the histiocytic nucleus has a smooth round or ovoid shape that is not indented by cytoplasmic vacuoles. Further, the vacuoles are not as sharply defined in histiocytes, conferring a foamy to granular quality to the cytoplasm. Atrophic muscle fibers have uniform round nuclei that do not manifest atypia or nucleoli.

Wakely and colleagues examined an aspiration series of 33 myxoid lesions of soft tissue origin.[24] Of these, 22 were cancer, whereas 11 were benign. This study analyzed semiquantitatively the amount of stroma within the smears, the degree of cellularity, and the density or opaqueness of the matrix material. Although arbitrary, at least one slide from each case had to have three or more intermediate-power fields occupied by matrix material in order to be included in the study. The matrix had a relatively watery or translucent appearance in the smears in many of the specimens derived from both benign and malignant lesions. The fragments of matrix had relatively poorly defined outlines that conferred an amorphous appearance. However, in many of the sarcomas, the matrix material had a different quality; specifically, it appeared much denser with sharply defined smooth edges. The latter was especially evident with the extraskeletal myxoid chondrosarcomas. For Gonzalez-Campora and colleagues, the most distinctive feature of their solitary example of an extraskeletal myxoid chondrosarcoma was the extreme

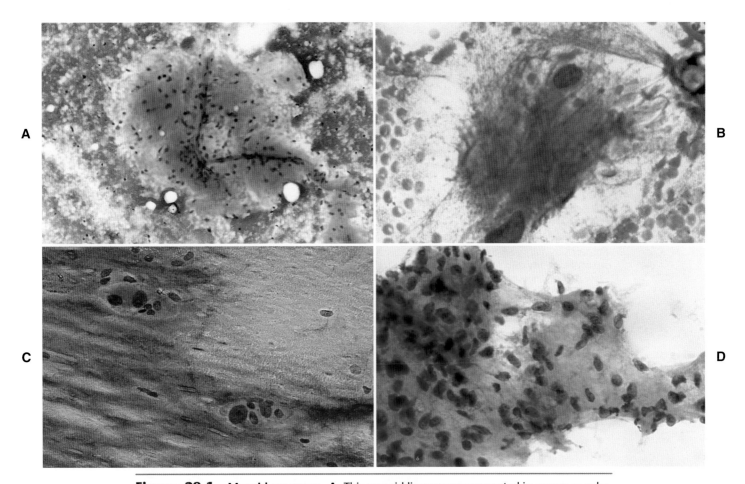

Figure 28-1 Myxoid sarcomas. **A,** This myxoid liposarcoma presented in smears as cohesive fragments of matrix material that contain moderate numbers of small homogeneous appearing neoplastic cells. The latter have solitary round or ovoid nuclei with darkly stained chromatin and generally high nuclear to cytoplasmic (N:C) ratios. Some cells demonstrate one or more cytoplasmic processes. In addition, delicate branched capillaries are evident. One or two neoplastic cells may possess cytoplasmic lipid vacuoles. **B** and **C,** Myxoid malignant fibrous histiocytoma (MFH). Solitary neoplastic cells are dispersed within the fibrillar-appearing metachromatic matrix. The neoplastic cells have solitary small to moderately sized nuclei with rather smooth round contours, finely reticulated chromatin, and inconspicuous to minute nucleoli. Cytoplasm is faintly basophilic and appears to blend with the adjacent matrix material. Pleomorphism and mitotic activity are absent. **D,** Myxoid MFH. With the Papanicolaou stain, the small solitary nuclei contain evenly dispersed, darkly stained chromatin and inconspicuous nucleoli. Cytoplasm is less distinct and blends more readily with the adjacent matrix material. However, a few cells do demonstrate distinct delicate cytoplasmic tails. Cellularity in this example is moderate. (**A-C,** Diff-Quik [DQ]; **D,** Papanicolaou [Pap])

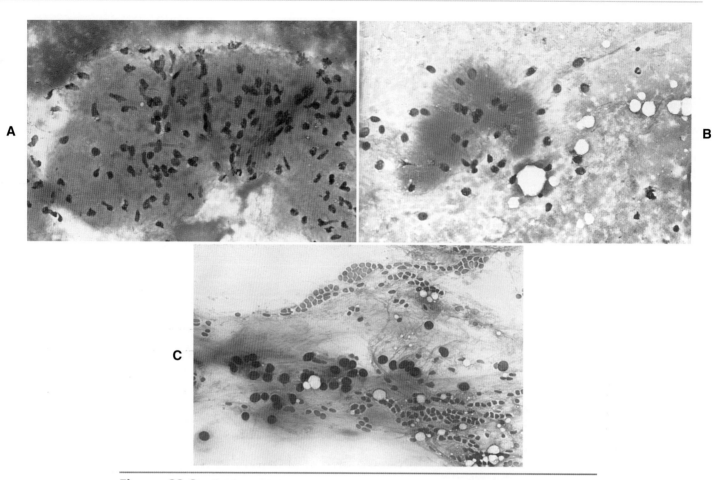

Figure 28-2 **A, Myxoid MFH.** The neoplastic cells have uniform sizes with round to ovoid to elongated nuclei with homogeneous-appearing chromatin. Nucleoli are lacking. Cytoplasm is indistinct, as it appears to blend with the adjacent matrix material. Note the absence of branched capillaries. **B, Myxoid liposarcoma.** A small fragment of homogeneous matrix material contains a few uniform neoplastic cells with solitary ovoid nuclei with even, smooth chromatin and apparently high N:C ratios. Also present are a few individually dispersed neoplastic cells with similar-appearing nuclei. **C, Myxoid liposarcoma.** Associated with delicate and somewhat stringy-appearing matrix are monotonous malignant cells with small round nuclei and high N:C ratios. A few neoplastic cells possess small to moderately sized univacuolated lipid droplets. **(A-C,** DQ)

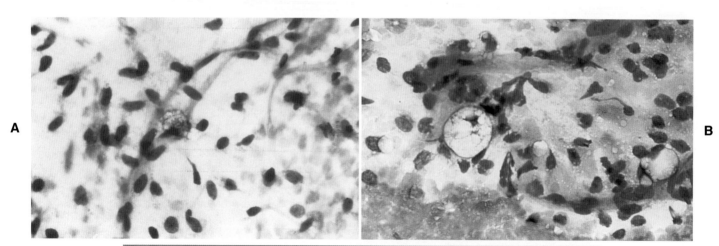

Figure 28-3   **Myxoid liposarcoma. A,** Most of the malignant cells have small ovoid to stellate nuclei with dense homogeneous chromatin, inapparent nucleoli, and high N:C ratios. Scanty rims of basophilic cytoplasm are apparent about many of the nuclei. A single neoplastic lipoblast is evident; it is characterized by a darkly stained and irregularly shaped nucleus and moderate volumes of cytoplasm with multiple lipid vacuoles. (Pap) **B,** A solitary neoplastic lipoblast is mixed with numerous small undifferentiated cells with ovoid to stellate nuclei and scanty cytoplasm. Although not readily apparent, capillaries are also present within the sample. (DQ)

metachromatic nature of the matrix material.[21] With the Romanowsky stain, it varied from brilliantly red to pink to intensely blue-red; it appeared violet to red with the Pap preparation (Figure 28-10). Dense stromal matrix was only very infrequently seen in aspirates of benign preparations.[24]

In this analysis, moderate to high levels of cellularity were found in 95% of the sarcomas, but only in 18% of the benign tumors.[24] Similarly, moderate to marked nuclear atypia was found in 59% of the malignant and 9% of the benign samples. The sole benign specimen with marked nuclear atypia was a pleomorphic lipoma. Malignant tumor giant cells, often multinucleated, were most characteristic of MFH. Five of the six myxoid chondrosarcomas contained neoplastic cells in spaces suggestive of lacunae. For the most part, the benign aspirates in the study of Wakely and colleagues were characterized by a combination of low smear cellularity and a lack of nuclear atypia.[24] Furthermore, the matrix had an amorphous semitransparent appearance that appeared not as fragments but as a thin diffuse film.

The differential diagnoses of the myxoid sarcomas include benign mxyoid soft tissue lesions and several other nonsarcomatous malignancies. Ganglion cysts may yield moderate amounts of viscous fluid on aspiration that may be difficult to smear on the slide. The smears are extremely hypocellular and are dominated by a granular appearing myxoid substance (Figure 28-11). The few cells that are present have a histiocytic appearance and are clearly benign.[30] Occasionally, mast cells may be seen. The combination of clinical and microscopic features allows for the recognition of this lesion and distinguishes it from myxoid sarcomas. As stated earlier, aspirates of myxomas of soft tissue are also characterized by low smear cellularity.[23,30] The cells are round to elongated with solitary small nuclei possessing bland chromatin. The abundant pale matrix material may appear granular or fibrillary. Thus, the aspiration appearance of ganglion cysts and true myxomas are morphologically indistinguishable. Although mitotic figures are often sparse in aspirates of the myxoid sarcomas, they would not be expected in aspirates of these benign entities. Furthermore, multinucleated tumor giant cells are not observed. Other benign soft tissue lesions that may have a myxoid background include nodular fasciitis and myxoid neurofibroma.[31-33] These entities are discussed in the differential diagnosis of lesions in the spindle cell category.

Once a myxoid neoplasm is identified as sarcoma, it is not always possible to subtype it histologically. On the other hand, some aspirates do provide histogenetic clues. Specimens that contain clearly identifiable lipoblasts and a well-defined branched capillary network within the matrix indicate a myxoid liposarcoma.[12,24-26,34] Although other sarcomas have tumor cells with cytoplasmic vacuoles, they should not be confused easily with those of a lipoblast. In the other myxoid sarcomas, the vacuoles are generally quite small and do not affect significantly the nuclear contour or position. In MFH, relatively easily isolated, obviously malignant, and even bizarre-appearing tumor giant cells can be found (see Figure 28-9).[24,28] The latter may possess one or

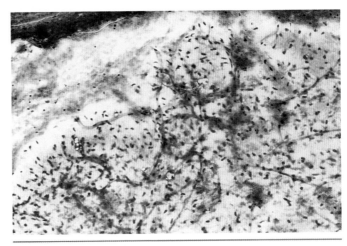

Figure 28-4 **Myxoid liposarcoma.** Complex branched small capillaries form a "chicken wire" network within the matrix material. This is the classic picture of myxoid liposarcoma. In addition, numerous undifferentiated malignant cells are evident within the smear; they have uniformly small to moderately sized nuclei and little in the way of obvious cytoplasm. Rare lipoblasts are also present. (DQ)

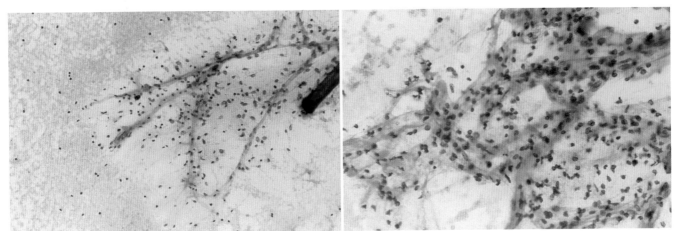

Figure 28-5 **Myxoid liposarcoma. A** and **B,** Little matrix is apparent in these fields. However, the complex delicate branched capillary arrays typical of this neoplasm are readily apparent. The external surfaces of the capillaries appear to be coated irregularly by malignant tumor cells. The latter have small- to medium-size round to elongated nuclei and high N:C ratios. Even at low magnification, hyperchromasia is readily apparent. Pleomorphism is slight. (Pap)

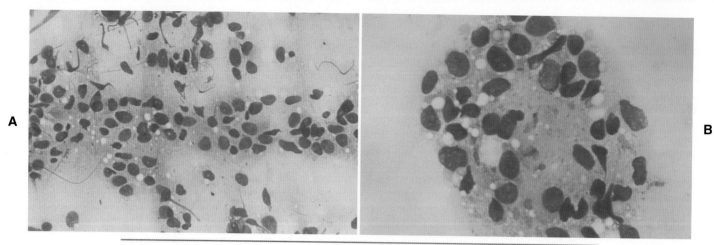

Figure 28-6 **Poorly differentiated (round cell) liposarcoma. A** and **B,** The malignant cells are larger than those seen in the low-grade myxoid fraction. The nuclei remain solitary with round to elongated contours, darkly stained chromatin, and evenly dispersed chromatin granules. A minority of the neoplastic cells possess one or more cytoplasmic lipid vacuoles. Note the absence of matrix material and branched capillaries. (DQ)

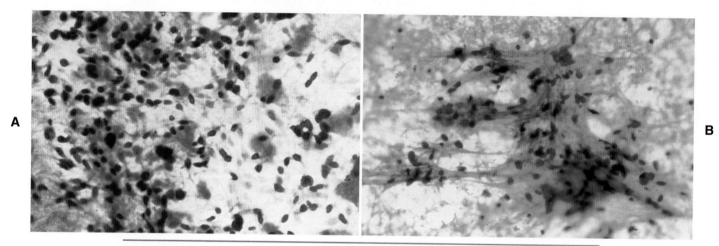

Figure 28-7 **Myxoid MFH. A** and **B,** This aspirate is characterized by a moderate level of smear cellularity, extracellular matrix material, and a moderate level of cellular and nuclear pleomorphism. The cells vary from small to moderately sized and generally possess a single nucleus. The latter range from round to ovoid to irregular in shape and have darkly stained, almost condensed chromatin. For the most part, nucleoli are not evident. The same can be said for cytoplasm. Thus, the N:C ratios are relatively high. The matrix has a stringy or linear appearance. Note the absence of branched capillaries and lipoblasts. (**A,** DQ; **B,** Pap)

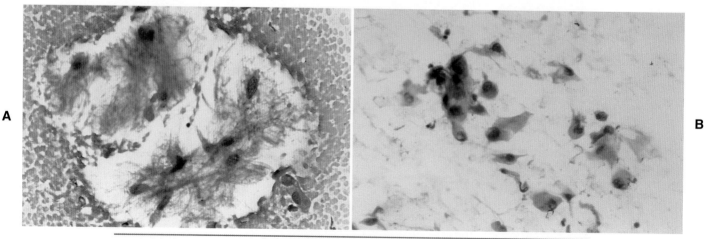

Figure 28-8 **Myxoid MFH. A** and **B,** Small homogeneous malignant cells are characterized by single hyperchromatic nuclei and high N:C ratios. Nuclei vary from round to elongated to irregular shape. Cytoplasm is faintly basophilic and blends imperceptibly with the metachromatic matrix material. In **B,** matrix is not apparent and cytoplasm is more obvious. The latter is dense and cyanophilic. (**A,** DQ; **B,** Pap)

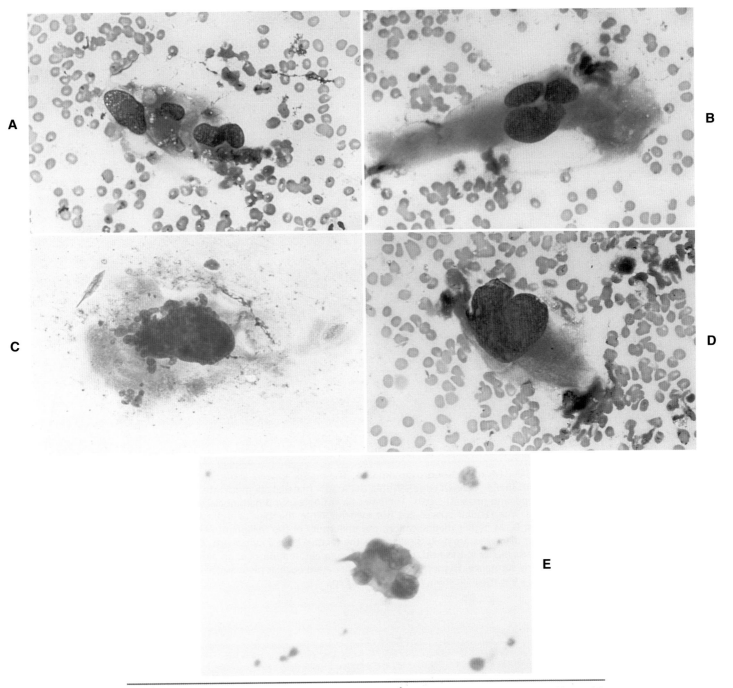

Figure 28-9 **Tumor giant cells in myxoid MFH. A-E,** Huge irregularly shaped and/or multiple nuclei characterize these neoplastic elements. Nucleoli vary from inconspicuous to large and are situated within darkly stained, finely granular (or reticulated) chromatin. Cytoplasmic volumes vary from relatively scanty to abundant. Cell borders are indistinct and appear to blend imperceptibly into the smear background. In **A,** small to moderately sized cytoplasmic vacuoles are evident but do not resemble those seen in lipoblasts. **(A-D,** DQ; **E,** Pap)

more huge nuclei with coarsely granulated chromatin and prominent nucleoli. Their N:C ratios may not be high because the cells may possess voluminous cytoplasm with indistinct borders that tend to blend imperceptibly into the smear background. In addition, large curvilinear blood vessels may be present at the periphery of matrix fragments in myxoid malignant fibrous histiocytoma. Myxoid chondrosarcomas may demonstrate cells within a dense and highly metachromatic matrix material.[24] Only rarely has

low-grade fibromyxoid sarcoma been reported in aspirates dominated by myxoid material and not by spindle-shaped tumor cells; the authors believe that they do not present a diagnostic picture[35] (Table 28-1).

Chordomas enter into the differential diagnosis of myxoid sarcomas occurring in the pelvis and retroperitoneum. Based purely on cytomorphologic attributes, chordomas may be difficult or even impossible to distinguish from the myxoid sarcomas (Figures 28-12 and 28-13). These smears

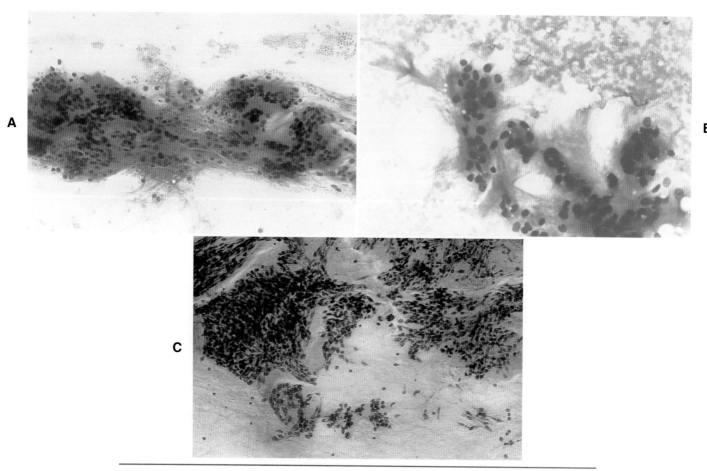

Figure 28-10 **Myxoid chondrosarcoma. A,** The matrix appears extremely dense and homogeneous with sharply defined edges. Within the matrix material are moderate numbers of homogeneous-appearing neoplastic cells. The latter have single round dark nuclei and inconspicuous cytoplasm. True lacunar spaces are not evident. Note the lack of individually dispersed neoplastic cells. **B,** At higher magnification, the uniformity of the malignant cells is readily apparent. Nuclear diameters are quite similar as is the relative lack of cytoplasm. **C,** Although the cellularity appears higher in this field, matrix is less apparent. It appears as an almost transparent watery pale grey substance. Hyperchromasia and moderate nuclear pleomorphism are apparent even at this very low magnification. (**A, B,** DQ; **C,** Pap)

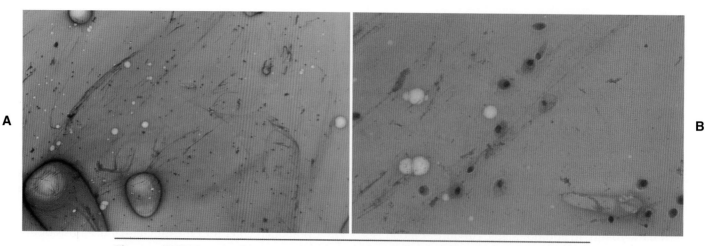

Figure 28-11 **Ganglion cyst. A,** Small numbers of lesional cells are present in voluminous watery matrix substance. **B,** Each cell is small with a solitary dark nucleus that is probably degenerated. Their cytoplasm is moderate, pale, and focally vacuolated. Nuclei are often eccentrically located. (DQ)

TABLE **28-1**

Differential Diagnosis of Myxoid Sarcomas

FEATURE	TUMOR		
	Liposarcoma	Malignant Fibrous Histiocytoma	Chondrosarcoma
Lipoblasts	+	−	−
Plexiform capillaries	+	−	−
Pleomorphic tumor giant cells	+	+++	+
Very dense matrix	+	+	+++

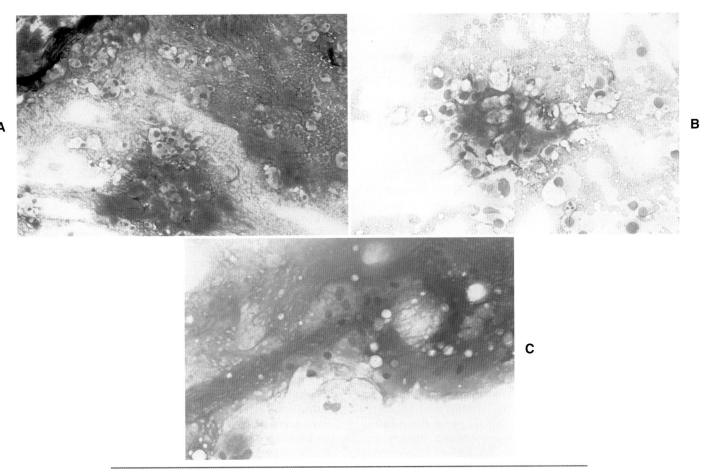

Figure 26-12 **Chordoma.** **A,** Neoplastic cells are intimately admixed with extracellular dense matrix material. Even at this rather low magnification, the neoplastic cells are larger than those expected in the myxoid sarcomas. They have more abundant, relatively pale cytoplasm and large round nuclei with finely reticulated chromatin. In addition to being embedded within the matrix material, clusters of tumor cells appear to abut on the external edges of these matrix fragments. **B,** The chordoma cells have one or two ovoid nuclei with delicate smooth membranes, finely reticulated chromatin, and generally inconspicuous nucleoli. The N:C ratios are relatively low compared with the myxoid sarcomas because of the moderate to abundant faintly basophilic cytoplasm. **C,** The matrix of chordomas appears extremely dense and relatively homogeneous, although a faint suggestion of a fibrillary appearance is present focally. The edges of the matrix are relatively sharply defined from the adjacent smear background. Overall, this matrix material is indistinguishable from that of the myxoid sarcomas. The neoplastic cells, however, are larger and have bigger nuclei, finely reticulated chromatin and lower N:C ratios. Note the occasional binucleated neoplastic cell. (DQ)

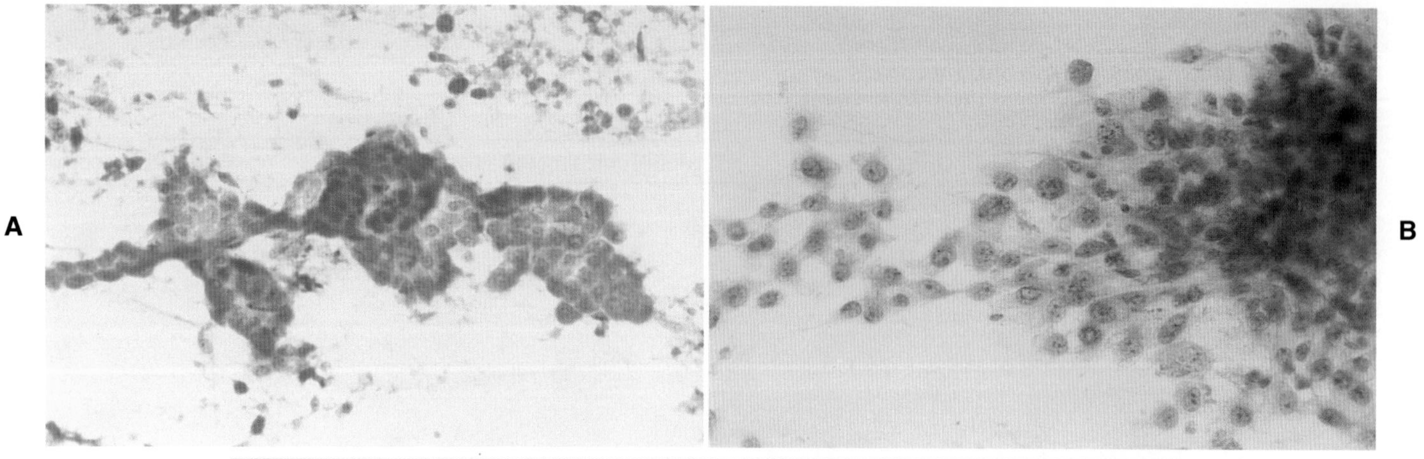

Figure 28-13 Chordoma. **A,** The epithelial-like nature of the chordoma cells is more readily apparent in this Pap-stained aspirate. Tumor cells are present in a large cohesive aggregate with well-defined borders. Furthermore, the nuclei appear to be fairly evenly dispersed in the fragment and cell borders are distinct. **B,** The tumor cells have one or two nuclei with round to ovoid contours, delicate membranes, and fine even chromatin; the latter appears relatively pale which allows the small nucleoli to stand out. Such cells would not be expected in aspirates of myxoid sarcomas of soft tissue. (Pap)

are characterized by moderate cellularity and abundant extracellular matrix material.[36] However, several potential microscopic clues suggest the correct diagnosis. In chordomas, the neoplastic cells tend to be larger, have more abundant cytoplasm, and a relatively epithelial appearance. Although their nuclei may be larger than those expected in the majority of the tumor cells from myxoid sarcomas, their N:C ratios are relatively low. Furthermore, in chordomas, a more distinct separation of tumor cells and matrix may be seen. Immunocytochemistry can be definitive; chordoma tumor cells are positive for cytokeratin, unlike the myxoid sarcomas.

Spindle Cell Sarcomas

This category includes fibrosarcoma, leiomyosarcoma, synovial sarcoma, malignant peripheral nerve sheath tumors, Kaposi's sarcoma, and some forms of MFH and angiosarcoma.[12,37-40] This group of malignancies poses the greatest diagnostic difficulties in FNA biopsy and has the highest potential for both false-positive and false-negative diagnoses because of the difficulty of distinguishing benign and low-grade tumors. The two major attributes that allow an aspirate to be designated as sarcoma are a moderate to high smear cellularity and hyperchromatic nuclei in almost all sampled cells.[12] Based purely on the cytomorphology, however, it may be difficult to distinguish among the different sarcomas and grade the neoplasm accurately.

In general, aspiration biopsies yield moderately to highly cellular smears (Figure 28-14).[12] The main feature of these smears is a predominance of cells with elongated nuclei paralleling the shape of the cell. The degree of intercellular cohesion may vary remarkably from patient to patient and among the different types of spindle cell sarcomas. Some specimens are dominated by individually dispersed neoplastic cells and small, loose aggregates, whereas in smears from other tumors large tissue fragments predominate. In the authors' experiences, the latter situa-

tion is most characteristic of leiomyosarcomas. The edges of the neoplastic fragments are often indistinct as the peripheral-most cells appear to be exfoliating from the surface of the fragment. This is in contrast with the sharply defined edges of cellular aggregates in aspirates of carcinomas. The sarcomatous cells are usually mononuclear, although multinucleated tumor giant cells may be seen in some of the more poorly differentiated sarcomas. Their chromatin is finely to coarsely granular and may be either evenly or irregularly distributed. Although nucleoli may be present, in general, they are neither large nor prominent. The volume of cytoplasm varies from scant to moderate; in some neoplasms the tumor cells possess long, tapering cytoplasmic tails. Although spindle cell sarcomas may be difficult to subclassify based purely on the cytomorphology, ancillary diagnostic procedures such as immunocytochemistry, cytogenetics, and molecular assays may help pinpoint a specific histologic type (Box 28-2).

Liu and colleagues have conducted two extensive logistic regression analyses of low-grade and high-grade spindle cell lesions, respectively, in aspiration biopsies.[38,39] In the study of low-grade lesions, 28 different cytomorphologic attributes were assessed in smears of 47 sarcomas (synovial sarcoma being the most common) and 52 benign proliferations (including 18 nerve sheath neoplasms).[38] The major criteria for interpreting an aspirate as malignant included the presence of high smear cellularity; short, spindled tumor cells; minute nucleoli; and an absence of a tissue culture appearance. However, the authors did not define specific criteria for evaluating each of these morphologic features. Furthermore, although most workers consider synovial sarcomas as high-grade sarcomas, in this study, Liu and colleagues included them among their low-grade lesions that we believe biased the results.[38] For the specific recognition of a synovial sarcoma, their primary criteria were high cellularity (75% of cases) and the presence of tissue fragments (80%). Two negative secondary criteria were the absence of both long filamentous tumor cells and a myxoid back-

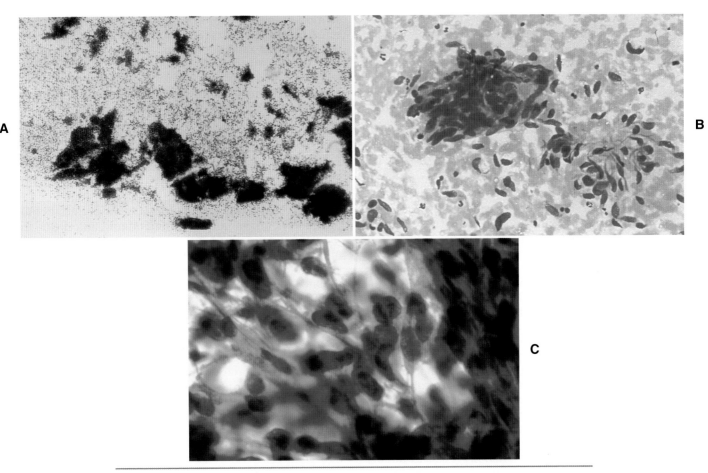

Figure 28-14 **Synovial sarcoma. A,** This scanning lens view demonstrates the high smear cellularity expected of most spindle cell sarcomas. Numerous individually dispersed tumor cells, small aggregates of cells, and large tumor fragments are present. The latter have fuzzy edges as the most peripherally oriented cells appear to be detaching from their surfaces. **B,** Individual neoplastic cells are relatively homogeneous in appearance. They possess solitary elongated nuclei with relatively smooth membranes and evenly dispersed chromatin without distinctive nucleoli. A minority of the nuclei have more irregular contours with central indentations. In many cells, delicate basophilic cytoplasm is also apparent as one or two blunt to long tapering tails. Within the cohesive fragments, cell borders are indistinct. (From Geisinger KR, Abdul-Karim F. Fine needle aspiration biopsies. In: Weiss SW, Goldblum JR, editors. Enzinger and Weiss's soft tissue tumors. 4th ed. St. Louis: Mosby; 2001.) **C,** At high magnification, the elongated nuclei appear homogeneous in that they have evenly dispersed, rather finely granular, and darkly stained chromatin. In fact, this is the hyperchromasia expected in aspirates of spindle cell sarcomas. Again, note the varying quantities of cyanophilic cytoplasm. (**A** and **C,** Pap; **B,** DQ)

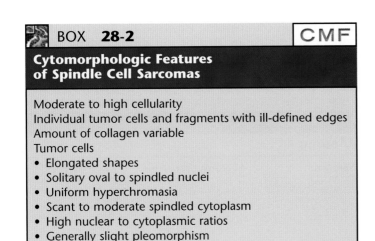

BOX **28-2**   CMF

Cytomorphologic Features of Spindle Cell Sarcomas

Moderate to high cellularity
Individual tumor cells and fragments with ill-defined edges
Amount of collagen variable
Tumor cells
- Elongated shapes
- Solitary oval to spindled nuclei
- Uniform hyperchromasia
- Scant to moderate spindled cytoplasm
- High nuclear to cytoplasmic ratios
- Generally slight pleomorphism

ground. The authors stated that nuclear morphology was not helpful in the diagnosis of synovial sarcomas.

The major purpose of another study by Liu and colleagues was to evaluate high-grade spindle cell neoplasms and attempt to identify criteria that could be used to distinguish the different tumors.[39] This study included leiomyosarcomas, liposarcomas, angiosarcomas, MFH, osteosarcomas, chondrosarcomas, and melanomas; it did not include synovial sarcomas. The authors evaluated 42 separate morphologic aspects of the smears, but again did not define specific morphologic guidelines for these different attributes. Although the definition of some of these features is inherently obvious, others are not; for example, the authors did not state how *short-spindled cells* were distinguished from *fibroblast-like cells*. According to Liu and colleagues, significant features for the diagnosis of MFH included the presence of fibroblast-like cells, multinucleated cells, and abundant myxoid matrix.[39] This is in contrast with the report of Berardo and colleagues in which no solitary cytomorphologic feature or constellation of attributes could be used to distinguish MFH reliably from other pleomorphic neoplasms.[41] The authors have found the combination of high smear cellularity, mostly single tumor cells, and marked pleomorphism characteristic of MFH. The last feature includes ovoid, spindled, and giant tumor cells. However, a similar picture may occur with pleomorphic liposarcoma and sarcomatoid carcinomas. According to Liu and colleagues, the most important feature for the diagnosis of leiomyosarcomas is the identification of fishhook nuclei.[39] In another study, however, the same investigators found fishhook nuclei in 30% of their synovial sarcomas.[38] Thus, their somewhat conflicting data supports our notion that nuclear configurations are of little value in distinguishing among different types of sarcomas, especially those of high grade. These authors found that the presence of intracytoplasmic iron deposits was the best criterion for the recognition of angiosarcomas. However, these deposits were found in only 57% of their angiosarcomas and an even lower proportion of angiosarcomas contained hemosiderin in the large series studied by Boucher and colleagues.[42] Aspirates of some angiosarcomas may manifest diagnostic clues such as primitive vessel formation and intracytoplasmic lumens with erythrocytes, but others are recognizable simply as sarcomas.[42] Immunocytochemistry is often far more specific, as outlined in Table 28-2.

The more commonly aspirated benign spindle cell soft tissue tumors are nerve sheath neoplasms and nodular fasciitis. Smear cellularity with benign nerve sheath tumors is generally low to moderate.[43-47] The most consistent feature of these specimens is that the vast majority of aspirated neoplastic cells is present in cohesive fragments of tumor tissue (Figure 28-15). These fragments have irregular contours and may consist of one or more interlacing fascicles of tumor cells. Most of the neoplastic cells possess a solitary elongated nucleus that often manifests relatively sharply pointed tips. Furthermore, some of the nuclei may possess a wavy or buckled contour. Their chromatin is usually finely granular and uniformly distributed. In some specimens, the chromatin appears very darkly stained. For the most part, nucleoli are not recognized, but intranuclear vacuoles may be common. Within the fragments, the neoplastic cells are embedded in collagenous matrix material that stains reddish-pink with Diff-Quik (DQ) and green with the Pap stain. The matrix material may have a fibrillar or granular appearance. The cytoplasm is generally inconspicuous because it appears to blend with the surrounding collagen.

In most examples, only a small number of individually scattered neoplastic cells are present. Many of these cells are not intact but rather consist of "stripped" nuclei without any visible attached cytoplasm. Within some aspirates, rows of parallel nuclei form palisades and rarely Verocay bodies can be recognized (see Figure 28-15). In neurofibromas, the neoplastic nuclei do not demonstrate any such orientation, but rather appear haphazardly scattered within the aspirated fragments of collagen. Mitotic figures are not expected in benign nerve sheath tumors. In the series of 29 benign nerve sheath neoplasms reported by Resnick and colleagues, 55% of the specimens were considered nondiagnostic.[44] The remaining 45% manifested attributes of a benign nerve sheath tumor, and four were specifically interpreted as neurilemmomas. An important clinical clue that the patient has a nerve sheath neoplasm is that the performance of the aspiration biopsy procedure elicits an intense pain at the site of the aspirate that often radiates distally.

One potential diagnostic pitfall for a false-positive interpretation of sarcoma in the FNA biopsy of benign nerve sheath tumors may be observed in the aspirates of ancient schwannomas.[46] Aspirated cells may be very large with one or more huge hyperchromatic and irregularly contoured nuclei (Figure 28-16). Careful attention to the chromatin structure is important because it appears completely homogeneous and smudged or pyknotic-like. These cells may be individually dispersed in the smears which otherwise completely resemble a typical schwannoma. These huge cellular elements should not be mistaken for malignant cells. Helpful clues for benignity include sparsity of such tumor giant cells, a degenerative chromatin pattern, lack of mitotic activity, and an overall preservation of cohesion. Cellular schwannomas represent another potential diagnostic problem (Figure 28-17). In the authors' limited experience, a major clue to recognizing the benign nature is the retention of almost all of the neoplastic cells within cohesive tumor fragments. The pattern of immunoreactivity for S100 protein is also useful; a malignant diagnosis is to be avoided if many of the cells are positive. Henke and colleagues have reported a patient in whom the preoperative aspiration biopsy was misinterpreted as sarcoma on the basis of high smear cellularity, mitotic activity, and focal necrosis.[45]

The differential diagnosis includes malignant peripheral nerve sheath tumors (MPNST).[48-50] Generally, smears from MPNST have a somewhat higher degree of cellularity than in the benign counterparts. However, the single most important discriminating attribute for distinguishing benign from malignant is the presence of a much greater propor-

---

TABLE 28-2

Differential Diagnosis of Spindle Cell Sarcomas: Ancillary Testing

Test	Fibrosarcoma	Synovial Sarcoma	Leiyomyosarcoma	MPNST*
Desmin	−	−	+	−
S100 protein	−	−	−	+
Cytokeratin	−	+	−	−
X,18 translocation	−	+	−	−

*MPNST, Malignant peripheral nerve sheath tumor.

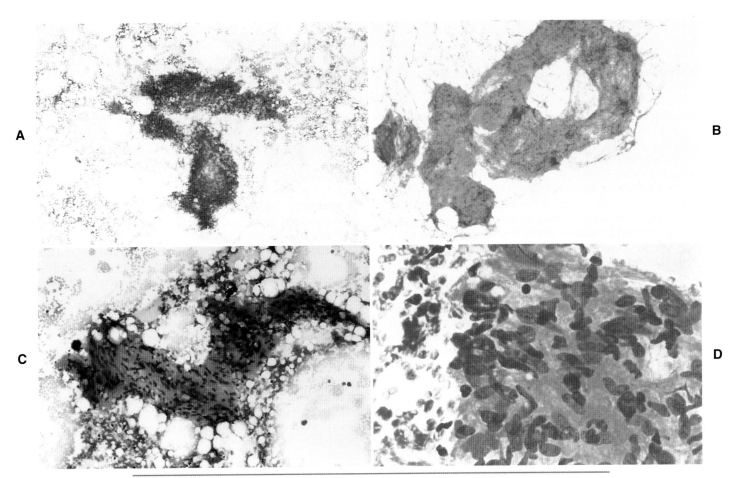

Figure 28-15 Schwannoma. **A** and **B,** Aspiration smears of this neoplasm are characterized by scant to moderate cellularity with essentially all of the neoplastic cells present within cohesive tissue fragments. Only very rare individually dispersed cells are evident. The fragments are composed of rather uniform spindle-shaped neoplastic cells and moderate collagenous matrix material. For the most part, the edges of these fragments appear well defined. In many examples, the matrix appears to dominate over the tumor cells. **C,** The uniformity of the tumor cells is readily apparent. They have solitary elongated nuclei with indistinct cytoplasm that blends with that of the neighboring cellular elements and the collagen. Again, note the sharply defined, smooth edge to these tumor fragments. **D,** Some of the elongated nuclei have wavy or serpentine contours. As seen in this example, the nuclei may line up in rows or palisades. (**A, B,** and **D,** DQ; **B,** Pap)

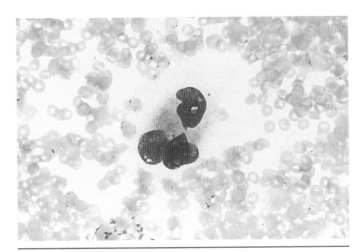

Figure 28-16 Ancient schwannoma. This solitary huge tumor giant cell is characterized by multiple variably sized and shaped nuclei situated within distinct cytoplasm. The nuclei have condensed chromatin and vacuoles. In aspirates of ancient schwannoma, such elements are usually sparse in number and overshadowed by the more characteristic features of the typical peripheral nerve sheath neoplasm. (DQ)

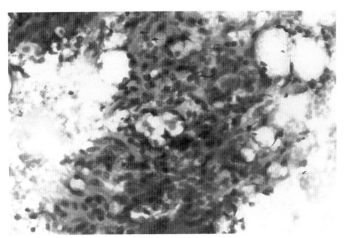

Figure 28-17 Cellular schwannoma. In comparison with the usual schwannoma, these uncommon neoplasms have a much more densely cellular population within the cohesive tissue fragments. Still, the cells remain rather uniform in appearance and are located almost exclusively within the cohesive tumor fragments. (DQ)

tion of individually dispersed neoplastic cells in the cancers (Figure 28-18). In the sarcomas that histologically are better differentiated, most neoplastic cells possess solitary uniform elongated nuclei, sometimes with a serpentine configuration. In less differentiated MPNST, a greater proportion of the cells is pleomorphic and may include multinucleated malignant tumor giant cells. As the histologic grade of these neoplasms increases, the amount of extracellular matrix material within the smears declines. Mitotic figures are usually readily recognizable. Jiménez-Heffernan and colleagues described aspiration biopsies from 10 malignant peripheral nerve sheath tumors.[50] Four of these were histologically relatively well differentiated; these smears could be recognized both as malignant and as derived from peripheral nerve sheath origin. Four others were high-grade spindle cell neoplasms that could be easily recognized as sarcomatous but did not manifest histogenetic clues. The remaining two cases had a more epithelioid appearance. In contrast with schwannomas, aspirated cellular material from malignant peripheral nerve sheath tumors are either negative or only focally and weakly positive for S-100 protein immunocytochemically.

Aspiration biopsies of synovial sarcomas yield moderately or more often highly cellular smears.[51-54] Each cell possesses a solitary ovoid nucleus with finely granular, evenly dispersed, hyperchromatic chromatin with inconspicuous nucleoli. Most neoplastic elements possess scanty cytoplasm resulting in high N:C ratios. A minority of the neoplastic cells in many cases possess more abundant cytoplasm which characteristically appears as bipolar tapered cytoplasmic tails. A proportion of these malignant cells are individually scattered, a manifestation of reduced intercellular cohesion, as are the frayed edges of many of neoplastic aggregates. The shapes of the individual neoplastic nuclei vary from blunt and ovoid to much more elongated. The number of mitotic figures in a given specimen is quite variable. Aspirates from histologically documented biphasic synovial sarcomas are dominated by these spindled neoplastic cells. However, in some examples malignant neoplastic elements manifest distinct epithelial-like differentiation (Figure 28-19). These consist of cohesive aggregates of cells with polygonal contours and solitary round hyperchromatic nuclei. The nuclei are either centrally or eccentrically positioned within the cytoplasm that may appear finely vacuolated. Mononucleated and multinucleated tumor giant cells are not usually seen.

The specific FNA biopsy diagnosis of synovial sarcoma is enhanced by the use of ancillary diagnostic procedures. By immunocytochemistry, positive reactivity for epithelial markers such as the various cytokeratins assists in the differential diagnosis with other spindle cell sarcomas.[12,51] Aspirated cellular material provides an excellent specimen for cytogenetic analysis, specifically to demonstrate the characteristic reciprocal translocation.[12,51] Using reverse transcription-polymerase chain reaction tests, Inauaki and colleagues were able to identify the specific SYT-SSX fusion products in aspiration specimens of synovial sarcomas.[55]

Similar to peripheral nerve sheath neoplasms, the authors believe that benign and malignant smooth muscle tumors can generally be distinguished from each other on the basis of smear cellularity and the presence or absence of well developed intercellular cohesion.[56-59] Smear cellularity

tends to be much higher with the sarcomas (Figure 28-20). In most aspiration biopsies of leiomyomas, the vast majority of the neoplastic cells are present in cohesive tissue fragments, whereas a larger proportion of the sampled tumor cells from leiomyosarcomas are individually dispersed or present in loosely cohesive clusters without much intervening matrix. In both benign and malignant neoplasms, the elongated nuclei may have a "cigar shape," whereas in others, nuclei have a nonspecific spindled contour. Cells possess eosinophilic cytoplasm, which appears to blend with the collagen-like matrix present in the aspirated tissue fragments of leiomyomas. Mitotic figures are not recognized in aspiration smears of these benign neoplasms.

Vascular neoplasms also need to be considered in the differential diagnosis of the spindle cell sarcomas.[42,60-64] This is especially true for Kaposi's sarcoma and hemangiopericytoma. In general, samples contain a prominent background of blood, and thus, smear cellularity may not be as high as is expected in many other sarcomas. Farshid and colleagues have recently demonstrated that many leiomyosarcomas arise from the walls of vascular vessels.[142]

Kaposi's sarcoma generally yields moderately cellular samples that are dominated by large tissue fragments comprised of homogeneous spindle shaped neoplastic cells.[62] Although matrix material may be seen within some of the fragments, especially in air-dried preparations, they are usually densely cellular with characteristically overlapping elongated neoplastic cells (Figure 28-21). The aspiration smears also contain smaller aggregates of loosely cohesive neoplastic cells. Individually scattered tumor cells and stripped elongated nuclei will also be present. The cells are characterized by ovoid to more elongated nuclei with finely granular evenly dispersed chromatin and inconspicuous nucleoli. According to Hales and colleagues, a characteristic morphologic attribute is nuclear fragility which manifests as streaks of chromatin material within the aggregates.[62] The neoplastic cells have scanty and weakly basophilic cytoplasm with poorly defined cell borders. Pleomorphism is minimal. Although the cytomorphologic findings are not specific, in the proper clinical setting, and in particular in a patient known to have acquired immune deficiency syndrome (AIDS), this picture is consistent with the diagnosis of Kaposi's sarcoma. The demonstration by immunocytochemistry of vascular differentiation markers such as CD31 and CD34 is useful is supporting the diagnosis. With PCR, Alkan and others demonstrated the presence of human herpes virus 8 in all aspiration biopsy specimens of Kaposi's sarcoma; aspirates of all other spindle cell proliferations were negative for this DNA marker.[65]

Similarly, hemangiopericytomas do not produce a specific diagnostic cytomorphologic picture in smears.[63,64] The specimens, however, may present a typical appearance. Smears are moderately to highly cellular with a bloody background (Figure 28-22). Similar to Kaposi's sarcoma, they are often predominated by cellular cohesive tissue fragments. A characteristic feature of some of the aspirated fragments is that they are traversed by endothelial cell lined capillaries. The neoplastic cells are larger and have plumper nuclei than the benign endothelial cells. This is in contrast to Kaposi's sarcoma in which capillaries do not course through the tumor fragments. According to some authors, "staghorn" vessels are not recognized within the neoplastic

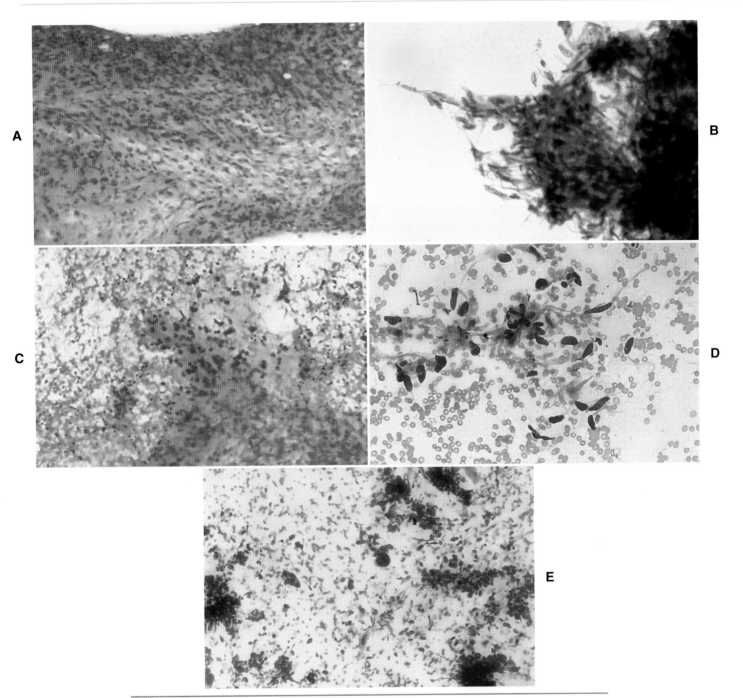

Figure 26-18   Malignant peripheral nerve sheath tumor. **A,** This low-magnification picture demonstrates a cohesive tissue fragment of an aspirate of a low-grade malignant peripheral nerve sheath neoplasm. This field is indistinguishable from that of a benign cellular schwannoma in that it contains a cohesive tissue fragment composed of relatively homogeneous cells with solitary elongated nuclei and moderate amounts of intercellular collagen. **B** and **C,** Reduced intercellular cohesion is manifested by individual cells "escaping" from the surface of the tissue fragments. At higher magnification, some variability in nuclear contours and sizes is apparent, as is hyperchromasia. This loss of cohesion is a very helpful feature in distinguishing benign from malignant nerve sheath tumors. **D,** Individual neoplastic cells are characterized by very elongated nuclei with delicate membranes, dense homogeneous chromatin, and inconspicuous nucleoli. The cells also possess variable amounts of cytoplasm, including long delicate tails. On a cell for cell basis, these might be indistinguishable from those of a benign nerve sheath neoplasm, but as seen in this field, they are individually dispersed and present in small loose clusters without associated matrix. **E,** Occasional malignant peripheral nerve sheath tumors include multinucleated tumor giant cells. As witnessed in this example, they may have one or more huge obviously malignant nuclei. (**A** and **C-E,** DQ; **B,** Pap)

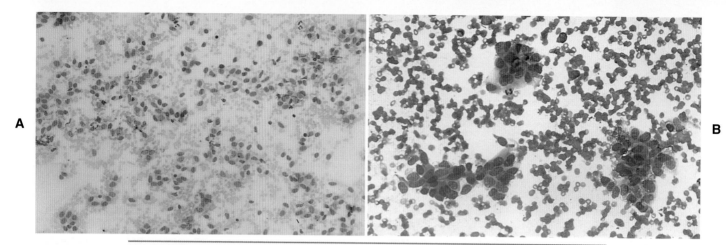

Figure 28-19 Biphasic synovial sarcoma. **A,** High cellularity characterizes this aspiration smear. Neoplastic cells are present individually and in small flat loose clusters. Some of the cells have elongated nuclei with overall spindled contours, whereas others have round to polygonal shapes. **B,** Some of the more cohesive aggregates have a distinct epithelial quality with polygonally shaped cells, somewhat distinct cell borders, and solitary ovoid nuclei that are either centrally or eccentrically positioned within the cytoplasm. (DQ)

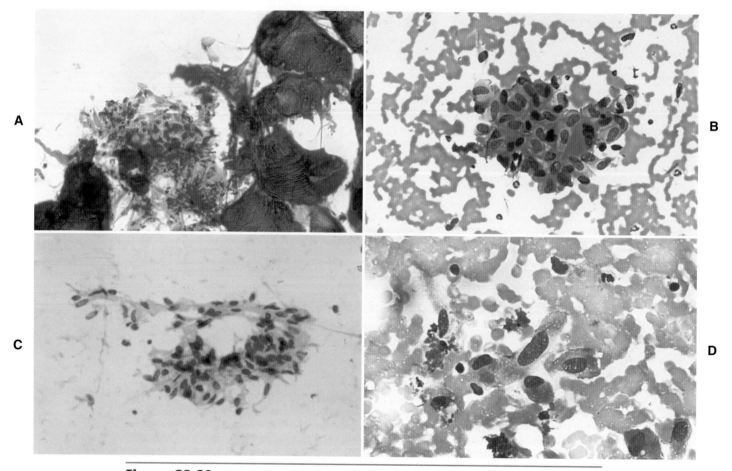

Figure 28-20 Leiomyosarcoma. **A,** This primary chest wall leiomyosarcoma demonstrates collections of obviously malignant cells within fragments of benign skeletal muscle. The neoplastic cells have single moderately to markedly enlarged nuclei and obviously darkly stained chromatin. Cell contours vary from round to quite spindled. **B,** This pelvic leiomyosarcoma is characterized by more homogeneous-appearing malignant elements. Each had a solitary ovoid nucleus of rather uniform contour and dimensions with evenly dispersed homogeneous chromatin and inconspicuous nucleoli. The cells possess moderate volumes of cytoplasm that again vary from round or polygonal to elongated. Compared with many other spindle cell sarcomas, leiomyosarcoma cells often have a greater volume of cytoplasm. **C,** This leiomyosarcoma is dominated by spindle-shaped cells with solitary elongated nuclei. Hyperchromasia is obvious, as is the lack of orientation of the cells within this fragment. **D,** The chromatin in these malignant nuclei is moderately clumped and rather uniformly distributed. Small nucleoli are evident within some, but not all, nuclei. The cells possess moderate volumes of cytoplasm and hence have relatively low nuclear-to-cytoplasmic ratios. Note the lack of true cohesion among these sampled neoplastic cells. (**A** and **C,** Pap; **B** and **D,** DQ)

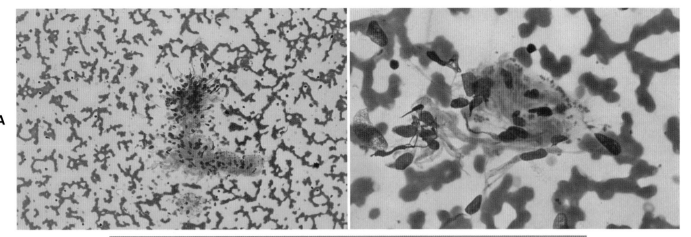

A

B

Figure 28-21 **Kaposi's sarcoma. A,** This cohesive fragment of neoplasm demonstrates a haphazard arrangement of the tumor cells and their nuclei. The cytoplasm of neighboring cells blend with each other, creating a syncytial appearance. The cells' spindled contours can be recognized focally at the fragment's edge. Such an aggregate could be mistaken for a granuloma. **B,** Nuclear contours vary from plump and oval to elongated. Their membranes may be either smooth or irregular with small indentations. Elongated cytoplasmic tails are evident in a few cells. (DQ)

fragments.[64] Furthermore, it is well known by histopathologists that "staghorn" blood vessels may be seen in other neoplasm (e.g., synovial sarcomas). The smears also contain smaller loosely cohesive monolayers of tumor cells and individually dispersed neoplastic cellular elements. Pleomorphism is mild to moderate, and most of the neoplastic cells possess solitary ovoid or somewhat more elongated nuclei with scanty, ill-defined cytoplasm. Their chromatin is finely granular, uniformly dispersed and variably stained. However, in most cases at least a portion of the nuclei appears hyperchromatic.

Aspiration biopsies of angiosarcomas present a more diverse cytomorphologic array.[19,42,61] Some tumors are dominated by distinctly spindle-shaped neoplastic cells, whereas in others, the malignant elements have rounded or polygonal contours (Figures 28-23 and 28-24). In addition, tumor fragments are less pervasive than in either Kaposi's sarcoma or hemangiopericytoma. Rather, a much greater proportion of the cells are either isolated or present in small loosely cohesive clusters. Distinct vasoformative channels are recognized in some samples. Individual cells typically have a solitary elongated or round nucleus with definite hyperchromasia and variably clumped chromatin granules. In general, prominent nucleoli are not evident, but examples with large macronucleoli have been seen. Pleomorphism may be greater than that seen in either Kaposi's sarcoma or hemangiopericytoma. Although some authors suggest that cytoplasmic hemosiderin is characteristic of angiosarcomas in aspiration biopsies, other authors have not found this to be helpful.[39,42] The use of immunocytochemistry to identify endothelial differentiation markers is more useful in confirming the diagnosis of angiosarcoma.

An FNA diagnosis of benign vascular tumors is generally uncommon because the smears are dominated by blood and in many cases do not demonstrate any other cell types.[60] An occasional aggregate of bland-appearing spindle-shaped endothelial cells and fibroblasts set within

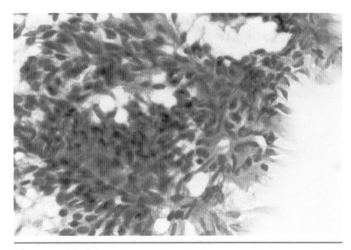

Figure 28-22 **Hemangiopericytoma.** Within this neoplastic fragment, elongated thin nuclei of benign endothelial cells are evident as a minority component. Most of the nuclei are larger, ovoid, and darkly stained. Most of the cells have high N:C ratios. No specific differentiation is evident. (Pap)

scanty collagenous matrix material may be randomly scattered within the specimen. In the aspiration biopsies from intramuscular hemangiomas, fragments of degenerating skeletal muscle fibers may also be recognized.[1]

The final group of soft tissue lesions that need to be entertained in the face of an aspiration smear dominated by spindle-shaped cells are the fibrous and fibrohistiocytic proliferations. The prototype, fibrosarcoma, has only rarely been described in cytologic samples.[1] Both the smear cellularity and the degree of pleomorphism depend largely on the histologic grade of the fibrosarcoma; in general, high cellularity and prominent anisonucleosis are associated with the poorly differentiated tumors. In smears, the cells are present both singly and in relatively loose clusters

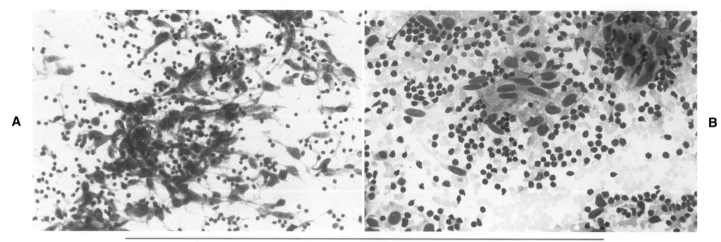

Figure 28-23 **Angiosarcoma metastatic to lymph node. A** and **B,** Loosely cohesive and individual tumor cells are present on a background of benign lymphocytes. The neoplastic cells possess solitary ovoid to elongated nuclei and bipolar cytoplasmic tails. The cytoplasm is delicate and cyanophilic. The nuclei have evenly dispersed, darkly stained chromatin and inconspicuous to small nucleoli. The production of vessels by the neoplastic cells is not apparent. (**A,** Pap; **B,** DQ)

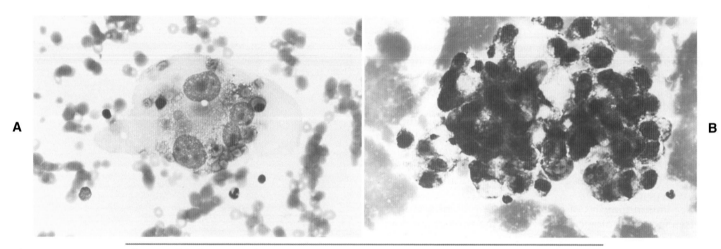

Figure 28-24 **Angiosarcoma. A,** It is not certain whether this represents a huge multinucleated tumor giant cell or a small cohesive cluster of malignant elements. This was derived from an angiosarcoma in which the majority of the tumor cells had an epithelioid appearance. The nuclei are variable in size but generally have ovoid contours with prominent nucleoli and finely reticulated chromatin. They possess abundant delicate to foamy cytoplasm. **B,** This loose, three-dimensional aggregate of angiosarcoma cells is derived from another neoplasm with largely epithelioid differentiation. The cells have large solitary nuclei with prominent nucleoli and scant to moderate volumes of cytoplasm. Some of the malignant cells have cytoplasmic vacuoles suggestive of intracytoplasmic lumina. Hemosiderin is not present within their cytoplasm. (DQ)

(Figure 28-25). In the better-differentiated neoplasms, the tumor cells are rather homogeneous in size and appearance. Most cells possess a solitary ovoid to elongated nucleus with evenly dispersed, finely granulated chromatin with small nucleoli. The neoplastic cells have variable amounts of cytoplasm ranging from scanty to moderate. Many possess a distinctly spindled contour with either unipolar or bipolar tails. Although it would be unusual to find multinucleated giant cells in aspirates of poorly differentiated fibrosarcomas, these neoplasms may yield moderate variability in nuclear sizes and contours. Mitotic figures are usually evident in the smears.

Based purely on cytomorphologic features, aspirates of well differentiated fibrosarcomas may be difficult or impossible to distinguish from the fibromatoses, dermatofibrosarcoma protuberans, synovial sarcomas, and well-differentiated peripheral sheath tumors.[1] The poorly differentiated fibrosarcomas need to be distinguished from MFH and high-grade leiomyosarcomas. Nonneoplastic proliferative lesions such as nodular fasciitis also fall into the differential diagnosis with fibrosarcoma.

The fibromatoses are characterized in smears by a variable cellularity, which tends to be low to moderate and therefore less than seen in frank sarcomas (Figure 28-26).[66,67] The pro-

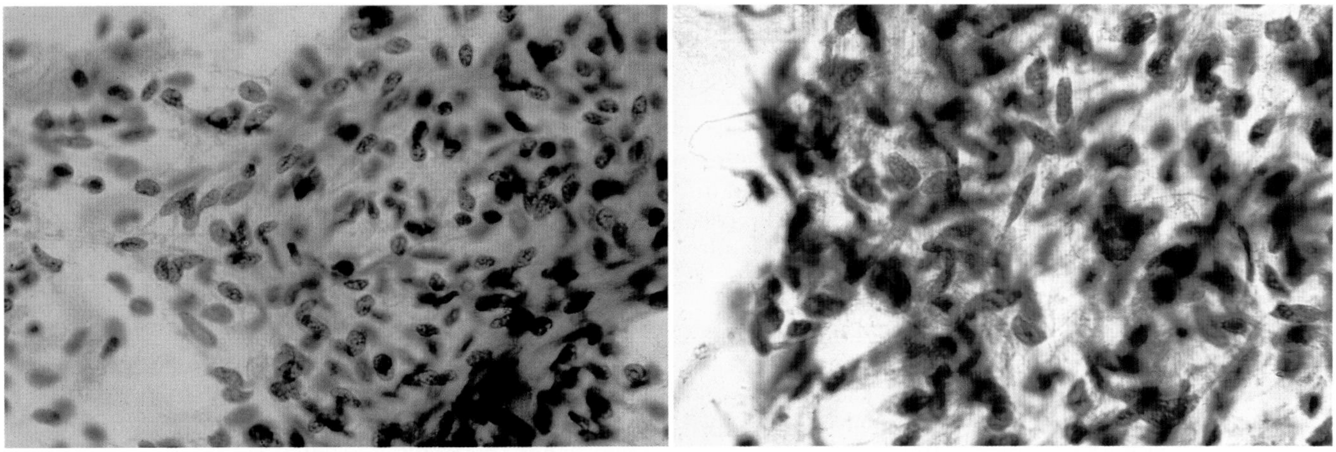

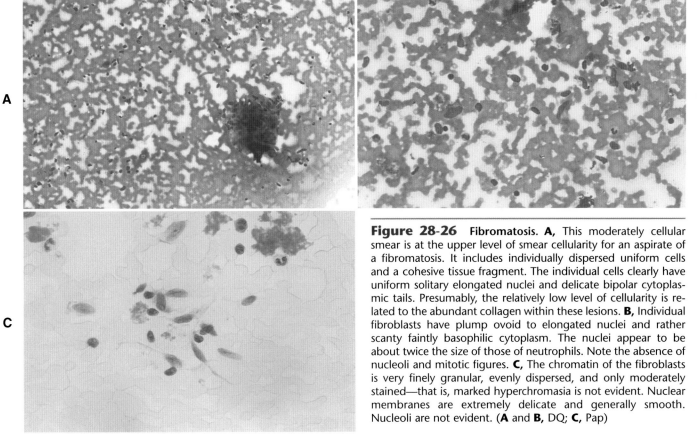

Figure 28-25 Fibrosarcoma. **A** and **B,** This aspiration biopsy of a fibrosarcoma is characterized by high smear cellularity, a striking monotony among the neoplastic cells, and obvious hyperchromasia. Each tumor cell possesses a single nucleus that varies from ovoid to elongated with relatively finely granular and uniformly dispersed chromatin and inapparent nucleoli. Their cytoplasm is indistinct and appears to blend with that of the adjacent collagenous matrix. Within the smears, the neoplastic cells appear to be randomly or haphazardly patterned. (Pap) (From Geisinger KR, Abdul-Karim F. Fine needle aspiration biopsies. In: Weiss SW, Goldblum JR, editors. Enzinger and Weiss's soft tissue tumors. 4th ed. St Louis: Mosby; 2001.)

Figure 28-26 Fibromatosis. **A,** This moderately cellular smear is at the upper level of smear cellularity for an aspirate of a fibromatosis. It includes individually dispersed uniform cells and a cohesive tissue fragment. The individual cells clearly have uniform solitary elongated nuclei and delicate bipolar cytoplasmic tails. Presumably, the relatively low level of cellularity is related to the abundant collagen within these lesions. **B,** Individual fibroblasts have plump ovoid to elongated nuclei and rather scanty faintly basophilic cytoplasm. The nuclei appear to be about twice the size of those of neutrophils. Note the absence of nucleoli and mitotic figures. **C,** The chromatin of the fibroblasts is very finely granular, evenly dispersed, and only moderately stained—that is, marked hyperchromasia is not evident. Nuclear membranes are extremely delicate and generally smooth. Nucleoli are not evident. (**A** and **B,** DQ; **C,** Pap)

liferating fibroblasts present with solitary uniform elongated nuclei with delicate membranes; fine, even chromatin; and inconspicuous nucleoli. Similar to fibrosarcoma, the predominant cellular contour is spindled, and the volume of cytoplasm is variable. Characteristically, one may find bipolar tapering long cytoplasmic tails. Importantly, mitotic figures should not be identified. The cells occur both singly and in small loose aggregates; at times, they are situated within collagenized stromal tissue. A similar cytomorphologic picture has been reported in idiopathic retroperitoneal fibrosis.[68]

In aspiration smears, dermatofibrosarcoma protuberans may be considered a bridge between the fibrous and fibrohistiocytic neoplasms.[69] Smears are moderately to highly cellular and contain both individually dispersed and loosely aggregated spindled cells. The smears also usually contain the neoplastic cells within fragments of stroma. The individual cells have solitary ovoid nuclei with delicate chromatin, which may appear darkly stained. Nucleoli are small and inconspicuous. Typically, the cells possess moderate volumes of pale basophilic cytoplasm, which may present as long bipolar tails. The presence at low magnification of a whorled or storiform arrangement of the cells and infiltration of fatty tissue by the proliferating spindle cells are useful in rendering a specific diagnosis.[69] The cytomorphologic features of MFH, another neoplasm that may possess a storiform pattern, is presented in the discussion of the pleomorphic sarcomas.

Although not pathognomonic, the distinctive cytomorphology of nodular fasciitis, in conjunction with the appropriate clinical presentation, can allow for a confident diagnosis of this lesion.[31-33] The smears are moderately to frequently highly cellular and are composed of singly dispersed cells, loose aggregates, and tissue fragments, all set within a highly characteristic metachromatic myxoid background (Figure 28-27). The matrix is better appreciated with the Romanowsky stain, where it appears red to violet; with the Pap stain, it appears pale green. Within the fragments, the proliferating cells appear loosely and haphazardly arranged, creating the characteristic tissue culture pattern. Although cellular contours are variable, most of the lesional cells are spindle shaped with moderate volumes of faintly basophilic cytoplasm and one or two blunt to long cytoplasmic tags (see Figure 28-27). Small amounts of the proliferating cells have ovoid, stellate, or polygonal contours with similar appearing cytoplasm. The majority of the cells possess a solitary nucleus, but binucleation also occurs. The nuclei are characteristically perfectly round with distinct thin membranes, generally vesicular chromatin, and distinct small to large nucleoli. The latter vary in shape from smooth and round to angulated. Nucleolar prominence results from both their large sizes and from the pale-stained chromatin. Mitotic figures may be evident within the smears and in some examples are numerous. Thus, the fibroblastic cells have a reparative look.[70] The cytologic picture is rounded out with an admixture of predominantly mononuclear inflammatory cells in the background (Box 28-3).

Nonsarcomatous malignancies must also be considered in the differential diagnosis of spindle cell sarcomas. Sarcomatoid carcinomas and mesotheliomas may present in smears as predominantly elongated neoplastic cells with obviously malignant nuclear attributes. In a minority of malignant melanomas, most of the sampled cells have distinctly spindled contours and thus closely simulate a sarcoma

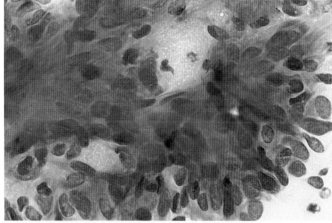

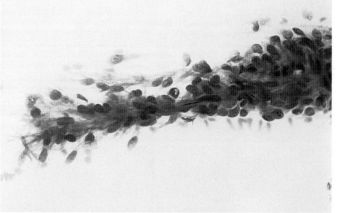

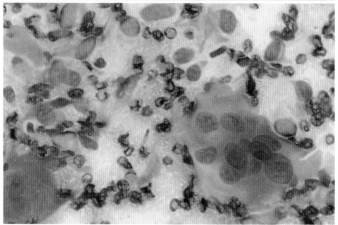

Figure 28-27 Nodular fasciitis. **A,** Small highly uniform-appearing fibroblastic cells are associated with a myxoid matrix material. The proliferating cells have solitary ovoid to slightly elongated nuclei with delicate membranes, finely reticulated chromatin, and small but distinct nucleoli. Cytoplasm is indistinct as it appears to blend with that of its neighbors and matrix material. **B,** A cohesive fragment of uniform cells is present in this sample. Each fibroblast has a single ovoid nucleus with delicate membranes; fine, even chromatin; and inconspicuous nucleoli. Many of the cells have long cytoplasmic tails and pale cytoplasm. No evidence of pleomorphism is present. **C,** The nuclei of the fibroblastic cells have very finely reticulated chromatin and distinct nucleoli. Although cellularity may be high and nucleoli may be well developed, in the proper clinical context, this should not be mistaken for a malignancy. (**A** and **C,** DQ; **B,** Pap)

(Figure 28-28). Appropriate immunocytochemical stains can often clarify this issue. The patient's previous medical history may also be most helpful. A proportion of non-Hodgkin's lymphomas may present, at least focally, in smears as a spindle cell proliferation. This typically occurs in mediastinal and retroperitoneal lymphomas associated with dense sclerosis. The collagenous material compresses some of the lymphoma cells creating elongated contours that may persist in aspiration smears. However, the characteristic lymphoid features of the cells aspirated from a non-Hodgkin's lymphoma are seen elsewhere in the sample, allowing for the correct diagnosis. Again, immunocytochemistry is helpful.

Pleomorphic Sarcomas

In aspiration smears, the pleomorphic sarcomas are almost always readily recognized as malignant and often as sarcomatous at low magnification.[12] The direct smears are usually highly cellular with little tendency for malignant cells to aggregate (Figure 28-29). Within a single field an admixture of small rounded cells with high N:C ratios, larger

polygonal or spindled cells with scant to moderate volumes of cytoplasm, and numerous bizarre tumor giant cells may be observed. The latter are characterized by one or more large hyperchromatic nuclei that may possess huge nucleoli (Figures 28-30 to 28-34; see Figure 28-29). Some nuclei appear irregularly contorted or polylobated. These cells typically possess moderate to abundant cytoplasm with cell borders that appear to blend imperceptibly into the background that often contains necrotic debris. Pleomorphic MFHs and liposarcomas account for almost all of the neoplasms in aspiration smears from this category. In many instances, it may not be possible to distinguish between these two tumors on the basis of cytomorphology, but this does not appear to be highly relevant clinically in most patients.[26,34,71,72] However, if lipoblasts (cells with cytoplasmic lipid vacuoles that indent the nucleus) are identified, then a specific diagnosis may be offered[34,71] (Box 28-4).

In smears of MFH, the cells are dispersed singly and present within loose clusters (see Figures 28-29 to 28-32).[41,73] The finding of a distinct storiform arrangement of aggregated tumor cells may be the most helpful feature in ren-

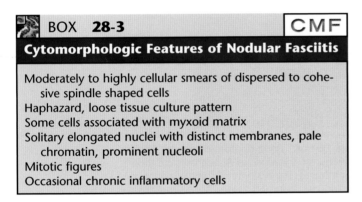

BOX 28-3 | CMF

Cytomorphologic Features of Nodular Fasciitis

Moderately to highly cellular smears of dispersed to cohesive spindle shaped cells
Haphazard, loose tissue culture pattern
Some cells associated with myxoid matrix
Solitary elongated nuclei with distinct membranes, pale chromatin, prominent nucleoli
Mitotic figures
Occasional chronic inflammatory cells

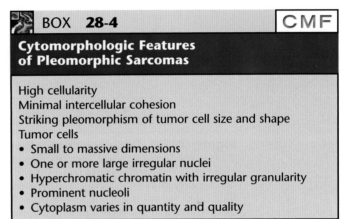

BOX 28-4 | CMF

Cytomorphologic Features of Pleomorphic Sarcomas

High cellularity
Minimal intercellular cohesion
Striking pleomorphism of tumor cell size and shape
Tumor cells
- Small to massive dimensions
- One or more large irregular nuclei
- Hyperchromatic chromatin with irregular granularity
- Prominent nucleoli
- Cytoplasm varies in quantity and quality

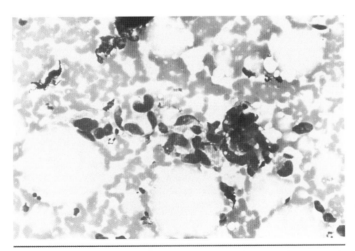

Figure 28-28 Spindle cell melanoma. This is from a primary aspirate of a large cutaneous melanoma mistaken by the clinician for a soft tissue neoplasm. The smears were moderately cellular and included both individual and loosely clustered malignant cells characterized by solitary elongated nuclei. Many of the nuclei possess small but distinct nucleoli. In addition, many of the cells had blunt to long cytoplasmic tails. (DQ)

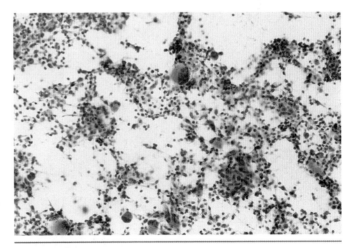

Figure 28-29 Malignant fibrous histiocytoma. This is the characteristic aspiration picture of the pleomorphic sarcomas. It includes a high level of cellularity, little in the way of intercellular cohesion among the sampled malignant cells, and striking variability in the contours and sizes of the neoplastic elements. The majority of the cells are relatively small with solitary hyperchromatic nuclei and rather high N:C ratios. At the opposite end of the spectrum, one may recognize huge tumor giant cells that may be mononucleated or multinucleated. Nucleoli are often prominent. (Pap)

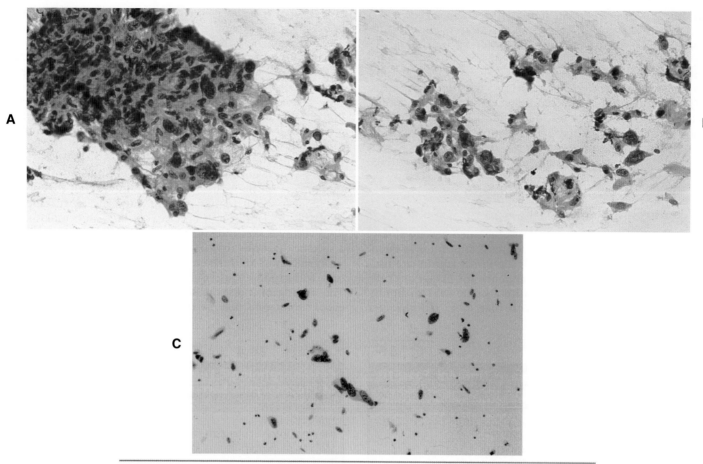

Figure 28-30   Malignant fibrous histiocytoma. **A** to **C,** These photomicrographs demonstrate a spectrum of cellular sizes, appearances, and loss of cohesion. In **A,** the cells are loosely clustered within a collagenous fragment and in all instances, the majority of the malignant cells are relatively small with round or ovoid solitary nuclei and inconspicuous cytoplasm. A progressive increase in the tumor cell size terminates in the presence of massive multinucleated tumor giant cells. Hyperchromasia is obvious and nucleoli are variably prominent. (Pap)

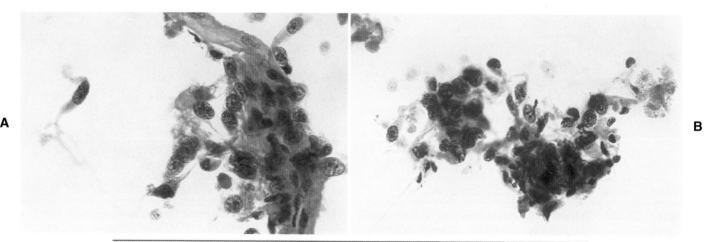

Figure 28-31   Malignant fibrous histiocytoma. **A** and **B,** The majority of the malignant cells in these neoplasms are relatively homogeneous. They possess solitary round or ovoid nuclei with smooth to irregular membranes of variable thicknesses, finely to coarsely granular chromatin, and small distinct nucleoli. The N:C ratios appear variable with some cells having cytoplasmic tails, whereas others possess polygonal contours. One constant is the striking hyperchromasia. (Pap)

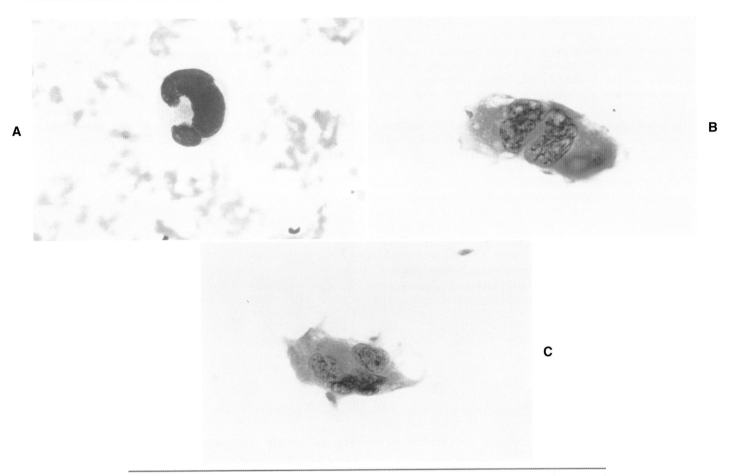

Figure 28-32   **Tumor giant cells in pleomorphic sarcomas. A** to **C,** Although many of these tumor cells are mononucleated, a proportion are multinucleated or have highly lobulated nuclei. Nuclear contours vary from smooth to irregular; the latter is better appreciated in alcohol-fixed preparations. Nucleoli may be inconspicuous or massive. The volume of cytoplasm possessed by the cells is also quite variable, although it is often abundant. Cell borders are indistinct, characteristic of mesenchymal cells. The malignant cells in **A** to **C** are from malignant fibrous histiocytomas. (**A,** DQ; **B** and **C,** Pap)

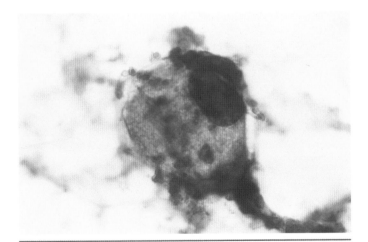

Figure 28-33   **Pleomorphic liposarcoma.** This huge tumor cell has a massive hyperchromatic nucleus which is displaced to the periphery by cytoplasmic lipid. (Pap)

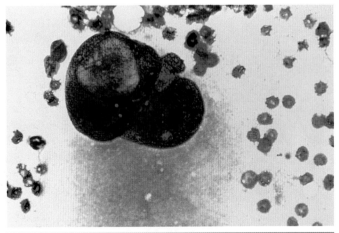

Figure 28-34   **Pleomorphic liposarcoma.** The huge nucleus contains a large cytoplasmic pseudoinclusion; some authors have suggested that this is characteristic of liposarcoma. (DQ)

dering a specific diagnosis (Figure 28-35). Liu and colleagues identified the combination of fibroblastic cells, multinucleated cells, and abundant myxoid matrix material as features supporting the interpretation of MFH.[39] However, Berardo and colleagues did not find a single cytomorphologic feature that allowed them to distinguish reliably MFH from other cytologically high grade pleomorphic neoplasms.[41]

Although most of the entities that fall into the differential diagnostic list with the pleomorphic sarcomas are other forms of cancer, a few benign proliferations also need to be considered. Examples include pleomorphic lipoma, giant cell tumors, ancient schwannoma, and proliferative fascitis/myositis. The aspiration cytomorphology of pleomorphic lipoma has only rarely been described.[24,34,74] According to Akerman and Rydholm, the smears consist largely of tissue fragments and aggregates indicating that intercellular cohesion is relatively well preserved.[34] The smears contain an admixture of bland to reactive fibroblasts-like spindled cells, unremarkable adipocytes, multinucleated tumor giant

cells, and lipoblasts (Figure 28-36). The lipoblasts typically possess a centrally or eccentrically located solitary hyperchromatic nucleus, the contours of which are deformed by the lipid vacuoles which impinge on it. Although these pleomorphic cells may simulate those of a sarcoma, strikingly bizarre and obviously malignant tumor giant cells are absent, smear cellularity is relatively low, and intercellular cohesion is preserved. The giant cells in aspirates of tenosynovial giant cell tumors also should not be mistaken for the anaplastic giant cells of sarcomas (Figure 28-37).[75,76,145,146]

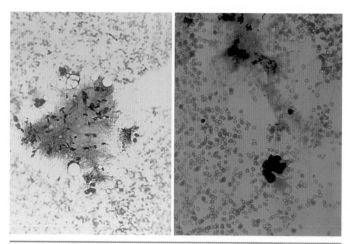

Figure 28-36   Pleomorphic lipoma. A key factor in the correct recognition of pleomorphic lipoma is the clinical history, namely a superficial soft tissue mass that is characteristically located in the posterior portion of the upper back. Another important clue is the relatively low level of smear cellularity. Thus, despite the presence of atypical lipoblasts and multinucleated tumor giant cells, the correct interpretation may be achieved. Note the dense homogeneous almost smudgy-appearing chromatin in the nuclei of the lesional cells. (DQ) (From Geisinger KR, Abdul-Karim F. Fine needle aspiration biopsies. In: Weiss SW, Goldblum JR, editors. Enzinger and Weiss's soft tissue tumors. 4th ed. St Louis: Mosby; 2001.)

Figure 28-35   Malignant fibrous histiocytoma. A cartwheel or storiform arrangement of spindled tumor cells is evident. (Pap)

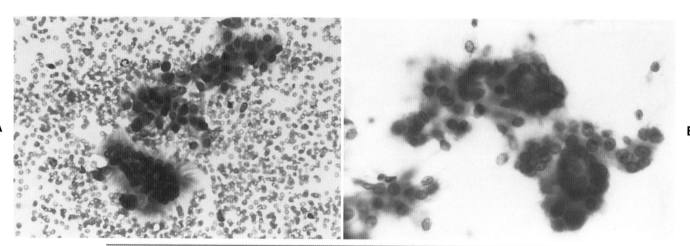

Figure 28-37   Tenosynovial giant cell tumor. A and **B,** Smear cellularity tends to be moderate or even high in aspirates and includes numerous small mononucleated tumor cells and scattered large multinucleated cells. The latter may have numerous nuclei and voluminous cytoplasm. It is important to recognize that the nuclei in the smaller cells completely resemble those in the giant cells. Furthermore, nuclei are bland with delicate membranes, very fine pale chromatin, and minute nucleoli. The strikingly bizarre, irregular, and hyperchromatic nuclei of the pleomorphic sarcomas are distinctly lacking. (**A,** DQ; **B,** Pap)

The authors have examined a striking example of proliferative myositis (Figure 28-38). Admixed with reactive fibroblasts and muscle fragments were dispersed giant cells, some of which clearly resembled ganglion cells, but others had large irregular dark nuclei. Their homogeneous smudged chromatin was diagnostically helpful, as was the recognition of the benign and mixed nature of most of the aspirated cells. Similar to many examples of nodular fasciitis, the mass resolved spontaneously after the biopsy procedure.

The most common entities in the differential diagnosis of pleomorphic sarcomas are cytologically high-grade carcinomas that may arise in many body sites.[77] Notable examples include giant cell or sarcomatoid carcinomas of the lung, thyroid, kidney, and pancreas. Some aspirates may be completely indistinguishable from sarcomas on the sole basis of cytomorphology. In addition to the clinical history, the smears should be carefully searched for the presence of residual epithelial differentiation in the form of cohesive aggregates of carcinoma cells with polygonal to columnar configurations. In most but not all examples, some of the neoplastic cells express the epithelial markers cytokeratin and epithelial membrane antigen.

Rare examples of sarcomatoid mesothelioma in FNA biopsy may completely simulate a pleomorphic soft tissue sarcoma (Figure 28-39). Positive immunostaining for cytokeratin and calretinin are the only pathologic clues to the ap-

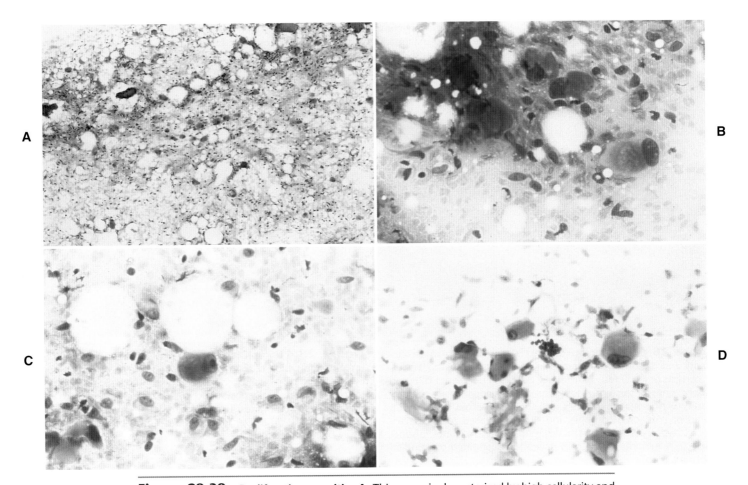

Figure 28-38   Proliferative myositis. **A,** This smear is characterized by high cellularity and a complete lack of cohesion among the sampled cells. Undoubtedly, the overwhelming majority of the cells present are small fibroblastic elements which have small elongated nuclei and apparently high N:C ratios. At this very low magnification, their cytoplasm is inapparent or may be discerned as delicate pale cytoplasmic tails. Although much less numerous, large ganglion-like cells are present and are characterized by abundant cytoplasm and eccentrically nuclei. The third component consists of fragments of unremarkable skeletal muscle. **B** to **D,** At high magnification, the fibroblastic or myofibroblastic cells are better seen. Their chromatin is finely reticulated and evenly dispersed within nuclei with smooth delicate membranes. For the most part, nucleoli are inconspicuous. Their cytoplasm is scanty and faintly basophilic. In sharp contrast the much more voluminous and deeply basophilic cytoplasm of the ganglion cells is obvious. These cells have large rounded contours with sharply defined cell borders and eccentrically placed nuclei. The latter are relatively large, have very fine even chromatin, and distinct nucleoli. Although these ganglion-like cells have large nuclei, their N:C ratios are low. In the proper clinical context, it is this combination of numerous small spindle-shaped cells and large ganglionic cells, in a background of skeletal muscle that allows one to render an interpretation of proliferative myositis. (**A** and **D,** Pap; **B** and **C,** DQ)

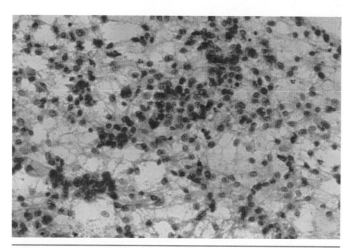

Figure 28-39   Sarcomatoid mesothelioma. A, Much of this aspirate consists of haphazardly arranged huge spindle-shaped malignant cells with solitary irregular and elongated nuclei and indistinct spindle-shaped cytoplasm. **B,** Scattered throughout the specimen were individually dispersed mononucleated and multinucleated tumor giant cells, at times with huge nucleoli. (DQ)

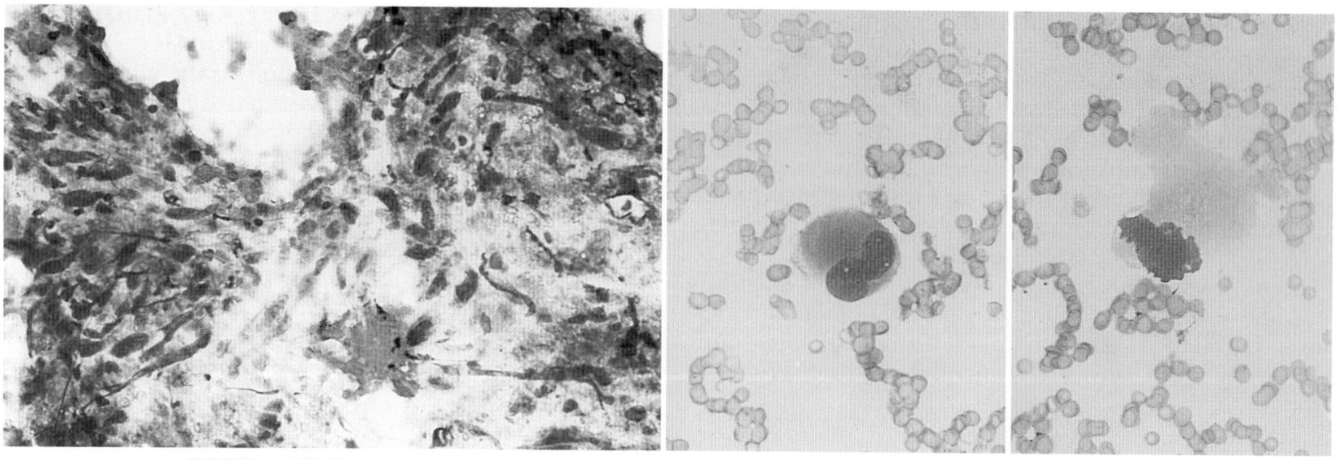

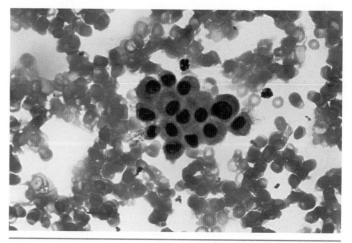

Figure 28-40   Alveolar soft part sarcoma. High smear cellularity and discohesive pattern characterize this aspirate. The latter consists of numerous individually dispersed neoplastic cells and loosely cohesive clusters. Also typical of this neoplasm are the uniformity of the malignant cells and their epithelioid quality with round or polygonal contours and centrally placed round nuclei. The latter possess hyperchromatic chromatin and at times, distinct nucleoli. A minority of the cells have more elongated or spindled contours. (Pap)

Figure 28-41   Epithelioid sarcoma. The neoplastic cells are uniform and typical of this neoplasm in that they possess abundant cytoplasm, distinct cell borders, round to polygonal cellular contours, and eccentrically positioned nuclei. The latter are round with well-defined membranes, hyperchromatic chromatin, and prominent nucleoli. Without an appropriate clinical history, this could easily be mistaken for a carcinoma. (DQ)

propriate diagnosis. Melanomas may simulate not only spindle cell sarcomas but also the pleomorphic variants. Although cytoplasmic melanin pigment is not usually recognized, the clinical history of a prior melanoma and/or immunostaining for melanoma-related antigens, especially HMB-45, allows one to render the correct diagnosis.

Anaplastic large cell lymphomas, especially those positive for Ki-1, may simulate pleomorphic sarcomas in aspiration smears. These specimens are generally highly cellular with a strikingly dissociative pattern and marked variability in size and shape of the cells, including multinucleated tumor giant cells. Characteristic wreath cells and the presence of lymphoglandular bodies may suggest the correct neoplasm. However, in contrast with most lymphomas, the latter bodies may not be easily found in smears. Rarely, gran-

ulocytic sarcomas, especially those of the M₇ type, resemble a pleomorphic sarcoma.[78,79] The finding of smaller malignant cells characteristic of myeloblasts may facilitate the proper interpretation as may the recognition of precursors of eosinophils.

Polygonal Cell Sarcomas

The least common of the FNA biopsy categories of soft tissue sarcomas is the polygonal or epithelial-like group.[12] This includes epithelioid sarcoma, alveolar soft part sarcoma, clear cell sarcoma, and the predominantly epithelioid types of other sarcomas. Although smear cellularity is variable, it is usually moderate to high, often with a largely dissociative pattern (Figures 28-40 to 28-42). These smears contain nu-

A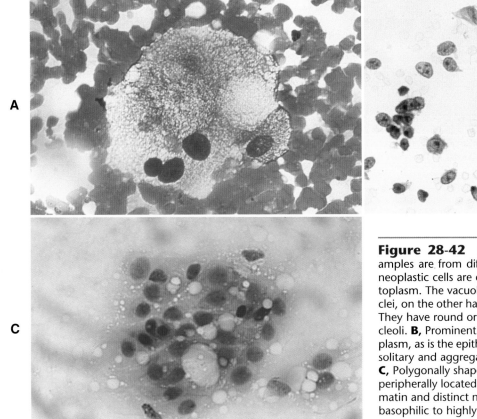

B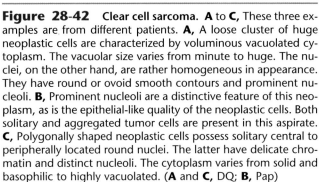

C

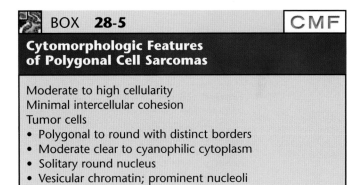

Figure 28-42 **Clear cell sarcoma. A to C,** These three examples are from different patients. **A,** A loose cluster of huge neoplastic cells are characterized by voluminous vacuolated cytoplasm. The vacuolar size varies from minute to huge. The nuclei, on the other hand, are rather homogeneous in appearance. They have round or ovoid smooth contours and prominent nucleoli. **B,** Prominent nucleoli are a distinctive feature of this neoplasm, as is the epithelial-like quality of the neoplastic cells. Both solitary and aggregated tumor cells are present in this aspirate. **C,** Polygonally shaped neoplastic cells possess solitary central to peripherally located round nuclei. The latter have delicate chromatin and distinct nucleoli. The cytoplasm varies from solid and basophilic to highly vacuolated. (**A** and **C,** DQ; **B,** Pap)

merous individually dispersed malignant cells and small generally flat aggregates. The malignant cells possess round or polygonal shapes, well-defined cellular borders, and at least moderate volumes of cytoplasm. Typically, they have a solitary, often eccentrically positioned round nucleus with a thick distinct membrane, vesicular chromatin, and one or more large nucleoli. In any of the polygonal cell sarcomas, some neoplastic cells may be binucleated or even multinucleated. A minority of the tumor cells may possess spindled shapes (Box 28-5).

The aspiration cytomorphologic attributes of epithelioid sarcoma, alveolar soft part sarcoma, and clear cell sarcoma are quite overlapping.[80-86,141] However, certain features may point to a specific lesion. The finding of optically clear cytoplasm and well-developed intranuclear cytoplasmic pseudoinclusions supports a clear cell sarcoma (see Figure 28-42).[84-86] In alveolar soft part sarcoma, some of the neoplastic cells may possess linear striations or distinct vacuoles in their abundant finely granulated cytoplasm.[82,83] Benign and malignant granular cell tumors may also be considered in this category, as the neoplastic cells possess voluminous, distinctly granular cytoplasm (Figure 28-43).[87,88] A panel of antibodies may allow for the separation of these neoplasms immunocytochemically (Table 28-3).

The differential diagnosis of the polygonal cell sarcomas in FNA biopsy is relatively limited. In the appropriate clinical scenario of a soft tissue mass in an extremity of a relatively young adult patient, a diagnosis of a polygonal cell sarcoma can be rendered. Although unlikely, a metastatic carcinoma or melanoma mimicking a primary soft tissue sar-

---

BOX   28-5   CMF

**Cytomorphologic Features
of Polygonal Cell Sarcomas**

Moderate to high cellularity
Minimal intercellular cohesion
Tumor cells
• Polygonal to round with distinct borders
• Moderate clear to cyanophilic cytoplasm
• Solitary round nucleus
• Vesicular chromatin; prominent nucleoli

---

coma needs to be excluded. In general, a greater degree of intercellular cohesion and three-dimensional aggregates favor metastatic carcinoma. Clinical data including past medical history and imaging studies should assist in this differential diagnosis. Based solely on the findings of a single aspiration biopsy, however, it may be impossible to distinguish a clear cell sarcoma from a metastatic melanoma. Renal and extrarenal rhabdoid tumors should also be considered in the differential diagnosis of some of these neoplasms.[89]

Round Cell Sarcomas

Although most soft tissue sarcomas occur predominantly in adult patients, the round cell sarcomas largely affect the pediatric population.[12] The most common of these is rhab-

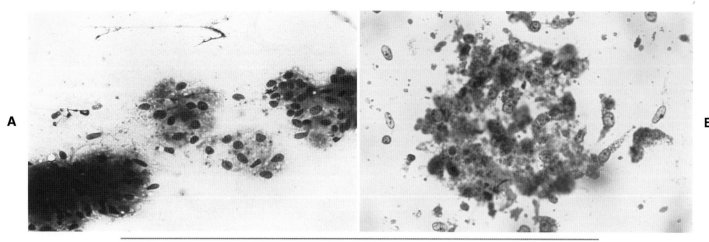

Figure 28-43   Granular cell tumor. A and **B**, Loosely clustered and individual cells are characterized by solitary small round or ovoid nuclei with inconspicuous nucleoli and by abundant cytoplasm. Although the granularity is evident with the Romanowsky stain in **A**, it is more readily apparent with Pap stain in **B**. Nuclei are not hyperchromatic and nucleoli are minute. This was derived from a benign granular cell tumor.

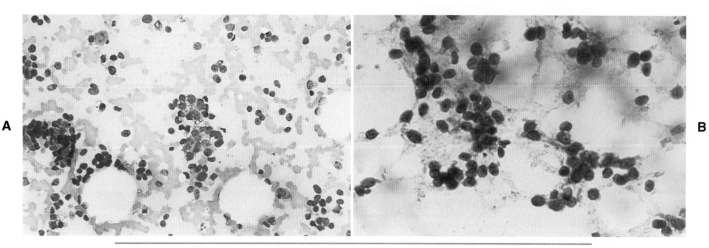

Figure 28-44   Ewing's sarcoma. A and **B**, The round cell sarcomas typically yield highly cellular smears which include both numerous individually dispersed malignant cells and small to large cohesive aggregates. Ewing's sarcoma is the prototype of this neoplasm in that it is composed of cells with solitary round nuclei and scanty cytoplasm. The nuclei typically have finely reticulated, evenly dispersed chromatin and lack well-developed nucleoli. In **A**, a minority of the neoplastic cells have small sharply punched out vacuoles that are positive for glycogen. In **B**, it is obvious that the nuclei are hyperchromatic and the N:C ratios are extremely high. (**A**, DQ; **B**, Pap)

TABLE 28-3				
Differential Diagnosis of Polygonal Cell Sarcomas: Immunocytochemistry				
	Clear Cell Sarcoma	**Epithelioid Sarcoma**	**Alveolar Soft Part Sarcoma**	**Granular Cell Tumor**
S-100 protein	+	−	−	+
HMB-45	+	−	−	−
Cytokeratin	−	+	−	−

domyosarcoma. Other entries in this category include extraskeletal Ewing's sarcoma/primitive neuroectodermal tumors and intraabdominal desmoplastic small round cell tumors. Aspiration biopsies of round cell sarcomas typically yield extremely cellular smears composed of relatively small, homogeneous malignant cells.[12,90-91] These neoplastic elements typically possess a solitary nucleus with high N:C ratios (Figure 28-44). The major exception to this is embryonal rhabdomyosarcoma in which a proportion of the neoplastic cells may have abundant cytoplasm and multiple

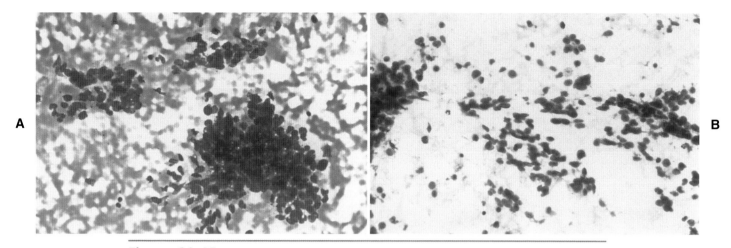

Figure 28-45 **Embryonal rhabdomyosarcoma. A** and **B,** This neoplasm is composed of primitive rhabdomyoblasts which show little in the way of specific differentiation. They possess solitary round to ovoid nuclei and have scanty cytoplasm resulting in high N:C ratios. Nucleoli are evident in some of the cells, but more striking are the marked uniformity of the cells and prominent hyperchromasia. (**A,** DQ; **B,** Pap)

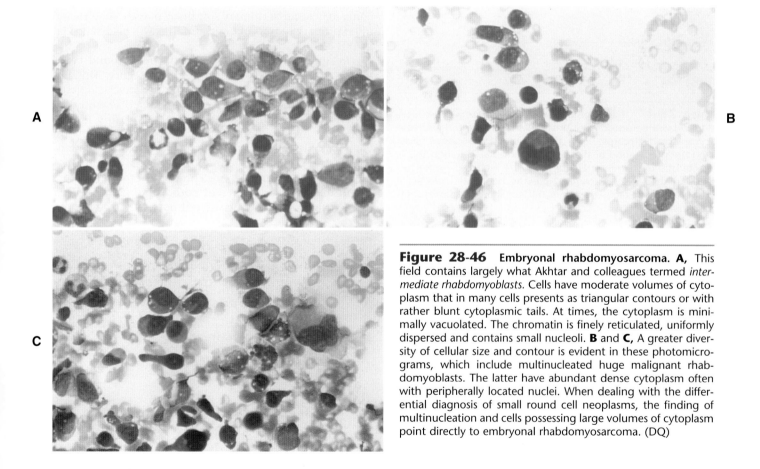

Figure 28-46 **Embryonal rhabdomyosarcoma. A,** This field contains largely what Akhtar and colleagues termed *intermediate rhabdomyoblasts.* Cells have moderate volumes of cytoplasm that in many cells presents as triangular contours or with rather blunt cytoplasmic tails. At times, the cytoplasm is minimally vacuolated. The chromatin is finely reticulated, uniformly dispersed and contains small nucleoli. **B** and **C,** A greater diversity of cellular size and contour is evident in these photomicrograms, which include multinucleated huge malignant rhabdomyoblasts. The latter have abundant dense cytoplasm often with peripherally located nuclei. When dealing with the differential diagnosis of small round cell neoplasms, the finding of multinucleation and cells possessing large volumes of cytoplasm point directly to embryonal rhabdomyosarcoma. (DQ)

nuclei.[92-95] Nuclear chromatin is generally hyperchromatic and nucleoli may or may not be prominent.

Aspiration biopsies of rhabdomyosarcoma yield moderately to very highly cellular samples (Figures 28-45 to 28-48).[92-96] The appearance may depend partly on the histologic subtype. A large proportion of the cells are individually dispersed with no evidence of intercellular cohesion. However, in alveolar rhabdomyosarcoma, it is more likely that a proportion of the neoplastic cells are present in large loosely cohesive aggregates (see Figure 28-48). Although some authors have suggested that these aggregates manifest a pseudoalveolar arrangement, the authors of this text believe this pattern may be exceedingly difficult to recognize in smears.[96] A large proportion of the neoplastic cells appear quite primitive in that they possess a solitary round nucleus and a high N:C ratio with no evidence of specific differentiation (see Figure 28-45). The chromatin is finely granular, evenly dispersed, and very darkly stained. Nucleoli tend to be small and inconspicuous but may be large. In a study of 15 aspirated rhabdomyosarcomas, Akhtar and colleagues divided the aspirated tumor cells into three categories: early, intermediate, and late rhabdomyoblasts.[92] These authors stated that in alveolar rhabdomyosarcoma, most of the neoplastic cells were early rhabdomyoblasts, resembling the undifferentiated cells described above. The intermediate rhabdomyoblasts had more abundant cytoplasm that tended to be pale stained and at times vacuolated. Voluminous, rela-

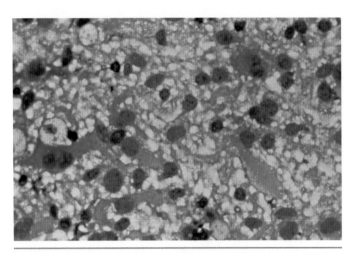

Figure 28-47 **Embryonal rhabdomyosarcoma.** The lace-like reticulated background of this smear results from the release of cytoplasmic glycogen from the malignant rhabdomyoblasts during the preparation of the aspiration smears. Although this is characteristic of germinomas, they may be seen with some frequency in rhabdomyosarcoma. Note the neoplastic cells have dense cytoplasmic tails, prominent nucleoli, and occasional multinucleation. (DQ)

tively opaque cytoplasm characterized the late rhabdomyoblasts. Cell contours varied from round to highly elongated. With the Romanowsky stain, some of the neoplastic elements possessed dense inclusion-like foci in the cytoplasm that corresponded ultrastructurally to concentrated aggregates of sarcomeres. A proportion of these cells were multinucleated and sometimes included very pleomorphic nuclei with prominent nucleoli. Embryonal rhabdomyosarcoma contained varying admixtures of rhabdomyoblasts with the three levels of differentiation (see Figures 28-45 and 28-46). However, these categories are artificial with no distinct lines of separation. Thus, in an individual patient, the distinction can be difficult. Clinical data and karyotypic analysis are more useful. More importantly, it is the presence of the relatively large cells with abundant dense cytoplasm and multinucleation that allows the pathologist to separate the rhabdomyosarcomas from the other small round cell tumors in FNA biopsy. This is supported by the recent logistic regression analysis of Layfield and colleagues in which the presence of strap or "tadpole-shaped" cells correlated well with the interpretation of rhabdomyosarcoma among small round cell tumors.[91] The smear background may have a tigroid appearance (see Figure 28-47). Although Ewing's sarcoma may occur as primary soft tissue masses, they are more often primary tumors of bone and thus will be detailed later in this chapter.

The intraabdominal desmoplastic small round cell tumor is another consideration in this category. This high-grade and generally fatal cancer typically affects adolescent males as a primary mass involving the peritoneum or the omentum. Very infrequently, these neoplasms have occurred in extraabdominal locations. Aspiration biopsies yield variably cellular smears, which presumably is a reflection of the prominent desmoplastic stroma within the tumor.[97,98,147] These smears are composed of uniform small round malignant cells present both as individual cells and in aggregates. Each neoplastic cell possesses a single round

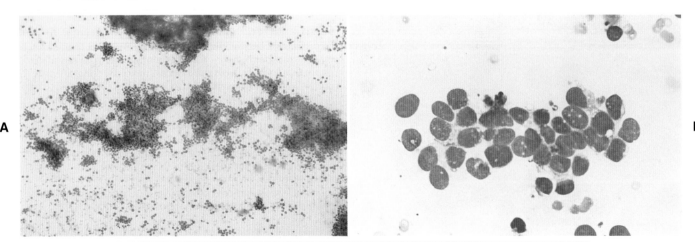

Figure 28-48 **Alveolar rhabdomyosarcoma. A,** In this scanning lens view, cohesive clusters of tumor cells appear to anastomose with one another with central spaces, perhaps recapitulating the histologic pseudoalveolar arrangement. Even at this low magnification, one may recognize the striking uniformity of the cells with solitary round nuclei and high N:C ratios. (From Geisinger KR, Abdul-Karim F. Fine needle aspiration biopsies. In: Weiss SW, Goldblum JR, editors. Enzinger and Weiss's soft tissue tumors. 4th ed. St. Louis: Mosby; 2001.) **B,** The malignant cells are strikingly uniform with solitary ovoid or round nuclei with smooth outlines, very finely reticulated chromatin, and minute but distinct nucleoli. For the most part, cytoplasm is minimal and thus the cells possess high N:C ratios. No specific differentiation is evident. (DQ)

nucleus with hyperchromatic chromatin and inconspicuous nucleoli (Figure 28-49). Generally, cytoplasm is scanty. Thus, in smears, the cells resemble those of Ewing's sarcoma. The smears may also show fragments of cellular collagen. If this diagnosis is considered, the results of immunocytochemistry on aspirated material may be quite supportive. These neoplastic cells manifest multidirectional differentiation, typically being positive for cytokeratin, desmin, and neuron-specific enolase. Material obtained by FNA biopsy may demonstrate an 11;22 reciprocal translation by cytogenetics or a specific gene fusion product by the polymerase chain reaction.

In intraaspiration biopsies, three other entities need to be entertained in the differential diagnosis: neuroblastoma, Wilms' tumor, and Burkitt's lymphoma. The last of these is detailed in Chapter 24, whereas nephroblastoma is considered in Chapter 22. Aspirates of neuroblastoma yield moderately to highly cellular samples dominated by small primitive malignant cells characterized by solitary nuclei and extremely high N:C ratios.[91,99] Each nucleus has a round, ovoid, or slightly irregular contour with even, fine chromatin that is very darkly stained. Nucleoli are either absent or small and inconspicuous. Although many of the neoplastic cells may not show any specific differentiation, the smears may demonstrate important diagnostic clues. One of these is the presence of pseudorosettes.[91,99] These consist of one or more layers of nuclei surrounding central fibrillar material. True lumens are not evident. Similar filamentous material corresponding to the neuropil may be present within the smear background and a large proportion of the cells may appear embedded within this material. With the DQ stain, it appears pink to gray, and with the Pap stain it is green. Another potentially helpful diagnostic clue is the presence of neoplastic ganglion cells that are characterized by much larger sizes, polygonal contours, voluminous basophilic cytoplasm and one or more nuclei. The latter often appear perfectly round,

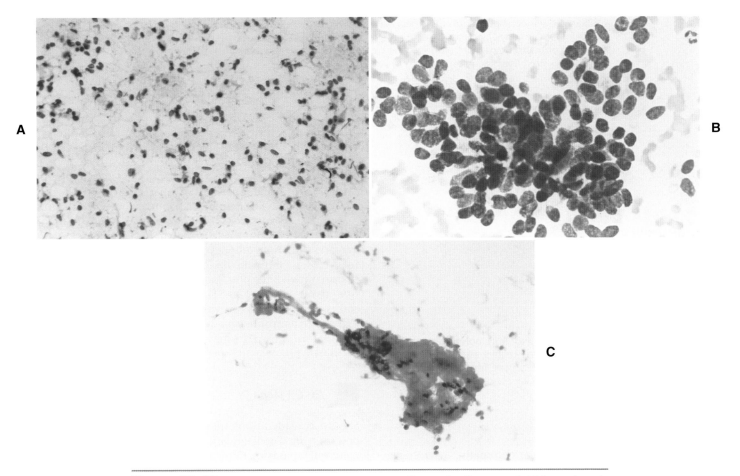

Figure 28-49 **Intraabdominal desmoplastic small round cell tumor. A,** This moderately cellular aspirate shows individually dispersed and very small loosely cohesive clusters of homogeneous malignant cells on a clean background. Each cell possesses a single hyperchromatic round nucleus and very little in the way of cytoplasm. No distinct differentiation is apparent. **B,** This undifferentiated appearance is confirmed at higher magnification. The cells have relatively small nuclei with finely reticulated chromatin that is evenly distributed and inconspicuous nucleoli. The N:C ratios are extremely high. In addition to the appropriate clinical and radiographic data, the results of ancillary diagnostic studies are crucial to the accurate interpretation of this sample. **C,** A fragment of poorly cellular dense collagenized stroma dominates this field. Although totally nonspecific, it is a characteristic component of aspirates of this neoplasm. This would be expected from the underlying histopathology. (**A** and **C,** Pap; **D,** DQ).

A   **B**

Figure 28-50 Well-differentiated liposarcoma. **A,** This scanning lens view demonstrates adipocytes with varying appearances; most are completely unremarkable with a huge solitary cytoplasmic lipid vacuole and a small, barely perceptible, peripherally located, and darkly stained nucleus. However, a minority of the neoplastic cells have moderately sized nuclei that are also darkly stained and at times, irregular in shape. The latter's contours may result from indentation by the cytoplasmic lipid vacuoles. A few cells possess relatively scanty cytoplasmic lipid. Several capillary vessels course through the smear background. **B,** Although most of the adipocytes in this field appear normal, at least two contain nuclei that are much larger than normal and have variably corrugated external contours. Their cytoplasm appears to contain multiple small to moderately sized lipid vacuoles. (**A,** DQ; **B,** Pap)

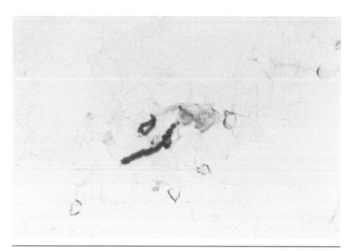

Figure 28-51 Elastofibroma. No cells are present in this field, which was derived from a poorly cellular aspirate of an interscapular soft tissue mass. This elastic tissue fiber stain highlights the classic appearance of thick, irregular elastic fibers typical of this lesion.

have distinct membranes, vesicular chromatin, macronucleoli, and eccentric locations. Cells with smaller sizes may represent partially differentiated neuroblasts.

Miscellaneous Sarcomas

One neoplasm that does not neatly fit into any of the above categories is the well-differentiated liposarcoma. Only rarely has the aspiration cytomorphology of this tumor been detailed.[26,34,71] Smears are only moderately cellular at best and may be mistaken for benign adipose tissue due to the presence of mostly (or exclusively) mature-appearing fat

cells, often in fragments (Figure 28-50). The latter are huge univacuolated cells with small, dark, round, peripheral nuclei. The diagnosis of liposarcoma requires finding unequivocal lipoblasts. Complex arrays of branching capillaries may be evident.

The major entity in this differential diagnosis is benign fat, either normal tissue or lipoma. These latter two are morphologically indistinguishable in aspirates. To diagnose a lipoma, a distinct mass must be detected clinically. Smears contain variable numbers of flat to three-dimensional aggregates of benign adipocytes.[26,34] In smears, elastofibromas may closely simulate lipomas as they contain clusters of mature adipocytes plus small fragments of fibrous connective tissue (Figure 28-51). With conventional cytologic stains, the characteristic thick elastic fibers are not evident. When an elastofibroma is clinically suspected (an interscapular mass), smears may be destained and then restained for elastic fibers, which permits an accurate diagnosis.[100]

 ## ACCURACY

Several considerations must be taken into account before determining the diagnostic accuracy of FNA biopsy of musculoskeletal masses. Only a relatively small number of series with large numbers of patients have been published.* Furthermore, there is a lack of standardization among these reports. Some studies have included patients with both benign and malignant neoplasms,† whereas others address only sarcomas.[8,13] A number of series are dedicated to the primary diagnosis of a mass, whereas others include many patients with recurrent sarcomas. Several studies have in-

---

*References 2, 3, 5, 6, 8, 13, 15-17, 20, and 101.
†References 2, 3, 5, 6, 16, 17, and 20.

TABLE 28-4

Diagnostic Accuracy in Fine-Needle Aspiration Biopsy of Soft Tissue Tumors

Reference	Number of Benign Tumors	Number of Sarcomas	False-Positive Rate (%)	False-Negative Rate (%)
3	315	202	4	7
6	149	151	2	5
101	17	25	0	6
17	34	60	4	0
15	63	51	2	4
5	16	37	0	0
8	*	41	8	7
13	†	68	†	3

*Not clear from published date.
†Only examined sarcomas.

cluded aspiration biopsies of both bone and soft tissue lesions.[8,16] The manner in which the data is analyzed is also variable from series to series. Some authors provide only the number of cases, whereas others have published levels of diagnostic sensitivity and specificity and/or their rates of false-negative and false-positive diagnoses. Several excellent studies detail the cytomorphologic features of aspirates of soft tissue lesions, but provide little or no numerical data on accuracy.

Akerman and colleagues from Sweden have described the largest series of FNA biopsy of soft tissue lesions.[3] Over a 20-year period, these investigators evaluated 517 patients undergoing an aspiration biopsy for the primary diagnosis of a soft tissue neoplasm; of these, 315 were benign, and 202 were sarcomas. The authors were able to distinguish benign from malignant in 94% of the patients.[3] Their errors were equally divided between 14 false-negative interpretations and 14 false-positive diagnoses (Table 28-4). Among the latter, two patients underwent excessive surgical therapy. In their experience, the area of greatest difficulty in morphologic interpretation was the spindle cell neoplasms, followed by lipomatous tumors.[3]

Also from Sweden, Brosjo and colleagues evaluated 342 patients with a relatively equal distribution between benign and malignant soft tissue tumors.[6] In 300 of these patients (88%), the FNA biopsy diagnosis was conclusive. Of the 153 benign cytologic diagnoses, there was a 5% false-negative rate. Of the 147 malignant cytologic diagnoses, a 2% false-positive rate resulted. Accordingly, a correct diagnosis was rendered in 97% of this population.

From Israel, Oland and colleagues reported their experience with 196 patients, including children, who underwent FNA biopsy of a soft tissue mass.[101] Of the patients, 132 had a benign cytologic diagnosis (either tumor or inflammation) and were followed medically. Sixteen additional patients had a diagnosis of metastatic carcinoma without subsequent surgery. Forty-eight patients had a histologic examination of their masses after the FNA biopsy, and all 25 patients with an FNA biopsy diagnosis of frank sarcoma were confirmed. Thus, there were no false-positive interpretations. Of the 17 individuals who had a benign soft tissue tumor diagnosed by cytology, one had a false-negative interpretation; a diagnosis of fibroma was rendered in an individual who was proven to have a fibrosarcoma. The final

six patients had an FNA biopsy diagnosis that did not commit between benign and malignant; their subsequent histologic evaluations all proved to be benign.[101]

Miralles and colleagues published a series of 117 soft tissue FNA biopsies from Spain.[17] Their patients were relatively evenly divided between having benign and malignant tumors. Unlike the above-cited studies in which FNA biopsy was used in the primary evaluation of a soft tissue mass, many individuals studied by Miralles and colleagues were clinically suspected recurrences or metastasis in patients with previously documented sarcomas.[17] These investigators had no false-negative interpretations but did experience a 4% false-positive diagnosis rate. One of the two patients with a false-positive had fat necrosis that was diagnosed in the smears as a liposarcoma; excessive surgery was the unfortunate result. Importantly, this manuscript contains a statement that makes us wonder whether the statistics are completely accurate. The authors stated in their discussion of pseudosarcomatous mass lesions that they encountered difficulties in the correct diagnosis of these lesions and thus recommended an open biopsy for their exact diagnosis.[17] None of the benign specimens in this series, however, are considered among the traditional pseudosarcomatous lesions. If the latter had been included in this series, we suspect that their false positive rate may have been higher.

In the United States, Layfield and colleagues and Bennert and Abdul-Karim have published series of similar sizes.[5,15] Layfield's series included 114 sufficient aspirates from patients with benign and malignant soft tissue lesions, including 51 individuals with histologically documented soft tissue sarcomas.[15] These authors had false-positive and false-negative rates of 2% and 4%, respectively. Two patients in whom lipomas were aspirated had a cytologic diagnosis of liposarcoma. The authors did not mention if there were any adverse clinical outcomes for these two patients. The study by Bennert and Abdul-Karim specifically compared the results of FNA biopsy and subsequent tissue core needle biopsies.[5] Of the 117 patients with soft tissue lesions, 38% of the aspirates were considered unsatisfactory for evaluation (insufficient cellularity), and 17% were inflammatory. The remaining 53 patients (45%) had aspirates that were considered diagnostic of a soft tissue tumor. All 16 benign aspiration interpretations were correct, as were the 37 aspiration diagnoses of sarcomas.

Although the needle core biopsies provided a more specific typing of the sarcoma than did the FNA biopsy in 19% of the malignant diagnoses, the overall clinical management of the patients was not improved by the tissue core biopsies. In their cases with histologic follow-up, the levels of diagnostic sensitivity and specificity were both 100% for the cytologic interpretations. The series by Costa and colleagues included a total of 52 FNA biopsies in patients with 46 soft tissue and six bone neoplasms.[8] Of these, 43 were for a primary diagnosis, whereas nine were for clinically suspected recurrences. They had a 7% false-negative rate and an 8% false-positive diagnostic rate; most of the latter occurred in the evaluation of potential recurrent tumors. This suggests that some pathologists may feel more comfortable in rendering a malignant interpretation in patients with a previous histologic diagnosis of sarcoma.[8] The same strict cytomorphologic criteria for recurrent sarcoma should be applied as in making a primary diagnosis of the same neoplasm.

Liu and colleagues systematically examined a series of 89 aspirates that included samples derived from 20 benign and 69 malignant masses including 11 metastatic melanomas.[16] Of the aspirates, 69 were soft tissue lesions. Each FNA biopsy was independently evaluated by four different pathologists who differed in their years of experience in performing and interpreting aspiration biopsies. Each pathologist evaluated these specimens in two separate settings, namely, without and then later with clinical history. In each of the two scenarios, each pathologist provided a precise cytopathologic diagnosis for the aspiration smears and also classified the smears into one of four categories: benign, probably benign, probably malignant, or definitely malignant. This data was used to create receiver operator characteristic (ROC) curves. Without the benefit of clinical history, the proportion of precise correct diagnoses ranged from 0.19 to 0.44. With the addition of clinical history, the proportions of precise interpretations improved to a range of 0.48 to 0.66, and the proportion of correct diagnoses improved for all four cytopathologists. These results strongly support our contention that one must integrate relevant clinical data and radiographic interpretations whenever evaluating aspiration biopsies of soft tissue lesions.[16] Without the addition of clinical history, the proportion of correct classifications, as measured by the area under the ROC curve, ranged from 0.81 to 0.9. The range of correct classification improved to 0.89 to 0.9 with the addition of clinical history. Difficulty was especially noted for benign spindle cell tumors including hemangiomas and nerve sheath neoplasms. The integration of clinical history with the cytomorphology proved to be most useful in the evaluation of lipomatous neoplasms, particularly in diagnosing liposarcomas as definitely malignant. In some cases, however, the clinical information was actually misleading in that the proportion of correct classifications declined for both hemangiomas and myositis ossificans. In these diagnostic exercises, the more experienced cytopathologists fared better in both designating a precise diagnosis and in the correct benign-to-malignant classification scheme. Overall, knowledge of the clinical history provided greater assistance for the less experienced pathologists. Again, this reiterates the crucial premise that FNA biopsy of soft tissue lesions should be interpreted in conjunction with the clinical and radiographic information.

Although the exact role to be played by FNA biopsy in the clinical evaluation of soft tissue mass lesions remains controversial, the authors believe that the bulk of published data and their own practices strongly support its ability to distinguish accurately between benign and soft tissue tumors (see Table 28-4). The levels of diagnostic specificity and sensitivity are approximately 95% in establishing a frank diagnosis of sarcoma.[3,12] In addition, FNA biopsy can accurately differentiate sarcomas from other forms of primary or metastatic malignancies involving the soft tissues.

It is also our opinion that FNA biopsy can accurately subclassify soft tissue tumors, especially sarcomas, into general, clinically relevant categories that permit the initiation of therapy in many patients. Specific subtyping along histologic grounds may not be necessary for many sarcomas with the obvious exception of the round cell tumors. Some pathologists are remiss to interpret a proportion of soft tissue tumors in histologic preparations as to specific subtypes without the aid of ancillary diagnostic procedures such as immunohistochemistry and cytogenetics. With few exceptions, these same procedures can be readily applied to aspirated material; thus, specific subtyping may be provided in a large proportion of non-pleomorphic sarcomas with the combination of cytomorphology and ancillary testing. A major limitation, however, may be retrieval of sufficient material to perform extensive testing. Preoperative grading of sarcomas by FNA biopsy may be problematic in a significant proportion of patients, but this is not prohibitive clinically. With greater experience by a larger proportion of practicing pathologists, FNA biopsy will become a well-accepted practice in the initial evaluation of superficial and deep soft tissue lesions. At the least, FNA biopsy will play an important triage role.

 ## GRADING OF SARCOMAS

Little attention has been paid to the ability to grade sarcomas in aspiration smears.[12,13,40,148] Willén and colleagues, for example, have discussed briefly dividing sarcomatous aspirates into low- and high-grade neoplasms.[20] However, actual application of their system appears to have been limited within their own study. With certain restrictions, many soft tissue sarcomas can be accurately graded in FNA biopsy in a clinically relevant manner.

Among prognostic factors in patients with soft tissue sarcomas, histologic grade consistently is one of the most significant.[102] Accordingly, it is important to consider the possibility of accurately grading soft tissue sarcomas in FNA biopsy. Although several different grading schemes exist for these neoplasms, most of them consistently incorporate several different microscopic attributes: mitotic activity, amount of necrosis, and degree of differentiation or histologic subtypes. In a recent manuscript, Guillou and Coindre have stated the following[102]:

> The risk of underestimating necrosis or mitotic activity is directly related to the low quantity of material provided. Grading sarcoma on fine needle or core biopsy should be discouraged. The risk of error is too high, and diagnosis of a histologic type of sarcoma is uncertain if not impossible.

According to these experts, the grading of sarcomas in aspiration smears cannot be accomplished accurately. The authors of this text do not totally agree.

These authors made this statement for several reasons.[102] First, mitotic figure counts in aspiration biopsies of any tumor types are not a standardized practice. Although mitotic figures can certainly be seen in direct smears, we are unaware of anyone who consistently and routinely uses mitotic figure counts in smears in any type of neoplasm. If for no other reason, the variability in cellularity from field to field would be prohibitive. Similarly, the proportion of the tumor that is necrotic before chemotherapy or radiotherapy cannot be predicted on the basis of aspiration biopsies. The cytologist can only state that necrotic debris is absent or present in scant or large amounts in the smears. A third feature, namely the degree of differentiation or histologic subtype, is somewhat different. In FNA biopsy, a specific cell type can be rendered in a large proportion of soft tissue sarcomas, especially if one uses ancillary diagnostic procedures such as immunocytochemistry and cytogenetics directly on aspirated cellular material.

Thus, many soft tissue sarcomas can be graded in a clinically relevant fashion in aspiration biopsies.[13,101a] Specifically, round cell sarcomas are almost always high-grade neoplasms. With the use of ancillary diagnostic testing, specific diagnoses can be rendered in a large proportion of these cases. Although the specific cell type of a pleomorphic sarcoma cannot always be determined, these neoplasms can almost always be recognized as high grade. Alternatively, if they can be identified accurately, well-differentiated liposarcomas are consistently low grade. Most myxoid sarcomas are either low- or intermediate-grade neoplasms. It is the polygonal cell and especially the spindle cell categories that pose the greatest difficulties.[13,40] In the latter type, if one can identify with certainty a synovial sarcoma by immunocytochemistry or cytogenetics, then the neoplasm can be given a high-grade automatically. In the authors' limited experiences, they do not believe that the polygonal

cell sarcomas can be stratified accurately into grades on the basis of aspiration biopsies.

Extracellular Deposits

Deposition of extracellular materials rarely may clinically and radiographically simulate a soft tissue neoplasm, particularly a sarcoma. Several patients have now been reported in which a gouty tophus was so large that it closely mimicked a soft tissue neoplasm.[103,104] In these instances, FNA biopsy provided the correct diagnosis potentially saving the patient undue surgery. Aspiration smears of these huge tophi are poorly cellular. The smears are dominated by long thin crystals with a uniform width and, at times, sharply pointed tips (Figure 28-52). With the Romanowsky stains, these appear as clear needles or crystal-like structures (crystaloid negative images). With the Pap stain, they present as pale brown colored crystals. These crystals typically appear haphazardly arranged both individually and in clusters. Occasional aggregates, however, resemble the sheaths of tyrosine crystals typical of aspirates of pleomorphic adenomas of salivary gland origin. These smears contain scattered, benign histiocytes and multinucleated inflammatory giant cells. The latter may appear to be phagocytizing some of these crystals. With a polarizing microscope, these crystals show weak negative birefringence. Similar-appearing benign giant cells may occur in soft tissue inflammatory masses but are not associated with crystals.[149]

An extremely unusual circumstance is when the deposition of amyloid in soft tissues is so extensive (and unassociated with an underlying gammopathy) that a soft tissue neoplasm is strongly suspected. Again, aspiration smears are poorly cellular and are dominated by variably sized but generally small fragments of amyloid (Figure 28-53). These fragments typically have sharply delineated edges that may appear straight or scalloped. With the Romanowsky stains, they are distinctly blue to purple in color. They appear variably pink to orange to green with the Pap preparation. Only

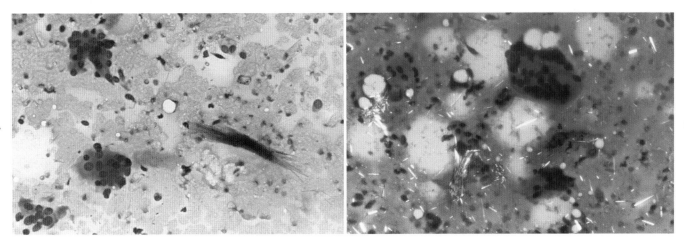

A **B**

Figure 28-52 **Gouty tophus. A,** These aspirates, as witnessed in this particular example, are generally poorly cellular and include scattered benign fibroblasts, mononucleated histiocytes, and multinucleated inflammatory giant cells. In addition, a yellow-brown–stained sheath of urate crystals is evident. In other instances, these needles create a negative image. **B,** Polarizing microscopy can be performed directly on the aspirated smears demonstrating the individual and clustered elongated urate crystals which manifest negative birefringence. (DQ)

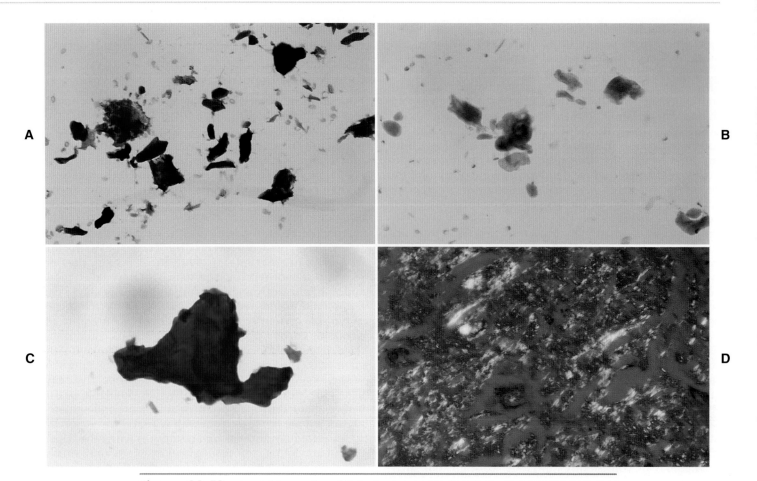

Figure 28-53   Amyloidoma. **A** and **B,** In these scanning lens views, the smear is extremely poorly cellular. Rather, irregularly contoured fragments of amyloid dominate the picture. Note the sharply defined relatively smooth edges to these collections of extracellular proteinaceous material. **C,** At higher magnification, the homogeneous appearance of the amyloid is evident as is again the rather sharply defined smooth external edges to the fragment. Note the lack of cells, including plasma cells, in the background. **D,** In the subsequently resected amyloidoma, the classic apple-green birefringence is evident in this section stained with Congo red. (**A** and **B,** DQ; **C,** Pap)

rare benign mesenchymal cells are present within the smears. In general, plasma cells are not expected in the smears to any extent.

NEOPLASMS AND OTHER LESIONS OF THE BONE

Unlike the authors' approach to FNA biopsy of soft tissue neoplasms where differential diagnoses are generated on the basis of the cytomorphologic patterns or categories of sarcomas, with bone neoplasms, a formal histopathologic classification is more closely followed.[105] Accordingly, lesions of bone are diagnosed and classified, in part, on their radiographic appearances. It is important for the pathologist to be aware of basic bone tumor radiology to render accurate and specific interpretations. In addition to patient age, such attributes include the exact location or specific bone involved and the portion (i.e., epiphyseal, metaphyseal, or diaphyseal) of that bone that is involved, along with the size of the lesion, the pattern of destruction of bone and its associated margins, the presence and type of matrix material evident, and the presence or absence of a periosteal reaction. In addition, this classification of bone tumors in aspiration biopsies incorporates the degree of smear cellu-larity, the type(s) of cells present, and the presence or absence of matrix material. Thus, the major categories include osseous, cartilaginous, cystic, lymphoreticular, and lesions of unknown origin. As with soft tissue neoplasms, some proliferations of bone do not readily fall into any of these categories. Finally, it is important to recognize that the most common malignant tumor of bone is metastases.

As is probably obvious from the above discussion, it is imperative for the pathologist to know at least rudimentary radiography of bone lesions to assess confidently these aspirates. No other organ or tumor type exists in which such knowledge is so important. In addition to tumor classification, this information allows general recognition of which bone lesions are accessible to FNA biopsy.

Mass lesions of bone for which aspiration biopsies are often achievable are large, destructive lesions that have markedly attenuated or traversed the cortical bone, those that may be associated with extension into the adjacent soft tissues, and those that may include only nonmineralized matrix and hence are softer. These attributes, of course, tend to correlate with malignant or at least locally aggressive neoplasms. However, some cancers such as low-grade central osteosarcomas are surrounded by thick cortex that does not readily permit sampling by FNA biopsy. Conversely, neoplasms that are confined beneath the cortex (intraosseous) are typically benign and do not lend themselves to sampling by a fine needle. The osteoid osteoma is a classic example.

Osteoid Osteoma

Osteoid osteomas are often benign bony proliferations that produce small well-delineated rounded areas of lucency in cortical bone. Radiographically, a dense sclerotic rim circumscribes the small mass. In some cases a small area of ossification is noted centrally. These tumors most commonly arise on the lower extremity, especially the femur. However, many bones including the vertebrae may be affected. Characteristically, the patient complains of pain of progressively increasing intensity. This pain, which is often reduced or alleviated by taking aspirin, is often accentuated at night.

Histologically, the central nidus is composed of anastomosing trabeculae of osteoid and woven bone situated within a prominently vascularized connective tissue stroma. Large osteoblasts typically line many of these interconnecting trabeculae. Because of sampling problems, a good example of an osteoid osteoma in direct smears has not been seen.[105] Rarely, however, such tumors have been examined in cell block preparations where the characteristic nidus may be identified. (Perhaps luck, more than anything else, was involved in these rare examples.) Perusal of many series does not reveal a single aspirated example.

Osteoblastoma

Osteoblastoma is another benign bony tumor that only infrequently has been sampled well by aspiration biopsy.[106-108] These neoplasms arise most commonly in the vertebrae, es-

pecially their dorsal components, and in the skull, most commonly in young adults. Radiographically, these neoplasms may resemble osteoid osteomas. Two potential major differences include a lack of a dense sclerotic rim and a greater likelihood of extensive ossification of the mass itself. In many cases, it is the presence of the latter element that precludes obtaining an adequate aspiration biopsy. Walaas and Kindblom have described two examples of osteoblastomas in FNA biopsy.[107] Most of the neoplastic osteoblasts contained a single round nucleus but a minority of the neoplastic cells were binucleated (Figure 28-54). Because the presence of voluminous cytoplasm, the N:C ratios are not high. The majority of the tumor cells had plump epithelioid configurations. Typically, the round nucleus is peripherally situated within the cytoplasm that may show a zone of clearing that is distinctly not perinuclear in location. The anaplasia and polymorphism of osteosarcomas are lacking.[107] In addition, the aspiration biopsies may sample a portion of the vascular fibroblastic connective tissue; thus, spindle-shaped fibroblasts with ovoid nuclei with distinct nucleoli also may be present. Individually dispersed cells predominate the smears, but small clusters are also present. In their experiences, the aspirates had some morphologic overlap with chondroblastomas.[107] The presence of many spindle-shaped cells favored osteoblastoma.

Osteosarcoma

The most common nonhematopoietic primary cancer of bone is osteosarcoma. Generally, these malignancies occur in young individuals with a peak incidence in the second decade. Osteosarcomas may present uncommonly, however,

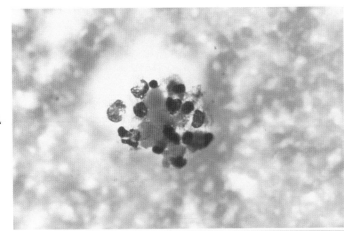

A

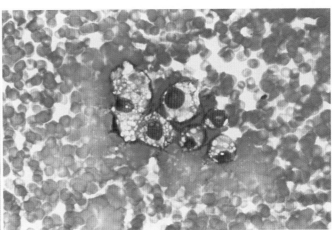

B

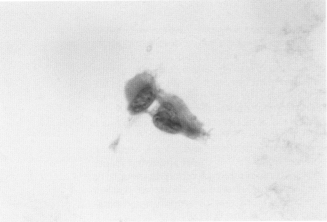

C

Figure 28-54 Osteoblastoma. **A,** Moderately sized and uniform-appearing osteoblasts are associated with small deposits of osteoid in this poorly cellular sample. The cells have solitary round or ovoid nuclei with delicate membranes; fine, even chromatin; and small nucleoli. Cytoplasm is polygonal in contour and delicately basophilic with fine vacuoles. No evidence of pleomorphism is present. **B,** Additional neoplastic cells have solitary round nuclei that are eccentrically located within the vacuolated cytoplasm. Small nucleoli are evident, but again, no evidence of anaplasia or pleomorphism is present. **C,** The nuclei have delicate, fine chromatin that is generally pale. Nucleoli are lacking. Note the eccentric location of the nuclei. (**A** and **B,** DQ; **C,** Pap)

in older individuals, especially those arising in preexisting Paget's disease, and to a lesser degree, as the periosteal type of osteosarcoma. Although almost any bone may at least rarely be affected, a large proportion of osteosarcomas arise in the extremities, especially the lower one; the area of the knee (distal femur and proximal tibia) is the major target. Clinically, these neoplasms typically occur as a painful mass that is often palpable. Several histologic variants exist, but the majority are conventional intramedullary osteosarcomas, a high-grade neoplasm. These tumors occur most commonly in the metaphysis. With routine skeletal radiographs, the lesion may appear lytic, blastic (sclerotic), or mixed. Typically, destruction of both cortical and trabecular bone is evident as is periosteal osteoneogenesis, classically resulting in Codman's triangle. In larger osteosarcomas, extension of the tumor into the adjacent soft tissue is expected.

Histologically, the conventional osteosarcoma is characterized by marked pleomorphism. All osteosarcomas have in common the production of osteoid by obviously malignant mesenchymal cells. This matrix often appears as a delicate lacelike arrangement about the malignant osteoblasts. The latter vary tremendously in size and shape; they may be spindled, polygonal, or round. Usually these cells are large with one or more clearly malignant and often eccentrically placed nuclei and moderate to abundant cytoplasm, the latter of which may vary from dense to highly vacuolated. Some of the neoplastic cells may show features characteristic of osteoblasts, namely, a large clear zone in the cytoplasm at some distance from the nucleus. Although cartilaginous matrix may not be present in some tumors, others are dominated by this material.

The cellularity of aspiration smears of osteosarcomas depends in part on the degree of bone formation within the neoplasm itself (Figures 28-55 to 28-57).[105-115] In highly sclerotic masses and those with relatively little in the way of soft tissue extension, smear cellularity may be rather low.

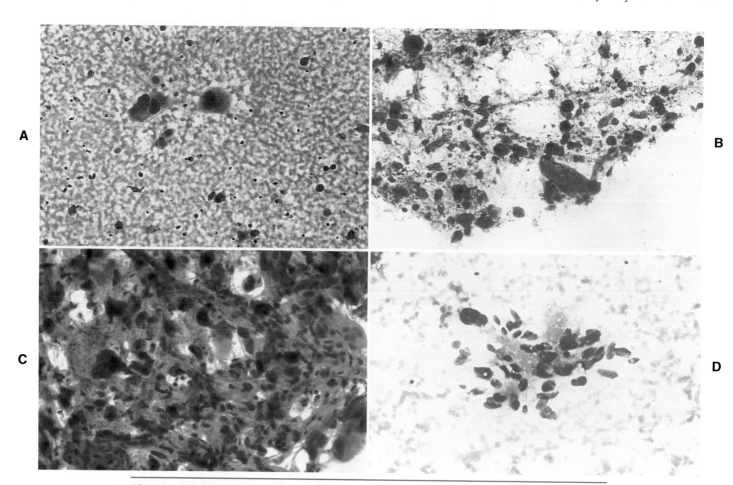

Figure 28-55 Osteosarcoma. **A,** This relatively poorly cellular aspirate does demonstrate striking pleomorphism of the malignant cells. Many are small with solitary round nuclei and high N:C ratios. However, one can recognize a spectrum of progressively larger cells with greater amounts of cytoplasm. This includes multinucleated tumor giant cells with irregularly shaped nuclei, distinct nucleoli, and moderate to abundant cytoplasm. The latter typically has a lacy appearance because of minute vacuoles. **B,** In addition to the attributes demonstrated in **A,** hyperchromasia is readily apparent among the malignant cells of all sizes. **C,** This aspirate is much more cellular with tumor cells embedded within collagenous and osteoid matrix materials. Again, moderate to marked variability in nuclear and cellular contours and sizes is apparent. Although some of the nuclei have smooth round outlines, many have irregular angulated shapes in addition to the dense dark chromatin. **D,** In this field, moderately pleomorphic neoplastic cells, including a binucleated tumor cell, is associated with a small amount of osteoid. Nuclear contours vary from round to elongated. Although necrotic debris may be seen in smear backgrounds, in this particular example, it is clean. (**A** and **D,** DQ; **B** and **C,** Pap)

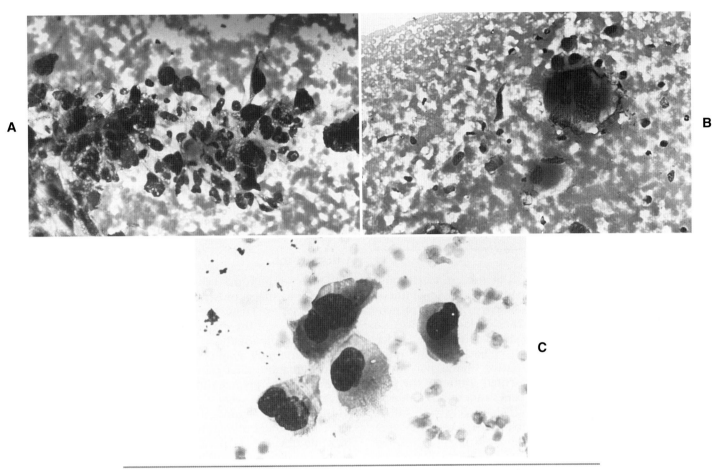

Figure 28-56 Osteosarcoma. **A,** A greater proportion of the malignant cells have moderate to large sizes. Although many of the cells have a round or polygonal shape, others are spindled. Overall, the N:C ratios are high; cytoplasm appears delicately vacuolated. A small amount of osteoid is also evident. **B,** Striking pleomorphism is evident in this rather scantily cellular field. Tumor cell sizes range from small to massive. The latter include multinucleated tumor giant cells. Note that the nuclei in the largest cell are huge, have coarsely granular chromatin and irregular contours, and vary from one to the other. **C,** At high magnification, the chromatin appears clumped and irregularly distributed within the variegated nuclei. Cytoplasm is moderate to abundant in amount; nuclei vary from centrally positioned to eccentric. These cells are obviously malignant. (DQ)

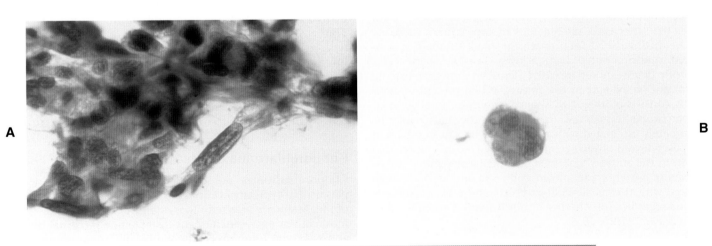

Figure 28-57 Osteosarcoma. **A** and **B,** With the Pap stain, the chromatin is more readily analyzed. It varies from finely granular to coarsely granular and clumped with an irregular distribution. Uniformly, however, hyperchromasia is the rule. Nucleoli may be prominent in a proportion of the malignant cells. In **A,** a huge spindle-shaped malignant osteoblast is present with a solitary large elongated nucleus, whereas in **B,** a polygonal multinucleated tumor giant cell is evident.

BOX 28-6   CMF

Cytomorphologic Features of Osteosarcoma

Variable but generally moderately cellular smears with individual tumor cells and small flat neoplastic aggregates

Variably pleomorphic tumor cells ranging from small to huge and from polygonal to round to spindled with moderate volumes of homogeneous cytoplasm

Obviously malignant nuclei with thick, smooth to irregular membranes, coarse chromatin with irregular distributions, and prominent nucleoli

In some cases, bizarre multinucleated tumor giant cells

Thin strands of dense matrix (osteoid); cartilaginous matrix with lacunae possible

Scattered benign osteoclasts

However, in general, cellularity is at least moderate and may be striking. The smears contain both individual tumor cells and small rather loosely cohesive aggregates of neoplastic cells (see Figures 28-55 to 28-57). Many instances are characterized by marked pleomorphism of both cellular size and contour. The cells, although characteristically quite large, also may be relatively diminutive. Round, polygonal, and spindled shapes are all represented, although the proportion of the different cellular shapes varies from tumor to tumor. Overall, polygonal or epithelioid cells with rather well-defined cell borders dominate most aspirates (see Figures 28-55 and 28-56). Most neoplastic cells possess one or two obviously malignant nuclei. Although some cells have central nuclei, eccentric positions are more typical. In the giant cell variant, the neoplastic cells possess four, five, or more nuclei. Some of the nuclei are round or ovoid with smooth contours, whereas others have highly irregular membranes. The chromatin tends to be coarsely and irregular granular and definitely hyperchromatic. Nucleoli usually are well-developed and may be multiple and/or very large. The polygonal shaped cells in particular have moderate to abundant cytoplasm that is relatively homogeneous, although small vacuoles may be prominent in some examples. Most specimens include at least a small proportion of huge and bizarre-appearing multinucleated tumor giant cells that are clearly sarcomatous in appearance. These are to be distinguished from relatively small numbers of scattered multinucleated benign osteoclast-like giant cells. Mitotic figures should be easily identified; however, osteoid may not be evident in the smears. When present, it typically consists of irregularly shaped strands of homogeneous metachromatic material. In some foci, the matrix may be intimately associated with malignant cells, but in others, it appears devoid of such elements. It needs to be emphasized that, in the authors' opinions, in a pediatric patient, an aspirate of a high-grade, pleomorphic sarcoma of bone associated with the classic radiographic features is an osteosarcoma regardless of whether or not osteoid is recognized in the smears[105] (Box 28-6).

Osteochondroma

Osteochondroma is the most common benign proliferation of bone. In a proportion of patients, a palpable mass is present. The most common sites include the distal femur, the proximal humerus, and the proximal tibia. Radiographically, the mass may be either pedunculated or sessile. These lesions arise in the metaphyses of long bones and characteristically demonstrate a continuity of the lesional cortical and trabecular bone with that of the underlying normal bone. In the long bones, the mass typically projects in a direction opposite of the joint. Histologically, osteochondromas are composed of a covering layer of hyaline cartilage that resembles the normal epiphyseal plate which coats and merges into normal-appearing trabeculae of bone. Between the trabeculae, one may find normal cellular marrow or fat. The authors of this text have not personally witnessed an aspiration biopsy of an osteochondroma. Furthermore, they are unaware of a well-described reported example. One case was misdiagnosed as a chondroma in smears.[110]

Chondroma

Although chondromas are fairly common benign neoplasms of cartilage, only rarely are they examined by aspiration biopsies. These neoplasms arise most often in the tubular bones of the digits, especially the hands. Most patients are asymptomatic with the mass being discovered on an incidental radiograph. These neoplasms are centered in the medulla and radiographically present as an expansive mass that is sharply marginated. Within the mass, small calcifications may be seen.

Histologically, chondromas (enchondromas) are characterized by lobules of mature hyaline cartilage. The neoplastic chondrocytes are present within lacunae and possess solitary uniform and darkly stained nuclei. Binucleation is unexpected and mitotic figures should not be seen.

Only a few examples of FNA biopsy of chondromas have been seen by the authors of this text. Aspirates of these benign cartilaginous neoplasms have occasionally been reported.[110,112,116,117] The smears are dominated by masses of normal-appearing hyaline cartilage (Figure 28-58). These fragments, which have sharply defined edges, appear bluish purple with the Romanowsky stains and eosinophilic with the Pap stain. The cartilaginous matrix may be so thick as to obscure the cytologic detail of the few neoplastic chondrocytes that are present. In thinner portions of the fragments, the chondrocytes are found within lacunar spaces. The cells have a single, small, often perfectly round nucleus with hyperchromatic chromatin, an inconspicuous nucleolus, and scanty or nondiscernable cytoplasm. The lacunar spaces appear as sharply punched-out circles that are unstained. The smears show only rare individually dispersed chondrocytes, infrequent binucleated chondrocytes (or two cells within the same lacunar space) and no mitotic figures.

Chondroblastoma

Chondroblastomas are benign cartilage-producing neoplasms that typically occur in patients in the second decade of life. Males are affected more often than are females. The most common sites include the distal femur, proximal tibia, and proximal humerus. Radiographically, these present as lytic lesions that are sharply delineated by a sclerotic margin. In some instances, punctate calcifications can also be seen within the mass. The young age of the patient and the epiphyseal location are key clinical factors that should suggest the possibility of chondroblastoma.

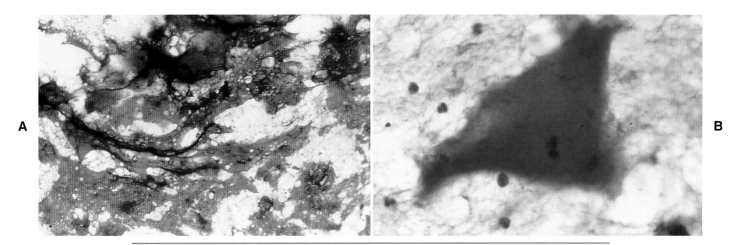

Figure 28-58 Enchondroma. **A** and **B,** Smears are dominated by fragments of cartilage that have well-defined peripheral borders and appear rather homogeneous. In **A,** neoplastic chondrocytes are not evident; however, the lacunar spaces in which they reside persist. In **B,** rare tumor cells are characterized by small round nuclei with fine even moderately stained chromatin and inapparent nucleoli. Cytoplasm is also not obvious. (**A,** DQ; **B,** Pap)

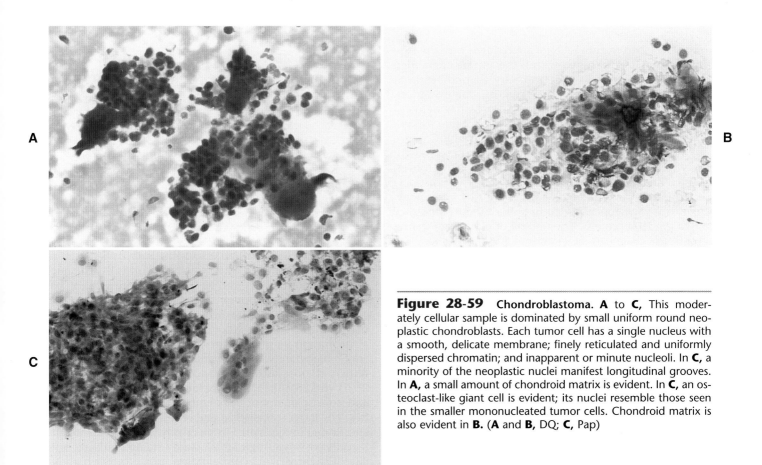

Figure 28-59 Chondroblastoma. **A** to **C,** This moderately cellular sample is dominated by small uniform round neoplastic chondroblasts. Each tumor cell has a single nucleus with a smooth, delicate membrane; finely reticulated and uniformly dispersed chromatin; and inapparent or minute nucleoli. In **C,** a minority of the neoplastic nuclei manifest longitudinal grooves. In **A,** a small amount of chondroid matrix is evident. In **C,** an osteoclast-like giant cell is evident; its nuclei resemble those seen in the smaller mononucleated tumor cells. Chondroid matrix is also evident in **B.** (**A** and **B,** DQ; **C,** Pap)

Histologically, the predominant neoplastic cell is a primitive chondroblast. Although these mononucleated cells are usually polygonal or spindle-shaped neoplastic elements may also be recognized. Scattered randomly throughout the proliferation of these small cells are two other elements. The first of these are multinucleated osteoclast-like giant cells. The second consists of small foci of chondroid material. Neoplastic cells may be present within this fibrochondroid matrix.

Aspiration biopsies of chondroblastomas typically yield highly cellular smears.[116,118,119] These smears are dominated by homogeneous, polygonal to round neoplastic chondroblasts that are scattered individually and in loose clusters (Figures 28-59 and 28-60). Each cell possesses a solitary nucleus with a delicate membrane, fine even chromatin, and inconspicuous nucleoli. Characteristically, a proportion of the neoplastic cells demonstrates longitudinal nu-

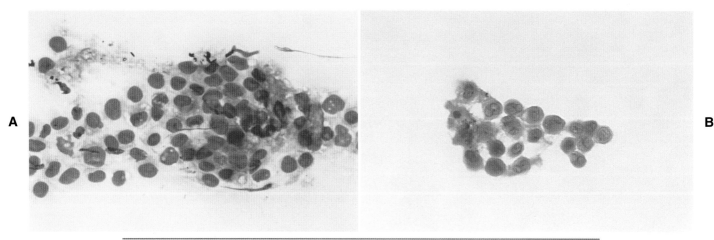

A   B

Figure 28-60   Chondroblastoma. **A** and **B,** A monotonous population of mononucleated chondroblasts dominate this sample. Nuclear membranes are generally smooth, the chromatin is very finely reticulated, and nucleoli are generally inconspicuous. Cytoplasm is scanty, resulting in relatively high N:C ratios in these rounded tumor cells. Rare nuclear grooves are evident. (**A,** DQ; **B,** Pap)

clear grooves; this feature is better appreciated with the Pap-stained material. Also noted within the smears are benign osteoclast-like giant cells that will vary in number from scanty to numerous (see Figure 28-59). In some instances, within the smears, rather sharply delineated fragments of chondroid matrix may also be found (see Figure 28-59). Inconspicuous cytoplasm results in high N:C ratios.

Because of the large number of small neoplastic cells with solitary nuclei, at times demonstrating prominent grooves, the differential diagnosis includes Langerhans' cell histiocytosis (eosinophilic granuloma). Furthermore, by immunocytochemistry, the neoplastic cells in both of these entities are positive for S100 protein. The finding of chondroid matrix supports the diagnosis of chondroblastoma, whereas the presence of numerous inflammatory elements, especially eosinophils, would support histiocytosis (Box 28-7).

Chondromyxoid Fibroma

This benign neoplasm occurs most commonly in the second and third decades with a slight male predominance. The proximal tibia is the most commonly involved site, but this neoplasm may involve many different bones of the body. By far, the most common clinical presentation is pain localized in the region of the neoplasm. Radiographically, the tumor has an eccentric location within the metaphysis. It demonstrates well-defined sclerotic margins that often have a scalloped appearance. Histologically, the neoplasm demonstrates a well-developed lobular growth pattern. These lobules consist of chondromyxoid matrix that varies somewhat in appearance. It may appear primarily as a loose myxoid tissue, a denser material, or even as hyaline cartilage. Within each lobule, a distinct gradient of cellularity is evident with the greatest concentration of tumor cells at the periphery. The neoplastic elements are generally small and homogeneous with stellate or spindled contours. Less frequently, they have more rounded shapes. The peripheral portions of the lobules are juxtaposed to a more richly cellular fibroblastic tissue that contains elongated mesenchy-

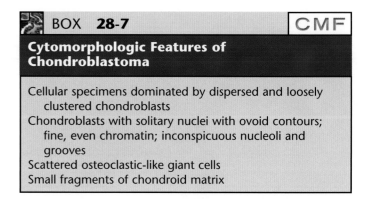

BOX 28-7   **CMF**

Cytomorphologic Features of Chondroblastoma

Cellular specimens dominated by dispersed and loosely clustered chondroblasts
Chondroblasts with solitary nuclei with ovoid contours; fine, even chromatin; inconspicuous nucleoli and grooves
Scattered osteoclastic-like giant cells
Small fragments of chondroid matrix

mal cells and scattered osteoclast-like giant cells. The nuclei of the neoplastic cells, for the most part, are solitary, have round to ovoid contours; smooth membranes; fine, dark chromatin; and minute nucleoli. Occasional tumor cells may manifest nuclear grooves.

Aspiration biopsies of chondromyxoid fibromas are generally moderately cellular and include both individually dispersed neoplastic cells and tumor fragments (Figures 28-61 and 28-62).[105,120,121] The latter vary from small to large and consist of tumor cells embedded within myxoid matrix. The latter stains green and reddish-purple with the Pap and Romanowsky stains, respectively. Most of the neoplastic cells possess a single small, darkly stained nucleus; a stellate or slightly ovoid configuration; and a rather high N:C ratio. At the edges of these fragments, somewhat larger spindled fibroblasts and osteoclast-like multinucleated cells may be present. The latter may also be individually dispersed within the smears. The authors have seen an example in which a large proportion of the aspirated tumor cells had round to polygonal contours, solitary round nuclei, and frequent nuclear grooves, simulating the tumor cells of chondroblastoma (see Figure 28-62). A recent case report describes a chondrosarcoma misdiagnosed as a chondromyxoid fibroma[122] (Box 28-8).

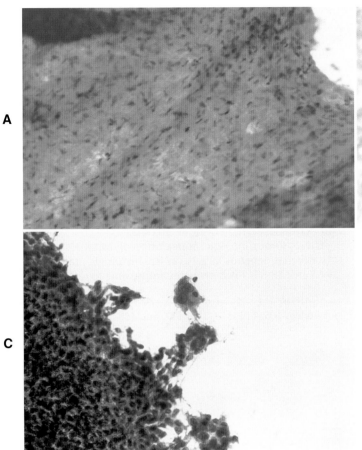

A

C

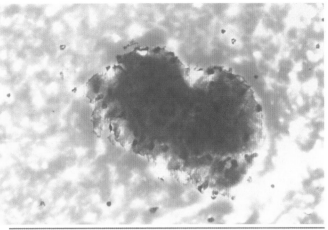

B

Figure 28-61 **Chondromyxoid fibroma. A,** This moderately cellular smear is dominated by small uniform neoplastic cells with solitary ovoid to elongated nuclei that are fairly darkly stained and evenly distributed within pale cyanophilic matrix material. Cytoplasm is indistinguishable because it appears to blend with the adjacent myxoid matrix material. No evidence of anaplasia or pleomorphism is found. **B,** This fragment of cellular matrix has sharply defined smooth edges and is composed of homogeneous metachromatic material. The neoplastic cells are uniform in appearance with solitary ovoid and darkly stained nuclei. Again, their cytoplasm is inapparent. **C,** At the periphery of one of these rather cellular fragments, individual cells are more readily apparent. They have solitary ovoid nuclei with rather smooth contours; fine, even chromatin; and inconspicuous nucleoli. Note the presence of multinucleated osteoclastic cells. (**A** and **C,** Pap; **B,** DQ)

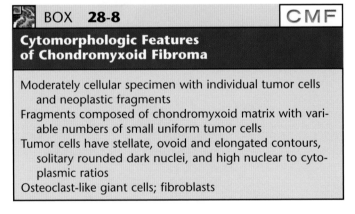

| BOX 28-8 | CMF |

Cytomorphologic Features of Chondromyxoid Fibroma

Moderately cellular specimen with individual tumor cells and neoplastic fragments

Fragments composed of chondromyxoid matrix with variable numbers of small uniform tumor cells

Tumor cells have stellate, ovoid and elongated contours, solitary rounded dark nuclei, and high nuclear to cytoplasmic ratios

Osteoclast-like giant cells; fibroblasts

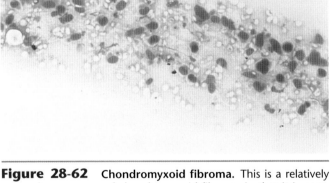

Figure 28-62 **Chondromyxoid fibroma.** This is a relatively unusual appearance of chondromyxoid fibroma in that it is composed of individually dispersed small neoplastic cells. They have polygonal contours with solitary round and bland nuclei and scanty eccentrically located basophilic cytoplasm. Some of the cells have longitudinal nuclear grooves. (DQ)

Chondrosarcoma

Chondrosarcomas are primary malignant neoplasms in which the neoplastic cells produce chondroid matrix but do not produce osteoid. Although young adults may be affected by conventional chondrosarcomas, most patients are adults who are between the ages of 30 and 60 years. Men are affected more often than are women. The single most common involved site is the acetabulum. The majority of these malignancies arise in the proximal femur, proximal humerus, and the central trunk bones. The most common symptom is pain localized to the region of the neoplasm. In some, but not all, patients a mass may be palpable with associated tenderness. Radiographically, these tumors affect the diaphysis or metaphysis of the involved bone as a de-

structive lesion that breaks through the cortical bone and extends into the adjacent soft tissue. The majority of these show splotchy calcifications.

The histologic appearance of chondrosarcomas is quite variable. Among the conventional chondrosarcomas, histologic grading is of prognostic importance. Patients with low-grade chondrosarcomas tend to fare well, whereas

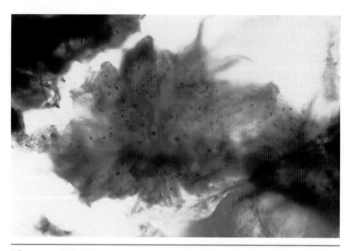

Figure 28-63   **Grade I chondrosarcoma.** This smear is dominated by fragments of poorly cellular chondroid matrix material that contains tumor cells present within distinct lacunae. Some of the chondrocytes have small uniform darkly stained nuclei without evidence of anaplasia. Note the sharply demarcated edges to the fragment and the lack of individually dispersed tumor cells. (Pap)

those with high-grade neoplasms often succumb to their malignancy. At low magnification, these neoplasms typically demonstrate voluminous chondroid matrix. Tumor cellularity varies tremendously, but overall, the cellularity is certainly higher than one would expect with chondromas. In general, the histologic grade correlates with the degree of cellularity, cellular pleomorphism and mitotic activity. The neoplastic cells characteristically possess a solitary and often centrally positioned round nucleus. The latter has a variably regular membrane, finely to coarsely granular and hyperchromatic chromatin, and at times, nucleoli. Not infrequently, binucleation of the neoplastic cells is present. Overall, markedly pleomorphic tumor cells are not expected in conventional chondrosarcomas. Clinical and histologic variants include mesenchymal, clear cell, myxoid, and dedifferentiated chondrosarcomas.

The cytomorphologic appearance of aspirates of chondrosarcomas depends largely on the histologic grade (Figures 28-63 and 28-64).* It is probably impossible to distinguish re-

*References 105, 110, 113, 116, 117, and 123.

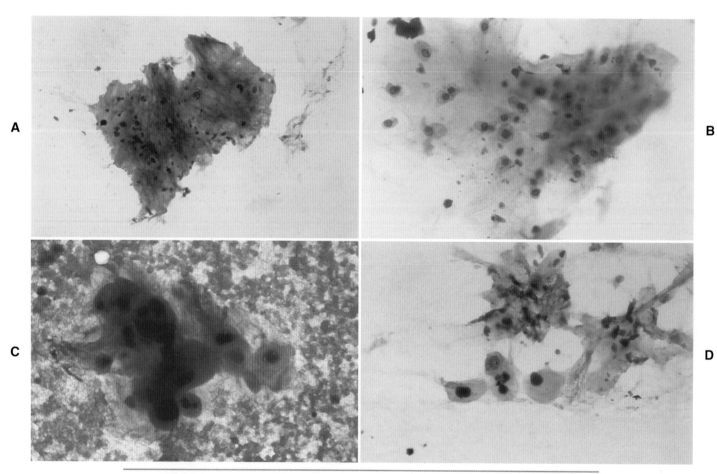

Figure 28-64   **Grade II chondrosarcoma. A,** This fragment of chondrosarcoma somewhat resembles that seen in Figure 28-63. However, it contains a greater number of malignant cells that demonstrate moderate nuclear pleomorphism. In addition, even at this low magnification, hyperchromasia is apparent. **B,** In addition to dense matrix, paler and looser myxoid matrix material is also evident in the smear associated with malignant chondrocytes. The latter typically have a solitary round nucleus with a thick membrane, evenly dispersed chromatin that varies in staining intensity, and an occasional small nucleolus. The cells have ovoid to round contours and have distinct cell borders (when individually dispersed) and pale cyanophilic cytoplasm. **C** and **D,** Among the neoplastic chondrocytes, an occasional binucleated tumor cell is evident. Again, note the variability in nuclear diameters and the hyperchromasia. (**A, B,** and **D,** Pap; **C,** DQ)

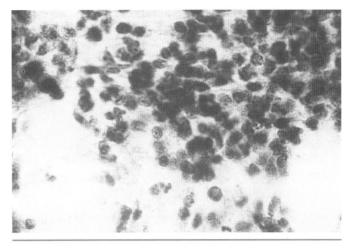

Figure 28-65 **Mesenchymal chondrosarcoma.** The poorly differentiated chondroblasts are characterized by small round or ovoid nuclei with hyperchromatic chromatin, inapparent nucleoli, and very scanty cytoplasm. The latter results in high N:C ratios. No evidence of specific differentiation is found. (Pap)

liably between a chondroma and a grade I chondrosarcoma solely on the basis of the aspiration cytomorphology (see Figure 28-63). One must incorporate clinical and radiographic data to achieve the correct diagnosis in this specific setting, and even then it may not be possible to be absolutely certain.[124] This is because the cellularity within the chondroid matrix of grade I neoplasms is relatively low and overlaps with that of a benign chondroma. These smears contain fragments of poorly cellular dense chondroid matrix and at times a less dense myxoid matrix material. In low-grade chondrosarcomas, the majority of the aspirated tumor cells may be present within lacunae in the fragments of cartilaginous matrix. In higher-grade chondrosarcomas, a much greater proportion of the cells is individually dispersed. Compared with osteosarcomas, the neoplastic cells in conventional chondrosarcomas are much more homogeneous in appearance. They are characterized by a large size, rounded contours often with well-defined cellular borders, one or two round nuclei, and moderate volumes of pale eosinophilic cytoplasm. The nuclei are often centrally located within the cytoplasm, again in contrast with the eccentric location of osteoblasts in osteosarcoma (Box 28-9).

Several morphologic and clinical variants of chondrosarcoma exist. One of these is the mesenchymal chondrosarcoma, which may also arise as a primary soft tissue malignancy. Mesenchymal chondrosarcoma of bone typically affects the central axial skeleton in patients who are younger than those developing conventional chondrosarcomas. Localized pain and a palpable mass are the major clinical features. Although the radiographic presentation points to a malignant neoplasm, no specific attributes are noted. A distinct biphasic histologic appearance is characteristic. The two components are mature-appearing cartilaginous areas and primitive, highly cellular, small round cell foci. The former consist of islands resembling hyaline cartilage, which vary both in contour and diameters and are surrounded by the second component, namely primitive chondroblasts. The latter cell type basically resembles other round small cell malignant neoplasms in that the neoplastic elements possess solitary round to ovoid, hyperchromatic nuclei and high N:C ratios.

The aspiration biopsy features of mesenchymal chondrosarcoma have only rarely been reported.[116] The primitive chondroblasts occupy most of the area of the highly cellu-

lar specimens (Figures 28-65 and 28-66). These neoplastic cells are characterized by solitary round nuclei with generally smooth contours, finely granular evenly dispersed and darkly stained chromatin, and scanty or inconspicuous cytoplasm. Nucleoli are generally not evident. These smears may also contain small fragments or islands of tumor showing definite cartilaginous differentiation. The latter is characterized by dense homogeneous matrix material that appears metachromatic with the Romanowsky stains. Within this matrix, relatively small and uniform chondrocytes are noted within distinct lacunae.

A much more common occurrence is the dedifferentiated chondrosarcoma. This consists of a neoplasm that is also biphasic.[105,125] The same can be said for the radiographic presentation that is composed of a mass typical of chondrosarcoma juxtaposed to a large radiolucent area, typically with production of a large soft tissue mass. One of the two major histologic components consists of a generally low-grade chondrosarcoma; the second population consists of an undifferentiated sarcoma that resembles either an MFH or a fibrosarcoma. At times, the sarcomatous elements may show foci of osteoid production. It is anticipated that the aspiration smears of a dedifferentiated chondrosarcoma contain solely the high-grade pleomorphic sarcomatous elements. Thus, a specific diagnosis of dedifferentiated chondrosarcoma is unlikely unless the aspiration specimen also yields definite chondrosarcomatous elements (Figure 28-67).

A rare neoplasm, the clear cell chondrosarcoma, typically occurs in patients who are younger than those with conventional chondrosarcoma. These neoplasms characteristically arise in or near the epiphysis of the long bones, especially the femur and humerus. Histologically, these neoplasms may show large variability from field to field microscopically. The most characteristic component is relatively large neoplastic cells that have solitary central nuclei and moderate to abundant cytoplasm that is optically clear. The nuclei have round or ovoid contours with smooth, delicate membranes; fine, evenly distributed and often pale-stained chromatin; and inconspicuous nucleoli. Cell borders are characteristically well defined. Elsewhere in the mass, distinct chondroid differentiation with dense matrix and tumor cells within lacunar spaces are evident. In addition, multinucleated giant cells may be present. As described by Walaas and colleagues, clear cell chondrosarcoma presents in smears as epithelial-like cells with distinct cell borders, abundant finely vacuolated cytoplasm, and generally a single central nucleus (Figure 28-68).[116] The latter may or may not be darkly stained.

Before leaving cartilaginous lesions, a rare primary proliferation needs to be mentioned. It is the infantile cartilaginous hamartoma of the rib that often presents in newborns or at least in young infants with a combination of respiratory difficulties associated with a chest wall mass. Recently, Rao and colleagues have reported the first instance of this hamartoma in an aspiration biopsy.[126] The authors warned that the highly cellular smears composed of primitive chondroblasts could mislead one into rendering a false-positive malignant diagnosis.

Ewing's Sarcoma

Although Ewing's sarcoma/primitive neuroectodermal tumor may present as a primary soft tissue tumor, it is much more commonly considered a primary neoplasm of bone.

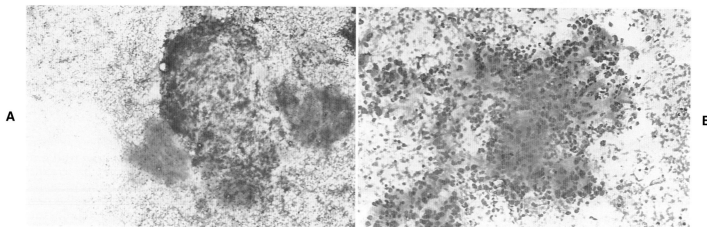

Figure 28-66 Mesenchymal chondrosarcoma. **A,** In this scanning lens view, most of the aspirate consists of loose clusters of individual primitive chondroblasts, as seen in Figure 28-65. Adjacent to them is a fragment of poorly cellular chondroid matrix in which lacunae but not neoplastic cells are readily apparent. **B,** A rather cellular fragment of chondroid matrix is present in this field. It is characterized by cells with small round homogeneous nuclei embedded within dense homogeneous chondroid matrix material. At the periphery, primitive tumor cells are also evident. (DQ)

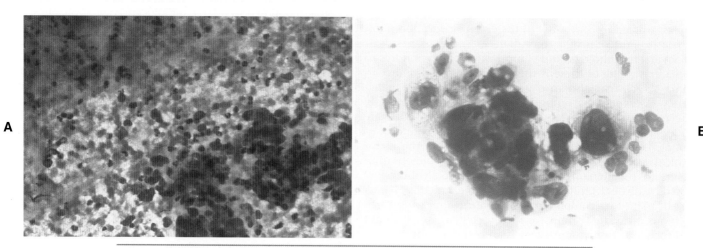

Figure 28-67 Dedifferentiated chondrosarcoma. **A,** In one corner of this field is a fragment of low-grade chondrosarcoma. It is characterized by cartilaginous matrix containing small, rather uniform-appearing cells with ovoid darkly stained nuclei. The remainder of this field is occupied by highly anaplastic malignant cells with large irregular and multiple nuclei, some of which contain prominent nucleoli. The latter represent the dedifferentiated portion of the neoplasm, which actually dominated this smear. **B,** The highly anaplastic component of this neoplasm consists of cells with huge nuclei, darkly stained chromatin, prominent nucleoli, and variable volumes of cytoplasm. No distinct chondrocytic differentiation was evident among this high-grade component. (DQ)

This tumor occurs most often in the second decade of life, affects males and females to a relatively equal extent, and is quite rare in the African-American population. Pain, localized to the region of the tumor, is the typical initial presentation. It is usually clinically associated with a palpable mass that is often tender. Not infrequently, fever is an accompanying symptom. This tumor characteristically involves the diaphysis of long bones, especially those of the lower extremities, and the pelvic bones. However, essentially any bone may be involved. Radiographically, a large lytic or sclerotic destructive lesion that is poorly delineated and associated with soft tissue extension is typical. Well-developed periosteal osteoneogenesis is characteristic.

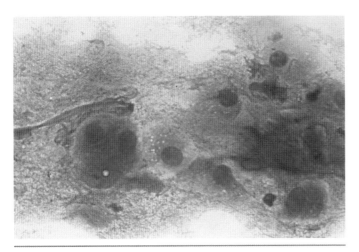

Figure 28-68 Clear cell chondrosarcoma. The neoplastic cells are relatively uniform and characterized by polygonal contours, abundant faintly basophilic and focally vacuolated cytoplasm, and solitary rounded nuclei. The latter have delicate membranes, fine even chromatin, and small nucleoli. Cell borders are distinct, although the cells are present within matrix material. (DQ)

Histologically, the neoplasm shows no specific differentiation. It is composed of small primitive cells with solitary round, hyperchromatic nuclei, inconspicuous nucleoli, and extremely high N:C ratios. Large areas of necrosis may be seen with only a thin collar of viable-appearing tumor cells situated immediately about blood vessels. Although an organoid arrangement of the cells is uncommon, pseudorosette-like structures may be seen.

Aspirates of Ewing's sarcoma/primitive neuroectodermal tumor present a much more homogeneous cytomorphologic picture (Figures 28-69 to 28-71; see Figure 28-44). Aspiration biopsies consistently yield high cellularity with numerous solitary mononucleated neoplastic cells.[105,127-129] The nuclei appear perfectly round with uniformly dispersed fine chromatin and inconspicuous nucleoli. For the most part, the N:C ratios are extremely high. Occasionally, cytoplasmic blebs or sharply "punched-out" glycogen vacuoles may be seen. Within cohesive monolayers of neoplastic cells, pseudorosettes may be evident. The smear background does not demonstrate matrix material or lymphoglandular bodies.

The differential diagnosis of Ewing's sarcoma in aspiration smears includes metastatic neuroblastoma, malignant lymphoma, small cell osteosarcoma, and mesenchymal chondrosarcoma. With the exception of mesenchymal chondrosarcoma, which may also be positive for CD99, immunocytochemistry should prove quite useful in this setting.[130] In addition, cytogenetic analysis of aspirated tumor cells may also prove quite beneficial by demonstrating the specific 11;22 reciprocal translocation.[131,132]

Plasmacytoma (Myeloma)

A fairly common primary neoplasm is the malignant plasmacytoma that typically occurs in middle-age or older adults. This is not a neoplasm expected in young individuals. Clearly, pain is the most common symptom at the time

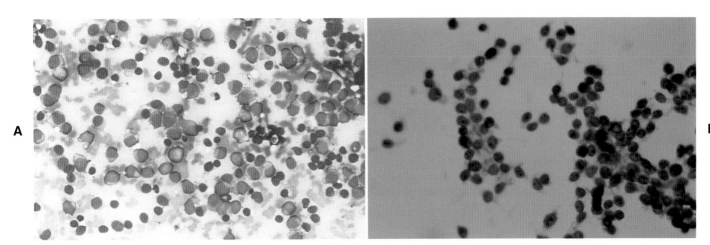

A   B

Figure 28-69 Ewing's sarcoma. **A,** This highly cellular aspirate is composed of monotonous-appearing tumor cells which are individually dispersed or present in small loose clusters. They have solitary round nuclei with finely reticulated, evenly dispersed chromatin and a distinct absence of nucleoli. Most cells possess only a scanty rim of cytoplasm and hence have high N:C ratios. The smaller cells in the background presumably represent degenerated malignant elements. **B,** The uniformity of the malignant cells is even more striking with alcohol fixation. In addition, the nuclear hyperchromasia is more apparent, as is the lack of nucleoli. Note the presence of true intercellular cohesion and lack of lymphoglandular bodies in the background. (**A,** DQ; **B,** Pap)

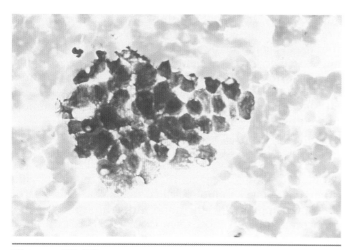

Figure 28-70 Ewing's sarcoma. Within the tumor fragment, the homogeneity of the malignant cells is readily apparent. A few possess sharply punched out cytoplasmic glycogen vacuoles. Again, note the smooth nuclear chromatin and the lack of nucleoli. (DQ)

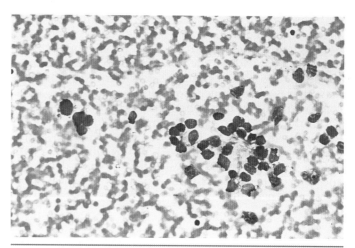

Figure 28-71 Ewing's sarcoma. Occasional pseudorosette-like structures may be evident in aspirates of this sarcoma. They are characterized by tumor cells in which the nuclei are peripherally oriented and surround central cytoplasm. This may be evidence of their primitive neuroectodermal derivation. (DQ)

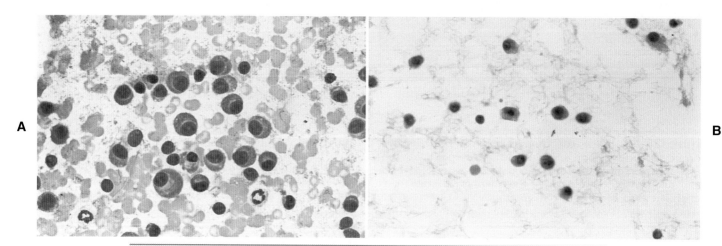

A

B

Figure 28-72 Plasmacytoma. **A** and **B,** Individually dispersed neoplastic plasma cells are essentially the only nucleated cells present in the smear. The cells are characterized generally by a single round nucleus that is eccentrically positioned within the cytoplasm. The chromatin is coarsely clumped. As seen in **A,** the cytoplasm is moderate to voluminous in amount, is basophilic, and has a distinct perinuclear clear zone. Such well-developed plasmacytic attributes are not as apparent with alcohol-fixed material as seen in **B.** Still, the plasmacytic nature of the malignant cells is evident. (**A,** DQ; **B,** Pap)

of initial diagnosis; if an abrupt initiation of pain occurs, this is usually related to a pathologic fracture. Typical laboratory findings include hypergammaglobulinemia, a monoclonal gammapathy, anemia, and hypercalcemia. The radiographic appearance is quite characteristic. Usually, one or more bones will show multiple well-delineated small lytic masses. The bones most commonly affected include the vertebrae, the skull, ribs, and those of the pelvic region.

If the tumor extends into the soft tissue or only a very thin layer of cortical bone persists, aspiration smears are highly cellular (Figures 28-72 to 28-74). For the most part, smears consist of individually dispersed plasma cells which vary tremendously in their degree of differentiation.[105,133,134] In some cases, almost all the malignant elements resemble normal plasma cells, whereas in other examples, marked

pleomorphism including tumor giant cells, multinucleation, and massive nucleoli are present. The typical cell possesses a single round nucleus that is peripherally located within moderate volumes of basophilic cytoplasm. With the Romanowsky preparations, a perinuclear "clear zone" may be evident. Although a single nucleus is typical, most aspirates show some cells with binucleation and multinucleation. Although a lack of cohesion among neoplastic cells is expected, a number of examples have been seen in which "pseudocohesion" among neoplastic cells is present as variably cohesive clusters of malignant plasma cells (see Figure 28-74). In the series by Wedin and colleagues, FNA biopsy of bony lesions was performed in 16 patients with myeloma.[134] The correct diagnosis was rendered in 15; in one patient, the aspirate yielded only necrotic neoplastic cells.

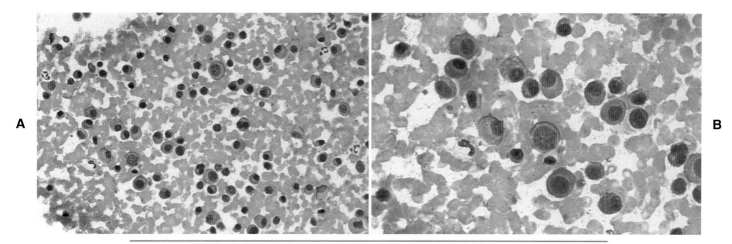

Figure 28-73 **Plasmacytoma. A** and **B,** Similar to Figure 28-72, the smear is dominated by isolated malignant plasma cells. Although many of the cells demonstrate typical plasmacytic attributes, others are less differentiated. They are characterized by greater N:C ratios, binucleation, and more primitive chromatin with prominent nucleoli.

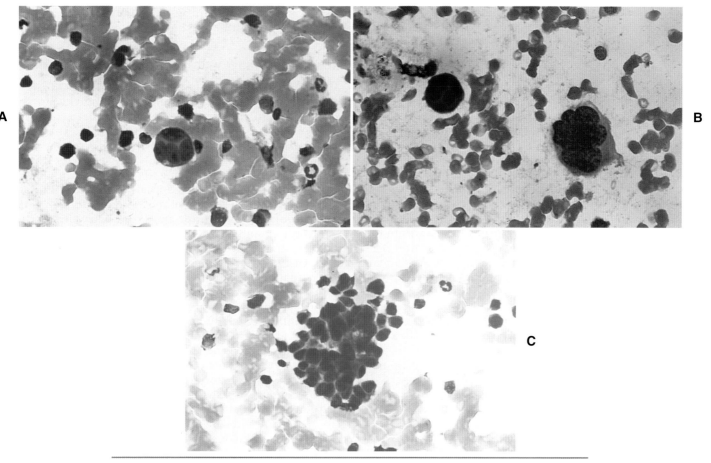

Figure 28-74 **Anaplastic plasmacytoma. A** to **C,** Although a minority of the neoplastic cells are clearly plasmacytic in nature, the spectrum of cellular appearances is striking. This includes the presence of multinucleated tumor cells with high N:C ratios and macronucleoli. In **C,** an area of pseudocohesion is evident. Although such foci may suggest an epithelial neoplasm, when the entire smear is examined, the hematopoietic, particularly the plasmacytic, nature is usually readily apparent. (DQ)

Chordoma

Chordomas typically present in middle-age or older individuals with a definite male predominance. The bones that are involved include the sacrum, clivus, and vertebrae. This central skeletal location reflects the presumed origin of these neoplasms in the notochord. Pain is the characteristic mode of presentation because of tumor entrapment of large nerves in the region of the tumor. For example, the spheno-occipital neoplasms most commonly affect the sixth cranial nerve. Neoplasms arising in the sacrum typically produce a presacral mass that may be palpable on a rectal examination. Radiographically, a lytic and calcified mass destroys the involved bone with extension into the adjacent soft tissue. Histologically, chordomas are characterized by a lobulated appearance. The lobules consist of neoplastic cells and matrix material. The latter has a myxoid or mucoid appearance. Epithelioid attributes characterize the neoplastic cells. The cells are typically present in linear arrays or cords but may also be individually dispersed and present in sheets. In some cases, especially in recurrent chordoma, a pleomorphic sarcomatoid component is evident. The neoplastic cells have moderate to voluminous eosinophilic cytoplasm that is variably vacuolated. Some neoplastic cells contain multiple large vacuoles that may indent the nucleus; these create the classic physaliferous tumor cell.

Aspiration biopsies are generally moderately cellular and dominated by the neoplastic cells.[36,105,108,110] The latter are characterized by one or at times more nuclei and voluminous cytoplasm that may appear dense, eosinophilic, and homogenous, or variably vacuolated (see Figures 28-12 and 28-13). The diameters of the vacuoles are also quite variable even within the same cell. The nuclei are generally round with a distinct membrane, variably stained and finely granular chromatin, and small but distinct nucleoli. Cellular borders are variably well defined. The tumor cells may be individually dispersed, present in sheets, or linear strands. In addition, variable amounts of matrix material may also be evident. The latter varies from dense and homogeneous to a fine granular film. In contrast with the myxoid sarcomas, the neoplastic cells are typically not located within the fragments of matrix. By immunocytochemistry, the neoplastic cells are positive for cytokeratin, epithelial membrane antigen, and S100 protein. They are negative for carcinoembryonic antigen. As with all other primary and secondary bone tumors, correlation with the clinical and radiographic features is essential to achieving the correct diagnosis. Knowing that a patient is an older adult with a central lesion in either the sacrum or the spheno-occipital area helps make a specific diagnosis of chordoma when presented with the expected aspiration cytomorphology.

Giant Cell Tumor

As with many other neoplasms of bone, pain often associated with a palpable mass lesion are the major features of the clinical presentation. Although patients of almost any age may be involved, it is uncommon in the second decade of life and almost unheard of in the first. The bones that are most commonly affected, in descending order of frequency, are the femur (distal), tibia (proximal), radius (distal), and sacrum. Radiographically, these neoplasms are centered in the epiphysis and are lytic in nature. The tumor typically does not induce either a periosteal reaction or peripheral sclerosis. Although giant cell tumor of bone is generally considered a benign entity, a minority of patients eventuate with metastases. Histologically, the neoplasms consist of an admixture of mononucleated and multinucleated neoplastic cells. The two cell types have similarly appearing nuclei that are round or ovoid with a delicate membrane, vesicular chromatin, and generally inconspicuous to small nucleoli. In contrast with many other bone lesions with multinucleated cells, two relatively distinctive features of giant cell tumor are evident. First, the absolute and relative numbers of the giant cells is markedly increased in this neoplasm. Secondly, the number of neoplastic nuclei per cell may be quite high, numbering 50 or more in some cells.

The aspiration cytomorphology reflects the underlying histopathology.[105,108109,135,136] Thus, the smears that are variably cellular and include both the mononucleated neoplastic cells and large numbers of multinucleated cells, some of which possess numerous nuclei (Figure 28-75). It is important to recognize that the nuclei in the two cell types resemble each other. The mononucleated cells have polygonal to ovoid to spindled contours. As in the histology, the nuclei have smooth membranes, finely granular, often pale-stained chromatin, and inconspicuous nucleoli. Matrix material is not evident in the smears.

Adamantinoma

Adamantinoma is a rare low-grade malignant neoplasm of bone which, although it may affect older individuals, usually presents in the first three to four decades of life. The vast majority of adamantinomas arise in the tibia. Occasionally, both the tibia and the fibula or the fibula alone are affected. Radiographically, the lesion presents as an eccentric lytic mass involving the diaphysis. The affected portion of the tibia or fibula appears expanded. Histologically, the dominant feature of most adamantinomas is the presence of sharply defined nests and aggregates and/or thin cords of epithelioid neoplastic cells. Typically, the tumor cells at the edges of the nests have a palisaded appearance. Occasional examples demonstrate distinct squamous differentiation. The epithelial nature of the cells is supported by positive immunostaining for cytokeratin. The strands and aggregates of epithelioid tumor cells are situated within a generally poorly cellular fibrous tissue with scattered fibroblasts. At higher magnification, the neoplastic cells have homogeneous and rather bland-appearing nuclei. The N:C ratios are often quite high. Only rarely have FNA biopsy of adamantinomas been reported.[105,108,137] The smears contain cohesive aggregates of uniform round to polygonal epithelial-like cells that have solitary nuclei. The latter have smooth, delicate membranes; finely granular chromatin; and inconspicuous nucleoli. Peripheral palisading may be evident in some of the sampled clusters. The smears also contain benign fibroblast-like cells. The major entity in the differential diagnosis is metastatic carcinoma. It is the bland nuclear features in conjunction with the relatively young age and the characteristic radiographic appearance that allows one to feel comfortable in distinguishing adamantinoma from the much more common metastatic carcinoma (Figure 28-76).

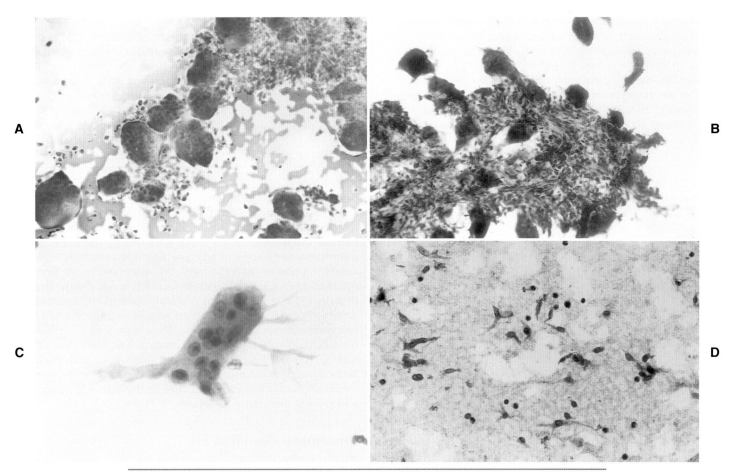

Figure 28-75 **Giant cell tumor. A** and **B,** Numerous massive giant cells dominate the fields that also include a large number of much smaller mononucleated neoplastic cells. Note that the nuclei in smaller neoplastic elements completely resemble those seen in the giant cells. Giant cell tumor should not be mistaken, on the one hand, for a sarcoma in that the nuclei appear bland and benign and no evidence of anaplasia is found. On the other hand, giant cell tumors should not be confused with granulomatous inflammation. In the latter, the number of giant cells is typically much fewer; these cells are generally smaller, and epithelioid histiocytes produce variably cohesive granulomas. **C,** The nuclei in this multinucleated tumor cell are strikingly uniform in appearance. They have slightly ovoid contours with delicate but distinct membranes; fine, pale chromatin; and minute nucleoli. They appear haphazardly arranged within the cytoplasm. **D,** When individually dispersed, the mononucleated neoplastic cells vary from round to elongated to stellate in contour. Their nuclei completely resemble those seen in the tumor giant cells. (**A,** DQ; **B** to **D,** Pap)

Langerhans' Cell Histiocytosis (Histiocytosis X)

Langerhans' cell histiocytosis occurs most commonly in the first decade of life with a progressive decline in incidence with increasing age. The bones of the skull are those that are most commonly involved, although essentially any bone may be affected. A distinct male predominance exists. Although variable, the characteristic radiographic presentation is that of a lytic mass centered in the medulla with sharply delineated margins. The disease may be multicentric at presentation. Histologically, a variable picture is also recognized. The neoplastic Langerhans' cells are present in small to large solid sheets and variably admixed with inflammatory elements including eosinophils, neutrophils, plasma cells, and multinucleated inflammatory giant cells. The most characteristic of these are the eosinophils that may be found in small collections. The neoplastic

Langerhans' cells are characterized by a solitary nucleus and a low N:C ratio resulting from voluminous eosinophilic cytoplasm. The nuclei have a characteristic appearance; they have a distinct nuclear membrane; pale, finely granulated chromati; inconspicuous nucleoli; and an indented configuration that may manifest as a characteristic longitudinal nuclear groove.

FNA biopsy of Langerhans' cell histiocytosis typically presents as highly cellular smears with large numbers of individually dispersed neoplastic cells (Figure 28-77).[105,138] With the Pap stain, the nuclear membrane is quite distinctive and often demonstrates the typical grooves. The chromatin is finely granular, evenly dispersed, and pale. Nucleoli are generally not evident. With alcohol-fixed preparations, cytoplasm is often barely visible. Conversely, nuclear attributes are less well recognized with the Romanowsky stains, but cytoplasm is more readily visualized. Smears also contain other inflammatory elements, notably eosinophilic leukocytes. In fact, the latter may be the initial clue to the appropriate diagnosis. However, we have seen several examples of aspirates of Langerhans' cell histiocytosis in which the smears contain almost pure populations of neoplastic cells. In this latter situation, the tumor cells may be difficult to distinguish, based purely on cytomorphology, from the neoplastic elements of chondroblastoma. With immunocytochemistry, the neoplastic cells in Langerhans' cell histiocytosis are positive for S100 protein and CD1a, whereas the cells of chondroblastoma are positive for the former and negative for the latter markers.

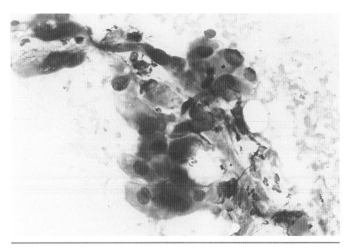

Figure 28-76 Adamantinoma. This was a relatively poorly cellular smear. However, the cells present were clearly malignant and appeared epithelial in quality. They had abundant, relatively dense cytoplasm; large solitary nuclei with prominent nucleoli; and relatively low N:C ratios. In some cells, the nuclei were centrally positioned, whereas in others they appeared at the periphery. (DQ)

Metastases

By far, the most common malignant neoplasm of bone is a metastasis, usually from a carcinoma. Although any cell type of carcinoma may spread to bone, the most common is adenocarcinoma. Primary neoplasms that metastasize with some frequency to bone include carcinomas of the lung, kidney, breast, and prostate.[108,134] In patients with a known primary neoplasm, it is important to review, if possible, the prior cytology or histology used to establish the initial diagnosis. Certain adenocarcinomas, especially those that are well differentiated, may show a characteristic cytomorphologic picture in smears allowing one to suggest a primary site in a patient without a prior diagnosis. Examples include renal cell adenocarcinoma, prostatic adenocarcinoma, follicular thyroid carcinoma, and ductal and lobular carcinomas of the breast. In some instances, immunocytochemistry can support the interpretation (cytokeratin, prostate specific antigen, prostatic acid phosphatase, thyroid transcription factor-1, gross cystic fluid protein-15, and E-cadherin). Several aspirates of metastatic renal cell carcinoma can simulate smears as a spindle cell or pleomorphic soft tissue sarcoma; these represent metastases from sarcomatoid renal cell carcinomas. The authors of this text agree with both Bommer and colleagues and Wedin and colleagues that aspiration biopsy is probably the most useful and cost-effective procedure in the initial workup of a suspected metastatic neoplasm.[108,134]

Unicameral (Simple) Cyst

Unicameral cysts are not true cysts in that they are not lined by epithelium. These benign, nonneoplastic lesions are discovered most often in the first two decades of life as asymptomatic lesions on incidental radiographs. They characteristically arise in the metaphysis, often against the epiphysis. They occur most often in the proximal humerus and proximal femur. Histologically, simple cysts are charac-

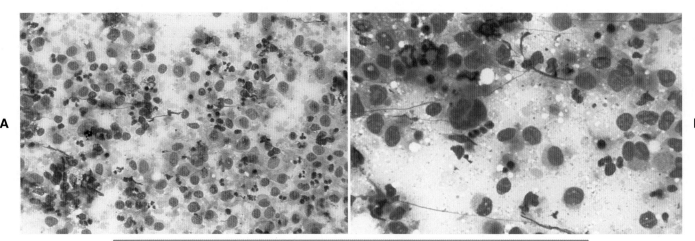

Figure 28-77 Langerhans' cell histiocytosis. A and **B,** Small, dispersed, uniform-appearing lesional cells dominate the smears. They are characterized by solitary ovoid nuclei with smooth contours; finely reticulated, uniformly dispersed chromatin; and inconspicuous nucleoli. The nuclei occasionally demonstrate well-developed longitudinal grooves. Also present are a sprinkling of eosinophilic leukocytes, as recognized by their bilobed nuclei, and scattered, multinucleated, osteoclast-like cells. The proliferating histiocytic elements have scant to moderate volumes of nonvacuolated, eosinophilic, and poorly defined cytoplasm. (DQ)

terized by fibrous connective tissue that may contain foci of multinucleated inflammatory giant cells, blood, fibroblastic proliferation, and other features that are essentially indistinguishable from those of an aneurysmal bone cyst. Aspiration biopsy of a unicameral cyst typically yields yellow, clear, or blood-tinged fluid. Even with concentration techniques, the specimens are so poorly cellular that the smears may be considered inadequate for diagnosis. However, in the proper clinical and radiographic setting, the gross and cytomorphologic presentation may be considered diagnostic of unicameral cyst.

Aneurysmal Bone Cyst

Similar to the unicameral cysts, aneurysmal cysts occur most often in the first two decades of life but can also be seen (although infrequently) in much older individuals.

The vertebral bones are most commonly involved by these lesions, followed by long bones of the lower extremity; however, in the authors' experience, it is the latter sites from which most aspirates of aneurysmal cysts have been seen. Clinically, pain is a common finding at the time of initial diagnosis. Radiographically, a lytic expansion of the affected bone involves the metaphysis and the dorsal portion of the vertebrae surrounded by a rim of sclerotic bone. The major histologic feature at low magnification consists of large cystic blood-filled spaces. The walls of these cysts contain an admixture of multinucleated inflammatory giant cells, fibroblasts, histiocytes, and possibly delicate trabeculae of bone.

FNA biopsy typically presents as a bloody fluid.[105,112] On the initial smears, the specimen may appear completely acellular or contain only rare individually dispersed benign mesenchymal cells (Figure 28-78). Concentration tech-

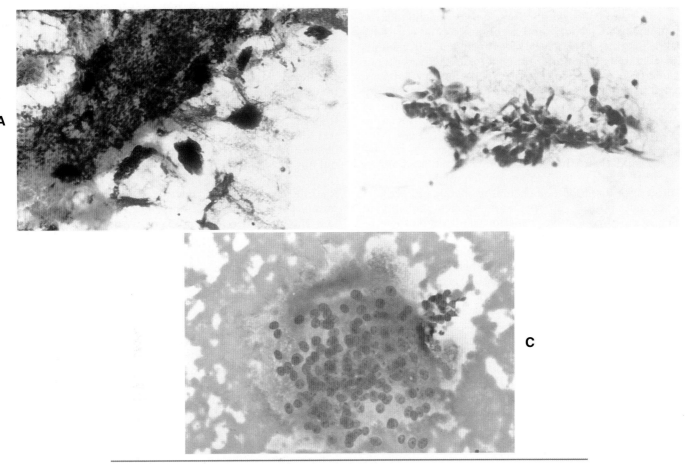

Figure 28-78 **Aneurysmal bone cyst. A,** This relatively cellular field demonstrates a fibrous septum that was captured by the needle. It consists of collagenous stroma that contains numerous benign spindle-shaped cells, presumably fibroblasts, and histiocytes. In addition, note the giant cells that coat the external surface of this septum. They have multiple nuclei and abundant dense cytoplasm. The background contains abundant blood. **B,** The individual fibroblasts are characterized by solitary elongated nuclei with delicate membranes; pale chromatin; inconspicuous nucleoli; and long, tapering cytoplasmic tails. The histiocytes have more round or ovoid nuclei with round or polygonal cellular contours and scant to moderate volumes of cytoplasm. No evidence of malignancy is found. **C,** The giant cells that may be sampled from these cysts may completely resemble those seen in giant cell tumors of bone—that is, they have voluminous generally nonvacuolated cytoplasm that may contain 40 or more nuclei. The latter are strikingly homogeneous in appearance with ovoid contours; smooth, delicate membranes; fine chromatin; and inconspicuous nucleoli. (**A** and **B,** Pap; **C,** DQ)

niques (e.g., cytocentrification), however, may yield cells derived from the septae of the aneurysmal cyst. Therefore, dispersed or loosely clustered spindle-shaped fibroblasts; histiocytes, the cytoplasm of which may contain hemosiderin granules; and multinucleated inflammatory giant cells may be found, along with collagen and possibly bone.

Accuracy

Compared with soft tissue neoplasms, it is more difficult to gauge the accuracy of aspirates of osseous preparations for several reasons. First, only a few large series have adequately addressed this question. Reflecting the real world to an extent, some series are heavily weighted to metastatic disease, whereas other studies from large referral centers concentrate on primary bone lesions. Additionally, some published studies do not include insufficient specimens in their statistical calculations. Another factor affecting accuracy is that primary neoplasms of bone, especially sarcomas, are even more rare than soft tissue tumors.

The single best discussion of accuracy may be the report of Layfield and colleagues.[112] These authors openly discuss the problems of accuracy and keenly review the earlier literature on this topic. Their series included 101 patients with primary bone lesions. Although many authors do not include their insufficient samples in the overall statistics, Layfield is more representative of daily practice as they include such information.[112] Their overall accuracy for the series was 62%, with a much higher level of diagnostic accuracy for malignant rather than benign lesions of bone (86% versus 41%). Seven patients potentially had an adverse outcome secondary to the cytologic interpretation. Cancers were misclassified in five of these, which might lead to the institution of inappropriate chemotherapeutic protocols. A solitary false-positive interpretation resulted probably in unnecessary preoperative radiation and chemotherapy. Granulomatous inflammation was not immediately recognized in the smears of a single patient, and thus, a delay occurred in the institution of antibiotic therapy.

Kreicbergs and colleagues evaluated accuracy prospectively in a series of 300 patients with bone lesions that had not been previously biopsied.[139] Cellular material sufficient to provide a diagnosis was obtained of 251 patients. Of these, the diagnosis of benign vs. malignant was accurate in 239 (95%). The false-positive and false-negative rates were 0.3% and 3%, respectively. Fortunately, no significant therapeutic problems related to these errors. The authors found the greatest difficulty in the diagnosis of chondrosarcomas. In the 49 patients in whom the diagnosis could not be rendered, 24 were the result of insufficient smear cellularity, and 25 aspirates had sufficient cellularity. The pathologists, however, were not able to provide an accurate diagnosis; most of the latter were associated with benign lesions.

Agarwal reported 69 patients with aspirates of primary lesions of bone.[109] No false-positive interpretations were in this series. Of the specimens, 83% were in complete agreement with the subsequent histologic diagnosis. The remaining 17 were insufficient because of poorly cellular samples. Also from India, Kumar and colleagues reported on FNA biopsy from 79 patients.[140] Again, no false-positive interpretations were noted. Subsequent examination of the bone lesion occurred in 37 patients. The cytologic diagnosis showed an accuracy rate of 94% in this subset. From China, Peng reported 53 patients, all but two of whom had

primary neoplasms of bone.[110] All patients had a subsequent histologic examination of the lesion. This series included five false-negative and two false-positive diagnoses.

Most of the work discussed above was done at institutions that have large numbers of primary bone tumors, especially sarcomas. A more realistic look at the world would be to examine aspiration biopsies of both primary and metastatic bone tumors. One of the larger series, which remains in abstract form, emanated from the MD Anderson Hospital in Houston more than a decade ago.[111] Over a 1-year experience, the authors evaluated 150 aspiration biopsies both benign and malignant primary and metastatic bone lesions.[111] Of the aspirates of benign bone lesions, 63% yielded the correct diagnosis; no false-positive interpretations were found. Of the malignancies, 90% were also correctly diagnosed by aspiration biopsies. Most of the false-negative interpretations appear to be the results of scant smear cellularity. There was one definite interpretive error. This was a failure to sample a MFH that appeared to arise in a giant cell tumor which was recognized in the smears. More recently, Bommer and colleagues published a substantial series.[108] This entailed 450 aspiration biopsies performed on 427 patients. It included benign and malignant primary metastatic lesions. Of the aspirates, 215 provided the frank diagnosis of cancer. Of these, 40 were primary bone neoplasms and 135 were metastases. The overall accuracy rate was 94%. A single false-positive diagnosis resulted from an overinterpretation of a scanty spinal aspirate that was diagnosed as malignant, but subsequent histology demonstrated a benign reactive proliferation. The authors did not include their unsatisfactory results in their calculations of a false-negative rate.[108] With this in mind, the rate was only 6%. Most of the unsatisfactory specimens were the result of sampling errors in that the aspirates did not contain the lesional cells. However, two interpretative false-negative diagnoses were also made.

SPECIMEN ADEQUACY

Most of the problems associated with insufficient specimens are not restricted to tumors of bone and soft tissue. Sampling problems occur when the needle is not placed in the most appropriate portion of the mass. In some cases, the tumor is completely missed. If the needle is placed in a portion that is necrotic, then the aspirate could not be positively interpreted. Finally, a proportion of soft tissue and bone neoplasms are quite heterogeneous from area to area; if the needle does not sample the least differentiated portion, then an underdiagnosis may result. Smear cellularity may be quite scanty for several reasons. This may include dense sclerosis, which may occur in both benign and malignant entities such as fibroma of tendon sheath, fibromatoses, and sclerosing liposarcomas. Tumors that are highly vascular including angiosarcomas may yield predominantly blood. This is also the case with aneurysmal bone cysts. Bone obviously is a very dense material, and it would be impossible to pass a fine needle through an intact normal bony cortex. Rather, the underlying lesions either have to break completely through or at least markedly weaken the bone for the needle to be able to sample the mass. This is a major reason that one finds a much higher satisfactory rate with malignant rather than benign osseous lesions. The reported insufficiency rates for aspiration biopsies of soft tissue neoplasms vary tremendously. The spectrum ranges from approximately 2% to 38% of all aspiration biopsies in different series. For aspiration biopsies of mass lesions of bone, the insufficiency has been reported to range from approximately 10% to 30%.

With any kind of aspiration sample, if the clinical data that was provided is incorrect or insufficient, this could lead one down the wrong diagnostic pathway. As has been emphasized, orthopedic lesions may be the area in which integration with clinical and radiographic features are the most important diagnostically.

 ## SUMMARY

FNA biopsy of soft tissue and osseous neoplasms has limitations that need to be recognized. Sampling of the neoplasm may be limited in cellularity to the point of being insufficient for diagnosis. Generally, soft tissue neoplasms possess several attributes that may lead to poor smear cellularity. This is even more relevant for tumors arising in bone. As with other tumor types, the pathologist should never feel compelled to make a diagnosis on limited samples. Certain neoplasms are evident for which a benign vs. malignant designation cannot be made with certainty in aspiration smears. In addition, it may be impossible to grade accurately some sarcomas in smears. Based purely on cellular morphology, the exact cell type of many neoplasms cannot be accurately stated. However, with the use of ancillary diagnostic procedures, many of these problems are resolved. Integration of radiographic data, especially for mass lesions of bone, may prove crucial. The need for a cytopathologist with interest and knowledge in bone and soft tissue pathology is obvious. Furthermore, the diagnostician must be willing to state in a proportion of cases that they simply do not know what is the correct diagnosis.

However, FNA biopsy possesses a number of advantages that overall outweigh their disadvantages. Aspiration biopsy provides a rapid and relatively nontraumatic procedure to sample both superficial and deep-seated mass lesions. With experience, orthopedic neoplasms can be recognized and accurately diagnosed in a large proportion of instances. Another advantage is that multiple samples may be obtained during a single clinic visit; this is especially relevant with the use of an on-site evaluation of the smears at the time of the biopsy. FNA biopsy is easily performed on these neoplasms in the outpatient setting. Finally, compared with other diagnostic procedures, FNA biopsy is relatively inexpensive. Thus, for many patients, an accurate typing and grading of the tumor can be performed with high levels of diagnostic sensitivity and specificity. At the very least, in other instances, FNA biopsy permits rapid triage of the patient for diagnosis by more traditional methods.

References

1. Abdul-Karim FW, Rader AE. Fine needle aspiration of soft-tissue lesions. Clinics Lab Med 1998; 18:507-540.
2. Akerman M, Rydholm A, Persson BM. Aspiration cytology of soft tissue tumors; the 10-year experience at an orthopaedic oncology center. Acta Orthop Scand 1985; 56:407-412.
3. Akerman M, Willen H. Critical review of the role of fine needle aspiration in soft tissue tumors. Pathol Case Rev 1998; 3:111-117.
4. Barth RJ, Merino MJ, Solomon D, et al. A prospective study of the value of core needle biopsy and fine needle aspiration in the diagnosis of soft tissue masses. Surgery 1992; 112:536-543.
5. Bennert KW, Abdul-Karim FW. Fine needle aspiration cytology vs. needle core biopsy of soft tissue tumors: a comparison. Acta Cytol 1994; 38:381-384.
6. Brosjö O, Bauer HCF, Kreisbergers A, et al. Fine needle aspiration biopsy of soft tissue tumors. Acta Orthop Scand 1994; 65(Suppl 256):108-109.
7. Cohen MB, Layfield LJ. Fine needle aspiration biopsy of soft tissue tumors. In: Schmidt WA, Miller TR, editors. Cytopathol annual. Chicago: ASCP Press; 1994. pp.101-132.
8. Costa MJ, Campman SC, Davis RL, et al. Fine-needle aspiration cytology of sarcoma: retrospective review of diagnostic utility and specificity. Diagn Cytopathol 1996; 15:23-32.
9. Finley JL, Silverman JF, Cappellari JO, et al. Fine needle aspiration cytology of gynecologic sarcomas and mixed tumors. In: Schmidt WA, Miller TR, editors. Cytopathol annual. Chicago: ASCP Press; 1996. pp.267-287.
10. Gonzalez-Campora R, Munoz-Arias G, Otal-Salaverri C, et al. Fine-needle aspiration cytology of primary soft tissue tumors: morphologic analysis of the most frequent types. Acta Cytol 1992; 36:905-917.
11. Hadju SI. Diagnosis of soft tissue sarcomas on aspiration smears. Acta Cytol 1996; 40:604-608.
12. Kilpatrick SE, Geisinger KR. Soft tissue sarcomas: the utility and limitations of fine needle aspiration biopsy. Am J Clin Pathol 1998; 110:50-68.
13. Kilpatrick SE, Ward WG, Cappellari JO, et al. Fine-needle aspiration biopsy of soft tissue sarcomas: a cytomorphologic analysis with emphasis on histologic subtyping, grading, and therapeutic significance. Am J Clin Pathol 1999; 112:179-188.
14. Kindblom L-G, Walaas L, Widelin S. Ultrastructural studies in the preoperative cytologic diagnosis of soft tissue tumors. Semin Diagn Pathol 1986; 3:317-344.
15. Layfield LJ, Anders KH, Glasgow BJ, et al. Fine needle aspiration of primary soft tissue lesions. Arch Pathol Lab Med 1986; 110:420-424.
16. Liu K, Layfield LJ, Coogan AC, et al. Diagnostic accuracy in fine-needle aspiration of soft tissue and bone lesions: influence of clinical history and experience. Am J Clin Pathol 1999; 111:632-640.
17. Miralles TG, Gosalbez F, Menéndez P, et al. Fine needle aspiration cytology of soft-tissue lesions. Acta Cytol 1986; 30:671-678.
18. Rydholm A. Centralization of soft tissue sarcoma: the southern Sweden experience. Acta Orthop Scand 1997; 68(Suppl 273):4-8.
19. Silverman JF, Lannin DL, Larkin EW, et al. Fine needle aspiration cytology of post-irradiation sarcomas, including angiosarcoma, with immunocytochemical confirmation. Diagn Cytopathol 1989; 5:275-281.
20. Willén H, Akerman M, Carlén B. Fine needle aspiration (FNA) in the diagnosis of soft tissue tumours; a review of 22 years experience. Cytopathology 1995; 6:236-247.
21. Nguyen GK. What is the value of fine needle aspiration biopsy in the cytodiagnosis of soft tissue tumors? Diagn Cytopathol 1988; 4:352-355.
22. Powers CN, Berardo MD, Frable WJ. Fine needle aspiration biopsy: pitfalls in the diagnosis of spindle-cell lesions. Diagn Cytopathol 1994; 10:232-241.

23. Gonzalez-Campora R, Otal-Salaverri C, Helvia-Vazquez A, et al. Fine needle aspiration in myxoid tumors of the soft tissues. Acta Cytol 1990; 34:179-191.

24. Wakely PE Jr, Geisinger KR, Cappellari JO, et al. Fine-needle aspiration cytopathology of soft tissue: chromyxoid and myoid lesions. Diagn Cytopathol 1995; 12:101-105.

25. Szadowska A, Lasota J. Fine needle aspiration cytology of myxoid liposarcoma: a study of 18 tumors. Cytopathology 1993; 4:99-106.

26. Nemanqani D, Mourad WA. Cytomorphologic features of fine-needle aspiration of liposarcoma. Diagn Cytopathol 1999; 20:67-69.

27. Pollono DG, Tomarchio S, Drut R, et al. Retroperitoneal and deep-seated lipoblastoma: diagnosis by CT scan and fine-needle aspiration biopsy. Diagn Cytopathol 1999; 20:295-297.

28. Merck C, Hagmar B. Myxofibrosarcoma: a correlative cytologic and histologic study of 13 cases examined by fine needle aspiration cytology. Acta Cytol 1980; 24:137-144.

29. Caraway NP, Staerkel GA, Fanning CV, et al. Diagnosing intramuscular myxoma by fine needle aspiration: a multidisciplinary approach. Diagn Cytopathol 1994; 11:255-261.

30. Dodd LG, Layfield LJ. Fine-needle aspiration cytology of ganglion cysts. Diagn Cytopathol 1996; 15:377-381.

31. Dahl I, Akerman M. Nodular fasciitis: a correlative cytologic and histologic study of 13 cases. Acta Cytol 1981; 25:215-233.

32. Azua J, Arraiza A, Delgado B, et al. Nodular fasciitis initially diagnosed by aspiration cytology. Acta Cytol 1985; 29:562-564.

33. Stanley MW, Skoog L, Tani EM, et al. Spontaneous resolution of nodular fasciitis following diagnosis by fine needle aspiration. Acta Cytol 1991; 35:616-617.

34. Akerman M, Rydholm A. Aspiration cytology of lipomatous tumors: a 10-year experience at an orthopedic oncology center. Diagn Cytopathol 1987; 3:295-301.

35. Lindberg GM, Maitra A, Gokaslan ST, et al. Low-grade fibromyxoid sarcoma: fine-needle aspiration cytology with histologic, cytogenetic, immunohistochemical, and ultrastructural correlation. Cancer Cytopathol 1999; 87:75-82.

36. Crapanzano JP, Ali SZ, Ginzberg M, Zakowski MF. Chordoma: a cytologic study with histologic and radiologic correlation. Cancer Cytopathol 2001; 93:40-51.

37. Ferretti M, Gusella PM, Mancini AM, et al. Progressive approach to the cytologic diagnosis of retroperitoneal spindle cell tumors. Acta Cytol 1997; 41:450-460.

38. Liu K, Dodge RK, Dodd LG, et al. Logistic regression analysis of low-grade spindle cell lesions. A cytologic study. Acta Cytol, 1999; 43:143-152.

39. Liu K, Dodge RK, Layfield LJ. Logistic regression analysis of high grade spindle cell neoplasms: a fine needle aspiration cytologic study. Acta Cytol 1999; 43:593-600.

40. Weir MM, Rosenberg AE, Bell DA. Grading of spindle cell sarcomas in fine-needle aspiration biopsy specimens. Am J Clin Pathol 1999; 112:784-798.

41. Berardo MD, Powers CN, Wakely P Jr, et al. Fine-needle aspiration cytopathology of malignant fibrous histiocytoma. Cancer Cytopathol 1997; 81:228-237.

42. Boucher LD, Swanson PE, Stanley MW, et al. Cytology of angiosarcoma: findings in fourteen fine-needle fluid specimens. Am J Clin Pathol 2000; 14:210-219.

43. Dahl I, Hagmar B, Idvall I. Benign solitary neurilemoma (schwannoma): a correlative cytological and histological study of 28 cases. Acta Pathol Microbiol Immunol Scand 1984; 92:91-101.

44. Resnick JM, Fanning CV, Caraway NP, et al. Percutaneous needle biopsy diagnosis of benign neurogenic neoplasms. Diagn Cytopathol 1997; 16:17-25.

45. Henke AC, Salomão DR, Hughes JH. Cellular schwannoma mimics a sarcoma: an example of a potential pitfall in aspiration cytodiagnosis. Diagn Cytopathol 1999; 20:312-316.

46. Dodd LG, Marom EM, Dash RC, et al. Fine-needle aspiration cytology of "ancient" schwannoma. Diagn Cytopathol 1999; 20:307-311.

47. Zbieranowski I, Bedard YC. Fine needle aspiration of schwannomas: value of electron microscopy and immunocytochemistry in the preoperative diagnosis. Acta Cytol 1989; 33:381-384.

48. Vendraminelli R, Cavazzana AO, Poletti A, et al. Fine needle aspiration cytology of malignant nerve sheath tumors. Diagn Cytopathol 1992; 8:559-562.

49. McGee RS Jr, Ward WG, Kilpatrick SE. Malignant peripheral nerve sheath tumor: a fine needle aspiration biopsy study. Diagn Cytopathol 1997; 17:298-305.

50. Jiménez-Heffernan JA, López-Ferrer P, Vicandi B, et al. Cytologic features of malignant peripheral nerve sheath tumor. Acta Cytol 1999; 43:175-183.

51. Akerman M, Ryd W, Skytting B. Fine needle aspiration of synovial sarcoma: criteria for diagnosis: retrospective re-examination of 37 cases, including ancillary diagnostics. A Scandinavian Sarcoma Group Study. Diagn Cytopathol 2003; 28:232-238.

52. Kilpatrick SE, Teot LA, Stanley MW, et al. Fine needle aspiration biopsy of synovial sarcoma. Am J Clin Pathol 1996; 106:769-775.

53. Ryan MR, Stastny JF, Wakely PE Jr. The cytopathology of synovial sarcoma: a study of six cases, with emphasis on architecture and histopathologic correlation. Cancer Cytopathol 1998; 84:42-49.

54. Viguer JM, Jiménez-Heffernan JA, Vicandi B, et al. Cytologic features of synovial sarcoma with emphasis on the monophasic fibrous variant: a morphologic and immunocytological analysis of bcl-2 protein expression. Cancer Cytopathol 1998; 84:50-56.

55. Inagaki H, Murase T, Otsuka T, et al. Detection of SYT-SSX fusion transcript in synovial sarcoma using archival cytologic specimens. Am J Clin Pathol 1999; 111:528-533.

56. Tao LC, Davidson DD. Aspiration biopsy cytology of smooth muscle tumors: a cytologic approach to the differentiation between leiomyosarcoma and leiomyoma. Acta Cytol 1993; 37:300-308.

57. Barbazza R, Chiarelli S, Quintarelli GF, et al. Role of fine-needle aspiration cytology in the preoperative evolution of smooth muscle tumors. Diagn Cytopathol 1997; 16:326-330.

58. Dahl I, Hagmar B, Agnervall L. Leiomyosarcoma of the soft tissue: a correlative cytological and histological study of 11 cases. Acta Pathol Microbiol Scand 1981; 89:285-291.

59. Smith MB, Silverman JF, Raab SS, Geisinger KR, et al. Fine-needle aspiration cytology of hepatic leiyomyosarcoma. Diagn Cytopathol 1994; 11:321-372.

60. Pérez-Guillermo M, Pérez JS, Rojo B, et al. FNA cytology of cutaneous vascular tumors. Cytopathology 1992; 3:231-244.

61. Abee J, Miller T. Cytology of well-differentiated and poorly differentiated hemangiosarcoma in fine needle aspirates. Acta Cytol 1992; 26:341-348.

62. Hales M, Bottles K, Muller T, et al. Diagnosis of Kaposi's sarcoma by fine-needle aspiration biopsy. Am J Clin Pathol 1987; 88:20-25.

63. Nickols J, Koivuniemi A. Cytology of malignant hemangiopericytoma. Acta Cytol 1979; 23:119-125.

64. Geisinger KR, Silverman JF, Cappellari JO, et al. Fine-needle aspiration cytology of malignant hemangiopericytomas with ultrastructural and flow cytometric analyses. Arch Pathol Lab Med 1990; 114:705-710.

65. Alkan S, Eltoum IA, Tabbara S, et al. Usefulness of molecular detection of human herpesvirus-8 in the diagnosis of Kaposi sarcoma by fine-needle aspiration. Am J Clin Pathol 1999; 111:91-96.

66. Wakely PE Jr, Price WG, Frable WJ. Sternomastoid tumor of infancy (fibromatosis colli): diagnosis by aspiration cytology. Mod Pathol 1989; 2:378-381.

67. Raab SS, Silverman JF, McLeod DL, et al. Fine needle aspiration biopsy of fibromatoses. Acta Cytol 1993; 37:323-328.

68. Stein AL, Bardawil RG, Silverman SG, et al. Fine needle aspiration biopsy of idiopathic retroperitoneal fibrosis. Acta Cytol 1997; 41:461-466.

69. Powers CN, Hurt MA, Frable JW. Fine needle aspiration biopsy: dermatofibrosarcoma protuberans. Diagn Cytopathol 1993; 145-150.

70. James LP. Cytopathology of mesenchymal repair. Diagn Cytopathol 1985; 1:91-104.

71. Walaas L, Kindblom LG. Lipomatous tumors: a correlative cytologic and histologic study of 27 tumors examined by fine needle aspiration cytology. Hum Pathol 1985; 16:6-18.

72. Geisinger KR, Naylor B, Beals TF, et al. Cytopathology, including transmission and scanning electron microscopy of pleomorphic liposarcomas in pleural fluids. Acta Cytol 1980; 24:435-441.

73. Walaas L, Angervall L, Hagmar B, et al. A correlative cytologic and histologic study of malignant fibrous histiocytoma: an analysis of 40 cases examined by fine needle aspiration cytology. Diagn Cytopathol 1986; 2:46-64.

74. Rigby HS, Wilson V, Cawthorn S, et al. Fine needle aspiration of pleomorphic lipoma: a potential pitfall of cytodiagnosis. Cytopathology 1993; 4:55-58.

75. Layfield LJ, Moffatt EJ, Dodd LG, et al. Cytologic findings in tenosynovial giant cell tumors investigated by fine-needle aspiration cytology. Diagn Cytopathol 1997; 16:317-325.

76. Yu GH, Staerkel GA, Kershnisnik MM, et al. Fine needle aspiration of pigmented villonodular synovitis of the temporomandibular joint masquerading as a primary parotid gland lesion. Diagn Cytopathol 1997; 16:47-50.

77. Silverman JF, Dabbs DJ, Finley JL, et al. Fine-needle aspiration biopsy of pleomorphic (giant cell) carcinoma of the pancreas: cytologic, immunocytochemical, and ultrastructural findings. Am J Clin Pathol 1988; 89:714-720.

78. Silverman JF, Geisinger KR, Park HK, et al. Fine-needle aspiration cytology of granulocytic sarcoma and myeloid metaplasia. Diagn Cytopathol 1990; 6:106-111.

79. Liu K, Mann KP, Garst JL, Dodd LG, et al. Diagnosis of posttransplant granulocytic sarcoma of fine-needle aspiration cytology and flow cytometry. Diagn Cytopathol 1999; 20:85-89.

80. Ahmen MN, Feldman M, Seemayer TA. Cytology of epithelioid sarcoma. Acta Cytol 1974; 18:459-461.

81. Pohar-Marinsek Z, Zidar A. Epithelioid sarcoma in FNAB smears. Diagn Cytopathol 1994; 11:367-372.

82. Kapila K, Chopra P, Verma K. Fine needle aspiration cytology of alveolar soft-part sarcoma. Acta Cytol 1985; 29:559-561.

83. Shabb N, Sneige N, Fanning CV, et al. Fine needle aspiration cytology of alveolar soft-part sarcoma. Diagn Cytopathol 1991; 7:293-298.

84. Caraway NP, Fanning CV, Wojeik EM, et al. Cytology of malignant melanoma of soft parts: fine needle aspirates and exfoliative specimens. Diagn Cytopathol 1993; 9:632-638.

85. Almeida MM, Nunes AM, Frable WJ. Malignant melanoma of soft tissue: a report of three cases with diagnosis by fine needle aspiration cytology. Acta Cytol 1994; 38:241-246.

86. Creager AJ, Pitman MB, Geisinger KR. Cytologic features of clear cell sarcoma (malignant melanoma) of soft tissue: a study of fine needle aspirates and exfoliative specimens. Am J Clinic Pathol 2002; 117:217-224.

87. Franzen S, Stenkvist B. Diagnosis of granular cell myoblastoma by fine needle aspiration biopsy. Acta Pathol Microbiol Scand 1968; 72:391-395.

88. Geisinger KR, Kawamoto EH, Marshall RB, et al. Aspiration and exfoliative cytology, including ultrastructure, of a malignant granular cell tumor. 1985; Acta Cytol 1985; 29:593-597.

89. Wakely PE Jr, Giacomantonio M. Fine needle aspiration cytology of metastatic malignant rhabdoid tumor. Acta Cytol 1986; 30:533-537.

90. Akhtar M, Ashraf AM, Sabbah R, et al. Small round cell tumor with divergent differentiation: cytologic, histologic and ultrastructural findings. Diagn Cytopathol 1994; 11:159-164.

91. Layfield LJ, Liu K, Dodge RK. Logistic regression analysis of small round cell neoplasms: a cytologic study. Diagn Cytopathol 1999; 20:271-277.

92. Akhtar M, Ali MA, Bakry M, et al. Fine needle aspiration biopsy of childhood rhabdomyosarcoma: cytologic, histologic, and ultrastructural correlations. Diagn Cytopathol 1992; 8:465-474.

93. Almeida M, Stastny JF, Wakely PE Jr, et al. Fine needle aspiration biopsy of childhood rhabdomyosarcoma: re-evaluation of the cytologic criteria for diagnosis. Diagn Cytopathol 1994; 11:231-236.

94. Pettinato G, Swanson PE, Insabato L, DeChiara A, Wick MR. Undifferentiated small round-cell tumors of childhood: the immunocytochemical demonstration of myogenic differentiation in fine needle aspirates. Diagn Cytopathol 1989; 5:194-199.

95. Seidal T, Walaas L, Kindblom LG, et al. Cytology of embryonal rhabdomyosarcoma: a cytologic, light microscopic, electron microscopic, and immunohistochemical study of seven cases. Diagn Cytopathol 1988; 4:292-299.

96. Seidal T, Mark J, Hagmar B, et al. Alveolar rhabdomyosarcoma: a cytometric and correlated cytological and histological study. Acta Pathol Microbiol Scand (A) 1982; 90:345-354.

97. Carraway NP, Fanning CV, Amato RJ, et al. Fine-needle aspiration of intra-abdominal desmoplastic small round cell tumor. Diagn Cytopathol 1993; 9:465-470.

98. Logrono R, Kurtycz DF, Sproat IA, et al. Diagnosis of recurrent desmoplastic small round cell tumor by fine needle aspiration: a case report. Acta Cytol 1997; 41:1402-1406.

99. Silverman JF, Dabbs DJ, Ganick DJ, et al. Fine needle aspiration cytology of neuroblastoma, including peripheral neuroectodermal tumor, with immunocytochemical and ultrastructural confirmation. Acta Cytol 1988; 32:367-376.

100. Pisharodi LR, Cary D, Bernacki EG Jr. Elastofibroma dorsi: diagnostic problems and pitfalls. Diagn Cytopathol 1994; 10:242-244.

101. Oland J, Rosen A, Reif R, Sayfan J, et al. Cytodiagnosis of soft tissue tumors. J Surg Oncol 1986; 37:168-170.

102. Guillou L, Coindre J-M. How should we grade soft tissue sarcomas and what are the limitations? Pathol Case Rev 1998; 3:105-110.

103. Liu K, Moffatt EJ, Hudson GR, et al. Gouty tophus presenting as a soft-tissue mass diagnosed by fine-needle aspiration: a case report. Diagn Cytopathol 1996; 15:246-249.

104. Nicol KK, Ward WG, Pike EJ, Geisinger KR, et al. Fine-needle aspiration biopsy of gouty tophi: lessons in cost-effective patient management. Diagn Cytopathol 1997; 17:30-35.

105. Kilpatrick SG, Geisinger KR. Bone. In: Geisinger KR, Silverman JF, editors. Fine needle aspiration cytology of superficial organs and body sites. New York: Churchill Livingstone: 1999. pp.157-181.

106. Dollahite HA, Tatum L, Moinuddin SM, et al. Aspiration biopsy of primary neoplasms of bone. J Bone Joint Surg 1983; 65A:1166-1169.

107. Walaas L, Kindblom L-G. Light and electron microscopic examination of fine needle aspirates in the preoperative diagnosis of osteogenic tumors: a study of 21 osteosarcomas and two osteoblastomas. Diagn Cytopathol 1990; 6:27-38.

108. Bommer KK, Ramzy I, Mody D. Fine-needle aspiration biopsy in the diagnosis and management of bone lesions: a study of 450 cases. Cancer Cytopathol 1997; 148-156.

109. Agarwal PK, Wahal KM. Cytopathologic study of primary tumors of bones and joints. Acta Cytol 1983; 27:23-27.

110. Xiaojing Peng, Xiangchang Y. Cytodiagnosis of bone tumors by fine needle aspiration. Acta Cytol 1985; 29:570-575.

111. Siddiqui S, Fanning CV. Fine needle aspiration of bone: a one-year experience. Acta Cytol 1988; 32:744-745.

112. Layfield LJ, Armstrong K, Zaleski S, et al. Diagnostic accuracy and clinical utility of fine-needle aspiration cytology: the diagnosis of clinically primary bone lesions. Diagn Cytopathol 1993; 9:168-173.

113. Koscick RL, Petersilge CA, Makley JT, et al. CT-guided fine needle aspiration and needle core biopsy of skeletal lesions. Complementary diagnostic techniques. Acta Cytol 1998; 42:687-702.

114. White VA, Fanning CV, Ayala AG, et al. Osteosarcoma and the role of fine-needle aspiration: a study of 51 cases. Cancer 1988; 62:1638-1646.

115. Kilpatrick SE, Ward WG, Bos Gary D, et al. The role of fine needle aspiration biopsy in the diagnosis and management of osteosarcoma. Ped Pathol Mod Med 2000; 19:323-335.

116. Walaas L, Kindblom L-G, Gunterberg B, et al. Light and electron microscopic examination of fine-needle aspirates in the preoperative diagnosis of cartilaginous tumors. Diagn Cytopathol 1990; 6:396-408.

117. Tunc M, Ekinci C. Chondrosarcoma diagnosed by fine needle aspiration cytology. Acta Cytol 1996; 40:283-288.

118. Fanning CV, Sneige NS, Carrasco CH, et al. Fine needle aspiration cytology of chondroblastoma of bone. Cancer 1990; 65:1847-1863.

119. Kilpatrick SE, Pike EJ, Geisinger KR, et al. Chondroblastoma of bone: use of fine needle aspiration biopsy and potential diagnostic pitfalls. Diagn Cytopathol 1997; 16:65-71.

120. Layfield LJ, Ferreiro JA. Fine-needle aspiration cytology of chondromyxoid fibroma: a case report. Diagn Cytopathol 1988; 4:148-151.

121. Gupta S, Dav G, Marya S. Chondromyxoid fibroma: a fine-needle aspiration diagnosis. Diagn Cytopathol 1993; 9:63-65.

122. Koh JS, Chung JH, Lee SY, et al. Chondrosarcoma of the proximal femur with myxoid degeneration mistaken for chondromyxoid fibroma in a young adult: a case report. Acta Cytol 2001; 45:254-258.

123. Abdul-Karim FW, Wasman JK, Pitlik D. Needle aspiration cytoloogy of chondrosarcomas. Acta Cytol 1993; 37:655-660.

124. Geirnaerdt MJ, Harmans J, Bloem JL, et al. Usefulness of radiography in differentiating enchondroma from central grade 1 chondrosarcoma. AJR 1997; 169:1097-1104.

125. Dee S, Meneses M, Ostrowski ML, Murakami M, et al. Pleomorphic ("dedifferentiated") chondrosarcoma: report of a case initially examined by fine needle aspiration biopsy. Acta Cytol 1991; 35:467-471.

126. Rao L, Kini AC, Valiathan M, et al. Infantile cartilaginous hamartoma of the rib. Acta Cytol 2001; 45:69-73.

127. Renshaw AA, Pérez-Atayde AR, Fletcher JA, et al. Cytology of typical and atypical Ewing's sarcoma/PNET. Am J Clin Pathol 1996; 106:620-624.

128. Mondal A, Misra DK. Ewing's sarcoma of bone: a study of 71 cases of fine needle aspiration cytology. J Indian Med Assoc 1996; 94:135-137.

129. Sahu K, Pai RR, Khadilkar UN. Fine needle aspiration cytology of the Ewing's sarcoma family of tumors. Acta Cytol 2000; 44:332-336.

130. Halliday BC, Slagel DD, Elsheikh TE, et al. Diagnostic utility of MIC-2 immunochemical staining in the differential of small blue cell tumors. Diagn Cytopathol 1998; 19:410-416.

131. Schlott T, Nagel H, Ruschenberg I, et al. Reverse transcriptase polymerase chain reaction for detecting Ewing's sarcoma in archival fine needle aspiration biopsies. Acta Cytol 1997; 41:795-801.

132. Udayakumar AM, Sundareshan TS, Gould TM, et al. Cytogenetic characterization of Ewing tumors using fine needle asiration samples: a 10-year experience and review of the literature. Cancer Genet Cytogenet 2001; 127: 41-48

133. Karmakar T, Dey P. Fine-needle aspiration of plasma cell disorders: special emphasis on plasma cell subtype. Diagn Cytopathol 1994; 11:119-123.

134. Wedin R, Bauer HC, Skoog L, et al. Cutologic diagnosis of skeletal lesion. Fine needle aspiration biopsy in 100 tumors. J Bone Joint Surg Br 2000; 82:673-678.

135. Sneige N, Ayala AG, Carraasco CH, et al. Giant cell tumor of bone: a cytologic study of 24 cases. Diagn Cytopathol 1985; 1:111-117.

136. Vetrani A, Fulciniti F, Boschi R, et al. Fine needle apsiration biopsy diagnosis of giant cell tumor of bone: an experience with nine cases. Acta Cytol 1990; 34:863-867.

137. Galero-Davidson H, Fernandez-Rodriguez A, Torres-Olivera FJ, et al. Cytologic diagnosis of a case of recurrent adamantinoma. Acta Cytol 1989; 33:635-638.

138. Elsheikh T, Silverman JF, Wakely PE Jr, et al. Fine-needle aspiration cytology of Langerhans' cell histiocytosis (eosinophilic granuloma) of bone in children. Diagn Cytopathol 1991; 7:261-266.

139. Kreicbergs A, Bauer HC, Brosjo O, et al. Cytological diagnosis of bone tumours. J Bone Joint Surg (Br) 1996; 78:258-263.

140. Kumar RV, Rao CR, Hazarika D, et al. Aspiration biopsy cytology of primary bone lesions. Acta Cytol 1993; 37: 83-89.

141. Cardillo M, Zakowski MF, Liu O. Fine-needle aspiration of epithelioid sarcoma: cytology findings in nine cases. Cancer Cytopathol 2001; 93:246-251.

142. Farshid G, Pradhan M, Goldblum J, et al. Leiomyosarcoma of somatitic soft tissues: a tumor of vascular origin with multivariate analysis of outcome in 42 cases. Am J Surg Pathol 2002; 26:14-24.

143. Geisinger KR, Abdul-Karim FW. Fine needle aspiration biopsies of soft tissue tumors. In: Weiss SW, Goldblum JR. Entinger and Weiss's soft tissue tumors. 4th ed. St Louis: Mosby; 2001. pp.147-188.

144. Sápi Z, Antal I, Pápai Z, et al. Diagnosis of soft tissue tumors by fine-needle aspiration with combined cytopathology and ancillary techniques. Diagn Cytopathol 2002; 26:232-242.

145. Wakely PE Jr, Frable WJ. Fine needle aspiration biopsy cytology of giant cell tumor of tendon sheath. Am J Clin Pathol 1994; 102:87-90.

146. Shapiro SL, McMenomey SO, Alexander P, Schmidt WA. Fine-needle aspiration biopsy diagnosis of "invasive" temporomandibular joint pigmented villonodular synotitis: clinical, imagine, and cytopathologic correlation. Arch Pathol Lab Med 2002; 126:195-198.

147. Crapanzano JP, Cardillo M, Lin O, et al. Cytopathology of desmoplastic small round cell tumor: a series including findings in ThinPrep. Cancer Cytopathol 2002; 96: 21-31.

148. Jones C, Liu K, Hirschowitz S, et al. Concordance of histopathologic and cytologic grading in musculoskeletal sarcomas: can grades obtained from analysis of the fine-needle aspirates serve as the basis for therapeutic decisions? Cancer Cytopathol 2002; 96:83-91.

149. Yamamoto T, Nagira K, Akisne T, et al. Aspiration biopsy of nodular sarcoidosis of the muscle. Diagn Cytopathol 2002; 26:109-112.

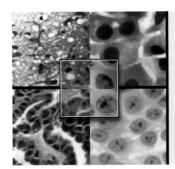

CHAPTER
29

Breast

Fine-needle aspiration (FNA) biopsy of the breast was first used in the 1930s by physicians at Memorial Hospital[1-3] but did not gain wide acceptance until Europeans reported their experience.[4-9] Currently, aspiration cytology of palpable breast lesions has gained wide acceptance,[10-16] whereas for mammographically evident, nonpalpable breast lesions, core biopsies are favored in most medical centers. The advantages of the FNA biopsy procedure include accurate diagnosis, low cost, excellent patient acceptance, and minimal to no morbidity.[14-18] However, reservations have been expressed about employing the FNA procedure because of a variety of factors including: concerns about needle tract seeding; the need for an experienced pathologist to interpret the aspirated material; potential for false-positive diagnosis with an unnecessary surgical procedure; the limitation of FNA biopsy in classifying proliferative breast disease; and FNA's inability to separate in-situ from invasive carcinoma.[10,17-25]

It has also been argued that FNA biopsy followed by excisional biopsy with frozen section for confirmation may actually increase the cost of the workup of a breast mass and that FNA and frozen section biopsy are mutually exclusive rather than complementary procedures.[24-28] Concerns about the accuracy of FNA biopsy and its limitations have contributed to the slow implementation of the procedure in centers having pathologists who are initially inexperienced with interpreting the material.[2] However, the authors and others have shown that FNA biopsy is cost effective by accurately assigning patients to either an outpatient or inpatient setting for the workup of their breast mass rather than eliminating the need for frozen section.[17] Cost analysis demonstrates considerable savings even when combined with the cost of frozen section.[29] Therefore, the authors believe that FNA biopsy has an important triage role for the workup of breast masses. Moreover, in a number of medical centers, FNA biopsy has compared quite favorably with core biopsy in terms of the diagnostic accuracy for palpable breast lesions.[30,31] Furthermore, in selected cases, FNA biopsy and core biopsy can be complementary.[32] When the lesion is small, dermal based, shallow, fibrotic or paucicellular, punch biopsies similar to what have been used by dermatologists to diagnose various skin lesions have also been employed by cytopathologists.[33]

FNA biopsy, combined with frozen section confirmation, can lead to a more accurate diagnosis, virtually eliminating false-positive diagnoses that could lead to an unnecessary surgical procedure such as a mastectomy.[29] Frozen section confirmation is especially needed when the clinical and mammographic findings are benign or when the FNA cytology is atypical or suspicious. The latter occurs when atypical cells are present in low numbers or when the smears are poorly prepared. Other scenarios in which FNA biopsy can be combined with frozen section confirmation is when pathologists are beginning to master the technique of FNA biopsy and smear interpretation, or when an insufficient number of cases is available to develop a sufficient level of expertise. FNA biopsy has also been used to evaluate accessory axillary breast tissue[34] and breast tissue margins after lumpectomy.[35]

 TECHNIQUE

For most FNA biopsies, 23 to 25 gauge 1.5-inch needles attached to a disposable 10 or 20 ml syringe fitted into a commercially available syringe holder are used. The nonaspiration technique is often employed, using a needle attached to the syringe from which the plunger has been removed, or even a needle to which no syringe is attached.[36] The majority of the smears are air-dried and stained by a modified rapid Romanowsky stain (Diff-Quik [DQ] stain). One or two smears can be selected for quick interpretation in the clinic or at the patient's bedside.[37,38] Some of the remaining smears are immediately spray fixed or wet fixed in 95% ethyl alcohol for Pap staining. Liquid-based preparations have also been effectively employed for preparing breast FNA specimens,[39] but direct smears are preferred because of greater preservation of architectural patterns.[40] However, if FNA biopsies are done off site by physicians unskilled in direct smear preparation, liquid-based techniques may be a preferred alternative to poorly prepared direct smears.[40]

Procedure Indications and Advantages

FNA biopsy is indicated for all palpable breast lesions and occasional nonpalpable mammographically evident le-

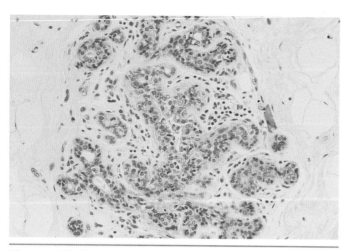

Figure 29-1 **Benign breast tissue.** The terminal-duct lobular unit (TDLU) consists of terminal ductules and acini surrounded by loose fibroconnective tissue. (Hemosiderin and eosin [H&E])

sions. Some recommend that a mammogram be obtained first to avoid any artifactual image changes secondary to the FNA biopsy procedure.[15] The procedure's major advantages are providing a rapid and accurate diagnosis and cost-effective triage in the workup of breast masses. FNA biopsy can also differentiate cysts from solid tumors; serve as a therapeutic procedure allowing evacuation of the cyst contents; provide prompt psychological relief of anxiety for patients having benign breast lesions; involve patients early in the decision making process when a malignancy is identified; evaluate local chest wall recurrences; and enable ancillary studies such as hormone receptor analysis, *Her-2neu,* DNA analysis to be performed on the aspirated material in selected cases such as metastatic disease, local recurrences, and in patients undergoing cytoreduction therapy before possible surgery.

Complications

Although unusual with the smaller 23- to 25-gauge needles, the most common complications of FNA biopsy are severe local pain and/or hematoma. The latter can be minimized if firm pressure is applied after performance of each biopsy. Pneumothorax is a very rare complication,[17,42-44] with an incidence of 1:470 aspirates in one series[45] and 0.18% of 74,000 fine-needle biopsies in another report.[46] For deep-seated lesions near the chest wall, a more lateral rather than a direct vertically approach is recommended to better avoid this complication. These issues are discussed more fully in Chapter 2.

The FNA procedure is usually well tolerated and causes little pain. However, percutaneous aspirations through the areolar skin for central lesions can be exceedingly painful. In this setting, either local anesthesia should be used or a lateral approach should be attempted through the nonareolar skin. Needle tract seeding has been reported with large core needle biopsies[47,48] but is exceedingly rare with FNA biopsy. In one study of 308 patients treated conservatively with local excision, no evidence of either increased local recurrence or decreased survival after FNA biopsy was shown.[49]

Other possible complications include a variety of histologic changes from the FNA biopsy procedure,[50] including extensive tissue necrosis, hemorrhage with or without organization, spindle cell nodules, and epithelial displacement.[50,51] The latter complication in cases of ductal carcinoma in situ (DCIS) may potentially cause simulation of an invasive carcinoma in the resected specimen.[53] Recognition of extensive hemorrhage, granulation tissue, and fibrin with or without fat necrosis near the layer of epithelial displacement should prompt consideration of this possibility and avoid an inappropriate diagnosis of invasive carcinoma.[16] However, the clinical significance of epithelial displacement remains unknown at the present time. These problems are not unique to FNA biopsy and in fact are seen more often in large core biopsies. Moreover, it has also been reported that dislodgment of benign and malignant cells with transport to the draining axillary lymph nodes can occur with large core biopsy.[53] This possibility should be suspected when epithelial cells are present in the subcapsular sinus of a draining lymph node associated with hemosiderin-laden macrophages and damaged red blood cells.[53] With preoperative diagnosis by either FNA or core biopsy as the norm and with highly sensitive cytokeratin immunostains applied to sentinel lymph nodes, it seems likely that epithelial displacement by needling procedures will continue to be an issue. This may complicate our ability to understand the true metastic potential of microscopic "metastases" identified only by special techniques.

 ANATOMY AND HISTOLOGY OF THE BREAST

The normal female breast is a modified sweat gland consisting of functional epithelial units and surrounding stroma. The breast is composed of 25 to 50 lobes or segments that radially converge on the nipple.[54] Each segment consists of a lactiferous duct, a lactiferous sinus, segmental collecting duct, subsegmental ducts, ductules (terminal duct), and acini (terminal ductules). The functional component of the breast is the terminal-duct lobular unit (TDLU), which is surrounded by a loose stroma (Figure 29-1). The TDLU responds to hormonal influences that are reflected by a variety of histologic changes related to the functional activity of the cells.

An aspirate of a nonlactating breast contains predominantly normal fat, fibrous tissue, and stromal cells with only a few scattered ductal or acinar cells. The glandular or ductal elements are arranged primarily in small, flat, honeycomb sheets (Figure 29-2). The myoepithelial cells are present as round to oval, naked nuclei without discernable cytoplasm. In the lactating breast, a greater amount of glandular tissue is aspirated, resulting in many epithelial cells with large nuclei with prominent nucleoli and coarsely vacuolated, pale cytoplasm (Figure 29-3). These changes are discussed more fully in the next section. In atrophic breast tissue, the involutionary changes result in replacement of the normal breast parenchyma by dense collagenized fibroconnective tissue. Aspirates from such a breast are generally paucicellular. It is important to recognize that after puberty, the breast will respond to minor stimulation associated with the menstrual cycle. It has been reported that nearly half of all the "atypical" findings of breast FNA biopsies

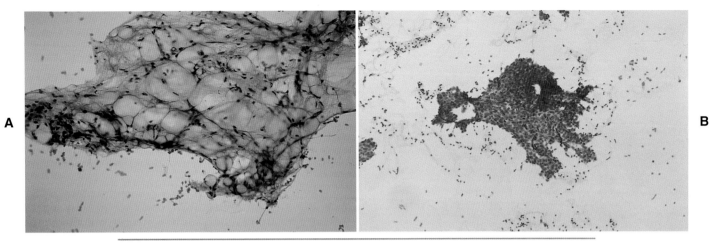

Figure 29-2   Adipose tissue and benign ductal cells. A, An aspirate of normal breast parenchyma consisting of fragments of benign adipose tissue. (Papanicolaou [Pap]) **B,** In this Diff-Quik (DQ)–stained smear, a flat sheet of ductal cells is present maintaining a honeycomb pattern, along with a few interspersed spindle-shaped bipolar naked nuclei in the background.

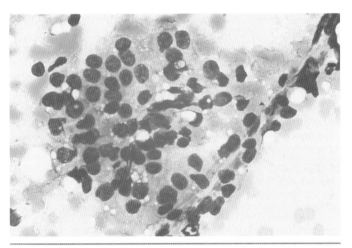

Figure 29-3   Lactating breast tissue. An aspirate of a lactating breast in which enlarged epithelial cells are present possessing prominent nuclei with clearly discernable nucleoli and coarsely vacuolated, pale wispy cytoplasm. (DQ)

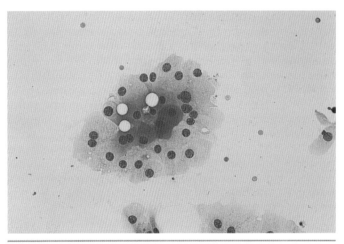

Figure 29-4   Benign cyst. An aspirate showing limited cellularity consisting of histiocytes (foam cells) and apocrine cells possessing small to enlarged nuclei having discernable nucleoli and abundant granular cytoplasm resulting in low nuclear to cytoplasmic (N:C) ratios. (DQ)

were the result of these benign secretory changes.[55] Therefore, when interpreting breast FNA specimens, it is important to take the patient's age and hormonal status into consideration.

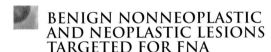

BENIGN NONNEOPLASTIC AND NEOPLASTIC LESIONS TARGETED FOR FNA

Cysts

The most common lesions of the female breast are solitary or multiple cysts. Aspiration of breast cysts is an excellent procedure for both diagnosis and treatment, although some have questioned the utility of cytologically examining all breast cyst fluid.[57-60] By definition, a *lesion* is a breast cyst when more than 1 ml of fluid is aspirated.[14] The cyst fluid

can be clear, opaque, or turbid and may be yellow, green, brown, or red (blood stained).[13] Clear or light yellow fluid is almost always acellular or limited in cellularity, consisting of only a few epithelial cells. The latter are often apocrine cells and foam cells, which are believed to be modified epithelial cells (Figure 29-4).[14] Following aspiration of the cyst, it is important to palpate the area again to determine whether a residual breast mass is present. If a mass is present, then additional aspirations of the residual solid component should be performed. In some cases, it is also advisable to repeat the mammogram if significant areas of breast tissue were obscured by cysts in previous studies.

Ciatto and colleagues reported the aspiration cytologic findings of 6782 breast cyst fluids.[59] These authors noted that intracystic carcinomas were almost always associated with blood-stained cyst fluid.[59] This is an important "gross" finding. Breast cysts may become inflamed, resulting in the patient's complaining of pain, swelling, and redness,

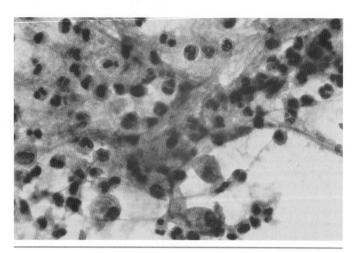

Figure 29-5 Acute mastitis. Aspirate containing numerous neutrophils and abundant granular background debris. (Pap)

especially if the cyst is superficial. Aspiration of these cysts generally yields turbid fluid with numerous neutrophils, in addition to the foam cells and degenerating ductal cells. A very uncommon finding in breast cysts are Liesegang rings, which are structures having a double layer outer wall with striations and an amorphous central nidus.[61,62] Liesegang rings are believed to form in supersaturated colloidal solutions and potentially can be confused with parasites.

Most surgeons aspirate breast cysts as a common office procedure and usually discard the fluid with no thought of cytologic preparations. In the case of the clear, yellow, or green fluid that is so often recovered, this is a safe practice. However, fluids that are turbid or bloody should be submitted for cytologic examination. This is also true for fluid from cysts that have refilled and enlarged within a few days or weeks of a previous drainage procedure.

Inflammatory Lesions Including Mastitis and Abscess Formation

Duct rupture with spillage of secretory material results in breast inflammation. Other examples result from bacterial infection. Although rare, tuberculous, fungal, filarial, and viral infections can cause inflammatory lesions.[63-65] Diabetic mastopathy also has a significant inflammatory component. There are a few cytologic reports of inflammatory breast lesions.[66-71]

FNA cytology of acute mastitis demonstrates yellowish or greenish fluid with numerous neutrophils and foamy macrophages, as well as abundant background debris (Figure 29-5). Epithelial atypia resulting primarily from the acute inflammatory process can occasionally be worrisome, but a conservative interpretative approach is important when one sees neutrophils surrounding and infiltrating the epithelial groups, especially when bipolar naked nuclei are also present (Figure 29-6). Atypical epithelial cells may also show features of regeneration and repair, characterized by the low-power appreciation of groups arranged in a flat, streaming pattern with maintenance of well-defined cell borders and polarity (Figure 29-7). In a benign repair reaction, the nuclear to cytoplasmic (N:C) ratios remain within normal limits and single atypical cells are not present or are few in number. It is only with high-power examination that these cells appear atypical because of their nuclear enlarge-

ment and prominent nucleoli. As with aspirates from other body sites, appreciation of architectural features at low magnification is crucial. In other words, it is important to study the overall smear pattern and not rush to high-power objectives. In any inflammatory lesion demonstrating atypical cells, the degree of atypia appears to be accentuated in the Romanowsky-stained smears because air drying with its attendant cell swelling accentuates real differences in cell size. Therefore, if inflammatory atypia is present, appreciation of the more benign appearance of cells in the alcohol-fixed Pap-stained preparations should prompt a conservative approach.

Plasma cell mastitis is a fairly common chronic inflammatory condition of the breast, characterized histologically by the presence of numerous lymphocytes and plasma cells surrounding ducts filled with inspissated secretions in the acute phase, and by fibrosis in the healing phase.[13] Most cases are probably caused by duct rupture. The cytologic findings reflect the stage of the process (Figure 29-8). A similar cytologic picture results from aspiration of a lymph node in the tail of Spence, as it will yield a polymorphic population of lymphoid cells ranging from small, mature lymphocytes to larger, more reactive-appearing lymphoid cells. Plasma cells and scattered tingible body macrophages will also be seen. The smears' background will show numerous lymphoglandular bodies. The differential diagnosis includes aspiration of a reactive lymph node in the axilla, since it may not be certain that the lymph node is actually in the nearby tail of Spence breast parenchyma. Intramammary lymph nodes may not be located in the axillary tail and present mammographically as similar to a fibroadenoma. Aspiration yields tissue identical to FNA of benign lymph nodes in other sites. Malignant lymphoma, either in the axillary lymph nodes or involving the breast, will consist of a uniform population of atypical lymphoid cells rather than of a polymorphic lymphoid population.

Subareolar Abscess

Subareolar abscess, a low-grade inflammation/infection involving the lactiferous ducts in the subareolar region, is a specific clinicopathologic entity that can be cytologically recognized.[72,73] This lesion begins as a localized area of inflammation, when the lactiferous duct undergoes squamous metaplasia resulting in duct obstruction with subsequent rupture and release of keratinous debris into the surrounding stroma. This induces a foreign body reaction, with acute and chronic inflammation, and possible formation of a sinus tract to the skin surface (Figure 29-9). A history of temporary relief after drainage is followed by partial healing, but characteristically, subsequent recurrences take place. The presence of a mass beneath the nipple and/or subareolar skin with or without nipple retraction can clinically simulate a neoplasm such as adenoma of the nipple or carcinoma. The FNA cytology smears, however, are diagnostic when anucleated squamous cells associated with numerous neutrophils, parakeratotic cells, cholesterol crystals, and even strips of squamous epithelium are found in the smears (Figure 29-10).[73] Foreign body reaction with sheets of histiocytes and multinucleated foreign body giant cells can also be present (Figure 29-11). Potential pitfalls for false-positive cytologic diagnosis occur when significant inflammatory atypia of ductal cells or a repair pattern is present, as well as squamous atypia and fragments of exuberant granulation tissue (see Figure 29-11).[18,73-75] The

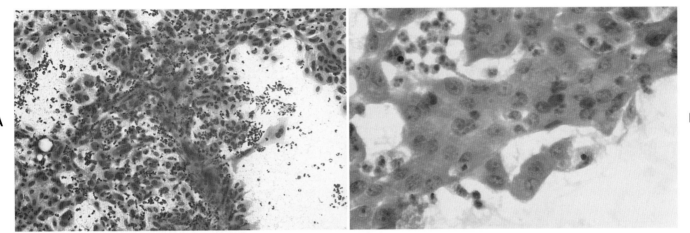

Figure 29-6   Acute mastitis with inflammatory atypia. In these aspirates of acute mastitis, atypical ductal cells are present, including some showing binucleation with nucleoli. Overlapping of the nuclei is evident, but a conservative diagnostic approach is warranted whenever neutrophils are present in the background and infiltrating the epithelial cell groups. (DQ)

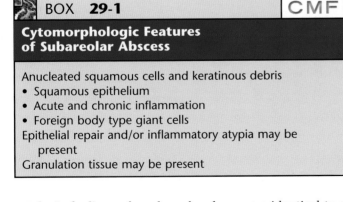

A

B

Figure 29-7   Acute mastitis with repair. In this aspirate of acute mastitis, some of the ductal cells show features of repair characterized by groups of cells arranged in flat streaming sheets with maintenance of cell borders and polarity. Occasional neutrophils are also seen intimately associated with the epithelial cells, prompting a conservative interpretation. (**A,** DQ; **B,** Pap)

BOX   **29-1**   C M F

**Cytomorphologic Features
of Subareolar Abscess**

Anucleated squamous cells and keratinous debris
• Squamous epithelium
• Acute and chronic inflammation
• Foreign body type giant cells
Epithelial repair and/or inflammatory atypia may be
   present
Granulation tissue may be present

---

cytologic findings of a subareolar abscess are identical to a ruptured epidermal inclusion cyst arising in a peripheral portion of the breast (Box 29-1). If a central subareolar lesion is aspirated, a definitive diagnosis of subareolar abscess should be made since the appropriate curative treatment is

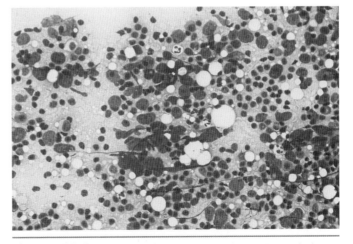

Figure 29-8   Plasma cell mastitis. In this aspirate of plasma cell mastitis, numerous lymphocytes of varying size are present along with a few scattered plasma cells. (DQ)

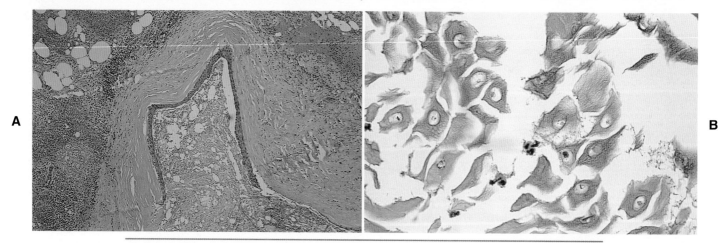

Figure 29-9 Subareolar abscess. **A,** Subareolar abscess is characterized by squamous metaplasia of the lactiferous ducts, which results in obstruction when the lumen is filled with keratinous debris. Subsequent rupture of the keratinous material into the surrounding stroma results in a foreign body reaction, along with acute and chronic inflammation and fibrosis. (H&E) **B,** Anucleated squamous cells in the lumen of a lactiferous duct. (H&E)

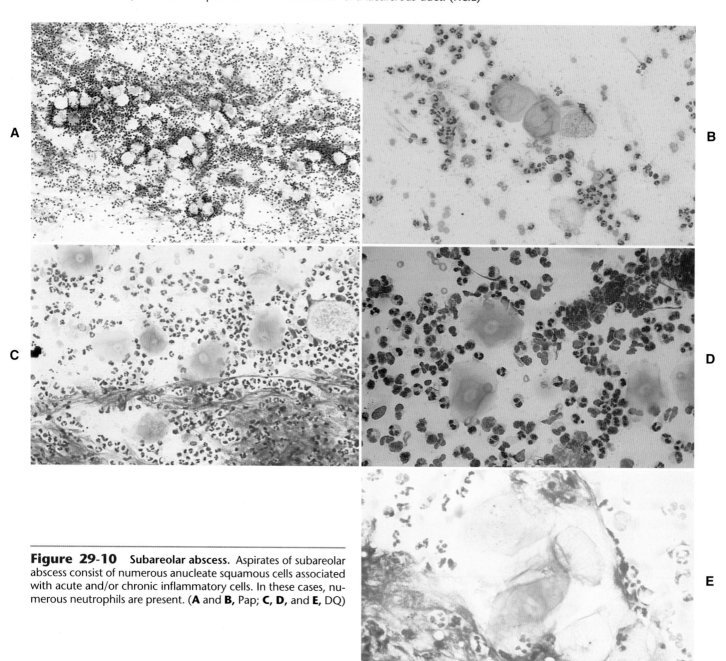

Figure 29-10 Subareolar abscess. Aspirates of subareolar abscess consist of numerous anucleate squamous cells associated with acute and/or chronic inflammatory cells. In these cases, numerous neutrophils are present. (**A** and **B,** Pap; **C, D,** and **E,** DQ)

complete surgical excision of the abscess, sinus tract, and dilated lactiferous duct, although early lesions may be treated by aspiration of the purulent material plus antibiotic therapy.[73]

Granulomas. Granulomatous lesions of the breast can be due to a variety of factors including sarcoidosis, infections (e.g., tuberculosis, fungi, leprosy, or brucellosis), reaction to tumor, fat necrosis, foreign body reaction and idiopathic granulomatous mastitis.[76-81] Rarely, a malignancy can elicit a granulomatous response. Granulomatous lesions can clinically and radiologically mimic carcinoma.[82] Aspiration cytology of granulomas is characterized by the presence of clusters of epithelioid histiocytes and multinucleated giant cells along with lymphocytes and plasma cells (Figure 29-12). Characteristically, epithelioid histiocytes have elongated, folded to bent nuclei with ill-defined cytoplasm. Specific clues to the origin of the granulomatous process

can occasionally be found in the smears. When anucleated squamous cells are present, subareolar abscess should be suspected. Lipophages are present in fat necrosis, whereas sarcoid-type granulomas usually show tight clusters of epithelioid histiocytes with peripherally located lymphocytes and no background necrosis. In addition to routine smears, special stains for fungi and mycobacteria can be useful in diagnosing a specific infectious cause, and obtaining material for culture is often of value. Our experience with fungal mastitis due to blastomycosis indicates that this condition can clinically and mammographically mimic breast carcinoma. Foreign body material associated with granulomatous inflammation can occasionally be appreciated with polarization. Silicone granulomas can be suspected when histiocytes are present and contain empty, perfectly round vacuoles and amorphous nonstaining material in DQ-stained smears.[76] However, a specific diagnosis cannot be rendered. It has been suggested that in cytologic reports the

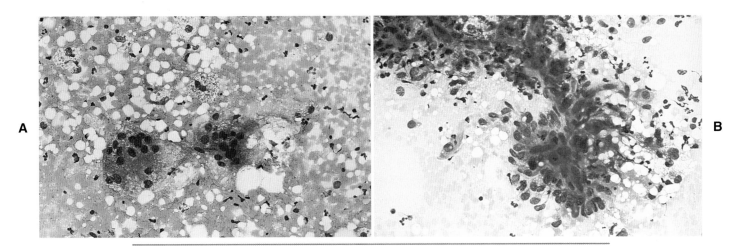

Figure 29-11 **Subareolar abscess with foreign body reaction and granulation tissue.** **A,** Aspirate of subareolar abscess in which multinucleated foreign body type giant cells reacting to keratinous material are seen along with scattered inflammatory cells in the background. (DQ) **B,** Fragment of inflamed granulation tissue consisting of capillary-type channels with swollen endothelial cells admixed with histiocytes and neutrophils. The enlarged endothelial cells can be a potential source for a false-positive diagnosis of malignancy. (DQ)

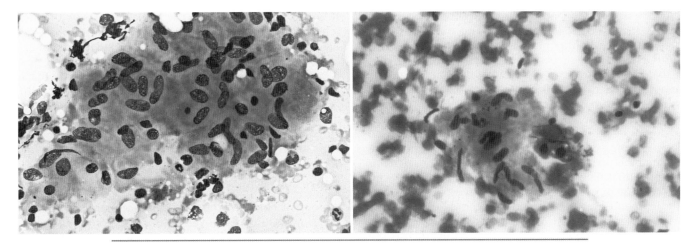

Figure 29-12 **Granuloma.** In these DQ-stained smears, clusters of epithelioid cells are arranged in a syncytial fashion and have oval to slightly bent nuclei and amphophilic cytoplasm.

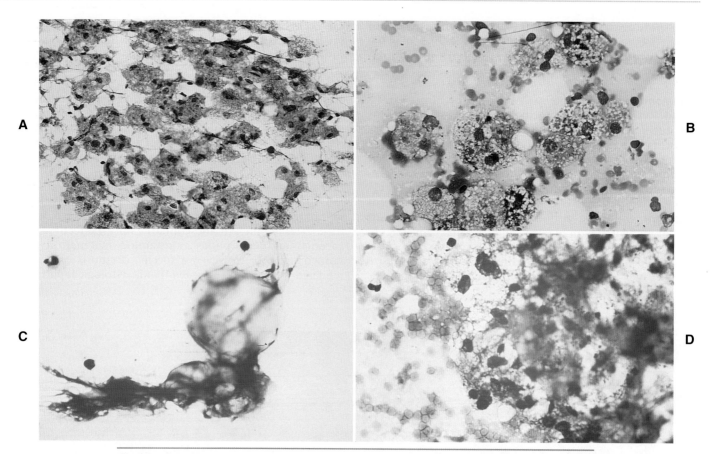

Figure 29-13 Fat necrosis. In aspirates of fat necrosis, necrotic and degenerating adipocytes are present along with numerous lipid-laden histiocytes. (**A**, Pap; **B**, **C**, and **D**, DQ)

term *granulomatous mastitis* should be avoided because a specific etiologic factor may not always be ascertained and the noncommittal term *granulomatous lesion of the breast* can be substituted.[83]

Fat Necrosis. Fat necrosis is another benign lesion that can radiologically, clinically, and histologically (especially at the time of frozen section) simulate malignancy. Only a minority of patients will give a history of trauma. With FNA biopsy, fat and amorphous debris, including degenerating adipocytes plus inflammatory cells such as neutrophils, plasma cells, lymphocytes, and numerous lipid-laden macrophages (lipophages) are seen (Figure 29-13). Multinucleated foreign body-type macrophages and spindle-shaped fibroblasts can also be present. The differential diagnosis of fat necrosis includes a breast carcinoma possessing cells with clear cytoplasm. However, lipophages have more delicate, eccentrically placed, reniform nuclei and do not tend to aggregate, in contrast with the more cohesive grouping of malignant epithelial cells in carcinoma. The rare hibernoma of the breast can also be considered in the differential diagnosis when finely and coarsely vacuolated cells are present in the smears.[84] Myospherulosis, possibly representing a sequela of fat necrosis, has been reported in FNA biopsy.[85] The diagnosis is made when a cluster of spherules measuring 4 to 7 microns each is present, simulating a "bag of marbles." These structures represent red blood cells altered by contact with lipid. The

spherules can be either scattered individually or arranged in characteristic saclike structures.

Lipomas

Adipocytes are the most common cellular elements appreciated in breast aspiration biopsies. This fact and the rarity of true lipomas of the breast should cause great reluctance in making an unequivocal diagnosis of a breast lipoma in FNA biopsy. The presence of only fat in the smears is usually due to inadequate sampling of the palpable mass, with the fat representing inadvertent aspiration of the surrounding non-diagnostic adipose tissue. Although individual adipocytes are present in smears, most are present in tight aggregates. It is only when a circumscribed, soft, freely movable mass is present, having mammographic features consistent with a lipoma, that this diagnosis should be suggested. The confidence level of making a diagnosis of lipoma is increased when the aspirator is the same person interpreting the cytologic material and evaluating the mammographic findings.

Fibrocystic Change

Fibrocystic change is the most common lesion to produce a breast mass in women over age 30. Up to 50% of American women have palpable "lumpiness" and up to 90% show histologic changes. The lesions are generally multifocal and bilateral. Fibrocystic change is much more commonly seen

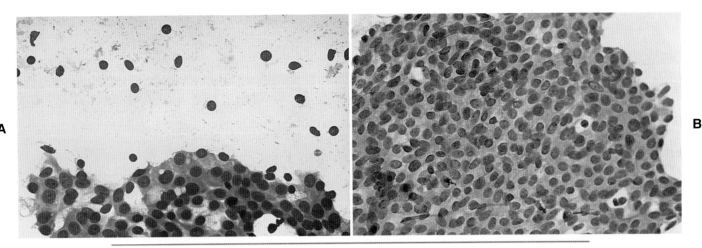

Figure 29-14 Fibrocystic change. **A,** In this DQ-stained smear, a flat sheet of epithelial cells is present having oval nuclei with a moderate amount of cytoplasm along with scattered oval, darkly staining, stripped nuclei (bipolar naked nuclei) derived from myoepithelial cells. **B,** In this Pap-stained smear, a flat sheet of uniform ductal cells is present having oval, finely granular cytoplasm without discernable nucleoli along with some interspersed, spindled, hyperchromatic smaller nuclei corresponding to the myoepithelial cells.

than cancer and thus is the most common palpable lesion sampled by either FNA or surgical biopsy. The histologic components of fibrocystic change includes dilatation of ducts, possibly resulting from periductal scarring, causing cysts associated with apocrine metaplasia, stromal fibrosis, chronic inflammation, and varying degrees of ductal hyperplasia.[64] Aspiration cytology of fibrocystic change often produces smears with limited cellularity because of the background fibrosis.[57] In Linsk and Franzen's FNA series of fibrocystic change, 82% of 210 cases showed few or no cells,[86] whereas Kline reported 47% of 214 cases having limited cellularity.[57]

In aspirates of fibrocystic change, the epithelial groups are arranged in flat, cohesive, honeycomb sheets of cells with round to oval nuclei, finely granular uniformly dispersed chromatin, and inconspicuous to very small nucleoli (Figure 29-14). Apocrine cells can be arranged in flat sheets, or occasionally, singly, and are characterized by abundant granular cytoplasm and larger, more hyperchromatic nuclei with prominent nucleoli (Figure 29-15). These cells might be potentially worrisome because of their larger nuclei and prominent nucleoli, but abundant granular cytoplasm and the resulting low N:C ratios, as well as preserved cohesion, should lead to recognition of benign apocrine cells. Foam cells and stromal fragments can also be present (Figure 29-16). An exceedingly important finding for the recognition of benign fibrocystic change and an excellent cytologic marker of benignity in general is the presence of stripped (naked) bipolar nuclei.[12,15,25] These cells have uniform hyperchromatic to smudged nuclear chromatin without nucleoli. Although some wispy bipolar cytoplasmic tags can be present, these cells are often completely stripped of cytoplasm (Box 29-2). Their nuclei are approximately 1½ times the size of a red blood cell.

Bipolar nuclei are often said to be derived from myoepithelial cells[87]; however, some consider them to be fibroblasts from the interlobular connective tissue because they do not react with antibodies specific for myoepithelial

> **BOX 29-2** CMF
>
> **Cytomorphologic Features of Nonproliferative Fibrocystic Change**
>
> Low epithelial cellularity
> Flat, honeycomb epithelial sheets with uniform small nuclei, low nuclear to cytoplasmic ratios, no loss of polarity, and distinct cell borders
> Bipolar stripped nuclei within epithelial groups and in background
> Foam cells and/or apocrine cells
> Fat and collagenous stromal tissue fragment

cells such as smooth muscle myosin and calponin.[88] However, because they are bereft of cytoplasm, tests for many markers of differentiation would be expected to give negative results. Conceptualizing these cells or myoepithelial is not without diagnostic utility, as any epithelial proliferation confined to a myoepithium-lined space cannot represent an invasive carcinoma. Further investigation of these cells' nature will depend on DNA analyses. We and others habitually refer to these naked nuclei as if their myoepithelial origin were proven. The presence of bipolar naked nuclei is not unique to fibrocystic change because they can be seen in a variety of other benign breast lesions and are especially numerous in fibroadenomas. Also present in fibrocystic change are fragments of fibrous tissue and adipocytes.

Various degrees of epithelial proliferation occur in fibrocystic change, reflecting ductal hyperplasia, sclerosing adenosis, collagenous spherulosis, and atypical ductal hyperplasia (ADH).[87-96] In FNA cytology of the proliferative lesions, increased numbers of cohesive ductal cell groups and bipolar naked nuclei are present (Figure 29-17 and

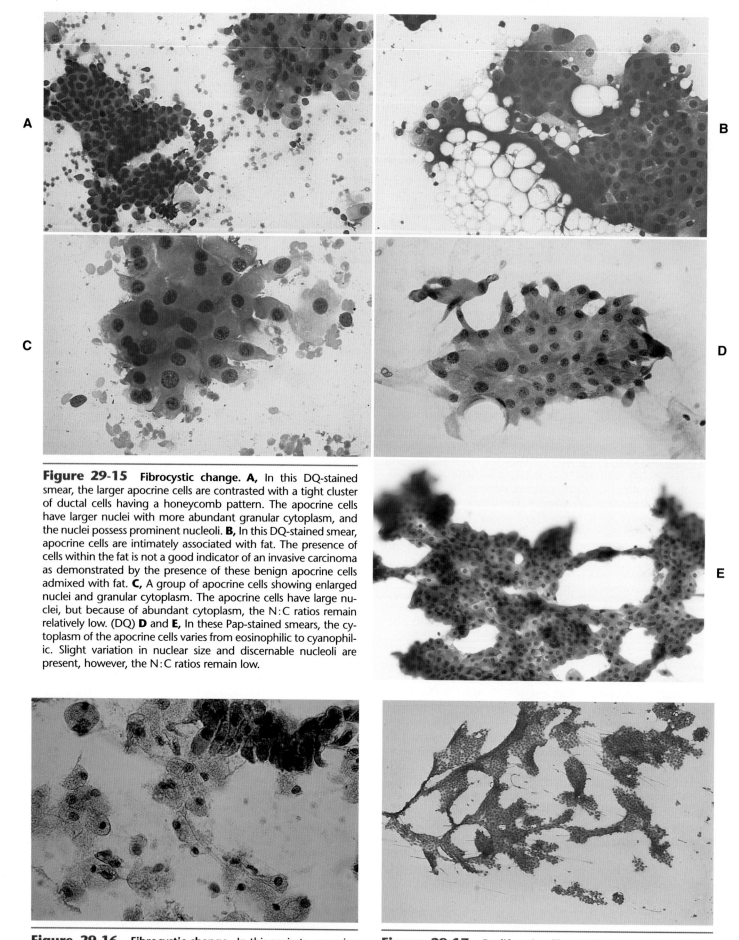

Figure 29-15 **Fibrocystic change. A,** In this DQ-stained smear, the larger apocrine cells are contrasted with a tight cluster of ductal cells having a honeycomb pattern. The apocrine cells have larger nuclei with more abundant granular cytoplasm, and the nuclei possess prominent nucleoli. **B,** In this DQ-stained smear, apocrine cells are intimately associated with fat. The presence of cells within the fat is not a good indicator of an invasive carcinoma as demonstrated by the presence of these benign apocrine cells admixed with fat. **C,** A group of apocrine cells showing enlarged nuclei and granular cytoplasm. The apocrine cells have large nuclei, but because of abundant cytoplasm, the N:C ratios remain relatively low. (DQ) **D** and **E,** In these Pap-stained smears, the cytoplasm of the apocrine cells varies from eosinophilic to cyanophilic. Slight variation in nuclear size and discernable nucleoli are present, however, the N:C ratios remain low.

Figure 29-16 **Fibrocystic change.** In this aspirate, apocrine cells have a more columnar shape and an eosinophilic hue to the cytoplasm. Numerous finely to coarsely vacuolated foam cells are also present. (Pap)

Figure 29-17 **Proliferative fibrocystic change.** In aspirates of proliferative fibrocystic change, numerous groups of ductal cells can be appreciated as demonstrated in this low-power view. (DQ)

Box 29-3). Aspirates of proliferative breast lesions can potentially serve as sources for false-positive diagnoses of malignancy when the smears are hypercellular and contain groups of ductal cells with mild nuclear overlap and slight loss of polarity.[74] Admixed apocrine cells demonstrating anisonucleosis and large nucleoli are additional sources of false-positive diagnoses. The benign nature of these proliferative breast lesions, however, should be suspected when a polymorphic population of cells is present, including apocrine, ductal, and histiocytic cells and especially numerous bipolar, naked nuclei in the background and within the cellular groups (Figure 29-18).[74] FNA cytology is generally limited in its ability to subclassify proliferative breast lesions and should not be used for risk assessment.[90,93]

Collagenous spherulosis is a benign breast lesion usually seen as an incidental finding associated with either intra-ductal papilloma, sclerosing adenosis, or radial scar.[15] Collagenous spherulosis is characterized histologically by the presence of acellular eosinophilic and fibrillary spherules, surrounded by a proliferation of bland, round to oval myoepithelial cells.[15] The aspirates contain scattered metachromatically staining hyaline globules, which are best seen in DQ smears, where they are associated with numerous benign ductal cells (Figure 29-19).[15] The major diagnostic entity in the differential diagnosis is adenoid cystic carcinoma (Figure 29-20).[91] The distinction between the benign collagenous spherulosis and the low-grade malignant adenoid cystic carcinoma is facilitated by knowledge of the clinical and histologic findings of these lesions. Collagenous spherulosis is usually an incidental finding of microscopic dimensions, and adenoid cystic carcinoma of the breast almost always presents as a suspicious palpable mass.[91] Collagenous spherulosis is confined to intralobular ductules, whereas adenoid cystic carcinoma is an invasive malignancy characterized by the presence of small duct-like spaces containing Alcian blue-positive material lined by epithelial cells. The extracellular basement membrane-type material of adenoid cystic carcinoma lacks the fibrillary appearance associated with collagenous spherulosis. The spherules of adenoid cystic carcinoma are surrounded by epithelial cells rather than the flattened myoepithelial cells in collagenous spherulosis.[91] Although a less likely consideration in the differential diagnosis, intracellular mucin in the rare intraductal signet ring carcinoma could be mistaken for the basement membrane material of collagenous spherulosis. Appreciation of the eccentrically placed atypi-

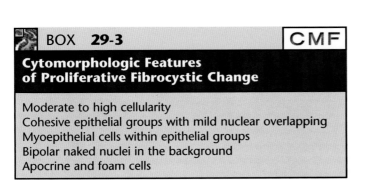

BOX 29-3   **CMF**

Cytomorphologic Features of Proliferative Fibrocystic Change

Moderate to high cellularity
Cohesive epithelial groups with mild nuclear overlapping
Myoepithelial cells within epithelial groups
Bipolar naked nuclei in the background
Apocrine and foam cells

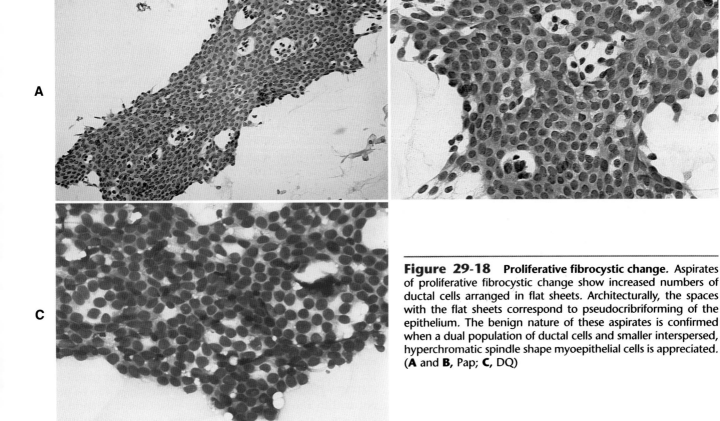

A   B   C

Figure 29-18 **Proliferative fibrocystic change.** Aspirates of proliferative fibrocystic change show increased numbers of ductal cells arranged in flat sheets. Architecturally, the spaces with the flat sheets correspond to pseudocribriforming of the epithelium. The benign nature of these aspirates is confirmed when a dual population of ductal cells and smaller interspersed, hyperchromatic spindle shape myoepithelial cells is appreciated. (**A** and **B**, Pap; **C**, DQ)

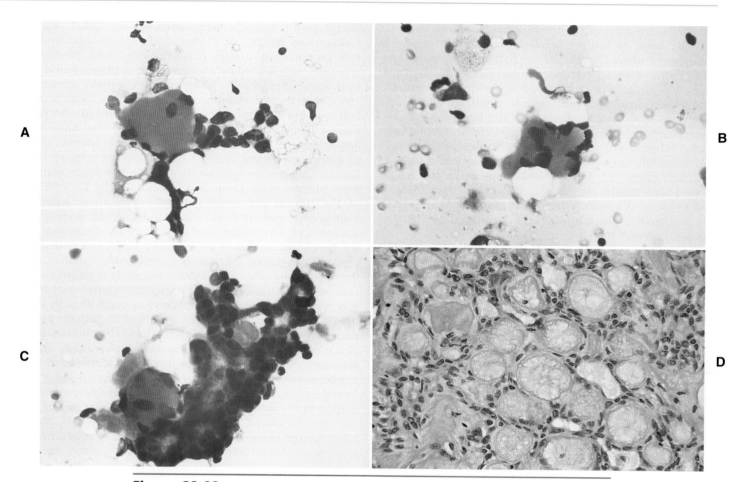

Figure 29-19 Collagenous spherulosis. **A** to **C,** In these DQ-stained smears, acellular eosinophilic hyaline globules are surrounded by spindle-shaped epithelial cells and some uniform ductal cells. **D,** Histologic examination of collagenous spherulosis demonstrates acellular eosinophilic and fibrillary spherules surrounded by a proliferation of bland, round to oval myoepithelial cells. (H&E)

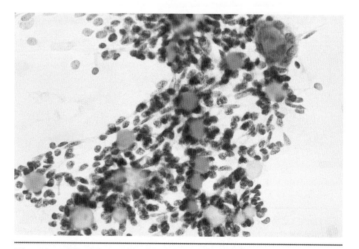

Figure 29-20 Adenoid cystic carcinoma. In this Pap-stained smear, small duct-like spaces are present containing amorphous cylinders surrounded by mildly atypical epithelial cells.

cal nuclei displaced by the intracellular mucin vacuole should allow a correct diagnosis of intraductal signet ring carcinoma. Secretory carcinoma of the breast contains grape-like clusters of vacuolated cells possessing inspissated, irregular-shaped mucus that could potentially be confused with the spherules of collagenous spherulosis.[92]

Atypical Ductal Hyperplasia

Intraductal epithelial proliferations of the breast represent a spectrum ranging from intraductal hyperplasia without atypia (conventional duct hyperplasia [CDH]) to atypical duct hyperplasia (ADH) to DCIS.[93] Quantitatively, CDH can be mild, moderate, or florid, depending on the degree of epithelioid proliferation and duct distension. Since Dupont and Page's studies correlating the relative risk of breast carcinoma with the degree of intraductal epithelial proliferation and atypia,[94-98] the ability of FNA cytology to identify and differentiate these lesions has been questioned.[19-22] The need to classify these proliferative breast lesions is more than an academic issue because of the increasing number of proliferative breast lesions detected with screening mammography.[97,98] It is generally agreed that aspirates from nonproliferative fibrocystic change are often scanty to mildly cellular, consisting of flat groups and sheets of uniform cells arranged in a honeycomb fashion and associated with bipolar nuclei within the groups and in the background.[93,99,100] Moderate and florid ductal hyperplasias are generally more cellular with cohesive crowded groups of epithelial cells showing regular to irregular cell spacing, but importantly, showing bipolar naked nuclei.[93,99,100] Some variations in cell size and shape can be present within the groups but single, intact atypical epithelial cells are generally not present or are very few in number. Although in one study a swirling pattern of the epithelial

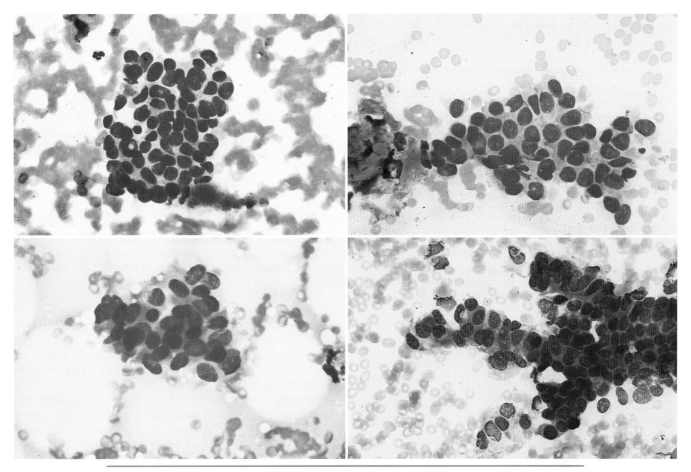

Figure 29-21 **Atypical ductal hyperplasia.** In these DQ-stained smears from aspirates of fibrocystic change having foci of atypical ductal hyperplasia, crowded groups of ductal cells show nuclear overlapping. Although the nuclei can have atypical features, the presence of interspersed smaller bipolar naked nuclei should prompt a benign diagnosis.

cells was more often seen in proliferative breast disease without atypia than in nonproliferative breast disease, no significant distinguishing features were identified between these two types of benign breast lesions.[19]

Aspirates of ADH are generally highly cellular and contain crowded groups of cells demonstrating both bland and atypical features (Figure 29-21).[93,99,100] The cells from aspirates of ADH tend to show considerable variation in cell size and shape as well as some loss of polarity within the groups. Some epithelial cell nuclei demonstrate a greater degree of hyperchromasia, and nucleoli can be appreciated. Occasional single atypical epithelial cells can also be present; however, in contrast with DCIS, bipolar naked nuclei are present in ADH (Box 29-4). Sneige and Staerkel[101] have presented criteria for the diagnosis of proliferative epithelial lesions of the breast, based on both architectural and cytologic features, in an attempt to separate CDH from ADH and ADH from DCIS. These investigators suggest that aspirates from CDH show groups of epithelial cells mixed with myoepithelial cells and stromal cells arranged in a complex or pseudocribriform pattern.[101] The epithelial cells have oval to round nuclei, with a bland chromatin pattern. Cell streaming, with overlapping nuclei and tapered intercellular bridges, was found to be a feature of ductal hyperplasia. A few single epithelial cells were also noted. In contrast, aspirates of ADH show a monotonous atypical epithelial cell population with hyperchromatic nuclei. A variable number

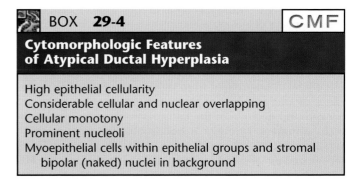

BOX 29-4 CMF

Cytomorphologic Features of Atypical Ductal Hyperplasia

High epithelial cellularity
Considerable cellular and nuclear overlapping
Cellular monotony
Prominent nucleoli
Myoepithelial cells within epithelial groups and stromal bipolar (naked) nuclei in background

of individually scattered atypical cells was noted in the background, but importantly, epithelial fragments containing myoepithelial cells in addition to the atypical cells were also found. Thus, in ADH, it has been suggested that a greater spectrum of appearances is seen than in CDH, but obvious malignant attributes are lacking. However, with few exceptions,[102] most experts believe that FNA cytology cannot reliably distinguish ADH from the noncomedo types of DCIS.[93,101] Whenever ADH or DCIS, noncomedo type is suggested by the cytologic findings, surgical biopsy confirmation is needed for definitive diagnosis because the cytologic features of both lesions overlap. Although most investigators believe that it is not possible to reliably distinguish

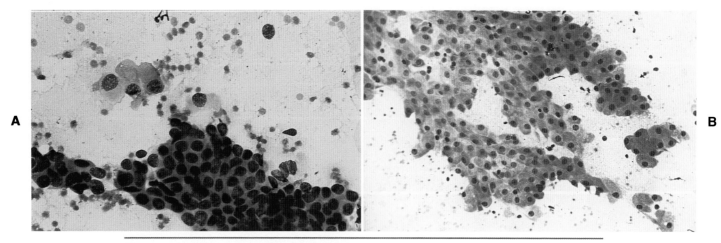

Figure 29-22 **Juvenile papillomatosis.** In this aspirate of a young patient with juvenile papillomatosis, numerous groups of both ductal cells and apocrine cells are seen along with a few scattered bipolar naked nuclei. (**A** and **B**, DQ)

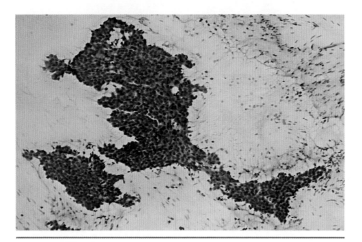

Figure 29-23 **Fibroadenoma.** In this aspirate, large flat sheets of ductal cells along with numerous bipolar naked nuclei are present. (Pap)

ADH from noncomedo types of DCIS,* both lesions can usually be differentiated from the comedo type of DCIS because of the presence of markedly pleomorphic cells and background necrosis in the latter.

In summary, cytology is not reliable for diagnosis and subclassification of proliferative breast disease. Aspirates recognized as "atypical" should lead to surgical biopsy. The physiologic variability in breast epithelial cells is too great for meaningful interpretation of minor alterations. In keeping with NCI guidelines, one may suggest that atypia is "probably benign" or "probably malignant." However, this does little to alleviate the need for surgical biopsy confirmation of worrisome cytologic findings.

Juvenile Papillomatosis

Juvenile papillomatosis is a proliferative breast lesion that occurs almost exclusively in young women from 10 to 40 years of age with a mean of 21 years.[15,103] In older individuals, its distinction from fibrocystic change may be prob-

lematic. Patients present with a discrete breast mass not unlike a fibroadenoma, but aspiration produces cyst fluid. Cytologic findings include moderately cellular smears containing numerous apocrine cells and bipolar naked nuclei in the background (Figure 29-22).[15] Juvenile papillomatosis is believed to be a marker of increased risk of breast carcinoma for the patient's family and indicates the need for continual long term follow-up of patients with this lesion.[103] Given one's expectations of high metabolic activity and cellularity in the breast tissue of young women, this diagnosis is likely to remain elusive in cytologic samples.

Clinical judgment regarding any mass that may represent must guide management decisions.

Benign Breast Neoplasms and Lesions that Simulate Benign Neoplasms

Fibroadenoma

Fibroadenoma is the most common breast neoplasm, occurring in all age groups, but it is especially seen in young women from 20 to 35 years of age.[104] In contrast with the ill-defined nature of fibrocystic change, fibroadenomas are movable, discrete tumors generally measuring less than 4 cm in maximum dimension. The term *breast mice* has been used to describe these highly mobile nodules. At the time of FNA, considerable effort may be required to stabilize the needle target. Although a single lesion is most often present, up to 20% of patients can have multiple lesions. Fibroadenomas often increase in size with pregnancy because of superimposed lactational changes.

FNA of a fibroadenoma generally produces hypercellular smears consisting of large groups of epithelial cells arranged in tightly cohesive, flat, honeycomb sheets and three-dimensional aggregates (Figure 29-23). An exception to this rule occurs when hyalinized. Lesions are encountered in older patients. Bottles and colleagues, using logistic regression analysis, found that cellular smears containing branching "stag horn" clusters of the epithelial cells associated with stromal fragments were highly characteristic but not totally specific for the diagnosis of fibroadenoma (Figure 29-24).[105] Within the sheets, epithelial cells are associated with numerous bipolar nuclei, and the naked nuclei are also found free in the background (Figure 29-25).[13,105]

*References 1, 23, 93, 99, 100, and 102.

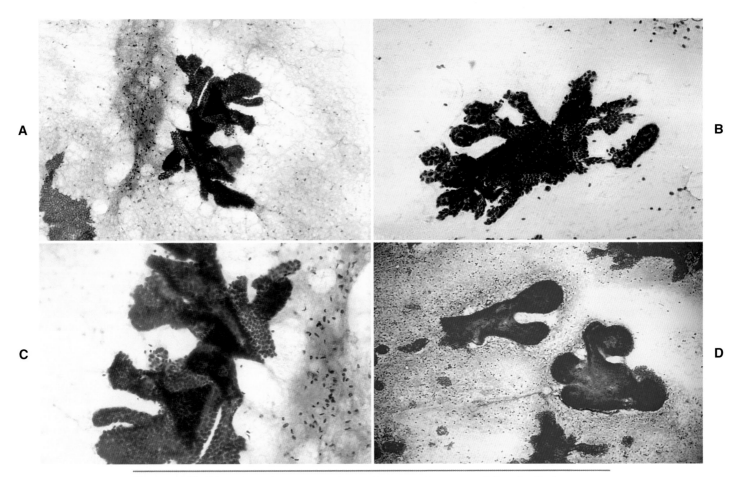

Figure 29-24   Fibroadenoma. Aspirates often contain groups of ductal cells demonstrating bulbous type branching, corresponding to a so-called "antler-horn" pattern. (**A, B,** and **C,** Pap; **D,** DQ)

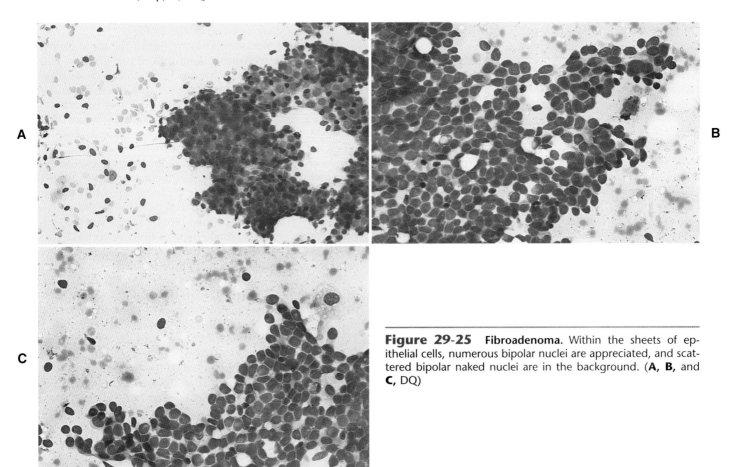

Figure 29-25   Fibroadenoma. Within the sheets of epithelial cells, numerous bipolar nuclei are appreciated, and scattered bipolar naked nuclei are in the background. (**A, B,** and **C,** DQ)

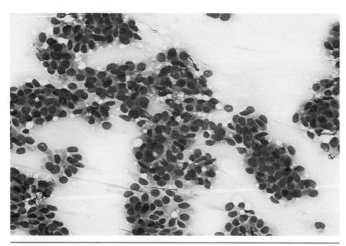

Figure 29-26 Fibroadenoma. In this low-power DQ-stained smear, the high cellularity in an aspirate of fibroadenoma can be a potential source for a false-positive diagnosis of malignancy.

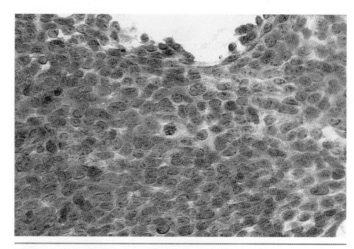

Figure 29-27 Fibroadenoma. In this aspirate, numerous ductal cells are present showing nuclear overlapping. A mitotic figure is present in the center of the field. However, the presence of scattered bipolar naked nuclei should prompt a benign interpretation. (Pap)

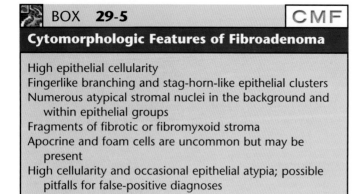

BOX 29-5   CMF

Cytomorphologic Features of Fibroadenoma

High epithelial cellularity
Fingerlike branching and stag-horn-like epithelial clusters
Numerous atypical stromal nuclei in the background and within epithelial groups
Fragments of fibrotic or fibromyxoid stroma
Apocrine and foam cells are uncommon but may be present
High cellularity and occasional epithelial atypia; possible pitfalls for false-positive diagnoses

Stromal fragments, stag horn clusters, and marked cellularity were the three most helpful cytologic features in distinguishing fibroadenoma from fibrocystic change in the analysis of Bottles and colleagues (Box 29-5).[105] Dejmek and Lindholm applied Bottles and colleagues' criteria to their series of fibroadenomas and found that stromal fragments were present in only 57% of the cases, stag horn clusters in 90%, and honeycomb sheets in 81%.[106]

Aspiration of fibrocystic change and fibroadenomas show the same range of cytologic findings. Most fibroadenomas give more cellular aspirates than most examples of fibrocystic change, but some overlap exists and occasional examples cannot be distinguished by cytology alone. However, as noted previously, the findings at physical examination (as well as the mammographic picture) are usually quite different.

Because of the high cellularity seen in some aspirates of fibroadenoma, a diagnosis of carcinoma may enter into consideration.[320] Again, honeycomb, stag horn clusters, and stroma were the most useful features in distinguishing fibroadenomas from ductal carcinoma (Figure 29-26).[105] Rarely, however, carcinoma can arise in a fibroadenoma and this seems to drive surgeons' enthusiasm for excising these otherwise innocuous lumps. Appreciation of two distinct cell populations, namely, benign-appearing ductal cells,

along with a second population of atypical pleomorphic cells, was noted in a small series by Gupta.[107] Conversely, fibroadenomas can demonstrate atypical features in FNA that could potentially mimic carcinoma.[108-110,320] Therefore, histologic examination of the fibroadenoma is necessary when atypical cells are present in smears that otherwise show cytologic features typical of fibroadenoma. The atypia, results from multifactorial causes including hormonal stimulation, inflammation, metaplastic changes, and preneoplastic atypia (Figure 29-27).[108] It has been suggested that carcinoma should only be diagnosed when multiple cytologic criteria of malignancy are satisfied in the smears.[108]

Aspirates of fibroadenomas are one of the more common sources for a false-positive diagnoses of malignancy. This is especially true when a hypercellular smear consisting of loosely cohesive cell groups shows anisonucleosis and nucleolar prominence.[74,110] The loose cohesion of the cells is often an artifact of vigorous smear preparation (Figure 29-28). However, if bipolar naked nuclei are present, especially when bordering or within the epithelial clusters, the benign nature of the lesion is suspected. Additional support for a benign cytologic diagnosis derives from correlation with the benign clinical and radiologic findings typical of fibroadenoma. A cytologic feature referred to as *benign pairs* characterized by doublets of stripped bipolar nuclei is another feature that some find characteristic of fibroadenomas.[111]

Other cytologic changes that can be appreciated in FNA smears of fibroadenomas include myxoid stroma, foam cells, apocrine cells, single cells with cytoplasm, and even mitotic figures (Figure 29-29). It has been noted that FNA of myxoid fibroadenomas often do not demonstrate groups showing the classic stag horn configuration. Therefore, the authors often integrate into their cytologic interpretations the clinical presentation of a freely movable, circumscribed, discrete mass characteristic of fibroadenoma, in contrast with the more indurated, ill-defined thickenings of fibrocystic change. These findings help us make a more specific diagnosis because both these lesions can have overlapping cytologic features. If the clinical features are not known at the time of evaluating the smears, the findings are reported

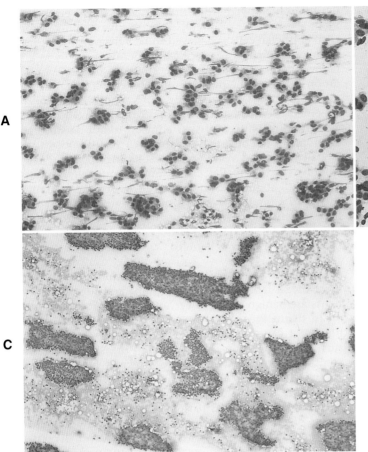

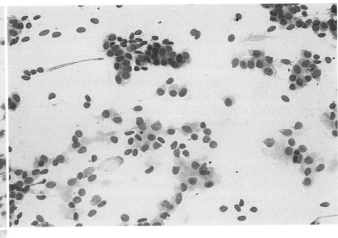

Figure 29-28   **Fibroadenoma with discohesion. A** and **B,** Vigorous smear preparation can artifactually cause cellular discohesion in aspirates of fibroadenoma, potentially leading to a false-positive diagnosis of malignancy. (DQ) **C,** In the paired smear from this aspirate, the cohesive nature of the benign epithelial cells is better appreciated. (DQ)

as benign ductal cells that are consistent with either fibroadenoma or fibrocystic change.

The stroma of myxoid fibroadenomas has been mistaken for the mucin of colloid carcinomas. The former is an organized connective tissue and the latter consists of pools of secretory material that are without form and void. Thus, in good samples, the stroma of myxoid fibroadenomas contains capillary-sized blood vessels and the mucinous lakes of colloid carcinoma do not. Because mucinous carcinomas often feature cells of very low nucleus grade, this diagnostic feature is helpful. It is also useful to recall that most patients with colloid carcinoma are considerably older than most women with fibroadenomas.

Sclerosing Adenosis and Adenosis Tumor.   Both of these lesions represent points along a spectrum of what is essentially a single pathologic process, with sclerosing adenosis appreciated as a microscopic finding and adenosis tumor forming a discrete palpable lesion. Adenosis tumor is an unusual breast mass that can be clinically and histologically confused with carcinoma, especially at the time of frozen section.[64,65] The lesion is seen in a wide age range, from 20 to 67 years with a mean of 37 years. The average size of adenosis tumor is approximately 2.5 cm. The histologic appearance of adenosis tumor recapitulates the findings seen in microscopic sclerosing adenosis. Treatment consists of local excision with close clinical follow-up.[65]

FNA cytology of adenosis tumor reveals changes of proliferative fibrocystic change with prominent stromal fibrosis.[321]

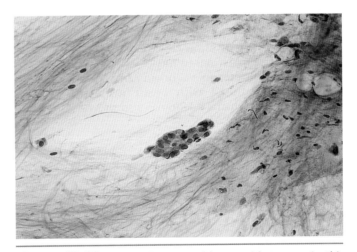

Figure 29-29   **Fibroadenoma with myxoid stroma.** In this aspirate of fibroadenoma, a benign group of epithelial cells is appreciated along with fibrillary myxoid stromal change that could potentially simulate an aspirate from a mucinous (colloid) carcinoma.

Numerous groups of uniform ductal cells, stromal fragments, and many bipolar naked nuclei are present.[65] Although a specific diagnosis of adenosis tumor is not possible in aspiration cytology, a correct interpretation of a benign proliferative breast lesion can be made. In fact, the benign nature of this lesion may be better appreciated in FNA cytology than at frozen section because of the marked distortion of the epithelial cells by the fibrous matrix in the latter preparation. Incidental sampling of sclerosing adenosis should show the same cytologic features as aspirates of adenosis tumor.[13,65]

FNA cytology of microglandular adenosis has been reported to consist of single and clustered epithelial cells with clear cytoplasm with spindled fibroblastic type cells. However, bipolar naked nuclei were not found in the two reported cases.[112] Aspirates of myoepithelioma of the breast contain cohesive clusters of spindle-shaped cells, but lack epithelial elements.[113] Adenomyoepithelioma can be a potential for a false positive diagnosis of malignancy because of the spectrum of atypical changes that can be present.[114,115] The aspirate smears are generally hypercellular and show discohesive groups of plasmacytoid-appearing cells characterized by eccentrically placed nuclei, inconspicuous nuclei, and vacuolated to clear cytoplasm. Surgical biopsy confirmation is recommended.[114,115,135] The myoepithelial nature of both myoepithelioma and adenomyoepithelioma can be confirmed with muscle actin stains.[16]

Adenomas of Several Types.   Only a few FNA reports describe tubular adenomas of the breast due to the uncommon nature of this lesion.[116,117] The cytologic features resemble a fibroadenoma[8,116,117] but may lack the stromal elements. Kumar and colleagues also noted that cohesive ball-like structures of epithelial cells and tubule formation can be present, potentially causing confusion with a tubular carcinoma.[116] However, the tubules in tubular carcinoma are more irregular in size and lack bipolar naked nuclei. In contrast, the tubules of tubular adenoma tend to be small, round, and uniform. Bipolar naked nuclei are always present.[116]

Adenomas of the nipple are benign lesions showing florid epithelial proliferation that demonstrates cytologic features identical to proliferative fibrocystic change. These cellular smear patterns show clusters of uniform ductal cells and numerous bipolar naked nuclei.[117-119]

Adenomas of skin adnexal origin can occur in the breast and can be confused with breast neoplasms. Eccrine spiradenoma and ductal adenomas also show features similar to proliferative fibrocystic change.[120] However, the intimate association of metachromatically staining stroma with epithelial cells is believed to be a diagnostic feature of ductal adenoma.[121] Clear cell hidradenoma occurs as a superficial tumor that can ulcerate the skin surface.[122] In aspiration cytology, the population of polygonal, clear to spindle-shaped cells, along with one's appreciation of the superficial dermal-based location of the lesion, should suggest the possibility of a skin adnexal tumor. Pleomorphic adenoma of the breast shows cytologic features identical to its salivary gland counterpart, including the presence of spindled myoepithelial cells, variable numbers of ductal cells, and abundant fibromyxoid matrix.[123] A common theme to aspiration cytology of all these unusual types of breast adenomas is that although a specific diagnosis cannot always be rendered, it is important to recognize these proliferative lesions as benign.

Pregnancy and Postpartum-Related Lesions.   Fortunately, most breast lesions seen in pregnant and postpartum patients are benign and result from hormonal stimulation of breast tissue. Pregnancy can produce *de novo* lactating adenomas or cause enlargement of preexisting breast lesions such as fibroadenomas. Most benign breast lesions associated with pregnancy completely regress by six months postpartum. The FNA cytologic features of lactating adenoma and fibroadenoma show similar changes, characterized by a cellular smear pattern in which a uniform population of epithelial cells is present as either individually scattered cells or as cell clusters.[13,124-129] However, in contrast with the lactating adenomas, fibroadenomas undergoing lactational change will also have numerous bipolar naked nuclei in the background, a feature not present in *de novo* lactating adenomas (Figure 29-30). The lactational change of epithelial cells in both lactating adenomas and fibroadenomas is characterized by cells having abundant, pale to vacuolated cytoplasm with frayed edges and numerous stripped epithelial nuclei (Figure 29-31). Many of the epithelial cells possess small but prominent nucleoli and the background has a dirty appearance because of the spillage of the lipid-rich secretory contents from the fragile cells. In contrast with the small bipolar, spindled, naked nuclei seen in fibroadenoma, larger, stripped, round to oval epithelial nuclei with obvious nucleoli are noted in lactating adenoma (Figure 29-32). The secretory fluid component can be demonstrated in air-dried smears or with periodic acid-Schiff (PAS) and lipid staining (Box 29-6).

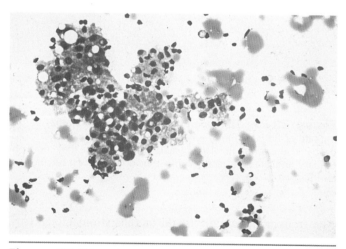

Figure 29-30   Fibroadenoma with lactational change. In this DQ-stained smear, besides the epithelial cells showing lactational changes, numerous stripped bipolar nuclei are present in the background, indicating that this is a fibroadenoma showing lactational change.

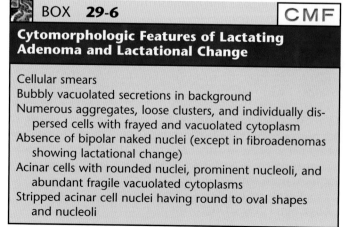

BOX 29-6   CMF

Cytomorphologic Features of Lactating Adenoma and Lactational Change

Cellular smears
Bubbly vacuolated secretions in background
Numerous aggregates, loose clusters, and individually dispersed cells with frayed and vacuolated cytoplasm
Absence of bipolar naked nuclei (except in fibroadenomas showing lactational change)
Acinar cells with rounded nuclei, prominent nucleoli, and abundant fragile vacuolated cytoplasms
Stripped acinar cell nuclei having round to oval shapes and nucleoli

A false-positive diagnosis of malignancy is possible in aspirates from lactating adenoma because of the prominent dissociative smear pattern of epithelial cells stripped of cytoplasm, coupled with large epithelial cells demonstrating nuclear enlargement and prominent nucleoli (Figure 29-33).[125] In this setting, it is important to recognize the presence of the abundant cytoplasmic secretions in the background and the lactational change of the cells reflected by cytoplasmic foaminess with fraying of the cytoplasmic borders to avoid a false-positive diagnosis of malignancy. The background material is very prominent in air-dried smears but is often nearly invisible in fixed preparations.

Second only to cervical cancer, breast carcinoma is the most commonly diagnosed malignancy in pregnant patients.[130] Although some have low-grade nuclear features, many ductal carcinomas show a greater degree of nuclear atypicality, hyperchromasia, loss of polarity, necrosis, and cellular discohesion with the presence of scattered intact abnormal cells than the atypical change in lactational lesions.[131] Galactocele consisting of abundant amorphous material with a few epithelial cells can also occur in this population. The authors encountered one case in which crystalline structures were also present in the aspirated fluid representing precipitation of protein and milk products.[15]

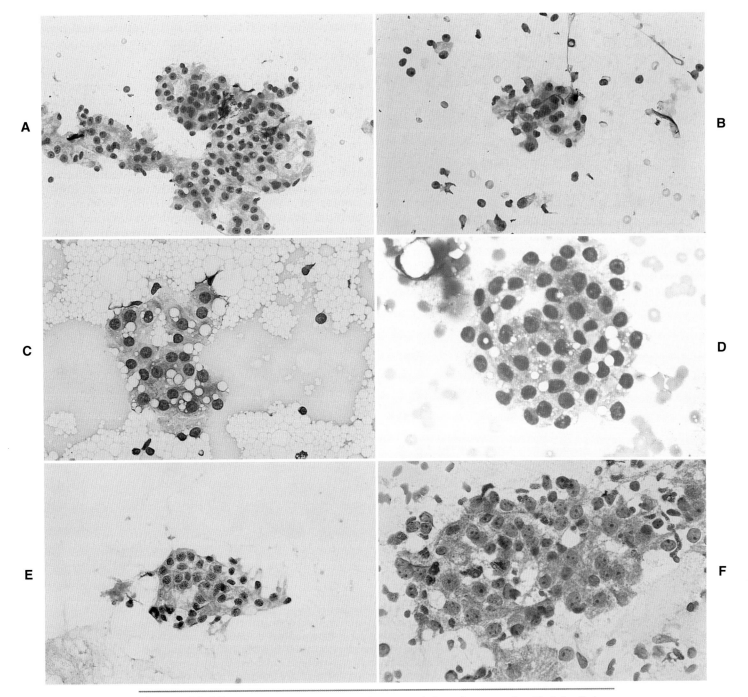

Figure 29-31 **Lactating adenoma.** Aspirates consisting of groups of epithelial cells having vacuolated, frayed cytoplasm. Coarse cytoplasmic vacuoles can be appreciated, and stripped epithelial nuclei and frothy material are in the background. (**A-C,** DQ; **D-F,** Pap)

The major advantage of FNA biopsy during pregnancy is the avoidance of surgical trauma and anesthesia, which can be an unnecessary risk to both the fetus and mother because surgery is sometimes followed by poor wound healing in the lactating breast. Another important advantage of breast FNA biopsy in the pregnant female is avoiding a delay in diagnosis, when malignancy is present.[125-132]

Granular Cell Tumor.   Granular cell tumor is an uncommon breast lesion seen more often in African-Americans

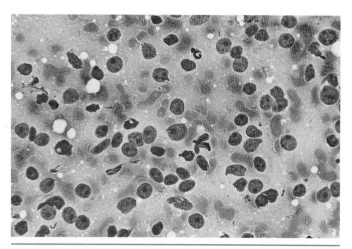

Figure 29-32   **Lactating adenoma.** Numerous stripped epithelial cell nuclei are present in this aspirate of a lactating adenoma. In contrast with naked bipolar nuclei, the stripped nuclei are derived from the epithelial cells of a lactating adenoma and are oval to round and possess prominent nucleoli. The background contains granular and frothy lipid material. (DQ)

and is often multifocal in nature.[133,134] Clinically, radiologically, and grossly granular cell tumor of the breast can mimic an infiltrating ductal carcinoma because of its ill-defined borders and associated stromal reaction. FNA cytology, however, will reveal a cellular population of scattered polygonal to spindled cells with abundant, distinctly granular cytoplasm and poorly delineated cell borders in the Romanowsky stains.[135] The tumor cells' nuclei vary from oval to round but are fairly uniform in shape, with evenly dispersed chromatin and generally inconspicuous nucleoli. The granular cells' cytoplasm stains red with the Pap stain and the granules can be accentuated with a PAS stain. A variety of immunoperoxidase stains can be used for confirmation, including S-100 and CD68 (KP-1).[136] The S-100 stain may be decreased in intensity in alcohol-fixed material.[10] Ultrastructural examination of the granules will demonstrate autophagosomes and angulate bodies.

Localized Amyloid Tumor.   Occurring predominantly in older women, localized amyloid tumor of the breast is an exceedingly rare lesion that can mammographically and clinically be confused with carcinoma.[137,138] Amyloid tumor of the breast usually occurs in three settings: secondary amyloidosis, systemic or multiple myeloma associated amyloid, or as a localized primary tumor having a benign course.[138] FNA can identify amyloid as irregular clumps of metachromatically staining homogeneous material present in the Romanowsky-stained smears and irregular cylindric fragments of refractile to glassy eosinophilic material in the alcohol-fixed Pap-stained smears. This is identical to the material illustrated in Chapter 16, in which localized pulmonary amyloidosis is considered. A few spindle-shaped cells can be present within the amyloid material and at the periphery.[138]

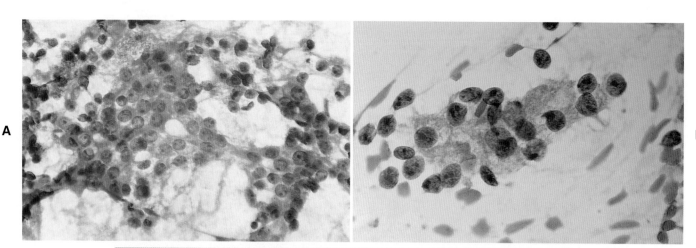

A   B

Figure 29-33   **Lactating adenoma. A,** In aspirates of some cases of lactating adenoma, the loosely cohesive nature of the epithelial cells and stripped epithelial cell nuclei possessing prominent nucleoli could be a potential source for a false-positive diagnosis of malignancy. However, the foamy vacuolated cytoplasm with frayed cytoplasmic borders of the cells and bubbly secretions in the background should prompt a benign diagnosis of lactating adenoma. (Pap) **B,** In this Pap-stained aspirate of a lactating adenoma, the nuclear enlargement with prominent nucleoli could be a potential source for a false-positive diagnosis of malignancy. However, the vacuolated frayed nature of the cytoplasm, the relatively low N:C ratios and the presence of stripped nuclei should prompt consideration for a benign diagnosis.

Osseous metaplasia and a foreign body reaction have been reported in the FNA smears of mammory amyloidosis.[139] The diagnosis can be confirmed with Congo red staining, with prior potassium permanganate incubation to identify the light chain type of amyloid. Immunofluorescence studies for immunoglobulins and electron microscopy can also be utilized.[138]

Papillomas. Solitary intraductal papillomas occur most often in women from 50 to 60 years of age. Patients often do not have a palpable mass, but rather present with a serous or bloody nipple discharge that is submitted for cytologic examination. If a papilloma is aspirated, epithelial cells arranged in tight clusters and three-dimensional groups with prominent depth of focus are appreciated (Figure 29-34). Individually scattered columnar-shaped cells and spindle-shaped stromal cells can also occasionally be present. As in histologic specimens, the major differential diagnosis is separation of a benign intraductal papilloma from a well-differentiated papillary carcinoma. Surgical excision is recommended for the definitive assessment of any papillary lesion, even those that are manifest in smear material only as a few columnar ("cyndrical") cells. Most papillary carcinomas are in-

tracystic, noninvasive, and prognostically favorable. Papillomas can also have a branching epithelial pattern in smears that prompts a differential diagnosis that includes fibroadenoma. Papillomas consist of columnar epithelial cells occasionally associated with stromal cores and increased numbers of foam cells, whereas fibroadenomas demonstrate numerous bipolar naked nuclei, a feature generally lacking in aspirates of papillomas. A rare potential source for a false-positive diagnosis of malignancy in FNA cytology is aspirates of an infarcted intraductal papilloma.[140]

Gynecomastia. Gynecomastia is a hormonally dependent mass lesion appearing most often in adolescent and older male patients. Although more often unilateral, bilateral examples occur. Gynecomastia can be classified as juvenile, idiopathic, or drug related. The latter is most often associated with digitalis, reserpine, and phenytoin-type agents. FNA cytology of gynecomastia shows changes similar to proliferative fibrocystic change with clusters of ductal and even apocrine type cells and naked bipolar nuclei (Figure 29-35).[15] The most cellular examples can mimic the FNA cytology of fibroadenomas. Aspirates from older lesions that have been present for several months may be very

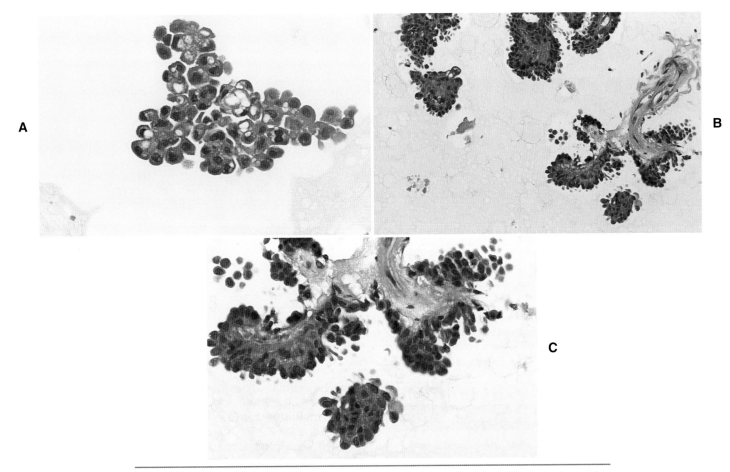

Figure 29-34 Papilloma. **A,** In this aspirate of an intraductal papilloma, a branching slightly three-dimensional cluster of benign cells is present. (Pap) **B** and **C,** Cell block from the breast aspirate reveals fibrovascular cores lined by benign ductal cells and myoepithelial cells. (H&E)

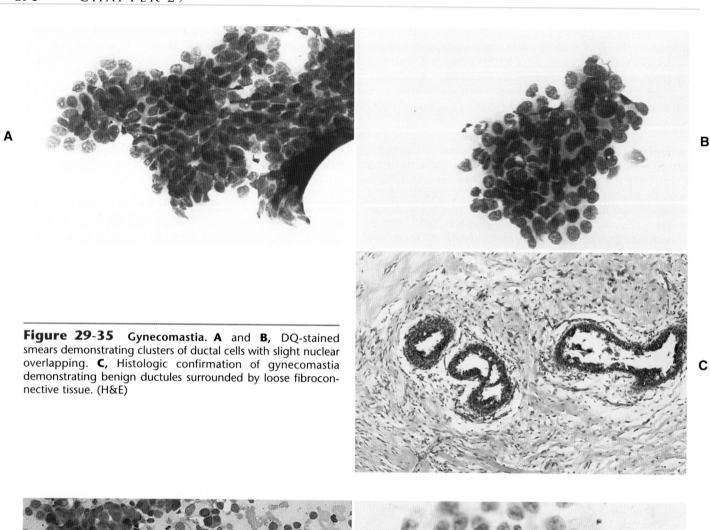

Figure 29-35 Gynecomastia. **A** and **B**, DQ-stained smears demonstrating clusters of ductal cells with slight nuclear overlapping. **C**, Histologic confirmation of gynecomastia demonstrating benign ductules surrounded by loose fibroconnective tissue. (H&E)

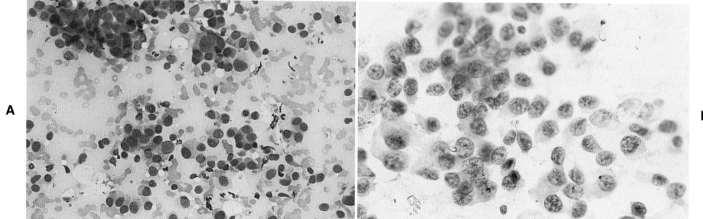

Figure 29-36 Male breast ductal carcinoma. Aspirate of ductal carcinoma from a male breast demonstrating unequivocal diagnostic features of malignancy such as individually scattered atypical cells having enlarged hyperchromatic nuclei and nucleoli. (**A**, DQ; **B**, Pap)

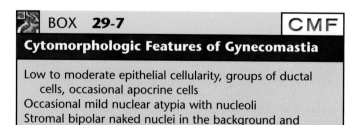

BOX **29-7**   CMF

Cytomorphologic Features of Gynecomastia

Low to moderate epithelial cellularity, groups of ductal cells, occasional apocrine cells
Occasional mild nuclear atypia with nucleoli
Stromal bipolar naked nuclei in the background and within groups of epithelial cells

sparsely cellular. The procedure will yield only a tiny droplet of clear fluid. Occasional cells may demonstrate atypia including nuclear molding and nucleolar prominence (Box 29-7).[322] A diagnosis of malignancy should be avoided in aspirates from male patients showing these atypical changes. Frankly malignant cytologic features are needed before an unequivocal diagnosis of breast cancer is made in a male patient (Figure 29-36).[141-146]

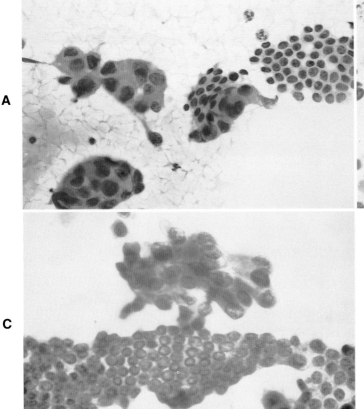

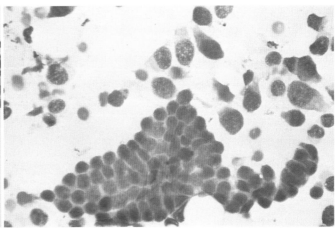

Figure 29-37 Ductal carcinoma. **A** and **B,** In these DQ-stained smears, an admixture of benign ductal cells and scattered clusters of malignant cells is present. Note the considerable enlargement of the nuclei and presence of the cells arranged in syncytial clusters and individually scattered. **C,** Comparison of benign ductal cells maintaining a honeycomb pattern with a loose cluster of malignant cells demonstrating nuclear enlargement and a syncytial arrangement of the cytoplasm with loss of polarity. (Pap)

MALIGNANT LESIONS

Ductal Carcinoma, Not Otherwise Specified

It is estimated that one in nine women will develop breast cancer and that approximately 45,000 to 50,000 women will die from this malignancy annually. Despite advances in detection and treatment, the 5-year survival for patients with established, invasive carcinoma has not significantly changed.[104] However, with the advent of mammography and radiology-guided biopsies of nonpalpable disease, approximately 20% to 30% of lesions currently detected are malignant and at least half of these are noninvasive. However, for palpable malignant lesions, the majority are invasive carcinomas. It is in this setting that FNA biopsy has its greatest value. Invasive ductal carcinoma is the most common histologic type of breast carcinoma, accounting for approximately 75% of all invasive carcinomas.[104] The 5-year survival is approximately 55% to 65%.

With few exceptions, aspirates of invasive ductal carcinoma, not otherwise specified (NOS) show cytologic features common to all breast carcinomas. Diagnostic malignant features usually include high smear cellularity with groups of loosely cohesive malignant cells and individually scattered, intact tumor cells that are usually much larger than benign ductal cells (Figure 29-37). The background can vary from bloody or necrotic to clean. The cellular smear pattern shows considerable variability with the malignant cells arranged in three-dimensional clus-

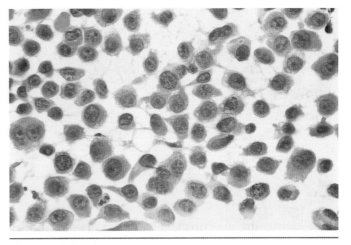

Figure 29-38 Ductal carcinoma. Numerous individually scattered malignant cells are present in this aspirate of a ductal carcinoma, not otherwise specified (NOS). (Pap)

ters, syncytial groupings, or occasionally, in acinar or gland-like patterns (Figures 29-38 and 29-39). The cells within the clusters demonstrate loss of polarity and nuclear molding. The tumor cells may show considerable variability, with most of the aspirates consisting of cells larger than normal ductal cells, but occasionally, small cancer cells can be present. The individual tumor cells demonstrate malignant cytologic features including elevated N:C ratios, hyperchromatic nuclei, nuclear mem-

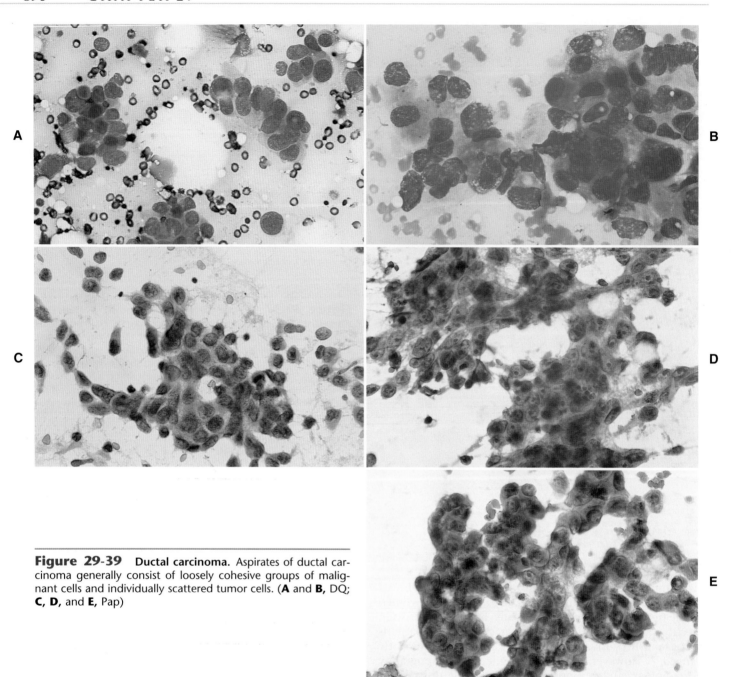

Figure 29-39 **Ductal carcinoma.** Aspirates of ductal carcinoma generally consist of loosely cohesive groups of malignant cells and individually scattered tumor cells. (**A** and **B**, DQ; **C, D,** and **E,** Pap)

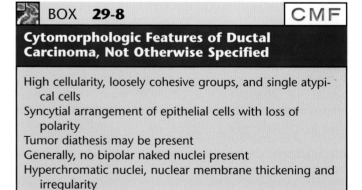

brane thickening and irregularity, and coarsely granular chromatin with small to prominent nucleoli (Box 29-8). The nuclei can be eccentrically arranged, importing a plasmacytoid appearance to the cells, which is best appreciated in DQ preparation (Figure 29-40). Although not specific, this pattern is most often seen in aspirates of ductal carcinoma from older women. In general, the cytoplasm of ductal carcinoma tends to be basophilic, finely to coarsely granular, or finely vacuolated. Occasional cases demonstrate coarse cytoplasmic vacuolization or intracellular lumina (Figure 29-41). Although seen more commonly in lobular carcinoma, signet ring cells can also be present in ductal carcinomas.[147] Occasionally, cells from infiltrating ductal carcinoma can be of a small size, overlapping with the size of cells seen in aspirates of lobular

BOX   29-8   CMF

Cytomorphologic Features of Ductal Carcinoma, Not Otherwise Specified

High cellularity, loosely cohesive groups, and single atypical cells
Syncytial arrangement of epithelial cells with loss of polarity
Tumor diathesis may be present
Generally, no bipolar naked nuclei present
Hyperchromatic nuclei, nuclear membrane thickening and irregularity
Nucleoli

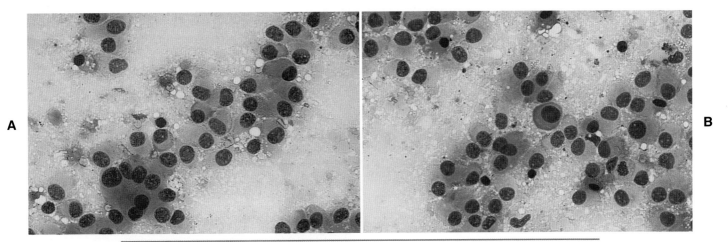

Figure 29-40   **Ductal carcinoma.** In aspirates of some cases of ductal carcinoma, the tumor cells can take on a uniform, plasmacytoid appearance best appreciated in DQ-stained smears. (**A** and **B**, DQ)

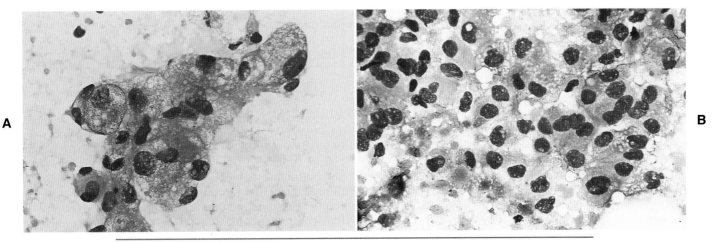

Figure 29-41   **Ductal carcinoma.** In aspirates of some examples of ductal carcinoma, the tumor cells can have a fine to coarsely vacuolated cytoplasm. (**A** and **B**, DQ)

carcinoma (Figure 29-42). However, FNA cytology can generally differentiate ductal from lobular carcinoma of the breast.[148] Usually, aspirates of infiltrating ductal carcinoma show greater cellularity with more significant pleomorphism, characterized by larger cells demonstrating hyperchromatic nuclei with more prominent nucleoli than cells of lobular carcinoma (Figure 29-43). Aspirates of poorly differentiated ductal carcinomas contain pleomorphic, bizarre cells, including multinucleated tumor cells. In general, bipolar naked nuclei and benign epithelial cells will not be seen in the smears unless the surrounding and/or admixed benign parenchyma has also been sampled. Rarely, aspirates from a carcinoma arising in a papilloma, fibroadenoma, or other benign lesions will contain both benign and malignant cellular elements.

Morphologic classification of breast carcinoma can be applied to FNA specimens. Using the classifications schema based on Fisher and World Health Organization (WHO) criteria, we advocate attempting to classify the various histologic types of invasive breast carcinoma by applying cytomorphologic criteria that parallel the histologic features.[104] We believe this is important since histologic classification

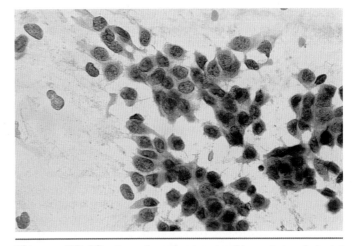

Figure 29-42   **Ductal carcinoma.** In this aspirate of ductal carcinoma, the tumor cells have a smaller size, which could cause potential diagnostic confusion with an infiltrating lobular carcinoma. However, the more hyperchromatic nature of the atypical nuclei should suggest that this is a ductal rather than a lobular carcinoma. (Pap)

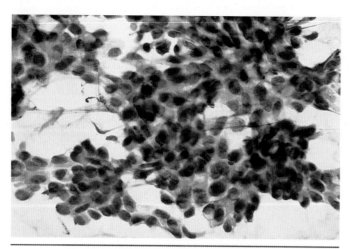

Figure 29-43 Ductal carcinoma. In this aspirate, the tumor cells have a smaller size with high N:C ratios. A diagnosis of lobular carcinoma should not be considered because of the greater degree of hyperchromasia and cellularity that is present, as demonstrated in this smear. (Pap)

---

has prognostic significance. Favorable breast carcinomas include pure mucinous (colloid) carcinoma, medullary carcinoma, tubular carcinoma, adenoid cystic carcinoma, papillary carcinoma, and secretory carcinoma. Unfavorable breast malignancies include metaplastic carcinoma, inflammatory carcinoma, pleomorphic lobular carcinoma, and sarcomas. In ductal carcinoma, NOS especially, prognostically significant nuclear grading can be applied in the cytologic material.[16] Although a morphologic classification can be suggested by the cytologic findings, final classification sometimes requires examination of the surgically resected specimen.

Intraductal Carcinoma (DCIS)

The cytology of DCIS varies according to whether a comedo or noncomedo type of DCIS has been aspirated. FNA cytology of comedo-type DCIS will reveal a cellular smear pattern consisting of loosely cohesive groups, as well as individually scattered malignant cells showing significant nuclear pleomorphism with large and multiple nucleoli as well as necrosis and mitotic figures (Box 29-9). In contrast, aspirates from noncomedo type of DCIS contain clusters and isolated single abnormal cells, and usually lack bipolar naked nuclei (Box 29-10). Surgical confirmation is required whenever ADH or DCIS, noncomedo type, is suggested by the cytologic findings.

In our experience, aspirates from the micropapillary type of DCIS often show a background of old blood and macrophages with hemosiderin. Small bits of calcified material may also be present. Rounded, three-dimensional clusters of small, uniform cells with low nuclear grade are set in this hemorrhagic background. These tissue particles are club-like, recapitulating this lesion's histology. True papillae with fibrovascular cores are not seen.

Most investigators believe it is not possible to separate in situ from invasive carcinoma definitively, but aspirates from invasive carcinoma are generally more cellular and demonstrate a greater loss of cellular cohesion (Figure 29-44).[93,149-151] Although cytologic evidence of infiltration of carcinoma into fat has been suggested as a diagnostic feature of invasion,[323] the authors concur with Maygarden and colleagues as well as others that it is not a reliable indicator but rather represents a mechanical artifact of aspiration and smear preparation.[152] Shin and Sneige reported that the presence of neoplastic tubules and stromal fragments associated with tumor cells are features of stromal invasion.[23] However, both attributes have too low an occurrence or specificity to reliably be used to separate invasive ductal carcinoma from DCIS.[23] Extensive necrosis associated with pleomorphic atypical cells is more often a feature of comedo-type DCIS than invasive ductal carcinoma, although large invasive breast carcinomas can often have extensive associated necrosis (Figure 29-45). With all of these limitations, breast malignancies of duct origin are reported as ductal carcinoma, and it is not specified whether invasive carcinoma or DCIS is present. Histologic examination is needed to distinguish reliably DCIS from an invasive ductal carcinoma.

Medullary Carcinoma

If strict diagnostic criteria are applied, medullary carcinoma is a rare entity. Medullary carcinoma usually occurs in patients in the fifth and sixth decade. Characteristically, it presents as a well-demarcated lesion. In our experience, it is this requirement of gross circumscription that keeps most high-grade, lymphocyte-rich carcinomas from meeting the definition of medullary carcinoma. Although medullary carcinoma has been thought to have a better 5- and 10-year survival than atypical medullary carcinoma or ductal carcinoma, NOS, recent studies have suggested that there is no

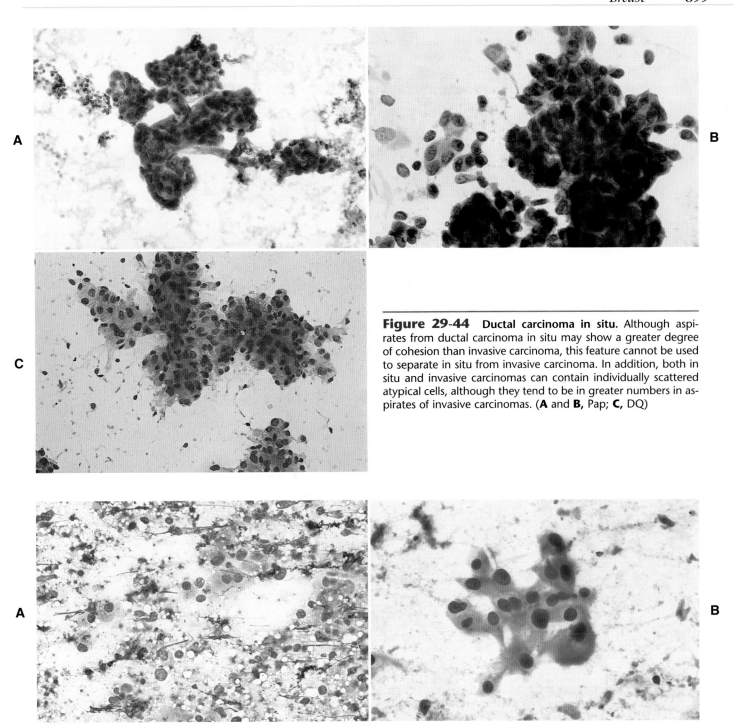

Figure 29-44 **Ductal carcinoma in situ.** Although aspirates from ductal carcinoma in situ may show a greater degree of cohesion than invasive carcinoma, this feature cannot be used to separate in situ from invasive carcinoma. In addition, both in situ and invasive carcinomas can contain individually scattered atypical cells, although they tend to be in greater numbers in aspirates of invasive carcinomas. (**A** and **B,** Pap; **C,** DQ)

Figure 29-45 **Ductal carcinoma in situ, comedo type.** In this aspirate from a comedo-type of ductal carcinoma in situ, loose clusters of individually scattered malignant cells are present along with extensive necrosis in the background. (**A,** DQ; **B,** Pap)

difference in prognosis.[153,154] The tumor is cytologically composed of syncytial sheets of poorly differentiated epithelial cells with high nuclear grade admixed with a lymphoplasmacytic infiltrate and occasionally focal necrosis (Figure 29-46). Besides the syncytial groupings of the pleomorphic cells, individually scattered malignant cells are also present. The tumor cells show considerable nuclear enlargement with variation in size and shape, thick nuclear membranes, and high N:C ratios. It is not unusual to see

tumor cells with multiple irregular macronucleoli. The cytoplasm of the malignant cells is basophilic to finely granular or can be vacuolated and can vary from scant to abundant. Large, stripped, bizarre tumor nuclei may occasionally be present (Figure 29-47). Besides the high-grade malignant cells, the other characteristic feature is an admixture of lymphocytes and some plasma cells in the smears. Occasional aspirates of medullary carcinoma may demonstrate a predominance of lymphocytes and plasma cells (Box 29-11).

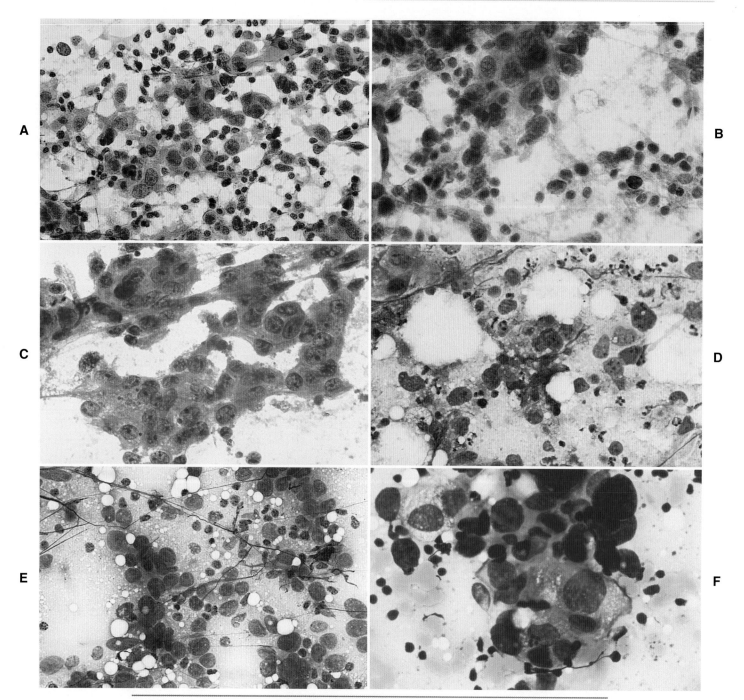

Figure 29-46   **Medullary carcinoma.** Aspirates of medullary carcinoma of the breast will consist of syncytial groupings of high nuclear grade ductal carcinoma admixed with numerous lymphocytes and plasma cells. (**A** to **C,** Pap; **D** to **F,** DQ)

Therefore, medullary carcinoma should be suspected whenever a circumscribed breast mass is aspirated, and both high-grade carcinoma cells and lymphocytes and/or plasma cells are present.[155] Finding fragments of desmoplastic fibrosis in the smears is not a feature of medullary carcinoma and should suggest that a ductal carcinoma, NOS, has been sampled in which medullary carcinoma-like features may be present. An unusual variant of medullary carcinoma is cystic medullary carcinoma, which has a potential to be misdiagnosed because it occurs in relatively young patients presenting with a cystic lesion in which there is a prominent inflammatory cell component.[156] Although medullary

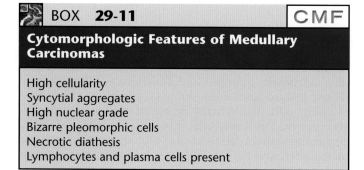

BOX   **29-11**   CMF

Cytomorphologic Features of Medullary Carcinomas

High cellularity
Syncytial aggregates
High nuclear grade
Bizarre pleomorphic cells
Necrotic diathesis
Lymphocytes and plasma cells present

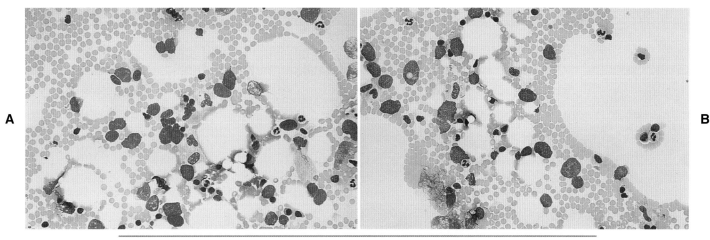

Figure 29-47 **Medullary carcinoma.** Stripped atypical nuclei in an aspirate from a medullary carcinoma. (**A** and **B**, DQ)

carcinoma can be suspected from the aspirate, the final classification should await surgical pathology examination of the resected specimen because a number of different types of breast carcinoma can have a prominent lymphoplasmacytosis in the background.[155]

Mucinous (Colloid) Carcinoma

Approximately 5% of all breast carcinomas are mucinous (colloid) carcinoma. They typically occur in older women and are associated with a better 5- to 10-year survival than the usual infiltrating duct carcinoma.[95] The three categories of mucinous carcinoma are pure, mixed, and signet ring carcinoma,[157] with the latter having the worst prognosis. Aspiration biopsy of mucinous carcinoma produces abundant gelatinous material with variable cellularity.[158-162] In the pure type of mucinous carcinoma, scattered three-dimensional clusters of tumor cells are surrounded by abundant extracellular mucinous material which stains metachromatically with the DQ stain and has an amorphous to fibrillary appearance with Pap stain (Figure 29-48). Generally, the malignant cells have low-grade (grade 1 and 2) nuclei, although tumor cells with high-grade nuclei (grade 3) can occasionally be present. Because of the relatively bland appearance of the tumor cells in some cases and the relatively low cellularity resulting from the abundant extracellular mucinous material, a false negative diagnosis is possible (Figure 29-49 and Box 29-12). The diagnosis should be suspected when extracellular mucinous material is recognized in the background and scattered mildly atypical malignant cells are present. Some connective tissue fragments may contain small vascular channels (Figure 29-50). The diagnosis is supported when the mammogram shows a smoothly outlined to lobulated mass with only a few irregularities, rather than the more stellate-shaped, infiltrating pattern of the usual type of breast cancer.[162] A corollary of this feature is that mucinous carcinoma feels soft when palpated and lacks the hard gritty texture usually encountered when needle aspiration is performed.

Mixed types of mucinous carcinoma show features of the pure variant along with cytologic findings of the more typical infiltrating ductal carcinoma.[163] The mucinous material can be highlighted with a variety of special mucin stains,

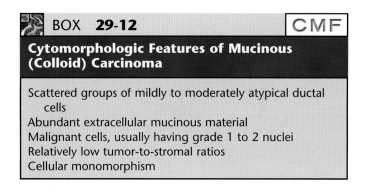

BOX 29-12 CMF

Cytomorphologic Features of Mucinous (Colloid) Carcinoma

Scattered groups of mildly to moderately atypical ductal cells
Abundant extracellular mucinous material
Malignant cells, usually having grade 1 to 2 nuclei
Relatively low tumor-to-stromal ratios
Cellular monomorphism

but this is usually not needed. Mixed carcinomas have the prognosis of infiltrating ductal carcinoma, NOS. It is not possible to completely exclude such elements at the time of FNA. Thus, it is our practice to report carcinoma with a mucinous component rather than to offer an unequivocal interpretation of mucinous carcinoma based solely on FNA.

The presence of extracellular mucin-positive material in FNA smears of the breast, however, is not a definitive feature of mucinous carcinoma because mucin and its simulators can be present in a variety of benign breast lesions. These mimics include fibroadenoma with myxoid stromal degeneration, cystic hypersecretory hyperplasia, benign breast cysts, lactating adenoma, and mucocele-like tumors of the breast.[164,165,331] Fibroadenomas generally occur in a younger age group and aspiration cytology reveals clusters of uniform, cohesive ductal-like cells with finger-like branching and many bipolar naked nuclei in the background. Benign breast cysts and mucocele-like tumors contain, in addition to the abundant mucinous material in the background, clusters of benign ductal cells that lack any significant nuclear atypicality.[165]

Tubular Carcinoma

Tubular carcinoma is a special type of breast carcinoma that usually measures 1 cm or less in diameter and has an excellent prognosis, even in the uncommon event of lymph node metastases. Wide application of screening mammography has led to a recent striking increase in its apparent

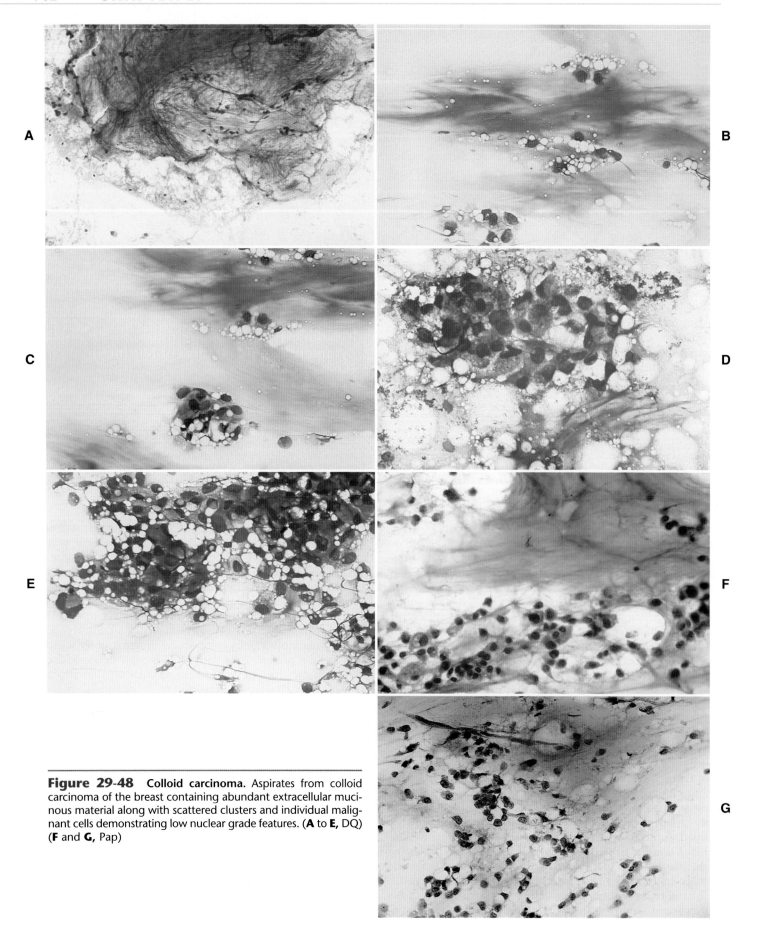

Figure 29-48   Colloid carcinoma. Aspirates from colloid carcinoma of the breast containing abundant extracellular mucinous material along with scattered clusters and individual malignant cells demonstrating low nuclear grade features. (**A** to **E**, DQ) (**F** and **G**, Pap)

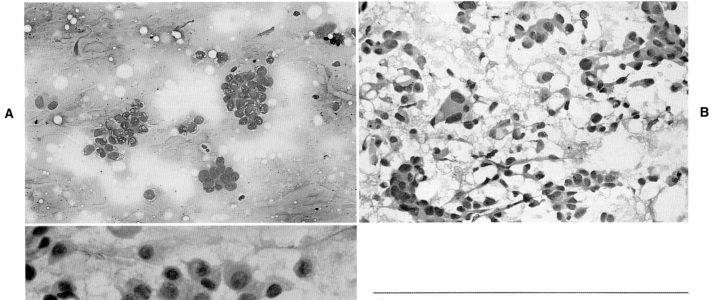

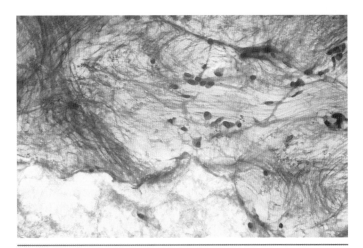

Figure 29-49 Colloid carcinoma. The relatively bland appearance of the tumor cells in some aspirates of colloid carcinoma could potentially lead to a false-negative diagnosis. The malignant diagnosis, however, should be suspected when mucinous material is seen elsewhere in the smears. (**A,** DQ; **B** and **C,** Pap)

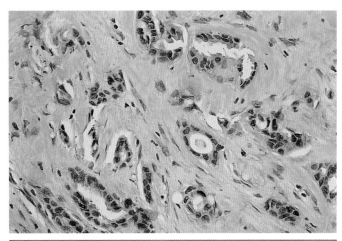

Figure 29-50 Colloid carcinoma. In aspirates of colloid carcinoma, vascularized connective tissue fragments can be appreciated. (DQ)

Figure 29-51 Tubular carcinoma. Histology of tubular carcinoma demonstrating angulated to comma-shape tubules consisting of relatively uniform malignant cells having low-grade nuclei set in a prominent desmoplastic fibrosis. (H&E)

prevalence. Histologic examination demonstrates infiltrating angulated to comma-shaped, tubular structures consisting of relatively small uniform cells with round, bland, low-grade nuclei (grade 1). Generally, prominent desmoplastic fibrosis is present (Figure 29-51). Because of the small size, bland-appearing nuclei and low epithelium to stroma ratio, this variant of breast cancer tends to be underdiagnosed in FNA biopsy.[46,166-168,332,333] Accordingly, a very high index of suspicion is needed when mildly atypical cells arranged in

angulated tubular structures or cores are encountered in the smears (Figure 29-52 and Box 29-13). Because of the relatively small size of tubular carcinoma, aspiration cytology often also samples both the tumor and the surrounding benign breast tissue, resulting in the presence of myoepithelial cells in some cases.[46,167] Therefore, the admixture of benign elements is another confounding feature that contributes either to an erroneously benign or equivocal diagnosis. When tubular carcinoma is suspected but a defini-

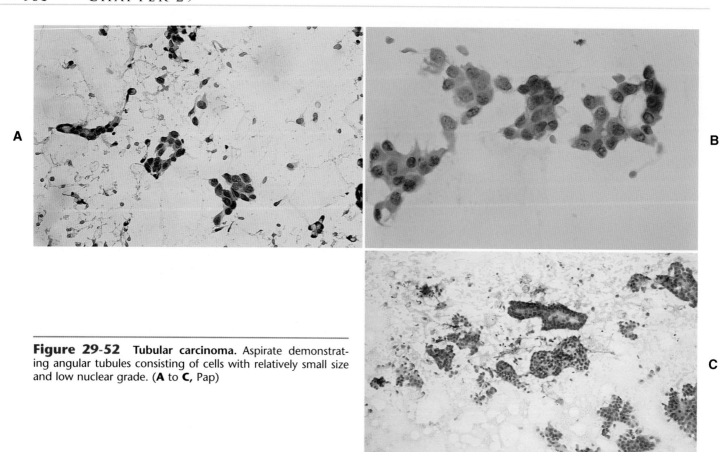

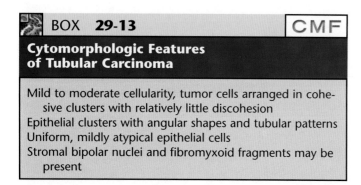

Figure 29-52   **Tubular carcinoma.** Aspirate demonstrating angular tubules consisting of cells with relatively small size and low nuclear grade. (**A** to **C,** Pap)

BOX   **29-13**   CMF

Cytomorphologic Features of Tubular Carcinoma

Mild to moderate cellularity, tumor cells arranged in cohesive clusters with relatively little discohesion
Epithelial clusters with angular shapes and tubular patterns
Uniform, mildly atypical epithelial cells
Stromal bipolar nuclei and fibromyxoid fragments may be present

---

tive diagnosis cannot be cytologically rendered, frozen section or biopsy confirmation may be recommended.

Adenoid Cystic Carcinoma

Adenoid cystic carcinoma is a rare variant accounting for approximately 0.1% of all breast carcinomas. This breast malignancy, which is associated with an excellent prognosis, usually does not result in lymph node metastasis. When metastases do occur, the lung is the preferred site. Hence, the vigor with which the axillary lymph nodes are pursued can be lessened to the patient's benefit. The cytologic features of adenoid cystic carcinoma of the breast are identical to the FNA findings of its more common salivary gland counterpart. The smears consist of nests of small uniform, basaloid cells intimately associated with metachromatically

staining matrix often forming three-dimensional spheres (Figure 29-53). Fragments of fibrillar stromal material, in close association with the epithelial cells and mucin-positive lumenal material can be present.[169] Although generally not needed for diagnosis, the matrix material can be immunohistochemically highlighted with applications of immunoperoxidase stains for collagen type IV.[170] The differential diagnosis of adenoid cystic carcinoma includes other salivary gland-type neoplasms that can occur in the breast such as pleomorphic adenoma. The cytologic features of these neoplasms are discussed in the salivary gland chapter. The differential diagnosis as discussed earlier in this chapter includes collagenous spherulosis, which has an admixture of benign relatively bland-appearing epithelial cells associated with cores of type IV collagen.[170] However, myoepithelial cells are also present in collagenous spherulosis, and the epithelial cells lack the nuclear atypicality that may be seen in adenoid cystic carcinoma.[15]

Papillary Carcinoma

Pure papillary carcinoma accounts for approximately 0.3% of all breast cancers, although a papillary component can be present in up to 3% to 4% of all mammary carcinomas.[171] Typically, this tumor occurs in postmenopausal, nonwhite patients. FNA cytology consists of three-dimensional papillary groupings of cells with scattered columnar tumor cells and a bloody diathesis with hemosiderin-laden macrophages in the background (Figure 29-54).[17,171] The mild nuclear atypicality seen in many cases

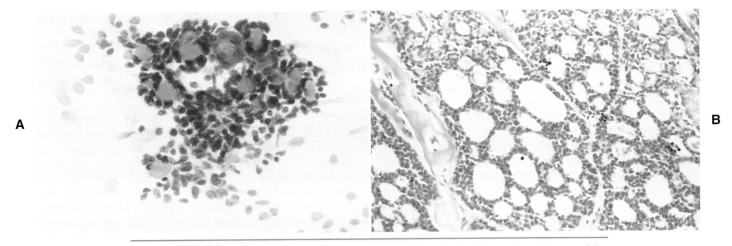

Figure 29-53 **Adenoid cystic carcinoma. A,** Aspirate of adenoid cystic carcinoma of the breast consisting of loose clusters of atypical cells surrounding round hyaline cylinders. (Pap) **B,** H&E confirmation of adenoid cystic carcinoma.

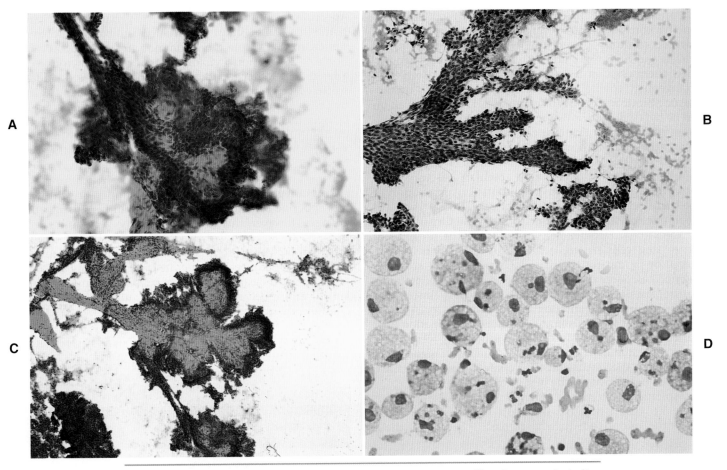

Figure 29-54 **Papillary carcinoma.** Aspirate demonstrating papillary fragments including some having fibrovascular cores, columnar-shaped cells, and numerous vacuolated histiocytes. (**A** to **D,** Pap)

is a potential source for a false-negative diagnosis of this breast carcinoma variant.[172] Its distinction from micropapillary DCIS was discussed previously.

The differential diagnoses of papillary carcinoma include fibroadenoma and papilloma.[57,172] Finger-like branching without a fibrovascular core and the presence of bipolar naked nuclei in the background favor a fibroadenoma. Although naked nuclei can be present in papillary carcinoma, they are often larger and more elongated than the small, uniform, bipolar naked nuclei of fibroadenoma. The more difficult differential diagnosis is separation of papillary carcinoma from a papilloma. This problem is not unique to aspiration cytology, as this diagnostic challenge can often occur at the time of frozen section and even permanent histologic examination. Invasive micropapillary carcinoma, an uncommon variant of breast cancer, has also been described in the FNA literature.[173,174,334] The smears tend to be cellular with numerous individually scattered cells and crowded clusters of cells with hyperchromatic irregular nuclei and peripherally located cytoplasm.[171-175] Fibrovascular cores are not seen, but psammoma bodies may be present (Box 29-14). Because of the difficulty of separating a benign papilloma from a well-differentiated papillary carcinoma, surgical excision is advised whenever a papillary neoplasm is encountered in aspiration cytology.[175] As discussed previously during our consideration of papillomas, this extends even to the finding of columnar cells ("cylindrical cells") that have no cytologic evidence of malignancy.

Lobular Carcinoma

Lobular carcinoma accounts for 5% to 10% of all invasive breast carcinomas.[104] This breast malignancy is often bilateral and/or multicentric. Histologically, classic lobular carcinoma consists of infiltrating, small, uniform cells that have eccentrically placed, mildly hyperchromatic, round nuclei, and high N:C ratios. The infiltrating cells tend to align themselves in a linear pattern or have a targetoid arrangement around ducts. Because a prominent desmoplastic fibrotic response is often present, FNA biopsy can often be hypocellular consisting of a sparse population of uniform, mildly atypical tumor cells arranged individually in small aggregates, thin strands, or cords (Figure 29-55). The cells are relatively small but have increased N:C ratios. The round nuclei tend to be finely granular and vary from hypochromatic to mildly hyperchromatic. Appreciation of the slight degree of nuclear irregularity and the presence of small nucleoli should alert one to the possibility of a lobular carcinoma. Another helpful feature is the presence of signet ring cells having eccentrically placed nuclei, displaced by prominent cytoplasmic vacuoles that can distort the nucleus. Some of these signet ring cells can contain intracytoplasmic target-like vacuoles, caused by inspissated mucin (Figure 29-56 and Box 29-15). The presence of 10% or more signet ring cells in the histologic examination may portend a poor prognosis for stage I infiltrating lobular carcinoma.[176] Studies correlating the number of signet ring cells in FNA specimens and their clinical significance have not been performed, to the best of our knowledge.

Aspiration of lobular carcinoma is the most common cause of a false-negative diagnosis of breast carcinoma when the lesion is adequately sampled.[177] Because of these bland features and the often low cellularity, the potential for a false-negative diagnosis is understandable. Kline and colleagues, however, identified lobular carcinoma in nearly 75% of their cases using strict cytologic criteria.[57,177] Potential exists to confuse lobular carcinoma with other types of breast carcinoma, especially when variants of lobular carcinoma are sampled, including the solid, alveolar, mixed, or pleomorphic types. These cases are often misclassified as ductal carcinoma because of greater cellularity and/or larger cells present in these variants of lobular carcinoma.[177-180] Analogous to the principles presented when interpreting smears of ductal carcinoma, distinguishing in situ from infiltrating lobular carcinoma is not possible.[181] However, Salhany and Page report that infiltrating lobular carcinomas are generally more cellular and discohesive with greater nuclear atypia and pleomorphism than aspirates of lobular carcinoma in situ.[181] Tissue evaluation is needed to confirm invasive lobular carcinoma.

Apocrine and Secretory Carcinoma Variants

Apocrine carcinoma is a morphologic variant of duct carcinoma that has a clinical presentation and biologic behavior similar to that of the more common invasive ductal carcinoma.[104] Aspiration cytology will reveal numerous cells arranged in syncytial fragments along with individually scattered cells.[15,16] The apocrine features are characterized by cells with abundant basophilic to eosinophilic granular cytoplasm and large nuclei with prominent nucleoli (Figure 29-57).[182,183] Thus, they share many features with atypical apocrine metaplasia, which therefore enters into the cytologic differential diagnosis. The greater cellularity, reduced cohesion, syncytial arrangements of cells, hyperchromasia, nuclear irregularity, and necrotic background should separate apocrine carcinoma from atypical but benign apocrine change. However, this can sometimes be very difficult because of the fact that we are accustomed to tolerating wide ranges of nucleolar prominence and nuclear pleomorphism in benign apocrine cells. Apocrine carcinoma may also contain cells with clear cytoplasm or cells that mimic a granular cell tumor because of coarsely granular cytoplasm.[104,182] Granular cell tumors lack the nuclear atypicality and larger cells of apocrine carcinoma. Further, immunocytochemical staining for cytokeratin confirms apocrine carcinoma,

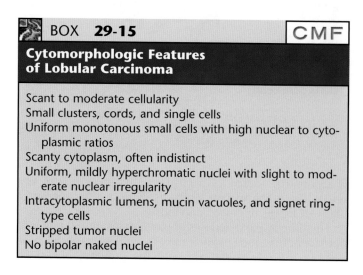

BOX   29-14   CMF

**Cytomorphologic Features
of Papillary Carcinoma**

Moderate cellularity
Three-dimensional papillary groups, fibrovascular cores
Atypical columnar cells
Naked epithelial nuclei rather than bipolar stripped nuclei
Hemosiderin-laden macrophages

BOX   29-15   CMF

**Cytomorphologic Features
of Lobular Carcinoma**

Scant to moderate cellularity
Small clusters, cords, and single cells
Uniform monotonous small cells with high nuclear to cytoplasmic ratios
Scanty cytoplasm, often indistinct
Uniform, mildly hyperchromatic nuclei with slight to moderate nuclear irregularity
Intracytoplasmic lumens, mucin vacuoles, and signet ring-type cells
Stripped tumor nuclei
No bipolar naked nuclei

whereas S-100 positive, cytokeratin-negative cells are features of a granular cell tumor.

Secretory carcinoma may also be considered in the differential diagnosis.[92,184-187] The aspirated smears consist of large irregular sheets of malignant polygonal cells with granular to vacuolated cytoplasm.[187] The presence of grape-like clusters of vacuolated cells may also be a helpful cytologic feature.[92] Other entities in the differential diagnosis include lipid-secreting carcinoma,[188] glycogen-rich clear cell carcinoma,[189] cystic hypersecretory carcinoma,[190] and secretory breast carcinoma simulating lactational changes.[191] A variant of apocrine carcinoma with lipid-rich giant cells has also been described.[182]

Squamous Cell Carcinoma

Pure squamous cell carcinoma of the breast is a very rare tumor, although a malignant squamous component can oc-

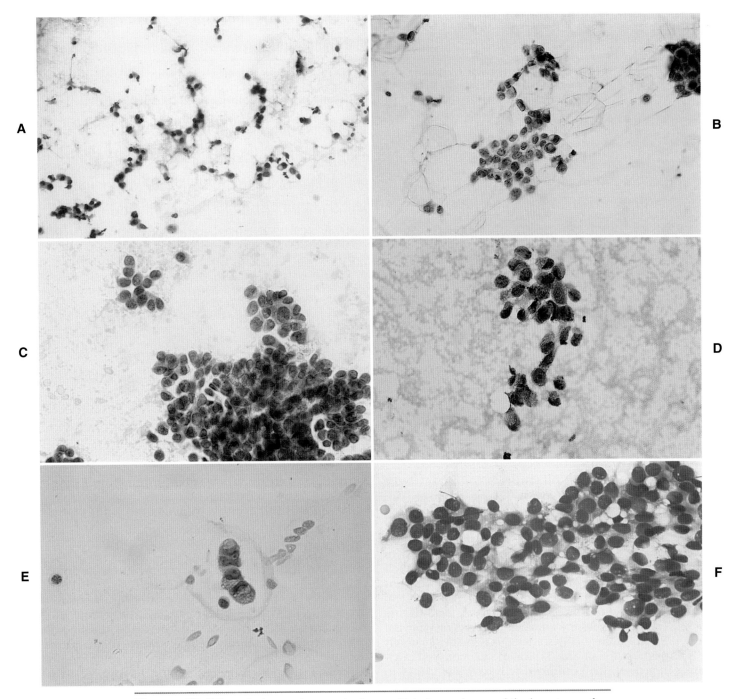

Figure 29-55 **Lobular carcinoma.** Aspirates of lobular carcinoma of the breast can often be hypocellular and consist of mildly atypical cells arranged in small aggregates, cords and linear arrays. The cells are relatively small with high N:C ratios and have low grade nuclear features. (**A** to **E**, Pap; **F**, DQ)

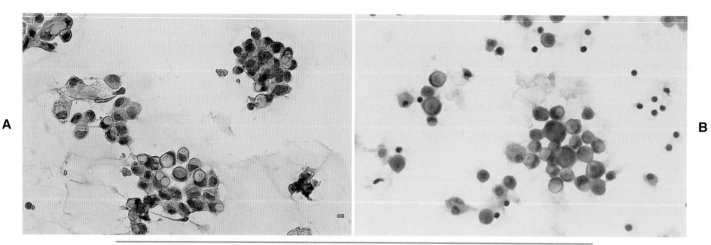

Figure 29-56   Lobular carcinoma. Signet ring cells, a feature of lobular carcinoma, are atypical cells having eccentrically placed nuclei displaced by prominent cytoplasmic vacuoles. Some of the signet ring cells can contain intracytoplasmic targetoid vacuoles caused by inspissated mucin. (**A,** Pap; **B,** DQ)

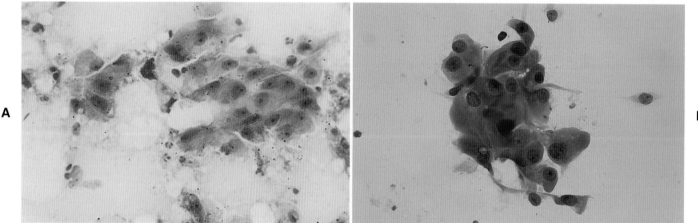

Figure 29-57   Apocrine carcinoma. Aspirate consisting of atypical cells having abundant basophilic to eosinophilic granular cytoplasm and large nuclei with prominent nucleoli. (**A,** Pap; **B,** DQ)

casionally be seen in an otherwise typical ductal carcinoma.[115,192,193] Some investigators classify squamous cell carcinoma as a type of metaplastic carcinoma with a better prognosis than metaplastic carcinomas demonstrating pseudosarcomatous features. The behavior and prognosis of pure squamous cell carcinoma of the breast are similar to those of usual, invasive ductal carcinoma.[194,195] FNA cytology reveals sheets of well to poorly differentiated malignant squamous cells, including evidence of cytoplasmic keratinization and the presence of intercellular bridges (Figure 29-58). The tumor cells are arranged in sheets or syncytial groupings with individually scattered malignant squamous cells throughout the smears. Typical of squamous cell carcinomas in general, the keratinized cells have a tendency to assume irregular pleomorphic to spindled shapes. Occasional examples of squamous cell carcinoma present as cystic masses. The major differential diagnosis of primary squamous cell carcinoma is a metastatic squamous cell carcinoma to the breast.[196] Squamous cells in breast aspirates can also be seen in a variety of benign lesions including epidermoid cysts, subareolar abscess, phyllodes tumor, fibroadenoma, and infarcted papillomas.[197]

Intracystic Carcinoma

Intracystic carcinoma is a very rare breast cancer accounting for less than 0.7% of all breast carcinomas.[198] The usual patient is an obese, elderly, African-American woman. The typical scenario is aspiration of hemorrhagic fluid from a cystic mass with persistence of the mass after the procedure. The cytologic findings include scanty cellularity with mildly atypical cells arranged in loosely cohesive groups and papillary clusters (Figure 29-59).[198,199]

Aspiration cytology of cystic hypersecretory duct carcinoma shows mildly atypical cells arranged singly and in small groups and sheets, set in a background of abundant, intensely staining, pink-to-purple, thyroid-like colloid material that imparts a bubbly, "cracked earth" artifact background.[198,199]

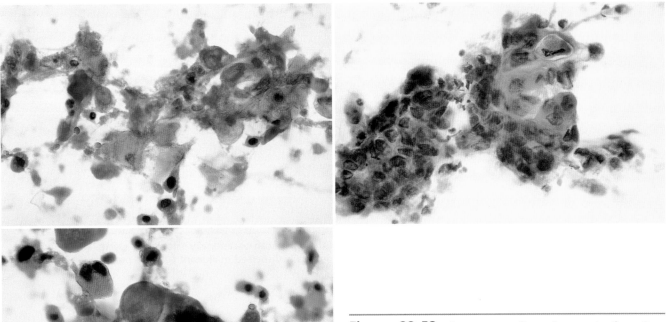

Figure 29-58 **Squamous cell carcinoma.** In these Pap-stained smears, malignant keratinized cells are present and consistent with a primary squamous cell carcinoma of the breast.

A

B

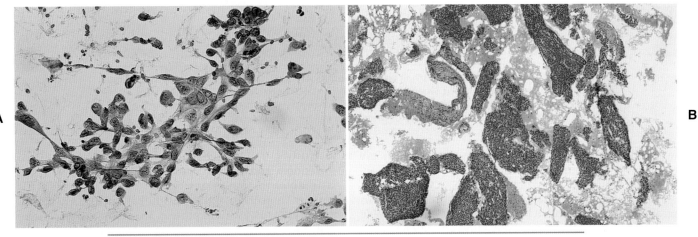

Figure 29-59 **Intracystic carcinoma.** **A,** Aspirate from intracystic carcinoma consisting of loose clusters of malignant cells in this Pap-stained smear. **B,** Cell block from another example of intracystic carcinoma consisting of clumps of tumor cells associated with proteinaceous material in the background and numerous red blood cells. (H&E)

Inflammatory Carcinoma

Inflammatory carcinoma of the breast is a relatively uncommon clinicopathologic entity that is suspected when a patient presents with a mass associated with redness and tenderness of the overlying skin. The simulation of an inflammatory process prompts a clinical differential diagnosis of mastitis. Palpation of the breast reveals a hyperemic, engorged, and edematous skin that can demonstrate "orange peel" skin changes. The histopathologic finding of malignant cells within dermal lymphatics satisfies the pathologic definition of inflammatory carcinoma. However, the clinical picture of inflammatory carcinoma is sometimes seen in the absence of this histopathologic feature. This type of breast carcinoma accounts for 2% to 4% of all breast cancers and carries a grave prognosis, with most patients dying within 2 to 3 years of diagnosis.[200] Aspiration of the underlying breast parenchyma generally reveals paucicellular smears that often contain fragments of fibrous and adipose tissue.[200] When a

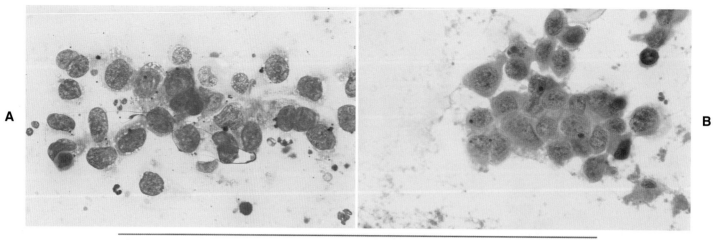

Figure 29-60   Paget's disease. Scraping of the nipple can occasionally establish the diagnosis of Paget's disease. Loosely cohesive and individually dispersed malignant cells are present in this example. (**A**, DQ; **B**, Pap)

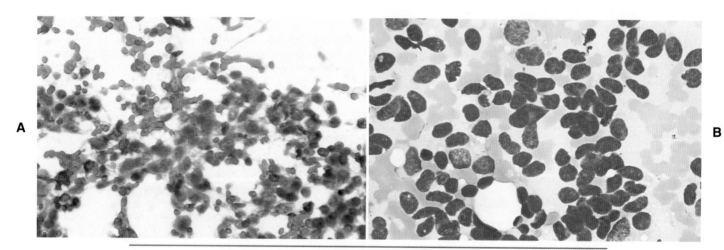

Figure 29-61   Metastatic small cell carcinoma. **A** and **B**, Metastatic small cell carcinoma to the breast was diagnosed when numerous small malignant cells with high N:C ratios were seen. The tumor cells have the characteristic salt-and-pepper chromatin pattern and lack nucleoli. The patient had a clinical history of prior small cell lung cancer. (**A**, Pap; **B**, DQ)

few malignant cells are sampled from the dermis, they are arranged in clusters, rather than individually dispersed, according to Dodd and Layfield's report of FNA cytology of inflammatory breast carcinoma.[200] Although mammograms typically reveal a mass or architectural distortion, a palpable mass may not be present. Therefore, blind aspirations of the dermis and underlying subcutaneous tissue may not adequately sample the tumor cells plugging the lymphatic spaces. When the diagnosis is clinically suspected but the cytology examination is nondiagnostic, multiple punch biopsies of the skin are recommended.

Paget's Disease

Paget's disease is an eczemal-like change of the nipple and areola usually associated with an underlying in situ or invasive breast carcinoma. The cytologic diagnosis can be made by either scraping the nipple or by FNA biopsy (Figure 29-60). Since the areolar skin has numerous nerve endings, aspiration can be quite painful; therefore, local anesthesia is recommended when either the nipple or areolar skin is biopsied. The tumor cells can be arranged individually and

in clusters. The differential diagnosis includes malignant melanoma and in situ squamous cell carcinoma. Positive staining of the malignant cells of Paget's disease for cytokeratin (especially CK7), epithelial membrane antigen, gross cystic disease fluid protein-15, carcinoembryonic antigen, and estrogen or progesterone receptors is confirmatory, whereas malignant melanoma will be positive for S-100, HMB-45, and melan A. In situ squamous cell carcinoma is negative for the melanocytic markers and CK7.

Metastatic Malignancies in the Breast

Metastatic malignancies to the breast are uncommon with an autopsy rate of approximately 1.4% to 6.6% of patients with cancer.[201] The clinically observed rate is much lower, accounting for only 0.4% to 2% of all breast malignancies.[201] In rare instances, cancers metastatic to the breast can be the initial presentation of the malignancy and therefore simulate a primary breast carcinoma. The most common malignancies metastatic to the breast in women are, in decreasing frequency, melanoma, lymphoma, lung cancer, ovarian cancer, and soft tissue sarcomas (Figures 29-61 to

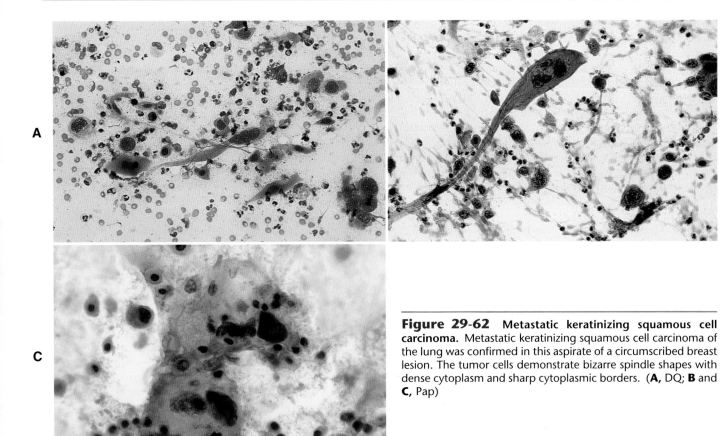

Figure 29-62 Metastatic keratinizing squamous cell carcinoma. Metastatic keratinizing squamous cell carcinoma of the lung was confirmed in this aspirate of a circumscribed breast lesion. The tumor cells demonstrate bizarre spindle shapes with dense cytoplasm and sharp cytoplasmic borders. (**A,** DQ; **B** and **C,** Pap)

29-63).[202] In men, a metastasis from a prostate carcinoma is the most common malignancy to secondarily involve the breast.[202]

In our FNA experience, less than 3% of all breast malignancies represent metastasis to the breast.[201] The authors' series consisted of 18 patients, in 16 of whom FNA biopsy confirmed metastatic malignancies in the setting of known extramammary cancers. However, importantly, the pre-biopsy clinical diagnosis in six of these patients was a benign breast lesion resulting from the superficial and circumscribed nature of many of these metastatic deposits. In two patients, FNA biopsy identified metastatic malignancy from an unsuspected extramammary primary. Therefore, it is important to be aware of this possibility, especially when an unusual cytologic presentation is encountered in a breast aspirate. There have been a number of other series and case reports documenting FNA cytology of metastatic malignancy to the breast.[15,16,203,204] With a correct diagnosis of a malignancy metastatic to the breast, an unnecessary mastectomy can be avoided and appropriate chemotherapy or radiation treatment can be given. In occasional cases, ancillary studies performed on the FNA material, including immunohistochemistry, and to a lesser extent, electron microscopy, can be useful in making a definite diagnosis.[201]

Confirmation of Metastatic Breast Carcinoma to Extramammary Sites

The most important prognostic parameter in breast cancer is the presence or absence of metastases. In addition to regional lymph nodes, metastatic disease can involve the

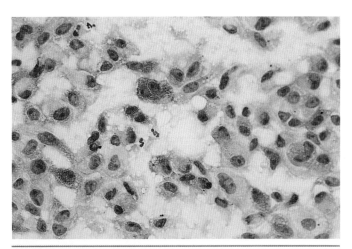

Figure 29-63 Metastatic malignant melanoma. Aspirate of metastatic malignant melanoma to the breast. Polygonal to spindle-shaped cells are seen with some cells demonstrating a slight brownish blush to the cytoplasm. The tumor cells have prominent nucleoli. (Pap)

same or contralateral breast and distant sites. More than 50% of women have distant metastasis as the first indicator of breast cancer recurrence.[95] Approximately 20% have bone involvement, 10% pulmonary disease, and 2% to 3% have liver involvement as the only sites of metastatic breast carcinoma.

It is important to recognize metastatic breast carcinoma because of recent improvements in treatment. In the differential diagnosis of metastatic breast carcinoma and a lung primary, Fabian and Dabbs[205] noted considerable overlapping of routine morphologic features between lung adenocarcinoma and metastatic breast carcinoma in pulmonary aspirates. In this setting, immunocytochemical studies can be extremely helpful. Although both lung and breast carcinomas are usually CK7 positive/CK20 negative, lung carcinomas often stain intensely for CEA-D14, whereas metastatic breast carcinomas are usually negative.[16] Breast carcinomas are usually positive for gross cystic disease fluid protein-15 antibody and can be estrogen (ER) and/or progesterone (PR) receptor positive. In contrast, lung cancers are believed to be negative for ER and PR proteins. However, when using the estrogen receptor antibody (6F11, Ventana), a significant percentage of adenocarcinomas of the lung were positive.[205,206] In contrast the 1D5 estrogen receptor antibody manufactured by Dako does not stain the nuclei of lung cancer cells.[206] Thyroid transcription factor-1, a specific antibody for thyroid and lung cancers, is negative in breast carcinoma but is expressed in approximately 75% of bronchogenic adenocarcinomas. Application of all of these stains, including ER and PR proteins, underscores the powerful diagnostic utility of paraffin-embedded cell block material.

Another important application of FNA is diagnosis of small dermal recurrences of breast cancer. This prognostically ominous finding presents as tiny "rice-grain" lumps. These are often easier to identify when the physician runs the fingertips lightly over the affected skin; they may be nearly invisible. Diagnosis is readily accomplished by FNA. The yield may be sparsely cellular, but in this clinical setting the diagnosis is usually clear.

Phyllodes Tumor

Phyllodes tumor (cystosarcoma phyllodes) is a biphasic epithelial and stromal neoplasm accounting for less than 0.3% of all breast tumors.[104] The malignant examples histologically resemble and clinically behave as sarcomas rather than as carcinomas. Patients are usually in their fourth to fifth decade, which is approximately 20 years older than patients with fibroadenomas.[63] Tumor size, mitotic activity, stromal atypia, stromal overgrowth, and the status of the excision margins are the most useful histologic guidelines for assessing the biologic potential of phyllodes tumor.[207,208] A phyllodes tumor with benign histologic features rarely metastasizes but often recur locally if not completely resected. Approximately 12% of histologically malignant phyllodes tumors metastasize. However, the behavior of an individual case is unpredictable. The clinical possibility of phyllodes tumor should be suspected whenever a large bulky breast tumor measuring greater than 4 cm in maximum dimension is encountered.

Mammographically, phyllodes tumors often show smooth, distinct borders.

Aspiration cytology of phyllodes tumor will show both epithelial and stromal components. The cytologic distinction of phyllodes tumor from fibroadenoma is based mainly on assessment of the cellularity of the stromal fragments.[209-214] Highly cellular stromal fragments favor phyllodes tumor in contrast with the relatively paucicellular stromal fragments of fibroadenoma in FNA specimens.[86,215] Within the stromal fragments of phyllodes tumor, the stromal cells have elongated nuclei with irregular nuclear membranes and occasional nucleoli, in contrast with the smaller, oval to round nuclei of bipolar cells in fibroadenoma (Figure 29-64 and Box 29-16).[149] This feature may even be more helpful than assessment of stromal cellularity because the latter can be overestimated from the thickness of stromal fragments in the smears. The separation of benign from malignant phyllodes tumors is based on the presence of atypical stromal cells and mitotic figures in the spindle cells adjacent to ducts. If the fragments consist of small spindle-shaped cells without significant atypia, the lesion is more likely benign. With increasing cellularity and atypia, malignant phyllodes tumor is favored.[13,216] However, final classification should always await review of the resected specimen because of morphologic heterogeneity occurring within any particular neoplasm. Furthermore, most of the prognostic factors noted previously cannot be assessed in smears.

A significant degree of epithelial proliferation can also occur in phyllodes tumors, including atypical epithelial hyperplasia that could potentially lead to a misdiagnosis of carcinoma (Figure 29-65).[211,217] This is not surprising because in the seminal study from the Armed Forces Institute of Pathology (AFIP), 15 of 94 phyllodes tumor had significant epithelial hyperplasia with varying degrees of atypia.[207]

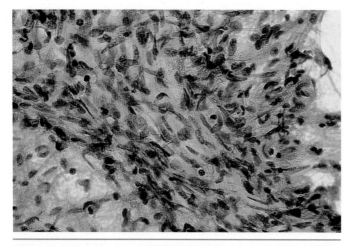

Figure 29-64 **Phyllodes tumor.** Hypercellular stromal fragment in an aspirate from phyllodes tumor. In contrast with the more oval bipolar nuclei seen in fibrocystic change and fibroadenoma, the spindle cells in phyllodes tumor take on a more elongated, irregular shape with pointed ends. The spindle cells are interspersed in a fibroconnective matrix. (Pap)

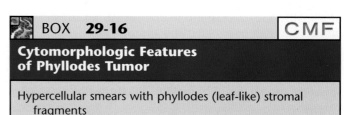

BOX **29-16**   CMF

**Cytomorphologic Features
of Phyllodes Tumor**

Hypercellular smears with phyllodes (leaf-like) stromal
   fragments
Numerous elongated and irregular spindled stromal cells
   with nucleoli
Fragments of metachromatically staining stroma
Epithelial hyperplasia may be present

When atypical epithelial hyperplasia is present, cytologic features to suggest the possibility of phyllodes tumor, rather than a breast carcinoma, are increased numbers of naked spindle-shaped nuclei and hypercellular stromal fragments, otherwise known as *phyllodes fragments*. However, because prominent epithelial hyperplasia can be seen in both benign and malignant phyllodes tumors leading to false-positive diagnoses of breast carcinoma, frozen section confirmation should be obtained in any case that is clinically or cytologically suspected to be a phyllodes tumor. Conversely, a potential for a false-negative diagnosis of fibroadenoma is possible because some aspirates of phyllodes tumors can be relatively hypocellular and some of the lesions are small.[13,211]

Metaplastic Carcinoma and True Sarcomas

Metaplastic carcinoma of the breast is a heterogenous group of breast malignancies characterized by the admixture of ductal carcinoma with areas of spindle, squamous, chondroid, or osseous metaplasia.[104,218-221] They account for only 0.2% of breast malignancies. Similar to the usual infiltrating ductal carcinoma, the average age of patients is 54.3 years. The overall survival is approximately 44% at 5 years. When a predominance of pseudosarcomatous metaplasia is evident, the survival decreases to 28% at 5 years.[220] However, matrix-producing metaplastic carcinoma may have a better prognosis, reflected in a 68% survival rate at 5 years, in contrast with the worse prognosis of metaplastic carcinomas with a predominantly spindle cell component.[221]

Primary pure sarcomas of the breast are even less common than metaplastic carcinoma, with malignant fibrous histiocytoma (MFH) the most common sarcoma encountered.[104,222,223] Breast sarcoma and the pseudosarcomatous component of metaplastic carcinomas have features similar to the more common sarcomas encountered in soft tissue as discussed in Chapter 28.[15,59,211,223-238] Aspiration cytology of mammary MFH is generally hypercellular consisting of cells with extreme pleomorphism, including numerous atypical mononucleated, binucleated, and multinucleated histiocyte-like and fibroblastic-like spindle cells. Occasionally, bland appearing, vacuolated, xan-thoma-type cells and Touton-like and osteoclast-like giant cells can be encountered.[228] Occasional aspirates can consist of atypical spindle-shaped, fibroblast-like cells arranged individually or in loose clusters. Metaplastic carcinomas with chondrosarcomatous differentiation have bizarre cells set in a chondromyxoid stroma (Figure 29-66). Other types of breast sarcomas reported in the FNA literature include osteogenic sarcoma,[10,210,213] primary rhabdomyosarcoma,[237] and angiosarcoma, including postirradiation epithelioid angiosarcoma.[232]

The differential diagnoses of metaplastic breast carcinoma include aspirates containing low-grade–appearing, spindle-shaped mesenchymal cells from nodular fasciitis; fibromatosis; myofibroblastoma; and adenomyoepithelioma.[223-235] FNA cytology of nodular fasciitis and fibromatosis can vary from hypocellular to hypercellular and consists of individually scattered spindle-shaped cells having a relatively bland appearance, along with occasional loose microtissue fragments of spindle-shaped cells (Figure 29-67). The cytologic features of these types of lesions are discussed in greater detail in Chapter 28.

Pleomorphic ductal carcinomas can be confused with pleomorphic metaplastic carcinomas and sarcomas such as MFH. Clinically, distinction from true sarcomas is important. Pleomorphic ductal carcinomas tend to have cells arranged in more cohesive sheets and clusters. Ancillary studies including immunocytochemistry for cytokeratin and other epithelial markers, specific immunocytochemical studies for various types of sarcomas, and myoepithelial differentiation can prove helpful in selected cases.[211,228,237,238] Lastly, osteoclast-like giant cells can occasionally be seen in metaplastic carcinomas, sarcomas, and ductal carcinoma.[239-242] The osteoclasts are generally large with centrally clustered nuclei within voluminous cytoplasm.

RADIATION AND CHEMOTHERAPY-INDUCED CHANGES

FNA cytology of radiated breast and patients receiving chemotherapy can be a diagnostic challenge. Histologic changes of irradiated breast include epithelial atypia in the

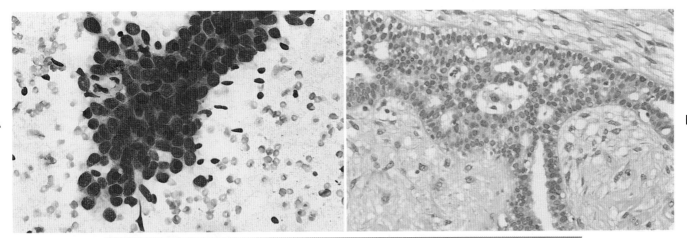

Figure 29-65 Phyllodes tumor. **A,** Epithelial proliferation can be present in aspirates of some cases of phyllodes tumor. (DQ) **B,** Resected phyllodes tumor with foci of epithelial hyperplasia. (H&E)

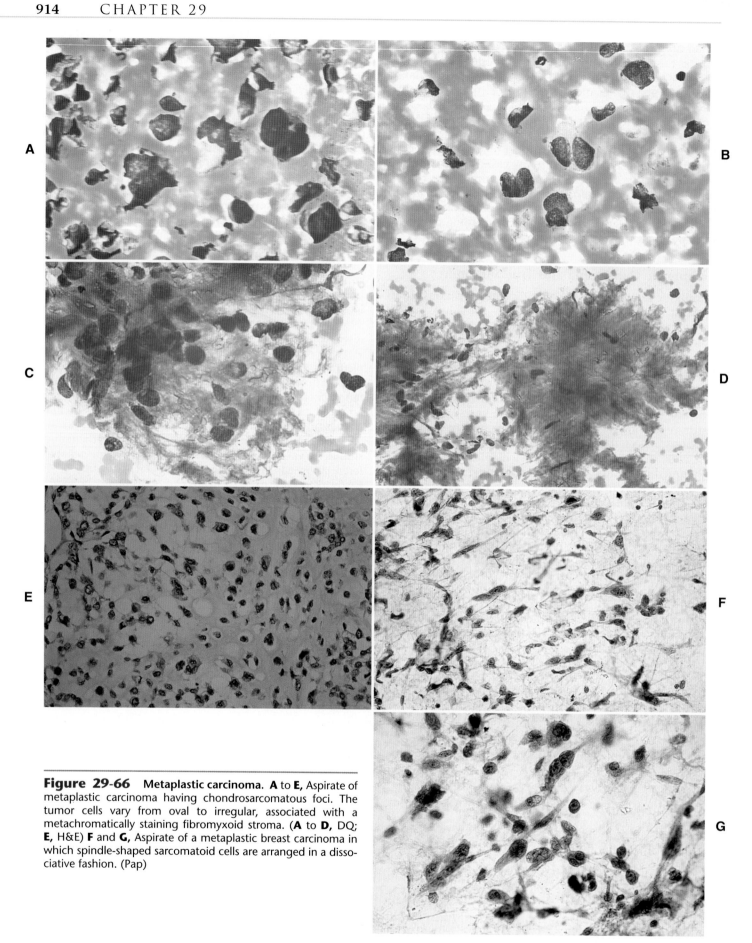

Figure 29-66   Metaplastic carcinoma. **A** to **E,** Aspirate of metaplastic carcinoma having chondrosarcomatous foci. The tumor cells vary from oval to irregular, associated with a metachromatically staining fibromyxoid stroma. (**A** to **D,** DQ; **E,** H&E) **F** and **G,** Aspirate of a metaplastic breast carcinoma in which spindle-shaped sarcomatoid cells are arranged in a dissociative fashion. (Pap)

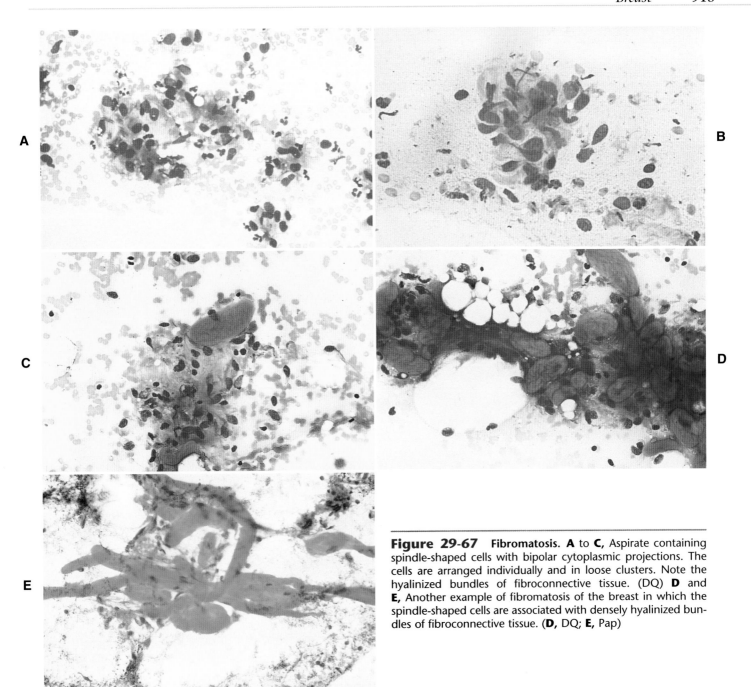

Figure 29-67 Fibromatosis. **A** to **C,** Aspirate containing spindle-shaped cells with bipolar cytoplasmic projections. The cells are arranged individually and in loose clusters. Note the hyalinized bundles of fibroconnective tissue. (DQ) **D** and **E,** Another example of fibromatosis of the breast in which the spindle-shaped cells are associated with densely hyalinized bundles of fibroconnective tissue. (**D,** DQ; **E,** Pap)

terminal duct-lobular units as well as in larger ducts. Prominent stromal and vascular changes may also be seen.[243]

FNA biopsy of an irradiated breast can sample severely atypical benign epithelium.[244] Therefore, having knowledge of prior irradiation therapy is crucial to avoid a false-positive diagnosis of malignancy in these patients presenting with a new breast mass after irradiation treatment.[244-246] Exercising caution when scattered atypical ductal cells are present in hypocellular smears from a patient with a history of prior irradiation is always prudent. Aspirates of cystic breast lesion can have atypical squamous metaplastic cells after breast irradiation.[247]

Reports of the histopathology and FNA cytology of chemotherapy-induced changes in carcinoma cells have been limited.[248-250] Postchemotherapy histologic changes described in the surgical pathology literature include extensive vacuolization of tumor cells imparting a histiocytic appearance to the cells.[250] Frierson and Fechner noted no significant difference in histologic grade induced by chemotherapy,[250] although Kennedy and colleagues reported severe degrees of epithelial atypia.[248] Brifford and colleagues reported the cytologic findings in postchemotherapy FNA biopsy specimens.[249] The smears contained tumor cells with enlarged nuclei and prominent nucleoli, nuclear vacuolization, chromatin clearing, and vacuolated cytoplasm (Figure 29-68).

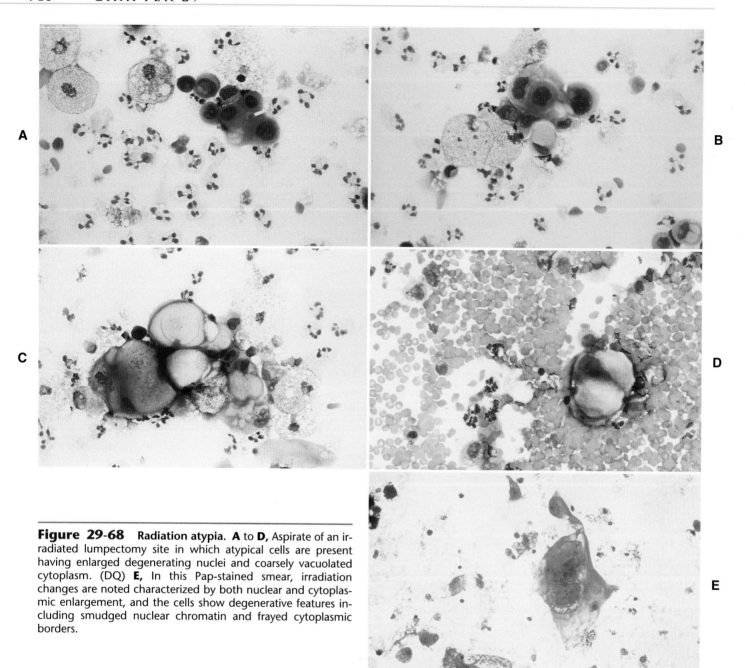

Figure 29-68 Radiation atypia. **A** to **D**, Aspirate of an irradiated lumpectomy site in which atypical cells are present having enlarged degenerating nuclei and coarsely vacuolated cytoplasm. (DQ) **E**, In this Pap-stained smear, irradiation changes are noted characterized by both nuclear and cytoplasmic enlargement, and the cells show degenerative features including smudged nuclear chromatin and frayed cytoplasmic borders.

FINE-NEEDLE ASPIRATION AND CORE BIOPSIES OF NONPALPABLE, MAMMOGRAPHICALLY EVIDENT LESIONS

Mammography is the best method for detecting nonpalpable breast lesions, having a sensitivity of up to 80%.[19] Ultrasound and stereotaxic-guided FNA biopsy of nonpalpable breast lesions have also been employed.[19,251-260] Although a number of studies compare tissue core biopsy with FNA biopsy of mammographically evident lesions, tissue core biopsy has recently gained ascendency and has become, with a few exceptions, the procedure of choice.

The death knell for FNA cytology of nonpalpable mammographically evident lesion occurred with the publication of a recent multiinstitutional study that reported the diagnostic superiority of core biopsies over FNA cytology.[269] This influential study has virtually ended the use of FNA biopsy for mammographically evident lesions in most medical centers because of the high inadequacy rate encountered.[269] This paper has implications that go beyond application of FNA to nonpalpable breast lesions. Perhaps the most interesting is the statement that "No special training for FNA or specimen preparation was provided to the clinicians as part of this study" (p. 269). The benefits of FNA in many clinical settings are obvious to all. However, in our opinion, the main reason for our failure to disseminate the method to the majority of practitioners and patients who might benefit from it is the fact that it does not work very well (and can even be diagnostically dangerous) in untrained or inexperi-

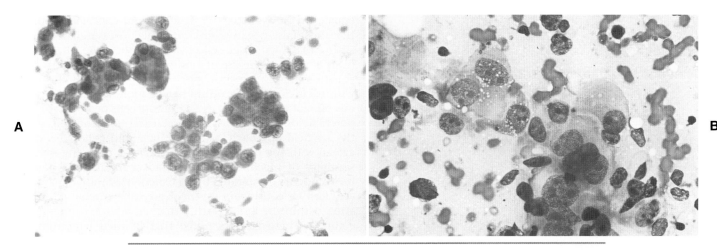

Figure 29-69 Nuclear grading. **A,** Ductal carcinoma, nuclear grade (NG) 1, having relatively small uniform nuclei without prominent nucleoli. (Pap) **B,** Ductal carcinoma, NG 3, showing considerable variation in nuclear size and shape with prominent nucleoli, readily seen at low power. (DQ)

enced hands. It is simply not as easy as it looks. For this reason, we would suggest that this study was fatally flawed from its conception and does not constitute a meaningful evaluation of FNA.

The authors believe that for experienced mammographers working with experienced pathologists, FNA biopsy of nonpalpable lesions can be quite accurate.[251] Despite the discontinuance of FNA cytology for mammographic-evident lesions, imprint cytology of the core needle biopsy specimens can be quite useful in assessing adequacy of the biopsies and rendering a preliminary diagnosis.[252,263]

For palpable lesions, it has been recommended that mammographic examination be obtained before the FNA biopsy because subsequent bleeding or edema can produce irregularities in an otherwise benign-appearing mammographic lesion leading to a false-positive mammographic diagnosis.[261,264] These changes appear to be accentuated within the first week after the aspiration biopsy. Therefore, it is recommended that the mammographic study be postponed for at least two weeks.[264] However, the studies on which these recommendations were based did not document needle size, which may have an influence on the occurrence of either hematoma or edema.[264] Additional studies are clearly needed because most medical centers now employ 23-gauge or smaller needles for the performance of FNA biopsy of palpable breast masses.

 ## ANCILLARY STUDIES INCLUDING NUCLEAR GRADING

It has now become the standard of practice to perform estrogen and progesterone receptor analysis, as well as *Her-2-neu* by immunocytochemical techniques, on tissue core biopsies and the resected breast carcinoma specimen. However, hormonal receptor protein analysis can also be employed on the aspirate smears with good results, in our experience, although *Her-2-neu* evaluation is still best performed on a paraffin-embedded specimen. These studies are most often performed in FNA specimens of metastatic breast carcinoma, rather than in the patient's primary le-

sion. DNA analysis using flow cytometry or image cytometry has also been employed on FNA biopsy specimens.[15] However, the value of DNA analysis as an independent prognostic factor in breast carcinoma has not been definitively established and currently is not requested by many oncologists.

Nuclear grading, however, can be readily accomplished with cytologic material and is considerably less labor intensive and costly than doing DNA analysis. Furthermore, it correlates quite well with tumor ploidy and other prognostic markers.[265-275] *Nuclear grade (NG)* 1 is defined as nuclei similar to those of normal duct epithelium demonstrating minimal enlargement with round, smooth nuclear contours, finely granular chromatin, and no obvious nucleoli.[16] NG 1 morphology is most commonly seen in tubular, papillary, and colloid carcinomas.[267,268] NG 2 morphology shows nuclei that are approximately twice the size of grade 1 nuclei, but maintain smooth nuclear membranes and uniform chromatin; a small nucleolus is usually present and moderate degree of anisonucleosis can be seen. NG 3 demonstrates marked anisonucleosis with nuclei showing more than threefold variation in nuclear diameter and increased hyperchromasia, irregular nuclear contours, coarse chromatin with chromatin clearing, and macronucleoli and/or multiple nucleoli.[267,268] Nuclear grading can be performed on both DQ and Pap-stained smears (Figure 29-69).[268] Nuclear grading applied to FNA specimens correlates quite well with histologic nuclear grading and flow cytometric studies.[16,267,268] Reporting of nuclear grading should be incorporated in any aspirate of a ductal carcinoma. It is not commonly reported when evaluating lobular carcinomas, but nuclear grading of pleomorphic lobular carcinoma is reasonable.[178] Nuclear grading is especially useful for patients receiving chemotherapy before resection of their tumors.[267] Other prognostic and predictive markers that have employed on breast FNA specimens include ER and PR proteins, *Her-2-neu* oncogene analysis, and proliferation studies including Ki-67 and MIB-1 (Figure 29-70).[273,276] Again, these studies are limited by the inability to differentiate invasive or in situ cancer in FNA biopsy.

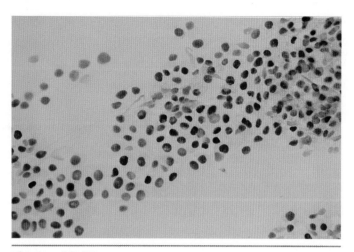

Figure 29-70 Estrogen. Immunocytochemical stain for estrogen receptor protein demonstrates strong and diffuse nuclear staining.

 ACCURACY, TRIPLE TEST, AND FALSE-NEGATIVE AND FALSE-POSITIVE RATES

FNA of the breast is a diagnostically accurate procedure with an average sensitivity of 87% (range of 72% to 99%), specificity of 98% to 100%, negative predictive value of 87% to 99%, and efficiency of 89% to 99%.[15,37,262,278] For palpable lesions, breast aspiration results compare favorably with Tru-Cut or other tissue core biopsy procedures.[279] The accuracy rate of FNA increases when the cytopathologist performs the aspiration and uses immediate assessment to determine specimen adequacy.[12,280,281] The false-negative rate varies from 1% to 31%[59] with a 10% average false negative rate.[15] The false-negative rate increases when aspirations are performed by inexperienced individuals.[278,280,282] Interpretative errors are less often responsible for false-negative results than technical errors.[278]

Less than optimal or unsatisfactory FNA biopsy technical results occur with both small and large breast lesions.[282] Breast masses smaller than 1 cm are associated with a false-negative rate in the range of 6% to 24% because of the greater potential of the aspirator to miss the lesion, whereas tumors larger than 4 cm can have a relatively high false-negative rate most likely resulting from the presence of necrosis, cystic degeneration, or hemorrhage.[5,278,282,283] Carcinomas that have the highest potential for false-negative diagnoses include those with low tumor cell–to–stroma ratios resulting from extensive desmoplastic fibrosis and low-grade malignancies characterized by bland cytologic features.[15,284] These cancers include lobular carcinoma, tubular carcinoma, colloid carcinoma, papillary carcinoma, and the monomorphic pattern of ductal carcinoma that typically occurs in older women. Careful attention to nuclear detail, appreciation of a monomorphic cell population, and the presence of individually scattered atypical intact cells should facilitate the recognition of these cells as malignant in FNA cytology.[15,284]

The false-negative rate is also conditional on whether the specimen has been adequately sampled. Considerable controversy is in the literature as to what constitutes an ad-

equate breast aspirate.[285-289] Layfield and colleagues found that most false-negative specimens had low cellularity consisting of six or fewer cell clusters.[289] Therefore, these authors advocated the use of a numerical cutoff point. An adequate aspirate may show either six or more cell clusters, with each cluster containing five or more cells, or numerous bipolar cells defined as 10 or more cells per 10 medium power fields. Sneige,[287] with some exceptions, agreed with the Layfield approach, whereas Abele and colleagues disagreed with the principal of epithelial cell counting for assessment of specimen adequacy, advocating that when a breast nodule is aspirated by an experienced individual, the cellularity is contingent on the degree of epithelial proliferation within the lesion, rather than an arbitrary numerical count.[290] These authors noted that in their community-based FNA practice, a high prevalence of fibrocystic change in a young patient population would mean that a large proportion of these cases would be considered unsatisfactory if based on a strict numerical adequacy criterion.[290] Supporting this idea is the observation that even with excellent screening, a large portion of the breast biopsies evaluated in surgical pathology consist almost exclusively of benign fibrofatty soft tissue. Such tissue would be expected to give a very sparsely cellular or even acellular aspiration specimen. Although the controversy will apparently not be settled in the near future, it is recommended that some statement of adequacy be presented in the FNA cytology report. If the aspirator is different from the individual interpreting the smears, then a negative diagnosis should not be rendered if very limited cellularity is available, but rather the specimen should be considered insufficient for definitive assessment.

Interpretative errors are responsible for essentially all false-positive diagnoses, with false-positive rates reported in the literature in the range of 0% to 4%.[10,15,59,278,291] Feldman and Covell reviewed 14 published series in which an average false-positive rate of 0.17% was found in more than 25,000 FNA biopsy of the breast.[10] This false-positive rate may be inflated because some series included suspicious diagnoses as malignant. Tissue confirmation is strongly recommended in any specimen suspected to be malignant but lacking either high cellularity or significant atypia to justify an unequivocal diagnosis of malignancy. Cytologic atypia can occur in a variety of benign breast lesions including fibrocystic change, fibroadenoma, inflammatory lesions, granulation tissue, gynecomastia, papilloma, hormonally related changes, and pregnancy-related hyperplasia.[15,16] Therefore, in any questionable aspirate, frozen section, or surgical biopsy confirmation is recommended.[15,16,278] The College of American Pathologists' retrospective assessment of breast FNA biopsy, as part of their quality assurance Q-probe program, evaluated more than 13,000 breast FNA biopsy specimens from 294 institutions.[292] Of the cases, 82% were deemed to be satisfactory for evaluation with one third having histologic correlation that served as the basis for determining diagnostic accuracy. In this retrospective review of primarily breast FNA in the community hospital setting, the sensitivity of the procedure compared quite well with results reported by expert cytopathologists at academic medical centers.

False-negative and false-positive diagnoses as well as other diagnostic errors can be decreased if physicians use the triple test approach that incorporates clinical examination, mammographic findings, and FNA cytology when evaluating breast lesions.[293-296] Although palpation, mammography, and FNA biopsy have their sets of limitations, by combining all three procedures, cumulative high levels of diagnostic sensitivity and specificity are achieved.[15,16,293-296] Layfield and colleagues and others have demonstrated that malignant FNA biopsy results, along with positive mammography and suspicious clinical examination, had a diagnostic accuracy exceeding 99% for breast carcinomas.[282] Breast carcinoma was found in palpable breast masses in only 0.6% of the cases when all three parameters were interpreted as benign.[282] When mammography and clinical findings are benign, but FNA cytology was suspicious for malignancy, the probability of cancer increased to 16%.[299] With a benign physical and mammographic examination, but a malignant FNA result, the probability of carcinoma was virtually 100%. Conversely, physical findings suspicious for malignancy associated with positive results of mammography examination resulted in the probability of cancer of only approximately 36% when coupled with a benign FNA diagnosis.[299] Therefore, clinical decisions should be based on all three parameters instead of relying exclusively on the FNA cytology results. Layfield and others advocate that when a discordant triple test result is encountered, surgical biopsy should be obtained.[282] Troxel and Sabella have reported that one of the more common areas for malpractice claims are problems related to FNA of the breast.[300] This further validates that strict adherence to the principles of the triple test is critical in making the most accurate diagnosis and avoiding both false-negative and false-positive diagnoses.

THE BREAST FINE-NEEDLE ASPIRATION CYTOLOGY REPORT

The National Cancer Institute sponsored a conference in 1996 in Bethesda, Md., advocating a uniform approach to the performance and reporting of breast fine-needle aspiration biopsy.[301] Guidelines for performance of FNA or core biopsies on palpable and nonpalpable breast masses, as well as training and credentialing, biopsy technique, diagnostic terminology, ancillary studies, and post-FNA follow-up recommendations were presented. The conference proposed classifying the cytologic findings into the following general categories: benign, atypical/indeterminate, suspicious/indeterminate, suspicious/probably malignant, malignant, and unsatisfactory, along with a detailed explanation of the microscopic findings that are diagnostically specific for each category. An important recommendation was to report the adequacy of the specimen and to note that an unsatisfactory specimen is present if the following conditions occurred: (1) scant cellularity, (2) air-drying (for those pathologists using fixed smears) or distortion artifact, and/or (3) obscuring blood, inflammation, or other factors. The prime importance of the latter recommendations is to classify these types of specimens as inadequate or unsatisfactory rather than as negative. This avoids falsely labeling these lesions as benign when the aspirated target was in fact not adequately sampled. Besides these general categories, a specific diagnosis can also be reported. This conference also recommended the use of cytologic nuclear grading corresponding to the grading system employed when evaluating

a histologic specimen. The authors of this text support the principles outlined by this conference, along with the need to standardize the reporting of breast FNA.[302]

Because of its importance in development of FNA technique and practice, breast aspiration is used extensively for our clinical and technical discussions in Chapter 2.

NIPPLE DISCHARGE CYTOLOGY

Nipple discharge, although relatively uncommon, is the second most common breast symptom after the presence of a lump. Nipple discharge can either be the result of physiologic or pathologic causes.[303] An abnormal nipple discharge is usually associated with underlying breast pathology and is usually spontaneous, persistent, unilateral, nonlactational, and especially seen in older patients. Other causes of nipple discharge include drugs and metabolic conditions such as hyper- and hypothyroidism, pituitary adenoma with elevated prolactin levels, or idiopathic pituitary adenoma. Physiologic nipple discharge occurs most often in young adult women because of hormonal fluctuations resulting from pregnancy or lactation.[304]

Approximately 3% of malignant breast lesions are associated with an abnormal nipple discharge.[303,305-309] Clinical features associated with malignancy in patients with an abnormal nipple discharge include male gender, older age (older than age 50), unilaterality, and a bloody appearance of the discharge.[304] In these patients, an abnormal mammogram and/or palpable breast mass is also often apparent. Bloody discharges can also be associated with intraductal papillomas.[304] Ciatto and colleagues recommended that cytologic examination should only be performed on bloody discharges, although others have cautioned that carcinoma can also be associated with a nonbloody discharge[310] that is often serous or watery.[311] However, purulent, milky and multicolored discharges are generally not related to breast cancer.[312]

Evaluation for occult blood and carcinoembryonic antigen (CEA) in nipple discharge fluid has been used as adjunctive tests in some centers. This may increase the sensitivity for finding occult nonpalpable breast cancer.[312] A variety of other biomarkers of breast cancer risk in nipple aspirate fluid has been investigated.[318]

In general, exfoliative cytology of nipple discharge fluid is a fairly insensitive but specific procedure for the diagnosis of an underlying nonpalpable breast carcinoma.[313] However, evaluation for mucin in the nipple discharge has not been useful.[314]

Cytologic examination of duct dilatation and stasis reveals predominantly foam cells ("histiocytes") having coarsely vacuolated cytoplasm together with occasional benign ductal cells.[303,315] The ductal cells are usually arranged in tightly cohesive, uniform groups and the cells show minimal to no variation in size. Although the cells may have high N:C ratios, hyperchromasia with coarse chromatin is not present. Occasionally, apocrine cells can be present. Intraductal papilloma will consist of three-dimensional clusters of cells in which considerable variation in cell size is evident (Figure 29-71). Although nuclear atypicality may be present within the clusters, single atypical cells, a useful feature of malignancy, are not seen with any significant frequency.[315] A malignant cytologic diagnosis should not be

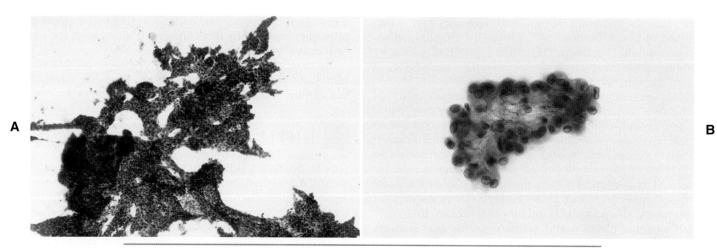

Figure 29-71   **Nipple discharge of intraductal papilloma. A,** Complex papillary group of benign ductal cells. (Pap) **B,** Three-dimensional papillary groups with fibrovascular cores. (Pap)

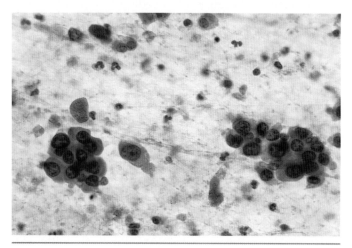

Figure 29-72   **Nipple discharge, ductal carcinoma of the breast.** Nipple discharge showing loosely cohesive clusters of malignant cells and individually scattered malignant cells. There was tumor necrosis in the background. (Pap)

rendered in a nipple discharge specimen unless many individually scattered atypical cells are present (Figure 29-72). In addition, it is also recommended that if a malignant diagnosis is made, histologic confirmation should be obtained before definitive treatment.[315]

Physiologic nipple discharge is generally paucicellular to acellular, consisting almost exclusively of proteinaceous background material (Figure 29-73). Inflammatory and infectious conditions can also result in a nipple discharge with the expected inflammatory cell exudate. A tuberculous etiologic factor for a nipple discharge can be suspected when the cytologic examination reveals epithelioid histiocytes and giant cells, in addition to neutrophils, foam cells, and necrotic debris. However, the definitive diagnosis needs to be confirmed by the presence of acid-fast bacilli.[303] Galactorrhea is characterized by numerous foam cells set in a prominent lipoproteinaceous smear background.[303] Other procedures used to evaluate a nipple discharge and nipple aspirate fluid[317,324] include intraductal aspiration.[316,317] Ductal lavage cytology is currently under investigation as a

tool for breast cancer screening, especially for those women having an increased risk of breast cancer.[324]

BREAST DUCT LAVAGE

The need to provide more specific prognostic information and to guide patients in consideration of various endocrine and surgical approaches to possible breast cancer prevention or early detection has driven searches for noninvasive detection of cellular abnormalities. The methods have included suction nipple aspiration, blind fine needle aspiration, and the recently described technique of ductal lavage (DL).[324-330] DL is safe, minimally invasive, and usually well accepted.

The initial studies are not large, and identification of atypical cells has lead to detection of otherwise occult in-situ or invasive breast carcinomas in less than 1% of DL from high-risk women. When unequivocally malignant cells are identified, this is a significant finding. Further investigation with tools such as ultrasound or MRI may then localize otherwise undetectable lesions.

However, the sensitivity and specificity of DL for diagnosis of carcinoma are not known. In one review, sparsely cellular nondiagnostic samples were common (22%) and only 6% of studies showed cells that were not diagnostic of carcinoma but that were considered to be markedly atypical. The ultimate significance of atypia below the level of frank malignancy and of benign DL findings is not known. Furthermore, the correlation of various cytologic abnormalities with specific histopathologic degrees of proliferative breast disease is very poor, making comparisons problematic at this time. It is hoped that identification of such cells will provide another component in a multifactorial patient data set used mostly in decision making about chemoprevention. A suggestion that atypical DL cytology may be a reason to consider prophylactic mastectomy[330] seems premature to us at the time of this writing.

We agree with Cangiarella and Masood that nuclear atypia is common and frequently because of factors other than malignancy including fibroadenoma, duct ectasia, papillomas, metaplasias of various types, inflammation, and infections as well as a range of endogenous and iatrogenic

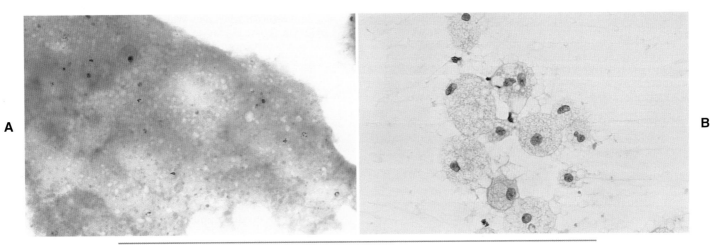

Figure 29-73 Nipple discharge, physiologic type. **A,** Physiologic nipple discharge showing the presence of background proteinaceous material with scant cellularity. **B,** Physiologic nipple discharge with numerous histiocytes and scattered acute inflammatory cells. (Pap)

hormonal states.[330] This suggests that the range of "normal" DL cytology in healthy women is probably very broad. Futhermore, a significant fraction of breast carcinomas shows little nuclear atypia, even with a palpable mass.

The current implications for risk assessment based on routine morphologic study of DL samples embody the following points: it is likely that we do not know enough about what constitutes normal cytology in such material; the implications of a sparsely cellular sample, the indications for repeat sampling, and the interval for repeat studies have not been investigated; the implications of completely benign cytology in high-risk women remain to be shown by follow-up studies; the reproducibility of atypical diagnoses is currently unknown; and the sensitivity and specificity of DL as a test for recognizing malignancy are unknown.

Perhaps application of molecular techniqiues to these samples will prove useful in ways that currently elude the morphologist. Our impression is that as a cytodiagnostic tool unembellished by ancillary methods, DL may be difficult to disseminate to the community from our academic centers. This has certainly been the case with community-based definitive cytologic diagnosis of even palpable, clinically malignant breast masses by FNA.

It is important to council patients that DL cannot be considered a replacement or a substitute for more established means of diagnosis and follow up, including periodic physical examination and mammography. Given the astounding success of uterine cervical cancer screening over several decades, suggestions that DL is a similarly efficacious procedure seem premature at this time.

References

1. Martin HE, Ellis EB. Biopsy by needle puncture and aspiration. Ann Surg 1930; 92:169-181.
2. Martin HE, Ellis EB. Aspiration biopsy. Surg Gynecol Obstet 1934; 59:578-589.
3. Stewart FW. The diagnosis of tumors by aspiration. Am J Pathol 1993; 9:801-812.
4. Franzen S, Zajicek J. Aspiration biopsy in diagnosis of palpable lesions of the breast: critical review of 3,479 consecutive biopsies. Acta Radiol Ther Phys Biol 1968; 7:241-262.
5. Zajdela A, Ghossein NA, Pilleron JP, et al. The value of aspiration cytology in the diagnosis of breast cancer: experience at the foundation curie. Cancer 1975; 35:499-506.
6. Zajicek J. Aspiration biopsy–cytology (Part II). Monogr Clin Cytol 1974; 7.
7. Zajicek J. Aspiration biopsy–cytology (Part I). Monogr Clin Cytol 1974; 4:136-195.
8. Zajicek J, Caspersson T, Jakobsson P, et al. Cytologic diagnosis of mammary tumors from aspiration biopsy smears: comparison of cytologic and histologic findings in 2,111 lesions and diagnostic use of cytophotometry. Acta Cytol 1970; 14:370-376.
9. Zajicek J, Franzen S, Jacobsson P, et al. Aspiration biopsy of mammary tumors in diagnosis and research: a critical review of 2,200 cases. Acta Cytol 1967; 11:169-175.
10. Feldman PS, Covell JL. Breast and lung. In: Fine needle aspiration cytology and its clinical application. Chicago: American Society of Clinical Pathologists Press; 1985. pp.27-43.
11. Frable WJ. Fine needle aspiration biopsy: a review. Hum Pathol 1983; 14:9-28.
12. Frable WJ. Needle aspiration biopsy: past, present, and future. Hum Pathol 1989; 20:504-517.
13. Koss LG, Woyke J, Olszewski W. Aspiration biopsy: cytologic interpretation and histologic bases. New York: Igaku-Shoin; 1984. pp.53-104.
14. Silverman JF: In: Bibbo M. Comprehensive cytopathology. 2nd ed. WB Saunders; 1997. pp.731-780.
15. Dabbs D, Silverman JF: Breast. In: Geisinger K, Silverman J, editors. Fine needle aspiration cytology of superficial organs and body sites. Edinburgh: Churchill Livingstone; 1999. pp.51-84.
16. Abele JS, Miller TR, Goodson WH III, et al. Fine-needle aspiration of palpable breast masses: a program for staged implementation. Arch Surg 1983; 118:859-863.
17. Langmuir VK, Cramer SF, Hood ME. Fine needle aspiration cytology in the management of palpable benign and malignant breast disease: correlation with clinical and mammographic findings. Acta Cytol 1989; 33: 93-98.
18. Kline TS, Joshi LP, Neal HS. Fine needle aspiration of the breast: diagnoses and pitfalls: a review of 3,545 cases. Cancer 1979; 44:1458-1464.
19. Lee GF. Fine-needle aspiration of the breast: the outpatient management of breast lesions. Am J Obstet Gynecol 1987; 156:1532-1537.

20. Frost AR, Aksu A, Kurstin R, et al. Can nonproliferative breast disease and proliferative breast disease without atypia be distinguished by fine-needle aspiration cytology? Cancer (Cancer Cytopathol) 1997; 81:22-28.

21. Sneige N, Staerkel GA. Fine-needle aspiration cytology of ductal hyperplasia with and without atypia and ductal carcinoma in situ. Hum Pathol 1994; 25:485-492.

22. Sidawy MK, Stoler MH, Frable WJ, et al. Interobserver variability in the classification of proliferative breast lesions by fine-needle aspiration: results of the Papanicolaou Society of cytopathology study. Diagn Cytopathol 1998; 18:150-165.

23. Shin HJC, Sneige N. Is a diagnosis of infiltrating versus in situ ductal carcinoma of the breast possible in fine-needle aspiration specimens? Cancer (Cancer Cytopathol) 1998; 84:186-191.

24. Bauermeister DE. The role and limitations of frozen section and needle aspiration biopsy in breast cancer diagnosis. Cancer 1980; 46:947-949.

25. Frable WJ. Needle aspiration of the breast. Cancer 1984; 53:671-676.

26. Griffith CN, Kern WH, Mikkelsen WP. Needle aspiration cytologic examination in the management of suspicious lesions of the breast. Surg Gynecol Obstet 1986; 162:142-144.

27. Norton LW, Davis JR, Wiens JL, et al. Accuracy of aspiration cytology in detecting breast cancer. Surgery 1984; 96:806-814.

28. Smallwood J, Herbert A, Guyer P, et al. Accuracy of aspiration cytology in the diagnosis of breast disease. Br J Surg 1985; 72:841-843.

29. Silverman JF, Lannin DR, O'Brien K, et al. The triage role of fine needle aspiration biopsy of palpable breast masses: diagnostic accuracy and cost effectiveness. Acta Cytol 1987; 31:731-736.

30. Scopa CD, Koukouras D, Spiliotis J, et al. Comparison of fine needle aspiration and tru-cut biopsy of palpable mammary lesions. Cancer Det Prevent 1996; 20(6):620-624.

31. Ballo MS, Sneige N. Can core needle biopsy replace fine-needle aspiration cytology in the diagnosis of palpable breast carcinoma: a comparative study of 124 women. Cancer 1996; 78:773-777.

32. Florentine BD, Cobb CJ, Frankel K, et al. Core needle biopsy: a useful adjunct to fine-needle aspiration in select patients with palpable breast lesions. Cancer (Cancer Cytopathol) 1997; 81:33-39.

33. Shin HJC, Sneige N, Staerkel GA. Utility of punch biopsy for lesions that are hard to aspirate by conventional fine-needle aspiration. Cancer (Cancer Cytopathol) 1999; 87:149-154.

34. Dey P, Karmakar T. Fine needle aspiration cytology of accessory axillary breasts and their lesions. Acta Cytol 1994; 38:915-916.

35. Ku NNK, Mela NJ, Fiorica JV, et al. Role of fine needle aspiration cytology after lumpectomy. Acta Cytol 1994; 38:927-932.

36. Zajdela A, Zillhardt P, Voillemot N. Cytological diagnosis by fine-needle sampling without aspiration. Cancer 1987; 59:1201-1205.

37. Silverman JF, Finley JL, O'Brien K, et al. Diagnostic accuracy and role of immediate interpretation of fine needle aspiration biopsy specimens from various sites. Acta Cytol 1989; 33:791-796.

38. Silverman JF, Frable WJ. The use of the Diff-Quik stain in the immediate interpretation of fine-needle aspiration biopsies. Diagn Cytopathol 1990; 6:366-369.

39. Bedard YC, Pollett AF. Breast fine-needle aspiration: a comparison of thin prep and conventional smears. Am J Clin Pathol 1999; 111:523-527.

40. Florentine BD, Wu NC, Waliany S, et al. Fine needle aspiration (FNA) biopsy of palpable breast masses: comparison of conventional smears with the Cyto-Tek MonoPrep System. Cancer (Cancer Cytopathol) 1999; 87:278-285.

41. The uniform approach to breast fine needle aspiration biopsy: a synopsis. (Developed and approved at an NCI-sponsored conference, Bethesda, Md, Sept. 9-10, 1996.) Acta Cytol 1996; 40:1120-1126.

42. Catania S, Boccato P, Bono A, et al. Pneumothorax: a rare complication of fine needle aspiration of the breast. Acta Cytol 1989; 33:140.

43. Gateley CA, Maddox PR, Mansel RE. Pneumothorax: a complication of fine needle aspiration of the breast. Br Med J 1991; 303:627-628.

44. Stevenson J, James AS, Johnston M, et al. Pneumothorax after fine needle aspiration of the breast. Br Med J 1991; 303:924.

45. Kaufman Z, Shpitz B, Shapiro M, et al. Pneumothorax: a complication of fine needle aspiration of breast tumors. Acta Cytol 1994; 38:737-738.

46. Bondeson L, Lindholm K. Aspiration cytology of tubular breast carcinoma. Acta Cytol 1990; 34:15-20.

47. Harter LP, Curtis JS, Ponto G, et al. Malignant seeding of the needle track during stereotaxic core needle breast biopsy. Radiology 1992; 185:713-714.

48. Stockdale FE. Questions and answers: mammography, needle biopsy, and tumor spread. JAMA 1994; 272:895-896.

49. Taxin A, Tartter PI, Zappetti D. Breast cancer diagnosed by fine needle aspiration and excisional biopsy: recurrence and survival. Acta Cytol 1997; 41:302-306.

50. Lee KC, Chan JKC, Ho LC, et al. Histologic changes in the breast after fine-needle aspiration. Am J Surg Pathol 1994; 18:1039-1047.

51. Gobbi H, Tse G, Page DL, et al. Reactive spindle cell nodules of the breast after core biopsy or fine-needle aspiration. Am J Clin Pathol 2000; 113:288-294.

52. Krasovec M, Golouh R, Avesperg M. Tissue damage after fine needle aspiration. Acta Cytol 1992;36:456-457.

53. Youngson BJ, Cranor M, Rosen PP. Epithelial displacement in surgical specimens following needling procedures. Am J Surg Pathol 1994; 18:896-903.

54. Raso DS. In: Herzberg AJ, Razo DS, Silverman JF. Color atlas of normal cytology. New York: Churchill Livingstone; 1999. pp.387-398.

55. Stanley MW, Henry-Stanley MJ, Zera R. Atypia in breast fine-needle aspiration smears correlates poorly with the presence of a prognostically significant proliferation lesion of ductal epithelium. Hum Pathol 1993; 24:630-635.

56. Carter BA, Jensen RA, Simpson JF, et al. Benign transport of breast epithelium into axillary lymph nodes after biopsy. Am J Clin Pathol 2000; 113:259-265.

57. Kline TS. Handbook of fine needle aspiration biopsy cytology. St Louis: Mosby; 1988.

58. Frable W. Major problems in pathology. In: Thin needle aspiration biopsy, vol 14. Philadelphia: WB Saunders; 1983.

59. Ciatto S, Cariaggi P, Bulgaresi P. The value of routine cytologic examination of breast cyst fluids. Acta Cytol 1987; 31:301-304.

60. Takeda T, Suzuki M, Sato Y, et al. Aspiration cytology of breast cysts. Acta Cytol 1982; 26:37-43.

61. Gupta RK, McHutchinson AGR, Fauck R. Liesegang rings in a needle aspirate from a breast cyst. Acta Cytol 1991; 35:700-702.

62. Raso DS, Greene WB, Finley JL, et al. Morphology and pathogenesis of liesegang rings in cyst aspirates: report of two cases with ancillary studies. Diagn Cytopathol 1998; 19:116-119.

63. Azzopardi JG. Problems in breast pathology. In: Bennington JL, editor. Major problems in pathology, vol II. Philadelphia: WB Saunders; 1979. pp.42-55, 346-378.

64. Haagensen CD. Diseases of the breast. Philadelphia: WB Saunders; 1986.

65. Silverman JF, Dabbs DJ, Gilbert CF. Adenosis tumor of the breast: cytologic, histologic, immunocytochemical and ultrastructural observations. Acta Cytol 1989; 33:181-187.

66. Bapat KC, Pandit AA. Filarial infection of the breast: report of a case with diagnosis by fine needle aspiration cytology. Acta Cytol 1992; 36:505-506.

67. Dey P, Walker R. Microfilariae in a fine needle aspirate from a skin nodule. Acta Cytol 1994; 38:114.

68. Epstein NA. Hydatid cyst of the breast: diagnosis using cytological techniques. Acta Cytol 1969; 13:420-421.

69. Farmer C, Stanley MW, Bardales RH. Mycoses of the breast: diagnosis by fine-needle aspiration. Diagn Cytopathol 1995; 12:51-55.

70. Govindarajan M, Verghese S, Kuruvilla S. Primary aspergillosis of the breast: report of a case with fine needle aspiration cytology diagnosis. Acta Cytol 1993; 37:234-236.

71. Jayaram G. Cytomorphology in tuberculosis mastitis: a report of nine cases with fine-needle aspiration cytology. Acta Cytol 1985; 29:974-978.

72. Galbum LI, Oertel YC. Subareolar abscess of the breast diagnosed by fine needle aspiration. Am J Clin Pathol 1983; 80:496-499.

73. Silverman JF, Lannin DR, Unverferth M, et al. Fine needle aspiration cytology of subareolar abscess of the breast: spectrum of cytomorphologic findings and potential diagnostic pitfalls. Acta Cytol 1986; 30:413-419.

74. Kline TS. Masquerades of malignancy: a review of 4,241 aspirations from the breast. Acta Cytol 1981; 25:263-266.

75. Oertel YC, Galblum LI. Fine needle aspiration of the breast: diagnostic criteria. Pathol Annu (Part I) 1983; 18:375-407.

76. Dodd LG, Sneige N, Reece GP, et al. Fine-needle aspiration cytology of silicone granulomas in the augmented breast. Diagn Cytopathol 1993; 9:498-502.

77. Doria MI, Tani EM, Skoog L. Sarcoidosis presenting initially as a breast mass: detection by fine-needle aspiration biopsy. Acta Cytol 1987; 31:378-379.

78. Houn H-YD, Granger JK. Granulomatous mastitis secondary to histoplasmosis: report of a case diagnosed by fine-needle aspiration biopsy. Diagn Cytopathol 1991; 7:282-285.

79. Macansh S, Greenberg M, Barraclough B, et al. Fine needle aspiration cytology of granulomatous mastitis. Report of a case and review of the literature. Acta Cytol 1990; 34:38-42.

80. Maygarden SJ, Novotny DB, Johnson DE, et al. Fine-needle aspiration cytology of suture granulomas of the breast: a potential pitfall in the cytologic diagnosis of recurrent breast cancer. Diagn Cytopathol 1994;10:175-179.

81. Oberman HA. Invasive carcinoma of the breast with granulomatous response. Am J Clin Pathol 1987; 88:718-721.

82. Gansler TS, Wheeler JE. Mammary sarcoidosis: two cases and literature review. Arch Pathol Lab Med 1984; 108:673-675.

83. Martinez-Parra D, Nevado-Santos M, Melendez-Guerrero B, et al. Utility of fine needle aspiration in the diagnosis of granulomatous lesions of the breast. Diagn Cytopathol 1997; 17:108-114.

84. Hashimoto CH, Cobb CJ. Cytodiagnosis of hibernoma: a case report. Diagn Cytopathol 1987; 3:326-329.

85. Shabb N, Sneige N, Dekmezian RH. Myospherulosis: fine needle aspiration: cytologic findings in 19 cases. Acta Cytol 1991; 35:225-228.

86. Linsk JA, Franzen S. Clinical aspiration cytology. Philadelphia: JB Lippincott; 1983. pp.105-137.

87. Schondorf H [translated by Schneider V]. Aspiration cytology of the breast. Philadelphia: WB Saunders; 1978, p.17.

88. Wang NP, Wan BC, Skelly VE, et al. Monoclonal antibodies to novel myoepithelium associated proteins can distinguish between benign and malignant lesions of the breast. Mod Pathol 1996; 9:26A.

89. Kreuzer G. Aspiration biopsy cytology in proliferating benign mammary dysplasia. Acta Cytol 1978; 22:128-132.

90. Lee WY, Wang HH. Fine-needle aspiration is limited in the classification of benign breast diseases. Diagn Cytopathol 1998; 18:56-61.

91. Stanley MW, Tani EM, Rutqvist L-E, et al. Adenoid cystic carcinoma of the breast: diagnosis by fine-needle aspiration. Diagn Cytopathol 1993; 9:184-187.

92. Shinagawa T, Tadokoro M, Kitamura H, et al. Secretory carcinoma of the breast: correlation of aspiration cytology and histology. Acta Cytol 1994; 38:909-914.

93. Silverman JF, Masood S, Ducatman BS. Can FNA biopsy separate atypical hyperplasia, carcinoma in situ, and invasive carcinoma of the breast? Cytomorphologic criteria and limitations in diagnosis. Diagn Cytopathol 1993; 9:713-728.

94. Dupont WD, Page DL. Risk factors for breast cancer in women with proliferative breast disease. N Engl J Med 1985; 312:146-151.

95. Page DL. Cancer risk assessment in benign breast biopsies. Hum Pathol 1986; 17:871-874.

96. Page DL, Dupont WD, Rogers LW, et al. Atypical hyperplastic lesions of the female breast: a long-term follow-up study. Cancer 1985; 55:2698-2708.

97. Rosen PP, Braun DW Jr, Kinne DE. The clinical significance of preinvasive breast carcinoma. Cancer 1980; 46:919-925.

98. Smart CR, Myers MH, Gloeckler LA. Implications from SEER data on breast cancer management. Cancer 1978; 42:787-789.

99. Thomas PA, Cangiarella J, Raab SS, et al. Fine needle aspiration biopsy of proliferative breast disease. Hum Pathol 1995; 6:130-136.

100. Thomas PA, Raab SS, Cohen MB. Is the fine-needle aspiration biopsy diagnosis of proliferative breast disease feasible? Diagn Cytopathol 1994; 11:301-306.

101. Sneige N, Staerkel GA. Fine-needle aspiration cytology of ductal hyperplasia with and without atypia and ductal carcinoma in situ. Hum Pathol 1994; 25:485-492.

102. Masood S, Frykberg E, McLellan GL, et al. Cytologic differentiation between proliferative and nonproliferative breast disease in mammographically guided fine-needle aspirates. Diagn Cytopathol 1991; 7:581-590.

103. Rosen PP, Cantrell B, Mullen DL, et al. Juvenile papillomatosis (Swiss cheese disease). Am J Surg Pathol 1980; 4:3-12.

104. Page DL, Anderson TJ. Diagnostic histopathology of the breast. New York: Churchill Livingstone; 1987.

105. Bottles K, Chan JS, Holly EA, et al. Cytologic criteria for fibroadenoma: a step-wise logistic regression analysis. Am J Clin Pathol 1988; 89:707-713.

106. Dejmek A, Lindholm K. Frequency of cytologic features in fine needle aspirates from histologically and cytologically diagnosed fibroadenomas. Acta Cytol 1991; 35:695-699.

107. Gupta RK. Fine-needle aspiration (FNA) cytology of concurrent breast carcinoma in fibroadenoma. Cytopathology 1995; 6:201-203.

108. Stanley MW, Tani EM, Skoog L. Fine-needle aspiration of fibroadenomas of the breast with atypia: a spectrum including cases that cytologically mimic carcinoma. Diagn Cytopathol 1990; 6:375-382.

109. Myers T, Wang HH. Fibroadenoma mimicking papillary carcinoma on ThinPrep of fine-needle aspiration of the breast. Arch Pathol Lab Med 2000; 124:1667-1669.

110. Al-Kaisi N. The spectrum of the "gray zone" in breast cytology: a review of 186 cases of atypical and suspicious cytology. Acta Cytol 1994; 38:898-908.

111. Sturgis CD, Sethi S, Cajulis RS, et al. Diagnostic significance of "benign pairs" and signet ring cells in fine needle aspirates (FNAs) of the breast. Cytopathology 1998; 9:308-319.

112. Gherardi G, Bernardi C, Marveggio C. Microglandular adenosis of the breast: fine-needle aspiration biopsy of two cases. Diagn Cytopathol 1993; 9:72-76.

113. Hock Y-L, Chan S-Y. Adenomyoepithelioma of the breast: a case report correlating cytologic and histologic features. Acta Cytol 1994; 38:953-956.

114. Nguyen G-K, Shnitka TK, Jewell LD. Aspiration biopsy cytology of mammary myoepithelioma. Diagn Cytopathol 1987; 3:335-338.

115. Stanley MW, Tani EM, Skoog L. Fine needle aspiration of the breast with atypia: a spectrum including cases that cytologically mimic carcinoma. Diagn Cytopathol 1990; 6:375-382.

116. Kumar N, Kapila K, Verma K. Characterization of tubular adenoma of breast: diagnostic problem in fine needle aspirates (FNAs). Cytopathology 1998; 9:301-307.

117. Shet TM, Rege JD. Aspiration cytology of tubular adenomas of the breast: an analysis of eight cases. Acta Cytol 1998; 42:657-662.

118. Stormby N, Bondeson L. Adenoma of the nipple. Acta Cytol 1984; 28:729-732.

119. Sood N, Jayaram G. Cytology of papillary adenoma of the nipple: a case diagnosed on fine-needle aspiration. Diagn Cytopathol 1990; 6:345-348.

120. Bosch MMC, Boon ME. Fine-needle cytology of an eccrine spiradenoma of the breast: diagnosis made by a holistic approach. Diagn Cytopathol 1992; 8:366-368.

121. Jensen ML, Johansen P, Noer H, Sorensen IM. Ductal adenoma of the breast: cytological features of six cases. Diagn Cytopathol 1994; 10:143-145.

122. Kumar N, Verma K. Clear cell hidradenoma simulating breast carcinoma: a diagnostic pitfall in fine needle aspiration of breast. Diagn Cytopathol 1996; 15:70-72.

123. Kanter MH, Sedeghi M. Pleomorphic adenoma of the breast: cytology of fine-needle aspiration and its differential diagnosis. Diagn Cytopathol 1993; 9:555-558.

124. Bottles K, Taylor RN. Diagnosis of breast masses in pregnant and lactating women by aspiration cytology. Obstet Gynecol 1985; 66:76S-78S.

125. Finley JL, Silverman JF, Lannin DR. Fine-needle aspiration cytology of breast masses in pregnant and lactating women. Diagn Cytopathol 1989; 5:255-259.

126. Grenko RT, Lee KP, Lee KR. Fine needle aspiration cytology of lactating adenoma of the breast: a comparative light microscopic and morphometric study. Acta Cytol 1990; 34:21-26.

127. Gupta RK, McHutchison AGR, Dowle GS, et al. Fine-needle aspiration cytodiagnosis of breast masses in pregnant and lactating women and its impact on management. Diagn Cytopathol 1993; 9:156-159.

128. Maygarden SJ, McCall JB, Frable WJ. Fine needle aspiration of breast lesions in women aged 30 and under. Acta Cytol 1991; 35:687-694.

129. Novotny DB, Maygarden SJ, Shermer RW, et al. Fine needle aspiration of benign and malignant breast masses associated with pregnancy. Acta Cytol 1991; 35:676-686.

130. Haas JF. Pregnancy in association with a newly diagnosed cancer: a population based epidemiologic assessment. Int J Cancer 1984; 34:229.

131. Mitre BK, Kanbour AI, Mauser N. Fine needle aspiration biopsy of breast carcinoma in pregnancy and lactation. Acta Cytol 1997; 41:1121-1130.

132. Gupta RK, Naran S, Buchanan A, et al. Fine-needle aspiration cytology of breast: its impact on surgical practice with an emphasis on the diagnosis of breast abnormalities in young women. Diagn Cytopathol 1988; 4:206-209.

133. DeMay RM, Kay S. Granular cell tumor of the breast. Pathol Annu 1984; 19:121-148.

134. Ingram DL, Mossler JA, Snowhite J, et al. Granular cell tumors of the breast: steroid receptor analysis and localization of carcinoembryonic antigen, myoglobin, and S100 protein. Arch Pathol Lab Med 1984; 108:897-901.

135. Lowhagen T, Rubio C. The cytology of the granular cell myoblastoma of the breast. Acta Cytol 1977; 21:314-345.

136. Sirgi KE, Sneige N, Fanning TV, et al. Fine-needle aspirates of granular cell lesions of the breast: report of three cases, with emphasis on differential diagnosis and utility of immunostaining for CD68 (KP1). Diagn Cytopathol 1996; 15:403-408.

137. Lew W, Seymour A. Primary amyloid tumor of the breast, case report and literature review. Acta Cytol 1985; 29:7-11.

138. Silverman JF, Dabbs DJ, Norris HT, et al. Localized primary (AL) amyloid tumor of the breast: cytologic, histologic, immunocytochemical and ultrastructural observations. Am J Surg Pathol 1986; 10:539-545.

139. Lynch LA, Moriarty AT. Localized primary amyloid tumor associated with osseous metaplasia presenting as bilateral breast masses: cytologic and radiologic features. Diagn Cytopathol 1993; 9:570-575.

140. Greenberg ML, Middleton PD, Bilous AM. Infarcted intraduct papilloma diagnosed by fine-needle biopsy: a cytologic, clinical and mammographic pitfall. Diagn Cytopathol 1994; 11:188-194.

141. Bhagat P, Kline TS. The male breast and malignant neoplasms: diagnosis by aspiration biopsy cytology. Cancer 1990; 65:2338-2341.

142. Gupta RK, Naran S, Simpson J. The role of fine needle aspiration cytology (FNAC) in the diagnosis of breast masses in males. Eur J Surg Oncol 1988; 14:317-320.

143. Johnson TL, Kini SR. Significance of bloody breast nipple discharge in men. ASCP Check Sample 1987; 15:C-87-11 (C-173).

144. Pinedo F, Vargas J, de Agustin P, et al. Epithelial atypia in gynecomastia induced by chemotherapeutic drugs: a possible pitfall in fine needle aspiration biopsy. Acta Cytopathol 1991; 35:229-233.

145. Russin VL, Lachowicz C, Kline TS. Male breast lesions: gynecomastia and its distinction from carcinoma by aspiration biopsy cytology. Diagn Cytopathol 1989; 5:243-247.

146. Skoog L. Aspiration cytology of a male breast carcinoma with argyrophilic cells. Acta Cytol 1987; 31:379-381.

147. Sethi S, Cajulis RS, Gokaslan ST, et al. Diagnostic significance of signet ring cells in fine-needle aspirates of the breast. Diagn Cytopathol 1997; 16:117-121.

148. Greeley CF, Frost AR. Cytologic features of ductal and lobular carcinoma in fine needle aspirates of the breast. Acta Cytol 1997; 41:333-340.

149. Sneige N, Singletary SE. Fine-needle aspiration of the breast: diagnostic problems and approaches to surgical management. Pathol Ann (Part I) 1994; 29:281-301.

150. Sneige N, Staerkel GA, Caraway NP, et al. A plea for uniform terminology and reporting of breast fine needle aspiration. MD Anderson Cancer Proposal. Acta Cytol 1944; 38:971-972.

151. Wang HH, Ducatman BS, Eick D. Comparative features of ductal carcinoma in situ and infiltrating ductal carcinoma of the breast on fine needle aspiration biopsy. Am J Clin Pathol 1989; 92:736-740.

152. Maygarden SJ, Brock MS, Novotny DB. Are epithelial cells in fat or connective tissue a reliable indicator of tumor invasion in fine-needle aspiration of the breast? Diagn Cytopathol 1997; 16:137-142.

153. Gaffey MJ, Mills SE, Frierson HF, et al. Medullary carcinoma of the breast. Interobserver variability in histopathologic diagnosis. Mod Pathol 1995; 8:31-38.

154. Ellis IO, Galea M, Broughton N, et al. Pathological prognostic factors in breast cancer (Part II). Histological type: relationship with survival in a large study with long-term followup. Histopathology 1992; 20:479-489.

155. Kleer CG, Michael CW. Fine-needle aspiration of breast carcinomas with prominent lymphocytic infiltrate. Diagn Cytopathol 2000; 23:39-42.

156. Howell LP, Kline TS. Medullary carcinoma of the breast: an unusual cytologic finding in cyst fluid aspirates. Cancer 1990; 65:277-282.

157. Silverberg SG, Kay S, Chitale AR, Levitt SH. Colloid carcinoma of the breast. Am J Clin Pathol 1971; 55:355-363.

158. Fanning TV, Sneige N, Staerkel G. Mucinous breast lesions: fine needle aspiration findings. Acta Cytol 1990; 34:754.

159. Gupta RK, McHutchinson AGR, Simpson JS, et al. Value of fine needle aspiration cytology of the breast, with an emphasis on the cytodiagnosis of colloid carcinoma. Acta Cytol 1991; 34:703-709.

160. Palombini L, Fulciniti F, Vetrani A, et al. Mucoid carcinoma of the breast on fine-needle aspiration biopsy sample: cytology and ultrastructure. Appl Pathol 1984; 2:70-75.

161. Stanley MW, Tani EM, Skoog L. Mucinous breast carcinoma and mixed mucinous-infiltrating ductal carcinoma: a comparative cytologic study. Diagn Cytopathol 1989; 5:134-138.

162. Dawson AE, Mulford DK. Fine needle aspiration of mucinous (colloid) breast carcinoma: nuclear grading and mammographic and cytologic findings. Acta Cytol 1998; 42:668-672.

163. Wall RW, Glant MD. The cytomorphology of mucinous carcinoma of the breast by fine-needle aspiration. ASCP Check Sample 1987; 15:C-87-12 (C-174).

164. Yeoh GPS, Cheung PSY, Chan KW. Fine-needle aspiration cytology of mucocele-like tumors of the breast. Am J Surg Pathol 1999; 23(5):552-559.

165. Simsir A, Tsang P, Greenebaum E. Additional mimics of mucinous mammary carcinoma. Fibroepithelial lesions. Am J Clin Pathol 1998; 109:169-172.

166. Dei Tos AP, Giustina DD, Martin VD, et al. Aspiration biopsy cytology of tubular carcinoma of the breast. Diagn Cytopathol 1994; 11:146-150.

167. de la Torre M, Lindholm K, Lindgren A. Fine needle aspiration cytology of tubular breast carcinoma and radial scar. Acta Cytol 1994; 38:884-890.

168. Fischler DF, Sneige N, Ordonez NG, et al. Tubular carcinoma of the breast: cytologic features in fine-needle aspirations and application of monoclonal anti-α smooth muscle actin in diagnosis. Diagn Cytopathol 1994; 10:120-125.

169. Culubret M, Roig I. Fine-needle aspiration biopsy of adenoid cystic carcinoma of the breast: a case report. Diagn Cytopathol 1996; 15:431-434.

170. Quinodoz IS, Berger SD, Schafer P, et al. Adenoid cystic carcinoma of the breast: utility of immunocytochemical study with collagen IV on fine-needle aspiration. Diagn Cytopathol 1997; 16:442-445.

171. Naran S, Simpson J, Gupta RK. Cytologic diagnosis of papillary carcinoma of the breast in needle aspirates. Diagn Cytopathol 1988; 4:33-37.

172. Kline TS, Kannan V. Papillary carcinoma of the breast: a cytomorphologic analysis. Arch Pathol Lab Med 1986; 110:189-191.

173. Wong S-I, Cheung H, Tse GMK. Fine needle aspiration cytology of invasive micropapillary carcinoma of the breast: a case report. Acta Cytol 2000; 44:1085-1089.

174. Kumarasinghe MP, Fernando MS, Sheriffdeen AH, et al. Cytohistologic features of invasive micropapillary carcinoma in a young female. Diagn Cytopathol 2000; 23:196-198.

175. Kumar PK, Talei AR, Malekhusseini SA, et al. Papillary carcinoma of the breast: cytologic study of nine cases. Acta Cytol 1999; 43:767-770.

176. Frost AR, Terahata S, Yeh IT, et al. The significance of signet ring cells in infiltrating lobular carcinoma of the breast. Arch Pathol Lab Med 1995; 119:64-68.

177. Kline TS, Kannan V, Kline IK. Appraisal and cytomorphologic analysis of common carcinomas of the breast. Diagn Cytopathol 1985; 1:188-193.

178. Dabbs DJ, Grenko RT, Silverman JF. Fine needle aspiration cytology of pleomorphic lobular carcinoma of the breast: duct carcinoma as diagnostic pitfall. Acta Cytol 1994; 38:923-926.

179. De las Morenas A, Crespo P, Moroz K, et al. Cytologic diagnosis of ductal versus lobular carcinoma of the breast. Acta Cytol 1995; 39:865-869.

180. Auger, Huttner I. Fine-needle aspiration cytology of pleomorphic lobular carcinoma of the breast: comparison with the classic type. Cancer (Cancer Cytopathol) 1997; 81:29-32.

181. Salhany KE, Page DL. Fine-needle aspiration of mammary lobular carcinoma in situ and atypical lobular hyperplasia. Am J Clin Pathol 1989; 92:22-26.

182. Duggan MA, Young GK, Hwang WS. Fine-needle aspiration of an apocrine breast carcinoma with multivacuolated lipid-rich giant cells. Diagn Cytopathol 1988; 4:62-66.

183. Gupta RK, Wakefield SJ, Naran S, Dowle CC. Immunocytochemical and ultrastructural diagnosis of a rare mixed apocrine-medullary carcinoma of the breast in a fine needle aspirate. Acta Cytol 1989; 33:104-108.

184. Craig JP. Secretory carcinoma of the breast in an adult: correlation of aspiration cytology and histology on the biopsy specimen. Acta Cytol 1985; 29:589-592.

185. d'Amore ESG, Maisto L, Gatteschi MB, et al. Secretory carcinoma of the breast: report of a case with fine needle aspiration biopsy. Acta Cytol 1986; 30:309-312.

186. Dominguez F, Riera JR, Junco P, et al. Secretory carcinoma of the breast: report of a case with diagnosis by fine needle aspiration. Acta Cytol 1992; 36:507-510.

187. Nguyen G-K, Neifer R. Aspiration biopsy cytology of secretory carcinoma of the breast. Diagn Cytopathol 1987; 3:234-237.

188. Aida Y, Takeuchi E, Shingawa T, et al. Fine needle aspiration cytology of lipid-secreting carcinoma of the breast: a case report. Acta Cytol 1993; 37:547-551.

189. Alexiev BA. Glycogen-rich clear cell carcinoma of the breast: report of a case with fine-needle aspiration cytology and immunocytochemical and ultrastructural studies. Diagn Cytopathol 1995; 12:62-66.

190. Kim MK, Kwon GY, Gong GY. Fine needle aspiration cytology of cystic hypersecretory carcinoma of the breast: a case report. Acta Cytol 1997; 41:892-896.

191. Vesoulis A, Kashkari S. Fine needle aspiration of secretory breast carcinoma resembling lactational changes: a case report. Acta Cytol 1998; 42:1032-1036.

192. Eggers JW, Chesney TM. Squamous cell carcinoma of the breast: a clinicopathologic analysis of eight cases and review of the literature. Hum Pathol 1984; 15:526-531.

193. Gubin N. A case of pure primary squamous-cell carcinoma of the breast diagnosed by fine needle aspiration biopsy. Acta Cytol 1985; 29:650-651.

194. Hsiu J-G, Hawkins AG, D'Amato NA, et al. A case of pure primary squamous-cell carcinoma of the breast diagnosed by fine needle aspiration biopsy. Acta Cytol 1985; 29:650-651.

195. Leiman G. Squamous carcinoma of the breast: diagnosis by aspiration cytology. Acta Cytol 1982; 26:201-209.

196. Macia M, Ces JA, Becerra E, et al. Pure squamous carcinoma of the breast: report of a case diagnosed by aspiration cytology. Acta Cytol 1989; 33:201-204.

197. Silverman J, Raso D, Elsheikh T, Lanin D. Fine needle aspiration cytology of a subareolar abscess of the male breast. Diagn Cytopathol 1998; 18(6):441-444.

198. Squires E, Betsill W. Intracystic carcinoma of the breast: a correlation of cytomorphology, gross pathology, microscopic pathology and clinical data. Acta Cytol 1981; 25:267-271.

199. Corkill ME, Sneige N, Fanning T, et al. Fine-needle cytology and flow cytometry of intracystic papillary carcinoma of the breast. Am J Clin Pathol 1990; 94:673-680.

200. Dodd LG, Layfield LJ. Fine-needle aspiration of inflammatory carcinoma of the breast. Diagn Cytopathol 1996; 15:363-366.

201. Silverman JF, Feldman PS, Covell JL, Frable WJ. Fine needle aspiration cytology of neoplasms metastatic to the breast. Acta Cytol 1987; 31:291-300.

202. Hajda SI, Urban JA. Cancers metastatic to the breast. Cancer 1972; 29:1691-1696.

203. Domanski HA. Metastases to the breast from extramammary neoplasms: a report of six cases with diagnosis by fine needle aspiration cytology. Acta Cytol 1996; 40:1293-1299.

204. Sneige N, Zachariah S, Fanning TV, et al. Fine-needle aspiration cytology of metastatic neoplasms in the breast. Am J Clin Pathol 1989; 92:27-35.

205. Fabian C, Dabbs DJ. The immunohistochemical profile of breast carcinoma metastatic in the lung. Breast J 1997; 3:98-103.

206. Dabbs DJ, Liu Y, Raab SS, Tung M, Silverman JF. Immunohistochemical detection of estrogen receptor adenocarcinoma is dependent upon the antibody used. Breast J 2000; 6:347.

207. Norris HG, Taylor HB. Relationship of histologic features to behavior of cystosarcoma phyllodes. Cancer 1967; 20:2090-2099.

208. Pietruzka M, Barnes L. Cystosarcoma phyllodes. Cancer 1979; 41:1974-1983.

209. Rao CR, Narasimhamurthy NK, Jaganathan K, et al. Cystosarcoma phyllodes: diagnosis by fine needle aspiration cytology. Acta Cytol 1992; 36:203-207.

210. Shimizu K, Masawa N, Yamada T, et al. Cytologic evaluation of phyllodes tumors as compared to fibroadenomas of the breast. Acta Cytol 1994; 38:891-897.

211. Silverman JF, Geisinger KR, Frable WJ. Fine-needle aspiration cytology of mesenchymal tumors of the breast. Diagn Cytopathol 1988; 4:50-58.

212. Simi U, Moretti D, Iacconi P, et al. Fine needle aspiration of cytopathology of phyllodes tumor: differential diagnosis with fibroadenoma. Acta Cytol 1988; 32:63-66.

213. Stanley MW, Tani EM, Rutqvist LE, et al. Cystosarcoma phyllodes of the breast: a cytologic and clinicopathologic study of 23 cases. Diagn Cytopathol 1989; 5:29-34.

214. Shabalova IP, Chemeris GJ, Ermilova VD, et al. Phyllodes tumour: cytologic and histologic presentation of 22 cases, and immunohistochemical demonstration of p53. Cytopathology 1997; 8:177-187.

215. Linsk J, Kruezer G, Zajicek J. Cytologic diagnosis of mammary tumors from aspiration biopsy smears (Part II): studies on 210 fibroadenomas and 210 cases of benign dysplasia. Acta Cytol 1972; 16:130-138.

216. Stawicki M, Hsiu J. Malignant cystosarcoma phyllodes. Acta Cytol 1979; 23:61-64.

217. Dusenbery D, Frable WJ. Fine needle aspiration cytology of phyllodes tumor. Potential diagnostic pitfalls. Acta Cytol 1992; 36:215-221.

218. Boccato P, Briani G, d'Atri C, et al. Spindle cell and cartilaginous metaplasia in a breast carcinoma with osteoclastlike stromal cells: a difficult fine needle aspiration diagnosis. Acta Cytol 1988; 32:75-78.

219. Huvos AG, Lucas JC, Foote FW. Metaplastic breast carcinoma: rare form of mammary cancer. NY State J Med 1973; 12:550-561.

220. Kaufman MW, Marti JR, Gallager HS, et al. Carcinoma of the breast with pseudosarcomatous metaplasia. Cancer 1984; 53:1908-1917.

221. Wargotz ES, Norris HJ. Metastatic carcinomas of the breast: matrix-producing carcinoma. Hum Pathol 1989; 20:628-635.

222. Langham MR, Mills AS, Demay RM, et al. Malignant fibrous histiocytoma of the breast. Cancer 1984; 54:558-563.

223. Stanley MW, Tani EM, Horwitz CA, et al. Primary spindle-cell sarcomas of the breast: diagnosis by fine-needle aspiration. Diagn Cytopathol 1988; 4:244-249.

224. Kim K, Naylor B, Han IH. Fine needle aspiration cytology of sarcomas metastatic to the lung. Acta Cytol 1986; 30:688-694.

225. Kline TS, Kline IK. Metaplastic carcinoma of the breast–diagnosis by aspiration biopsy cytology: report of two cases and literature review. Diagn Cytopathol 1990; 6:63-67.

226. Pettinato G, Manivel JC, Petrella G, et al. Primary osteogenic sarcoma and osteogenic metaplastic carcinoma of the breast. Immunocytochemical identification in fine needle aspirates. Acta Cytol 1989; 33:620-626.

227. Stanley MW, Tani EM, Skoog K. Metaplastic carcinoma of the breast: fine-needle aspiration cytology of seven cases. Diagn Cytopathol 1989; 5:22-28.

228. Walaas L, Angervall L, Hagmar B, et al. A correlative cytologic and histologic study of malignant fibrous histiocytoma: an analysis of 40 cases examined by fine needle aspiration cytology. Diagn Cytopathol 1986; 2:46-54.

229. Chhieng DC, Cangiarella JF, Waisman J, et al. Fine-needle aspiration cytology of spindle cell lesions of the breast. Cancer (Cancer Cytopathol) 1999; 87:359-371.

230. Bardales RH, Stanley MW. Benign spindle and inflammatory lesions of the breast: diagnosis by fine-needle aspiration. Diagn Cytopathol 1995; 12:126-130.

231. Mertens HH, Langnickel D, Staedtler F. Primary osteogenic sarcoma of the breast. Acta Cytol 1982; 26:512-515.

232. Vesoulis Z, Cunliffe C. Fine-needle aspiration biopsy of postradiation epithelioid angiosarcoma of breast. Diagn Cytopathol 2000; 22:172-175.

233. El-Naggar A, Abdul-Karim FW, Marshalleck JJ, et al. Fine-needle aspiration of fibromatosis of the breast. Diagn Cytopathol 1987; 3:320-322.

234. Fritsches HG, Muller EA. Pseudosarcomatous fasciitis of the breast: cytologic and histologic features. Acta Cytol 1983; 27:73-75.

235. Tani EM, Stanley MW, Skoog L. Fine needle aspiration cytology presentation of bilateral mammary fibromatosis: report of a case. Acta Cytol 1988; 32:555-558.

236. Kindblom LG, Walaas L, Widehn S. Ultrastructural studies in the preoperative cytologic diagnosis of soft tissue tumors. Semin Diagn Pathol 1986; 3:317-344.

237. Torres V, Ferrer R. Cytology of fine needle aspiration biopsy of primary breast rhabdomyosarcoma in an adolescent girl. Acta Cytol 1985; 29:430-434.

238. Lindhohm K, Nordgren H, Akerman M. Electron microscopy of the needle aspiration biopsy from a malignant fibrous histiocytoma. Acta Cytol 1979; 23:399-401.

239. Pettinato G, Petrella G, Manco A, et al. Carcinoma of the breast with osteoclast-like giant cells: fine-needle aspiration cytology, histology and electron microscopy of 5 cases. Appl Pathol 1984; 2:168-178.

240. Stewart CJR, Mutch AF. Breast carcinoma with osteoclast-like giant cells. Cytopathology 1991; 2:215-219.

241. Sugano I, Nagao K, Kondo Y, et al. Cytologic and ultrastructural studies of a rare breast carcinoma with osteoclast-like giant cells. Cancer 1983; 52:74-78.

242. Shabb NS, Tawil A, Mufarrij A, et al. Mammary carcinoma with osteoclast like giant cells cytologically mimicking benign breast disease: a case report. Acta Cytol 1997; 41:1284-1288.

243. Schnitt SJ, Connolly JL, Harris JR, et al. Radiation-induced changes in the breast. Hum Pathol 1984; 16:545-550.

244. Bondeson L. Aspiration cytology of radiation-induced changes of normal breast epithelium. Acta Cytol 1987; 31:309-310.

245. Gupta RK. Radiation-induced cellular changes in the breast: a potential diagnostic pitfall in fine needle aspiration cytology. Acta Cytol 1989; 33:141-142.

246. Pedio G, Landolt U, Zobeli L. Irradiated benign cells of the breast: a potential diagnostic pitfall in fine needle aspiration cytology. Acta Cytol 1988; 32:127-128.

247. Destouni CH, Skevoudi S, Varduli A, et al. Radiation-induced changes in FNA smear of the breast. Cytopathology 1995; 6:419-425.

248. Kennedy S, Merino M, Swain SM, et al. The effects of hormonal and chemotherapy on tumoral and nonneoplastic breast tissue. Hum Pathol 1990; 21:192-198.

249. Brifford M, Spyratos F, Tubiana-Huhn M, et al. Sequential cytopunctures during preoperative chemotherapy for primary breast cancer. Cancer 1989; 63:631-637.

250. Frierson HF, Fechner RE. Histologic grade of locally advanced infiltrating ductal carcinoma after treatment with induction chemotherapy. Am J Clin Pathol 1994; 102:154-157.

251. Boerner S, Fornage BD, Singletary E, et al. Ultrasound-guided fine-needle aspiration (FNA) of nonpalpable breast lesions: a review of 1885 FNA cases using the National Cancer Institute-supported recommendations on the uniform approach to breast FNA. Cancer (Cancer Cytopathol) 1999; 87:19-24.

252. Albert US, Duda V, Hadji P. Imprint cytology of core needle biopsy specimens of breast lesions: a rapid approach to detecting malignancies, with comparison of cytologic and histopathologic analyses of 173 cases. Acta Cytol 2000; 44:57-62.

253. Ciatto S, Del Turco MR, Bravetti P. Nonpalpable breast lesions: stereotaxic fine-needle aspiration cytology. Radiology 1989; 173:57-59.

254. Dowlatshahi K, Jokich PM, Schmidt R, et al. Cytologic diagnosis of occult breast lesions using stereotaxic needle aspiration: a preliminary report. Arch Surg 1987; 122:1343-1346.

255. Jackson VP. Mammographically guided fine-needle aspiration cytology of nonpalpable breast lesions. Curr Opin Radiol 1990; 2:741-745.

256. Horobin JM, Matthew BM, Preece PE, et al. Effects of fine needle aspiration on subsequent mammograms. Br J Surg 1992; 79:52-54.

257. Fornage BD, Coan JD, David CL. Ultrasound-guided needle biopsy of the breast and other interventional procedures. Radiol Clin North Am 1992; 30:167-185.

258. Klein DL, Sickles EA. Effects of needle aspiration on the mammographic appearance of the breast: a guide to the proper timing of the mammography examination. Radiology 1982; 145:44.

259. Sneige N, Fornage BD, Saleh G. Ultrasound-guided fine-needle aspiration of nonpalpable breast lesions: cytologic and histologic findings. Am J Clin Pathol 1994; 102:98-101.

260. Dowlatshahi K, Yaremko ML, Kluskens LF, Jokich PM. Nonpalpable breast lesions: findings of stereotaxic needle-core biopsy and fine-needle aspiration cytology. Radiology 1991; 181:745-750.

261. Svensson WE, Tohno E, Cosgrove DO, et al. Effects of fine-needle aspiration on the US appearance of the breast. Radiology 1992; 185:709-711.

262. Evans WP. Fine-needle aspiration cytology and core biopsy of nonpalpable breast lesions. Curr Opin Radiol 1992; 4:130-138.

263. Jacobs TW, Silverman JF, Schroeder B, et al. Accuracy of touch-imprint cytology of image-directed breast core needle biopsies. Acta Cytol 1999; 42(2):169-174.

264. Sickles E, Klein DL, Goodson WH, et al. Mammography after needle aspiration of palpable breast masses. Am J Surg 1983;145:395-397.

265. Bozzetti C, Nizzoli R, Naldi N, et al. Nuclear grading and flow cytometric DNA pattern in fine-needle aspirates of primary breast cancer. Diagn Cytopathol 1996; 15:116-120.

266. Cajulis RS, Hessel G, Hyang S, et al. Simplified nuclear grading of fine-needle aspirates of breast carcinoma: concordance with corresponding histologic nuclear grading and flow cytometric data. Diagn Cytopathol 1994; 11:124-130.

267. Dabbs DJ. Role of nuclear grading of breast carcinomas in fine needle aspiration specimens. Acta Cytol 1993; 37:361-366.

268. Dabbs DJ, Silverman JF. Prognostic factors from the fine-needle aspirate: breast carcinoma nuclear grade. Diagn Cytopathol 1994; 10:203-208.

269. Pisano ED, Fajardo LL, Tsimikas J, et al. Rate of insufficient samples for fine-needle aspiration for nonpalpable breast lesions in a multicenter clinical trial: the radiologic diagnostic oncology group 5 study. Cancer 1998; 82:679-688.

270. Dawson AE, Austin RE, Weinberg DS. Nuclear grading of breast carcinoma by image analysis. Am J Clin Pathol 1991; 95:S29-S37.

271. Howell LP, Gandour-Edwards R, O'Sullivan D. Application of the Scarff-Bloom-Richardson tumor grading system to fine-needle aspirates of the breast. Am J Clin Pathol 1994; 101:262-265.

272. Thor AD. Prognostic factors in breast cancer: Integrating the cytology laboratory. Diagn Cytopathol 1992; 8:319-321.

273. Corkill ME, Katz R. Immunocytochemical staining of c-erb B-2 oncogene in fine-needle aspirates of breast carcinoma: a comparison with tissue sections and other breast cancer prognostic factors. Diagn Cytopathol 1994; 11:250-254.

274. Dawson AE, Norton JA, Weinberg DS. Comparative assessment of proliferation and DNA content in breast carcinoma by image analysis and flow cytometry. Am J Pathol 1990; 136:1115-1124.

275. Kuenen-Boumeester V, Kwast THVD, Laarhoven HAJV, et al. Ki-67 staining in histological subtypes of breast carcinoma and fine-needle aspiration smears. J Clin Pathol 1991; 44:208-210.

276. Martin AW, Davey DD. Comparison of immunoreactivity of neu-oncoprotein in fine-needle aspirates and paraffin-embedded materials. Diagn Cytopathol 1995; 12:142-145.

277. Sinha SK, Singh UR, Bhatia A. *C-erb-B2* oncoprotein expression. Correlation with the Ki-67 labeling index and AgNOR counts in breast carcinoma on fine needle aspiration cytology. Acta Cytol 1996; 40:1217-1220.

278. Silverman JF. Diagnostic accuracy, cost-effectiveness, and triage role of fine-needle aspiration biopsy in the diagnosis of palpable breast lesions. Breast J 1995; 1:3-8.

279. Shabot M, Goldberg IM, Schick P, et al. Aspiration cytology is superior to Tru-Cut needle biopsy in establishing the diagnosis of clinically suspicious breast masses. Ann Surg 1982; 196:122-126.

280. Dixon JM, Lamb J, Anderson TJ. Fine needle aspiration of the breast: importance of the operator. Lancet 1983; 2:564.

281. Cohen MB, Rodgers RPC, Hales MS, et al. Influence if training and experience in fine-needle aspiration biopsy of breast: receiver operating characteristics curve analysis. Arch Pathol Lab Med 1987; 111:518-520.

282. Layfield LJ, Glasgow BJ, Cramer H. Fine-needle aspiration in the management of breast masses. Pathol Annu 1989; 24:23-62.

283. Beidrzycki T, Dabska M, Sikorowa L, et al. On cytologic vagaries in the diagnosis of breast tumors. Tumori 1980; 66:191-196.

284. Layfield LJ, Dodd LG. Cytologically low grade malignancies: an important interpretative pitfall responsible for false negative diagnoses in fine-needle aspiration of the breast. Diagn Cytopathol 1996; 15:250-259.

285. Abati A. To count or not to count? A review of the issue of adequacy in breast FNA. Diagn Cytopathol 1999; 21:142-147.

286. Boerner S, Sneige N. Specimen adequacy and false-negative diagnosis rate in fine-needle aspirates of palpable breast masses. Cancer (Cancer Cytopathol) 1998; 84:344-348.

287. Sneige N. Should specimen adequacy be determined by the opinion of the aspirator or by the cells on the slides? Cancer (Cancer Cytopathol) 1997; 81:3-5.

288. Eckert R, Howell LP. Number, size, and composition of cell clusters as related to breast FNA adequacy. Diagn Cytopathol 1999; 21:105-111.

289. Layfield LJ, Mooney EE, Glasgow B, et al. What constitutes an adequate smear in fine-needle aspiration cytology of the breast? Cancer (Cancer Cytopathol) 1997; 81:16-21.

290. Abele JS, Wager LT, Miller TR. FNA of breast: cell count as an illusion of adequacy: a clinicocytopathologist's point of view. Cancer Cytopathol 1998; 84:319-323.

291. Bell DA, Hajdu SI, Urban JA, et al. Role of aspiration cytology in the diagnosis and management of mammary lesions in office practice. Cancer 1983; 51:1182-1189.

292. Zarbo RJ, Howanitz PJ, Bachner P. Interinstitutional comparison of performance in breast fine-needle aspiration cytology. Arch Pathol Lab Med 1991; 115:743-750.

293. Hermansen C, Poulsen HS, Jensen J, et al. Diagnostic reliability of combined physical examination, mammography, and fine-needle puncture ("triple-test") in breast tumors. Cancer 1987; 60:1866-1871.

294. Martelli G, Pilotti S, de Yoldi GC, et al. Diagnostic efficacy of physical examination, mammography, fine needle aspiration cytology (triple-test) in solid breast lumps: an analysis of 1708 consecutive cases. Tumori 1990; 76:476-479.

295. Negri S, Bonetti F, Capitanio A, et al. Preoperative diagnostic accuracy of fine-needle aspiration in the management of breast lesions: comparison of specificity and sensitivity with clinical examination, mammography, echography, and thermography in 249 patients. Diagn Cytopathol 1994; 11:4-8.

296. Salami N, Hirschowitz SL, Nieberg RK, et al. Triple test approach to inadequate fine needle aspiration biopsies of palpable breast lesions. Acta Cytol 1999; 43:339-343.

297. Abele J, Kline T, Silverman JF, et al. What constitutes adequate sampling of breast lesions that appear benign by clinical and mammographic criteria? Diagn Cytopathol 1995; 13:473-485.

298. Lannin DR, Silverman JF, Walker C, et al. Cost effectiveness of fine needle aspiration of the breast. Ann Surg 1986; 203:474-480.

299. Donegan WL. Evaluation of a palpable breast mass. N Engl J Med 1992; 327:937-942.

300. Troxel DB, Sabella JD. Problem areas in pathology practice. Uncovered by a review of malpractice claims. Am J Surg Pathol 1994; 18:821-831.

301. The National Cancer Institute. The uniform approach to breast fine-needle aspiration biopsy—a synopsis: development of proof at a National Cancer Institute-sponsored conference. Bethesda, Md, December 9 and 10, 1996. Acta Cytol 1996; 40:1120-1126.

302. Bibbo M, Abati A, et al. The uniform approach to breast fine needle aspiration biopsy: a synopsis. Acta Cytol 1996; 40:1120-1126.

303. DeMay RM. The art and science of cytopathology, vol 1. Chicago:ASCP Press; 1966:293-294.

304. Johnson TL, Kini SR. Cytologic and clinicopathologic features of abnormal nipple secretions: 225 cases. Diagn Cytopathol 1991; 7:17-22.

305. Barnes AB. Diagnosis and treatment of abnormal breast secretions. N Engl J Med 1966; 275:1184-1187.

306. Leis HP. Management of nipple discharge. Br J Clin Pract 1989; 68(Suppl):58-65.

307. Leis HP. Management of nipple discharge. World J Surg 1989; 13:736-742.

308. Leis HP, Greene FL, Cammarata A, et al. Nipple discharge: surgical significance. South Med J 1988; 81:20-26.

309. Urban JA, Egel RA. Nonlactational nipple discharge. CA Cancer J Clin 1978; a28:130-140.

310. Ciatto S, Bravetti P, Cariagg P. Significance of nipple discharge clinical patterns in the selection of cases for cytologic examination. Acta Cytol 1986; 30:17-20.

311. Okazaki A, Hirata K, Okazaki M, et al. Nipple discharge disorders: current diagnostic management and the role of fiber-ductoscopy. Eur Radiol 1999; 9(4):583-590.

312. Leis HP, Jr. Management of nipple discharge. World J Surg 1989; 13:736-742.

313. Dunn JM, Lucarotti ME, Wood SJ, et al. Exfoliative cytology in the diagnosis of breast disease. Br J Surg 1995; 82(6):789-791.

314. Farkas AM, Nayar R, Chell S, et al. Positive stain for mucin in nipple discharge fluid: a mucin-producing lesion or not? Diagn Cytopathol 1998; 19:228.

315. Koss LG. Diagnostic cytology and its histopathologic bases, vol 1. Philadelphia: JB Lippincott; 1992.

316. Hou M-F, Tsai K-B, Lin H-J, et al. A simple intraductal aspiration method for cytodiagnosis in nipple discharge. Acta Cytol 2000; 44:1029-1034.

317. King EB, Chew KL, Petrakis NL, et al. Nipple aspirate cytology for the study of breast cancer precursors. JNCI 1983; 71:1115-1121.

318. Klein P, Glaser E, Grogan L, et al. Biomarker assays in nipple aspirate fluid. Breast J 2001; 7(6):378-387.

319. Das DK, Al-Ayadhy B, Ajrawi MTG, et al. Cytodiagnosis of nipple discharge: a study of 602 samples from 484 cases. Diagn Cytopathol 2001; 25:25-37.

320. Simsir A, Waisman J, Cangiarella J. Fibroadenomas with atypia: causes of under- and overdiagnosis by aspiration biopsy. Diagn Cytopathol 2001; 25:278-284.

321. Cho EY, Oh YL. Fine needle aspiration cytology of sclerosing adenosis of the breast. Acta Cytol 2001; 45:353-359.

322. Amrikachi M, Green LK, Rone R, et al. Gynecomastia. Cytologic features and diagnostic pitfalls in fine needle aspirates. Acta Cytol 2001; 45:948-952.

323. McKee GT, Tambouret RH, Finkelstein D. Fine-needle aspiration cytology of the breast: invasive vs. in situ carcinoma. Diagn Cytopathol 2001; 25:73-77.

324. O'Shaughnessy JA, Ljung BM, Dooley WC, et al. Ductal lavage and the clinical management of women at high risk for breast carcinoma: a commentary. Cancer 2002; 94:292-298.

325. Dooley WC, Ljung BM, Veronesi U, Cazzaniga M, Elledge RM, O'Shaughnessy JA, et al. Ductal lavage for detection of cellular atypia in women at high risk for breast cancer. J Natl Cancer Inst 2001; 93:1624-1632.

326. Masood S, Siddiqi AM, Payandeh F, Khalbuss W. Exfoliative breast cytopathology: an experience with ductal lavage. Lab Invest 2002; 82:79A.

327. King BL, Crisi GM, Tsai SC, Haffty BG, Phillips RF, Rimm DL. Immunocytochemical analysis of breast cells obtained by ductal lavage. Cancer 2002; 96:244-249.

328. Morrow M, Vogel V, Ljung BM, O'Shaughnessy JA. Evaluation and mangaement of the woman with an abnormal ductal lavage. J Am Coll Surg 2002; 194:648-656.

329. Noga CM, Brainard JA, Dietz JR, Kim JA, Dawson AE. Ductal lavage cytology: cytologic features in high-risk women versus women with known breast adenocarcinoma. Lab Invest 2002; 83A.

330. Cangiarella J, Masood S: New frontiers in cytopathology: ductal lavage. FOCUS 2002; 9:11-12.

331. Sohn JH, Kim LS, Chae SW, et al. Fine needle aspiration cytologic findings of breast mucinous neoplasms: differential diagnosis between mucocele-like tumor and mucinous carcinoma. Acta Cytol 2001; 45:723-729.

332. Dawson AE, Logan-Young W, Mulford DK. Aspiration cytology of tubular carcinoma. Diagnostic features with mammographic correlation. Am J Clin Pathol 1994; 101:488-492.

333. Cangiarella J, Waisman J, Shapiro RL, et al. Cytologic features of tubular adenocarcinoma of the breast by aspiration biopsy. Diagn Cytopathol 2001; 25:311-315.

334. Ng W-K, Poon CSP, Kong JHB. Fine needle aspiration cytology of invasive micropapillary carcinoma of the breast. Review of cases in a three-year period. Acta Cytol 2001; 45:973-979.

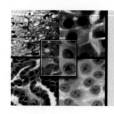

Index